Prescription Pharmacy

Contributors

GEORGE F. ARCHAMBAULT, PH.C., LL.B., LL.D., SC.D., PHARM.D.

Editor, Hospital Formulary Management, Washington, D.C.

THEODORE R. BATES, PH.D.

Associate Professor of Pharmacy, School of Pharmacy, University of Connecticut

SEYMOUR BLAUG, PH.D.

Professor of Pharmacy, College of Pharmacy, The University of Iowa

WILLIAM H. BRINER

Chief, Radiopharmaceutical Service Pharmacy Department, Captain, United States Public Health Service, The Clinical Center, National Institutes of Health, Department of Health, Education and Welfare, Bethesda, Md.

ROY C. DARLINGTON, PH.D.

Professor of Pharmacy and Chairman, Department of Pharmacy, College of Pharmacy, Howard University

ROBERT L. DAY, PHARM.D.

Assistant Dean and Lecturer in Pharmacy, School of Pharmacy, University of California

JERE E. GOYAN, PH.D.

Dean, Professor of Pharmacy and Pharmaceutical Chemistry, School of Pharmacy, University of California

PETER P. LAMY, PH.D.

Associate Professor of Pharmacy, School of Pharmacy, University of Maryland

GERHARD LEVY, PHARM.D.

Professor of Biopharmaceutics, School of Pharmacy, State University of New York at Buffalo

EUGENE L. PARROTT, PH.D.

Associate Professor of Pharmacy, College of Pharmacy, The University of Iowa

CHARLES F. PETERSON, PH.D.

Professor of Pharmacy, School of Pharmacy, Temple University

ELMER M. PLEIN, PH.D.

Coordinator of Pharmaceutical Services, Professor of Pharmacy, College of Pharmacy, University of Washington

JOSEPH R. ROBINSON, PH.D.

Assistant Professor of Pharmacy, School of Pharmacy, University of Wisconsin

JOHN J. SCIARRA, PH.D.

Director of Graduate Division and Professor of Pharmaceutical Chemistry, College of Pharmacy, St. John's University

WALTER SINGER, PH.D.

Professor of Pharmacy and Dean, Albany College of Pharmacy, Union University

DALE E. WURSTER, PH.D.

Professor of Pharmacy, School of Pharmacy, University of Wisconsin

VICTOR A. YANCHICK, PH.D.

Assistant Professor of Pharmacy, College of Pharmacy, The University of Texas at Austin

PRESCRIPTION PHARMACY

Dosage Formulation and Pharmaceutical Adjuncts

Edited By

Joseph B. Sprowls, Jr., Ph.D.

Dean and Professor of Pharmacy
College of Pharmacy
The University of Texas at Austin

SECOND EDITION

J. B. Lippincott Company

Philadelphia • Toronto

Preface to the Second Edition

The first edition of *Prescription Pharmacy* was planned and written in response to rapid changes which were then taking place in the profession of pharmacy and, particularly, in the curriculums designed for students of pharmacy. The Preface to the first edition took note of dramatic changes which have taken place in the art of therapeutics during recent decades and the consequent adjustments which have developed in the practice of pharmacy. The following sentence from the Preface to the first edition will bear repeating: "No longer is the dispensing of prescriptions a test of the pharmacist's compounding skills; rather, it is a challenge to his knowledge of dosage forms and his ability to interpret this knowledge for the best interest of the patient and the physician whom he serves."

During the years which have passed since publication of the first edition the pace of change in medical and pharmaceutical sciences has continued unabated, but some trends have become sufficiently evident to serve as guidelines in textbook development. Notable among these trends are the increasing significance of biopharmaceutical considerations in prescription drug design and control and a growing awareness of the need for the pharmacist to have a better understanding of the clinical applications of preparations which are dispensed or distributed. At the same time there has been a notable impetus in the development of programs which provide total health care on an interdisciplinary basis. Thus, there has been increasing urgency for the pharmacist to understand the total health care needs of patients as well as a greater need to understand the privileges and responsibilities of other professions which have a relation to the prescription distribution system. These trends seem to offer ample justification for those chapters which were innovative in the first edition and to affirm guidelines which have been followed in the preparation of the second edition. For the benefit of those who may not be familiar with the first edition, the list of innovative chapters will be repeated here:

"Biopharmaceutical Considerations in Dosage Form and Design"

"Services to the Allied Professions"

"Prescription Accessories and Related Items"

These chapters as well as all others have been completely revised and updated in the preparation of this second edition of the text.

In recognition of the growing consideration for biopharmaceutical data in the preparation and evaluation of dosage forms, the separate authors have extended their coverage of this information as it relates to the dosage forms which are under consideration. Significant attention has been given to the clinical aspects of prescription medication through the introduction of a chapter titled "Therapeutic Incompatibilities." This chapter not only presents a general discussion of the causes and classification of therapeutic incompatibility but also provides a single composite reference source of current information relating to drug-drug and drug-food interactions as well as the underlying phenomena which cause these reactions to occur.

Recognition was given in the first edition to the growing importance of institutional pharmacy through inclusion of a comprehensive chapter on hospital pharmacy practice.

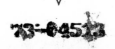

This chapter has been extensively revised by a new collaborator. Although this chapter retains the title "Hospital Pharmacy," the procedures and controls which it presents are applicable in all types of institutional pharmacy practice. For example, the pharmacist who serves as a consultant to nursing homes will benefit by studying the control and distributional systems which are described in this chapter as well as the discussion of the procedures and responsibilities of the Pharmacy and Therapeutics Committee.

It is anticipated that the revisions and additions as described will make the second edition of *Prescription Pharmacy* even more useful than the first in bridging the gap between basic pharmaceutical sciences and the clinical aspects of pharmacy. Thus, the text should be more useful to teachers of dispensing or clinical pharmacy (even biopharmaceutics) and to practitioners of pharmacy, who are continually faced with the challenge of providing information and interpretations relating to the products which they dispense.

JOSEPH B. SPROWLS
Austin, Texas
August, 1970

Contents

Chapter 1

The Prescription

Elmer M. Plein, Ph.D.*

HISTORY OF THE PRESCRIPTION

Until comparatively recently, it was commonly agreed that the art of prescription writing originated in the distant past. It was thought that the Egyptian priests practiced prescription writing because they engaged in treating the sick in addition to their religious duties. There are preserved in museums such Egyptian records as those cut on stone or written on papyrus which contain a variety of medical formulas. There are several formulas preserved in the British Museum which are said to date from the time of the Cheops, about 3700 B.C.[13]

The *Ebers Papyrus*, written in about the 16th century B.C., is considered to be an unofficial formulary or private recipe book.[13] It contains many invocations for driving away disease and specific recipes directing the use of drugs in common use today. Some of the formulas in the *Ebers Papyrus* tended toward polypharmacy. These recipes, calling for as many as 35 ingredients, were intended to treat the more complex illnesses. Each formula names the ingredients and the quantities to be used and gives directions for the preparation and the use of the medicines. It is thought possible that the preparation of the medicine in a form to be used by the patient was accomplished by a class of individuals corresponding to today's pharmacists.

According to these ideas, the separation of pharmacy and medicine as professions could have originated a few thousand years ago. However, the late Dr. George Urdang, who did considerable research on the history of the prescription, claimed that there could

not have been any prescriptions before about A.D. 1000, if by "prescription" we understand it to be a written order by a physician to a pharmacist. Dr. Urdang pointed out that, while it is true that these formulas have come down to us from Assyrian-Babylonian and Egyptian antiquity, the former written on clay tablets and the latter on stone and papyrus, they are not prescriptions as such. They are merely formulas or recipes to be used as guides by those mixing medicines. Nothing is known about individual prescription filling during that period.

Early pharmacy and medicine in Greece were centered around the supernatural. Though simple herb medicines were used, there was strong reliance on incantations and prayers. Greek physicians prepared their own medicines, although a special class of individuals, *rhizotomoi*, dug the medicinal plants.[13,21]

It was Hippocrates who was responsible for freeing medicine and surgery from the supernaturalistic basis. Alexandrian conquest of the Egyptians was responsible for the Egyptian influence on Greek pharmacy and medicine. The Greeks held strong contempt for labor and the specialization of functions was effected easily. Even the surgeon was placed outside the class in which the physician resided. Perhaps the manual nature of the duties of the *rhizotomoi* or the *pharmacopoloi* and the surgeon contributed to the rapid development of their skills.

Greek culture, including medical theories and practices, was passed on to the Romans as a result of the Roman conquest of Greece. Thus, while early Roman formulas were those built around mysticism, they soon became of a rational, naturalistic nature.

* Coordinator of Pharmaceutical Services, Professor of Pharmacy, University of Washington.

In Graeco-Roman times, according to Dr. Urdang, there were various groups of tradespeople who compounded medicines besides mixing and selling perfumes, fumigations, love potions, and fragrant oils and ointments for athletes and gladiators. However, those people could not be classified as pharmacists. Dr. Urdang also reminded us of the fact that Pliny (23-79) and Galen (131-201) admonished the physicians not to trust the *pigmentarii* (dealers in dyestuffs and medicinal drugs) or the *seplasarii* (importers of and dealers in drugs and oriental aromatics), but to prepare the medicaments to be applied in their practices themselves. These admonitions prove that dispensing by the physician was regarded as a medical ethical requirement, and that there had developed craftsmen to whom at least some of the physicians delegated the laborious task of mixing medicines according to their directions. Nevertheless, even in these cases the physician remained the one who applied the medicine or dispensed the product for application to the patient. The present established circuit by which the physician hands the patient a prescription that is brought to and filled by the pharmacist, who in turn hands the finished product to the patient, still did not exist as a matter of routine.

The history of pharmacy and medicine since the time of the great Roman Empire is not a story of steady advances. The teachings of such scientifically minded men as Hippocrates were replaced by magic and mysticism during the period immediately before the birth of Christianity. Prescriptions included amulets and charms to be worn by the patient. Certain words or phrases were spoken during the preparation of the medicine, and the patient was directed to face a certain direction (usually the east) when he used the medicine.

Throughout the Middle Ages, science remained on a lower plane than that developed by the Egyptians and the Greeks. Medicine during this period was largely in the hands of priests and monks, and their religious beliefs influenced medical practice. Astrologers and alchemists also influenced prescription writing. In their desire to hold the knowledge of the practice of pharmacy and medicine from the general populace, these individuals used symbols to indicate the medicinal ingredients.

It was the Arabians[13,21] who preserved the art of pharmacy and medicine. They kept in close contact with the classical traditions of the Egyptians and the Greeks, and, after their conquests in Europe, brought with them a revival of learning and science. The Mohammedan conquerors established on the Spanish peninsula such universities as those of Cordova, Murcia, Seville and Toledo. From these centers of learning, their influence slowly made itself felt over the rest of Europe.

During the Middle Ages, the status of the pharmacist was lowered because the physician tended to prepare his own medicines. Separation of pharmacy from medicine began to be felt in Europe during the 11th century, as a result of the influence of the Moors. In the *Statuta sive Leges* of the southern French town of Arles was a rule (supposed to have originated between 1162 and 1202) that the pharmacist should accurately fill the prescriptions of the physicians. In this ordinance, as well as in later similar ordinances, the physician was obligated to observe the compounding, or at least to be present until all individual ingredients were collected, by the pharmacist. These rules provided restrictions for both health professions, forbidding the pharmacist to counterprescribe and the physician to dispense.

In 1240, Frederick II of Hohenstaufen brought about legislation separating pharmacy and medicine in the Two Sicilies. From the 13th century on, pharmacists in some European countries had to swear to fill conscientiously the prescriptions of the physicians. This oath is still taken in some of those countries. Some time in the 14th century, specialization in the two professions began to appear in England. In 1683, the City Council of Bruges, Belgium, passed a law forbidding physicians to prepare their own medicines. Dr. John Morgan, in America, in 1765 proposed the separation of pharmacy and medicine.

Generally speaking, in Anglo-Saxon countries the right of the physician to dispense has been retained. In England, in 1911, the introduction of compulsory health insurance for employees within certain income brackets required prescriptions to be written for those

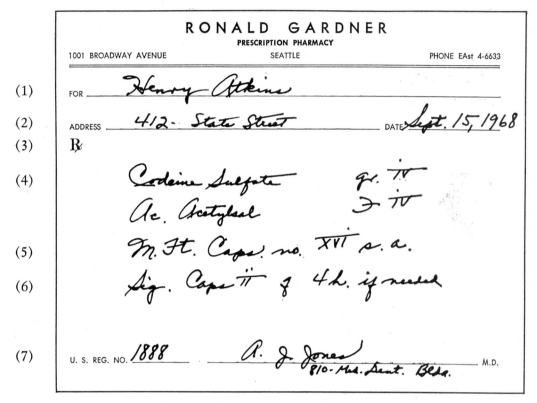

(1)
(2)
(3)
(4)
(5)
(6)
(7)

RONALD GARDNER
PRESCRIPTION PHARMACY
1001 BROADWAY AVENUE   SEATTLE   PHONE EAst 4-6633

FOR _Henry Atkins_

ADDRESS _412- State Street_   DATE _Sept. 15, 1968_

℞

Codeine Sulfate   gr. IV
Ac. Acetylsal   ℨ IV

M. Ft. Caps. no. XVI s. a.

Sig. Caps II q 4h. if needed

U. S. REG. NO. _1888_   _A. J. Jones_   M.D.
810-Med. Dent. Bldg.

FIG. 1-1. Typical prescription, properly written. See text for discussion of the various parts of the prescription.

people and hence limited the right of the physician to dispense. Certain rules and regulations (such as pension and workmen's compensation) in the United States also limit the right of the physician to dispense under certain conditions, though generally his right to dispense to his own patients is still unimpeded.

DEFINITION OF PRESCRIPTION

A prescription is an order for a medicine or medicines usually written as a formula by a physician, a dentist, a veterinarian or some other licensed health science practitioner legally entitled to prescribe. It contains the names and the quantities of the desired substances, with instructions to the pharmacist for the preparation of the medicine and to the patient for the use of the medicine at a particular time.

The prescription may be (1) a formula written on a piece of paper, usually a pre-scription blank, or (2) it may be written by the pharmacist pursuant to the telephoned dictation of the physician. It may be (3) oral instructions that direct the use of certain drugs or call for the use of some physical agent, such as heat. Therefore, oral prescriptions may or may not concern the pharmacist. The term prescription is extended also to include (4) the finished product, that drug or mixture of drugs compounded and dispensed by the pharmacist pursuant to the instructions of a prescriber.

According to Gosselin's National Prescription Audit[16] about 534 million new prescriptions valued at approximately 1.97 billion dollars were filled in the United States in 1968.

PARTS OF THE PRESCRIPTION

Figure 1-1 represents a typical prescription properly written on a printed blank of the type often used in pharmacies for telephoned prescriptions and for prescriptions which the physician may wish to write when he is in the pharmacy. It should be pointed out that it was formerly customary for the pharmacist to supply physicians with printed prescription blanks bearing the name of the pharmacy or the name of the pharmacy and the name of the physician. This custom originated as a form of advertising on the part of the pharmacist. Since such practice is apt to be interpreted as collusion between the pharmacist and the physician, and perhaps to interfere with the patient's free choice of pharmacy, it is now considered unethical for pharmacists to supply physicians with printed blanks (with the name of the pharmacy) for office use. Objections to the use of blanks bearing the name of the pharmacy have come from both the pharmaceutical and the medical professions. Some pharmaceutical organizations such as the King County Pharmaceutical Association (of Washington State) consider it unethical for pharmacists to supply physicians with such printed blanks[11] and the Judicial Council of the American Medical Association has adopted the policy that it is unethical for physicians to use prescription blanks with the name of the pharmacy imprinted thereon.[1]

Many pharmacists have continued to supply physicians with blanks imprinted with the physician's name, but the name of the pharmacy is not included.

Printed blanks like the one illustrated in Figure 1-1 are still used by many pharmacists for telephoned prescriptions, but some pharmacists use either blank pieces of paper cut to convenient size or the universal type prescription blank such as the one shown in Figure 1-3.

Along the side of Figure 1-1 are numbers indicating the various parts of the prescription.

1. **The name and the address of the patient** usually are supplied by the prescriber. If this information is lacking on the prescription, the pharmacist should add it to keep his records complete. Reasons for this are obvious. Federal regulations require this information on narcotic prescriptions. The laws of some states require the name of the patient on all prescriptions.

2. **The date on which the prescription is written** usually is supplied by the prescriber. According to Federal narcotic regulations, narcotic-containing prescriptions must be dated. The prescription illustrated in Figure 1-1 contains codeine sulfate and is subject to control by Federal narcotic regulations.

3. The **superscription** is written ℞ and is the symbol for the Latin word *recipe* ("take thou," or "you take"), the imperative form of the Latin verb *recipio*, "I take." It directs the pharmacist to take the drugs listed in (4) in the quantities given to prepare the medication. The ℞ (pronounced R-X) has become the symbol of pharmacy as well as the symbol of the prescription.

4. The **inscription** contains a list of the ingredients and their quantities to be used in compounding the prescription.

5. The **subscription** comprises the directions to the pharmacist for the compounding of the several ingredients into a form suitable for use by the patient. The class of the preparation (capsule) is noted and the number of doses (16) to be prepared is indicated.

6. The **transcription** gives the necessary directions to the patient for the use of the prescription: "(Take) two capsules every four hours if needed."

7. The **name of the prescriber** may be given as an official signature, which is required by Federal regulations on many narcotic-containing prescriptions. This prescription calls for a Class A narcotic, codeine sulfate, in a quantity not more than one grain per dose, which, when combined with a therapeutic dose of aspirin, is converted into a component of a Class B narcotic so that the official signature of the prescriber is not required. Any narcotic prescription falling within the definition of a Class B product may be accepted orally, in person or by telephone, by the pharmacist from a physician. Also necessary on a narcotic prescription, such as this, are the narcotic registry number of the prescriber and his office address.

While there is a decided tendency on the part of the medical practitioner to write simple, single-ingredient prescriptions, there are still some compound prescriptions such as the one illustrated in Figure 1-2.

The inscription of a typical compound prescription may contain 4 distinct portions, known as the **basis,** the **adjuvant,** the **correc-**

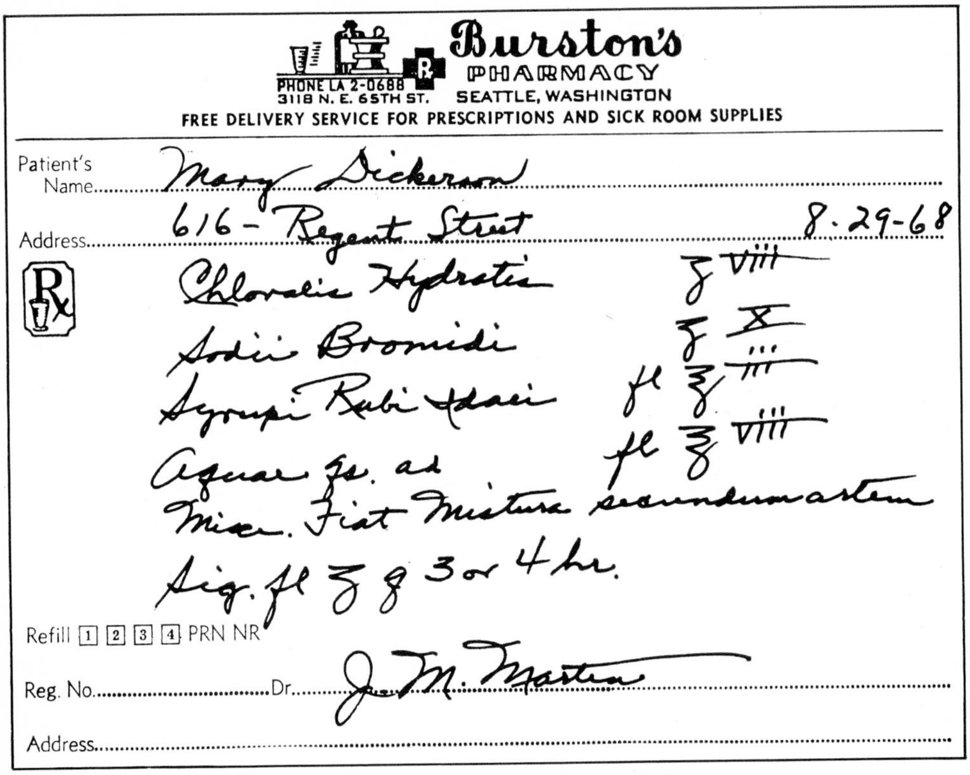

FIG. 1-2. Typical compound prescription.

tive and the **vehicle.** The basis is the chief active ingredient. In Figure 1-2, chloral hydrate is the basis, and from it the patient will derive a greater therapeutic effect than from any other ingredient. Chloral hydrate is a drug with hypnotic action. The adjuvant is that medicine included to aid or assist the basis. Sodium bromide is the adjuvant here; it has a sedative action due to the bromide ion. The corrective is that substance or those substances added to qualify the action of the basis and the adjuvant. Correctives are used to make other drugs less irritating or to serve as flavoring agents. The syrup of raspberry is added as a flavor. Finally, a vehicle (water in this prescription) is added to dilute the active constituents to a reasonable dose size.

This discussion of the portions of the inscription is of historical interest in that it fits the older prescriptions very well, but it can be applied to some modern prescriptions, too. The physician may only on occasion write such a compound prescription, but there are many commercial products prescribed by a single trade name that are actually in themselves compound prescriptions.

In a prescription requiring compounding by the pharmacist, the quantities of the ingredients and the total amount of the medication may be expressed in either apothecaries' or metric units. Occasionally, in certain types of formulas, the concentration of the active constituent is stated in percentage.

Figures 1-1 and 1-2 illustrate prescriptions in which quantities are expressed in the apothecaries' system. These units are still used in some prescriptions, but the proportion of metric prescriptions is in the majority and is increasing. Any table of units, whether it involves weights and measures or some other problem such as a monetary system, is more convenient to use if it is based on the decimal system. The use of the metric system in preference to the apothecaries' system is, in most instances, more convenient to the physician and the pharmacist.

The metric system is used for formulas and doses of products in the *U.S.P.,* the *N.F., New Drugs* and the *American Hospital Formulary Service.* The sizes of many products and the doses of practically all of the individual units of the newer products marketed by

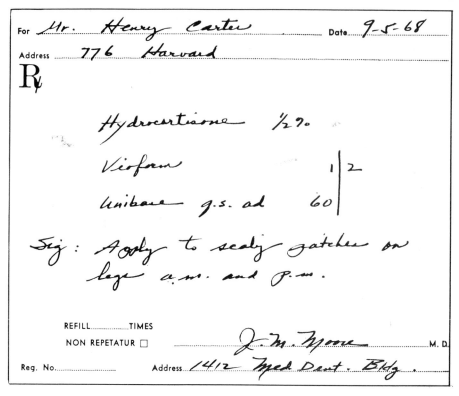

For *Mr. Henry Carter*   Date *9-5-68*

Address   *776 Harvard*

R

Hydrocortisone   ½%

Viofoam

Unibase — q.s. ad   60

Sig: Apply to scaly patches on legs a.m. and p.m.

REFILL............TIMES

NON REPETATUR ☐   *J. M. Moore*   M. D.

Reg. No................   Address *1412 Med Dent. Bldg.*

FIG. 1-3. Typical prescription employing the metric system.

drug manufacturers are given in the metric system. Sizes and doses of some new products and many of the older products are given in both the metric and the apothecaries' systems.

The following prescriptions indicate 2 methods by which metric quantities may be expressed:

R

Resorcin	2.4
Zinc Oxide	24.0
Talc	24.0
Sulfur	4.8
Acetone	12.0
Glycerin	12.0
Neutracolor	4.8
Isopropanol,	
Water, aa q.s. ad	240.0

Sig.—Apply thin coat after each washing.

In the prescription immediately preceding, the decimal points are placed properly one under the other, and it is understood that the dry, weighable substances are called for in grams, whereas the quantities following the liquids refer to milliliters. This prescription directs a total volume of 240 ml. of solution, a quantity which can readily be placed in an 8-fluidounce bottle. Volumes of 100 ml., 200 ml. and other amounts which do not approximate apothecary volumes for which containers are available are not dispensed so conveniently. Prescription bottles manufactured to contain convenient metric amounts are not available at present, although it is probable that, as the need becomes more apparent, they will be supplied. If a 100-ml. prescription is dispensed in a 4-oz. bottle, the container will be considerably less than full and the partially filled bottle must be explained to the average patient. The explanation can be accomplished by means of an "excuse label" which merely bears the statement that the prescription has been compounded according to the physician's directions, and, owing to the nature of the prescription, the bottle is not filled completely. A still simpler form of excuse label states: "Due to nature of contents, this bottle is not filled completely."

Ŗ

Codeine phosphate		48
Ammonium chloride	8	
Wild cherry syrup to make	120	

In the prescription immediately preceding, the vertical line serves as a decimal point. Every portion of the number to the left of the line indicates the whole number of grams or milliliters, while the figures to the right of the line indicate tenths, hundredths, etc., of a gram or milliliter. The amount of codeine phosphate usually would be read as 480 mg., although it might be expressed as 48 cg. or 0.48 Gm.

For convenience, the vertical line may be printed on the prescription blank. If it is not already on the blank, some physicians make a practice of drawing in the vertical line (as illustrated in Fig. 1-3) in order to eliminate misinterpretation of quantities. If the figures calling for a series of ingredients are made in such a manner that the decimal points do not fall one beneath the other, the pharmacist may have difficulty in interpreting the prescription.

Figure 1-4 illustrates a prescription in which the quantities are not written in a straight vertical line. The quantity of phenol (4 Gm.) easily could be read as 0.4 Gm. Not only is the 4 set over to the right toward the tenths position, but the dot over the *i* in

calcis is so located that it might be mistaken for a decimal point. The usual quantity of phenol in such a dermatologic preparation is between 1 and 2 per cent. However, since similar prescriptions written by this physician had been filled at this particular pharmacy, it was an easy matter for the pharmacist to interpret the prescription.

If there ever is any doubt on the part of the pharmacist as to the intentions of the physician, he should telephone the physician to have him clarify the prescriptions.

Figure 1-3 illustrates a prescription that necessitates calculation of the amounts of the active ingredients. Percentage strength in ointments is of the weight-in-weight type. Sixty Gm. is to be the total weight of the ointment. One-half per cent of 60 Gm. or 0.3 Gm. is the quantity of hydrocortisone required.

Calculations w/w in the apothecaries' system utilize the figure 480 (grains per ounce). If one were to make 1 ʒ of a 10 per cent ointment of ammoniated mercury in white ointment, he would use 10 per cent of 480 or 48 gr. of the active constituent and enough white ointment (432 gr.) to make the finished product up to a total of 480 gr.

As a general rule, Roman numerals are used with apothecaries' units and Arabic figures are used to designate quantities in the metric system. The prescription in Figure 1-5 is unusual in that Roman numerals are used with the metric volumetric unit, cc. In writing the directions to the patient, the physician used an Arabic figure for 2 drops rather than the Roman numeral generally employed with such abbreviations.

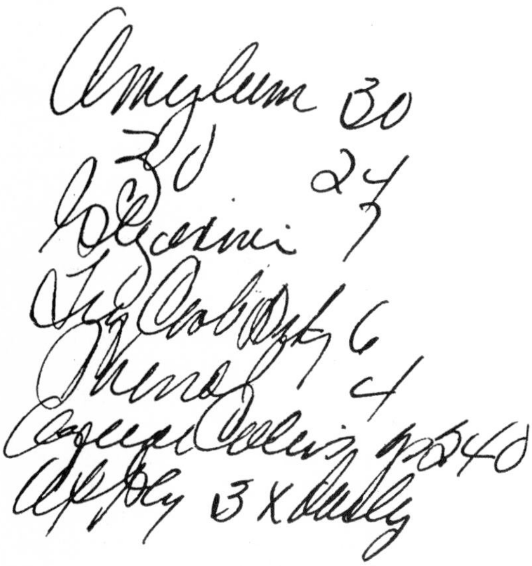

FIG. 1-4. Metric prescription.

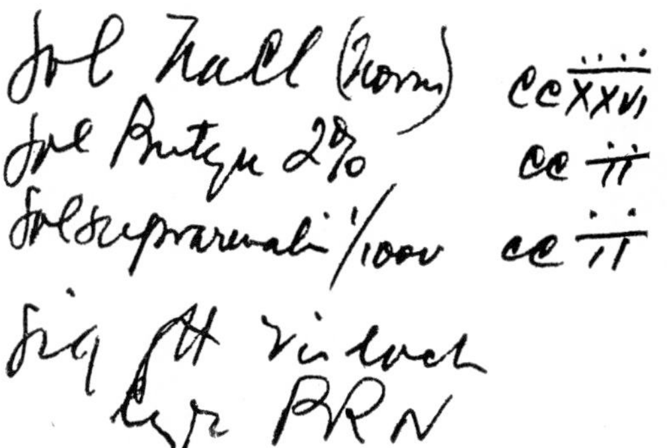

FIG. 1-5. Unusual modern prescription.

DOSAGE CALCULATIONS

The quantities of drugs in a prescription are occasionally written for a single dose with instructions to send a specific number of doses. In the following prescription, a 5-gr. quantity of potassium iodide is directed to be dissolved in enough cherry syrup to make 1 fluidram. Twenty-four such doses or 24 fluidrams (3 fluidounces) is the quantity to be dispensed. The dose (1 fluidram) is translated to the patient as 1 teaspoonful. Accordingly, the required 120 gr. or 2 drams of potassium iodide should be dissolved in enough of the syrup to make 3 fluidounces. However, the patient will very likely use a household teaspoon to measure his medicine; he will probably take close to 5 ml. at each dose and may get only 18 doses from his prescription. A practical solution to the problem would be to make the volume of the prescription up to 4 fluidounces (approximately 120 ml.) to assure 24 doses of 5 ml. each. In any event the problem should be discussed with the physician and with the patient.

℞
Potassii iodidi . . . . gr. v
Syrup cerasi, q.s. . . . . fl ℨ i

M. Ft. solutio. D.t.d. xxiv.

Sig.: fl ℨ i in aqua t.i.d. p.c.

It was assumed in discussing the preceding prescription that the likely size of the household teaspoon is 5 ml. Actually the size varies considerably, and a given teaspoon will yield different volumes of medicine dependent on the technic of the person measuring the powder or the liquid.[14] In a similar manner, the dessertspoon, the tablespoon and the teacup vary in size, depending on the measuring devices available in different households. *U.S.P. X* recognized the volumes of the teaspoon, the dessertspoon and the tablespoon to be "4 cc., 8 cc. and 15 cc.," or 1 fluidram, 2 fluidrams and 4 fluidrams, respectively. Some physicians continue to write prescriptions in the apothecaries' system (see preceding prescription); in such cases, wherever fluidram is employed it is assumed to mean teaspoonful. Medicine graduates, made of glass and standardized in terms of 8 teaspoonfuls to the fluidounce,

TABLE 1-1. APPROXIMATE EQUIVALENTS IN FLUID MEASURE

HOUSEHOLD MEASURE	APOTHECARIES	METRIC
Teaspoonful	fl. ℨ i	4 ml.
Dessertspoonful . .	fl. ℨ ii	8 ml.
Tablespoonful . . .	fl. ℨ iv	15 ml.
Wineglassful	fl. ℥ ii	60 ml.
Teacupful	fl. ℥ iv	120 ml.
Tumblerful	fl. ℥ viii	240 ml.
Cupful	fl. ℥ viii	236.6 ml.*

* American Standards Association, New York 17, N. Y.

are still in wide use. Accordingly, the household measures would have the values indicated in columns 2 and 3 of Table 1-1. The dessertspoon, wineglass and teacup listed in the table are now infrequently used in measuring doses of prescriptions.

In view of the fact that the American Standards Association has established an American Standard Teaspoon as containing 4.93 ± 0.24 ml., and recognizing that the majority of people will use teaspoons ordinarily available in the household for the administration of medicine, the U.S.P. Revision Committee specified in *U.S.P. XV* that the teaspoon may be regarded as being equivalent to 5 ml. Originally, the Committee added that the dessertspoon and the tablespoon may be regarded as representing 10 and 15 ml., respectively, but this last statement was not included in the *U.S.P.* text. *U.S.P. XVIII* specifies that the teaspoon is equivalent to 5 ml.

The American Standards Association recognized ⅙ fl. ℥ as the apothecaries' equivalent of the teaspoon. The American Standards tablespoon is 14.79 ± 0.73 ml. (½ fl. ℥) and the cupful is 236.6 ± 11.8 ml. (8 fl. ℥).

It should be pointed out that tables of household measurement in cookbooks also recognize 3 teaspoonfuls as being equal to 1 tablespoonful.

Some manufacturers, in labeling oral liquid preparations intended to be administered in teaspoonful quantities, specify the quantity of medicinal contained in 1 teaspoonful to be 5 ml. However, a few manufacturers specify the quantity of medicinal in a 4-ml. teaspoonful; accordingly, there are approximately 7½ such doses in each fluidounce of liquid.

Glass medicine graduates have already been mentioned. Disposable, plastic medicine graduates especially designed for use in hospitals are also available. Some manufacturers mark the graduates to contain 8 teaspoonfuls to the fluidounce and others mark them to conform to the 5-ml. teaspoonful and 15-ml. tablespoonful (3 teaspoonfuls to the tablespoonful). On the latter graduates dessertspoonfuls (10 ml.) are also marked.

Another unit of volumetric measure which varies considerably is the drop. This unit is used to measure doses of potent remedies and frequently is confused with the minim. The minim is always one sixtieth of a fluidram, but the drop varies in size depending on a number of factors. One factor contributing to the variability of the size of the drop is the surface from which the liquid is dropped, including the external diameter of the delivery end of the tube if a tube is used to produce the drops. Other factors affecting the size of the drop are surface tension, the density and the temperature of the liquid and the rate at which the drops are formed.

The *U.S.P.* defines the pharmacopeial medicine dropper as a tube of glass or other suitable transparent material that is generally fitted with a collapsible bulb. The tube is of varying capacity but is constricted at the delivery end to an external diameter of 3 mm. When held vertically the dropper will deliver water in drops which weigh between 45 and 55 mg. each. A dropper which delivers 20 drops per milliliter of water may deliver as many as 50 drops per milliliter of alcohol.

The pharmacist may prepare a number of stock solutions which commonly are used in such small quantities that it is desirable to express these quantities in terms of drops. Liquefied phenol, amaranth solution, solutions of other coloring agents and flavoring oils or alcoholic solutions thereof serve as examples. If these solutions are stored in dropper bottles, the dropper of which has been standardized for the particular liquid its bottle contains, the process of compounding can be facilitated.

PHARMACEUTICAL LATIN

Latin has been used as the language of the prescription because it is the language of scientific nomenclature and is used in the sciences in general. Since it is a dead language, it is less likely to be altered than are the modern languages. It is a universal language; Latin terms are definite, whereas the vernacular names of drugs are characteristic of certain localities. Latin was the language of official nomenclature until publication of *U.S.P. XIII* and *N.F. VIII,* when English titles were listed first and Latin titles were placed second. *U.S.P. XVIII* and *N.F. XIII* do not list Latin titles.

The majority of prescriptions today present a mixture of English and Latin. The names of the ingredients are usually in English or in an abbreviated form which may represent either English or Latin titles, while the directions to the pharmacist and to the patient commonly are in abbreviated Latin. Only very rarely is a prescription written entirely in Latin. There are many prescriptions calling for the specialty products of drug manufacturers which are designated by titles incapable of ready Latinization.

So long as any Latin words or abbreviations appear in prescriptions, the pharmacist must be able to interpret them correctly. This problem is not usually a difficult matter as the terms most commonly used are recognizable at a glance after sufficient experience has been gained.

The ability to explain why the various terms possess their particular grammatical construction is quite another story. One must have a knowledge of the various declensions of nouns and adjectives, the conjugation of verbs, the uses of prepositions and, occasionally, the interpretation of idiomatic expressions. Latin is a highly inflected language. The changes in the words, or inflections, are used in Latin to show case and number of nouns; case, number and gender of adjectives; and voice, tense, mood, person and number of verbs.

There are 6 cases for Latin nouns and adjectives, but only 2 of these are used extensively in pharmacy—nominative and genitive. The stem of the word is that portion which does not change in any of the various

TABLE 1-2. LATIN WORDS AND PHRASES

TERM OR PHRASE	ABBREVIATION	MEANING
acidum	acid, ac.	an acid
ad	ad	to, up to
adde, addatur	add.	add, let be added
ad libitum	ad lib.	at pleasure, as much as one pleases
admove, admoveatur	admov.	apply, let be applied
ad partes dolentes	ad part. dolent.	to the painful parts
agita, agitetur	agit.	shake, stir; let it be shaken or stirred
albus, -a, -um	alb.	white
ampulla	ampul.	an ampul
ana	aa, $\overline{aa}$	of each
ante	a.	before
ante cibos	a.c.	before meals
ante cibum	a.c.	before food
aqua	aq.	water
aqua bulliens	aq. bull.	boiling water
aqua destillata	aq. dest.	distilled water
balneum	baln.	bath
balneum vaporis	baln. vap.	a steam bath
bene	bene	well
bis in die	b.i.d.	twice a day
bis terve in die	b.t.i.d.	2 or 3 times a day
bromidum	brom.	a bromide
calcium	calc., Ca	calcium
capsula, capsulae	cap., caps.	a capsule, capsules
carbonas	carb.	carbonate
cataplasma	catapl.	a cataplasm, poultice
charta	chart.	paper, powder
charta cerata	chart. cerat.	waxed paper
chartae	chart.	papers, powders
chartula	chart.	(small) paper, powder
chloridum	chlorid.	chloride
cochleare amplum	coch. ampl.	tablespoonful
cochleare magnum	coch. mag.	tablespoonful
cochleare medium	coch. med.	dessertspoonful
cochleare parvum	coch. parv.	teaspoonful
collodium	collod.	collodion
collunarium	collun.	nasal douche
collyrium	collyr.	an eye lotion, an eyewash
compositus, -a, -um	comp., co.	compound
congius	cong., C.	a gallon
contusus, -a, -um	contus.	bruised
cum	c, $\overline{c}$	with
cum aqua	cum aq.	with water
da, detur, dentur	d., det.	give, let be given
decubitus	decub.	having gone to bed
dentur tales doses	d.t.d.	give of such doses
diebus alternis	dieb. alt.	on alternate days
dilutus, -a, -um	dil.	dilute (adj.), diluted
dimidius, -a, -um	dim.	one half
dividatur in partes aequales	div. in par. aeq.	let be divided into equal parts
doses	dos.	doses
dosis	dos.	a dose
durante dolore	dur. dol.	while pain lasts
elixir	elix.	an elixir
emplastrum	emp.	a plaster
emulsum	emuls.	emulsion
et	et	and

TABLE 1-2. LATIN WORDS AND PHRASES *(Continued)*   [11]

TERM OR PHRASE	ABBREVIATION	MEANING
ex aqua	ex aq.	in water
ex modo praescripto	e.m.p.	in the manner prescribed
extractum	ext.	an extract
fac	ft.	make
ferrum	ferr.	iron
fiant	ft.	let them be made
fiat	ft.	let it be made
fiat lege artis	f.l.a.	let be made according to the law of the art
filtra	filt.	filter
gargarisma	garg.	a gargle
gelatum	gel.	a gel, jelly
glyceritum	glycer.	a glycerite
glycerogelatinum	glycerogel.	glycerogelatin
granum, grana	gr.	a grain, grains
gutta, guttae	gtt.	drop, drops
guttatim	guttat.	drop by drop
hora decubitus	hor. decub.	at bed hour, at bedtime
hora somni	h.s.	at bedtime
hydrargyrum	hydrarg.	mercury
in	in	in, into, within
in aqua	in aq.	in water
in die	in d.	in a day
infusum	inf.	an infusion
inhalatio	inhal.	inhalation
in vitro	in vit.	in glass
iodidum	iodid.	an iodide
kalium	K	potassium
lavatio	lavat.	a wash
leviter	lev.	lightly
linimentum	lin.	a liniment
liquor	liq.	a liquor; solution
lotio	lot.	a lotion
magma	mag.	a magma; milk
magnus, -a, -um	mag.	large
mane primo	man. prim.	first thing in the morning
medius, -a, -um	med.	medium
misce	M.	you mix
mistura	mist.	a mixture
mitte talis, mitte tales	mitt. tal.	send such
modo dictu	m. dict.	as directed
modo praescripto	mod. praes., m.p.	in the manner prescribed
mollis	moll.	soft
more dicto	mor. dict.	in the manner directed
mucilago	mucil.	a mucilage
natrium	Na	sodium
nebula	nebul.	a spray
nihil album	nihil alb.	zinc oxide
nocte	noct.	at night
nocte maneque	noct. maneq.	night and morning
non repetatur	non rep.	do not repeat
numero	no.	number
octarius	O., oct.	a pint
oculo dextro	ocul. dext.	in the right eye
oculo sinistro	ocul. sinist.	in the left eye
oculo utro	o.u., ocul. utro, O_2	each eye
odontalgicum	odont.	toothache drops

TERM OR PHRASE	ABBREVIATION	MEANING
oleum	ol.	an oil
omni hora	omn. hor.	every hour
omni mane vel nocte	omn. man. vel noct.	every morning or night
omni quarta hora	omn. 4 hr.	every 4 hours
omnis	omn.	all; every
omni secunda hora	omn. 2 hr.	every second hour
omni tertia hora	omn. tert. hor.	every 3 hours, every third hour
optimus, -a, -um	opt.	the best
partes aequales	p.e.	equal parts
parvus, -a, -um	parv.	small
pasta	past.	a paste
pastillus	pastil.	lozenge, pastille
per diem	per diem	per day
per os	per os	by mouth
phosphas	phos.	a phosphate
pilula, pilulae	pil.	a pill, pills
placebo	placebo	I please
ponderosus	pond.	heavy
pone	pone	put, place
post cibum, post cibos	p.c.	after food, after meals
praecipitatus	ppt.	precipitated
pro dose	pro dos.	for a dose
pro ratione aetatis	pro rat. aetatis	according to age
pro recto	pro rect.	rectally
pro re nata	p.r.n.	as occasion arises
pro urethra	pro ureth.	urethral
pro usu externo	pro us. ext.	for external use
pro vagina	pro vagin.	vaginal
pulvis, pulveres	pulv.	a powder, powders
quantum libet	q.l.	as much as you wish
quantum sufficit	q.s.	as much as suffices
quantum vis	q. vis	as much as you wish
quaque hora	qq. hor.	every hour
quater in die	4 i.d., q.i.d.	4 times a day
recipe	℞	take thou
ruber, rubra, rubrum	rub.	red
sal	sal	salt
saturatus, -a, -um	sat.	saturated
secundum artem	s.a.	according to art
semel	semel	once
semi, semis	ss, s̄s̄	one half
semihora	semihor.	half hour
sesqui	sesq.	one and one half
signa, signetur	sig.	write, let be written
simul	simul	at the same time
sine	s.	without
sine aqua	sine aq.	without water
si opus sit	si op. sit, s.o.s.	if there is need
sodium	sod., Na	sodium
solutio	sol.	a solution
solutio saturata	sol. sat.	a saturated solution
spiritus	sp.	a spirit
spiritus vini rectificatus	sp. vin. rect., s.v.r.	alcohol
spiritus vini tenuis	sp. vin. ten., s.v.t.	proof spirit, diluted alcohol
statim	stat.	immediately
sulfas	sulf.	a sulfate
sume, sumendus	sum.	take, to be taken

TABLE 1-2. LATIN WORDS AND PHRASES *(Continued)*   [13]

TERM OR PHRASE	ABBREVIATION	MEANING
suppositoria	suppos.	suppositories
suppositoria rectalia	suppos. rect.	rectal suppositories
suppositorium	suppos.	a suppository
syrupus	syr.	a syrup
tabletta	tab.	tablet
tales doses	tal. dos.	such doses
talis, tales, talia	tal.	such
ter	t.	3 times, thrice
ter in die	t.i.d.	3 times a day
ter quaterve in die	t.q.i.d.	3 or 4 times a day
tinctura	tr., tinct.	a tincture
trituratio	trit.	a trituration
trochiscus, trochisci	troch.	a troche, troches
uncia	oz., ℥	ounce
unguentum	ungt.	an ointment
ut dictum	ut dict.	as told, as directed
vaccinum	vac.	a vaccine
vel	vel	or
vinum	vin.	a wine
viridis, -e	vir.	green
unus, -a, -um	i, I	1
duo, duae, duo	ii, II	2
tres, tria	iii, III	3
quattuor	iv, IV	4
quinque	v, V	5
sex	vi, VI	6
septem	vii, VII	7
octo	viii, VIII	8
novem	ix, IX	9
decem	x, X	10
undecim	xi, XI	11
duodecim	xii, XII	12
tredecim	xiii, XIII	13
quattuordecim	xiv, XIV	14
quindecim	xv, XV	15
sedecim	xvi, XVI	16
septendecim	xvii, XVII	17
duodeviginti	xviii, XVIII	18
undeviginti	xix, XIX	19
viginti	xx, XX	20
viginti unus	xxi, XXI	21
viginti duo	xxii, XXII	22
trigenta	xxx, XXX	30
quadraginta	xl, XL	40
quinquaginta	l, L	50
sexaginta	lx, LX	60
septuaginta	lxx, LXX	70
octoginta	lxxx, LXXX	80
nonaginta	xc, XC	90
centum	C	100

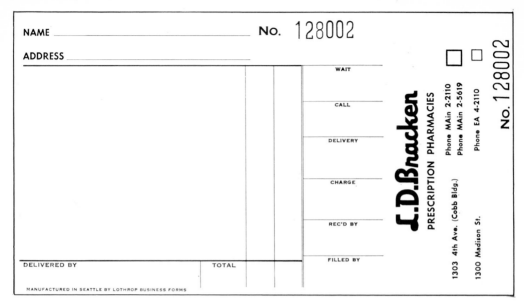

NAME _____ No. 128002

ADDRESS _____

WAIT

CALL

DELIVERY

CHARGE

REC'D BY

FILLED BY

DELIVERED BY   TOTAL

MANUFACTURED IN SEATTLE BY LOTHROP BUSINESS FORMS

J.D.Bracken
PRESCRIPTION PHARMACIES

Phone MAin 2-2110
Phone MAin 2-5619

Phone EA 4-2110

No. 128002

1303 4th Ave. (Cobb Bldg.)

1300 Madison St.

FIG. 1-6. A combination claim check and pilot sheet which is useful for recording necessary information and will help avoid errors in processing information.

inflected forms. To the stem is added the necessary ending to form each case. One example will suffice at this point. The Latin for tincture is *tinctura* (nominative case) and the Latin for belladonna is *belladonna* (nominative case). The stems of the words are *tinctur* and *belladonn,* respectively. The prescription form for tincture of belladonna is *tincturae belladonnae* (both words in the genitive case for limitation).

For a complete discussion of the subject, the student is referred to one of the textbooks devoted entirely to pharmaceutical Latin.[15] in Table 1-2 are listed pharmaceutically useful Latin words and phrases with their abbreviations and meanings.

PRESCRIPTION PROCEDURE

RECEIVING THE PRESCRIPTION

In the majority of pharmacies, it is the practice to have a registered pharmacist personally receive the prescription from the patient or the person who presents the prescription for the patient. The pharmacist can serve in this capacity in a more dignified and a more efficient manner than can some other employee of the pharmacy. There may be questions asked by the patient which need the attention of the pharmacist. Also this

patient contact offers the pharmacist the opportunity to practice one phase of clinical pharmacy. The use of family prescription records is discussed later in this chapter.

If the patient's name and address do not appear on the prescription, the receiver should obtain this information. If the prescription is intended for a child, the age of the patient for whom the medicine is intended should be recorded on the prescription. Some physicians supply this information on the order.

The receiver of the prescription should ascertain whether the patient (or his agent) wishes to wait for the medicine, return for it at some specified time or have it delivered. On this information will depend the order in which the prescriptions then in the pharmacy will receive the attention of those compounding and dispensing. Well-designed pharmacies have waiting areas provided for those who wait for their prescriptions.

PROCESSING THE PRESCRIPTION

Some of the larger pharmacies use a claim-check system to prevent mistakes in the identity of prescriptions. A combination claim check and pilot sheet such as that illustrated in Figure 1-6 may be used. This sheet has a space for the patient's name and address and spaces where the receiver can place his own identity and note whether the patient will wait for his prescription or return for it later. The pilot sheet is divided into 2 parts, designed so that the smaller part can be torn off and can be used as a claim check. The major portion of the sheet carries the same number as the claim check and follows the written order through the pharmacy while the medicine is prepared. This claim-check number, of course, bears no relationship to the serial number that will be assigned to the prescription and the finished product. Most pharmacists using the pilot-sheet system stamp the current date on both the claim-check portion and the remainder of the pilot sheet. Sometimes this date is of value in keeping records.

The pilot sheet and the prescription are taken by some compounder who puts his initials in the space provided for his identity and then proceeds to fill the prescription. When the prescription is labeled, the serial number of the prescription is stamped on the pilot sheet as well as on the label and the pharmacist sets down in the space provided the fee to be charged for the prescription. The pilot sheet is attached to the finished product and these are laid aside to be claimed. Space is provided on the sheet for the listing of additional purchases. If the bill is paid, the cash register stamps the amount paid on the pilot sheet. If the bill is to be charged, the pilot sheet is so marked and is sent to the bookkeeper, who makes the proper charges.

Many prescriptions are received from the physician by telephone. Usually, the pharmacist taking the dictated prescription over the telephone will first write it out in abbreviated form on scratch paper and in a few moments write out the good copy which is to be kept on file. The pharmacist must use care in taking prescriptions by telephone that he gets them correctly. If any question arises about the physician's wishes, the pharmacist should hold the conversation open until he is sure he has the prescription correctly in mind and enough of it on paper to transfer that information in its entire intent to the good copy.

One real advantage of the telephone to both the pharmacist and the physician is that it develops a good interprofessional relationship. While the pharmacist has the physician on the telephone, he can question any possible incompatibilities. Many times, the physician inquires about new drugs or new forms of administration. The pharmacist can be of real service as a consultant to the physician if he studies the new products and is alert in answering the physician's questions.

DISPENSING THE PRESCRIPTION

Dispensing includes reading the prescription, checking the prescription for safety, compounding and/or measuring the medication, packaging the medication, labeling the prescription, checking the prescription, recording information on the prescription, filing the prescription and talking with the patient.

Dispensing pharmacy is the final step in the presentation of medicaments in a form suitable for administration to the patient. Although dispensing pharmacy is based on sound scientific principles, it is described as an art, and much of the personality of the pharmacist is evidenced by the prescriptions which he compounds.

Neatness, accuracy and speed are 3 qualities that must be developed by the individual who wishes to become a pharmacist. Neatness and accuracy must be developed first; speed comes with experience.

Nothing can impede the progress of a pharmacist as much as a disarranged counter on which to compound his prescriptions. A slovenly dispenser will never become a good one. The habit of leaving bottles and utensils in disorder on the counter, or of allowing dirty apparatus and containers to collect on or in the prescription case, indicates an undisciplined attitude which will not express itself in accuracy.

In many smaller pharmacies, only a small part of the pharmacist's time is spent in the compounding of prescriptions. Whatever the ratio of professionalism to merchandising, a portion of the pharmacy should be set apart wherein the compounding of prescriptions can be conducted without interruption.

During the time a pharmacist is compounding any one prescription, that prescription should be given his undivided attention. When his attention is not devoted entirely to the prescription, errors are likely to creep in. For this reason, it is a good

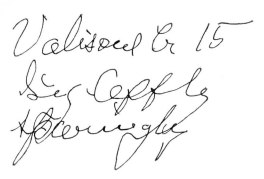

FIG. 1-7. Prescription presenting a problem in legibility.

policy to keep the prescription room clear of everyone except the pharmacist. If visitors do happen to come in, the pharmacist should complete his visiting and then return to his work.

READING THE PRESCRIPTION

The legibility of a prescription depends on the experience of a pharmacist as well as the penmanship of the medical practitioner. A pharmacist who is accustomed to handling prescriptions written by certain physicians will experience no difficulty in reading them, whereas another pharmacist may have trouble with portions of the orders. As the pharmacist becomes more experienced in recognizing certain drug combinations and characteristic directions for the compounding and the uses of those combinations, he finds it easier to read prescriptions.

A pharmacist with experience in reading the penmanship of the physicians who wrote the prescriptions in Figures 1-7 and 1-8 would probably have little difficulty in interpreting their intentions. The inexperienced pharmacist, however, might have considerable trouble in reading them, and might even find it necessary to consult the physicians.

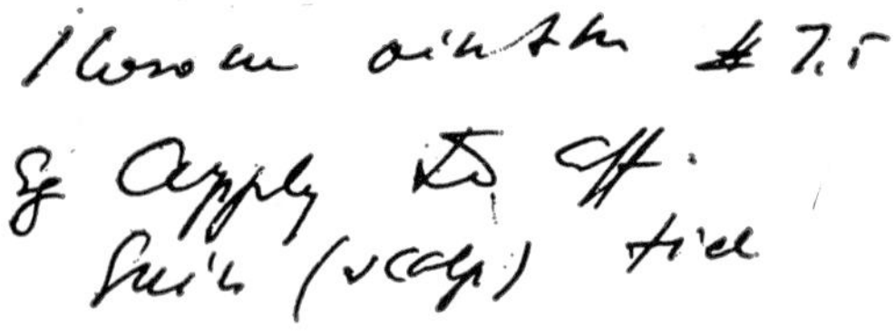

FIG. 1-8. Prescription presenting problems in legibility and in product identity.

The prescription in Figure 1-7 calls for 15 Gm. of Valisone* Cream; the directions are to apply sparingly.

The prescription in Figure 1-8 is written for 7.5 Gm. of Ilosone* ointment with the directions, apply to affected skin (scalp) three times a day. Actually there is no such product as Ilosone ointment; what the physician wanted whenever he wrote for such was Ilotycin* ointment.

CHECKING THE PRESCRIPTION FOR SAFETY

Before a pharmacist attempts to compound a prescription, he must understand all of it thoroughly. He must be satisfied that there are no dangerous overdoses or incompatibilities. If any portion of the prescription is not understood, or if he has detected an incompatibility, he should consult the physician who wrote the order. Some pharmacists hesitate to call the medical practitioner about these matters, but, if the calls are executed tactfully, there is no reason why they should not create a better understanding between the practitioners of both professions.

The dose of each drug in a prescription should be checked carefully by the pharmacist before he proceeds to fill the prescription. It should be emphasized that, in the event of injuries or fatalities from prescriptions containing overdoses of drugs, *the pharmacist can be held criminally liable.*

Those factors which the pharmacist should take into account in judging the danger or the safety of a dose of medicine follow.

Age, Weight or Body Surface Area of the Patient. There are a number of methods for calculating the fractional part of the average adult dose which an infant or a child can take safely. One method (*Dr. Fried's Rule*) which has been recommended for calculating doses for infants younger than 1 year of age is based on the assumption that an adult dose of a drug can be tolerated safely by a child when he reaches the age of 150 months. Therefore,

$$\frac{\text{Age (in months)}}{150} \times \text{Adult dose} = \text{Infant's dose}$$

Two other formulas which are based on age of the patient and which have been used

* Trade mark.

FIG. 1-9. West's nomogram for the estimation of body surface area. Prepared by C. D. West. (From Shirkey, H. C., and Barba, W. P., II: Drug Therapy. *In:* Nelson, W. E. (ed.): Textbook of Pediatrics. ed. 9. Philadelphia, W. B. Saunders, 1969.)

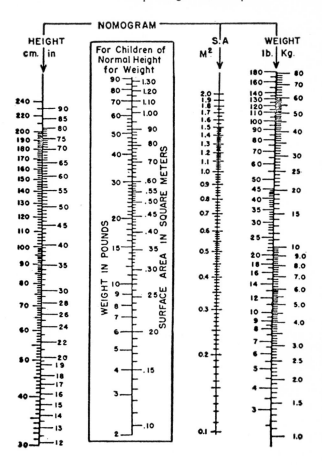

for calculating doses for children 2 years of age or older are *Dr. Young's Rule* and *Dr. Cowling's Rule.*

By Dr. Young's Rule:

$$\frac{\text{Age}}{\text{Age} + 12} \times \text{Adult dose} = \text{Child's dose}$$

Dr. Cowling's Rule is based on age in years at next birthday (present age + 1):

$$\frac{\text{Age} + 1}{24} \times \text{Adult dose} = \text{Child's dose}$$

Dr. Clark's Rule assumes the average weight of an adult to be 150 pounds. Therefore,

$$\frac{\text{Weight of child in pounds}}{150} \times \text{Adult dose} = \text{Child's dose}$$

As a general rule, a naturally heavy individual can withstand larger doses of medicines than a person of less weight.

According to Shirkey[19] and Done[10] many physiological factors, including blood volume, oxygen consumption, glomerular filtration and body organ growth as well as requirements for fluids, electrolytes and calories are more closely related to body surface area (BSA) than they are to body weight, and use of BSA in calculation of pediatric dosage as a fraction of the usual adult dosage is preferable to calculations on the basis of body weight. The following formula can be used to calculate pediatric doses from the usual adult dose:

$$\frac{\text{BSA in M}^2 \text{ of child}}{\text{BSA in M}^2 \text{ of adult}} \times \text{usual adult dose} = \text{child's dose}$$

$$\frac{\text{BSA in M}^2 \text{ of child}}{1.7} \times \text{usual adult dose} = \text{child's dose}$$

The formula is based on the 100 per cent adult dose for an individual weighing about 140 lb. and having a BSA of about 1.7 M². The BSA of an individual can be estimated from his height and weight by reference to the nomogram shown in Figure 1-9. A straight edge is placed from the patient's height in the left column to his weight in the right column, and the intersect on the body-surface-area column indicates his body surface area. For children of average build, the surface area may be estimated from the weight alone by reference to the enclosed area in the left center of the figure.

Particular caution should be exercised in estimating doses of drugs for premature and full-term newborn infants. Some of the enzyme systems and organ functions of these infants are not completely developed and these babies are not able to metabolize and excrete certain drugs in the same manner as do older children and adults. Consequently, a toxic reaction may occur from a dose of medicine which would be expected, on a size-of-the-patient basis, to be a safe dose.

Geriatric patients also may lack ability to metabolize and excrete certain drugs because of impaired organ function. Hence, dosage of certain drugs for these patients must be carefully considered.

Route of Administration. Comparison of the oral doses of drugs with the intravenous, the intramuscular, the subcutaneous or the rectal doses of the same drugs shows that no valid rule can be established for predicting the parenteral or the rectal dose of a drug from the oral dose. Drugs which are absorbed completely from the gastrointestinal tract will probably have equal parenteral and oral doses, whereas drugs which are poorly absorbed by the oral route will have smaller doses parenterally than orally. The pharmacist must know the range of safe and effective doses for the prescribed drug when administered by the prescribed route. Since many drugs cannot be administered safely by all parenteral routes, the pharmacist should also make certain that the prescribed route of administration is safe for the particular drug.

Pharmaceutical Dosage Form. The vehicle of a prescription or the degree of subdivision of a solid drug in the particular dosage form affects the safety and the therapeutic efficacy of the prescription. If polyethylene glycol is used as the base for an ointment containing benzoic acid and salicylic acid, the concentrations of the acids should be only half what they would be if a hydrocarbon ointment base were employed, because the acids are more active in the polyethylene glycol base than they are in the hydrocarbon base. The degree of subdivision of an active drug also may affect its therapeutic activity and potential toxicity. Again using an ointment as an example, if polysorbate 80 is mixed with coal tar prior to incorporation of coal tar into the ointment base, a lower concentration of coal tar must be prescribed. This is due to the fact that the subdivision of coal tar brought about by prior mixture with the polysorbate 80 results in a more pronounced action on the skin.

Frequency of Administration. If the drug has a fleeting action, there should be little concern about the short intervals of time between doses. On the other hand, many potent drugs have a cumulative action. If the frequency of administration is too great, toxic manifestations may appear, even though the individual dose appears to be safe. There should be more concern about these drugs when prescriptions of large quantity are ordered which make possible a large number of doses over a short time. Among such cumulative drugs are bishydroxycoumarin, digitoxin and thyroid.

Sometimes, the author of a prescription has a particularly good reason for the apparent overdose of a drug and he perhaps intends the dose he has prescribed, but the pharmacist nevertheless should consult the practitioner to satisfy himself that the dose is correct.

There are many factors involved concerning the safety of a given dose which the physician alone has the opportunity of knowing. A nervous person usually requires a greater quantity of sedative than a normal person, whereas a phlegmatic person usually requires a quantity of stimulant that seems abnormally large. The patient may have developed a tolerance for certain drugs and consequently needs abnormally large doses for the desired effect. Gross tolerances may exist in the patient who may have been taking one sedative for some time and has developed a tolerance for other member sedatives of the group as well as the one taken. Pathologic conditions sometimes demand larger doses of certain drugs. There may be an unusually large amount of pain accompanying the condition and abnormally large doses of narcotic may be required. These are some of the characteristics pertaining to the patient which only the physician knows. When he writes the prescription, he could underline the drug and the quantity to direct the pharmacist's attention to the fact that he is aware of the unusual dose he has called for. The letters Q.R. (*quantum rectum,* quantity verified or correct), both apothecaries' and metric systems or both Arabic figures and Roman numerals may be used for the same purpose.

COMPOUNDING THE PRESCRIPTION

A number of years ago the majority of prescriptions required compounding; that is, the pharmacist weighed or measured several drugs and combined them into one compatible, easily administered dosage form. Today, relatively few prescriptions involve compounding (as few as 1 per cent in some localities), but the pharmacist must still possess the knowledge and the skills in compounding that he formerly did, so that he can prepare the prescriptions and special formulations that are called for. In fact, with the development of new pharmaceutical aids — surface active agents, suspending agents, preservatives, synthetic flavors—today's pharmacist has more opportunity to use his specialized skills than did his predecessor. We now know that the excipients and the procedures he uses in compounding may have a pronounced effect on the therapeutic efficacy of the drug.

No one set procedure can be designed for compounding all prescriptions. Each class of prescription and, oftentimes, each prescription within the class requires its own characteristic procedure. The properties of the ingredients and even their quantities alter the methods that should be employed to fill the prescription. For a complete discussion of prescriptions representing each of the various classes of pharmaceutical preparations,

see the respective chapters in which they are treated.

Two essential factors in the compounding of prescriptions are qualitative and quantitative accuracy. Qualitative accuracy is probably the more important of the two, but results of either qualitative or quantitative inaccuracy are obvious. The most important precaution to be observed in the achievement of qualitative accuracy is to check the labels of the containers of stock drugs.

After the pharmacist has read and thoroughly understands the prescription, he should assemble all the ingredients on the prescription case, placing them on the left side of the balance and in the order in which they will be used. As this procedure is carried out, he compares the labels of the containers with the names of the drugs on the prescription. When he weighs or measures the prescribed quantity of each ingredient, he should place the stock bottle on the right side of his balance, again comparing the labels of the containers with the names of the drugs on the prescription. Then he is ready to mix the ingredients in the proper order to make the finished prescription.

As soon as the pharmacist is through with the stock containers, he should return them to their proper storage places, and, in so doing, he should again read the inscription of the prescription, as well as the label on the stock bottle. By following such a procedure, the pharmacist reads the label on each stock container 3 times and reads the inscription of the prescription 3 times while he is filling the prescription—once when the bottle is taken from the shelf and placed on the prescription case, again when the weighing or the measurement is made and, finally, when the stock bottle is returned to its proper place on the shelf.

Much has been written on the subject of prescription tolerances. Prescriptions have been analyzed and attempts have been made to establish legal tolerances. Regardless of what tolerances eventually may be established, the pharmacist should make every effort to compound his prescriptions accurately.

The *U.S.P.* and the *N.F.* have established individual standards for official preparations, and most of them seem to approximate a permitted error of $\pm$ 5 per cent. This degree of accuracy is sufficiently precise for nearly all therapeutic purposes and can be achieved with equipment ordinarily available in the pharmacy; in fact, with care, it is possible to compound with a greater degree of quantitative accuracy than an error of 5 per cent. Nevertheless this value will be selected for the discussion which follows.

It should be understood clearly that nothing should ever be said or done to pardon inaccuracy. On no account are carelessness and any tendencies to approximate to be permitted in any of the acts of dispensing. It must be emphasized that accurate compounding cannot be achieved by considering it a procedure to be practiced only under certain circumstances. It can be achieved only by developing an exacting technic and by rigidly adhering to such technic regardless of the pharmacist's opinion of the necessity for accuracy in any particular prescription. He cannot decide to compound carefully and exactly one time and to approximate on the next occasion.

In maintaining a satisfactory degree of accuracy in compounding, not only must the medicinal substances be weighed or measured with care, but also these ingredients must be handled in a manner to prevent losses of drugs and diluent in completing the prescription. Care must be exercised in transferring weighed materials and in pouring viscous fluids from graduates to make certain all of each ingredient is present in the final mixture. Furthermore, if the prescription calls for individual doses, each dosage form must contain an accurate fraction of the total medicinal products present. The dosage form may be either a weighable quantity or a measured volume. Most of the potent medicinal substances are solids. Therefore discussion of weighing will precede that of measurement of volume.

A prescription balance in good condition is usually sufficiently accurate to weigh fairly large quantities within the limits of $\pm$ 5 per cent, but its ability to weigh small quantities within these limits depends on its sensitivity. By one definition the sensitivity of a balance is the smallest weight which will disturb the equilibrium of the balance and is determined in the following manner.

Carefully adjust the balance to equilibrium and arrest the beam. Place the smallest weight on a pan and release the beam. If the equilibrium is undisturbed, arrest the beam and replace the weight with the next larger weight. If this weight does not upset the equilibrium, repeat the process until the minimum weight which will do so is found. This minimum weight designates the sensitivity of the balance and may be as little as 1 or 2 mg. (high sensitivity). Wear on the bearings and corrosion of knife edges cause a progressive decline in sensitivity and it is not unusual to find a balance with a sensitivity as low as 10 mg. Torsion balances of 120-Gm. capacity have a sensitivity of 2 mg. when new and, with proper care and technic in use, decline little in sensitivity because of lack of bearing surfaces.

It should be pointed out that interpretation of the end point "disturbs the equilibrium of the balance" can easily vary from one person's technic to the next. For this reason a sensitivity determination such as sensibility involving a definite scale on the balance is preferred. The sensibility reciprocal or sensitivity reciprocal of a balance is the amount of weight which must be added to one pan in order to produce a change of one division on the index plate in the rest point of the balance. The sensitivity reciprocal will be greater than the sensitivity determination previously described. A careful pharmacist should certainly be able to achieve an equilibrium with each weighing so that there is no greater deflection from the zero point of the balance than one division on the index scale. In fact, it should be possible for the pharmacist to duplicate weighings within one-half division or less of deflection.

The sensitivity of the balance is important when determining possible errors in weighing small quantities. For example, if 100 mg. is weighed on a balance having a sensitivity of 2 mg., the actual weight will be between 98 mg. and 102 mg., a possible error of $\pm$ 2 per cent. If the sensitivity of the balance is 5 mg., the actual weight will be between 95 mg. and 105 mg., a possible error of $\pm$ 5 per cent. If the sensitivity of the balance is 10 mg., the actual weight will be between 90 mg. and 110 mg., a possible error of $\pm$ 10 per cent. If one wished to achieve an accuracy of ± 5 per cent, he would have to weigh a minimum of 20 times the sensitivity of the balance. Since there are often other operations subsequent to the initial weighing, it is not good policy to weigh the minimum, but rather to weigh 30 or even 40 times the sensitivity of the balance. When more than one operation is involved in compounding, possible errors may cancel each other or they may be additive. In the latter case it is obvious why more than 20 times the sensitivity of the balance should be weighed.

When the desired quantity of medicinal is too small to be weighed with the selected accuracy, the pharmacist can follow one of several procedures. Tablets of the medicinal substance may be used, provided that they are available in such strength that a number of them will contain exactly the quantity needed for the prescription and, also, provided that excipients and fillers in the tablets are not objectionable ingredients in the prescription.

Tablet triturates or hypodermic tablets of the medicinal may be available for use in the prescription. However, it is quite unlikely that the quantity of medicinal needed would be exactly satisfied by one or a segment of the tablet. Furthermore, even if a segment contained exactly the desired quantity, it would be difficult to procure a segment which would be an accurate fraction of the tablet.

A third possibility is the use of triturations of potent medicinals prepared in quantities large enough to maintain accuracy of the product. These triturations vary in strength (usually from 1% to 10%) depending on the requirements for these dilutions and are kept in stock for compounding prescriptions which call for small quantities of potent drugs.

Aliquot Method of Weighing and Measuring. A fourth procedure for weighing or measuring very small quantities of drug is known as the aliquot method. An excess of the drug equal to a multiple of the quantity needed is weighed or measured, and is diluted to a convenient weight or volume. Then the aliquot, or part of the dilution which represents the desired quantity of drug, is used in the prescription. This method is illustrated by the following example.

℞
Atropine sulfate . . . . gr. ¼
Dist. water q.s. ad . . . . f℥ i
M. et Ft. Sol.
Sig. Gtt. ii ex. aq. 10′ before feeding

The sensitivity of the balance is 3 mg.; therefore, in order to have an error no greater than ± 5 per cent at least 60 mg. must be weighed. The pharmacist may weigh 1 gr. of atropine sulfate (four times the amount needed), place the drug in a small graduate and add enough distilled water to give a volume of 4 fluidrams. Since he has weighed four times the amount of atropine sulfate needed, he then uses ¼ of the solution (which then contains ¼ gr. of atropine sulfate) in the prescription. To the 1 fluidram of atropine sulfate concentrated solution he adds sufficient distilled water to make 1 fluidounce. This prescription could be filled just as well (or probably better) by weighing six times the amount of atropine sulfate actually needed, placing it in sufficient distilled water to give a volume of 6 fluidrams of solution and then using 1/6 of the concentrated atropine sulfate solution in the prescription. There are several correct methods of filling each prescription when using the aliquot method. The important rule is, the particular mutiple of the amount needed which is weighed or measured is the same factor by which the resulting powder or solution must be divided in order to obtain the quantity of diluted drug to use in the prescription. The pharmacist chooses a quantity of diluent which will give him a volume or weight of diluted drug which can be divided conveniently by the multiple he has chosen for the pure drug and which will give an aliquot large enough to be measured accurately. The pharmacist must at all times keep in mind the limitations of his balance, graduates, and pipets. Other examples and explanations follow.

℞
Benzalkonium chloride 1:5000
in sterile buffer solution q.s. ad . . . . 30 ml.
M. & Sig.: gtt. i O.U. q. 4 hr.

Benzalkonium chloride concentrate solution is 17 per cent in strength. A volume of 0.035 ml. of the concentrate is needed for this prescription. This volume cannot be measured accurately, even with a pipet graduated in 0.01 ml. However, a volume 10 times that needed, or 0.35 ml., can be measured accurately with this pipet. A volume of 0.35 ml. of the concentrate (ten times the amount needed) is added to enough sterile buffer solution to give a volume of 10 ml. Then 1/10 of this volume (1.0 ml., which contains 0.035 ml. of the benzalkonium chloride concentrate) is placed in a 30-ml. graduate, and sufficient sterile buffer solution is added (slowly, to prevent foaming) to give a volume of 30 ml. If the pharmacist wished, he could measure 100 times the volume of benzalkonium chloride concentrate needed (3.5 ml.), add sufficient sterile buffer solution to make 100 ml. and then use 1/100 of this solution or 1 ml. in the prescription. The 0.035 ml. of concentrate could also be measured by preparing a 1:500 solution (1 ml. of benzalkonium chloride concentrate and enough sterile buffer solution to make 85 ml.) and then using 3 ml. of the 1:500 solution with a sufficient quantity of sterile buffer solution to make 30 ml. of the 1:5000 solution called for in the prescription.

An important consideration in the use of volumetric graduates is the degree of accuracy with which they can be read. It is assumed that a pharmacist can read a graduate at the volume markings within ± 1 mm.[12] The measured internal diameter at the marking can be used to calculate the volume of fluid contained in 1 mm. of the graduate, using the formula,

$$V = \pi r^2 h$$

in which V is the volume of fluid, r is the radius and h is the height of fluid (1 mm.). If this volume is made equal to 5 per cent of the total volume, the minimum volume of liquid that could be measured with no greater than ± 5 per cent error can be determined. As an example, a 10-ml. graduated cylinder has an internal diameter of 1.18 cm.

$$V = (3.1416) \ (0.59)^2 (0.1) = 2.18 \ ml.$$

The smallest volume which can be measured with this cylinder and maintain an accuracy within ± 5 per cent is 2.2 ml. (the cylinder is graduated in 0.2-ml. increments).

℞

Belladonna ext.	0.004
Pentobarbital sodium	0.010
Acetylsalicylic acid	0.150

M. Ft. Cap. i d.t.d. No. IV
Sig. 1 Capsule 1 hr. before each dental appointment

The pharmacist should prepare enough powder for 5 capsules to prevent the necessity of recovering minute quantities from the mortar in order to bring each capsule to the exact weight. Using a balance with a sensitivity of 2 mg., at least 40 mg. must be weighed to assure accuracy within ± 5 per cent. This degree of accuracy could be achieved by weighing two times the 20 mg. of belladonna extract needed in the prescription, but, since there are several manipulations to be performed in compounding this prescription, four times the necessary quantity is prepared. The 80 mg. of belladonna extract is thoroughly mixed with a sufficient quantity of powdered diluent—lactose, sucrose or starch—so that one fourth the total mixture will weigh at least 40 mg. (the minimum quantity which can be weighed on this balance with an accuracy of ± 5 per cent). If a weight of 300 mg. were selected for the mixture, the weight of the diluent in this case would be: 300 mg. − 80 mg. = 220 mg. After thorough mixing, an aliquot consisting of one fourth of the 300 mg., or 75 mg., is weighed and placed in a mortar to be mixed with the pentobarbital and the acetylsalicylic acid. Fifty mg. of pentobarbital sodium can be weighed on this balance with an accuracy of better than ± 5 per cent.

The dosage in each capsule is to be adjusted by weight. Since an aliquot of 75 mg. of belladonna extract mixture was weighed for the five capsules, each capsule should contain 15 mg. of the dilution. Therefore, the total weight of medicinal in each capsule is 175 mg.

LABELING

The completed prescription should be placed in an appropriate-sized container and the label attached. The size of label will depend on the style and the size of the container selected. It often has been suggested that the label should be typed before the prescription is compounded. Typewriters are

RONALD GARDNER
Prescription Pharmacy
EA 4-6633 1001 BROADWAY AT MADISON . SEATTLE
No. N 38421 Dr. A. J. Jones
Med. Dent. Bldg.
Reg. No. 8149 Reg. No. 1888
Take two capsules every four hours
if needed.
Henry Atkins
412 State Street 9-15-68 DMG

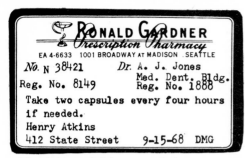

FIG. 1-10. Label for prescription shown in Figure 1-1.

now standard equipment in pharmacies and labels should always be typed. Figure 1-10 illustrates a typical label.

It is customary to include on the label such information as the serial number of the prescription, the patient's name, directions for use of the medicine, the date and the prescriber's name. Each printed label for the pharmacy bears the name and the address of the pharmacy. Some states require the initials of the compounder to appear on the label also. Labels of prescriptions that contain narcotics have already been discussed.

Labels should be placed properly on the container, should be smoothed out and should not be smudged. The directions for the use of the medicine should be clear and concise. As a double check on the class of preparation dispensed, the pharmacist should list that class of product in the directions to the patient: "Take one capsule three (3) times a day," instead of "one 3 times a day." This form of double check is particularly of value for those products marketed in more than one form—e.g., in tablets and capsules. This procedure also makes for a more complete and more professional label. The word "take" indicates an internal preparation, although some physicians emphasize the mode of administration by directing the patient to take one capsule "by mouth" three times a day.

In addition to directions for use of a medication, physicians frequently ask the pharmacist to place the name of the medication on the label. Physicians may do this by adding to the directions, "Label as such." Occasionally, they use along with directions some identifying terms such as "allergy medicine," "sleep tablets," or "blood pressure

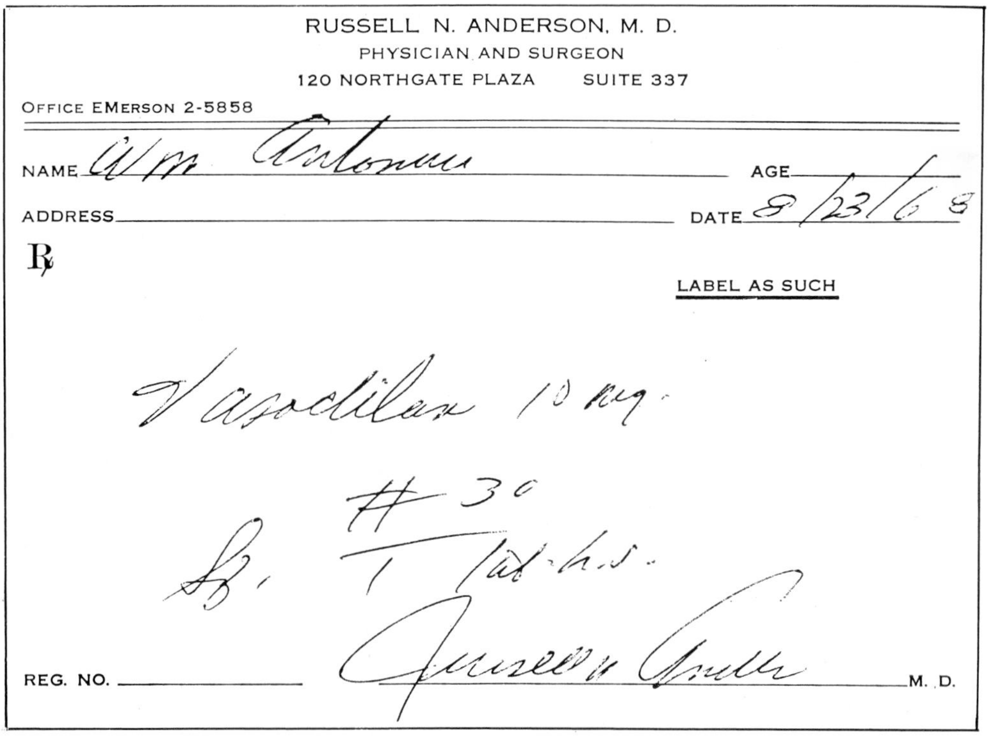

RUSSELL N. ANDERSON, M. D.
PHYSICIAN AND SURGEON
120 NORTHGATE PLAZA SUITE 337
OFFICE EMERSON 2-5858
NAME Wm Antonucci AGE
ADDRESS DATE 8/23/68
℞
LABEL AS SUCH
Vasodilan 10 mg.
#30
Sig. 1 tab. h.s.
REG. NO. Russell Anderson M. D.

FIG. 1-11. Prescription with directions to identify the medication on the label.

tablets." These latter general terms may be directed to be used along with the name of the drug or used in place of it. There are probably very few instances where the patient should not know the identity of his medication and there are many advantages to having the name and strength of the drug on the label of his prescription. The ready availability of this information is obviously of great help if the patient develops symptoms of untoward reactions or of too high dosage. The name of the drug on the label saves time in treating cases of attempted suicide, accidental overdose or accidental poisoning of children. The information can also be used to advantage in the event the patient contacts another physician as in moving to another locality.

The Council on Drugs of the American Medical Association has resolved[2,3] that it favors labeling the prescription with the name and strength of the drug and it suggests that physicians use two sets of prescription blanks, one of which is for routine use

and is imprinted with an order to label (see Fig. 1-11.). The other blank, without the imprint, would be used in writing prescriptions for those patients for whom the physicians felt it was inadvisable to identify the drug. The Council recognizes it is the physician[2] and not the pharmacist[7] who should make the decision about labeling the prescription with the name of the drug.

Additional qualifying labels besides the one carrying the information listed above occasionally may be necessary. Lotions and mixtures should have "Shake Well" directions, and prescriptions not intended for internal use should bear directions "For External Use Only."

The patient probably has no means of judging the quality of his prescription except by the appearance of the product. A good impression will be made on the patient if his powder papers, for example, are folded neatly and are placed in a container of good quality.

Properly finishing the prescription includes the wrapping or the placing of the product in a prescription envelope for delivery to the patient. One type of prescription envelope is shown in Figure 1-12.

CHECKING THE PRESCRIPTION

In some large pharmacies prescription labels are typed by nonprofessional help. A pharmacist checks these labels, prices the prescription and serves as a checker of the prescriptions. In other pharmacies a pharmacist is the labeler as well as the checker. His checking may be based on the appearance of the finished product only, unless he considers it necessary to call in the compounder for his explanation of the procedure employed. If a pharmacist works alone, as is frequently the situation where only one pharmacist is on duty at a time, he must serve as his own checker. Whatever the method of checking, every step which can be taken to prevent errors is to be regarded as an essential.

INFORMATION TO BE RECORDED ON THE PRESCRIPTION

When a prescription is compounded, certain information should be recorded on it for easy reference in refilling the prescription.

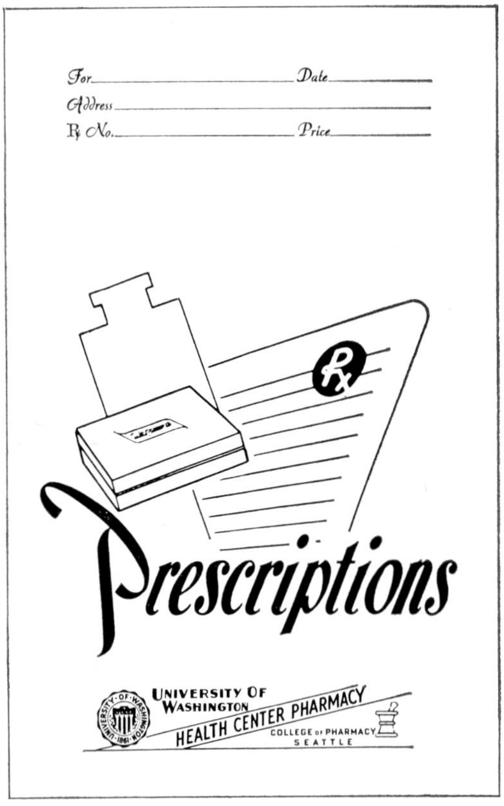

FIG. 1-12. Prescription envelope.

Such information includes the serial number of the prescription, the date on which it was dispensed, the cost price, the selling price, the size and the type of container used, and special procedures. The serial number usually is stamped on the prescription with an automatic numbering machine, such as one of those made by the Bates Manufacturing Co. Such machines can be set to number consecutively, in duplicate, in triplicate or in quadruplicate, or to repeat. Duplicate numbering allows for numbering the prescription and the label with the same number. If a pilot-sheet system and a daily work sheet are kept, the numbering machine should be set to number in quadruplicate in order to put the same number on these records as appears on the prescription and the label. The date on which the prescription is filled is stamped on the prescription with a rubber stamp. Usually, this dating is done for the day's prescriptions when they are assembled on the prescription file. Often it is necessary to know when the prescription was filled originally, and the presence of the date on the prescription is a convenient reference. The cost of the constituents, including the container, generally is marked on the prescription in some code which the pharmacist has worked out. The N.A.R.D. code is PHARMOCIST, where the first nine letters are assigned the numbers 1 through 9 and T is 0. RMT, therefore, would mean $4.50.

Any convenient combination of 9 or 10 different letters will serve as a code. If 9 letters are used, zero may be designated by X. In a 10-letter code, X is used to designate a repeat figure—e.g., PTX means $1.00 in the N.A.R.D. code. REPUBLICAN, DEMOCRATS, WELD COUNTY, BLACK HORSE and BLACK HOUSE are a few examples of codes which might be used.

A code system is used for the cost of the constituents because that is the pharmacist's personal information. The fee charged (selling price) is recorded in Arabic figures because it is announced to the patient and there would be no point in using a code system for it. It is recorded on the prescription so the same fee can be charged for refills.

Although the majority of pharmacists determine the selling price of prescriptions by a certain percentage mark up on the cost of the medication or by use of a pricing schedule which they have developed, the tendency now is toward the use of a fee system. To the cost of the medication is added a professional fee of about $2.00. Under the fee system the price of prescriptions for relatively inexpensive drugs or for small quantities will be higher, whereas the price of prescriptions for the more expensive drugs or for larger quantities will be lower, than the same prescriptions priced by a percentage mark-up system. The use of the fee system in pricing prescriptions is more in keeping with a professional atmosphere in the pharmacy. The fee is for a professional service like other members of the health care team charge, whereas percentage mark-ups and pricing schedules emphasize products and the economics thereof.

The size and the type of container, especially if it is an unusual one, special procedures employed in mixing the ingredients, the size and the color of the capsule used if the medicine was encapsulated and any other pertinent information that will enable the pharmacist to make the medication look exactly like the original product—all are valuable bits of information in case a refill is called for. If, on refill, the medication does not look exactly like the original product the patient obtained, he sometimes becomes apprehensive for fear some error has been made in compounding his medication. Even a container of a style different from that originally used, or differently worded directions, cause some patients to ask questions about the "different" medicine.

In some pharmacies, it is the policy also to mark on the prescription the identity of the original compounder and the checker of the prescription. In addition, if the pharmacist found it necessary to check with the physician concerning authorization to refill the prescription, this information is included.

The Daily Work Sheet

The daily work sheet is a daily record of the prescriptions filled and usually is designed to include such information as that shown in Figure 1-13. The prescriptions are recorded in serial number order, except for the refills which are recorded in the order in which they are dispensed. If a large num-

Serial Number	Patients Name	Doctors Name	Com-pounder	Checker	Cost Price	Selling Price

FIG. 1-13. Daily work sheet.

ber of prescriptions is filled, one record is kept for original prescriptions and one for refills. If only a few prescriptions are filled in a day, an extra column can be introduced into the table to indicate whether the prescription is new or refilled.

Another form of daily work sheet is the Lokato System,* a portion of which is shown in Figure 1-14. In this system both the new and the refilled prescriptions are recorded under the letter of the alphabet corresponding to the first letter of the patient's name. Thus if the pharmacist was for some reason searching for Mrs. William Jones' prescription originally dispensed within some specified time interval, he would refer to the "J" pages and take into consideration also those dates between which it was thought the prescription had been filled.

The importance of the daily work sheet in the pharmacy is obvious. It shows the pharmacist at a glance the number of new prescriptions filled, the number of refills and the total cost and income from his prescriptions each day. Occasionally, the daily work sheet helps to identify a prescription for a patient in the event that the label on the container has been obliterated partially or wholly during his use of the medicine.

FAMILY PRESCRIPTION RECORD

Some pharmacists are now keeping separate records of prescriptions filled for each patient or for each family on forms similar to the one shown in Figure 1-15. With such a system a complete drug profile could be developed for each patient, with some definite advantages — for example, in advising the patient concerning his requests for over-the-counter purchases and in consulting with the physician about the patient's medications. The pharmacist would find such records valuable in pursuing his efforts in clinical pharmacy.

* Trade mark.

FILING THE PRESCRIPTION

Stringing the prescriptions on wires, pasting them in books and pasting them on filing cards are procedures which are practically obsolete. Some pharmacists tie the prescriptions in bundles of 500 and place 2 bundles in a box, thus filing the orders in boxes of 1,000.

Another effective method of filing prescriptions is to bind them in books of 500 each and keep the books in a steel filing cabinet of the size intended for 4 by 6 inch index cards. The books are formed by loosely tying the prescriptions in a cover of lightweight cardboard and covering the back of the book and the string with binding tape. The range of serial numbers is indicated by large numbers on the back of the book. The books are placed in the cabinets numerically and with the number side (back) up so as to be easily visible when the drawer is opened.

There are on the market a number of prescription files of different styles. Each will hold from 500 to 1,000 prescriptions usually on a pair of wires or on a rod. The files generally are contained in a cardboard or metal box or a cabinet of appropriate size.

Some pharmacists use a microfilming device to photograph each prescription and thus file the prescriptions on reels of 16-mm. film. This system is used conveniently, and conserves space in preserving the records. It is especially valuable for filing the older prescriptions, which are not used so frequently as are those filled more recently.

REFILLED PRESCRIPTIONS

Narcotic prescriptions cannot be refilled under any circumstances. In order to obtain more of the medicine, the patient must present a new prescription, or if the narcotic drug is in the oral classification (Class B), the physician can give the pharmacist a new prescription by telephone.

According to the Federal Food, Drug and Cosmetic Act of 1938, prescriptions calling for such drugs as barbiturates, chloral hydrate and other hypnotics and the sulfonamides cannot be refilled without the consent of the prescriber. However, the provisions of the Act were not enforced rigidly until much later, when the authority of the Food

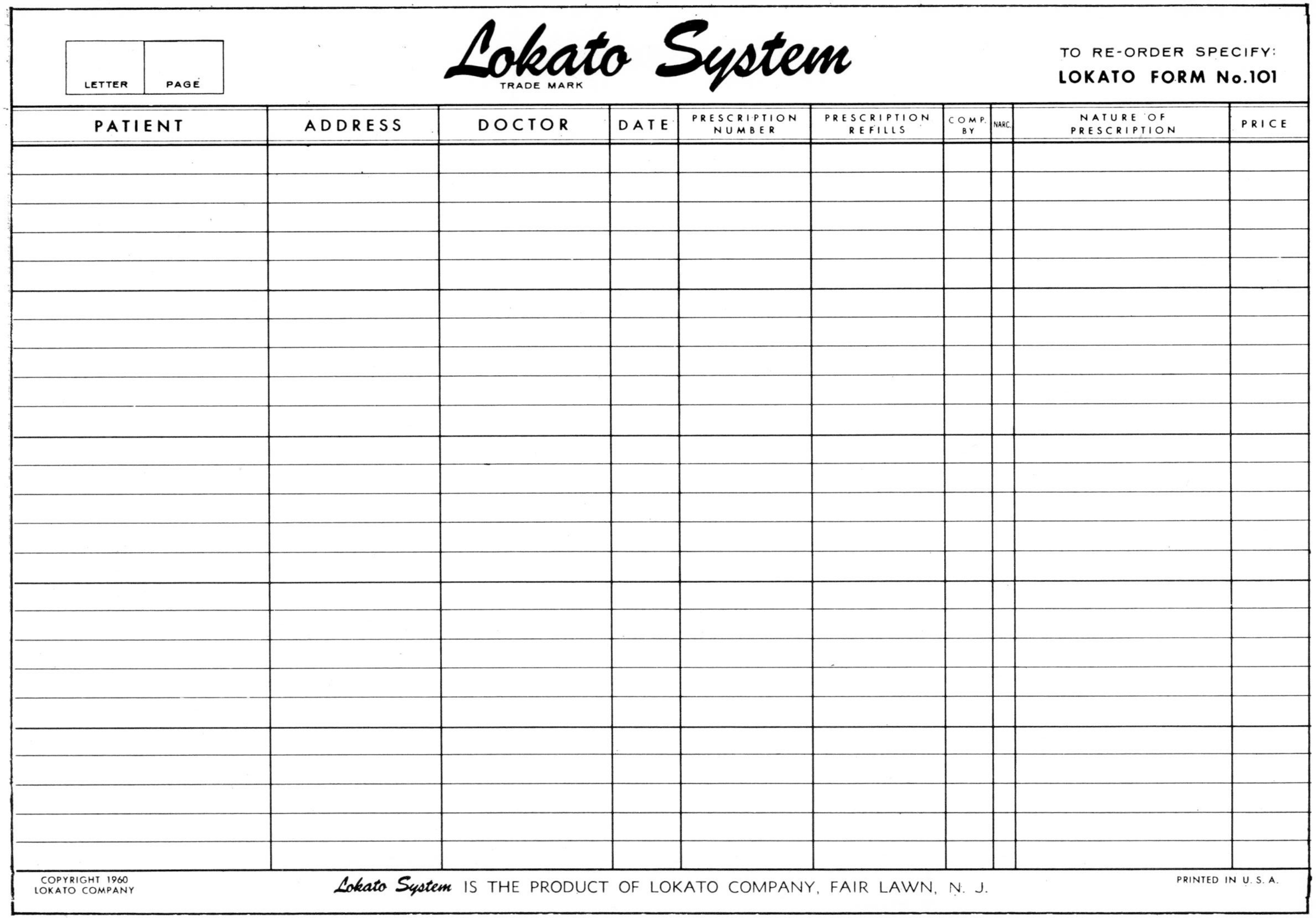

Lokato System
TRADE MARK

LETTER | PAGE

TO RE-ORDER SPECIFY:
LOKATO FORM No. 101

PATIENT	ADDRESS	DOCTOR	DATE	PRESCRIPTION NUMBER	PRESCRIPTION REFILLS	COMP. BY	NARC.	NATURE OF PRESCRIPTION	PRICE

Lokato System IS THE PRODUCT OF LOKATO COMPANY, FAIR LAWN, N. J.

PRINTED IN U.S.A.

Fig. 1-14. Lokato System prescription record. (Lokato Company, Fair Lawn, N.J.)

L. D. BRACKEN PHARMACY

FAMILY PRESCRIPTION RECORD

LAST NAME FIRST NAME & INITIAL ____________ TO ____________

ADDRESS CITY & STATE PHONE

PATIENTS NAME	REMARKS AGE · SENSITIVITY · REACTION	PATIENTS NAME	REMARKS AGE · SENSITIVITY · REACTION

DATE	NUMBER	PATIENT	FEE	PHYSICIAN	DRUG

Fig. 1-15. Family prescription record.

and Drug Administration was defined by decisions from court cases and the Durham-Humphrey Amendment (October 26, 1951) to the Act. A prescription for any drug that bears the prescription legend, *"Caution: Federal Law prohibits dispensing without prescription"* or *"Caution:* To be dispensed only by or on the prescription of a physician, dentist or veterinarian,"* cannot be refilled unless the prescriber has authorized such action. (Any drug the label of which bears the above caution is a "legend" drug.) The prescriber can authorize a reasonable number of refills on the original prescription or he can authorize them by written request or by telephone. The act of dispensing a drug contrary to the provisions of the amendment shall be deemed to be an act which results in the drug being misbranded.

If a physician does not want a prescription to be refilled, he may so indicate by writing on the prescription *non rep.* or *non repetatur*—"not to be repeated." He may direct that the prescription can be refilled only once by so marking it.

Figure 1-16 illustrates a prescription blank printed to include a convenient method by which the prescriber can indicate the number of times he wishes the prescription to be refilled. Simply by encircling the appropriate square or set of letters in the lower left-hand corner, the prescriber can convey his wishes to the pharmacist. The prescription in Figure 1-16 may be refilled three times.

Some physicians insist that none of their prescriptions be refilled without their authorization, desiring to have the patients return to their offices for examination to determine whether the same prescriptions should be continued. It may be pointed out that, according to our definition of the word prescription, it is an order for a medicine to be used by the patient *at a particular time.* Therefore, it follows that, as the condition of the patient changes, his requirements for a medicine also may change.

In labeling refilled prescriptions, most pharmacists supply the date on which the prescription was filled originally instead of the date of refill. Such procedure keeps the serial number and the date on the same basis, and, should the serial number be obliterated, it is an easy task to find the patient's prescription in the files. However, those phar-

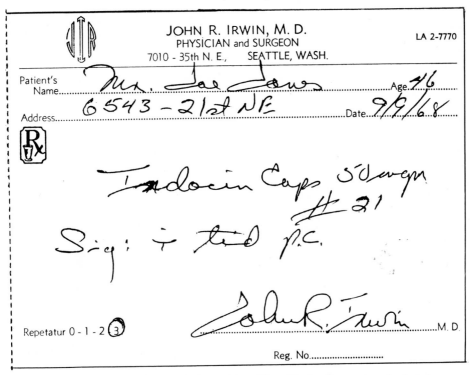

FIG. 1-16. Typical prescription with refill authorization system included.

macists who date the label as of the day on which the prescription was refilled can still trace the patient's original prescription number from the daily work sheet.

When a prescription is refilled, it carries its same serial number regardless of the number of times the order has been repeated. The advantages of this system are obvious. In order to incorporate the refills into the serial numbering, some pharmacies follow the policy of setting the numbering machine ahead each day by an amount corresponding to the number of old prescriptions refilled on the particular day. There may be 100 new prescriptions and 85 refills dispensed on a certain day. If the numbering machine is advanced for only the new prescriptions, it will register 100 more at the close of the day than it registered at the beginning of the day. However, there were actually 185 prescriptions (100 new ones and 85 refills) dispensed. Therefore, some pharmacies believe they are justified in advancing the numbering machine by the amount (85 in this illustration) equal to the refills. This is accomplished simply by setting the numbering machine on "consecutive" and stamping a number on each of the lines used for the refills in the daily work sheet. These numbers are not used to identify any of the prescriptions.

The number of times a particular prescription is refilled and the dates on which those refills are made is important information which should be recorded on the prescription. This can be accomplished effectively by stamping the refill date on the reverse side of the prescription. Opposite the date should also be included some simple note to indicate the authorization of the prescriber to refill the order, if such authorization is necessary, and the initials of the pharmacist who dispensed the refill. These data are an indication of extent of use of the medicine by the patient and are valuable for discussion of the refill problem with the prescriber and the patient. Refill information is occasionally of value in preventing a person from having certain of his prescriptions filled oftener than proper dosage warrants and in preventing neighbors and friends of the patient from obtaining the prescription for their own use.

While it is true that some physicians keep a record on each patient's chart of requests for authorization to refill a prescription, in the majority of cases this information is either incomplete or entirely lacking in the physicians' offices. This of course refers to "legend" drugs. Since most of the drugs currently prescribed are "legend" drugs, it is necessary for the pharmacist to obtain authorization from the medical practitioner to refill the prescription in the majority of instances. In those cases where legend drugs are not involved the pharmacist can exercise his own judgment in deciding to refill the prescription. It should be pointed out, however, that a pharmacist who refills a prescription for the original patient, or for anyone else, without the authority of the prescribing physician, does so on his own responsibility. As far as the physician is concerned, the transaction is complete when the pharmacist compounds and delivers the original prescription. Even unauthorized sales of quantities larger than that called for by the prescription are the responsibility of the pharmacist.

SOME LEGAL ASPECTS OF PHARMACY

Various state and Federal laws govern the right of certain individuals to dispense drugs pursuant to medical practitioners' prescriptions. Registered pharmacists generally are designated as the persons directly or indirectly responsible for the handling of the various drugs. The pharmacist should be thoroughly familiar with the laws of his state. Usually, pamphlets of state pharmacy laws are furnished by the state board on request. When the provisions of state and Federal regulations are not identical, the more stringent of the two must be observed.

NARCOTIC PRESCRIPTIONS

According to the Federal Narcotic Law and Regulations,[22] a narcotic is any drug derived from opium or coca or any of its natural or synthetic derivatives or drugs which have narcotic properties similar to those of morphine or of drugs expressly mentioned in the Law. Narcotic prescriptions must include the name, the address and the registry number of the prescriber, the date when written, and the name and the address of the patient. Prescriptions for Class A narcotics must be signed by the prescriber. On the label of a narcotic prescription must appear the name, the address and the registry number of the prescriber, the name and the address of the patient, directions for use of the drug, the date on which the prescription was filled and the name, the address and the registry number of the pharmacy. Narcotic prescriptions must be kept in a separate file and may not be refilled.

The U.S. Bureau of Narcotics now categorizes narcotics in four classes—A, B, X, and M. Class A includes the narcotics which are considered to be highly addicting, Class B includes the drugs which are thought to possess relatively little addiction liability, Class X narcotics are so-called "exempt" narcotics and Class M narcotics are "especially exempt."

Class A narcotics include: opium and its derivatives and compounds; phenanthrene opium alkaloids, their salts, derivatives and compounds; coca leaves, their alkaloids, derivatives, extracts and compounds; meperidine, its salts, compounds and preparations; and opiates, their salts, derivatives and compounds.

Medical practitioners' prescriptions for narcotics in Class B may be accepted by the pharmacist orally or by telephone and no signature is required. The prescriptions are filed on the narcotic file and the label of the finished product must have the same information as Class A narcotic prescriptions.

Class B narcotics include the following substances and any of their salts:
1. Isoquinoline alkaloids of opium (cotarnine, narceine, noscapine and papaverine)
2. Apomorphine
3. Nalorphine
4. (a) Methylmorphine (codeine) with one or more active, non-narcotic ingredients in therapeutic amounts where the codeine content does not exceed 8 grains per fluid ounce or, 1 grain per dosage unit such as Empirin* Compound with Codeine, Edrisal* with Codeine, Trigesic* with Codeine.
(b) Compounds of codeine with equal or greater quantity of isoquinoline alkaloid where the codeine content does not exceed 8 grains per fluidounce or 1 grain per dosage unit (Copavin*).

* Trade mark.

5. (a) Compounds of hydrocodone with one or more active non-narcotic ingredients in therapeutic amounts where the hydrocodone content does not exceed $1\frac{1}{3}$ grains per fluidounce or $\frac{1}{6}$ grain per dosage unit (Tussionex*).
(b) Compounds of hydrocodone with a fourfold quantity of any isoquinoline alkaloid where the hydrocodone does not exceed $1\frac{1}{3}$ grains per fluid ounce or $\frac{1}{6}$ grain per dosage unit.
6. Compounds of dihydrocodeine with one or more active non-narcotic medicinal ingredients in therapeutic amounts where the diydrocodeine does not exceed 8 grains per fluid ounce or 1 grain per dosage unit.
7. Compounds of ethylmorphine (Dionin) with one or more active non-narcotic ingredients in therapeutic amounts where the ethylmorphine content does not exceed $1\frac{1}{3}$ grains per fluid ounce or $\frac{1}{6}$ grain per dosage unit.

Class X narcotic drugs may be dispensed without prescription but a record of each transaction must be kept in a registration book.

Preparations of this group contain in each fluidounce or avoirdupois ounce, along with therapeutically active non-narcotic ingredients, not more than 2 grains of opium, $\frac{1}{4}$ grain of morphine or any of its salts, 1 grain of codeine or any of its salts, $\frac{1}{2}$ grain of dihydrocodeine or any of its salts, or $\frac{1}{4}$ grain of ethylmorphine or any of its salts. Also included in Class X are diphenoxylate preparations in solid forms containing not more than 2.5 mg. of diphenoxylate and not less than 25 micrograms of atropine sulfate per dosage unit.

Class M products are exempt from stamp tax when dispensed as medicines and records of disposition are not required.

Class M narcotic drugs contain one of the following drugs, without limit in quantity, along with either active or inert non-narcotic ingredients of the type used in medicinal preparations: noscapine, papaverine, narceine, cotarnine and nalorphine.

DRUG ABUSE CONTROL AMENDMENTS OF 1965

The Drug Abuse Control Amendments of 1965 (DACA), known also as H. R. 2 or as the Harris Bill[18] amends the Federal Food, Drug and Cosmetic Act by placing additional

* Trade mark.

controls (intrastate as well as interstate) over drugs which, because of their central nervous system stimulant or depressant effects or their hallucinogenic activity have been found to have potential for abuse. Such drugs[4,18] as the barbiturates, amphetamines, chloral hydrate, ethchlorvynol, ethinamate, glutethimide, methyprylon, paraldehyde, methamphetamine and its salts, desoxyephedrine and its salts and certain combinations[6] of these drugs with other substances are included. Some drug combinations containing small amounts of depressants and stimulants have been exempted after consideration by the FDA. These exemptions are published periodically in the *Federal Register*. A recent list of combinations not exempted[5] has been published.

The law specifies those persons who may manufacture, sell or possess drugs covered by this act and the records which must be kept, and it provides for inspection of the records. The pharmacist is the one primarily concerned in keeping records of procurement and disposition of the drugs, but physicians and dentists must also keep records of the drugs they use on their patients. Prescriptions for drugs covered by H. R. 2 may not be dispensed or renewed more than 6 months after the date on which they are issued and prescriptions for these drugs may not be refilled more than five times.

COMMON LAW AND THE PHARMACIST

Besides the Federal Narcotic Act, other Federal laws govern the quality of drugs, the handling of caustic poisons and the handling of alcohol for medicinal purposes.

Many responsibilities of the pharmacist are controlled by common law. The courts often refer to the degree of care and skill exercised by the pharmacist and require him to conduct his practice with "ordinary care." The pharmacist is responsible, for example, for the proper interpretation of the prescription and the dispensing of a product which, when used according to the directions of the order, will not prove injurious or poisonous to the patient. He is responsible for and should detect therapeutic incompatibilities involving overdoses.

The pharmacist may be held responsible for the mistakes of his employees caused by neglect or incompetence. For this reason, the owner of a pharmacy should buy liability insurance to protect himself in case a damage suit is filed as a result of the negligence of one of his pharmacists.

Before a pharmacist can be held liable in court action, it must appear that he was negligent in his duties as a pharmacist and that such negligence was responsible for the plaintiff's injury. The defense to such accusation attempts to show that the pharmacist did exercise "ordinary care," that the plaintiff contributed negligence or that the pharmacist's negligence was not the real cause of injury of the plaintiff.

In an Illinois case,[17] substitution of a drug in a prescription was considered as negligence on the part of the pharmacist. The prescription called for "Strontium Salicylate, Wyatt." The pharmacist, because he could not find Wyatt in his manufacturer's catalog, dispensed pure strontium salicylate instead of the intended "Effervescent Strontium Salicylate, Wyeth." The patient, injured by excessive quantities of strontium salicylate, recovered damages from the pharmacy because the pharmacist did not understand the prescription. The court ruled that he should have consulted the physician for proper interpretation of the order.

The pharmacist is guilty of negligence if he labels a prescription incorrectly. In a Michigan case,[17] the pharmacist's label directed the patient to take his prescription, Fowler's solution, in teaspoonful quantities instead of 3-drop doses.

OWNERSHIP OF THE PRESCRIPTION

Ownership of the prescription has always been a moot question. It is a problem worthy of consideration at this point because, whatever document the pharmacist keeps for filing purposes, whether it be the original prescription written by the physician or a copy of that prescription, there are certain data— such as the serial number of the prescription, the cost price and the selling price—that the pharmacist will want to record on it and preserve among his records.

The original prescription is, of course, more valuable to the pharmacist than is a copy of a prescription in the event such a document is used in court proceedings. In the case of *Humber v. State* (1926), 21 Ala. App. 378, 108 So. 646,[8] the court declined to allow the doctor to read what he claimed was a copy of the prescription. Under the "best evidence" rule, the highest degree of proof possible must be produced and no evidence shall be received if the court thinks that the person offering it can secure better. In this case, the original prescription was considered to be the best authority as to its contents and also the highest degree of proof possible.

The original prescription written by a medical practitioner and given to the patient is the patient's property until he presents it to a pharmacist for compounding purposes. Then there are various factors which determine who the owner may be.[9]

A patient may submit his prescription to a pharmacist for compounding without asking the price of the finished product. Even after the medicine is prepared, the patient has a right to recover his original prescription if he refuses to pay the price asked for the medicine or refuses to comply with the terms the pharmacist has set. In the case of *White v. McComb City Drug Store,* Supreme Court of Mississippi, 1905, 86 Miss. 498, 38 So. 739, 4 Ann. Cos. 518,[8,17] the court decided that the apothecary, after compounding a prescription and delivering the finished product, might have the right to retain the original prescription as a record of his business, but that he had no right to retain the original prescription in that instance where the sale of the medicine was not completed because the patient could not or would not comply with the terms the apothecary had set. If the medicine is not delivered, the pharmacist has no need of the prescription as a record of his business or as an instrument of evidence. Hence, the written prescription should be returned to the patient for whom it was written.

The ownership of the prescription is controlled by laws in some states which require a pharmacist who compounds and dispenses any medicine on a written prescription to preserve the original prescription for a specified length of time (1 to 5 years). In other states, there are no such laws designating ownership of the prescription.

Regardless of the existence of such state laws, a pharmacist who fills a prescription that contains a drug classed as a narcotic drug must retain the original prescription for a stated time. The Harrison Narcotic Act (Federal law) requires a pharmacist who compounds and dispenses any of the drugs covered by the act (namely, opium, coca leaves and their derivatives and compounds) to preserve the original prescription on file for a period of at least 2 years from the date on which it was compounded. The pharmacist is the legal custodian of such prescriptions, but he cannot refill any of them lawfully.

If the pharmacist is not required by law (either Federal or state) to retain the original written prescription, qualified ownership of the prescription may be determined by an expressed agreement[9] between the pharmacist and the patient. Such an agreement (oral contract) is often entered into by the pharmacist and the patient. This problem is presented most frequently by those persons who have some unusual prescription, such as one that may have been written in a foreign country while that person was on a vacation or a business trip. Perhaps he wishes to keep the original prescription as a souvenir of his trip. If it is decided that the patient will retain the original prescription, then the pharmacist must file a copy. Such agreement, of course, should be entered into before the prescription is dispensed. Another problem which the pharmacist should consider before filling this prescription is whether dispensing this particular product or mixture is contrary to any U. S. law or regulation.

Ownership of the prescription may be determined also by implied contract,[9] provided, of course, that no laws govern ownership of the prescription. If, in any given community, it is the prevailing custom for the pharmacist to retain the original prescription, it is assumed that all patients will leave their prescriptions to be filed in the pharmacy where they have their prescriptions dispensed. On the other hand, if it is the prevailing custom for the patient to retain the original prescription, then the pharmacist should retain a copy for his files. Expressed agreement seems to hold precedence over implied contract, and, in localities where the latter is the general rule, the pharmacist and the patient can still determine ownership of the prescription by expressed contract.

The fact that a physician has devised a formula for a drug or drugs to be compounded and dispensed in the form of a medicine does not give him exclusive right to his prescriptions.[9] Unless he patents it, any person may use the formula and dispense the medicine under his own name or a fanciful name, provided, of course, that the law does not restrict the sale of the constituents (narcotics, for example). However, he may not attach the originator's name to the product unless he has the author's consent to do so. A pharmacist legally can convert the formula to his own commercial purposes even without the originator's consent, but there would be a more pleasant feeling between the two if the pharmacist first obtained permission from the physician to use his formula than if he neglected to do so.

The responsibility for diagnosing disease and prescribing medications lies with the medical practitioner. The pharmacist is not qualified to accept this responsibility and is prohibited by law, ethics and professional training from practicing medicine. He should therefore refer persons requiring such services to appropriate practitioners. However, the pharmacist does have an important responsibility as a consultant to the public in supplying them with information about over-the-counter remedies. He should not diagnose, but he should make available those remedies which can legally and safely be used by the patient in autotherapy. Also the pharmacist should discourage the use of products which are of questionable value.

The ownership of the medicine dispensed in accordance with the terms of a prescription passes into the hands of the patient when he pays for the product.[9] If the medicine does not include ingredients the sale of which is regulated by law, he may use it or dispose of it by sale or gift. If it is a narcotic-containing prescription, he cannot give it away or sell it, since the medicine is intended only for his use.

Very few pharmacies refuse to give copies of prescriptions filled to the person for whom they were written. Such refusal usually is made at the request of the physician who wrote the prescription—the physician wishing to handle the problems of copies himself. In a Texas case,[17] *Stuart Drug Co. v. Hirsch,* 50 S.W. 583, it was indicated that the customer had a qualified right to the use of the prescription after it was deposited with the pharmacist. A pharmacist probably has no right to give copies to anyone other than the original purchaser, the prescribing physician and duly authorized officers of the law. If a pharmacist gives a copy of a prescription to a person not entitled to it, and the act of giving said copy discloses the fact that the patient for whom the prescription was written is suffering from a disorder hurtful to him socially or in his business, the pharmacist can be held accountable.

Occasionally, a person will bring to a pharmacist a container bearing a prescription number and a label from another pharmacy, with the request that the prescription be filled by the second pharmacist. In most instances, it is possible for the pharmacist to obtain a copy of the prescription from the first pharmacy merely by telephoning for it. Of course, the prescription must be one that can be legally refilled, and if "legend" drugs are prescribed, permission of the physician to refill the order must be obtained.

REFERENCES

1. Anon: Annual Report of the Judicial Council of the American Medical Association. J.A.M.A., *194*:419, 1965.
2. ———: Council on Drugs, A. M. A. To label or not to label. J.A.M.A., *194*:1311, 1965.
3. ———: Editorial. Labeling of prescription drugs. J.A.M.A., *316*:(July 27), 1963.
4. ———: FDA's Drug Abuse Regulations. J. Am. Pharm. Ass., [*NS*]6:11, 1966.
5. ———: Latest drug control advice. J. Am. Pharm. Ass., [*NS*]7:165, 1967.
6. ———: Updated List, Stimulant and Depressant Drugs. J. Am. Pharm. Ass., [*NS*] 7:577, 1966.
7. Apple, W. S., and Abrams, R. E.: Problems in prescription order communications. J.A.M.A., *185*:291, 1963.
8. Arthur, W. R.: The Law of Drugs and Druggists. St. Paul, West, 1955.
9. Bureau of Legal Medicine and Legislation: Ownership of prescriptions. J.A.M.A., *109*:19B, 1937.

10. Done, A. K.: Drugs for Children. *In* Modell, W. (ed.): Drugs of Choice 1968-1969. St. Louis, C. V. Mosby, 1967.

11. Duckering, R. E.: Private communication, August 20, 1968.

12. Goldstein, S. W., and Mattocks, A. M.: Professional equilibrium and compounding precision. Part I, Part II, Part III, Part IV. J. Am. Pharm. Ass. [Pract. Ed.],*12*:214, 293, 362, 421, 1951.

13. LaWall, C. H.: The Curious Lore of Drugs and Medicines (Four Thousand Years of Pharmacy). Philadelphia, J. B. Lippincott, 1927.

14. Morrell, C. A., and Ordway, E. M.: The capacity and variability of teaspoons. Drug Standards, *22*:216, 1954.

15. Muldoon, H. C.: Pharmaceutical Latin. 4th ed. New York, John Wiley & Sons, 1946.

16. National Prescription Audit, National Hospital Survey. 7th ed. Dedham, Massachusetts, R. A. Gosselin and Company, 1968.

17. O'Connell, C. L., and Pettit, W.: A Manual on Pharmaceutical Law. Philadelphia, Lea & Febiger, 1938.

18. Public Law 89-74, 89th Congress, H. R. 2, July 15, 1965.

19. Shirkey, H. C.: Drug dosage for infants and children. J.A.M.A., *193*:443, 1965.

20. Shirkey, H. C., and Barba, W. P., II: Drug Therapy. *In:* Nelson, W. E. (ed.): Textbook of Pediatrics. 8th ed. Philadelphia, W B. Saunders, 1964.

21. Sonnedecker, Glenn: Kremers and Urdang's History of Pharmacy. Philadelphia, J. B. Lippincott, 1963.

22. United States Treasury Department, Bureau of Narcotics, Internal Revenue Service: Regulations No. 5, Opium, Coca Leaves, Isonipecaine or Opiates, 1964.

Chapter 2

Biopharmaceutical Considerations in Dosage Form Design and Evaluation

Gerhard Levy, Pharm. D.*

What is meant by "dosage form"? In the narrow sense, it refers to the gross physical form in which a drug is administered to or used by a patient: tablet, capsule, powder, solution, suspension, ointment, aerosol, etc. The term will be used here in a more comprehensive manner to include also dosage form characteristics such as particle size, salt form, solvent type and dissolution rate, as well as consideration of effects due to additives. These additives may be pharmacologically inert in the amounts used (tablet fillers and lubricants, preservatives, stabilizing agents), or they may have the function of modifying the absorption, the biotransformation, or the excretion of the primary therapeutic agent.

Assessment of the desirable or undesirable effects of a dosage form on the therapeutic efficacy of the active ingredient and development of superior dosage forms require consideration of many physical, chemical and biologic factors. The utilization of knowledge and technics derived from such diverse disciplines as physics, chemistry, mathematics, physical chemistry, physiology, biochemistry, pharmacology and pharmaceutical technology toward the development and the evaluation of pharmaceutical formulations and dosage forms is embodied in a new area of knowledge and research named biopharmaceutics. Such a far-reaching and inclusive subject can hardly be covered in detail within one chapter, and it is intended here only to present an overview. Much additional information and stimulation can be obtained by

reading the papers cited as references, and in particular the reviews by Wagner,[206] Nelson,[138] Harper,[81] Bousquet[27] and Lazarus and Cooper.[104] The biopharmaceutical approach to pharmaceutical problems is characterized by simultaneous consideration of both physicochemical and biologic factors and recognizes their interaction. The reader should guard against compartmentalized thinking and, rather, draw on the totality of his previously acquired knowledge and apply it to the present subject. The discussion to follow will be concerned mainly with oral dosage forms excluding sustained release medication (which is considered in Chapter 3), but many of the factors described here are also applicable to dosage forms administered by other than the oral route.

INTRODUCTION

The therapeutic efficacy of a drug is not due solely to its inherent chemical constitution nor is the quality of a compounded prescription necessarily reflected only by its elegance and lack of visible signs of incompatibility. The pharmacologic effect elicited by a therapeutic agent is influenced and modified by the physical form in which it is administered, by the nature and the concentration of various additives used as pharmaceutical formulation aids and by the physicochemical and pharmacologic properties of other drugs with which it may be combined. Important and potentially life-saving drugs may be rendered practically useless by poor formulation. Prescriptions compounded conscientiously by pharmacists who are unaware

* Professor of Biopharmaceutics, School of Pharmacy, State University of New York at Buffalo.

of the adverse effect of certain pharmaceutical manipulations may fail to elicit the expected therapeutic results.

Recognition of the importance of proper pharmaceutical formulation and the role of the dosage form in therapeutics has only evolved in recent years. The modern pharmacist must become thoroughly familiar with the subject if he is to fulfill his proper function as a member of the health team. Research directed toward acquiring greater understanding and additional knowledge of this field has become an important and exciting new frontier of pharmacy.

KINETICS OF DRUG ABSORPTION AND ELIMINATION

The intensity of the pharmacologic effect elicited by a drug is usually some function of the concentration of this drug at its site of action in the body. In general, it is not possible to measure drug concentration at this site, but a relative measure as well as an indication of the change of concentration with time can often be obtained by determining the concentration of drug in the blood as a function of time after drug administration. After a drug has entered the bloodstream, it diffuses to other fluids of distribution (lymph, spinal fluid, etc.), organs and tissues. Pseudo distribution equilibrium is usually reached fairly rapidly and, from then on, any change in drug concentration in the blood is indicative of concentration changes of diffusable drug in other tissues. Despite certain complications which may arise due to drug binding and slow back diffusion from some sites, it has been found that the drug concentration in the blood reflects the intensity of the pharmacologic effect of many therapeutic agents. It is appropriate, therefore, to consider the various processes which

affect the direction and the magnitude of the concentration changes of drug in the blood.

The transfer of a drug from the site of absorption to the bloodstream and from there to other body tissues, and its subsequent biotransformation and excretion can be represented schematically by the diagram shown in Figure 2-1. This scheme is simplified considerably, since it should be noted that each process depicted by an arrow is actually a series of consecutive processes. However, each series may be represented as one overall process. Furthermore, some of the single arrows which indicate a unidirectional, irreversible process actually should be replaced by a pair of arrows pointing in opposite directions to reflect the reversibility of these processes. The single arrows are used where the transfer of drug occurs solely or predominantly in one direction, so that transfer in the opposite direction may be neglected.

The transfer of most drugs across biologic membranes occurs by passive diffusion from a region of higher concentration to a region of lower drug concentration. Fick's law of diffusion relates diffusion rate to the concentration gradient across the real or the imaginary boundary between two regions in the following manner:

$$\frac{da}{dt} = - K_d \, A \, \frac{dD}{dx} \qquad (1)$$

where da/dt is the diffusion rate across a plane of area A, which is perpendicular to the direction of diffusion, dD/dx is the concentration gradient and K_d is a proportionality constant known as the coefficient of diffusion. The negative sign on the right side of the equation indicates that the drug is diffusing from a region of high concentration to one of lower concentration. Thus the concentration gradient is negative in the direc-

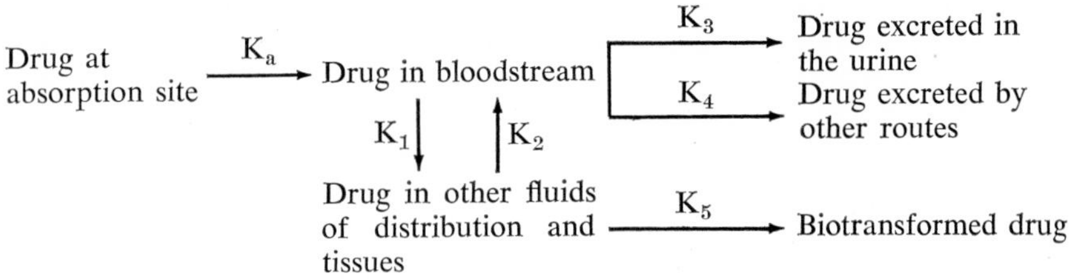

FIG. 2-1. Schematic representation of drug disposition after absorption. (The rate constant K_5 represents processes occurring primarily in the liver.)

tion in which diffusion proceeds.* The concentration gradient may be expressed as $(D - D_1)/(X - X_1)$, where D and D_1 refer to drug concentration on the high and the low concentration sides of the membrane, respectively, and $(X - X_1)$ indicates the distance between the two regions. Then,

$$\frac{da}{dt} = - K_d \, A \, \frac{D - D_1}{X - X_1} \qquad (1a)$$

In the case of many diffusion processes occurring in the body, this relationship may be simplified by incorporating the area term A and the distance expression $(X - X_1)$ in the proportionality constant. Furthermore, the concentration gradient expression $(D - D_1)$ may be replaced by D, the term representing drug concentration in the region from which diffusion is taking place. The latter simplification is justified when the drug concentration in the region of lower concentration (i.e., the region toward which diffusion is taking place) is very low and negligible compared with the concentration in the region from which diffusion occurs. The simplified equation then takes the form

$$\frac{da}{dt} = - K_t D \qquad (2)$$

where D is the drug concentration in the region from which diffusion is taking place and K_t is a proportionality or rate constant. Equation (2) indicates that the diffusion or transfer rate is proportional to the concentration of drug at the originating site. In kinetic terms, this is a first-order rate process as opposed to a zero-order rate process (where the rate is constant and independent of concentration). In the discussion to follow, all the processes depicted in Figure 2-1 by arrows are considered to be first-order processes, and the K's with various subscripts are the first-order rate constants for the indicated processes. This means that not only rates of transfer, but also rates of other processes, such as biotransformation, are considered to be proportional to concentration. Such is the case with many drugs when administered in therapeutic dosage.[138, 193] In

* Actually, diffusion occurs in both directions. We are concerned here with net diffusion, where diffusion rate in one direction is greater than in the other.

such circumstances a generalized consideration of drug absorption and elimination is feasible.

Apparent Volume of Distribution. The various fluids of distribution, tissues, glands and organs of the body may be considered as real or imaginary body compartments and will be referred to as such. At pseudo distribution equilibrium, the concentration of an administered drug is not the same throughout the body. There may be compartments into which the drug may not be able to penetrate and other compartments with high affinity and binding capacity for the drug, where drug concentration is very high. The drug concentration in the blood reflects these factors. It will be relatively high if the drug cannot penetrate into a number of body compartments and low if certain body compartments have a high affinity for the drug. The distribution of a drug between the blood and the rest of the body compartments at apparent equilibrium is reflected by its apparent volume of distribution. In the simplest case,

$$V_b = \frac{a_B}{D_b} \qquad (3)$$

where V_b is the apparent volume of distribution, D_b the concentration of drug in the blood, and a_B the total amount of drug in the body (exclusive of the gastrointestinal tract and the bladder) at the time D_b was measured. Knowing V_b, which is a characteristic property of the drug, under defined conditions, it is possible to determine the total drug content of the body by measuring drug concentration in the blood, since equation (3) may be re-arranged as follows:

$$a_B = V_b \, D_b \qquad (4)$$

It is important to realize that this relationship holds true only during apparent distribution equilibrium.* The apparent volume of distribution does not represent the volume of body space actually containing drug. Rather, it is an apparent value which reflects the distribution of drug between the blood and the rest of the body, and permits calculation of transfer rates on the basis of

* This equilibrium is only apparent, but it permits determinations of values suitable for practical purposes.

drug concentration changes in the blood. In many cases it is necessary to treat the body as a multi-compartment system, with hypothetical volumes, characteristic of each drug, assigned to each compartment. It is preferred, however, to quantitate the drug in these compartments in terms of amount rather "concentration." The only "real" drug concentrations are those determined by actual measurement in blood, spinal fluid, etc.

Changes in Body Drug Content and Drug Concentration in the Blood. Referring again to Figure 2-1, it can be seen that any change in body drug content is due to the relative magnitude of absorption rate, on the one hand, and excretion and biotransformation rates, on the other. The excretion and the biotransformation processes designated by the rate constants K_3, K_4 and K_5 may be considered together as one elimination process with a first-order rate constant K_e where

$$K_e = K_3 + K_4 + K_5 \qquad (5)$$

The rate of change of body drug content is equal to the rate of absorption minus the rate of elimination, which may be expressed in the language of calculus as

$$\frac{da_B}{dt} = \frac{da_A}{dt} - \frac{da_E}{dt} \qquad (6)$$

where da_B represents the change in amount of drug in the body during time interval dt, da_A/dt is the absorption rate, and da_E/dt is the elimination rate. This may be related to the drug concentration changes in the blood by making use of equation (4), substituting for a_B and transposing the term V_b to the right side of the resulting equation:

$$\frac{dD_b}{dt} = \left(\frac{da_A}{dt} - \frac{da_E}{dt} \right) \frac{1}{V_b} \qquad (7)$$

Accordingly, the drug concentration in the blood, as well as the total amount of drug in the body, increases when absorption rate is higher than elimination rate, decreases when elimination rate is higher than absorption rate and remains the same ($dD_b/dt = 0$) when the absorption and the elimination rates are equal. The latter consideration is the basis of sustained release medication, where the dosage form is designed to release

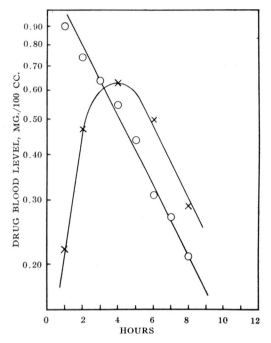

FIG. 2-2. Average theophylline blood levels for 11 human subjects receiving 0.5 Gm. of aminophylline by rapid intravenous injection ($\bigcirc$) and 1 subject receiving 0.5 Gm of aminophylline orally ($\times$). (From Swintosky, J. V.: Illustrations and pharmaceutical interpretations of first order drug elimination rate from the bloodstream. J. Am. Pharm. Ass. [Sci. Ed.], *45*:395)

initially, and permit the rapid absorption of, an amount of drug which is sufficient to exert the desired pharmacologic effect and then to release slowly additional drug so as to bring about absorption at a rate which is just sufficient to replace the amount of drug being eliminated from the body.

When a drug is administered by rapid intravenous injection, the maximum concentration in the blood is reached at once and begins immediately to decline, while upon oral administration drug levels first increase, reach a peak and then decrease. This is illustrated in Figure 2-2, which shows blood levels of theophylline after oral and after intravenous administration. It should be noted that the peak concentration after oral administration is considerably lower than after intravenous injection of an equal dose.

After the absorption process has been completed, the drug disappears from the body at a rate reflected by the first-order rate constant of elimination, K_e, as shown:

$$-\frac{da_B}{dt} = K_e\, a_B \qquad (8)$$

where the negative sign indicates that body drug content is decreasing with time. As a_B decreases, the *rate* of decrease also diminishes, but the *fraction* of drug eliminated in a given time period remains constant. The elimination rate of theophylline as indicated by the data shown in Figure 2-2 can be described by the elimination rate constant $K_e = 0.23$ hrs.$^{-1}$. This means that the elimination rate at time t is 23 per cent of the amount of drug in the body at that time, per hour. Figure 2-2 actually represents drug *concentration* changes in the blood rather than changes in amount of drug in the body. By substituting V_bD_b for a_B (equation (4)) in equation (8) and dividing each side by V_b the expression

$$-\frac{dD_b}{dt} = K_eD_b \qquad (9)$$

is obtained. This shows that the rate of decline of drug concentration in the blood (after absorption has been completed) is proportional to concentration, just as the rate of decline in total body content of drug at time t is proportional to the amount of drug in the body at that time. The urinary excretion rate of the drug can be related similarly to K_e and D_b by incorporating V_b and a factor f which reflects the fraction of the total amount of drug eventually eliminated by urinary excretion without prior biotransformation[138]:

$$\frac{da_E}{dt} = K_eV_bfD_b \qquad (10)$$

Integration of equation (9) results in

$$\log D_b = \log D_o - \frac{K_e}{2.303}\,t \qquad (11)$$

where D_b is the drug concentration in the blood at time t, K_e is the elimination rate constant (in time^{-1}) and D_o is a constant.*

* Log D_o is the intercept on the concentration axis at zero time upon extrapolation of the linear portion of the descending blood concentration curve when log D_b is plotted as a function of time after intravenous administration. (See Fig. 2-3.)

In theoretic terms, D_o is the hypothetic drug concentration in the blood immediately after drug administration, if absorption and equilibration with other tissues were to be instantaneous and no elimination had occurred. It can be seen from equation (11) that when the logarithm of D_b is plotted against t, a straight line with a slope of $-K_e/2.303$ is obtained after absorption is complete. This is the reason why blood level data are presented advantageously in the form of semilogarithmic graphs whenever elimination rate is proportional to drug concentration. The value of D_o can be employed to determine V_b, since

$$V_b = \frac{\text{Dose of drug}}{D_o} \qquad (12)$$

in cases where the body can be treated as a single compartment system. From equation 11 it can be deduced that

$$t_{\frac{1}{2}} = \frac{0.693}{K_e} \qquad (13)$$

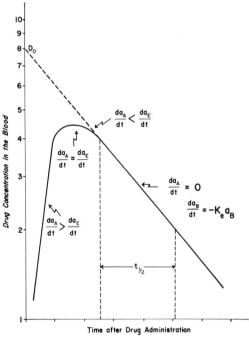

FIG. 2-3. Schematic representation of drug concentration changes as a function of time after oral administration. Symbols are explained in the text. (D_o ordinarily should be determined from blood levels obtained after intravenous administration of drug and is shown here only for illustrative purposes.)

where $t_{\frac{1}{2}}$ is the biologic half-life of the drug (the time required for a given drug concentration to be decreased by 50%). This value can be obtained experimentally from blood level data after absorption has been completed (Fig. 2-3), and from it K_e may be calculated by use of equation (13). Consideration of biologic half-life is of importance in establishing a proper dosage schedule such that neither drug accumulation to the point of toxicity nor periods when drug levels are below the minimum required for effective therapy will occur.

The complete time course of drug levels in the body after oral administration of a single dose, when absorption and elimination are both apparent first-order processes and the body can be considered as a single compartment, is given by the expression

$$a_B = \frac{K_a \text{ Dose}}{K_e - K_a} (e^{-K_a t} - e^{-K_e t})$$

$$(14)$$

If a drug is given in equal doses at constant intervals Δt, and if absorption is very rapid relative to elimination, the amount of drug in the body after n doses is

$$a_{B(n)} = \frac{\text{Dose } (1 - r^n)}{1 - r} \qquad (15)$$

where $r = e^{-K_e \Delta t}$. After a large number of doses, body levels become essentially constant, since equation 15 reduces to

$$a_{B(\infty)} = \frac{\text{Dose}}{1 - r} \qquad (16)$$

when n is large (r is always less than unity, and r^n in equation 15 approaches zero when n is large). A further discussion of the applications of these equations may be found in the review paper by Nelson.[138]

One now may identify certain factors which can affect the concentration of a drug at its site of action and thus modify the intensity and duration of the pharmacologic effect elicited by it. These are primarily rates of absorption, excretion and biotransformation and the nature of the distribution equilibrium between the site of action and other body compartments. How these characteristics may be modified quantitatively by various physiologic, pharmacologic and physicochemical factors will be discussed in the following sections.

A more extensive review of the kinetics of drug absorption, distribution, biotransformation and excretion is that by Nelson.[138] The application of kinetic considerations to the study of a given drug and to the design of dosage forms is exemplified in a series of papers by Swintosky and co-workers.[143, 164, 194-197]

KINETICS OF PHARMACOLOGIC EFFECTS

Our interest in the time course of drug levels in the body is due mainly to the realization that the intensity of pharmacologic effects is related in some manner to drug concentration at the site of action. It is appropriate therefore to consider the kinetics of pharmacologic effects in relation to the principles already presented concerning drug absorption and elimination.

The intensity of the pharmacologic effect (E) of many drugs is related linearly, over a considerable range, to the logarithm of the amount of drug in the body (a_B), such that

$$E = m \log a_B + e \qquad (17)$$

where m is the slope of the line obtained when E is plotted against log A, and e (which is usually a negative number) is the intercept of the line on the E axis. Rearrangement of equation 17 yields

$$\log a_B = \frac{E - e}{m} \qquad (18)$$

If a drug is eliminated from the body by an apparent first-order process,

$$\log a_B = \log a_B^o - \frac{K_e}{2.303} t \qquad (19)$$

which is identical to equation 11, except for the use of amount instead of concentration terms. Substitution of equation 18 in equation 19, and rearrangement, yields

$$E = E - \frac{K_e m}{2.303} t \qquad (20)$$

Equation 20 predicts that the pharmacologic effect of a drug declines at a constant rate while the amount of drug in the body decreases exponentially. An example of such kinetics is shown in Figure 2-4, which depicts the exponential decrease of tubocurarine concentration in the plasma some time after intramuscular administration to a human subject, while the pharmacologic effect of the drug (skeletal muscle relaxation) decreased linearly. Equation 20 may be expected to apply if a drug is pharmacologically active as such and its metabolites are inactive, and if the intensity of the pharmacologic effect at any time is a function of the amount of drug in the body at that time according to equation 17. It is of interest that the biologic half life of the drug will be independent of the size of the administered dose whereas the time required for the pharmacologic effect to decrease to one half of its highest observed magnitude will increase with increasing dose.

The duration of a pharmacologic effect is equal to the time during which the drug level in the body exceeds the minimum effective level. If, in equation 19, a_B is defined as the minimum effective amount of drug $a_{B(min)}$, then t becomes the duration of the pharmacologic effect. Thus, by rearrangement of equation 19,

$$t = \frac{2.303}{K_e} \log a_B^o - \frac{2.303}{K_e} \log a_{B(min)} \quad (21)$$

This equation predicts that a plot of the duration of action of a drug, when plotted against the logarithm of the administered dose (a_B^o), yields a straight line with the slope $2.303/K_e$. It is assumed that drug absorption is rapid relative to elimination. An example of the predicted relationship is presented in Figure 2-5, in which the duration of general anesthesia in man is plotted against the administered intravenous dose (log scale) of the general anesthetic CI-581.

It is often necessary or desirable to maintain a particular pharmacologic effect, such as general anesthesia or muscle relaxation, by administering another dose of the drug as soon as the effect of the preceding dose has worn off. Under these conditions it has often been observed that the effect of the second dose is more intense and longer lasting than the effect of the first dose. The reason for this apparent potentiating effect of the second dose is readily apparent in Figure 2-5. If a dose of 1 mg./Kg. CI-581 is administered, the patient will be unconscious for 6 minutes, at which time the amount of drug in the body has declined to the minimum effective level (0.39 mg./Kg.). If at this time another 1 mg./Kg. dose is administered, the amount of drug in the body is now 1.39 mg./Kg. and the effect of this second dose is therefore more intense and longer lasting than that of the first dose. In Figure 2-5, the effect of the first and the second 1 mg./Kg. dose is plotted (solid symbols) at 1 mg./Kg. and 1.39 mg./Kg. respectively, and these data fit perfectly the relationship obtained by injecting only single doses of different amounts of drug (open

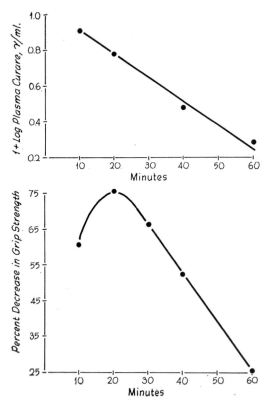

FIG. 2-4. Disappearance of tubocurarine from the plasma (logarithmic concentration scale) and decline of muscular relaxation effect (linear scale) in a human subject as a function of time after intramuscular injection of 12 mg. of tubucurarine. (Data from Belville, J. W., Cohen, E. N., and Hamilton, J.: The interaction of morphine and d-tubucurarine on respiration and grip strength in man. Clin. Pharmacol. Ther., 5:35, 1964)

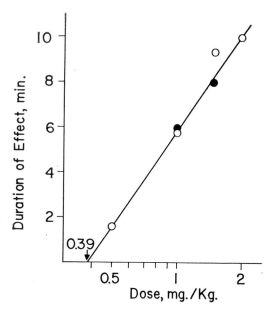

FIG. 2-5. Relationship between intravenous dose of CI-581 and duration of general anesthesia in human subjects. Open circles, single doses. Closed circles, single 1 mg./Kg. dose, followed immediately upon recovery by another 1 mg./Kg. dose (plotted at 1.39 mg./Kg. to account for the amount of drug remaining from the first dose). (Data from Domino, E. F., Chodoff, P., and Corssen, G.: Pharmacologic effects of CI-581, a new dissociative anesthetic, in man. Clin. Pharmacol. Ther., 6:279, 1965)

symbols). Since the more pronounced effect of second and subsequent doses is often undesirable, they may be reduced by an amount equal to the minimum effective dose so that the effect of these doses will be the same as that of the first dose. For additional reading on the kinetics of pharmacologic effects, see the review by Levy.[109]

EFFECT OF ABSORPTION RATE ON DRUG ACTION

When dosage form properties account for some modification of the pharmacologic activity of a therapeutic agent, the reason is most commonly that the inherent absorption pattern of the drug has been altered to some extent. Therefore, it is appropriate to consider in some detail the effect of changes in absorption rate on pharmacologic activity. Figure 2-6 represents in schematic form the drug concentration in the blood as a function of time after oral administration of a given amount of drug in three different dosage forms. These dosage forms, designated A, B, and C, cause the drug to be absorbed at different rates. The resulting drug concentration vs. time patterns will serve to illustrate the modifications in pharmacologic activity which may be brought about when a drug is absorbed at different rates.

A therapeutic agent usually must attain some minimum concentration at its site or sites of action before it elicits a given pharmacologic response. At apparent distribution equilibrium, there is frequently a corresponding minimum drug concentration in the blood which is referred to as the "therapeutic blood level" or the "minimum effective concentration" of the drug for a specified therapeutic

purpose. Such a concentration is indicated in Figure 2-6 by a stippled horizontal line. Since the *onset of therapeutic activity* occurs at the time the drug concentration has reached this level, it is apparent that a therapeutic effect is elicited most rapidly upon administration of dosage form A. A longer time is required to obtain a similar effect when the drug is administered in dosage form B, while absorption from dosage form C is so inadequate that the drug concentration never reaches the level of effectiveness. It is evident that dosage form A would be the one of choice when rapid onset of therapeutic effect is desired—for example, in the case of analgesics. On the other hand, dosage

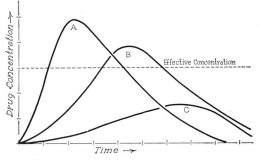

FIG. 2-6. Schematic representation of blood levels obtained after oral administration of equal amounts of a drug in three conventional dosage forms with different release characteristics.

form C is so poorly formulated that ordinarily it must be considered to be unacceptable as a medicinal preparation.

The *intensity of the pharmacologic effect* is usually some function of drug concentration. Thus, the higher peak concentration of drug when administered in dosage form A generally will be accompanied by a more intensive pharmacologic response than that obtained after administration of the drug in dosage form B. When the peak concentration due to A is sufficiently high to cause *undesirable systemic side-reactions or toxic effects*, it may be preferable to use a dosage form yielding the absorption pattern of B. Alternatively, a lower dose of drug may be administered in dosage form A with the possible added advantage over B of a more rapid onset of action.

The higher the maximum or peak concentration, the longer may be the time required for the drug concentration to decline to a subtherapeutic level. The duration of the pharmacologic effect frequently is reflected by the length of time during which the drug concentration in the blood is equal to or higher than the minimum effective concentration. When this is the case, dosage form A will bring about a longer duration of pharmacologic activity than dosage form B.

The total amount of drug absorbed may be ascertained by measuring the area under the drug concentration vs. time curve.[208] The areas under the curves for dosage forms A and B, respectively, are about equal. This means that although the drug is more rapidly absorbed when administered in dosage form A, the total amount absorbed is the same with both dosage forms. The area under the concentration versus time curve obtained after administration of the drug in dosage form C is about 60 per cent smaller than the area under the other two curves. Assuming that the drug is completely absorbed when administered in dosage form A or B, it may be stated that the biologic availability of the drug when administered in dosage form C is only 40 per cent. The absorption rate is so low in the latter case that, evidently, 60 per cent of the drug is propelled past the absorption sites and excreted in the feces before it can be absorbed.

Faulty formulation of dosage forms resulting in reduced biologic availability of the active constituents is a serious problem because it may cause patients to be undermedicated on a dosage regimen thought to be adequate by the physician who prescribed it. A number of reports concerning incomplete biologic availability of drugs due to poor formulation have appeared in the literature.[6] Some of these involve very potent substances, such as anticoagulants, and other drugs that are used to treat serious diseases, such as tuberculosis. Figure 2-7 shows differences in blood levels after administration of equal doses of phenylindanedione in two different tablet preparations. A patient requiring anticoagulant therapy after a stroke, on switching from one tablet preparation to the other, either could be subject to serious hemorrhages due to overdosage, or could be exposed to the danger of further infarctions because of inadequate lowering of prothrombin levels. Similar formulation problems have occurred with the anticoagulants dicumarol[126] and warfarin.[14] Blood levels of para-aminosalicylate after administration of equal doses of the tuberculostatic agent sodium para-aminosalicylate in two different tablet preparations are shown in Figure 2-8 and demonstrate the inadequate biologic avail-

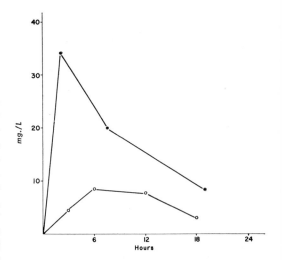

FIG. 2-7. Plasma levels of phenylindanedione following administration of 0.4 Gm. in two types of tablets (after Schulert, A. R., and Weiner, M.: The physiologic disposition of phenylindanedione in man. J Pharmacol. Exp. Ther., *110*:451).

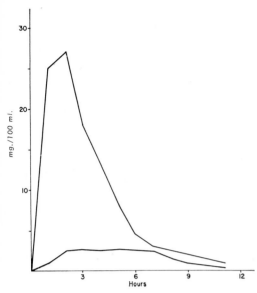

FIG. 2-8. Blood levels of para-amino-salicylate after administration of 12 Gm. of sodium para-aminosalicylate in two types of tablets (after Frostad, S.: Continued studies in concentration of para-aminosalicylic acid (PAS) in the blood. Acta tuberc. pneumol. scand., *41*:68).

ability of this drug from one of these preparations. It must be realized that it is not sufficient for a dosage form to contain the labeled amount of drug; it is equally important that full biologic availability of the drug be assured by proper formulation.

A number of drugs can cause gastrointestinal irritation such as localized erosions of the mucosa and hemorrhages, or gastrointestinal distress such as nausea, vomiting and diarrhea. Salicylates represent the best-documented example of a drug capable of contact irritation,[114] but there are other medicinal agents which appear to have similar liabilities.[77,175] Tetracyclines have a selective inhibitory effect on certain micro-organisms usually found in the intestinal tract and, therefore, can disturb the normal balance of the microbial flora. The resulting overgrowth of certain molds and fungi may cause nausea, vomiting, pruritus ani and diarrhea. It is desirable that such antibiotics be as completely absorbed as possible so that there is not a large unabsorbed portion in the large bowel, because the incidence and the severity of *local side-effects* caused by them is usually

proportional to the concentration of the drugs in the large bowel. Accordingly, prompt absorption will tend to diminish these side-effects while slow and incomplete absorption would have the opposite effect.

One of the desirable attributes of a pharmaceutical preparation intended for oral administration is that it be absorbed in a consistent and predictable manner, since this is a necessary prerequisite for obtaining a reasonably consistent therapeutic response. The more rapidly a drug is absorbed from the gastrointestinal tract, the less likely it is that physiologic variables such as gastric emptying rate, intestinal motility, diet and pH cause this drug to be absorbed incompletely or erratically. This is apparent from absorption studies with sulfadiazine,[160] sodium para-aminosalicylate[38] and many others.[110] On the other hand, delayed absorption, such as is encountered with sustained release dosage forms, is frequently more erratic[58] and sometimes incomplete.[182] A possible exception to this generalization concerns drugs that are unstable in gastric fluids. It may be preferable to formulate such drugs in a manner which prevents or retards their dissolution in the stomach and thereby minimizes their degradation due to gastric enzymes or low pH. While it is evident that usually the most reliable way of introducing a given amount of a drug into the body is the parenteral route, the research pharmacist must consider it a challenge to develop oral dosage forms which approach as much as possible the reliability of parenteral medication in this respect.

On the basis of this generalized and, of necessity, oversimplified discussion, it can be seen that modifications in the inherent absorption rate of medicinal agents due to properties of their oral dosage forms can affect the onset, the intensity, and the duration of pharmacologic activity and the incidence and severity of toxic reactions and systemic and local side-effects.

BIOLOGIC FACTORS

ABSORPTION PROCESSES: PASSIVE DIFFUSION VS. ACTIVE TRANSPORT

Most drugs are absorbed from the gastrointestinal tract by a process of passive diffusion, but some are absorbed by means of an active transport mechanism. The absorption of a drug is affected differently by various biologic and physicochemical factors, depending on the type of absorption process involved. Since this must be taken into consideration when designing and evaluating pharmaceutical dosage forms, a short review of absorption processes is in order.

Passive diffusion refers to the movement of molecules from a region of relatively high concentration to one of lower concentration. It also includes the movement of ions from a region having the same charge to a region of lesser or opposite charge. Absorption by passive diffusion does not require expenditure of energy by the organism; it is due entirely to the concentration or the electrical gradient existing across the membrane which separates the gastrointestinal lumen from the surrounding tissues. From equation 2 on page 38 it is apparent that in the case of passive diffusion, gastrointestinal absorption rate is directly proportional to the concentration of drug in the gastrointestinal fluids. This is true so long as the drug concentration in the surrounding tissues and the bloodstream is very low compared with that in gastrointestinal fluids. Accordingly, the *per cent* or *fraction* of drug absorbed per unit time is independent of concentration, while the *amount* absorbed over a given time is directly proportional to initial concentration. This is one of the criteria used to establish whether absorption is occurring by passive diffusion.[173]

Apart from the concentration gradient, diffusion rate depends also on the permeability characteristics of the membrane separating the two body compartments. These are reflected in equation 2 (p. 38), by the value of K_t, all other conditions being equal. The gastrointestinal membrane acts like a lipid barrier which permits the ready passage of lipid-soluble drugs, but across which large lipid-insoluble substances diffuse only with difficulty or not at all. Smaller lipid-insoluble, but water-soluble substances may pass across the membrane through numerous pores which are too small to be seen even with the aid of the electron microscope, but for which strong though indirect evidence exists. When absorption occurs by passive diffusion,

the rate of absorption per unit of mucosal surface area depends mainly on the concentration of the absorbable form of the drug in gastrointestinal fluids, the rate of diffusion through gastrointestinal fluids toward the mucosal surface and the relative permeability of the membrane with respect to the drug. These factors are influenced by a number of dosage form properties which will be discussed in subsequent sections of this chapter.

Absorption by active transport is a specialized process which requires the expenditure of energy. The various active transport processes found in the gastrointestinal tract are relatively structure-specific and serve primarily for the absorption of natural substrates, such as monosaccharides, L-amino acids, pyrimidines, bile salts and certain vitamins. However, there is evidence that certain drugs also may be absorbed by one of these active transport processes, if their chemical structures are sufficiently similar to that of the natural substrate. The anticancer drug 5-fluorouracil is an example of an actively transported drug.[171] It is similar in structure to the natural substrate uracil, which is absorbed by means of the pyrimidine transport system. 5-Fluorouracil is absorbed by the same specialized process. Active transport is relatively specific not only in terms of chemical structure but also with respect to direction. For example, it may function only in the movement of a substance from the mucosal to the serosal side of the gastrointestinal tract and not in the reverse direction. Absorption by active transport can take place against a concentration gradient, that is, from a region of low concentration to one of higher concentration. The process becomes saturated at high concentrations of the substance which is being transported, and one substance can compete with and depress the absorption of another if both are transported by the same process. Since active transport processes consume energy, they can be inhibited by various metabolic poisons, such as fluoride and dinitrophenol, and by lack of oxygen. Some natural substrates and drugs can be absorbed by both active transport and passive diffusion processes. Absorption by the former process is usually much more rapid at sufficiently low concentrations. Absorption by passive diffusion becomes important at concentrations that are high enough to saturate the active transport process. From the biopharmaceutical point of view, it must be recognized that a drug which can be absorbed by active transport will be absorbed relatively more rapidly at low concentration than at higher concentrations where the active process is more or less saturated and the slower passive diffusion process predominates. Furthermore, in the case of active transport, dietary conditions can influence absorption rate of drugs through the competitive effect of natural substrates ingested as part of the normal food intake.

There are some variants of the two major types of transport processes described thus far. Water flux can increase the diffusion rate of a substance across the gastrointestinal membrane in the same direction; this is known as *solvent drag*. Some substances are transported by a process which does not require energy and cannot take place against a concentration gradient, but which is subject to competition by other substances of similar structure. This absorption process appears to be an active one and is called *facilitated transport*. Another mechanism of absorption is that of *pinocytosis* ("cell-drinking"), where particulate matter such as oil droplets is brought into the cell by being engulfed in a membrane invagination which is subsequently pinched off and moved into the interior of the cell.

The various absorption and transfer processes have been reviewed in greater detail by Laster and Ingelfinger[103] and by Schanker.[170] Interesting descriptions of cell membrane permeability characteristics written in popular fashion are those by Holter[89] and Solomon.[188]

ROLE OF VARIOUS REGIONS OF THE GASTROINTESTINAL TRACT IN ABSORPTION

As an ingested drug descends through the gastrointestinal tract, it encounters different environments with respect to pH, enzymes and fluidity, as well as anatomic regions with different surface characteristics. All of these variables can affect the rate of absorption of the drug. It has been stated in the previous subsection that absorption by passive diffusion across the gastrointestinal membranes is restricted primarily to lipid-soluble drugs and that the rate of absorption per unit of mucosal surface is proportional to the concentration of the *absorbable form* of the drug in gastrointestinal fluids. Accordingly, weak acids and weak bases are absorbed predominantly in lipid-soluble, un-ionized form.[87] Their rate of absorption depends not on their total concentration in gastrointestinal fluids but on the concentration of the absorbable (un-ionized) species, which, in turn, is a function of dissociation constant and of the pH of their immediate environment. Thus, weak acids are readily absorbed from the stomach, since they exist in essentially un-ionized form in the acidic gastric fluids. Weak bases are largely ionized in gastric fluids and are, therefore, absorbed very slowly or not at all from the stomach. This situation is reversed in the fluids of the small intestine which are either only mildly acidic, neutral or even somewhat basic. Such an environment favors, relatively speaking, the absorption of drugs that are weak bases. Under these circumstances it is apparent that a weakly acidic drug, when administered in solid form, must dissolve readily in gastric fluids if rapid absorption is desired. Unfortunately, weak acids generally do not dissolve as rapidly in acidic fluids as do weak bases. The reverse would be much more desirable, since rapid dissolution of weakly basic drugs in gastric fluids is not as important because weak bases are not absorbed to any significant extent from the stomach.

It is enlightening to consider the change in the degree of ionization of two weak acids, differing in K_a value, as they are exposed to an environment of increasing pH (which would be the case when they descend through the gastrointestinal tract). Both substances essentially are un-ionized at very low pH and dissociate to an increasing degree as they encounter regions of higher pH. The weaker acid will ionize to a lesser degree at a given pH than the stronger acid, and the concentration *ratio* of the un-ionized (absorbable) species of the two drugs will increase in favor of the weaker acid at higher pH.

This is shown in Figure 2-9 for two weakly acidic drugs, benzoic acid and salicylic acid. It is to be expected that the weaker acid

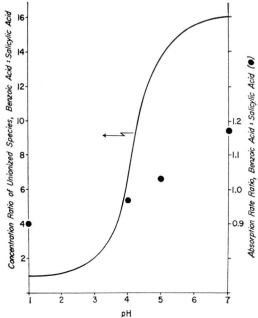

FIG. 2-9. Change in the ratio of un-ionized benzoic acid ($pK_a = 4.2$) to un-ionized salicylic acid ($pk_a = 3.0$) and in the ratio of their absorption rates from the gastrointestinal tract of the rat, as a function of pH (assuming equimolar concentration of total drug). Absorption data from Schanker, L. S., et al.: J. Pharmacol. Exp. Ther. *120*:528; and Hogben, C. A. M., et al.: J. Pharmacol. Exp. Ther., *125*: 275.

(benzoic acid) is relatively better absorbed than the stronger acid as the pH increases. This is indeed the case, as evidenced by the absorption data also shown in Figure 2-9. A more extensive tabulation demonstrates that this relationship holds also for other weakly acidic drugs.[113] However, in all instances, the relative increase in absorption rate ratio was not as great as the increase in the concentration ratio of the un-ionized form of the two drugs. This is probably due to the fact that the pH at the gastrointestinal membrane is not necessarily the same as the pH of the gastrointestinal fluids, since it has been found that the intestinal membrane has a somewhat acidic zone.[86] While this acidic pH apparently can be modified in either direction by changing the pH of the gastrointestinal fluids, the magnitude of the membrane pH change is not necessarily the same

as that of the pH change of the gastrointestinal fluids. It should be pointed out that in the intact animal the small intestine strongly resists alteration in the pH of its luminal contents.[32] Hence, it is not practical to modify the pH of intestinal fluids under clinical conditions. The pH of gastric fluids can be increased by antacids and other suitable alkaline substances, and the absorption rate of weak acids and weak bases can be decreased and increased, respectively, in the human under these circumstances.[88]

While the differences between the pH of the gastric and the intestinal fluids account to some extent for the different rates of absorption of certain drugs from these two areas, the main reason is the difference in the absorptive surface areas. Anatomically, the small intestine is much better designed for absorption than the stomach. The intestinal mucosa is covered by numerous villi and provides a very large surface for absorption. The ratio of mucosal surface area/serosal surface area (MA/SA) is highest in the proximal region of the small intestine and decreases toward the more distal regions. MA/SA ratios of the upper, the middle and the lower segments of the rat small intestine are 11.3, 9.8 and 4.3, respectively.[76] It is known that the decrease in MA/SA ratio as one descends the human intestine is also rather large.[209] Furthermore, the electrical potential across the small intestine, which is positive on the serosal side, is higher in the jejunum than in the ileum.[40] The pH of the intestinal fluids also increases in the distal direction.[102] Thus, there exists a duodenal, jejunal to ileal gradient with respect to absorptive surface area (MA/SA), electrical gradient and pH. The large intestine presents much less favorable anatomic conditions for absorption: a larger lumen and no villi. The effect of the latter will be appreciated by the fact that the presence of villi in the human small intestine increases the surface area from seven to eighteen times over what it would be without villi.[64]

Most of the water absorption from the gastrointestinal tract occurs in the small intestine.[45] As the gastrointestinal content passes through the small intestine, it changes from fluid to pasty consistency. Drug solids which have not been dissolved in the stomach or the small intestine may not encounter sufficient fluids for dissolution in the large intestine. Diffusion of dissolved drug to the intestinal mucosa also is hindered by the inspissation (thickening) of the contents of the large intestine. Thus pH, surface area, availability of aqueous fluids to dissolve ingested drug solids and consistency of intestinal contents are some of the factors which differ in various regions of the gastrointestinal tract. They can account for differences in the absorption rate of a drug from these regions.

The existence of optimal regions for absorption is even more clear-cut with respect to substances that are absorbed by means of an active transport mechanism. It has been established that iron absorption occurs mainly in the proximal part of the small intestine and decreases progressively in the more distal intestinal segments,[57, 75] while the absorption of bile salts is limited to the distal ileal segment.[101] Riboflavin apparently is absorbed only from the upper regions of the intestine[131] and thiamine absorption also occurs mainly in the proximal regions. Under equal conditions of supply, the absorption of thiamine in the distal sections of the intestine is only 20 per cent of that found in the proximal sections.[72] The site of active vitamin B_{12} absorption in man is the ileum, and there may be a specific vitamin B_{12} receptor mechanism in this part of the small intestine.[26] The colon apparently lacks certain specific transport processes present in some or all of the regions of the small intestine; namely, those for glucose and galactose, L-tyrosine, and vitamin B_{12}.[43] This suggests that the rectal route of administration is not satisfactory for substances which are absorbed by one of several active transport processes.

The existence of specialized absorption sites and regional differences with respect to pH, surface area and other properties in the gastrointestinal tract implies that orally administered drugs should be in physiologically available form (for example, in solution rather than in solid form) by the time they reach their respective optimum absorption sites. Only limited time is available for the dissolution of a solid medicament, the modification of an unabsorbable molecule to an absorbable one by hydrolysis, and similar transformations of drugs to their physiologically available forms in the gastrointestinal tract, especially if the optimum absorption site is the proximal section of the small intestine. The rate of passage of intestinal contents through the upper small intestine is higher than it is through the lower part. For example, it has been found that the transit time of a balloon through the duodenum is 5 minutes, through the jejunum, 2 hours, and through the ileum, 3 to 6 hours.[91] Drugs that are not in absorbable form within indicated time limits may be propelled past their absorption sites and excreted totally or in part in the feces.

GASTRIC EMPTYING RATE

In view of the qualitative and the quantitative differences between the absorption properties of the stomach and the intestine, any delay in the transfer of a drug from stomach to intestine may affect absorption rate and, thereby, the onset of therapeutic activity. For instance, a weak base such as codeine will be absorbed primarily from the small intestine rather than from the stomach, and any delay in gastric emptying will tend to delay the onset of analgesia. Slow gastric emptying can also affect the biologic availability of drugs that are unstable in gastric fluids, the extent of degradation being proportional to the time during which such drugs are exposed to low pH or gastric enzymes. The effect of pharmaceutical formulation variables on the dissolution rate of weakly acidic drugs often will be most noticeable while the drugs are in the stomach, where ordinarily they dissolve relatively slowly. Such differences may disappear when the drugs reach the small intestine, where dissolution is usually more rapid and less affected by differences in dosage form properties.[113] Consequently, the results of absorption studies and certain other types of clinical evaluations, both comparative and absolute, can be affected by the gastric emptying rate of the experimental subjects. This is one reason why absorption studies often yield more consistent results when carried out on fasted subjects. Type of food, volume, osmotic pressure, pH and buffer capacity, temperature and viscosity of gastric contents, age and state of health of the subjects and environmental circumstances during the study are typical factors which can influence gastric emptying rate.[49] Gastric content leaves the stomach by a first-order process, i.e., at a rate which is proportional to volume. With small volumes, there is an initial lag time before gastric emptying begins, while with higher volumes there is an initial phase of more rapid emptying. Thus, ingestion of large volumes of liquid may favor drug absorption by increasing the initial rate of transfer of drug to the small intestine. Liquids of low viscosity are emptied more rapidly than liquids of high viscosity. Solutions or suspensions of fine particles leave the stomach at a higher rate than lumpy substances. Hence, enteric coated tablets, which do not disintegrate in gastric fluids, often remain in the stomach for a considerable length of time.[24] Liquids having a high osmotic pressure are emptied more slowly than pure water or solutions of lower osmotic pressure. Fats slow gastric emptying rate considerably, proteins have a lesser effect, and starch retards gastric emptying the least.[13] Gastric emptying also is retarded by increased acidity of the duodenal contents, which, in turn, is related to the acidity of the gastric fluids.[102] It has been found that subjects with duodenal ulcers and gastric hyperacidity have a higher gastric emptying rate than healthy subjects, while those suffering from gastric achylia have a lower emptying rate.[102]

A number of drugs are capable of affecting gastric emptying rate, usually by some central mechanism but, in some instances, apparently by means of a local effect. Aspirin, morphine and codeine are among those drugs which delay gastric emptying.[12, 176] Posture also can affect the rate of gastric emptying. For certain individuals, gastric emptying is facilitated by lying on the right side and delayed by lying in supine position.[13] Since gastric emptying can be a major limiting factor with respect to the rate of absorption of certain drugs, it will be appreciated that the variables described in the preceding paragraphs can have a significant effect on drug absorption. It has been pointed out recently that it may even make a difference whether a subject is standing or sitting, since this can affect the rapidity and completeness of absorption of orally administered drugs.[122] Dis-

regard for these considerations could introduce considerable bias in the clinical testing and evaluation of dosage forms.

INTERACTION OF DRUGS WITH COMPONENTS OF GASTROINTESTINAL MUCOSA

Interaction of drugs with substances present in or secreted by the gastrointestinal mucosa can be of considerable consequence in the absorption of such drugs. This may be illustrated by a consideration of the gastrointestinal absorption of quaternary ammonium compounds, many of which are used as anticholinergic and hypotensive agents. It is known that many of these drugs are absorbed poorly and irregularly from the gastrointestinal tract.[106] While this probably is related to some extent to their poor lipoid solubility, it has been shown that quaternary ammonium compounds form nonabsorbable complexes with polysaccharide acids of intestinal mucin.[106] Once the mechanism for the poor absorption of quaternaries had been elucidated, formulation adjustments to circumvent this problem and to facilitate absorption could be made.[36] A physiologically inert quaternary was coadministered, which either interacted preferentially or competed with the pharmacologically active quaternary for interaction sites. This resulted in less binding and greater physiologic availability of the drug, as shown in both animals and humans.[36, 37] The more complete gastrointestinal absorption of hypotensive quaternaries thus attained permitted a reduction of the administered dose, which is desirable not only for economic reasons but also because some of these drugs exhibit undesirable local actions on the gastrointestinal tract.[37] The use of pharmacologically inert quaternaries to enhance drug absorption is not limited to hypotensives but is also applicable to other quaternaries such as cholinergics and antispasmodics.[37] Of interest with respect to the previous discussion concerning regions of optimum absorption in the gastrointestinal tract is the observation that the drug-mucin interaction decreases at lower pH.[36] It has been suggested that for this reason absorption of quaternaries may be most rapid from the upper part of the gastrointestinal tract. Delayed drug release from dosage forms could, under such circumstances, have serious consequences. One might also speculate that coadministration of antacids could interfere with the absorption of these drugs due to increased drug binding at higher pH.

Along with a consideration of those types of interactions which cause inhibition of drug absorption, it is appropriate to mention interactions leading to opposite effects. Obviously, this encompasses all instances of active transport, for which the interaction of drug with a "carrier" is often postulated.[185] Of greater interest to biopharmaceutics are interactions with compounds which can be isolated and reasonably defined, such as the well-known interaction of vitamin B_{12} with intrinsic factor and the more recently reported interaction of quaternary ammonium compounds with a phosphatido-peptide fraction of intestinal tissue.[107] Since these physiologic materials can be isolated, they can be employed as dosage form additives to enhance the absorption of certain drugs. Little published work is as yet available in this area, but it would seem that it represents a unique and perhaps fruitful approach to improved drug formulation.

Biotransformation and Biologic Half-life

The subject of biotransformation, which is also called detoxication or drug metabolism, is so extensive as to constitute almost a separate discipline. It will be discussed here only in a limited manner, primarily with respect to its relationship to the biologic half-life or elimination rate of drugs. More extensive and detailed information can be obtained from the book *Detoxication Mechanisms* by R. T. Williams[214] and from a review article on the subject.[27]

Williams[215] has classified the metabolic changes undergone by drugs and other foreign compounds in the body from a pharmacologic aspect as follows: (1) reactions in which biologically inactive compounds are converted into active metabolites; (2) reactions in which biologically active compounds are converted into active metabolites with the same or different activity; (3) reactions in which biologically active compounds are converted into inactive metabolites by oxidation, reduction or hydrolysis; (4) detoxication mechanisms, i.e., reactions between foreign

compounds and body carbohydrates or amino acids to yield inactive and nontoxic excretory products; and (5) lethal syntheses, i.e., reactions between the foreign compound and a body constituent to produce an injurious product. The discussion to follow will be concerned primarily with reactions of types (3) and (4) which involve the conversion of pharmacologically active compounds to essentially inactive metabolites. It has already been pointed out that the elimination rate of a pharmacologically active compound depends on its rate of biotransformation to inactive metabolites and the rate of excretion of its unchanged (active) form. The elimination rate, which is often expressed in terms of the biologic half-life of the drug involved, determines the persistence time of drug present in the body. The persistence time frequently can be related to the duration of pharmacologic activity.

A rational dosage regimen must be based on a consideration of a drug's biologic half-life. Too frequent administration of additional (maintenance) doses after the initial dose, or maintenance doses which are too high, may cause drug accumulation and toxic reactions. On the other hand, maintenance doses which are too low or which are spaced too far apart result in a decline in the total amount of drug in the body and may cause the treatment to be ineffective. Frequently, it is necessary to administer a relatively high initial or priming dose, followed by lower maintenance doses at appropriate intervals. The shorter the time intervals between doses, the lower is the amount of drug required to maintain the drug content of the body in the desired range. Furthermore, the magnitude of the fluctuations of drug concentration in various body compartments diminishes as the frequency of administration of appropriate maintenance doses increases until, when the frequency becomes infinitely large (i.e., on continuous administration), the drug concentration in the body remains constant (assuming the dosage or rate of drug administration to be correct). Continuous drug administration can be achieved by intravenous drip or by means of properly designed oral sustained release dosage forms.

In certain instances it may be possible to achieve much better therapeutic results by continuous drug administration (thereby maintaining a constant drug concentration in fluids of distribution) than are obtained with periodic drug administration and the associated fluctuations of drug concentration in the fluids. The reader may recall that drug diffuses from blood to the tissues when the concentration of drug in diffusible form is higher in the blood and that drug leaves the tissues and diffuses back into the blood when the concentration gradient is reversed. If the rate of diffusion of a drug to the site of action is very low,* it may be impossible to achieve diffusion equilibrium between the particular site and the fluids of distribution in the course of conventional drug therapy, particularly if the drug is rapidly eliminated. Under such circumstances it becomes necessary to establish a relatively high drug concentration in the bloodstream in order to attain a considerably lower concentration at the site of action. This may be undesirable, not only for economic reasons but also because of possible toxic reactions which could occur, especially when there is a separate site of action with respect to the toxic activity and when diffusion to that site can occur quite rapidly. On reflection, one is struck by the question of how many potentially useful drugs may have been overlooked during a pharmacologic screening process or clinical trial because neither biologic half-life nor diffusion problems were taken into consideration adequately in establishing the dosage schedule. It has been reported that the blood supply to cancerous tissue is quite limited,[78] which suggests that failure of chemotherapy of malignancies may, in some instances, be due to an inadequacy of the drug concentration obtained in tumor tissue. Based on considerations outlined in the preceding paragraphs, it would seem to be advisable to administer certain anticancer drugs in a manner which leads to relatively constant drug levels in the fluids of distribution. Indeed, it has been observed that

---

* For example, the rate of diffusion of sulfa-diazine from blood to cerebrospinal fluid is so low that 6 to 8 hours are required for the concentration of drug in cerebrospinal fluid to reach half the free drug concentration in blood plasma (under conditions where drug-plasma concentration is constant).[158]

TABLE 2-1. DOSAGE INTERVALS (T) AND RATIOS OF INITIAL DOSE TO MAINTENANCE DOSE (D*/D) FOR MAINTAINING CONSTANT DRUG CONCENTRATION*

DRUG	AVERAGE $t_{\frac{1}{2}}$ (hours)	T (hours)	D*/D
Sulfathiazole	3.5	4	1.8
Sulfisoxazole	6.1	6	2.0
Sulfanilamide	8.8	8	2.1
Acetyl sulfisoxazole	13.1	12	2.1
Sulfadiazine	16.7	24	1.6
Sulfamerazine	23.5	24	2.0
Sulfadimethoxine	41.0	24	3.0

* Part of a tabulation by Krüger-Thiemer, E., and Bünger, P.: Arzneim-Forsch., *11*:867.

administration of the anticancer drug amethopterin by continuous intravenous drip was more effective than administration of the same amount of drug in a single daily dose.[123] Apparently, this is due to the sustained drug levels achieved by the former procedure.

How important it is for rational therapy to consider the biologic half-life of a drug when establishing its dosage schedule may be shown in the tabulation by Krüger-Thiemer and Bünger,[99] who calculated for a number of sulfa drugs the ratio of initial dose:maintenance dose (D*/D) and the time intervals (T) between doses necessary to maintain drug levels in the body within a constant range (Table 2-1).

According to the data in Table 2-1, it is necessary to administer one half the initial dose of sulfisoxazole every 6 hours to maintain constant body concentration of the drug, while in the case of sulfadimethoxine one would give one third the initial dose every 24 hours. The differences in biologic half-life between the various sulfa drugs were not generally appreciated in the early days of sulfonamide therapy, and it has been pointed out that sulfa drugs with a long half-life (such as sulfadiazine and sulfamerazine) became discredited because of frequent toxic reactions. These latter were actually due to too frequent dosage and the resulting drug accumulation.[55] The combination of two or more sulfonamides in one dosage form also has been criticized, since most of such combinations involve substances that differ significantly in biologic half-life.[99] Rational adjustment of dosage regimen is impossible under such circumstances; maintenance dosage based on the half-life of the most rapidly eliminated component leads to accumulation of the other component, while dosage based on the longer half-life results in ineffective concentration levels of the sulfonamide with the shorter half-life during much of the time.

The effect of dosage regimen also has been related directly to the magnitude of a pharmacologic response. The diuretic effect of chlorothiazide, a widely used diuretic, is considerably greater when the drug is administered in divided doses than in a single daily dose.[133] This is understood easily in view of the very short half-life of chlorothiazide; practically all of an intravenously administered dose is excreted within 5 hours.[29] The foregoing comments amply illustrate the importance of biotransformation processes and their kinetic aspects in dosage form design and evaluation. This should become even more evident in the following paragraphs which deal with the effect of various factors on the biotransformation of drugs. The other process involved in drug elimination, excretion of unmodified drug, will be discussed separately in another section.

Effect of Dosage. Man has a limited capacity to metabolize certain drugs. When this capacity is approached, drug metabolism no longer proceeds by apparent first-order kinetics, but begins to approach a constant maximum rate. A case in point is the metabolism of ethanol, which occurs in man at a maximum rate of about 100 mg./Kg./hour. A classic example of saturable drug metabolism is the conversion of salicylate to its major metabolite, salicyluric acid. When the dose of salicylate in adult humans exceeds about 200 or 300 mg., the kinetics of its

elimination begin to deviate from that of an apparent first-order process. The biologic half-life of salicylate is only about 3 hours at the low (less than 300 mg.) doses, but it takes about 6 hours to eliminate 50 per cent of a one gram dose,[121] and about 19 hours to eliminate 50 per cent of a very large dose (10 Gm. and above).[193] This saturation effect is evident in Figure 2-10, which shows the time course of elimination of different doses of salicylate in the same subject. Note that the elimination curves become exponential only when drug levels in the body are less than 300 mg., and that from then on the half-lives are the same regardless of the size of the original dose. The increasingly longer time required to eliminate larger doses of salicylate causes this drug to be accumulated easily during therapy. There have been many cases of salicylate intoxication due to its accumulation in the body during therapy, particularly in the case of infants. Some other drugs, for example, bishydroxycoumarin, apparently inhibit their own metabolism at higher doses. This self-inhibition is not a saturation effect, and elimination is essentially exponential, except that the half-life increases with increasing dose. It is very difficult to design proper dosage regimens for drugs with these characteristics.

Effect of Age. A number of drugs are eliminated much more slowly by infants than

FIG. 2-10. Elimination of different doses of salicylate by the same human subject. Plotted are the amounts of salicylate remaining in the body as a function of time. Vertical arrows on the time axis indicate the time necessary to eliminate one half of the respective dose. (Levy, G.: Pharmacokinetics of salicylate elimination in man. J. Pharm. Sci., 54:959, 1965)

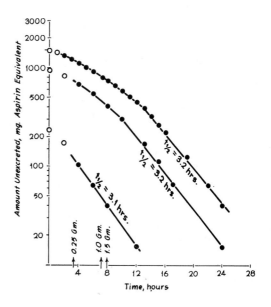

they are by adults. This phenomenon is apparently due to the fact that the activity of enzymes such as those involved in glucuronide formation is very low in the first few weeks of life.[212] A number of deaths of infants have occurred as a consequence of chloramphenicol administration, since this drug is detoxified by transformation to glucuronide and was accumulated in the very young who are deficient in this mechanism for its rapid elimination.[192] The biologic half-life of sulfonamides also is longer at birth than at subsequent times.[53] Other studies have established that the activity of drug-metabolizing enzymes in aged individuals also differs from that of average-age adults. For example, the biologic half-life of barbiturates appears to be longer in subjects older than 55 years than in younger adults.[30]

Effect of Disease. Various pathologic conditions, particularly those involving the liver, affect the biotransformation rate of drugs. For example, glucuronide formation is impaired during acute infectious hepatitis, as evidenced by decreased formation of N-acetyl-p-aminophenol glucuronide after administration of N-acetyl-p-aminophenol.[204] Thus, the half-life of the drug has been found to average 178 minutes in subjects with hepatitis and only 134 minutes in healthy controls. As a further example, the acetylation of p-aminobenzoic acid[35] is affected in various metabolic disorders. Subjects with uncontrolled diabetes show increased acetylation, while low acetylation is found in hyperthyroidism. Obese subjects show higher acetylation than lean ones.[145] In guinea pigs it has been found that the biologic half-lives of aniline, antipyrine and acetanilide are increased when the animals are depleted of ascorbic acid.[11] It must be noted that what may appear to be an altered rate of biotransformation could in some cases be the result of changes in the excretion rate of the drug or one or more of its metabolites. Determination of the respective excretion rate constants will indicate whether this is, indeed, the case.

Effect of Drugs. Administration of N-acetyl-p-aminophenol together with hydrocortisone or prednisolone results in a marked increase of steroid plasma levels.[44] This is due evidently to an inhibition of steroid glucuronide formation as a result of the competition by N-acetyl-p-aminophenol for available glucuronide-forming enzyme. Other phenolic compounds, such as various bioflavonoids, are also capable of prolonging the half-life of hydrocortisone.[210] Similar retardation of drug elimination is achieved for salicylic acid by coadministration of p-aminobenzoic acid, since both substances are conjugated to some extent with glycine and thus compete for the same biotransformation system. This mechanism was indicated by the marked decrease in the amount of excreted salicyluric acid when p-aminobenzoic acid was administered together with the salicylate.[167] These observations exemplify a possible pharmacologic approach to the prolongation of the therapeutic effect of certain drugs. Opposite effects, namely more rapid inactivation, have been achieved by administration of potential conjugating substrates.

Glycine administration increases the elimination of large doses of benzoic acid[5] because the rate-limiting factor in the formation of hippuric acid (the glycine conjugate of benzoic acid) is the availability of glycine. On the other hand, glycine does not increase the rate of formation of salicyluric acid (the glycine conjugate of salicylic acid) from salicylic acid in man, since another step in this process is rate limiting. Administration of sulfate (as such or in the form of a precursor such as L-cysteine) increases the rate of formation of salicylamide sulfate from salicylamide and thereby increases the rate of elimination of the latter.[117]

There has been a great deal of interest in the effect of preadministered barbiturate on the biotransformation rate of a number of different types of drugs.[27] Barbiturates apparently cause increased synthesis of drug-metabolizing enzymes. Pretreatment with a barbiturate has been found to accelerate the elimination and decrease the pharmacologic activity of the coumarin anticoagulants dicumarol, biscoumacetate and acenocoumarin,[51] which led the investigators to caution that "it may be necessary in the future to pay more attention to the mutual influence of concomitant therapy on the physiological disposition of the drugs employed." *

* Dayton, P. G., et al.: The influence of barbiturates on coumarin plasma levels and prothrombin response. J. Clin. Invest., 40:1797, 1961.

The various reports cited here are indicative of the fact that some drugs can stimulate or inhibit the metabolism of other drugs. Additional examples of such activities are described and discussed by Bousquet[27] and Conney.[41] While these properties of drugs cause problems and complications in chemotherapy, they can be utilized also in prolonging the duration of drug action or in terminating it more rapidly where necessary.

It has recently been demonstrated that enzyme inducers may be used as therapeutic tools in the treatment of certain enzyme deficiencies. For example, phenobarbital has been found to enhance the glucuronide formation capacity of an infant who was severely jaundiced due to an inability to effectively metabolize bilirubin to bilirubin glucuronide.[221] The phenobarbital treatment not only lowered bilirubin levels in the plasma but also normalized the infant's ability to form the glucuronide of the drug salicylamide.

Intersubject Variation. The biologic half-life of drugs as reported in the literature represents an average value for the type of subject in which it was established. However, even within a group of individuals relatively standardized with respect to age, state of health, therapeutic regimen and similar potential variables, the biologic half-life varies significantly. Such intersubject variation is as characteristic as that of other biologic parameters, such as weight, height and color of the eyes. Krüger-Thiemer and Bünger found twofold differences in the biologic half-life of each of a number of sulfonamides in different individuals all of whom were healthy and of similar age.[99] These authors cite similar experiences of other investigators with streptomycin, kanamycin, isoniazid and pyrazinamide. Another report indicates eightfold differences in rates of metabolism of dicumarol and ethylbiscumacetate.[31] Also, there may be occasional intrasubject variations due to changes in dietary habits, fluid intake and physical activity. Such variations, regardless of cause, can represent serious problems in chemotherapy due to the danger of undertreatment or drug accumulation and the attendant toxicities. Fortunately, it is often possible to "titrate" patients, using lack of clinical response and onset of side effects

as indicators of underdosage and overdosage, respectively. Such technic may not be useful with drugs having unfavorable therapeutic ratios or insidious or delayed toxic reactions. Often, it may be desirable actually to determine the biologic half-life of a drug in a given patient at the start of therapy and to adjust the subsequent dosage regimen accordingly. Alternatively, it has been suggested that daily blood samples be drawn during the course of therapy just prior to administration of the next dose in order to establish the minimum concentration of drug in the blood and, then, to note whether accumulation or concentration decline is occurring in the course of therapy.[99] These considerations are also indicative of some serious fundamental limitations of sustained release dosage forms, since the release characteristics of such forms must, of necessity, be based on requirements related to the half-life of a drug in the average individual. Moreover, such dosage forms permit no adjustments of dosage regimen other than to increase or decrease the *amount* of administered drug; the *rate* of release or drug supply to the body (which is analogous to the frequency of administration of drug in conventional form) cannot be changed.

Biotransformation During Gastrointestinal Absorption. Some recent work points to the gastrointestinal wall as a site of biotransformation of certain drugs. Thus, a drug may be partially inactivated even before it enters the fluids of distribution unless, for example, its conjugated form is fully hydrolyzed and reverted to free drug at the serosal side of the gastrointestinal membrane. A consideration of possible biotransformation of drugs during their gastrointestinal absorption is therefore pertinent before considering, in a following section, the effect of route of administration on drug activity.

Formation of drug glucuronides, until recently thought to be limited to the liver and (to a lesser extent) the kidneys, takes place also in the mucous membranes of the gastrointestinal tract.[82] In fact, animal data suggest that synthesis of glucuronides in the fetal stomach is already at the adult level, whereas hepatic conjugation with glucuronides is known to be very low in the newborn.[190] Thyroxine, triiodothyronine and certain thyroxine analogs which are absorbed by an active transport process are also changed to glucuronic acid conjugates during absorption.[84]

Whether biotransformation of drugs in the gastrointestinal tissues is reversible and primarily a mechanism for active transport (the glucuronide cannot diffuse back into the lumen due to its lipoid insolubility), or whether it is irreversible in the body and thus serves as part of the detoxication process, has not as yet been established. Most drug conjugates are so rapidly eliminated that their in-vivo hydrolysis to the original active form is probably negligible. It is important that the possibility of biotransformation during gastrointestinal absorption be considered as one possible cause for differences between the pharmacologic results obtained from oral and parenteral dosage forms, since drug plasma levels and therapeutic response after parenteral administration often serve as the standard of comparison for evaluation of oral dosage forms.

URINARY EXCRETION

It has been explained previously that drug elimination is the result of biotransformation and excretion of unchanged drug. In most cases, the urinary route is the major excretory pathway, although some drugs are excreted primarily in the bile. Biliary excretion becomes an important means of drug removal from the body only if subsequent gastrointestinal reabsorption of a drug thus excreted does not occur to any major degree. Urinary excretion of drugs can involve three processes: glomerular filtration, active tubular excretion of organic acids or bases in ionic form and passive back diffusion (reabsorption) of part of such acids or bases in nonionic form from the lower tubular regions.[156] Since the rate of reabsorption is proportional to the concentration of drug in un-ionized form, it is possible to modify this rate by changing the pH of the urine. In this way one may either increase or decrease the urinary excretion rate and, therefore, the elimination rate of drugs which are weak acids or weak bases.

The urinary excretion rate of salicylic acid can be decreased and higher salicylate blood levels achieved by acidifying the urine with ammonium chloride.[184] An opposite effect is obtained by administration of sodium bicarbonate, and this technic has been used to treat cases of salicylate poisoning, since it achieves rapid removal of the drug from the body. Similarly, Kostenbauder and co-workers have shown that the elimination rate of the sulfonamide sulfaethidole can be changed by urinary pH adjustment.[98] When the urine was maintained at a pH of 4.8 to 5.2, the average biologic half-life of the drug was 11.4 hours. Upon adjustment of urinary pH to 7.9 to 8.1, the half-life was shortened to an average of only 4.2 hours. Sulfaethidole is a weak acid with a pK_a of 5.5, and it may be calculated that 76 per cent of the drug is in un-ionized form at pH 5.0, while only about 1.5 per cent is un-ionized at pH 7.8.[98]

The urinary excretion of drugs can also be retarded by administration of agents capable of inhibiting their tubular secretion. For example, probenecid prolongs the biologic half-life of penicillins by such a mechanism.[83] The state of health, particularly with respect to kidney function, can be a factor in the urinary excretion of drugs. Thus, the average excretion rate constant for exogenous hippuric acid was found to be 2.7 hours^{-1} in normal subjects, but only 1.2 hours^{-1} in subjects with renal disease.[219]

ROUTE OF ADMINISTRATION

Quantitative differences in the pharmacologic activity of drugs as a function of route of administration are observed frequently and can be related usually to differences in rates of absorption and drug concentration maxima. One ordinarily expects a drug to have the same qualitative effect regardless of route of administration, but there is a sufficient number of exceptions to justify special consideration. A case in point is magnesium sulfate, which acts as a laxative when taken orally but is a powerful central nervous system depressant when administered parenterally.[213] The laxative effect and absence of systemic activity on oral administration is due to the very limited absorption of magnesium sulfate from the gastrointestinal tract. Drugs that are absorbed from the gastrointestinal tract enter the portal circulation and are channeled immediately to the liver, which is the major site of biotransformation. On the other hand, drugs do not pass directly to the liver when administered parenterally, sublingually or rectally. Consequently, the tissue distribution pattern of drugs may differ considerably, depending on route of administration. This, in turn, can result in the predominance of one or another pharmacologic effect. Certain monamine oxidase inhibitors, namely pheniprazine, phenelzine and, to some extent, isocarboxazid, give rise to greater brain monoamine oxidase inhibition than liver monoamine oxidase inhibition when administered subcutaneously. On oral administration, these drugs exert a more pronounced liver monoamine oxidase inhibition than brain monoamine oxidase inhibition.[90] This is considered to be due to the drug passing directly to the brain on subcutaneous administration, while passing first through the liver when given orally. A difference in tissue distribution pattern as a function of route of administration has also been observed with griseofulvin; the drug was concentrated in the lungs and the skin after intravenous administration and in liver, skin, skeletal muscle and fat after oral administration.[19] Pretreatment with barbiturates accelerates the elimination of orally administered biscoumacetate, but barbiturates have no appreciable effect on the elimination of intravenously administered biscoumacetate. This suggests differences in the metabolic pathway of this anticoagulant as a function of route of administration[51]—or, more likely, that the barbiturate affects the absorption of biscoumacetate.

The activity ratios between several opiates vary with different routes of administration.[59] This is also true for the active constituents of thyroid, namely triiodothyronine and thyroxine. The latter instance can be related to the incomplete gastrointestinal absorption of thyroxine. Since triiodothyronine is well absorbed, the activity ratio between the two compounds differs depending on route of administration.[115]

In some instances, the differences in drug effects associated with different routes of administration may be related to different biotransformation patterns as a consequence of differences in rates of absorption. In these cases, similar effects can be observed by administering the drug at different rates by any one route. The metabolism of 5-hydroxy-tryptamine is thus affected. Rapid intravenous injection of this compound causes greater formation of its O-glucuronide than subcutaneous administration or slow intravenous infusion.[2] The phenolic conjugation of 5-hydroxytryptamine, therefore, is considered to be an emergency route for its elimination. However, the most intense phenolic conjugation occurs after oral administration, despite the slower rate of drug entry into the body.[2] This may be due to partial conjugation in the gastrointestinal wall, as described in a previous section. Opposite rate effects are found with respect to the biotransformation of the antitubercular drug p-aminosalicylic acid. This drug is inactivated primarily by acetylation. Administration of a daily dose in several small increments causes the greatest degree of acetylation, while giving the drug in a single large daily dose causes the least acetylation[68] probably due to saturation of the acetylation process in the body. Consequently, the use of single daily doses is preferred and considered to be more effective.

The hormonal activity of Δ^4-3-ketosteroids is affected in a paradoxical manner by enol etherification: parenteral activity is decreased while oral effectiveness is increased.[60] The investigators feel that this is due to differences in biotransformation, but it has also been suggested that differences in rates of hydrolysis of these compounds in the gastrointestinal tract compared with the rates in parenteral depots can account for the observed effects.[206] Another example concerns 3-phenyl-1,2,4-triazole, which produces strong central nervous system stimulation when injected intravenously and pronounced depression when administered intraperitoneally.[61]

The examples cited so far demonstrate that some drugs exhibit not only quantitative but also qualitative differences in activity as a function of route of administration. These differences may be due to differences in tissue distribution patterns, biotransformation and physiologic availability from the gastrointestinal tract. Relative drug stability in different body compartments may also be involved and will be discussed in a following section. Such effects must be considered in any attempt to extrapolate pharmacologic data obtained after drug administration by one route to instances where the drug is administered by another route. This is obviously pertinent to the intelligent interpretation of literature data and to rational development of dosage forms.

BLOOD LEVELS AND PLASMA PROTEIN BINDING

Blood level data are widely employed to evaluate the absorption rate of drugs as a function of dosage form, route of administration and similar variables. This involves no unusual complications in the majority of individual cases, since the biologic properties of a drug such as apparent volume of distribution, elimination rate and activity are usually unchanged so that differences in blood levels are a direct reflection of differences in absorption rate. (Many of the possible complications discussed in previous sections can be avoided in a clinical evaluation by proper experimental design.) The utilization of blood levels as criteria of the comparative absorption efficacy and activity of a series of derivatives or homologs is not as simple, and such data can easily be misinterpreted. The various compounds, despite basic structural similarities, may differ considerably in activity, distribution pattern and biologic half-life, among other things. In such cases, blood levels can be interpreted rationally only if the dissimilarities mentioned above are considered concurrently. Many drugs are bound partially to plasma proteins and exist in the blood in part as free drug and in part as drug-protein complex. Only the free drug can diffuse to other tissues; the protein-bound portion does not pass across blood vessel walls in the healthy individual. The greater the degree of protein binding, the smaller the amount of the drug which is available to extravascular sites, since the driving force for diffusion from blood stream to other tissues is the concentration gradient of diffusible (not total) drug.

Obviously, even an inherently active chemotherapeutic agent cannot be effective unless it reaches its site of action in sufficient concentration. Some drugs are relatively ineffective because they are highly protein-bound, while appropriately modified derivatives may be quite active because of their lesser affinity for plasma proteins. The higher blood levels obtained after administration of one compound, as compared with the blood levels resulting from administration of another derivative, may mean either that the former is more rapidly absorbed or that it is more extensively bound to plasma proteins. In the latter case, the higher blood levels would be indicative of low availability to extravascular tissues and, probably, of low therapeutic effectiveness.

The generalities mentioned so far may be discussed more specifically, using the sulfonamides and tetracyclines as examples. Both types of compounds are active only in unbound (diffusible) form. The binding of sulfonamides to plasma proteins can be described by the equation,

$$D_p = K D_f^a \qquad (22)$$

where D_p is the concentration of bound drug, D_f is the concentration of free drug and K and a are constants characteristic of a particular sulfonamide.[177] This equation is analogous to the Freundlich adsorption isotherm, which characterizes many adsorption processes. It indicates that the degree of protein binding is a function of concentration.

This important point has been overlooked by the many investigators who determined the degree of protein-binding at only one drug concentration. Equation 22 is handled more easily in logarithmic form.

$$\log D_p = \log K + a \log D_f \qquad (23)$$

In this form, there exists a linear relationship between $\log D_p$ and $\log D_f$, with $\log K$ as the intercept and a as the slope. Such a log-log plot, representing the degree of protein binding of a number of sulfonamides in human serum as a function of drug concentration, is shown in Figure 2-11. Several of the lines intersect, which indicates that one drug may be more extensively bound than another at a low concentration, while the reverse is true at higher concentrations. In general, the degree of protein-binding of any one sulfonamide decreases with increasing drug concentration, as exemplified by the data shown in Table 2-2. Only sulfadiazine and sulfamerazine do not show this relationship; the interaction of these compounds with plasma proteins is practically independent of concentration. The sulfonamide B5254 is almost

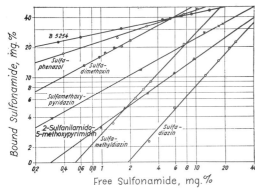

FIG. 2-11. Protein binding of various sulfonamides in human blood serum (from Scholtan, W.: Die Bindung der Langzeit-Sulfonamide an die Eiweiss Körper des Serums. Arzneim.-Forsch., *11*:707).

TABLE 2-2. THE RELATION BETWEEN FREE SULFONAMIDE CONCENTRATION* AND TOTAL SULFONAMIDE CONCENTRATION IN HUMAN BLOOD SERUM†

TOTAL SULFONAMIDE CONCENTRATION (mg. %):	100	10	1
B 5254‡	44.0	0.04	< 0.01
Sulfaphenazole	31.0	0.63	0.01
Sulfadimethoxine	20.5	3.5	0.42
Sulfamethoxypyridazine	45.0	13.5	2.1
Sulfamerazine	25.5	27.0	28.5
2-Sulfanilamido-5-methoxypyrimidine	55.0	31.0	12.7
Sulfadiazine	52.0	55.0	59.0

* Expressed as per cent of total concentration.
† Scholtan, W.: Arzneim.-Forsch. *11*:707.
‡ 5-sulfanilamido-3-ethyl-1,2,4-thiadiazole.

totally protein-bound at concentrations of 10 mg. % or less. It yields high blood levels but has no bacteriostatic effect in vivo[177] because of its extremely low availability to extravascular areas. The degree of plasma-protein binding of sulfonamides differs considerably between various animal species. Moreover, the various species cannot be grouped in any distinct order with respect to the relative magnitude of plasma-protein binding; a different sequence is obtained with different sulfonamides.[177] Therefore, animal data have limited value in assessments of the activity of sulfonamide drugs.

When the degree of plasma-protein binding of a drug decreases at higher blood levels, the apparent volume of distribution of the drug will increase with increasing dose. Accordingly, doubling an intravenous dose may not double D_o, the value obtained by extrapolating the drug concentration decay curve to zero time (cf. p. 40). For example, D_o after intravenous administration of 10 Gm. of sodium salicylate (which is partially bound to plasma proteins) was 40 mg. %; after intravenous administration of 20 Gm., D_o increased to only about 55 mg. %.[193] As the relative intravascular retention of such drugs decreases, a greater fraction reaches biotransformation sites. This can result in higher biotransformation rates and smaller half-lives at higher doses, provided that there is no saturation of the conjugating system as previously described. Such

effects have been observed with iophenoxic acid*[177] and phenylbutazone.[9] It is of interest that there is little correlation between the degree of plasma-protein binding and the excretion rate of sulfonamides.[142, 177] The kidneys evidently are capable of dissociating the drug-protein complex. Various pathologic conditions cause changes in the composition of plasma proteins and can affect the degree of drug binding. Scholtan[177] reports cases of nephrosis, diabetes and cirrhosis where the degree of plasma-protein binding of a sulfonamide was considerably lower than in healthy subjects.

Another mechanism by which the degree of protein binding of drugs can be reduced and drug availability to extravascular areas increased is displacement of the drug from its adsorption site by another substance. This approach can be an effective one for enhancing drug action. Anton found that sulfinpyrazone, ethyl biscoumacetate, iophenoxic acid and other substances displace sulfonamide from plasma proteins, resulting in a decrease of total drug plasma concentration and an increase of sulfonamide concentration in the tissues.[9]

Effective displacing agents are substances highly bound to plasma proteins, but certain structural characteristics are also required, probably for adsorption site specificity. Dis-

* This highly plasma-protein bound compound can have a half-life as long as 2½ years in humans!

placement agents have not yet been tried in chemotherapy as drug potentiating agents, but unintentional displacement effects have been observed clinically. The protein binding of 2-sulfanilamido-5-methoxy-pyrimidine was very much decreased in a patient with high serum bilirubin concentration due to cirrhosis of the liver; bilirubin was found to displace the sulfonamide from plasma proteins also in vitro.[177] On the other hand, there are indications that several fatal cases of kernicterus in premature babies were due to the displacement of protein-bound bilirubin by sulfisoxazole, a sulfonamide which was used prophylactically for its antibacterial effect. The freed bilirubin accumulated in the central nervous system of these infants and reached toxic levels there.[148, 183] It is likely that in vivo equilibrium between drugs or physiologic substances and plasma proteins is a function of concentration and respective stability constants, precisely like the equilibria of other types of reactions. Thus, it is not surprising that a sulfonamide can displace protein bound bilirubin in one instance, while bilirubin replaces a sulfonamide in another instance. Actually, both of these effects occur concurrently. Their relative magnitude depends on the concentrations of bilirubin and drug, and on the relative affinity of these compounds for plasma proteins.

The use of blood level data to judge the relative merits of antibiotics such as the penicillins and the tetracyclines is associated with considerable difficulty and chance of misinterpretation. Both broth dilution and agar diffusion assay methods tend to minimize the effect of protein binding and do not reflect the concentration of diffusible drug alone.[100] Since different homologs may differ considerably in their affinity to plasma proteins, it is not appropriate to base judgment solely on total drug levels in the blood. This is exemplified by the data in Table 2-3, which show that the greater in vitro activity of demethyl-chlortetracycline as compared with tetracycline (which is less protein-bound) is nullified and actually reversed in the presence of serum.[163] Moreover, different tetracycline homologs differ in their activity against a given micro-organism.

Concentrations of various tetracyclines in the blood, as determined by microbiologic

TABLE 2-3. EFFECT OF SERUM ON ANTIBACTERIAL ACTIVITY OF DEMETHYLCHLORTETRACYCLINE AND TETRACYCLINE*

	MINIMAL INHIBITORY CONCENTRATION (mcg./ml.)	
	DEMETHYL-CHLORTETRA-CYCLINE	TETRA-CYCLINE
Streptococcus—9282		
Broth	0.05	0.08
50% Serum	0.98	0.70
Streptococcus—CL-25		
Broth	0.5	4.0
50% Serum	32.0	64.0
Staphylococcus—P		
Broth	0.1	0.2
50% Serum	0.8	0.8
Staphylococcus—T		
Broth	0.05	0.2
50% Serum	3.2	1.6
Coli—Aerogenes—119		
Broth	0.5	1.0
50% Serum	4.0	2.0

*Roberts, C. E., et al.: Demethylchlortetracycline and tetracycline. Arch. Intern. Med., 107:204.

assay, can be expressed either in terms of the antibiotic ingested or in terms of a reference compound, such as tetracycline itself. The two methods yield different results and may show either one or another tetracycline derivative to be the most useful (see Fig. 2-12). Since we are interested in the activity of such drugs against a particular pathogen and not in their activity with respect to the micro-organism used in the bioassay, it is apparent that this type of study may not be very helpful in the choice of the most useful tetracycline derivative for treating a particular infection.

In summary, it may be stated that blood level data alone offer an insufficient basis on which to judge the relative merits of structurally and pharmacologically related compounds such as the sulfonamides, the penicillins and the tetracyclines. Differences in plasma-protein binding, antibacterial spectrum and peculiarities of assay methods must also be taken into account. High blood levels may be indicative of low drug concentration in extravascular tissues and low chemotherapeutic effectiveness. Pharmacists should

FIG. 2-12. Serum levels of 4 tetracyclines expressed in terms of the administered homolog (*above*) and in terms of tetracycline activity (*below*). (From Kunin, C. M., and Finland, M.: Clinical pharmacology of the tetracycline antibiotics. Clin. Pharmacol. & Therap., 2:51)

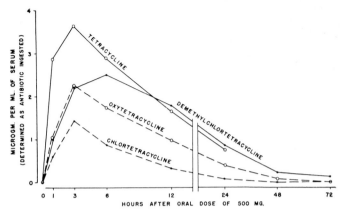

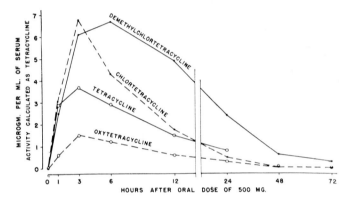

view the "battle of blood levels" waged by the sales promotion departments of some pharmaceutical manufacturers with a good deal of reservation and realize that there may be a great deal more to the issue than that which meets the eye.

PHYSICAL AND CHEMICAL FACTORS

LIPOID SOLUBILITY AND DISSOCIATION CONSTANT

The gastrointestinal epithelium acts as a lipidlike barrier to most drugs. It permits the absorption of lipoid-soluble substances from the gastrointestinal tract by a process of passive diffusion, while lipoid-insoluble substances can diffuse across this barrier only with considerable difficulty, if at all.[170] Many drugs are either weak organic acids or bases. Depending on their dissociation constants and on pH, they exist in solution partly ionized and partly in undissociated form. Only the undissociated form is lipoid-soluble,

and diffusion of drug across the gastrointestinal membrane is restricted essentially to this form. Since the rate of diffusion is proportional to the concentration gradient of diffusible drug across the membrane, it is possible to increase the absorption rate of weak acids and weak bases by appropriate pH adjustments. As the pH is decreased, the concentration of the undissociated form of a weak acid increases and, therefore, the rate of gastrointestinal absorption also is increased.

The same effect is obtained by increasing pH in the case of weak bases. The experimental data in support of these statements have been summarized by Hogben[87] and by Schanker.[170]

When the pH's of fluids on opposite sides of a membrane differ, it is possible for a weak acid or base to concentrate on one side. Diffusion equilibrium involves only the unionized portion of such substances; it will be present on each side of the membrane in equal concentration at equilibrium. The concentration of total (dissociated and undissociated) drug will differ if the pH's on the opposite sides of the membrane are not the same. As an example, one may consider the diffusion equilibrium of a weak acid ($pK_a = 4.0$) between gastric fluids ($pH \simeq 1$) and blood ($pH \simeq 7$). Employing the Henderson-Hasselbalch equation

$$pH = pK_a + \log \frac{\text{salt concentration}}{\text{acid concentration}} \quad (24)$$

it may be calculated that at pH 7 the ratio of undissociated to ionized drug is 1:1,000 while at pH 1 the ratio is 1:0.001. Thus, when the concentration of un-ionized drug is equal on both sides of the gastric membrane, the concentration ratio of total drug (gastric fluids:blood) will be 1.001:1,001 or, roughly, 1:1,000. These considerations provide explanations for the passive diffusion of weakly acidic or basic drugs against what appears to be a concentration gradient (but is not), and for the "trapping" of such drugs in certain fluids or tissues which differ in pH from that of their environment.

Gastrointestinal absorption of weakly acidic or basic drugs is affected not only by their degree of ionization but also by the lipid solubility of their un-ionized forms. The relative affinity of a drug for lipids and for water may be estimated on the basis of its partition coefficient between a lipidlike solvent and water. The effect of partition coefficient is illustrated in Table 2-4, in which are listed partition coefficients and degrees of absorption of a series of barbiturates from the colon of the rat. The various barbiturates have about the same dissociation constants, so that differences in their gastrointestinal absorption can be related directly to partition coefficients.

The physicochemical factors of importance in the gastrointestinal absorption of weakly acidic or basic drugs suggest several methods which may be used to increase absorption.† These involve either modifications in environmental pH or structural modifications of the drug itself. The pH of gastric fluids can be increased by administration of sodium bicarbonate or other antacids. This increases the absorption of weak bases and decreases the absorption of weak acids. However, it is important to consider also several other possible consequences of antacid administration including modifications of urinary pH and drug excretion rate, gastric emptying rate and the dissolution rate of administered drug solids. Changes in the pH of intestinal fluids are difficult to bring about under clinical conditions. Less difficult are temporary pH modifications at more accessible sites, such as the eye. Basic buffer solutions have been employed successfully to obtain increased pharmacologic response from alkaloidal ophthalmic solutions.[25]

It is often possible to make minor structural modifications in drugs (and thus to obtain compounds with greater lipid solubility and more favorable dissociation constants) without affecting significantly their intrinsic pharmacologic properties. Such an approach has resulted in the development of propionyl erythromycin ester lauryl sulfate, a compound which is considerably better absorbed than the weak base erythromycin itself. The pK_a of erythromycin is 8.6; that of the ester is 6.9. Furthermore, the lipid partition coefficient of the ester is about 180 times larger than that of erythromycin.[8] Another example is the weak acid heparin, which is not absorbed at a pH above 4; esterification with methanol yields a partially methylated compound with unimpaired anticoagulant ac-

TABLE 2-4. COMPARISON BETWEEN COLONIC ABSORPTION OF BARBITURATES IN RATS AND CHLOROFORM: WATER PARTITION COEFFICIENT OF THE UNDISSOCIATED DRUG*

BARBITURATE	PARTITION COEFFICIENT	PER CENT ABSORBED
Barbital	0.7	12
Aprobarbital	4.9	17
Phenobarbital	4.8	20
Allylbarbituric acid	10.5	23
Butethal	11.7	24
Cyclobarbital	13.9	24
Pentobarbital	28.0	30
Secobarbital	50.7	40
Hexethal	> 100	44

* Schanker, L. S.: Absorption of drugs from the rat colon. J. Pharmacol. Exp. Ther., *126*:283.

†Compare Chapter 4, p. 169, for specific applications.

tivity, which is absorbed at pH's 5, 6 and 7.[166]

These physicochemical considerations with regard to the passage of drugs across the gastrointestinal membrane are also applicable to other biologic barriers, including the one between blood and brain.[159] The factors which favor drug penetration through biologic membranes in general are a high degree of lipoid solubility, a low degree of ionization, and lack of plasma protein binding.[159]

DISSOLUTION RATE

Drugs which are administered orally in solid form first must dissolve in gastrointestinal fluids before they can be absorbed. Dissolution takes time and frequently is the rate-limiting step in the absorption process. The dissolution of a substance in a nonreacting solvent may be described by the Noyes-Whitney law:[147]

$$\frac{dC}{dt} = KS\,(C_s - C) \qquad (25)$$

where dC/dt is the rate of dissolution, S is the surface area of the dissolving solid and K is the dissolution rate constant (which includes several factors such as intensity of agitation of the solvent and diffusion coefficient of the dissolving drug). C is the concentration of drug in the dissolution medium at time t and C_s is the concentration of drug in the diffusion layer surrounding the solid material. This diffusion layer is a thin film saturated with the drug, so that C_s is essentially equivalent to the concentration of a saturated solution. The rate of dissolution is governed by the rate of diffusion of solute molecules through the diffusion layer into the body of the solution.

Equation (25) indicates several ways by which the dissolution rate of a drug may be increased. Since dissolution rate is directly proportional to surface area, one may decrease particle size. The greater surface area of drug in contact with dissolution medium then will bring about more rapid dissolution and thereby more rapid gastrointestinal absorption, provided that absorption is rate-limited by the dissolution process. In instances where the intrinsic dissolution rate is so low that the drug is ordinarily not completely absorbed when administered in solid form, the more rapid absorption attained by increasing the specific surface area will cause also an increase in the total amount of drug absorbed from a given dose.

As an example, sulfadiazine, when given as a fine particle suspension, is absorbed more rapidly and more completely than when administered as a suspension of larger particles.[160] The gastrointestinal absorption rate of sulfaethylthiadiazole also is increased when this drug is administered in smaller particle size.[95]

One of the most striking examples of the role of dissolution rate and the effect of surface area concerns the antifungal drug griseofulvin. This substance is absorbed incompletely because of its very low dissolution rate, which is probably related to its poor solubility in gastrointestinal fluids. It has been found that the absorbability of griseofulvin increases linearly with the logarithm of specific surface area, as shown in Figure 2-13. By using 0.5 Gm. of finely micronized drug it was possible to obtain the same blood levels as those following administration of 1.0 Gm. of the then available commercial form of the drug.[10] As a result of such studies, manufacturers now market griseofulvin in finely micronized or microcrystalline form,

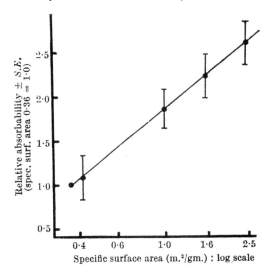

FIG. 2-13. Effect of specific surface area on absorbability of griseofulvin (from Atkinson, R. M., *et al.*: Effect of particle size on blood griseofulvin levels in man. Nature, *193*:588).

which permits dosage reduction by 50 per cent.

An interesting particle size effect has been observed in veterinary practice with respect to the anthelmintic activity of phenothiazine preparations.[56] The activity of these slowly dissolving substances against parasites in the small intestine of lambs increases with increasing surface area, as would be expected from dissolution rate theory. However, it has been found that larger particles are more effective against parasites inhabiting the large intestine. This is due apparently to the smaller particles being dissolved and absorbed before reaching the large intestine, while larger particles, because of their smaller specific surface area, reach the large intestine and are able to exert an anthelmintic effect there. Obviously, this approach can also be used in human chemotherapy where necessary.

The dissolution rate of drugs may also be increased by increasing their solubility in the diffusion layer. This would be reflected by an increase in the value of the C_s term in the Noyes-Whitney equation. In the case of weakly acidic or basic drugs, C_s can be increased by modifying the pH of the diffusion layer. Considering a weak acid HA as an example, its total solubility C_s is the sum of the concentrations of un-ionized acid HA and the anion A^-:

$$C_s = [HA] + [A^-]. \tag{26}$$

The total solubility of a weak acid in aqueous media at any pH usually is limited by the solubility of its un-ionized form. Since

$$K_a = \frac{[H^+][A^-]}{[HA]}, \tag{27}$$

$$[A^-] = K_a \frac{[HA]}{[H^+]} \tag{28}$$

where K_a is the dissociation constant of the weak acid and the brackets refer to the concentrations of the indicated species in solution. Substitution for $[A^-]$ in equation 26 results in

$$C_a = [HA] + K_a \frac{[HA]}{[H^+]}. \tag{29}$$

When $[H^+] << K_a$,

$$C_s = K_a \frac{[HA]}{[H^+]} \tag{30}$$

and, expressed in logarithmic form,

$$\log C_s = \log [HA] - pK_a + pH. \tag{31}$$

From the last equation it can be seen that the solubility C_s of a weak acid in the diffusion layer increases with increasing pH. There are several ways of increasing pH of the diffusion layer. One may (1) increase the pH of the entire dissolution medium as such, (2) mix a basic substance such as sodium bicarbonate or sodium citrate with the weak acid or (3) use a highly water-soluble salt of the weak acid instead of the weak acid itself.

Using the first method listed and considering physiologic conditions, one may administer antacids and thereby raise the pH of gastric fluids in order to enhance the dissolution of weak acids. The high acidity of the gastric fluids of course favors the dissolution of weak bases and has an opposite effect on weak acids. The second approach, that of adding solid basic substances to a weak acid, serves to increase pH in the immediate environment of the weak acid solids. This is the basis of the so-called buffered aspirin tablets and of combinations of other weak acids, such as PAS, with calcium carbonate, magnesium oxide and similar basic substances. In combinations such as these, there probably exists an optimum ratio of the two components which is related, among other things, to the strength of the weak acid and the decreasing fraction of total surface occupied by it as the proportion of additive in the mixture is increased.[135]

The most effective means of attaining higher dissolution rates is to use a highly water-soluble salt of the weak acid instead of the free acid itself. The salt acts as its own buffer and markedly raises the pH of an acidic dissolution medium in the immediate environment surrounding the dissolving drug solids. The dissolution rate of the sodium salt of a weak acid in an acidic dissolution medium under certain circumstances may be 1,000-fold higher than the dissolution rate of the weak acid itself.[134] Even if the sodium salt precipitates subsequently as the free acid in the bulk phase of an acidic solution such as gastric fluid, it will do so usually in the form of very fine particles. The large surface area of the drug thus precipitated favors rapid dissolution as additional fluid becomes available or as some of the dissolved drug is removed by absorption. The intrinsically more

TABLE 2-5. EFFECT OF DISSOLUTION RATE ON GASTROINTESTINAL ABSORPTION AND
BLOOD SUGAR LOWERING ACTIVITY OF TOLBUTAMIDE*
(Administered in Pure Form as Nondisintegrating Pellets)

FORM OF TOLBUTAMIDE	IN VITRO DISSOLUTION RATE†		AMOUNT OF DRUG IN BODY‡	LOWERING OF BLOOD SUGAR LEVEL§
	0.1 N HCl	pH 7.2 BUFFER		
Acid	.21	3.1	14	5.2
Sodium salt	1069	868	251	19.1

* Nelson, E., et al.: Influence of the absorption rate of tolbutamide on the rate of decline of blood sugar levels in normal humans. J. Pharm. Sci., *51*:509.

† In mg. of tolbutamide (acid form)/cm^2/hr.

‡ In mg. of tolbutamide (acid form) 1 hour after oral ingestion of 500 mg. of tolbutamide (or equivalent); average of four subjects.

§ In mg. per cent, 1 hour after drug administration.

rapid dissolution of salts of most weak acids as compared with that of weak acids themselves may be overshadowed, of course, by other factors, such as differences in particle size and in the physical properties of their dosage forms.

The dosage form and the surface area factors have been kept essentially constant in a comparative study of the absorption and resultant blood sugar lowering activity of the weak acid tolbutamide and several of its salts.[139] This was accomplished by the use of nondisintegrating pellets containing only the respective drug and no additives. In this way it was possible to establish the effect of dissolution rate on the absorption rate and the pharmacologic activity of the drug. Part of the results of this study are summarized in Table 2-5. The greater activity of the sodium salt as compared with the acid form of tolbutamide is readily apparent.

Differences in in-vivo dissolution rate between weak acids and their water-soluble salts are greatest at low pH and often diminish at higher pH. Thus, such differences would show up most prominently in gastric fluids.[108] This is well illustrated by the findings of Lee et al.,[105] who have studied the absorption of penicillin V when administered as the free acid and as the sodium salt, respectively, from the stomach and the small intestine of the dog. The results, depicted in Figures 2-14 and 2-15, show that drug absorption from the stomach was much more rapid after administration of the sodium salt but that there was essentially no difference when the two forms were introduced directly into the

duodenum. The role of gastric motility in clinical evaluations becomes apparent here; prolonged retention of the drugs in the stomach will accentuate the differences in absorption rate, while clinical conditions which favor rapid stomach emptying will tend to diminish the differences between the two forms.

Correlation between intrinsic dissolution rate and gastrointestinal absorption has been demonstrated also in model experiments using tetracycline and some of its salts.[136] These studies also have shown that the absorption rate of the slowly dissolving tetra-

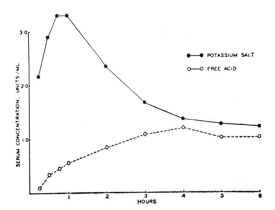

FIG. 2-14. Serum levels of penicillin V in dogs, resulting from gastric absorption of drug administered as the free acid and the potassium salt, respectively, to animals whose stomachs were sectioned from the duodenum. (From Lee, C. C., et al.: Gastric and intestinal absorption of potassium penicillin V and the free acid. Antibiot. Chemother., *8*:354)

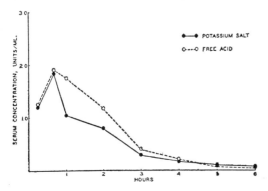

FIG. 2-15. Serum levels of penicillin V in fistular dogs after intraduodenal administration of free acid and potassium salt, respectively. (From Lee, C. C., *et al.*: Antibiot. Chemother., *8*:354)

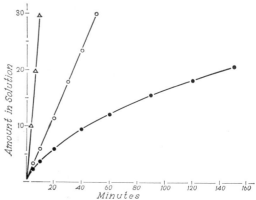

FIG. 2-16. Dissolution of aspirin and aluminum aspirin in 0.1 M Tris buffer of pH 8.0. ($\triangle$) aspirin: ($\bullet$) aluminum aspirin: ($\bigcirc$) aluminum aspirin with 1% EDTA added to dissolution medium. Amounts are expressed in terms of mg. of salicylic acid. (From Levy, G., and Prockfnal, J. A.: Unusual dissolution behavior due to film formation. J. Pharm. Sci., *51*: 294)

cycline was increased by using drug having a greater specific surface area (smaller particles). However, this effect was not noted with the much more rapidly dissolving tetracycline hydrochloride, thus indicating that dissolution rate was no longer the rate-determining factor in gastrointestinal absorption when tetracycline was administered as the hydrochloride. The observations with tetracycline hydrochloride should be expected, since this drug is absorbed mainly from the intestine and only slightly from the stomach.[157] Unless dissolution is extremely slow, the rate of transfer of the drug from stomach to intestine, rather than the dissolution rate, would be rate-limiting in the absorption process.

In considering the importance of specific surface area with respect to dissolution rate, one must distinguish between surface area as determined by standard methods such as nitrogen adsorption and what will be designated here as effective surface area. The latter term refers to the area which is in actual contact with solvent and which is subjected to the agitation conditions prevailing in the dissolution medium. The difference in meaning between the two terms will become apparent on description of the following experiment. Wurster and Seitz have prepared cylindrical pellets and have drilled several pores of about 1 mm. diameter into some of these.[220] Although the surface area of the pellets was thereby increased 20 per cent,

dissolution rate increased by only 4 per cent as compared with the pellets without pores. Clearly, the surface in the pores was not fully available to the solvent. Also, the intensity of agitation could not be the same in the pores as at the external surface of the pellets. The limited availability of the pore surface was due, in part at least, to occlusion by air. Better penetration of solvent was obtained when its surface tension was lowered by addition of sodium lauryl sulfate.[220] The surface of the granules liberated by the disintegration of tablets and the surface of other aggregates of drug solids are also somewhat irregular, presenting crevices and pores to the dissolution medium. It will be explained in the section devoted to pharmaceutical formulation factors that the approach described on p. 75 may be used to increase the dissolution rate of drugs contained in such forms.

Another surface effect that is rather interesting has been observed. This involves the deposition of a water-insoluble film on the surface from which dissolution is taking place.[120] When aluminum aspirin was dissolved in a medium of pH 8 under conditions which were such that dissolution should take place at a constant rate (negligible drug concentration in the dissolution medium and constant surface area), it was found that the rate of dissolution actually decreased with time. This did not occur with plain aspirin or when the aluminum complexing agent ethylenediamine tetraacetic acid was added to the medium (Fig. 2-16). It was established that, at basic pH, a water-insoluble basic aluminum compound was formed and deposited on the solid surface, thus retarding further dissolution. Similar effects evidently occur in the intestine, because the absorption of aspirin from aluminum aspirin seems to diminish considerably once the drug leaves the stomach and enters the intestine.[120, 121] Salts of a base and a poorly soluble acid may exhibit similar effects upon dissolution in acidic media, where a film of the acid may deposit on the drug surface.[129]

This discussion of dissolution rates and their biopharmaceutical importance cannot be concluded without making the simple but critical distinction between solubility and dissolution rate. The former refers to an equilibrium condition while the latter involves a kinetic situation. Saturation is rarely reached in gastrointestinal and other biologic fluids since absorption, distribution and other processes constantly remove dissolved drug. The important factor is how rapidly solid drug dissolves and thus converts into absorbable and diffusable form, because dissolution rate, rather than saturation of biologic fluids with respect to the drug, is usually the absorption- or diffusion-limiting factor.

CRYSTAL FORM

Many drugs can exist in two or more crystalline forms with different space-lattice arrangements. This property is known as polymorphism. The various polymorphic forms usually exhibit different x-ray diffraction patterns, infrared spectra, densities, melting points and solubilities. As a result of different solubilities, the polymorphic forms may also differ with respect to their intrinsic dissolution rates. For this reason, one polymorph may be more effective in chemotherapy than another polymorphic form of the same drug.

Many drugs may be prepared in a particular polymorphic form by appropriate choice of crystallization conditions (solvent, temperature and crystallization rate), by melting and subsequent cooling at particular rates, by use of pressure or by the intentional addition of impurities. Only one form of the pure drug is stable at a given temperature and pressure (other than the transition point). The other forms will convert in time to the stable one. This transformation may be quite rapid or very slow. A polymorph which, though thermodynamically unstable, transforms only slowly to the stable form, is referred to as metastable. Many metastable polymorphs can be considered stable in terms of pharmaceutical use, on the basis of the usual shelf-life of pharmaceutical products. The stable polymorph usually has the highest melting point, the greatest chemical stability and the lowest solubility. Metastable forms are sometimes preferred in pharmaceutical preparations in view of their higher solubilities and dissolution rates. For example, riboflavin can exist in three different polymorphic forms, having a solubility in water at 25° of 60 mg., 80 mg., and 1,200 mg. per liter, respectively.[47] It is evident that the most soluble form of this vitamin can be particularly useful in certain pharmaceutical products, such as powdered parenteral formulations that are constituted before use by addition of water.

The rate of absorption of drugs administered in solid form may be increased by use of the most rapidly dissolving polymorph. In the case of methyl prednisolone, which was administered to rats by subcutaneous implantation, it could be shown that the mean absorption rate from the more soluble polymorphic form II was about 1.7 times as high as that from the stable and less soluble polymorph I.[16] This difference reflects the difference in dissolution rate between the two forms.[79]

Though primarily of toxicologic interest, it may be pointed out that the various polymorphic forms of silica differ in their tendency to cause silicosis, a condition involving the formation and progressive growth of collagenous nodules in the lungs due to inhalation of finely powdered silicas.[21] However, there seems to be no correlation between fibrogenic effect and dissolution rate. Rather, the toxic effect appears to be related to crystal structure as such.

The different polymorphic forms of a drug exhibit difference in their properties only in the solid state. It is believed that, once in solution, the polymorphs lose their identity and become indistinguishable from one another. However, there have been reports from Russian workers that different polymorphic forms of certain organic acids may exhibit different dissociation constants in solution.[200, 201] The differences are more pronounced at higher concentrations of solute and in solvents of low polarity. These observations refer perhaps to nonequilibrium conditions, and their biopharmaceutical significance is yet to be assessed. The reported differences in dissociation constants may mean that different polymorphs can have different oil:water partition coefficients, a possibility that has already been suggested.[67] This may have pertinence to the formulation of parenteral products containing an oil as the vehicle.

In view of the possible effect of crystal form on absorption rate and thereby on pharmacologic activity, it is necessary to consider this property as an additional variable in pharmaceutical formulation and evaluation. It has been estimated that at least one third of all organic compounds are polymorphic.[28] About one half of 22 barbituric acid derivatives and 11 of 16 sex hormones were found to have polymorphic forms. Some of these drugs have as many as four or five polymorphic modifications.[28] Cortisone acetate occurs in at least five distinct crystalline forms, and an examination of 4 brands of cortisone acetate tablets has revealed that 2 contained Form I and the others Form II of the drug.[34] Future revisions of official compendia may be expected to incorporate standards that will distinguish between polymorphs in cases where the various forms may exhibit significantly different pharmacologic activities due to differences in dissolution rate and other physical properties.

Since metastable modifications of a drug are often absorbed more rapidly, it becomes desirable to determine rates of transformation to the stable form and to find means of retarding this transformation. An example of such a rate study is that by Tamura and Kuwano,[199] who determined the transition velocity of chloramphenicol palmitate from the amorphous and the α-forms to the β-form. A number of polymorphic transformation studies with nondrugs are described by Van Hook.[202] An otherwise unstable polymorphic form may be stabilized by the intentional inclusion of impurities.[33] This is possible when the dimensions of the atoms of the impurity are such that they can fit only into a particular lattice arrangement of the polymorphic compound. Rearrangement of the lattice into another, perhaps more stable, polymorphic form may then become impossible because the voids in the stable lattice arrangement cannot contain the impurity without the lattice being subjected to very high stress. Polymorphic transformation in suspensions may also be retarded by increasing the viscosity of the medium or by addition of substances that are capable of adsorbing on the crystals.[85]

From the point of view of physical and chemical stability, it is often advantageous to use a drug in its thermodynamically most stable polymorphic form. The latter is usually most resistant to chemical degradation, and this advantage is increased further in the case of suspensions by the lower solubility of the stable polymorph.[67] In addition, the conversion of one polymorphic form to another in suspensions may be accompanied by caking and, in the case of parenteral suspensions, by poor syringeability.[127] Thus, the greater physical and chemical stability of one polymorph may have to be weighed against the greater physiologic availability of another form.

There are factors other than polymorphism which can account for differences in physicochemical properties of drug solids. Such factors include modifications of crystal habit, formation of hydrates or other solvates and the property of a drug to exist in either crystalline or amorphous form. The growth rate of a crystal may be modified by certain additives and by pH. An additive may retard the growth of the several faces of a crystal to different extents, thereby causing modifications of crystal habit.[127] In this manner, one may obtain a drug in the form of either fine needles or thin plates, for example. Since the rates of dissolution from the various faces may differ,[203] it is possible to modify overall dissolution rates by crystal habit changes which are accompanied by changes in surface area ratios between the various crystal faces.

A significant number of organic medicinals can form solvent addition compounds or solvates.[181] Quinine, sulfonamides, steroids, barbiturates, xanthines and tetracyclines can form hydrate structures. These can differ markedly from their anhydrous equivalents with respect to dissolution rate. The anhydrous forms of caffeine, theophylline and glutethimide have higher dissolution rates than their respective hydrates, while organic solvates (n-amylate and ethyl acetate) of fludrocortisone acetate dissolve much more rapidly than the nonsolvated form of the drug.[181] This presents another method for modifying dissolution rates of pharmaceuticals.

Finally, it is of importance to consider the case in which a drug can exist in either crystalline or amorphous form. The amorphous form is always more soluble than the corresponding crystalline form[85] and, therefore, may exhibit quantitatively different pharmacologic properties. The antibiotic novobiocin, for example, is not absorbed to any significant extent when administered in crystalline form and, thus, is therapeutically inactive. However, the amorphous drug is absorbed readily and is therapeutically effective.[132] Amorphous novobiocin is at least ten times more soluble initially than the crystalline drug and exhibits similar differences in dissolution rate. Although amorphous novobiocin tends to crystallize in suspension, it is possible to retard this transformation considerably by addition of methylcellulose. One may thereby prepare a suspension dosage form of adequate stability and therapeutic efficacy.[132]

One of the most striking and potentially most critical differences in therapeutic activity between crystalline and amorphous drug pertains to chloramphenicol, an antibiotic which is usually reserved for the treatment of serious and potentially life-threatening infections. It has been found that the crystalline forms of chloramphenicol stearate and chloramphenicol palmitate are therapeutically inactive and that only the amorphous forms of these two compounds are hydrolyzed in the gastrointestinal tract to yield absorbable chloramphenicol.[4]

DRUG STABILITY IN GASTROINTESTINAL FLUIDS

Drugs must remain sufficiently stable not only during storage (subject to appropriate storage conditions and limitations of shelf-life) but also in gastrointestinal fluids. Any chemical change due to pH or enzymic action and resulting in a product that is pharmacologically inactive or less active than the administered substance should be prevented or minimized. This may be accomplished sometimes by chemical modification of the parent molecule to yield new derivatives. This approach is exemplified by the greater efficacy of orally administered penicillin V as compared with orally administered penicillin G, due to the greater acid stability of the former. Enteric coatings, if properly formulated, can prevent exposure of a drug to gastric pH and enzymes and minimize degradation due to one of these factors. The oral inefficacy of drugs because of acid hydrolysis in gastric fluids generally should be predictable by formal kinetic studies, as was done with p-chlorobenzaldoxime.[71] This muscle relaxant, though active parenterally, is ineffective when administered orally. It has a stability half-life of less than 20 minutes in the stomach and thus is largely hydrolized to the aldehyde before being absorbed.[71] The low potency of orally administered nitroglycerin and erythrol tetranitrate is also believed to be due to the instability of these drugs in the gastrointestinal tract.[162] Some compounds, though unstable in acidic solution, are protected from the destructive effect of gastric fluids by their hydrophobic surface. Such compounds are poorly wetted by aqueous fluids, and chemical interaction is decreased by the restricted contact. Esters of chloramphenicol and erythromycin exhibit this property.[74, 189] In the case of chloramphenicol esters, hydrolysis in the intestine, being a prerequisite for absorption of the parent drug, can be promoted by use of surfactants and by administering the drug in finely divided form.[74] Erythromycin and its esters are inactivated by gastric fluids, and low wettability is in this case a desirable protective feature. Stephens and co-workers have shown that although propionyl erythromycin yields satisfactory blood levels when administered in capsule form, addition of a wetting agent (5% polyoxyethylene sorbitan mono-oleate) to the contents of the capsule results in much lower blood levels, evidently due to greater degradation of the drug in gastric fluids.[189]

Degradation of slowly dissolving drugs in gastric fluids can also be minimized by administering such drugs in the form of relatively large particles. Dissolution rate is thereby reduced, less of the drug dissolves in the stomach and less is therefore destroyed by gastric fluids. However, if the particles are too large, they may dissolve so slowly that they are not fully biologically available. Optimum particle size, therefore, is in some intermediate range where dissolution is slow enough to prevent extensive degradation of drug in the stomach and yet sufficiently rapid to assure complete dissolution before the drug passes absorption sites. This balance of relatively low dissolution rate in acidic fluids (to minimize degradation in the stomach) and relatively high dissolution rate in slightly basic media (to assure rapid and complete absorption in the intestine) sometimes may be achieved by appropriate chemical modification. Nelson has shown this elegantly for erythromycin and several of its esters.[140] He has demonstrated an inverse relationship between the dissolution rate of the erythromycin compounds in 0.1 N hydrochloric acid and the amount absorbed from the gastrointestinal tract (Fig. 2-17), and a direct relationship between dissolution rate at pH 7.4 and amount absorbed (Fig. 2-18).

COMPLEXATION

Drugs may interact reversibly to form complexes with substances occurring in the body, with other drugs and with pharmacologically inert components of pharmaceutical dosage forms. The stability of these complexes under defined conditions can be described by a stability constant K_m, where

$$K_m = \frac{[\text{Drug—Complex}]}{[\text{Free Drug}][\text{Free Complexing Agent}]} \quad (32)$$

Equation 32 refers to a 1:1 complex; the bracketed terms indicate molar concentrations. Equilibria involving complexes of different stoichiometry can be described by simi-

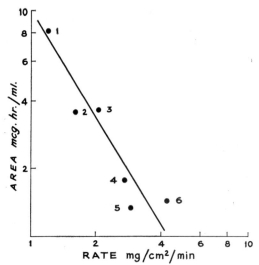

Fig. 2-17. Relationship between area beneath erythromycin blood level curves and dissolution rate of various forms of erythromycin in 0.1 N HCl. Erythromycin (E.) propionate, 1; E. acetate, 2; E. acrylate, 3; E. isobutyrate, 4; E. n-butyrate, 5; free E., 6. (From Nelson, E.: Physicochemical factors influencing the absorption of erythromycin and its esters, Chem. Pharm. Bull., 10:1099)

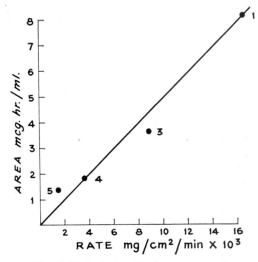

Fig. 2-18. Relationship between area beneath erythromycin blood level curves and dissolution rate of various forms of erythromycin in 0.1 M borate buffer of pH 7.4. Numbers designate various compounds as listed under Figure 2-17. (From Nelson, E.: Physicochemical factors influencing the absorption of erythromycin and its esters, Chem. Pharm. Bull., 10:1099)

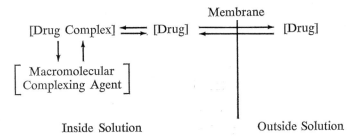

FIGURE 2-19

lar expressions. Equation 32 is based on the equilibrium

$$\text{Drug} + \text{Complexing Agent} \rightleftharpoons \text{Drug Complex} \tag{33}$$

The drug complex differs from the free drug with respect to solubility, diffusivity, partition coefficient and other properties. More important, drug contained in a complex is usually pharmacologically ineffective. The complex ordinarily must dissociate at some stage in the body before the drug can exert its usual pharmacologic effect.

The drug complex will usually differ from the free drug itself with respect to its ability to penetrate biologic membranes. This may be due to differences in physicochemical properties between the two forms, or because the molecules of complexing agent are so large that they cannot pass through biologic membranes.

It is important to distinguish between the equilibrium and the kinetic aspects of drug complexes. This may be done by considering the interaction of a drug with a macromolecular substance, resulting in a drug complex which, due to its large size, cannot penetrate biologic membranes or artificial membranes with fine pores (such as dialysis membranes). If one places an aqueous solution of both drug and complexing agent into a dialysis

bag, immerses the latter in a beaker of water and permits the system to come to equilibrium, the species distribute in the manner shown in Figure 2-19. The double arrows across the membrane indicate that free drug is diffusible and that it exists in essentially equal concentration on both sides of the membrane. The drug complex and the complexing agent cannot pass through the membrane and remain inside the dialysis bag.

If the drug in the outside solution is constantly removed by some mechanism, the situation may be depicted as in Figure 2-20. Here there exists a nonequilibrium condition, where the drug complex eventually dissociates completely and all of the drug passes across the membrane. In the equilibrium case, only part of the ordinarily available drug is available to the environment outside the membrane. In the nonequilibrium case, all of the drug is available but not as rapidly as it would be in the absence of complexing agent. This follows from the fact that the rate of diffusion from the inside solution is a function of the concentration gradient of *diffusible* drug across the membrane and not of total drug. The problem of drug binding by plasma proteins (which has been discussed in a previous section) is represented essentially by the nonequilibrium model described here. Suitably modified to account

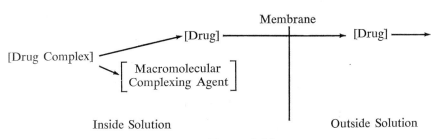

FIGURE 2-20

for penetrable complexes which differ from the free drug with respect to *rate* of membrane penetration and considering possible competition by other substances for both drug and complexing agent, the model can represent the conditions which may be found in the body.

Drug complexation with nonabsorbable macromolecules can be a useful method of retarding drug absorption and thereby reducing toxicity. Polyvinylpyrrolidone can reduce the oral toxicity of iodine, nicotine, potassium cyanide and other drugs in this manner.[7] Where the free drug is a local irritant, complexation may prevent or reduce irritation by keeping the concentration of free drug low. This approach has been used to reduce the skin irritation liability of iodine[42] and the gastrointestinal and tissue irritation caused by iron compounds.[65] On the other hand, nonintended complexation of a drug with other components of its pharmaceutical dosage form may reduce the effectiveness of the preparation due to the slower absorption of the drug. Many suspending, emulsifying and solubilizing agents form complexes with certain drugs, but, fortunately, most of these complexes are not very strong and dissociate readily on dilution of the preparation in the gastrointestinal tract. The problem is more acute in animal experiments, where comparative dosages and actual concentrations may be much higher than in ordinary human chemotherapy. This is particularly pertinent in animal toxicity studies and in the interpretation of certain other pharmacologic data obtained from animal experiments. For example, it has been stated that solubilizers have occasionally interfered with the biologic activity of riboflavin.[20]

Complexation often serves as a means of increasing the solubility of a drug. Compared with a suspension, a solution containing drug, a portion of which is complexed, may be more effective (or more toxic) because dissociation of the complex can occur almost instantaneously on dilution, whereas dissolution of suspended drug solids occurs at much lower rates. This aspect has been discussed in greater detail by Weiner with respect to LD_{50} determinations in rats.[211]

Some drug complexes penetrate biologic barriers more readily than the free drug itself. This may be a means of obtaining increased drug activity, provided that the drug is released from the complex at or prior to reaching its site of action. The gastrointestinal absorption of iron has been increased by complexation with citrate, pyrophosphate and EDTA, but the amount of iron actually remaining in the body was less than when the drug was administered alone, because the complexes did not dissociate significantly and also were excreted much more rapidly than iron itself.[62] The degree of dissociation of a metal complex in the body depends to some extent on the concentration of the metal in body fluids. Animals deficient in calcium are more capable of taking calcium from the complex than normal, "calcium-saturated" animals. The same appears to apply to iron.[211] This follows from considerations of the physical-chemical equilibrium involved.

Complexation may also reduce the absorbability of a drug considerably, as in the case of the tetracyclines.[100] The complexes formed by these drugs with divalent and trivalent cations are absorbed much less efficiently than are uncomplexed tetracyclines. The binding of tetracyclines by protein macromolecules appears to be mediated by the metal ions, which apparently serve as a connecting bridge between the drug and the protein molecules.[97] Such an interaction could be the one responsible for the poor absorption of tetracycline complexes from the gastrointestinal tract.

Calcium apparently plays an important role in the normal physiology of gastrointestinal membranes. The chelating agent sodium ethylenediamine tetraacetate (EDTA) causes mucosal cells to become detached from the remaining tissue due to removal of calcium.[80] The permeability of the membrane to passively diffusing substances is increased in the presence of EDTA, perhaps because the "pores" in the membrane are increased or spaces between epithelial cells are widened through removal of calcium.[172] Thus, the absorption of several neutral, acidic and basic lipid-insoluble organic compounds from the gastrointestinal tract is increased by EDTA.[172] These substances, which include mannitol, inulin, a quaternary ammonium compound and sulfanilic acid, are very poorly absorbed under ordinary circumstances.

Heparin, which normally is not absorbed at all from the gastrointestinal tract, is absorbed in the presence of EDTA.[217] In some instances, however, EDTA and other calcium-binding substances may reduce gastrointestinal absorption. Evidently this involves more complicated mechanisms, such as reduced utilization of glucose and inhibition of transmucosal transport of glucose and water. These factors in turn may inhibit the absorption of certain drugs, including barbiturates, strychnine and sulfonamides.[186, 187] The use of EDTA to obtain the effects described in these paragraphs is thus restricted to investigational purposes. It is unlikely that this agent will be used in chemotherapy to achieve similar results, in view of the deleterious effects of removing essential trace metals from the body. However, the experiments referred to are useful for obtaining a better understanding of the effects to be anticipated following the administration of drugs or additives which are effective complexing agents. Such effects would be most noticeable in instances where the drug is not significantly diluted by body fluids in the course of administration, as, for example, on application to the cornea, or by the rectal route. For additional discussion of the pharmaceutical and pharmacologic aspects of complexation, the reader may refer to review articles by Marcus[128] and by Weiner.[211]

SURFACE-ACTIVE AGENTS

Surface-active agents (surfactants) are used so widely as emulsifiers, solubilizers and formulation adjuncts that their effect on drug absorption requires careful consideration. Since these substances can affect the integrity of biologic membranes, it has been thought that they might be effective absorption-enhancing agents. However, reports concerning the usefulness of surface-active agents in enhancing the gastrointestinal absorption of drugs have been conflicting. Enhancement as well as inhibition of the gastrointestinal absorption and the pharmacologic activity of drugs has been observed when surface-active agents were added to a medication. Many of these reports have been reviewed and summarized by Blanpin.[23] Much of the difficulty with some of the studies probably has been due to the different types of effects which

surface-active agents can exert. Briefly, they may act on the biologic membrane, the drug, or the dosage form as such. Some surface-active agents also have pharmacologic properties specific to their particular chemical structure and not related to their surfactant property in general. Several of the listed effects may be operative at the same time, the magnitude of each being dependent on concentration to a different degree. This complexity can make proper assessment of surfactant effects very difficult and indicates the need for careful experimental design of studies concerned with the biopharmaceutical and pharmacologic effects of surface-active agents.

The two major mechanisms of surfactant activity with respect to drug absorption are described comprehensively in a series of reports dealing with the kinetics of rectal absorption.[161] The rate of absorption of sodium iodide was found to be accelerated 4 to 5 times by small amounts of polysorbate 20 and sodium lauryl sulfate, while the rate of absorption of iodoform and triiodophenol was retarded by the same agents. The accelerated absorption of sodium iodide was attributed to the surface tension lowering and mucous peptizing action of the surface-active agents, which results in greater contact of drug with the absorbing membrane. On the other hand, the retarding effect in the case of iodoform and triiodophenol evidently is due to the entrapment of these drugs in surfactant micelles. (Sodium iodide is not affected in this manner.) This type of interaction is a special case of complexation, as described in the previous subsection. Aggregates of surface-active agent molecules (micelles) are too large to pass through biologic membranes, and drug molecules bound in these micelles cannot be absorbed. The low absorption rate of iodoform and triiodophenol in the presence of surface-active agents is a reflection of the lowered concentration gradient of diffusible drug across the membranes. Micelle formation does not take place until the concentration of surface-active agent exceeds a certain value known as the critical micelle concentration (CMC). Surfactants can thus exert a two-phase effect which is a function of concentration. Below the CMC, absorption of drugs may be enhanced due to better contact of drug solution with the membrane;

this is a "wetting" or spreading effect resulting from a decrease in the surface tension of the solution. There may also be a direct effect of the surfactant on the permeability of the biologic membranes.

Above the CMC, a portion of the drug molecules may become entrapped in micelles and, as such, be unavailable for absorption. The net effect (absorption enhancement or retardation) depends to some degree on the relative magnitude of interaction between drug and surfactant. The absorption-retarding effect usually predominates at higher surfactant concentrations because a larger fraction of the drug is bound to micelles. However, repeated or prolonged exposure to high doses of a surface-active agent may lead to partial disruption of biologic membranes and thereby reduce their barrier effect significantly.

The concentration-dependent activity of surfactants is well illustrated by their effect on the bactericidal activity of phenols. The effectiveness of the phenols is increased with increasing surfactant concentration until the CMC is reached. At this point the bactericidal activity is at its maximum. As additional surfactant is added, the activity of the phenols is successively reduced until they become practically inactivated.[18] In more complex environments such as the gastrointestinal tract, one must also consider the competition by certain physiologic substances with the drug molecules for micellular binding sites. Thus, it is evident that the nature and the magnitude of the effect exerted by surface-active agents can be highly dependent on concentration. It should not be considered unusual for different groups of investigators to attribute absorption enhancing and absorption retarding activity, respectively, to a particular surface-active agent, even with respect to the same drug, since the different workers could have employed different concentrations of surfactant or different experimental procedures.

Anionic surfactants can form insoluble precipitates with large drug cations, and cationic surfactants can interact similarly with large drug anions. The insoluble compounds thus formed are often not absorbable and combinations leading to this type of reaction should be avoided in pharmaceutical practice.

Fats and fat-soluble vitamins are usually dispersed in fine globules in the small intestine by the emulsifying action of bile salts. This dispersion is a prerequisite for adequate absorption. Patients who are unable to absorb fats properly may be aided by administration of surface-active agents. Emulsification and dispersion of fats and lipoid substances such as vitamin A are thereby promoted and absorption is enhanced.[93]

Some apparently pharmacologic effects of surfactants actually are due to a modification of the physical properties of the dosage forms in which they and the medicament are contained. For example, a group of investigators have found that coadministration of polysorbate 80 with spironolactone yielded blood levels of the latter which were as much as four times higher than when spironolactone was administered alone.[69] Since the biologic half-life of the drug remained the same, it was concluded that polysorbate 80 promoted the intrinsic gastrointestinal absorption of spironolactone. However, this conclusion proved to be erroneous in subsequent experiments and had to be withdrawn, since mere modification of the physical properties of the tablets had similar effects.[70] The surfactant acted in this instance on the dosage form itself and modified its drug release properties. (This example will be discussed further in the section devoted to pharmaceutical formulation factors.)

Some effects that are apparently specific and limited to particular surface-active agents deserve mention. It had been found that polysorbate 80, polysorbate 85 and G-1096 (polyoxyethylene sorbitan hexaoleate), when administered undiluted in high doses, enhanced the gastrointestinal absorption of Vitamin B_{12} by rats.[149] A number of other surfactants did not have this enhancing effect. Further examination revealed that the three effective agents formed a highly viscous mass when mixed with gastric fluids, while the ineffective surfactants did not. The absorption-enhancing activity of the three "effective" surfactants could be attributed to retardation of gastric emptying, as shown by additional experiments. Naturally, the conditions of the experiments were completely unphysiologic and are not applicable to human therapy. Many of the pharmacologic investigations of surface-active agents involve the administration of extraordinarily high doses, and the results should not be extrapolated routinely to clinical conditions. In interpreting laboratory observations, particular emphasis must be placed on the doses or the concentrations employed, especially if the surfactant effect is on the biologic membrane.

Dioctyl sodium sulfosuccinate is another surfactant which exerts a pharmacologic effect which is apparently specific to this particular agent rather than being shared by all other surfactants. It retards gastric emptying and has a powerful inhibitory effect on gastric secretions, even when administered in relatively low doses.[124] Interestingly enough, inhibition of gastric secretions occurs when the drug is administered intraduodenally, but there is no effect when contact of the drug is limited to the lumen of the stomach or when it is administered parenterally. It has been suggested that the inhibitory effect of dioctyl sodium sulfosuccinate is mediated by a hormone released from the intestinal mucosa, e.g., enterogastrone.[124]

Dioctyl sodium sulfosuccinate as well as another anionic surfactant, sodium lauryl sulfate, enhances the absorption of the anionic dye phenol red from the colon of the rat, while a nonionic surfactant does not. None of the three surfactants influenced the absorption of a cationic dye, methyl violet.[125] The mechanism of this effect is not quite clear, since it could be inhibited by a ganglionic blocking agent or an anticholinergic drug. This suggests that an active biologic process may be involved.[125]

In evaluating the effect of surface-active agents on the absorption rate of a drug, it is essential to establish whether this effect is mediated through an alteration of the absorbing membrane, an interaction with the drug or a modification of the physical properties of the dosage form. A change in the permeability characteristics of the absorbing membrane may be noted by any change in the absorption of substances which are known not to interact with the surfactant (provided that dosage form effects are ruled out by administering the drug in solution). Micellular solubilization is determinable by equi-

librium dialysis[155] and solubility methods,[1] while dosage form effects can be established by means of dissolution rate studies. In this manner it is generally possible to obtain an understanding of the nature of the surfactant effect and thereby utilize surfactants intelligently to enhance the activity of drugs or to avoid inhibitory effects by removing the surfactant from a formulation where this becomes necessary. As in the case of complexation reactions in general the absorption-inhibiting effects of surfactants can be expected to be most noticeable in dosage forms which are not diluted extensively by body fluids on administration.

PHARMACEUTICAL FORMULATION FACTORS

The pharmacologic and physical-chemical considerations concerning the development and the evaluation of pharmaceutical dosage forms, which have been outlined in the previous sections, represent the necessary foundation for a review of pharmaceutical formulation factors. Many of the subjects discussed in the previous section could as readily be included here, but they have been grouped separately for better clarity of presentation. This section deals primarily with a consideration of biopharmaceutical aspects of the more important classes of pharmaceutical preparations and outlines some of the problems that may be encountered with certain

TABLE 2-6. GASTROINTESTINAL ABSORPTION OF CALCIUM BY NORMAL SUBJECTS AND BY ANACID SUBJECTS AFTER ADMINISTRATION OF CALCIUM CARBONATE POWDER AND CALCIUM CITRATE SOLUTION IN EQUIVALENT DOSES*

	AVERAGE AREA UNDER SERUM LEVEL VS. TIME CURVE (in mg. % · hr.)	
	CALCIUM CARBONATE	CALCIUM CITRATE SOL.
Normal subjects	4.47	4.77
Anacid subjects	0.87	2.75†

* Niepmann, W.: Klin. Wochenschr. *39*:1064.

† Average of 13 subjects; all other values are averages of 10 subjects.

of these. The effect of pharmaceutical formulation factors on the therapeutic efficacy of drugs has been reviewed and illustrated recently by examples from clinical and scientific literature.[6, 118, 119] It is hoped that the reader will refer to these articles, because the present section will be more concerned with the reasons why and the mechanisms by which pharmaceutical formulation factors can modify the therapeutic efficacy of drugs.

The major classes of pharmaceutical dosage forms designed for internal use may be listed in a sequence representing the order of rate of release of their active ingredients:

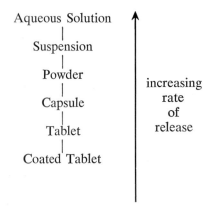

This sequence is based on the usual properties of the listed classes of preparations, and it should be clear that exceptions may occur in specific instances. Emulsions, nonaqueous solutions, sustained release dosage forms, aerosols and suppositories are not listed, because they represent more complicated systems which do not lend themselves to ready classification and which must be assessed individually.

LIQUIDS

Drugs are absorbed from the gastrointestinal tract most promptly when administered in aqueous solution. Solubility limitations, poor stability, objectionable taste and economic considerations may require the use of other dosage forms, but, in the absence of such deterrents, aqueous solutions represent the dosage form of choice when rapid and predictable absorption is desired. Homologs, when administered in tablet form, may differ in rate of absorption because of differences in their intrinsic rate of dissolution, but these

differences are not operational when the compounds are administered already in solution. For example, potassium penicillin V gave higher blood levels than benzathine penicillin V when both were administered in tablet form, but solutions of the two drugs yielded essentially equal blood levels of penicillin.[94] This could be attributed to differences in the dissolution rates of these substances and to their apparently similar intrinsic absorption rates.

It is obvious that liquids are easier to swallow than solid dosage forms and that, for this reason, solutions are often preferred in pediatric and geriatric medicine. However, there is an interesting example of a case in which the solution dosage form is particularly indicated in a certain type of pathology. The gastrointestinal absorption of calcium after administration of calcium carbonate and a solution of calcium citrate, respectively, was compared in healthy subjects and in anacid subjects.[144] The results of the study are summarized in Table 2-6, where the area under the calcium serum level vs. time curve is indicative of the relative amounts of calcium absorbed.

Calcium carbonate dissolves in acidic gastric fluids to yield calcium ion in absorbable form. Individuals who do not produce gastric hydrochloric acid are unable to dissolve significant amounts of the drug. This accounts for the very poor absorption of calcium by anacid subjects after administration of calcium carbonate powder. When calcium was administered in the form of calcium citrate solution, the gastrointestinal absorption by anacid subjects was considerably increased. However, it was not as high as in normal subjects, probably because some of the drug precipitated in the absence of an acidic environment in the stomach and the proximal small intestine of the anacid subjects. Chelation of calcium with citrate had no apparent effect as such on absorption rate, as evidenced by essentially identical serum levels at all times after administration of the two forms of calcium to normal subjects. These observations should apply also to other acid-soluble drugs which are insoluble or poorly soluble in neutral or alkaline fluids.

Viscosity-enhancing agents are sometimes included in solutions to modify consistency

TABLE 2-7. EFFECT OF DOSAGE FORM ON GASTROINTESTINAL ABSORPTION
OF SALICYLATES BY RATS*†

	ACETYLSALICYLIC ACID SUSPENSION WITH 2% METHYLCEL-LULOSE	SODIUM ACETYLSALICYLATE SOLUTION	SODIUM SALICYL-ATE SOLUTION WITH 2% METHYLCEL-LULOSE	SODIUM SALICYLATE SOLUTION
Plasma concentration‡	132	201	162	208
Brain concentration§	11.6	19.6	13.3	21.1

* Dose: 0.72 mmol./kg.; data are averages of 12 rats per group.
† Davidson, C., et al.: J. Pharmacol. Exper. Therap. 134:176.
‡ In mcg./ml. as salicylic acid; ½ hour after drug administration.
§ In mcg./Gm. as salicylic acid; ½ hour after drug administration.

and pourability. Of course, they are routinely used in suspensions to obtain greater physical stability. If the concentrations of suspending agent and the administered dose are sufficiently high so as to maintain a relatively high viscosity even on dilution of the preparation in the gastrointestinal tract, drug absorption may be retarded. This is shown by the data in Table 2-7, which lists plasma and brain concentrations of salicylate after oral administration of sodium salicylate solution with and without 2 per cent methylcellulose, sodium acetylsalicylate solution, and acetylsalicylic acid suspension containing 2 per cent methylcellulose.[50] The volume administered in each case was 0.2 ml. per 100 Gm. of body weight. It is likely that high viscosity was the major reason for the lower blood levels obtained with the sodium salicylate solution containing methylcellulose, although some complexation cannot be ruled out. In the case of acetylsalicylic acid suspension, viscosity as well as dissolution rate would be a factor limiting absorption. The viscosity effect is due to the inverse relationship between the rate of diffusion of drug molecules to absorption sites and the viscosity of the fluids in which diffusion takes place.

Suspensions rank next to solutions with respect to the rate of release of their active ingredients because of the large surface area of the dispersed solids. Particle size is a critical factor, faster dissolution and absorption being achieved by use of finer particles. The particle size of drug solids in suspensions tends to increase with time, due to dissolution of the smaller particles and deposition of drug from solution on the larger particles.

Such particle growth should be prevented or retarded by means which have been described.[85] The advantage of administering poorly soluble drugs dispersed in suspension rather than compacted in tablets is exemplified by a study of sulfadimethoxine absorption. (See Fig. 2-21.) The drug was absorbed much more rapidly and more completely when administered in microcrystalline suspension.[165]

Interactions between active ingredients and pharmaceutical adjuncts are particularly difficult to notice in opaque suspensions, and the possibility of such occurrences must be considered carefully. For example, sodium carboxymethylcellulose reacts with amphetamine to form an even less soluble and less rapidly available substance than amphetamine itself.[206] The use of sodium carboxymethyl-

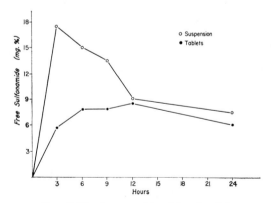

FIG. 2-21. Average blood levels of free sulfonamide in children following oral administration of sulfadimethoxine (1 Gm./M²) in tablets and in suspension. (After Sakuma, T., et al.: Am. J. Med. Sci., 239:142)

cellulose to suspend amphetamine would therefore be contraindicated. The same may apply to many other weak organic bases.

There is sometimes the choice either of formulating a sparingly water soluble drug in aqueous suspension or of dissolving it in an organic solvent. If the organic solvent is water-miscible, such as glycerin, dilution of the solution with gastrointestinal fluids may not cause precipitation of drug because of the increased total volume of liquid. Precipitation can occur if the drug is very insoluble in water and the administered dose is high, but the precipitate is usually of very small particle size, which favors rapid dissolution as some of the dissolved drug is removed by absorption. Dissolved drug is not as readily available if the solvent is immiscible with water (i.e., an oil). The comparative efficacy of an aqueous suspension and a solution of drug in an oil depends on the dissolution rate of the drug, its oil-water partition coefficient and the ease with which the oil tends to disperse in the gastrointestinal fluids (the latter factor relates to the interfacial area between oil and water phase; larger contact area promotes diffusion of drug from one phase to another). In one study, the investigators found that the activity of various esters of testosterone, androstanolone, prednisone and prednisolone on oral administration, as well as the activity of the respective free steroids, was greater when these drugs were administered in sesame oil solution than when given in aqueous suspension.[3] While the investigators were unable to offer an adequate explanation for their findings, it appears that the rate of drug release from the oil to the gastrointestinal fluids was higher than the rate of dissolution of the solid drug particles contained in the aqueous suspensions.

The availability of drugs contained in emulsion dosage forms depends on whether the drug is present primarily in the aqueous or the oil phase and whether the emulsion is an oil-in-water or a water-in-oil system. It may also depend on the particle size of the dispersed phase. The latter factor is also of importance in the absorption of poorly absorbable lipids. In one study, for example, less than 10 per cent of unemulsified liquid paraffin was absorbed, but more than 30 per cent was absorbed when the oil was administered in emulsified form.[66]

SOLIDS

The major factors that can influence the biologic availability of drugs from powders are readily identifiable: particle size, dissolution rate and possible interaction with other medicinal components or with diluents present in the powder dosage form. Significant particle growth on aging does not occur unless the drug has a high vapor pressure or the dosage form is exposed to moisture. Dissolution rate may be modified by appropriate choice of crystal form or solvate type, where indicated. The most common type of interaction of drug with diluent involves adsorption of the former on the latter. The availability of adsorbed drug can be reduced markedly if the diluent is water-insoluble and a powerful adsorbent.

A previously cited example, namely that of spironolactone, may be enlarged on to illustrate the effect of particle size on the biologic availability of a drug with low intrinsic dissolution rate. A recent study[17] permits comparison of the relative biologic availability of spironolactone when administered as a loose, encapsulated powder or when compacted in highly-compressed tablets. The amount of spironolactone absorbed from powdered drug mixed with lactose and encapsulated in gelatin capsules was found to be 6.6 times as large as the amount absorbed from highly compressed commercial spironolactone tablets. Administration of micronized spironolactone resulted in the absorption of 10 times as much drug as from the commercially available tablets. Thus, micronization improves the absorption from the gastrointestinal tract so that 40 mg. give the same blood level · time values as 400 mg. in the form of conventional tablets. Some of these data are shown in Figure 2-22.

A unique technic has been developed by Japanese pharmaceutical scientists, to cause sparingly water-soluble drugs to become dispersed finely in gastrointestinal fluids.[180] This technic involves the formation of a eutectic mixture of the drug and a pharmacologically inactive, readily soluble compound. The eutectic mixture must have a melting point that is higher than room tem-

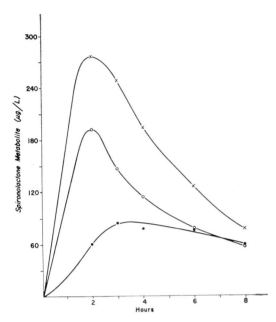

FIG. 2-22. Plasma levels of spironolactone metabolite after administration of
400 mg. of spironolactone in commercially
available tablets (●); 100 mg. of powdered
drug in gelatin capsules (○); and 100 mg.
of micronized drug in gelatin capsules
(X). (After Bauer, G., *et al.:* Arzneim.-
Forsch., *12*:487)

perature. The two substances are melted and
mixed; the mixture is cooled until it solidifies
and then is finely powdered. When placed in
water, the readily soluble carrier substance
dissolves rapidly and releases extremely fine
particles of the drug. By using a eutectic mixture of sulfathiazole and urea, it was possible
to achieve higher blood levels and earlier
concentration peaks of the sulfonamide than
are obtained by administration of ordinary
sulfathiazole.[180]

Retardation of drug release and a resulting decrease in biologic availability due to
adsorption of the drug on diluents has been
observed with thiamine as well as other drugs.
Some years ago, an acid-clay adsorbate of
thiamine served as an international standard
for the bioassay of this vitamin. Subsequent
studies revealed that the adsorbate actually
contained twice as much thiamine as was believed to be present on the basis of its anti-

neuritic activity in rats.[152] In other words,
only one half of the adsorbed vitamin was
biologically available under the experimental
conditions. In another study, only 40 per cent
of the thiamine and 79 per cent of the riboflavin in Vitamin B complex capsules containing fuller's earth were available to human
test subjects.[152] Adsorption of vitamins
on insoluble diluents can reduce their availability so seriously that several scientists
associated with the Food and Drug Administration have suggested that the vitamin content of pharmaceutical products be evaluated
for labeling purposes on the basis of physiologic availability.[52]

All the factors mentioned above also apply
to capsule dosage forms. An additional factor in the case of capsules is the dissolution
rate of the capsule shell. Hard gelatin capsules dissolve quite readily in gastrointestinal
fluids, but a small difference between the absorption rate of drugs administered in powder
form, on one hand, and in gelatin capsules,
on the other, has been observed.[111] Soft gelatin capsules often dissolve more slowly than
hard gelatin capsules. The former, if poorly
formulated, may interfere with the prompt
absorption of their active ingredients. In one
study, vitamin B_{12} was less completely absorbed from soft gelatin capsules than from
solution.[39] This may have been due to the
slow dissolution of the capsule shells. Adsorption of drug on fillers and diluents can occur
with capsules as well as with powders. Chemical interaction between components, though
rare in the absence of moisture, can occur
during dissolution. This accounted for the
absorption retarding effect of dicalcium phosphate when this substance was used as a
diluent in commercial tetracycline capsules.

Compressed tablets, which are the most
widely used dosage forms, also present some
of the most difficult problems with respect
to the biologic availability of their active ingredients. In commenting on the marked
effect of tablet properties on the rate of absorption of various penicillins, Juncher and
Raaschou concluded that "many published
studies that do not describe the pharmaceutical properties of the preparations used can
hardly be considered indicative of an estimate of the resorption of the penicillin com-

pounds concerned." * They point out that "this affords an explanation of many discrepant results and conclusions in studies on the oral administration of penicillin." *

The major problem encountered with compressed tablets is due to the decrease in the effective surface area of the active ingredients as a result of granulation and compression of the drug particles. Availability of drugs in tablets can be affected seriously unless this process of compaction is readily reversible when the tablets come into contact with gastrointestinal fluids. This reversal involves usually the disintegration of compressed tablets into their constituent granules, followed by disintegration of the granules into primary particles. The primary particles dissolve at a rate which is a function of their specific surface area, their intrinsic dissolution rate and the nature of their immediate environment. If a tablet fails to disintegrate, the surface available for dissolution is limited to the surface area of the tablet as such. Disintegration of the tablets but not of the constituent granules yields an available surface area which, though larger than that of the intact tablets, is considerably smaller than that obtainable by complete disintegration of the tablet and its constituent granules into primary particles.

The foregoing comments should indicate to the reader that the intentions of those who recommended adoption of the presently official tablet disintegration test (namely, "to insure to the user of the tablet the ultimate availability of the medication and in such reasonable time as the nature of the medication might warrant"†) cannot be realized by such a test. The fact that a tablet disintegrates promptly into granules does not assure subsequent disintegration of the granules and dissolution of the primary drug particles. It is not too difficult to prepare tablets out of crushed glass particles, for instance, in a manner which permits such tablets to pass the *U.S.P.* tablet disintegration test. This test, though it represents a commendable attempt to establish minimum availability standards for compressed tablets,

can no longer be considered useful for this purpose in the light of present knowledge.

Tablet disintegration may determine dissolution rate if it is the slowest process in the sequence: tablet disintegration $\longrightarrow$ granule disintegration $\longrightarrow$ particle dissolution. A tablet disintegration test could be indicative of the release rate of the active constituents under these relatively rare conditions. Such a case has been reported by Juncher and Raaschou, who found that the absorption of potassium penicillin V administered in compressed tablets was influenced markedly by the disintegration time of the tablets.[94] Using these data, and assuming complete availability of the drug from the most rapidly disintegrating tablets, Nelson constructed the graph shown as Figure 2-23.[137] It indicates that, in this instance, potassium penicillin V tablets could pass the U.S.P. tablet disintegration test even when one third of their drug contents was not biologically available.

The more commonly occurring lack of correlation between tablet disintegration time and rate of gastrointestinal absorption of the active ingredient is shown in Table 2-8 for a series of commercial aspirin tablets. These studies, carried out in the author's laboratory, demonstrate that dissolution rate, rather than disintegration time, is indicative of the rate of absorption of aspirin from compressed tablets.[108]

Schroeter and colleagues undertook an extensive study of the possible relationship between rate of dissolution and disintegration time of compressed tablets.[178] They found

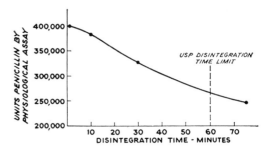

INFLUENCE OF DISINTEGRATION TIME OF TABLETS ON AVAILABILITY OF PENICILLIN V FOR ABSORPTION

FIG. 2-23. From Nelson, E.: Therapeutic considerations of generic name prescriptions, Western Pharm., *73*:9.

* Juncher, H., and Raaschou, F.: The solubility of oral preparations of penicillin V. Antibiot. Med. Clin. Ther., *4*:497, 1957.

† Vliet, E. B.: Tablet disintegration tests. Drug & Allied Ind., *42*:17, 1956.

TABLE 2-8. DISINTEGRATION, DISSOLUTION AND GASTROINTESTINAL ABSORPTION VALUES FOR A SERIES OF COMMERCIAL ASPIRIN TABLETS*

PRODUCT	AVERAGE U.S.P. DISINTEGRATION TIME (SECONDS)	AVERAGE AMOUNT DISSOLVED IN 10 MINUTES (MG.)	AMOUNT EXCRETED IN URINE† (MG.)	
A	256	242	24.3	
C	< 10	165	18.1	Study I‡
E	< 10	127	15.9	
B	35	205	18.5	
D	13	158	13.6	Study II‡
E	< 10	127	12.1	

* Levy, G.: Comparison of dissolution and absorption rates of different commercial aspirin tablets, J. Pharm. Sci. *50*:388.

† In terms of apparent salicylic acid, 1 hour after administration of two 0.3-Gm. tablets.

‡ Studies I and II were carried out with different test subjects and under somewhat different conditions.

some cases where a relationship exists and others where it does not. Correlations found were highly specific and depended not only on the type of drug but, in some cases, also on the nature of pharmaceutical adjuvants in the tablets. These considerations limit the tablet disintegration test to manufacturing control purposes only and preclude its rational use as an official availability test.

Recognition of dissolution rate rather than disintegration time as the tablet property of importance with respect to drug availability from compressed tablets required re-examination of certain aspects of tablet formulation. It became necessary to determine the effect of formulation factors, such as the type and the concentration of disintegrant, binder, filler and lubricant, and the compression pressure, on tablet dissolution rate.

Dissolution rate usually is decreased when tablet compression pressure is increased.[112] This is due to the more difficult disintegration of highly compressed particle aggregates. However, dissolution rate actually may be increased when the drug solids are exposed to extremely high pressure, because of fracturing of drug particles and the resultant increase in their specific surface area.[141] Compression pressure has no effect on the dissolution rate of nondisintegrating drug solids.[154]

Dissolution rate is increased as the concentration of starch, the most commonly used disintegrant, is increased.[112] Tablet binders ordinarily tend to retard dissolution, because they delay disintegration and form a layer of viscous solution around dissolving drug

solids. Dissolution rate is also inversely proportional to granule size if the granules are nondisintegrating.[112] Certain vitamins are prepared in coated granules for inclusion in conventional and "chewable" tablets. These granules are coated with lipid or other materials to overcome stability problems or objectionable taste. Unfortunately, it has been found that a number of commercial vitamin products containing this type of granules did not release their full contents of vitamins on oral ingestion.[130] Caution and adequate invivo evaluation of coated granules and of preparations containing these is indicated.

Tablet lubricants are substances which are mostly water-insoluble and water-repellent. They can prevent adequate contact between drug solids and dissolution medium. One of the few good water-soluble tablet lubricants is sodium lauryl sulfate. It has the further advantage of being a surface-active agent that actually promotes contact between drug solids and aqueous medium and furthers penetration of solvent into agglomerates of solid particles. The dissolution-retarding effect of a hydrophobic tablet lubricant (magnesium stearate) and the pronounced dissolution-enhancing effect of sodium lauryl sulfate is evident in Figure 2-24, which is based on results of studies carried out in the author's laboratory.[112] It is this type of effect, rather than the proposed absorption enhancement, which undoubtedly accounted for the greater absorption of spironolactone from tablets containing polysorbate 80,[69] as already indicated in the subsection on surface-active agents.

Considerable research effort is still needed to obtain a greater understanding of the various formulation factors that can affect the therapeutic efficacy of drugs contained in compressed tablets. Currently, pharmaceutical scientists are particularly concerned with the development of suitable in-vitro dissolution tests and their correlation with in-vivo results. An interesting and unique approach to the study of dissolution of drugs from tablets is the use of thermal analysis which permits continuous monitoring of the total surface area of a dissolving tablet on the basis of the heat evolved due to the dissolution process.[146]

The biopharmaceutical problems associated with coated tablets are so numerous and so complex that they cannot be dealt with adequately in a general review of this type. An excellent presentation of the subject is available elsewhere.[207]

CORRELATION OF IN-VITRO DISSOLUTION AND GASTROINTESTINAL ABSORPTION

Since it is now generally appreciated that the rate-limiting factor in the gastrointestinal absorption of most drugs from solid dosage forms is their dissolution in gastrointestinal fluids, various in-vitro tests are being used to determine the dissolution characteristics of drugs in different dosage forms. Unless these in-vitro tests have been calibrated against in-vivo measurements, the data obtained cannot be used to predict in-vivo performance. This is so because the dissolution rate of drugs in dosage forms may be highly dependent on such variables as stirring rate, pH, and composition of the dissolution medium. Different formulations can be affected by these variables to a different extent, and one often finds that a certain rank order of dosage forms obtained on the basis of their dissolution characteristics under certain test conditions may be reversed entirely when the tests are carried out under different conditions. Take, for example, the case of three different aspirin tablet preparations with widely different absorption characteristics (Fig. 2-25). In-vitro dissolution tests at various stirring rates revealed that the dissolution of the most slowly absorbed preparation made from microencapsulated particles was relatively insensitive to changes

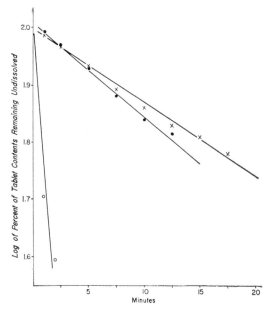

FIG. 2-24. Effect of lubricant on dissolution rate of salicylic acid from compressed tablets. (X) Magnesium stearate 3%: (●) no lubricant; (○) sodium lauryl sulfate 3%. (From Levy, G., et al.: Effect of certain tablet formulation factors on dissolution rate of the active ingredient, J. Pharm. Sci., 52:1140, 1963)

in stirring rate while that of the other tablets was highly sensitive to such changes (Fig. 2-26). At low stirring rates, aspirin dissolution from the more rapidly absorbed regular aspirin tablets was actually slower than from the much more slowly absorbed microencapsulated preparation! To find the proper stirring conditions for a suitable in-vitro test, the ratio of in-vitro dissolution rates of the two preparations was calculated as a function of stirring rate. The ratio of absorption rates of these preparations as obtained from clinical tests was three, and this same ratio of dissolution rates was obtained at 50 rpm in the in-vitro test (Fig. 2-27). An excellent correlation between the absorption and in-vitro dissolution data for all three preparations was obtained when the stirring rate of the dissolution test was 50 rpm (Fig. 2-28). No such correlation was found with in-vitro data obtained at other stirring rates.[116] Similar problems arise in the choice of pH[151] and other variables of the in-vitro dissolution test. These considerations should be kept in mind when assessing the suitability of various in-vitro dissolution tests, be they "official" or not, for evaluating the absorption characteristics of pharmaceutical dosage forms.

CLINICAL EVALUATION OF DOSAGE FORMS

Pharmacists must be aware of the more important aspects of clinical evaluation of drugs and particularly of the evaluation of new formulations and dosage forms. The community and the hospital pharmacist will have to be able to read critically and judge the significance of research reports which appear in the clinical literature or are incorporated in manufacturers' brochures, if they want to assist physicians in the choice of dosage form and manufacturers' brand of

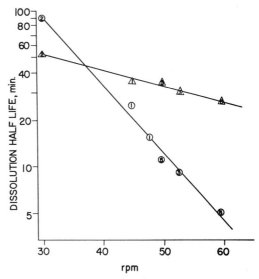

FIG. 2-26. Effect of stirring rate on in-vitro dissolution rate of aspirin from plain tablets (O) and microencapsulated particles (Δ). Numbers within symbols indicate number of tablets tested. (Levy, G., Leonards, J. R., and Procknal, J. A.: J. Pharm. Sci., *54*:1719, 1965)

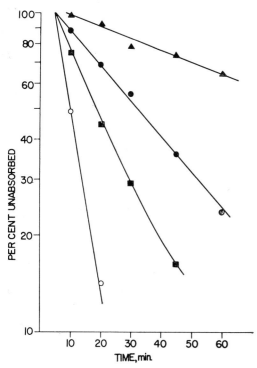

FIG. 2-25. Absorption of 0.65 Gm. of aspirin from solution (O), from tablets containing buffering agents (■), plain tablets (●), and microencapsulated particles (▲). Average of 12 subjects. (Levy, G., Leonards, J. R., and Procknal, J. A.: J. Pharm. Sci., *54*:1719, 1965)

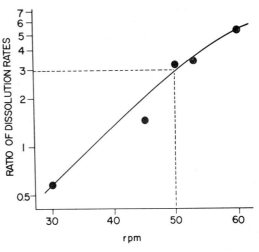

FIG. 2-27. Ratio of dissolution rates, plain tablets:microencapsulated particles, as a function of stirring rate. Broken line indicates the ratio found in vivo and the corresponding in-vitro stirring rate. (Levy, G., Leonards, J. R., and Procknal, J. A.: J. Pharm. Sci., *54*:1719, 1965)

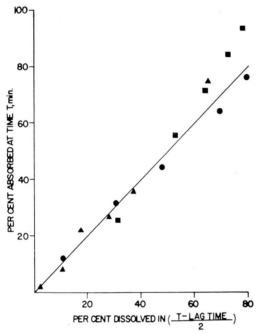

FIG. 2-28.   Plot of per cent of dose of aspirin absorbed at time T after drug administration vs. per cent dissolved in vitro at time (T = lag time)/2. (Levy, G., Leonards, J. R., and Procknal, J. A.: J. Pharm. Sci., *54*:1719, 1965)

therapeutic agents. This requires knowledge of the fundamentals of experimental design and statistical methodology. Pharmacists can also play an important part in the design of clinical studies and in the evaluation of results derived from such studies, if pharmaceutical factors are involved to the extent that the clinical data may be significantly influenced by them. It is up to the pharmacist to point out certain variables which may not be considered ordinarily by the clinical investigators, such as differences in salt form, particle size, vehicle and other formulation and dosage form properties of the therapeutic agents to be studied. Similarly, pharmacists should be able to aid physicians in the evaluation of research reports where biopharmaceutical factors may have affected the results. The research and the manufacturing pharmacist is even more directly concerned with clinical evaluation, since new dosage forms and formulations developed by him usually require clinical trial to assess their efficacy or deficiencies.

There is no standard methodology which is applicable to the clinical evaluation of every conceivable drug and its several dosage forms. The purpose of the study, as well as the known or the expected pharmacologic and pharmaceutical properties of a given drug or formulation, will dictate the experimental design. Therefore, the research pharmacist must be involved directly in both the design and the interpretation of results of clinical studies of dosage forms and formulations. He will have to acquire competence much beyond that which can be obtained from the following paragraphs, which can provide only an outline of the subject.

OBJECTIVE VS. SUBJECTIVE TEST METHODS

Fortunately, most aspects of dosage form evaluation permit the use of objective methods such as the determination of drug concentration in various body fluids. This is so because the therapeutic efficacy of the drug as such has usually been established, and the main purpose is to determine the degree to which intrinsic absorption rate, availability and elimination rate of the drug may have been modified by the dosage form. Whenever possible, it is desirable that dosage form evaluation be based on quantitative determination of the drug and/or its metabolites in the blood, the tissues or the urine. Such procedures are least subject to bias and differences in interpretation. In some instances, no specific assay method is available, or the concentration of drug in the biologic fluids is too low for quantitative measurement. Various pharmacologic parameters may then be used as indices of drug concentration, provided that the intensity of the pharmacologic effect is known to be a function of drug concentration. Thus, the physiologic availability of a diuretic agent may be assessed by the volume of urine voided, and the absorption of a mydriatic by determination of pupil diameter, but such values are subject to considerable variation. Therefore, these indirect methods are used only when direct methods are not available. Evaluations based on subjective methods are much more complicated because the results depend to a considerable degree on environmental and personal factors which may affect both investigator and subject. It is difficult to quantitate in a reproducible manner such conditions as pain, itching or nervousness and to evaluate dosage form effects on the basis of analgesia, relief of itching and degree of tranquility.

EXPERIMENTAL DESIGN

Selection of Subjects. Pharmacodynamic properties of drugs may often be studied in healthy subjects, while determinations of therapeutic efficacy require subjects suffering from the disease for which the drug is considered to be indicated. Thus, one may use healthy subjects to determine the gastrointestinal absorption of an antibiotic, but studies with anemic individuals are required to verify the anti-anemia activity of liver extract. It is fortunate that dosage forms usually can be evaluated on healthy subjects, because studies which require the use of patients suffering from certain illnesses are often complicated by factors such as fluctuations in the severity of their condition, the self-limiting nature of certain diseases and the difficulty of assembling a sufficient number of patients with similar pathologic involvements. However, some drugs are too toxic to be evaluated in healthy volunteers. For instance, many cytotoxic agents used in the treatment of malignancies have extremely unfavorable therapeutic indices so that their pharmacodynamic evaluation in normal subjects cannot be justified. Absorption, biotransformation and elimination data obtained from studies using healthy subjects can provide useful comparative information about certain dosage form effects, but it must be recognized that these values frequently may not be applicable in the quantitative sense to subjects suffering from gastrointestinal, hepatic or renal disease.

Where the purpose of a study is the determination of absolute rather than comparative values, such as the biologic half-life of a given drug, the selection of a representative population sample becomes important. While the sample may be restricted arbitrarily to a certain specified age, racial or geographic group, the selection of subjects who are to constitute this sample must be randomized by means of available statistical technics so that it may be representative of that total population group.

Controls. The purpose of using controls as part of the experimental design is to isolate the variable to be studied and to provide a sound basis of comparison. A potential sustained release medicament must be compared with a conventional dosage form of the same drug at the same dose if the sustained release effect is to be demonstrated. The effectiveness of a topical antipruritic agent can be assessed meaningfully only by comparison with the effect obtained from the ointment or the lotion base alone, because the latter may exert a soothing, cooling or protective effect and, thus, account entirely for the efficacy of the preparation. The use of controls may not be possible if it requires that some severely ill patients remain unmedicated, or if only a small number of unusual cases are available, but, even then, an admittedly less satisfactory "historical" control is implied, i.e., the recollection of previous cases treated differently. However, in the majority of instances and, particularly, in the clinical evaluation of dosage forms, the use of adequate controls must be considered mandatory, and their absence will usually invalidate the results of the study. Despite this, pharmacists will frequently find reports of clinical studies which are devoid of adequate controls, as indicated by a recent assessment of research methods used in 103 scientific studies reported in Canadian medical journals: 35.5 per cent had no controls, 12.5 per cent had inadequate controls and only 25.1 per cent of the studies were considered to have been well controlled. The balance of the articles dealt with studies where control was impossible or inapplicable.[15]

Placebos. Placebos are pharmacologically inert substances which are administered to subjects who believe that they are receiving an active drug. This permits distinguishing between the effects of the drug proper and the effects due to the act of administering it. Placebos are used primarily in therapeutic trials which are based on an assessment of subjective responses. In dosage form evaluation, placebos are necessary controls when the incidence and the severity of side effects such as gastrointestinal irritation, nausea and vomiting are to be established. Without controls, one may get a false impression of a large number of side effects when, actually,

TABLE 2-9. SIDE EFFECTS IN A 16-WEEK DOUBLE-BLIND TRIAL OF GRISEOFULVIN*

SYMPTOMS	PATIENTS RECEIVING GRISEOFULVIN (37)	PATIENTS RECEIVING INERT TABLETS (39)
Headache	3	1
Dyspepsia	1	1
Abdominal discomfort	1	2
Vomiting + nausea	0	2
Diarrhea	1	2
Ulcers in mouth	0	1
Cramps in limbs	2	0
Flushing of face	0	1
Drowsiness	0	1
Fever	1	0
Lassitude	1	0
Brittle nails	0	1
Rashes or itching	3	4

* Frain-Bell, W., and Stevenson, C. J.: Report on a clinical trial with griseofulvin. Trans. St. John Hosp. Derm. Soc., 45:47.

most of these are not directly due to the drug, as shown in Table 2-9.[63]

While the substance constituting the placebo may be pharmacologically inert, the process of administering this substance as a medicament may have both subjective and objective pharmacologic effects, such as increased gastric hydrochloric acid secretion, analgesia, relief of allergic symptoms, etc.[218] The quantitative and the qualitative nature of the placebo effect is largely influenced by environmental conditions, including the attitude of the investigator and the hopes, the apprehensions and the past experiences of the patient.

Experimental Technics. In addition to the use of controls and placebos where indicated, there are several experimental technics which are utilized to overcome extraneous factors which could affect the experimental results. In the *single-blind technic,* the patient does not know the identity of the medication so that his response is not influenced by preconceived notions or previous experiences. In dosage form evaluation, this requires that the various preparations should not be readily differentiable on the basis of appearance, taste and similar properties. Thus, two tablet formulations should not differ in size, shape

or imprint. When comparing a parenteral form of a drug with a tablet form, it may be necessary to administer the parenteral medicament and a placebo tablet in one instance, and the tablet containing drug together with a placebo injection such as sodium chloride solution in the other instance. The single-blind technic is applicable when the subject's response may be affected by bias or suggestive influences. If the drug evaluation is based on objective parameters such as drug concentration in the blood, the single-blind technic is not usually indicated.

Where the pharmacodynamic properties and effects of a drug cannot be measured readily by objective methods but are based on impressions and qualitative assessments by the investigator (for example, reduction of inflammation, improvement of a skin condition or degree of tranquility), it is desirable that neither the subject nor the investigator know the identity of the medicament. This is known as the *double-blind technic,* in which all medications are coded and the code is not broken until the study is concluded and the data have been analyzed. Unfortunately, some drugs have side effects, taste or other properties so characteristic and impossible to conceal that the patient soon learns to recognize them and only the investigator remains "blind."

There are considerable differences between subjects with respect to such physiologic factors as gastrointestinal motility, body weight, blood volume, etc. If two dosage forms were to be compared by administering them to two different groups of individuals, the possible physiologic differences between these two groups can complicate interpretation of the experimental data. Therefore, it is desirable to administer both dosage forms to each subject. This is known as the *cross-over* technic and establishes a better control. A more sophisticated design is the *double cross-over* technic, which involves a repetition of the cross-over procedure so that each subject receives both dosage forms twice. The double cross-over technic permits determination of reproducibility and indicates the degree of intrasubject variation. It thereby results in more valuable information and permits more meaningful conclusions.

Further refinements of the cross-over tech-

TABLE 2-10. SEQUENCE OF DRUG ADMINIS-
TRATION ACCORDING TO A LATIN-SQUARE
DESIGN

1. EVALUATION OF TWO DRUGS OR DOSAGE
FORMS (DESIGNATED A AND B):

	First Period	Second Period
Patient Group 1	A	B
Patient Group 2	B	A

2. EVALUATION OF THREE DRUGS OR DOSAGE
FORMS (A, B AND C):

	First Period	Second Period	Third Period
Patient Group 1	A	C	B
Patient Group 2	B	A	C
Patient Group 3	C	B	A

nics are obtained by means of a *latin-square design,* in which the sequence of drug administration is varied. Consider an experiment in which dosage form A is to be compared with dosage form B. One may first administer A to all subjects and, after an appropriate time interval, follow it with B. This constitutes a cross-over. Alternately, one may divide the experimental subjects into two groups, with Group 1 receiving A and Group 2 receiving B. After an interval of time, drug B is administered to Group 1 and drug A to Group 2. In this way the two groups receive the drugs in different order. This design can be extended to more than two drugs or dosage forms as shown schematically in Table 2-10. In this way, the order of drug administration is eliminated as an experimental variable which, potentially, could influence the results. For instance, A may cause gastrointestinal irritation which makes the mucosa sufficiently sensitive to react adversely to B despite the fact that B ordinarily does not affect the gastrointestinal mucosa to any significant degree. The latin-square design also serves to equalize certain unrecognized factors which may influence the experimental results, such as an unusually hot day, a malfunctioning analytic instrument or a different laboratory technician.

Experimental Conditions. Various experimental conditions can either enhance or suppress differences between dosage forms, so that it is important to be aware of the mech-

anisms which account for particular advantageous or undesirable properties of the dosage forms studied. If a drug is absorbed more rapidly when administered in tablet formulation A than in tablet formulation B because the former tablets disintegrate more rapidly, this effect will be noticeable only when the tablets are swallowed whole and not chewed. If an alkaline additive enhances the gastrointestinal absorption of a weakly acidic drug by increasing the rate of dissolution of the latter, the enhancing effect will occur only if the drug-additive combination is administered in solid form and not in solution. Many similar examples may be cited, but they all indicate merely that the choice of experimental conditions as well as conclusions drawn from the results of a clinical evaluation of dosage forms must be based on a thorough understanding of the biopharmaceutical factors and mechanism involved in the dosage form effects.

Dietary factors can influence markedly the gastrointestinal absorption of certain drugs. Apparently, the amount of griseofulvin absorbed following oral administration can be increased markedly by giving the patient a meal high in fat.[45] This is shown in Figure 2-29. Success of therapy may be affected decisively by the patient's dietary regimen, since inadequate absorption of griseofulvin

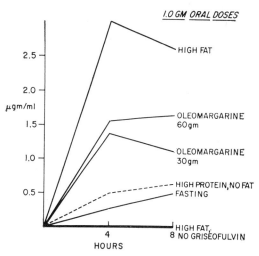

FIG. 2-29. Effects of different types of food intake on the serum griseofulvin levels following a 1.0 Gm. oral dose. (From Crounse, R. G.: J. Invest. Dermat., *37*:529)

appears to be one of the mechanisms of clinical unresponsiveness to therapeutic doses of this drug. The gastrointestinal absorption of 7-chloro-6-demethyltetracycline and other tetracyclines is seriously impaired by simultaneous ingestion of milk, milk products or aluminum hydroxide gel.[174] Milk and antacids have been prescribed by physicians to reduce gastrointestinal complaints associated with tetracycline therapy. Such practice and the lower tetracycline blood levels resulting therefrom (Fig. 2-30) may be responsible for some of the therapeutic failures encountered with these antibiotics.[174]

METHODS OF DOSAGE FORM EVALUATION

Dosage forms and formulations are evaluated usually with respect to one or more of the following properties: absorption rate, stability in the gastrointestinal tract, physiologic availability of the therapeutic agent and incidence and severity of side effects caused by the drug or other constituents of the dosage form. In certain more specialized cases it may be necessary to extend the scope of

the evaluation process to such matters as tissue distribution, elimination kinetics, plasma binding and sensitization liability, but these will not be discussed here.

Gastrointestinal Absorption Rate. This may be studied by determining the concentration of the drug in the blood as a function of time after drug administration. In a comparative study, it may only be necessary to compare the blood levels of drug when the latter is administered in a given dosage form with a suitable standard, such as the blood levels obtained after administration of the drug in aqueous solution. In an absolute study, such as estimation of the inherent absorption rate of a new compound, the time of peak drug concentration or the initial rate of increase of drug concentration in the blood are useful indicators of absorption rate. When the urinary excretion rate of the drug or its major metabolite is a function of drug concentration in the blood, it is feasible to study drug absorption by means of the urinary excretion method.[108,138] This involves collection of total urine at regular intervals after drug administration, and quantitative assay of each portion with respect to the drug or the major metabolite. A cumulative plot of amount excreted versus time may then be constructed, from which average excretion rates may be estimated by graphic methods (Fig. 2-31). Excretion rates can also be obtained from the experimental data by mathematical technics.[150] If in a comparative study different dosage forms affect urinary pH, urine flow rate and drug biotransformation to different degrees, utilization of either blood sampling or urinary excretion methods as sole indices of drug absorption may not be sufficient, and both technics may have to be used together.

The onset of a characteristic pharmacologic effect, such as reduced salivary flow, can serve as an index of drug absorption rate. Some drugs, such as potassium iodide, are concentrated in saliva in which they may be determined chemically or by taste, so that the time interval between drug administration and its appearance in the saliva can be a useful indicator of absorption rate. Sometimes isotope-labeled drugs may be administered and their appearance and concentration build-up monitored by measurements

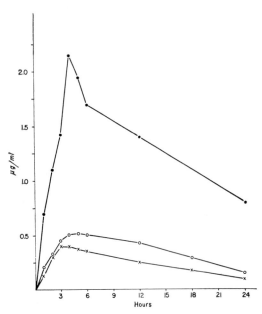

FIG. 2-30. Serum concentrations after a single oral dose of 300 mg. of 7-chloro-6-demethyltetracycline. (●) on empty stomach; (○) with 20 ml. of aluminum hydroxide gel; (X) with ½ pint of whole milk. (After Scheiner, J., et al.: Surgery, *114*:9)

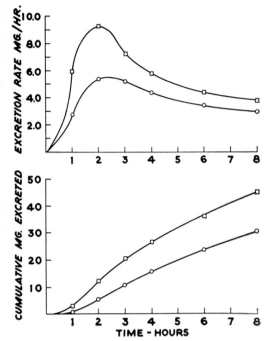

FIG. 2-31. Excretion rate vs. time plot (*above*), obtained by graphical determination of average hourly excretion rates from a graph of cumulative amount excreted vs. time (*below*). (○) tetracycline hexametaphosphate complex; (□) tetracycline hydrochloride. (From Nelson, E.: J. Am. Pharm. Ass. (Sci.), *48*:96)

Biologic Availability. When drugs are administered orally, it is always important to determine whether they are absorbed completely. The degree to which an orally administered drug is absorbed into the system is referred to as its biologic availability. As mentioned previously, a therapeutic agent may not be fully biologically available for reasons such as a low inherent absorption rate, slow dissolution rate, slow release from a tablet matrix, or because it is bound to some nonabsorbable macromolecule. Several technics, both absolute and comparative, are available for the determination of biologic availability. If a drug is stable in the gastrointestinal tract and is inherently well absorbed, it is possible to determine the possible adverse effect of slow dissolution rate or other dosage form factors on biologic availability by using a solution of the drug as the standard for comparison. The areas under the blood level vs. time curves obtained after administration of the drug in solution and in a given dosage form should be equal if availability is not reduced by dosage form effects.* If only a fraction of the drug is absorbed when administered in a particular dosage form, the per cent absorbed may be estimated by the ratio of the respective areas under the concentration vs. time curves. When there is some question concerning the biologic availability of a drug even when given in solution, it may be necessary to use a parenterally administered dose as the basis of comparison. If tissue distribution or biotransformation of the drug differs with route of administration, such comparison of areas under the blood level vs. time curves is not justified and can lead to erroneous conclusions. Biologic availability is estimated most commonly and readily by determining the amount of drug and its biotransformation products which are excreted in the urine. This also requires a standard of comparison in most instances, because urinary recovery is seldom quantitative, since some of the drug may be eliminated by other routes (pulmonary, skin, biliary) or metabolized to the point where it can no longer be identified as to its origin. Quantitative recovery is sometimes possible by means of

of isotope activity at an extremity, such as the hand, or at a site where the drug may become localized, such as the thyroid gland (in the case of certain iodinated compounds).

Drug Stability in the Gastrointestinal Tract. The efficacy of certain dosage forms depends on protecting the therapeutic agent from the degradative effect of acidic gastric fluids or various enzymes that are present in the gastrointestinal tract. In such studies it is particularly necessary that the drug assay method be sufficiently specific so that it will distinguish between the drug and its breakdown products. It is often possible to obtain at least comparative information concerning the protective effect of dosage forms by in-vitro experiments, since degradative conditions such as pH and enzyme concentration can be duplicated relatively easily in the laboratory and since primarily physicochemical rather than biologic processes are involved.

* This is true if drug elimination is not a saturable or otherwise dose-dependent process.

isotopic labeling and analysis of urine, sweat, expired air and feces, but this complicated methodology is rarely indicated or applicable to human subjects. In urinary recovery studies it is necessary to continue collection of urine samples for a sufficient time to assure complete recovery of whatever fraction is eliminated by this route. This may require a number of days or even weeks, depending on the rate of elimination. Another technic which may have to be used if the rate of elimination is very low or if little or no characteristic excretion products appear in the urine, is the fecal recovery method. Obviously, drug which is not absorbed will appear in the feces and may be determined by suitable assay methods. The feces also may contain some drug and, particularly, biotransformation products that were excreted in the bile and not reabsorbed. This possibility must be considered in the choice of the assay method and in the analysis of the experimental data.

Side-Effects. Therapeutic agents may elicit both systemic and local side-effects. Systemic effects are usually some function of drug concentration in the body, while local effects may have various causes, some of which are related to the dosage form in which the drug is administered. If the dosage form can affect the incidence and the severity of side effects such as nausea, vomiting, gastrointestinal bleeding or diarrhea, it is mandatory that these effects be considered in any evaluation of new dosage forms. The control in such studies is usually a placebo, although one dosage form may be compared with another. When evaluation is based on objective parameters, such as fecal blood content, it may be feasible to use the unmedicated subject as his own control without administering placebos. Assessment of subjective side effects usually is extremely difficult, due to placebo effects and many other extraneous influences, and represents a challenge of great magnitude to the clinical investigator who undertakes the study, to the statistician trying to analyze the significance of the data and to the pharmacist and the physician who must utilize this information intelligently in daily practice.

Sensitivity of the Experimental Method. The success of many research efforts depends largely on the specificity and the sensitivity of the technics used. Subtle differences may not be apparent, or the data may show so much variation that observed differences are statistically insignificant when the experimental methods or conditions are inadequate or inappropriate. Assay procedures may often be made more specific by proper utilization of separatory procedures such as solvent extraction, chromatography and ion exchange. Adequate recovery of drug from the biologic specimen must be demonstrated. The actual assay must be sufficiently discriminating to keep blank values low. When pharmacologic criteria rather than chemical assays are used in the study, it is desirable to choose a dosage which is in the sensitive range of the dose-response curve. The relationship between dose and response must be established experimentally in order to indicate the sensitivity of the method. When a therapeutic agent is absorbed both by an active process and by diffusion, different dosage forms should be compared at the same dosage level, since lower doses may be absorbed more rapidly than higher doses. Greater uniformity among the experimental subjects often reduces the degree of variation in the experimental results. It may be necessary to use the same technician for all analyses and clinical procedures. Last but not least, an increase in number of subjects will usually lead to more representative and significant results.

EVALUATION OF EXPERIMENTAL DATA

Statistical Analysis. Once the clinical observations and measurements have been completed, it is necessary to assemble and summarize the data, analyze the significance of any differences between dosage forms or other variables studied and derive conclusions. It is important that the results of the investigation be described in sufficient detail to permit others to judge for themselves whether the investigator's conclusions are justified. Often it is not feasible to report every single observation or analytic result. Instead, these are usually summarized in terms of measures of central tendency, such as the average or the mean, the mode and/or the median values. However, measures of central tendency do not indicate the variation within the group of individual data so summarized. Various measures of variation or dispersion are used for this purpose. The simplest measure of variation is the range, i.e., the difference between the highest and the lowest values. A more useful measure of variation is the standard deviation, since it notes not merely the extreme (highest and lowest) values but gives an indication of the way in which the total number of individual values are distributed around the average. If the individual values are normally distributed around the average (i.e., the number and the magnitudes of positive differences from the average are the same as the number and the magnitude of negative differences), then the range of values encompassed by the average $\pm$ one standard deviation includes about two thirds of the total number of values which make up the group. The average $\pm$ two standard deviations will include about 95 per cent of all values. Another commonly used measure of variation is variance, which is the square of the standard deviation.

Without information concerning the variations of values within each group, it is impossible to come to a reasonable judgment concerning the significance of an average value or the significance of differences between two or more average values. A small difference between two averages may be more meaningful than a large difference, if the internal variations are very small in the first pair and very large in the second pair.

Any differences in results obtained from different dosage forms, modes of treatment or other variables may be either "real" or due to chance. Various statistical technics (such as Student's "t" test, the chi-square test and analysis of variance) are used to determine the likelihood that observed differences are due to chance. This is expressed in terms of a probability or "P" value. A "P" value of 0.05 or 95 per cent signifies that in only 1 out of 20 cases will a difference have occurred by chance alone. A "P" value of 0.1 or 90 per cent shows that in 1 out of 10 cases the difference will have been due to chance. In most instances, experimental differences are considered significant if the calculated "P" value is less than 0.05. Thus, statistics cannot "prove" differences to be real or fortuitous; it can only establish the odds concerning their "realness." The con-

verse is also true: lack of statistically significant difference between two groups does not prove that these groups are equal or identical. More refined experimental technics and/or a larger number of measurements may well establish differences that are statistically significant. On the other hand, negative data (i.e., the absence of any significant differences) acquire validity primarily on the basis of the demonstrated sensitivity of the experimental method used. It is not intended here to describe in detail various statistical technics or designs. Numerous excellent books on statistics are available for this purpose.

Validity of Conclusions. Even the most sophisticated statistical analyses cannot guard against wrong interpretation of the experimental data and unjustified conclusions. The mathematical manipulations cannot ordinarily cause an unrecognized variable to be uncovered, nor can they prevent an overenthusiastic investigator from extrapolating his results far beyond the confines of his experimental system. It is at this point that the reader of any published research paper or manufacturer's brochure must be especially on guard. A few hypothetic examples may help to illustrate the problem.

Example No. 1. It has been found that stilbestrol administered orally in the form of a given brand of enteric-coated tablets is fully physiologically available, and it is concluded that enteric-coated tablets may be used without concern as to the possibility of incomplete absorption of stilbestrol. *Comment:* This conclusion is unjustified because there are large differences between brands with respect to types of coating and stability of the latter in gastrointestinal fluids. The conclusions apply only to the particular brand of tablets used or even only to the particular lot, if large lot-to-lot differences exist.

Example No. 2. It is shown that salicylate absorption is more rapid after oral administration of tablets containing aspirin and phenacetin than after administration of an equal dose of aspirin in the form of plain aspirin tablets. It is concluded that phenacetin enhances the gastrointestinal absorption of aspirin. *Comment:* This conclusion is incorrect because the more rapid absorption from the aspirin-phenacetin tablets may be due to tablet formulation factors. Perhaps aspirin particle size, lubricants, compression pressure and disintegrant were such as to result in much more rapid dissolution of aspirin from the aspirin-phenacetin tablets than from the plain aspirin tablets.

Example No. 3. The relative effectiveness of cortisone and hydrocortisone as topical anti-inflammatory agents was studied by comparing results obtained from lotions containing various concentrations of these agents suspended in the same vehicle. According to the experimental data, a 1 per cent cortisone lotion is equal in effectiveness to a 2 per cent hydrocortisone lotion, and it is concluded that cortisone is twice as effective as hydrocortisone. *Comment:* This unusual result may be due to a difference in particle size between the two drugs; cortisone may have been in micronized form while hydrocortisone was of relatively large particle size. The conclusions are not justified because the variable to be evaluated (the drug) was not isolated since an additional variable (particle size) was overlooked.

Example No. 4. A new derivative of tetracycline is shown to yield considerably higher blood levels on oral administration than tetracycline itself. On this basis, it is claimed that the new derivative is better absorbed and that, at equal doses, it would be more effective than tetracycline. *Comment:* The higher blood levels may be due to greater plasma-protein-binding, and drug concentration in the tisues may actually be lower when the derivative is used. Similarly, the total amount of drug absorbed from the gastrointestinal tract may be the same in each case, or may even be greater after administration of the less plasma-protein-bound tetracycline. It must be demonstrated, among other things, that the new derivative is not bound to plasma proteins to a greater extent than tetracycline itself, before the conclusions can be accepted.

The hypothetic examples cited above illustrate some (but not all possible) reasons why certain conclusions derived from experimental data may be unjustified. There may be other reasons, such as experimental conditions and doses or modes of administration being "unphysiologic." They may differ so much from the usual clinical conditions that results of the study may not be applicable to normal therapeutics.

Finally, assuming that experimental design was flawless and that the significance of observed differences is demonstrated impressively by means of highly sophisticated statistical methods, one must still decide as to the practical significance of the data. For example, there may be very little advantage associated with a new derivative, 1 mg. of which is as active as 5 mg. of the parent compound. After all, both substances probably end up in tablets of equal size. However, if the data also show that the new derivative has a more more favorable therapeutic index, then the differences between parent compound and derivative are significant not only in the statistical sense but also in terms of practical application.

SOURCES OF INFORMATION

The body of knowledge in the general area of biopharmaceutics is growing so rapidly that regular and intensive perusal of the current literature is necessary to keep up with new developments. Judgments and evaluations of dosage forms and formulations must be based on established facts, and these too can only be obtained through a consistent review of the literature. For this purpose, the pharmacist requires sources of information quite different from and additional to those that only list composition, indications, dosage schedules, side effects, etc. of proprietary products. Among the journals, books and services which could serve as the basis for a continuing program of acquiring information which is helpful in evaluating and designing dosage forms are the following:

Journal of Pharmaceutical Sciences. Issued monthly by the American Pharmaceutical Association, this journal contains many original research papers dealing with the pharmaceutical aspects of drug efficacy. A regular feature of each issue is a review article in which the more recent advances in an area such as kinetics of drug absorption, sustained release medication or antibiotics is summarized by an authority in the field.

Clinical Pharmacology and Therapeutics. This is the official publication of the American Therapeutic Society, the American Society for Pharmacology and Experimental Therapeutics, and the American Society of Clinical Pharmacology and Chemotherapy. It is issued bimonthly. The journal contains articles on aspects of clinical pharmacology, experimental design and evaluation of new drugs, and a *Current Drug Therapy Section* in which a given pharmacologic class of drugs is reviewed critically, as well as a section entitled *Diseases of Medical Progress* which contains abstracts of papers on adverse drug reactions. There is also a section of official literature on new drugs.

Journal of the American Medical Association. Through the pages of this publication, the Council on Drugs of the American Medical Association attempts to provide authoritative and unbiased information on drugs and drug therapy. As soon as practicable after a drug is marketed, the Council issues a detailed, descriptive monograph. This monograph is known as the *Preliminary Statement*. As additional information about the drug becomes available, it is published in a column entitled *New Drugs and Developments in Therapeutics*. The journal also contains Council-sponsored articles on the current status of therapy in the treatment of various diseases, as well as articles on pre-compounded combinations of two or more active ingredients in which pros and cons concerning their appropriate role in therapy are discussed. In addition, the journal features an *Annual Therapeutic Number* containing summaries of additions to therapeutic knowledge accumulated in the previous year, articles on the more fundamental aspects of drug therapy and a review of information derived from the Registry of Adverse Reactions. A considerable number of the articles and monographs mentioned above are reprinted in the *American Journal of Hospital Pharmacy*.

Drugs of Choice (C. V. Mosby Co., St. Louis, Mo.), edited by Walter Modell, is published every 2 years. In this book, the authors try to present a comprehensive and critical appraisal of all drugs in current use. Included in the discussions are results of clinical tests and data concerning relative potency, toxicity, modes of administration, onset and duration of effect and side effects.

One chapter deals with physical and chemical considerations in the choice of drugs.

Year Book of Drug Therapy (Year Book Medical Publishers, Inc., Chicago 11, Ill.), edited by Harry Beckman, consists of clinical and experimental evaluations of drugs and includes a chapter on drug reactions as well as a special section in which the year's new drugs are evaluated critically.

Current Contents (published weekly by the Institute for Scientific Information, Philadelphia, Pa. 19106) represents a unique service which helps to overcome the difficulty inherent in the fact that research papers dealing with topics of biopharmaceutical interest are scattered throughout numerous scientific journals. In this publication, the tables of contents of over 700 foreign and domestic chemical, biologic and pharmaco-medical journals are reproduced regularly. Any article of interest can be looked up in the appropriate journal which may be available in the libraries of universities or hospitals in the area, or reprints may be requested directly from the authors. For this purpose, *Current Contents* contains in each issue a listing of authors' addresses. The journal also provides an original article tear sheet service through which any of the articles listed may be purchased directly from the Institute for Scientific Information.

International Pharmaceutical Abstracts (published biweekly by the American Society of Hospital Pharmacists, 4630 Montgomery Avenue, Washington, D. C. 20014) is a very useful compilation of abstracts of papers on pharmacy, pharmaceutics, biopharmaceutics, drug metabolism, drug evaluations, adverse reactions, and similar subjects. This publication permits the reader to scan rapidly a considerable number of titles of potentially interesting papers. The short abstracts help in the selection of those papers that should be reviewed in detail. The listing of authors' addresses makes it possible to write for reprints. *International Pharmaceutical Abstracts* should be particularly valuable to pharmacists who have no ready and regular access to an extensive health sciences library.

The Medical Letter on Drugs and Therapeutics (published biweekly by Drug and Therapeutic Information, Inc., New York

22, N. Y.) can be likened to a physician's "Consumer's Digest." It incorporates critical comments concerning claims made in manufacturers' advertisements and brochures, evaluations of new products as compared with more established drugs and assessments of the significance of published studies concerning the efficacy of pharmaceutical products. The publishers periodically acquire various brands of generically identical drugs and have these assayed by an independent laboratory. The results are published in the form of a tabulation listing manufacturer's name, assay data and price. Since a drug may adhere to all official standards and still be therapeutically inadequate,[119] it should be appreciated that the above tabulation is most useful in revealing definitely unreliable brands without necessarily providing an indication of therapeutic equivalence for those brands that are found to satisfy official standards.

The above-mentioned sources can be used readily as the core of a regular information-gathering program by community and hospital pharmacists. These sources should be supplemented with standard and well-known reference texts, such as the *United States Dispensatory* and *Remington's Practice of Pharmacy*. The reader also is referred to the Special Literature Number of the *American Journal of Hospital Pharmacy* (Vol. 18, January 1961), which features articles on utilization of literature, classification and filing, as well as a comprehensive guide to information sources for pharmacists.

Apart from the need to keep abreast of scientific developments in his field, the pharmacist must be able to utilize the literature in order to find specific information concerning stability, compatibility, pharmacologic properties, assay methods and similar aspects of a given drug. This may require a formal search covering the literature of the past 10 years or more. Usually, such a search is undertaken with the aid of indices and abstract journals which are available in the libraries of universities and in larger public libraries. The more important among these are *Chemical Abstracts, Index Medicus* and *Biological Abstracts*. Readers interested in learning more about the subject are referred to *A Key to Pharmaceutical and Medicinal*

Chemistry Literature, a book published as No. 16 of the Advances in Chemistry Series by the American Chemical Society.

REFERENCES

1. Ahsan, S. S., and Blaug, S. M.: Interaction of Tweens with some pharmaceuticals. Drug Stand., *28*:95, 1960.
2. Airakinen, M. M.: Effect of route of administration on the metabolism of 5-hydroxytryptamine. Biochem. Pharmacol., *8*:245, 1961.
3. Alibrandi, A., Bruni, G., Ercoli, A., Gardi, R., and Meli, A.: Factors influencing the biological activity of orally administered steroid compounds: Effect of the medium and of esterification. Endocrinology, *66*:13, 1960.
4. Almirante, L., DeCarneri, I., and Coppi, G.: Rapporto tra attivita terapeutica e stato cristallino e amorfo dello stearato del cloramfenicolo. Il Farmaco, Ed. Prat., *15*:471, 1960.
5. Amsel, L. P., and Levy, G.: Drug metabolism interactions in man. II. A pharmacokinetic study of the simultaneous conjugation of benzoic and salicylic acids with glycine. J. Pharm. Sci., *58*:321, 1969.
6. Anonym.: Bibliography on Biopharmaceutics. Pharm. Manufacturers Assoc., Washington, D. C., 1968.
7. Anonym.: PVP brochure. Antara Chemicals, N. Y., 1959.
8. Anonym.: The easy way in on the absorption of drugs. Time & Till, *47*:94, 1961.
9. Anton, A. H.: A drug-induced change in the distribution and renal excretion of sulfonamides. J. Pharmacol. Exp. Ther., *134*:291, 1961.
10. Atkinson, R. M., Bedford, C. B., Child, K. J., and Tomich, E. G.: Effect of particle size on blood griseofulvin levels in man. Nature, *193*:588, 1962.
11. Axelrod, J., Udenfriend, S., and Brodie, B. B.: Ascorbic acid in aromatic hydroxylation. J. Pharmacol. Exp. Ther., *111*:176, 1954.
12. Baas, K. H.: Ueber die Resorption von Jodkalium im menschlichen und tierischem Magen und ueber den hemmenden Einfluss des Morphius auf die Magenentleerung. Deutsch. Arch. klin. Med., *81*:455, 1904.
13. Bachrach, W. H.: Physiology and pathologic physiology of the stomach. CIBA Clin. Sympos., *11*:3, 1959.

14. Back, N., and Levy, G.: Unpublished data.

15. Badgley, R. F.: An assessment of research methods reported in 103 scientific articles from two Canadian medical journals. Canad. M. A. J., *85*:246, 1961.

16. Ballard, B. E., and Nelson, E.: Physicochemical properties of drugs that control absorption rate after subcutaneous implantation. J. Pharmacol. Exp. Ther., *135*:120, 1962.

17. Bauer, G., Rieckmann, P., and Schaumann, W.: Einfluss von Teilchengrosse und Losungsvermittlern auf die Resorption von Spironolacton aus dem Magendarmtract. Arzneimittel-Forsch., *12*:487, 1962.

18. Bean, H. S.: Solubilisation by surface active agents. Pharm. acta helv., *35*:512, 1960.

19. Bedford, C., Busfield, D., Child, K. J., MacGregor, I., Sutherland, P., and Tomich, E. G.: Studies on the biological disposition of griseofulvin, an oral antifungal agent. A. M. A. Arch. Derm., *81*: 5, 1960.

20. Beinert, H.: *In:* P. D. Boyer *et al.* (eds.): The Enzymes. ed. 2. p. 351. New York, Acad. Press, 1960.

21. Bergman, I., and Paterson, M. S.: Silica powders of respirable size. I. Preliminary studies of dissolution rates in dilute sodium hydroxide. J. Appl. Chem., *11*: 369, 1961.

22. Biles, J. A.: Crystallography. Part II. J. Pharm. Sci., *51*:601, 1962.

23. Blanpin, O.: Modifications de l'intensité d'action pharmacodynamique par les substances dites mouillantes. Prod. Pharm., *13*:425, 1958 (available in English as manuscript No. 16 in S.K.F. Selected Pharmaceutical Research References).

24. Blythe, R. H., Grass, G. M., and Mac-Donnell, D. R.: The formulation and evaluation of enteric coated aspirin tablets. Am. J. Pharm., *131*:206, 1959.

25. Boberg-Ans, J., Grove-Rasmussen, K. V., and Hammarlund, E. R.: Buffering technique for obtaining increased physiological response from alkaloidal eyedrops. Brit. J. Ophthal., *43*:670, 1959.

26. Booth, C. C., and Mollin, D. L.: The site of absorption of vitamin B_{12} in man. Lancet, *1*:18, 1959.

27. Bousquet, W. F.: Pharmacology and biochemistry of drug metabolism. J. Pharm. Sci., *51*:297, 1962.

28. Brandstätter-Kuhnert, M.: Polymorphism in drugs. Oester. Apoth. Ztg., *13*:297, 1959.

29. Brettell, H. R., Aikawa, J. K., and Gordon, G. S.: Studies with chlorothiazide tagged with radioactive carbon (C^{14}) in human beings. Arch. Int. Med., *106*:57, 1960.

30. Brilmayer, H., and Loennecken, S. J.: Die Eliminationsgeschwindigkeit von Barbiturat aus dem Blut akut intoxizierter Patienten. Arch. int. Pharmacodyn., *136*: 137, 1962.

31. Brodie, B. B.: Difficulties in extrapolating data on metabolism of drugs from animal to man. Clin. Pharmacol. Ther., *3*:374, 1962.

32. Broitman, S. A., and Zamcheck, N.: Influence of pH on glucose absorption in the rat *in vivo*. Fed. Proc., *21*:259, 1962.

33. Buerger, M. J.: Polymorphism and phase transformations. Fortschr. Miner., *39*:9, 1961.

34. Callow, R. K., and Kennard, O.: Polymorphism of cortisone acetate. J. Pharm. Pharmacol., *13*:723, 1961.

35. Careddu, P., Mereu, T., and Apollonio, T.: Glucuronic acid conjugation in infectious hepatitis. Minerva Pediat., *13*: 1614, 1961 (through Chem. Abstr.).

36. Cavallito, C. J., and O'Dell, T. B.: Modification of rates of gastrointestinal absorption of drugs. II. Quaternary ammonium salts. J. Am. Pharm. Ass. [Sci.], *47*:169, 1958.

37. Cavallito, C. J., and O'Dell, T. B.: Oral pharmaceutical composition for enhanced absorption of the therapeutically active quaternary ammonium salt ingredient. U. S. Patent 2,899,357, August 11, 1959.

38. Chapman, D. G., Crisafio, F., and Campbell, J. A.: The relation between *in vitro* disintegration time of sugar-coated tablets and physiological availability of sodium p-aminosalicylate. J. Am. Pharm. Ass. [Sci.], *45*:374, 1956.

39. Chow, B. F., Hsu, J. M., Okuda, K., Grasbeck, R., and Horonick, A.: Factors affecting the absorption of Vitamin B_{12}. Am. J. Clin. Nutr., *6*:386, 1958.

40. Clarkson, T. W., Cross, A. C., and Toole, S. R.: Electrical potentials across isolated small intestine of the rat. Am. J. Physiol., *200*:1233, 1961.

41. Conney, A. H.:. Pharmacological implications of microsomal enzyme induction. Pharmacol. Rev., *19*:317, 1967.

42. Connor, J. J.: Chemistry and uses of iodophors. Amer. Perf., *75*:44, 1961.

43. Cordero, N., and Wilson, T. H.: Comparison of transport capacity of small and large intestine. Gastroenterology, *41*:500, 1961.

44. Corte, G., and Johnson, W.: Effect of N-acetyl-para-aminophenol on plasma levels of 17-hydro-corticosteroids. Proc. Soc. Exp. Biol. Med., *97*:751, 1958.

45. Crounse, R. G.: Human pharmacology of griseofulvin: the effect of fat intake on gastrointestinal absorption. J. Invest. Derm., *37*:529, 1961.

46. Cuenca, E., Costa, E., Kuntzman, R., and Brodie, B. B.: The methyl ether of methyl reserpate; a prototype of reversible short-acting tranquilizing agents. Med. Exp., *5*:20, 1961.

47. Dale, J. K.: Crystalline form of riboflavin. U. S. Patent 2,603,633, July 15, 1952.

48. Davenport, H. W.: Physiology of the Digestive Tract. p. 162. Chicago, Year Book Pub., 1961.

49. ——: Ibid., pp. 50 ff., 149 ff.

50. Davison, C., Guy, J. L., Levitt, M., and Smith, P. K.: The distribution of certain non-narcotic analgetic agents in the CNS of several species. J. Pharmacol. Exp. Ther., *134*:176, 1961.

51. Dayton, P. G., Tarcan, Y., Chenkin, T., and Weiner, M.: The influence of barbiturates on coumarin plasma levels and prothrombin response. J. Clin. Invest., *40*:1797, 1961.

52. Deutsch, M. J., Schiaffino, S. S., and Loy, H. W.: Experience with an extraction method for thiamine. J. Ass. Off. Agr. Chemists, *43*:55, 1960.

53. Dietel, V., and Walther, G.: Experimentelle Untersuchungen über Ausscheidung und Verteilungs Volumen von Sulfonamiden bei Frühgeborenen. Z. ges. inn. Med., *16*:567, 1961.

54. Doluisio, J. T., and Swintosky, J. V.: In: Martin, E. W. (ed.): Remington's Pharmaceutical Sciences. p. 380. Easton, Pa., Mack Publishing Co., 1965.

55. Domagk, G.: Twenty-five years of sulfonamide therapy. Ann. N. Y. Acad. Sci., *69*:380, 1957.

56. Douglas, J. R., Baker, N. F., and Longhurst, W. M.: Further studies on the relationship between particle size and anthelmintic efficiency of phenothiazine. Am. J. Vet. Res., *20*:201, 1959.

57. Dowdle, E. B., Schachter, D., and Schenker, H.: Active transport of iron-59 by everted segments of rat duodenum. Am. J. Physiol., *198*:609, 1960.

58. Dragstedt, C. A.: Oral medication with preparations for prolonged action. J.A.M.A., *168*:1652, 1958.

59. Ercoli, N., and Lewis, M. N.: Studies on analgesics. J. Pharmacol. Exp. Ther., *84*:301, 1945.

60. Ercoli, A., and Gardi, R.: Δ^4-3 Keto steroidal enol ethers. Paradoxical dependency of their effectiveness on the administration route. J. Am. Chem. Soc., *82*:746, 1960.

61. Erdman, C. J., Gibson, W. R., Martin, J. W., and Meyers, D. B.: The pharmacology of 3-phenyl-1,2,4-triazole. Paper presented at National Meeting of American Pharmaceutical Association, Chicago, April 1961.

62. Forth, W., and Seifen, E.: Der Einfluss von Komplexbildnern auf die ^{59}Fe-Resorption am isolierten Darm der Ratte. Naunyn-Schmiedeberg's Arch. exp. Path., *241*:556, 1961.

63. Frain-Bell, W., and Stevenson, C. J.: Report on a clinical trial with griseofulvin. Trans. St. John Hosp. Derm. Soc., *45*:47, 1960.

64. Francis, C. C., and Knowlton, G. C.: Textbook of Anatomy and Physiology. ed. 2. p. 479. St. Louis, C. V. Mosby, 1950.

65. Franklin, M., Rohse, W. G., Huerga, J., and Kemp, C. R.: Chelate iron therapy. J.A.M.A., *166*:1685, 1958.

66. Frazer, A. C.: Lipide absorption. Voeding, *16*:535, 1955 (through Chem. Abstr.).

67. Frederick, K. J.: Performance and problems of pharmaceutical suspensions. J. Pharm. Sci., *50*:531, 1961.

68. Frostad, S.: Continued studies in concentrations of para-aminosalicylic acid (PAS) in the blood. Acta tuberc. pneumol. scand., *41*:68, 1961.

69. Gantt, C. L., Gochman, N., and Dyniewicz, J. M.: Effect of a detergent on gastrointestinal absorption of a steroid. Lancet, *1*:486, 1961.

70. ——: Gastrointestinal absorption of spironolactone. Lancet, *1*:1130, 1962.

71. Garrett, E. R.: Facile hydrolysis of p-chlorobenzaldoxime and its oral inefficacy. J. Pharm. Sci., *51*:410, 1962.

72. Gassmann, B., Lexow, D., and Ehrt, D.: Zum Ablauf der Vitamin-B_1-Resorption bei der Ratte. Biochem. Z., *332*:449, 1960.

73. Ghazal, A., and Wright, H. N.: Glycine and glucuronic acid in salicylate intoxication. Paper presented at First Inter-

natl. Pharmacol. Mtg., Stockholm, Sweden, August 22-25, 1961.

74. Glazko, A. J., Dill, W. A., Kazenko, A., Wolf, L. M., and Carnes, H. E.: Physical factors affecting the rate of absorption of chloramphenicol esters. Antibiot. Chemother. (Wash.), 8:516, 1958.

75. Goodman, L. S., and Gilman, A.: The Pharmacological Basis of Therapeutics. ed. 2. p. 1455. New York, Macmillan, 1955.

76. Gordon, H. A., and Bruckner-Kardoss, E.: Effect of normal microbial flora on intestinal surface area. Am. J. Physiol., 201:175, 1961.

77. Grossman, M. I., Matsumoto, K. K., and Lichter, R. J.: Fecal blood loss produced by oral and intravenous administration of various salicylates. Gastroenterology, 40: 383, 1961.

78. Gullino, P. M., and Grantham, F. H.: Studies on the exchange of fluids between host and tumor. J. Nat. Cancer Inst., 27: 1465, 1961.

79. Hamlin, W. E., Nelson, E., Ballard, B. E., and Wagner, J. G.: Loss of sensitivity in distinguishing real differences in dissolution rates due to increasing intensity of agitation. J. Pharm. Sci., 51:432, 1962.

80. Hansen, I. A.: Bivalent metal ion effects on rat ileum in vitro. J. Sci. Indust. Res. [Biol.], 18C:84, 1959.

81. Harper, N. J.: Drug latentiation. J. Med. Pharm. Chem., 1:467, 1959.

82. Hartiala, K.: Experimental studies of gastrointestinal conjugation functions. Biochem. Pharmacol., 6:82, 1961.

83. Henderson, W. R., Carleton, J., and Hamburger, M.: The effect of probenecid upon serum levels of methicillin. Am. J. Med. Sci., 243:489, 1962.

84. Herz, R., Jr., Tapley, D. F., and Ross, J. E.: Glucuronide formation in the transport of thyroxine analogues by rat intestine. Biochim. Biophys. Acta, 53:273, 1961.

85. Higuchi, T.: Some physical chemical aspects of suspension formulation. J. Am. Pharm. Ass. [Sci.], 47:657, 1958.

86. Hogben, C. A. M., Tocco, D. J., Brodie, B. B., and Schanker, L. S.: On the mechanism of intestinal absorption of drugs. J. Pharmacol. Exp. Ther., 125: 275, 1959.

87. Hogben, C. A. M.: The first common pathway. Fed. Proc., 19:864, 1960.

88. Hogben, C. A. M., Schanker, L. S., Tocco, D. J., and Brodie, B. B.: Absorp-

tion of drugs from the stomach. II. The human. J. Pharmacol. Exp. Ther., 120: 540, 1957.

89. Holter, H.: How things get into cells. Sci. Am., 205(3):167, 1961.

90. Horita, A.: The route of administration of some hydrazine compounds as a determinant of brain and liver monoamine oxidase inhibition. Toxicol. Appl. Pharmacol., 3:474, 1961.

91. Ingelfinger, F. J., and Abbott, W. O.: Intubation studies of the human small intestine: the diagnostic significance of motor disturbance. Am. J. Dig. Dis., 7: 468, 1940.

92. Jaques, L. B.: Anticoagulants, physiology and pharmacology. Il Farmaco, Ed. Scient., 17:266, 1962.

93. Jones, C. M., Culver, P. J., Drummey, G. D., and Ryan, A. E.: Modification of fat absorption in the digestive tract by the use of an emulsifying agent. Ann. Int. Med., 29:1, 1948.

94. Juncher, H., and Raaschou, F.: The solubility of oral preparations of penicillin V. Antibiot. Med., 4:497, 1957.

95. Kakemi, K., Arita, T., and Koizumi, T.: Relation of particle size to blood concentration following oral administration of N^1-(5-Ethyl-1,3,4-thiadiazol-2-yl) sulfanilamide. Yakugaku Zasshi, 82:261, 1962.

96. Kakemi, K., Arita, T., and Ohashi, S.: Absorption and excretion of chloramphenicol. Preprint B-IV in booklet of symposium papers presented at the National Meeting of the American Pharmaceutical Association, Las Vegas, March 1962.

97. Kohn, K. W.: Mediation of divalent metal ions in the binding of tetracyclines to macromolecules. Nature, 191:1156, 1961.

98. Kostenbauder, H. B., Portnoff, J. B., and Swintosky, J. V.: Control of urine pH and its effect on sulfaethidole excretion in humans. J. Pharm. Sci., 51:1084, 1962.

99. Krüger-Thiemer, E., and Bünger, P.: Kumulation und Toxizität bei falscher Dosierung von Sulfanilamiden. Arzneimittel-Forsch., 11:867, 1961.

100. Kunin, C. M., and Finland, M.: Clinical pharmacology of the tetracycline antibiotics. Clin. Pharmacol. Ther., 2:51, 1961.

101. Lack, L., and Weiner, I. M.: In vitro absorption of bile salts by small intestine of rats and guinea pigs. Am. J. Physiol., 200:313, 1961.

102. Lagerlöf, H. O., Rudewald, M. B., and

Perman, G.: The neutralization process in duodenum and its influence on the gastric emptying time in man. Acta med. scand., *168*:269, 1960.

103. Laster, L., and Ingelfinger, F. J.: Intestinal absorption—Aspects of structure, function and disease of the small-intestine mucosa. New Engl. J. Med., *264*: 1138, 1192, 1961.

104. Lazarus, J., and Cooper, J.: Absorption, testing, and clinical evaluation of oral prolonged-action drugs. J. Pharm. Sci., *50*:715, 1961.

105. Lee, C. C., Froman, R. O., Anderson, R. C., and Chen, K. K.: Gastric and intestinal absorption of potassium penicillin V and the free acid. Antibiot. Chemother., *8*:354, 1958.

106. Levine, R. M., Blair, M. R., and Clark, B. B.: Factors influencing the intestinal absorption of certain monoquaternary anticholinergic compounds with special reference to benzomethamine. J. Pharmacol. Exp. Ther., *114*:78, 1955.

107. Levine, R. R., and Spencer, A. F.: Effect of a phosphatido-peptide fraction of intestinal tissue on the intestinal absorption of a quaternary ammonium compound. Biochem. Pharmacol., *8*:248, 1961.

108. Levy, G.: Comparison of dissolution and absorption rates of different commercial aspirin tablets. J. Pharm. Sci., *50*:388, 1961.

109. ———: Kinetics of pharmacologic effects. Clin. Pharmacol. Therap., *7*:362, 1966.

110. ———: The effect of absorption rate upon inter-subject variation in drug absorption from the gastrointestinal tract. Unpublished data.

111. ———: Unpublished research data.

112. Levy, G., Antkowiak, J. M., Gumtow, R. H., and Procknal, J. A.: Effect of certain tablet formulation factors on dissolution rate of the active ingredient. J. Pharm. Sci., *52*:1039, 1047, 1140, 1963.

113. Levy, G., Gumtow, R. H., and Rutowski, J. M.: The effect of dosage form upon the gastrointestinal absorption rate of salicylates. Canad. M. A. J., *85*:414, 1961.

114. Levy, G., and Hayes, B. A.: Physicochemical basis of the buffered acetylsalicylic acid controversy. New Engl. J. Med., *262*:1053, 1960.

115. Levy, G., and Knox, F. G.: The biological activity of orally administered desiccated thyroid. Am. J. Phcy., *133*: 255, 1961.

116. Levy, G., Leonards, J. R., and Procknal, J. A.: Development of in vitro dissolution tests which correlate quantitatively with dissolution rate-limited drug absorption in man. J. Pharm. Sci., *54*:1719, 1965.

117. Levy, G., and Matsuzawa, T.: Pharmacokinetics of salicylamide elimination in man. J. Pharmacol. Exp. Therap., *156*: 285, 1967.

118. Levy, G., and Nelson, E.: Pharmaceutical formulation and therapeutic efficacy. J.A.M.A., *177*:689, 1961.

119. ———: United States Pharmacopeia and National Formulary Standards, Food and Drug Administration regulations, and the quality of drugs. N. Y. State J. Med., *61*: 4003, 1961.

120. Levy, G., and Procknal, J. A.: Unusual dissolution behavior due to film formation. J. Pharm. Sci., *51*:294, 1962.

121. Levy, G., and Sahli, B. A.: Comparison of the gastrointestinal absorption of aluminum acetylsalicylate and acetylsalicylic acid in man. J. Pharm. Sci., *51*: 58, 1962.

122. Lewis, R. A., and Said, D.: Influences of posture on gastric function: Absorption of glucose and production of acid. Paper presented at First Internatl. Pharmacol. Mtg., Stockholm, Sweden, August 22-25, 1961.

123. Liguori, V. R., Giglio, J. J., Miller, E., and Sullivan, R. D.: Effects of different dose schedules of amethopterin on serum and tissue concentrations and urinary excretion patterns. Clin. Pharmacol. Ther., *3*:34, 1962.

124. Lish, P. M.: Some pharmacologic effects of dioctyl sodium sulfosuccinate on the gastrointestinal tract of the rat. Gastroenterology, *41*:580, 1961.

125. Lish, P. M., and Weikel, J. H., Jr.: Influence of surfactants on absorption from the colon. Toxicol. Appl. Pharmacol., *1*: 501, 1959.

126. Lozinski, E.: Physiological availability of dicumarol. Canad. M. A. J., *83*:177, 1960.

127. Macek, T. J.: *In*: Remington's Practice of Pharmacy. ed. 12. pp. 335-336. Easton, Mack, 1961.

128. Marcus, A. D.: Complexation incompatibilities. Drug Cosm. Ind., *79*:456, 1956.

129. Morozowich, W., Chulski, T., Hamlin, W. E., Jones, P. M., Northam, J. I.,

Purmalis, A., and Wagner, J. G.: The relationship between *in vitro* dissolution rates, solubilities and LT$_{50}$'s in mice of some salts of benzphetamine and etryptamine. J. Pharm. Sci., *51*:993, 1962.

130. Morrison, A. B., and Campbell, J. A.: Physiologic availability of riboflavin and thiamine in "Chewable" vitamin products. Am. J. Clin. Nutr., *10*:212, 1962.

131. Morrison, A. B., Perusse, C. B., and Campbell, J. A.: Physiologic availability and *in vitro* release of riboflavin in sustained-release vitamin preparations. New Engl. J. Med., *263*:115, 1960.

132. Mullins, J. D., and Macek, T. J.: Some pharmaceutical properties of novobiocin. J. Am. Pharm. Assoc. [Sci.], *49*:245, 1960.

133. Murphy, J., Casey, W., and Lasagna, L.: The effect of dosage regimen on the diuretic efficacy of chlorothiazide in human subjects. J. Pharmacol. Exp. Ther., *134*:286, 1961.

134. Nelson, E.: Comparative dissolution rates of weak acids and their sodium salts. J. Am. Pharm. Ass. [Sci.], *47*:297, 1958.

135. ———: Dissolution rate of mixtures of weak acids and tribasic sodium phosphate. J. Am. Pharm. Ass. [Sci.], *47*:300, 1958.

136. ———: Influence of dissolution rate and surface on tetracycline absorption. J. Am. Pharm. Ass. [Sci.], *48*:96, 1959.

137. ———: Therapeutic considerations of generic name prescriptions. Western Pharmacy, *73*:9, 1961.

138. ———: Kinetics of drug absorption, distribution, metabolism, and excretion. J. Pharm. Sci., *50*:181, 1961.

139. Nelson, E., Knoechel, E. L., Hamlin, W. E., and Wagner, J. G.: Influence of the absorption rate of tolbutamide on the rate of decline of blood sugar levels in normal humans. J. Pharm. Sci., *51*:509, 1962.

140. Nelson, E.: Physicochemical factors influencing the absorption of erythromycin and its esters. Chem. Pharm. Bull., *10*:1099, 1962.

141. ———: Personal communication.

142. Newbould, B. B., and Kilpatrick, R.: Long-acting sulfonamides and protein binding. Lancet, *1*:887, 1960.

143. Nicholson, A. E., Tucker, S. J., and Swintosky, J. V.: Sulfaethylthiadiazole VI. Blood and urine concentrations from sustained and immediate release tablets. J. Am. Pharm. Ass. [Sci.], *49*:40, 1960.

144. Niepmann, W.: Experimentelle Untersuchungen zur intestinalen Calcium-Resorption in Abhängigkeit von der Magenacidität beim Menschen. Klin. Wschr., *39*:1064, 1961.

145. Nikkilä, E. A.: Acetylation of p-aminobenzoic acid in metabolic disorders. Ann. med. intern. Fenn., *49*:269, 1960.

146. Nogami, H., Hasegawa, J., and Nakai, Y.: Studies on powdered preparations. II. Studies on tablet disintegration of calcium carbonate by thermal analysis. Chem. Pharm. Bull., *7*:331, 1959.

147. Noyes, A. A., and Whitney, W. R.: The rate of solution of solid substances in their own solutions. J. Am. Chem. Soc., *19*:930, 1897.

148. O'Dell, G. B.: Studies in Kernicterus. I. The protein binding of bilirubin. J. Clin. Invest., *38*:823, 1959.

149. Okuda, K., Duran, E., and Chow, B. F.: Effects of physicochemical state of Vitamin B-12 preparation in digestive tract on its absorption. Proc. Soc. Exp. Biol. Med., *103*:588, 1960.

150. O'Reilly, I., and Nelson, E.: Urinary excretion kinetics for evaluation of drug absorption. IV. J. Pharm. Sci., *50*:413, 1961.

151. O'Reilly, R. A., Nelson, E., and Levy, G.: Physicochemical and physiologic factors affecting the absorption of warfarin in man. J. Pharm. Sci., *55*:435, 1966.

152. Oser, B. L., Melnick, D., and Hochberg, M.: Physiological availability of the vitamins. Ind. Eng. Chem., Analyt. Ed., *17*:405, 1945.

153. Otobe, S.: Conjugation of glucuronic acid with morphine. Jap. J. Pharmacol., *9*:100, 1960.

154. Parrott, E. L., Wurster, D. E., and Higuchi, T.: Investigation of drug release from solids. J. Am. Pharm. Ass. [Sci.], *44*:269, 1955.

155. Patel, N. K., and Kostenbauder, H. B.: Interaction of preservatives with macromolecules. I. J. Am. Pharm. Ass. [Sci.], *47*:289, 1958.

156. Peters, L.: Urinary excretion of drugs. Paper presented at First Internat. Pharmacol. Mtg., Stockholm, Sweden, August 22-25, 1961.

157. Pindell, M. H., Cull, K. M., Doran, K. M., and Dickison, H. L.: Absorption and excretion studies on tetracycline. J. Pharmacol. Exp. Ther., *125*:287, 1959.

158. Rall, D. P., Moore, E., Taylor, N., and Zubrod, C. G.: The blood-cerebrospinal

fluid barrier in man. Arch. Neurol., *4*:318, 1961.

159. Rall, D. P., and Zubrod, C. G.: Passage of drugs in and out of the central nervous system. Ann. Rev. Pharmacol., *2*:109, 1962.

160. Reinhold, J. G., Phillips, F. J. Flippin, H. F., and Pollack, L.: Comparison of the behavior of microcrystalline sulfadiazine with that of ordinary sulfadiazine in man. Am. J. Med. Sci., *210*:141, 1945.

161. Riegelman, S., and Crowell, W. J.: The kinetics of rectal absorption. I.-III. J. Am. Pharm. Ass. [Sci.], *47*:115, 123, 127 (1958).

162. Riseman, J. E. F., Altman, G. E., and Koretsky, S.: Nitroglycerin and other nitrites in the treatment of angina pectoris. Circulation, *17*:22, 1958.

163. Roberts, C. E., Perry, D. M., Kuharic, H. A., and Kirby, W. M.: Demethyl chlortetracycline and tetracycline. Arch. Int. Med., *107*:204, 1961.

164. Robinson, M. J., and Swintosky, J. V.: Sulfaethylthiadiazole. V. Design and study of an oral sustained release dosage form. J. Am. Pharm. Ass. [Sci.], *48*:473, 1959.

165. Sakuma, T., Daeschner, C. W., and Yow, E. M.: Studies on the absorption, distribution excretion, and use of a new long-acting sulfonamide (sulfadimethoxine) in children and in adults. Am. J. Med. Sci., *239*:142–92, 1960.

166. Salafsky, B., and Loomis, T. A.: Intestinal absorption of a modified heparin. Proc. Soc. Exp. Biol. Med., *104*:62, 1960.

167. Salassa, R. M., Bollman, J. L., and Dry, T. J.: The effect of para-aminobenzoic acid on the metabolism and excretion of salicylate. J. Lab. Clin. Med., *33*:1393, 1948.

168. Schanker, L. S., Shore, P. A., Brodie, B. B., and Hogben, C. A. M.: Absorption of drugs from the stomach. I. The rat. J. Pharmacol. Exp. Ther., *120*:528, 1957.

169. Schanker, L. S.: Absorption of drugs from the rat colon. J. Pharmacol. Exp. Ther., *126*:283, 1959.

170. ———: On the mechanism of absorption of drugs from the gastrointestinal tract. J. Med. Pharm. Chem., *2*:343, 1960.

171. Schanker, L. S., and Jeffrey, J. J.: Active transport of foreign pyrimidines across the intestinal epithelium. Nature, *190*:727, 1961.

172. Schanker, L. S., and Johnson, J. M.: Increased intestinal absorption of foreign organic compounds in the presence of ethylenediamine tetraacetic acid. Biochem. Pharmacol., *8*:421, 1961.

173. Schanker, L. S., Tocco, D. J., Brodie, B. B., and Hogben, C. A. M.: Absorption of drugs from the rat small intestine. J. Pharmacol. Exp. Ther., *123*:81, 1958.

174. Scheiner, J., and Altemeier, W. A.: Experimental study of factors inhibiting absorption and effective therapeutic levels of Declomycin. Surgery, *114*:9, 1962.

175. Schloss, E. M.: Drugs and the gastroenterologist. Am. J. Gastroent., *35*:437, 1961.

176. Schnedorf, J. G., Bradley, W. B., and Ivy, A. C.: Effect of acetylsalicylic acid upon gastric activity and modifying action of calcium gluconate and sodium bicarbonate. Am. J. Dig. Dis. Nutr., *3*:239, 1936-7.

177. Scholtan, W.: Die Bindung der Langzeit-Sulfonamide an die Eiweiss Körper des Serums. Arzneimittel-Forsch., *11*:707, 1961.

178. Schroeter, L. C., Tingstad, J. E., Knoechel, E. L., and Wagner, J. G.: The specificity of the relationship between rate of dissolution and disintegration time of compressed tablets. J. Pharm. Sci., *51*:865, 1962.

179. Schulert, A. R., and Weiner, M.: The physiologic disposition of phenylindanedione in man. J. Pharmacol. Exp. Ther., *110*:451, 1954.

180. Sekiguchi, K., and Obi, N.: Studies on absorption of eutectic mixture. I. A comparison of the behavior of eutectic mixture of sulfathiazole and that of ordinary sulfathiazole in man. Chem. Pharm. Bull., *9*:866, 1961.

181. Shefter, E., and Higuchi, T.: Dissolution behavior of crystalline solvated and nonsolvated forms of some pharmaceuticals. J. Pharm. Sci., *52*:781, 1963.

182. Shenoy, K. G., Chapman, D. G., and Campbell, J. A.: Sustained release in pelleted preparations as judged by urinary excretion and *in vitro* methods. Drug Stand., *27*:77, 1959.

183. Silverman, W. A., Andersen, D. H., Blanc, W. A., and Crozier, D. N.: A difference in mortality rate and incidence of kernicterus among premature infants allotted to two prophylactic antibacterial regimens. Pediatrics, *18*:614, 1956.

184. Smith, P. K., Gleason, H. L., Stoll, C. G., and Orgorzalek, S.: Studies on the pharmacology of salicylates. J. Pharmacol. Exp. Ther., *87*:237, 1946.

185. Snell, F. M., Shulman, S., Spencer, R. P., and Moos, C.: Biophysical Principles of Structure and Function. p. 23. Buffalo, University of Buffalo, 1961.

186. Sögnen, E.: Effects of calcium-binding on orally induced chloralose and barbiturate anesthesia. Acta Pharmacol. (Kbh.), 18:38, 1961.

187. ———: Intestinal absorption influenced by calcium-binding substances. Paper presented at First Internatl. Pharmacol. Mtg., Stockholm, Sweden, August 22-25, 1961.

188. Solomon, A. K.: Pores in the cell membrane. Sci. Am., 203(6):146, 1960.

189. Stephens, V. C., Conine, J. W., and Murphy, H. W.: Esters of erythromycin. IV. Alkyl sulfate salts. J. Am. Pharm. Ass. [Sci.], 48:620, 1959.

190. Stevenson, I. H., and Dutton, G. J.: Glucuronide synthesis in kidney and gastrointestinal tract. Biochem. J., 82:330, 1962.

191. Sturtevant, F. M.: Mydriatic half-life of a new anti cholinergic as affected by dose, route, quaternization. Proc. Soc. Exp. Biol. Med., 104:120, 1960.

192. Sutherland, J. M.: Fatal cardiovascular collapse of infants receiving large amounts of chloramphenicol. J. Dis. Child., 97:761, 1959.

193. Swintosky, J. V.: Illustrations and pharmaceutical interpretations of first order drug elimination rate from the bloodstream. J. Am. Pharm. Ass. [Sci.], 45:395, 1956.

194. Swintosky, J. V., Bondi, A., Jr., and Robinson, M. J.: Sulfaethylthiadiazole. IV. Steady state blood concentration and urinary excretion data following repeated oral doses. J. Am. Pharm. Ass. [Sci.], 47:753, 1958.

195. Swintosky, J. V., Foltz, E. L., Bondi, A., Jr., and Robinson, M. J.: Sulfaethylthiadiazole. III. Kinetics of absorption, distribution and excretion. J. Am. Pharm. Ass. [Sci.], 47:136, 1958.

196. Swintosky, J. V., Robinson, M. J., Foltz, E. L., and Free, S. M.: Sulfaethylthiadiazole. I. Interpretations of human blood level concentrations following oral doses. J. Am. Pharm. Ass. [Sci.], 46:399, 1957.

197. Swintosky, J. V., Robinson, M. J., and Foltz, E. L.: Sulfaethylthiadiazole. II. Distribution and disappearance from the tissues following intravenous injection. J. Am. Pharm. Ass. [Sci.], 46:403, 1957.

198. Swintosky, J. V., and Sturtevant, F. M.: Note on the disappearance of pharmacologic activity. J. Am. Pharm. Ass. [Sci.], 49:685, 1960.

199. Tamura, C., and Kuwano, H.: Polymorphism of long-chain esters of chloramphenicol. I. On transition. Yakugaku Zasshi, 81:755, 1961.

200. Urazovskii, S. S., Kotlyarenko, I. P., and Kuris'Ko, A. I.: Difference in the dissociation constants for polymorphic modifications of acids in nonaqueous solutions. Zhur. Fiz. Khim., 33:2732, 1959 (through Chemical Abstracts).

201. Urazovskii, S. S., and Kuris'Ko, A. I.: Potentiometric study of the molecular polymorphism of monochloracetic and glycolic acids. Trudy Khar'Kov, 26:11, 1959 (through Chemical Abstracts).

202. Van Hook, A.: Crystallization: Theory and Practice. p. 68-69. New York, Reinhold, 1961.

203. ———: Ibid., pp. 65-68.

204. Vest, M. F., and Fritz, E.: Studies on the disturbance of glucuronide formation in infectious hepatitis. J. Clin. Path., 14:482, 1961.

205. Vliet, E. B.: Tablet disintegration tests. Drug Allied Ind., 42:17, 1956.

206. Wagner, J. G.: Biopharmaceutics: absorption aspects. J. Pharm. Sci., 50:359, 1961.

207. Wagner, J. G.: Coating of tablets, capsules, and pills. In: Remington's Practice of Pharmacy. ed. 12. p. 476. Easton, Mack, 1961.

208. Wagner, J. G., Carpenter, O. S., and Collins, E. J.: Sustained action oral medication. I. A quantitative study of prednisolone in man, in the dog and in vitro. J. Pharmacol. Exp. Ther., 129:101, 1960.

209. Warren, R.: Serosal and mucosal dimensions at different levels of the dog's small intestine. Anat. Rec., 75:427, 1939.

210. Weichselbaum, T. E., and Margraf, H. W.: Effect of citrus bioflavonoids on metabolism of hydrocortisone in man. Proc. Soc. Exp. Biol. Med., 107:128, 1961.

211. Weiner, M.: The influence of the physiologic disposition of chelates on their use in medicine. Ann. N. Y. Acad. Sci., 88:426, 1960.

212. Weiss, C. F., Glazko, A. J., and Weston, J. K.: Chloramphenicol in the newborn infant. New Engl. J. Med., 262:787, 1960.

213. Wells, J. A.: In: Drill, V. A. (ed.): Pharmacology in Medicine. ed. 2. p. 7. New York, McGraw-Hill, 1958.

214. Williams, R. T.: Detoxication Mechanisms. New York, John Wiley and Sons, 1959.

215. Williams, R. T.: Detoxication mechanisms *in vivo*. Paper presented at First Internatl. Pharmacol. Mtg., Stockholm, Sweden, August 22-25, 1961.

216. Wilson, A., and Schild, H. O.: Applied Pharmacology. ed. 9. p. 518. Boston, Little, Brown & Co., 1959.

217. Windsor, E., and Cronheim, G. E.: Gastrointestinal absorption of heparin and synthetic heparinoids. Nature, *190*: 263, 1961.

218. Wolf, S.: The pharmacology of placebos. Pharmacol. Rev., *11*:689, 1959.

219. Wu, H., and Elliott, H. C., Jr.: Urinary excretion of hippuric acid by man. J. Appl. Physiol., *16*:553, 1961.

220. Wurster, D. E., and Seitz, J. A.: Effect of changing surface-weight ratio on the dissolution rate. J. Am. Pharm. Ass. [Sci.], *49*:335, 1960.

221. Yaffe, S. J., Levy, G., Matsuzawa, T., and Baliah, T.: Enhancement of glucuronide-conjugating capacity in a hyperbilirubinemic infant due to apparent enzyme induction by phenobarbital. New Engl. J. Med., *275*:1461, 1966.

Chapter 3

Solid Dosage Forms

Eugene L. Parrott, Ph.D.*

Approximately two thirds of all preparations dispensed are solid dosage forms. Current solid dosage forms consist of powders, divided powders, dusting powders, insufflation powders, granules, capsules and tablets. With the exception of the compressed tablets, which are prescribed in approximately 50 per cent of all prescriptions, these solid dosage forms may be prepared extemporaneously at the prescription counter. Although each form has distinctive characteristics, solid dosage forms have several general advantages over liquid medication.

Solid dosage forms have a small bulk and are easy to package, transport and store. The patient finds them convenient to carry on his person in small containers. A gallon of phenobarbital elixir is not portable from the viewpoint of the patient; however, 505 30-mg. tablets containing the same amount of the drug may be carried without any serious objection. For administration of a liquid medication a troublesome teaspoon is required.

Compounds must be in solution to elicit the sensation of taste; consequently, taste is more pronounced in a liquid than in a solid medication. Unpleasant tasting drugs are administered most easily in the solid state because the dosage form can be swallowed rapidly before a significant amount of the drug can dissolve in the oral cavity to produce an unpleasant taste. With the use of confectionary bases, flavors and sweetening excipients in solid dosage forms, there is less rejection of obnoxious tasting drugs in solid dosages than in a flavored liquid preparation.

Many solid dosage forms enclose the drug within a shell or a coating which acts as a mechanical barrier between the drug and the taste buds, so that the flavor of the drug is never experienced by the patient.

Predivided solid dosage forms provide an accurate dose, since each dosage form represents one dose. With liquid medication the patient inadvertently introduces variance in dose due to the lack of uniformity in the size of the teaspoon and in the extent to which he fills each teaspoon.

Solid dosage forms may be prepared of many drugs that cannot be satisfactorily dispensed in a liquid form. Aspirin is rapidly hydrolyzed in the presence of moisture, and, to date, no satisfactory liquid preparation of aspirin has been developed. Because chemical reactions at room temperature normally occur in solution, a drug in the dry solid state has a greater shelf-life or stability than in the liquid state. Incompatibilities are less evident in the dry state. For example, in Alka-Seltzer and Seidlitz powders acidic substances are blended with a bicarbonate, and no reaction occurs while the mixture is dry. When the consumer places the medication in water, a reaction occurs rapidly.

Sustained release and delayed release of medication has become popular in the past several years. The vast majority of sustained release products marketed are solid dosage forms because controlled release technics generally are more applicable to solid than to liquid medication.

PARTICLE SIZE

In preparing a prescription for a solid dosage form, all drugs must be reduced to a

* Associate Professor of Pharmacy, University of Iowa.

fine state of subdivision before mixing. The fine particle size facilitates mixing and permits a more homogeneous preparation, assuring the patient of a uniform dose.

Therapeutic efficacy of a drug may be affected by the particle size. Microcrystalline sulfadiazine given orally appears more rapidly and in higher concentrations in the blood than ordinary sulfadiazine powder.[47] As the particles of sulfadiazine are reduced in size, there is a greater specific surface area. Since the solution of a given weight of the sulfadiazine is proportional to the exposed surface, with an increased surface area there is more rapid solution and increased absorption from the gastrointestinal tract, as shown in Figure 3-1.

The effect of particle size of chloramphenicol administered as an oral suspension to rabbits is shown in Figure 3-2.[2] With the smaller particles of 50 to 200 microns the maximum blood level is obtained in one hour, with a marked lowering of blood level after two hours. With the larger particles of 800 microns the blood level rises slowly to a maximum value at three hours and a prolonged effect is provided. The blood-level–time curve of the 400-micron particles is intermediate. In all cases the total amount of the chloramphenicol absorbed is the same.

Novobiocin also shows the effect of particle size on solution and absorption.[39] When the crystalline, acid form of novobiocin is given orally, practically no absorption occurs as indicated by blood levels. If this antibiotic is micronized or precipitated in a finely divided amorphous form, it becomes an effective oral drug. The more effective absorption of finer particles is especially important with sparingly soluble drugs such as corticosteroid and sulfa drugs. This effect has been demonstrated with calomel,[62] Lente Iletin,[37] griseofulvin,[3] oxytetracycline,[40] procaine penicillin G,[10] spironolactone[5] and Theelin.[52]

In the subsieve ranges, physical properties of solids are a function of particle size. In the colloid range, there is a decrease in melting point and an increase in solubility and vapor pressure.[21] A particle must be in the order of 10^{-6} cm. before it has appreciable surface energy. Since the reality of increased solubility is evident only in the colloidal range or less than 0.1 micron, for practical purposes solubility remains unchanged with a change in particle size.

A change of color with a change in particle size may be seen by the pharmacist. Red mercuric oxide becomes yellow when triturated to a finer state.

The particles of a powdered substance may appear uniform to the naked eye; yet

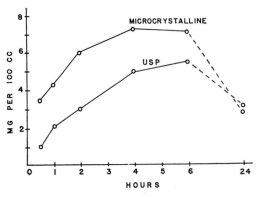

FIG. 3-1. Serum levels in humans after one 3-Gm. dose of sulfadiazine. Microcrystalline sulfadiazine with the smaller particle size produces a higher serum level. (Reinhold, J. G., Phillips, F. J., Flippin, M. F., and Pollack, L.: Am. J. Med. Sci., *210*:141, 1945)

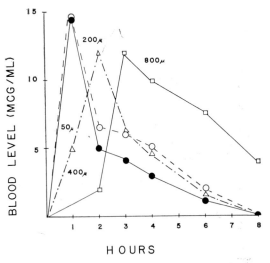

FIG. 3-2. Effect of particle size on absorption of 200 mg. of chloramphenicol administered to rabbits as an aqueous oral suspension. (Kakemi, K., Arita, T., and Ohashi, S.: J. Pharm. Soc. Japan, *82*: 1468, 1962)

there is a wide variation in the size of the particles. Most of the particles will fall within a narrow range about the average particle size, but there will be some much smaller and some much larger. The per cent frequencies of the various particles plotted against the mean of a group size forms a "size frequency curve." An average of the particle size would not indicate if the particles were adequately reduced, for there could be an equal number of very large particles and very small particles which would produce the desired average size; however, the subdivision would not be acceptable. By complex and varied means, pharmaceutical industry determines size frequency distributions whenever essential to the production of an elegant product.

The dispensing pharmacist cannot carry out elaborate measurements, but, as a good procedure, he can pass all powders through a sieve to make sure that all macroparticles have been pulverized and to establish the upper limits of particle size in the prescription.

Mechanical subdivision is accomplished industrially by attrition, hammer or high speed mills.[28] Solid drugs to be used for insufflation, parenteral or ophthalmic use must be of size ranging from 1 to 5 microns. At times comminution is carried out at low temperatures to facilitate fracture and passage of elastic solids such as proteins and methylcellulose. Very small particle size has been attained experimentally by applications of freeze drying, spray drying, ultrasonics and impingement procedures. Since specialized and expensive equipment is not available to the practicing pharmacist, he commonly reduces particle size by triturating a substance in a mortar with a pestle and/or by passing the substance through a sieve.

In the process of trituration, the pestle is given a circular motion beginning on the drug and extending in larger circles until the side of the mortar is touched. The pestle should be held in the palm so that the four fingers and the thumb are wrapped about the handle allowing the application of downward pressure. The powder should be scraped frequently from the sides of the mortar with a spatula. The time required to pulverize a crystal depends on the individual chemical; however, a minimum of 5 minutes of trituration should be employed by the compounding pharmacist.

Porcelain and Wedgwood mortars are usually found in the pharmacy. The pestle should fit the mortar so that it permits a maximum contact between the surfaces of the mortar and the pestle. The efficiency in trituration depends on the area of contact between the grinding surfaces as well as on the pressure applied. A rounded pestle in a flat-surfaced mortar wastes energy and does not reduce particle size effectively. Glass mortars and pestles are not used for trituration because of their smooth surfaces. A glass mortar is used for dissolving substances, since it is easy to know when solution has been completed. A glass mortar is used in mixing chemicals, such as iodine and dyes, which would stain a porcelain mortar.

After a solid has been reduced in size from the original granule or crystal, it may be brushed through a sieve to further reduce particle size or to make certain the proper degree of subdivision has been obtained. The fineness of pharmaceutical powders is expressed by the *U.S.P.* in terms of a precise range. It is interesting to note that the classification of powder by fineness is different for chemical and for vegetable and animal drugs.

All dosage forms must be uniform to ensure that the proper dose of medication is given to the patient. Blending of the various ingredients is most readily accomplished when each ingredient is in powdered form before mixing. V-blenders, double conical and ribbon blenders are used in pharmaceutical industry to blend tons of powders. The dispensing pharmacist utilizes mortar and pestle and sieves to mix a prescription intimately.

After each ingredient has been pulverized and then weighed, the drug called for in the smallest amount is placed in a mortar and an equal volume of the drug next in quantity is added. The two drugs are triturated until intimately mixed. Then, twice as much of the third ingredient, again the drug next in quantity, is added and triturated. This is repeated until all drugs have been mixed. This method is known as mixing by geometric dilution. Although the use of geometric dilution is essential when a prescription contains a small amount of a potent drug, geometric dilution may well be used in all blending procedures.

POWDERS

Powders are mixtures of drugs and chemicals in a dry, fine state of subdivision. Powders are compounded as bulk powders and as divided powders (chartulae). They are used internally or externally. There are powders for preparing douches, dusting and dental powders, and there are insufflations to be blown into body cavities.

Powders have certain inherent advantages. The small particle size of powders permits greater and more rapid dispersion of drugs than do drugs given in compacted form. Capsules and tablets containing very soluble drugs, such as chloral hydrate, bromides and iodides, often irritate the gastrointestinal tract locally. Irritation and nausea are caused by the high concentration of drug in contact with a small portion of the stomach mucosa.[8,20,36] The more rapid diffusion of powders lessens local irritation.

Powders give the physician free choice of drugs, dose and bulk. While many dosage forms are prefabricated, it would be impossible to have all combinations and strengths of drug in ready-made dosage forms. Extemporaneously prepared powders allow the physician to prescribe any combination of drugs in any dosage best for the individual patient.

Powders permit the administration of a large bulk of medicinals which would be prohibitive in size for tablets or capsules. Children and some adults have difficulty in swallowing a tablet or a capsule. For such persons, the powder form may be used to advantage. Powders are administered orally by being stirred in part of a glass of water and swallowed immediately. Some persons prefer to place the powder on the tongue and follow with a drink of water. Taste of the medicine may be improved by mixing the powder with fruit juice or honey.

Powders are not the dosage form of choice for ill-tasting drugs. Drugs which deteriorate readily on exposure to the atmosphere should not be dispensed as powders with their large surface area but in a dosage form protected from the air. Ferrous iron salts are easily oxidized and should be dispensed as a coated tablet.

Medicinal agents administered as solids must be reduced to powders and thoroughly mixed with the other ingredients to ensure uniformity, eliminate grittiness and prepare an elegant dosage form.

Mixing of coarse and fine particles results in stratification. The coarse particles collect near the top and the fine particles slip through the void spaces and collect at the bottom. For this reason, all drugs and chemicals should be reduced to approximately the same size before weighing and mixing. Even with such precautions, the particles of the greatest density tend to settle.

In the pharmacy powders are most efficiently mixed with mortar and pestle. Gentle trituration produces a light, fluffy powder. Heavy and prolonged trituration reduces granules and crystals to a fine powder or changes a bulky powder to a more compact one. Heavy trituration causes undesirable caking of resinous vegetable powders. Routine sifting is excellent to ensure the proper mixing and reduction of particle size.

When a prescription contains a potent drug, it is especially important that a uniform powder be prepared.

1. ℞
   Belladonna extract 0.5
   Phenobarbital 0.4
   Bismuth subnitrate 24.0
   Kaolin 45.0
   Peppermint oil 0.12

   Sig.: ℥ i a.c. until diarrhea has subsided.

The belladonna extract, the phenobarbital and the peppermint oil are triturated in a porcelain mortar until the mixture is homogeneous. One, 2, 4 and 8 Gm. of bismuth subnitrate are added in sequence with trituration after each addition. The remainder of the bismuth subnitrate and 10 Gm. of kaolin are added and triturated until the mixture is homogeneous. On the addition of and trituration with the remainder of the kaolin, a uniform powder is obtained.

2. ℞
   Hard soap   50
   Precipitated calcium carbonate   935
   Saccharin sodium   2

Peppermint oil	4
Cinnamon oil	2
Methyl salicylate	8

Sig.: N. F. Tooth Powder.

The saccharin sodium, the oils and the methyl salicylate are blended with about one half of the precipitated calcium carbonate. The soap is mixed with the remainder of the precipitated calcium carbonate. The two powders are mixed thoroughly and passed through a fine sieve.

No mixing procedure is universal. Each prescription must be considered as an individual challenge. The method and the order of mixing is determined by the chemical and the physical properties of the ingredients and the intent of the physician.

BULK POWDERS

Bulk powders are restricted to those powders that are nonpotent and can be measured safely in a spoon by the patient. Antacids, laxatives or powders for the preparation of douches fall in this category.

The usual containers for bulk powders are pasteboard boxes or wide-mouth, screw-cap glass jars. The opening should be large enough for convenient use of a spoon. Bottles are preferred in order to protect the prescription from moisture and to retard the loss of volatile components. Powders for external use should be dispensed with EXTERNAL USE labels.

3. ℞

Bismuth subcarbonate	
Calcium carbonate	
Light magnesium oxide, aa	30
Peppermint oil	0.1
Sodium bicarbonate q. s.	180

M. ft. powder.

Sig.: Take as directed (Alkaline Powder)

4. ℞

Magnesium carbonate	12
Bismuth subcarbonate	3
Calcium carbonate	9
Sodium bicarbonate	30
Taka-Diastase	2

Sig.: ℥ i in H_2O t. i. d.

DUSTING POWDERS

A single therapeutic agent may be a medicated dusting powder, but, more often, a base is used as a means to apply a therapeutic agent and maintain it in contact with the skin. Aluminum stearate, kaolin, magnesium stearate, zinc oxide and zinc stearate impart adhesiveness to a powder. Zinc stearate, starch and talc impart an easy flow to powders so that they spread uniformly.

Dusting powders are applied to intertriginous areas as a covering which protects the skin from the chafing of friction and moisture. Vehicles such as bentonite, kaolin, kieselguhr, magnesium carbonate and starch absorb secretions with a resultant drying action that relieves congestion and imparts a cooling effect. The cooling effect is due to the greatly increased surface for evaporation and radiation of heat.

Dusting powders possess the characteristics of all properly prepared powders. Dusting powders are generally for dermatologic use, but they are sometimes applied to wounds and mucous membranes. Since dusting powders are applied to traumatic areas, they must be grit-free. All extemporaneous dusting powders should be passed through a 100-mesh sieve. Dusting powders are dispensed in sifter-top cans or boxes with appropriate directions and auxiliary labels.

5. ℞

Boric acid	6
Starch	10
Salicylic acid	2
Talc	78

Sig.: Apply to feet morning and night.

The salicylic acid is triturated to a fine powder in a porcelain mortar. The correct weight of salicylic acid is triturated with the boric acid until the mixture is homogeneous. The starch and approximately one third of the talc are added and triturated. The remainder of the talc is added and, after trituration, the blend is passed through a 100-mesh sieve. The foot powder is dispensed in a sifter-top can.

6. ℞

| Paraformalin | 3 |
| Talc | 60 |

Sig.: Apply to feet h. s.

7. ℞
   Acetarsone   4
   Kaolin   14
   Sodium bicarbonate   14

   M. Dusting Powder

   Sig.: Sprinkle on affected area.

8. ℞
   Tannic acid   10
   Bismuth tribromphenate   10
   Powdered boric acid   30

   Sig.: Use as directed.

9. ℞
   Boric acid
   Sulfathiazole, aa   60

   Sig.: Use as a dusting powder.

10. ℞
    Zinc oxide   2
    Calamine   30
    Starch 1.5

    M. Dusting Powder

    Sig.: Apply to feet h. s.

11. ℞
    Talc
    Starch, aa   30
    Lavender oil q. s.

    Sig.: Use on moist areas.

12. ℞
    D. D. T. Powder 10%
    Talc, q. s.   120

    Sig.: Apply locally b. i. d.

13. ℞
    Menthol 0.2
    Camphor 0.5
    Zinc oxide 5.0
    Talc
    Starch, aa q. s.   60

    Sig.: Apply to affected areas p. r. n.

14. ℞
    Menthol 0.25
    Thymol 0.25
    Monobasic sodium phosphate . .   5.0
    Magnesium carbonate 5.0
    Talc, q. s.   100

    Sig.: Apply as foot powder.

DOUCHE POWDERS

In community pharmacy douches are limited to aqueous solutions for irrigation of the vaginal tract. In general, the pH ranges from 3.5 to 5. Douche solutions for the vagina are introduced by means of a suitable rubber syringe with a specially designed nozzle. Frequently, the physician prescribes an individual formula as a powder such that one teaspoonful dissolved by the patient in a specified volume of water provides the desired concentration of drugs.

Aromatics such as methyl salicylate, peppermint oil, thymol, menthol and eucalyptol are often present in douche powders for their fragrance, freshness and possible antiseptic action. Deodorization is effected by peroxides and perborates. Alums, tannic acid, zinc sulfate and zinc phenosulfonate are used as astringents.

15. ℞
    Powdered alum
    Zinc oxide, aa   30
    Oil of peppermint   1

    Sig.: Use ℥ i in 1 qt. H_2O as a douche.

16. ℞
    Lead acetate
    Powdered borax, aa   60

    Sig.: Alkaline Douche: use as directed.

17. ℞
    Citric acid   10
    Lactose   20
    Zinc sulfate   10
    Ammonia alum   10
    Dried magnesium sulfate   10

    Sig.: Use as douche ut dict.

18. ℞
    Aluminum acetate
    Boric acid, aa   30

    Sig.: One tablespoonful in 1 qt. H_2O. Use as douche q. P.M.

19. ℞
    Boric acid powder   15
    Tannic acid   15
    Peppermint oil 0.1

    Sig.: ℥ i in 1 qt. H_2O as a douche.

INSUFFLATIONS

Occasionally, finely divided powders are introduced into cavities such as tooth sockets, ears, nose, vagina and the throat. The powder is placed in the chamber of an insufflator, and, when the bulb is pressed, the air current carries the fine particles through the nozzle to the area for which the medication is intended.

Disadvantages of the insufflator are the difficulty of obtaining a uniform dosage and the tendency of the particles to stick to each other and the walls of the insufflator because of electrostatic attraction. The newer aerosols have overcome these difficulties and have largely replaced the insufflator (see Chap. 8).

20. ℞

    Tricofuron Vaginal Powder ... 15

    Sig.: ut dict.

21. ℞

    Vioform Insufflate 30

    Sig.: Cleanse before insufflation.

22. ℞

    Floraquin Powder 30

    Sig.: Use as insufflation b. i. d.

23. ℞

    Norisodrine cartridges 10%

    Dispense Aerohaler and 12 cartridges

    Sig.: Inhale at start of asthmatic attack

24. ℞

    Penicillin Inhaler with 3 cartridges.

    Sig.: Inhale orally as directed.

DIVIDED POWDERS

The procedure for mixing the ingredients in the usual prescription for divided powders differs in no manner from that followed, and previously described, whenever dry substances are to be mixed by the pharmacist. Briefly, all drugs are reduced to a fine state of subdivision before weighing. The weighed powders are blended by geometric dilution or by mixing in ascending order of amount.

The reason for dividing the prescription into individual doses is to present the patient with an accurate dose; therefore, the powder to be dispensed in each paper is weighed separately. Because of variation in weights of powder papers, a pair of counterbalanced weighing papers are used and each weighed portion of the powder is transferred to the paper in which it is to be wrapped.

Loss of material during compounding may make the last powder deficient in weight. To compensate for the loss of material, the ingredients for one powder more than the number prescribed may be prepared if the drugs are neither expensive nor narcotic drugs. A meticulous pharmacist will not find this procedure necessary. Generally ± 5 per cent has been accepted as a reasonable error permissible in compounded prescriptions.

There are three types of powder papers marketed. Vegetable parchment and glassine are relatively impermeable and water repellent. They are used for volatile and hygroscopic substances. Lightweight bond paper is commonly used although it is not moisture-proof.

Hygroscopic and volatile drugs should be double-wrapped with a paraffin and a bond paper. A pharmacist may have his name printed on the bond paper so it appears on the top of the paper after the paper is folded.

Colored papers, such as used in Seidlitz powders, are used to distinguish powders. Colored papers are not readily available and often must be cut by the pharmacist.

Powder papers are available in a number of sizes designated by numbers, but, unfortunately, there is no standardized numbering system. The correct size of paper depends on the amount of powder to be dispensed and the size of the powder box. The most popular sizes are 2¾ x 3¾ inches, 3 x 4½ inches, 3¾ x 5 inches, and 4½ x 6 inches.

With a little practice the traditional way of folding powders provides a neat dosage form.

1. Fold over approximately ½ inch of the long edge of the paper. This fold will be the top of the finished powder paper. Several papers should be folded at once to save time and to obtain a uniform fold.

2. With the folds distal, lay the powder papers side by side so they overlap slightly.

3. Place the weighed powder in the center of each paper.

4. Bring the lower edge up and fit it into the top fold. (Care should be taken to avoid powder in the fold or beyond it.)

5. Pull the top fold toward you until it divides the remainder of the paper approximately in half.

6. Pick up the folded paper with the thumb and index finger of each hand and fold the ends over a powder box so that the finished paper will just fit into the box. The ends of the paper should be folded uniformly. Press the end folds firmly with a spatula to produce sharp creases. The spatula should not be passed over the full length of the folded paper as this tends to cause some powdered material to cake and it ruins the appearance of the papers by flattening the rolled edges.

Divided powders are dispensed in hinged-cover cardboard boxes with the label pasted inside the cover. The most common practice is to face all powder papers in the same direction with the top fold uppermost. A second method is to alternate the powders by placing half of them with the top folds upward and half with the top folds downward. This method does not result in as neat an appearance but it permits the fitting of more divided powders into a box.

The hinged-cover box presents a better appearance than the outmoded telescope powder box. With the hinged-cover box, the label is an integral part of the prescription, and the hinged-cover box eliminates the possibility of the accidental interchange with the lid from another box.

The shouldered box is made so that the folded powders project slightly above the edges of the base without being crushed when the cover is closed. By so projecting, a powder may be easily removed from the box.

Cellophane or plastic envelopes may be used instead of powder papers for enclosing the individual dose. Cellophane envelopes, which are made of seamed cellophane tubing, have a closed and an open end. The correct weight of medicament is placed into the cellophane envelope using the weighing paper as a funnel and taking care that no powder collects at the opening of the envelope. As the envelopes are filled they are set upright. The open end of the filled envelope is folded over approximately ½ inch and is creased sharply. The folded envelope is laid on a pill tile and it is sealed by passing a heated spatula over the creased end. Since the envelopes are too wide to be placed on edge in an ordinary powder box, they are dispensed by stacking them one on top of another in the box.

Packaging in cellophane envelopes takes less time than traditional powder folding and makes differences in skill between pharmacists less apparent. Dispensing hygroscopic drugs in cellophane envelopes protects them from atmospheric moisture.

25. ℞
Potassium acetate 1.0

M. Ft. Chart. tales No. XV.

Sig.: One powder t. i. d.

Potassium acetate is a deliquescent substance. It is usually recommended that potassium acetate be dispensed in a liquid form such as an elixir. If the physician insists on a solid dosage form, the dried potassium acetate may be sealed in cellophane envelopes. The powder will remain dry for two weeks.

26. ℞
Sodium sulfocyanate 0.3

Make 30 powders

Sig.: One three times daily.

Sodium sulfocyanate is hygroscopic and it is normally administered as an elixir. If the dried sodium sulfocyanate is sealed in cellophane envelopes, the powder remains dry for several months.

27. ℞
Acetophenetidine 4.0
Acid acetylsalicylic 7.5

M. ft. chart. #24

Sig.: One q. 4 hr. in milk.

28. ℞
Acetanilid 0.10
Caffeine citrate 0.03
Sodium bicarbonate 0.20

D. T. D. #12

Sig.: Headache powders.

29. ℞
Extract of belladonna 0.02
Bismuth subcarbonate 0.60
Sodium bicarbonate 0.30

Tales Chart #1. Dispense XXIV

Sig.: One p. r. n.

TABLE 3-1. SPECIALTY NAMES OF SOLIDS IN POWDERED FORM

SPECIALTY	COMPANY	DESCRIPTION
Duchette	Purdue Frederick	Individual packette of douche powder
Envule	Glenwood	Sealed container of powdered drug
Niphanoid	Winthrop	Instantly soluble dry powder
Spersoid	Lederle	Soluble or dispersible powder
Sterap	Lilly	Sterile powder in envelope for topical use
Sterilope	Abbott	Sterile powder in envelope for topical use

30. ℞
    Bismuth subcarbonate 0.30
    Bismuth subgallate 0.30
    Powdered opium 0.06

    Make powders # 30

    Sig.: One powder as directed.

31. ℞
    Menthol 0.4
    Salicylic acid 2
    Sodium chloride 60
    Zinc sulfate 65
    Alum 65
    Boric acid q. s. 500

    Ft. Chart. No. XV

    Sig.: Ut dict.

GRANULES

Granulated medication consists of small irregular particles ranging from 4-mesh to 10-mesh size. Granules are measured by a teaspoon, and, as the patient does the measuring, granules seldom are used for potent medicaments. Granules may be dietary supplements such as Somagen. Pasara Calcium Granulate and Aureomycin Spersoids are examples of medicinal granules to be taken by the spoonful. Some products such as Panalba KM and Sugracillin Flavored Granules exist as granules which are to be suspended in water by the pharmacist before the prescription is dispensed to the patient.

Effervescent granulations are mixtures of medicinal agents with citric acid, tartaric acid or sodium biphosphate and a bicarbonate. They are dissolved in water and taken immediately after effervescence subsides. The carbonated solution is a pleasant vehicle for bitter and saline salts such as magnesium sulfate. Observation of the effervescence may be of some psychological benefit to the patient.

The evolution of carbon dioxide occurs very rapidly when the granules are added to water. If powders were added, the violent effervescence would spill the solution from the container. The granules are made to retard solution and effervescence. With the larger sized granule, effervescence is slower and less violent. The rapidity of solution also depends on the temperature of the water. The slow reaction in cold water results in a more complete carbonation.

The two methods for the preparation of effervescent granulations are the fusion method and the wet method. In the fusion method, the blended powders are moistened by heating in an oven or over a water bath. The wet method consists of moistening the mixed powders with some nonsolvent moistening agent. In both methods, the moistened mass is passed through a sieve and the granules are dried at low temperatures before packaging. For detailed process and formulations the reader may consult *American Pharmacy.**

32. ℞
    Magnesium sulfate 50
    Sodium bicarbonate 40
    Tartaric acid 21
    Citric acid 14

    Sig.: One tablespoonful in water.

The uneffloresced crystals of citric acid are powdered and mixed intimately with the

* Sprowls, J. B.: American Pharmacy. 6th ed. Philadelphia, J. B. Lippincott, 1966.

magnesium sulfate and the dry, powdered sodium bicarbonate and tartaric acid. The mixed powders are placed on a plate of glass or in a suitable dish in an oven previously heated to approximately 100°C. The mixture is carefully blended and, when it becomes moist, it is rapidly rubbed through a 6-mesh sieve. The granules are immediately dried at 50°C.

The pharmacist rarely has occasion to prepare effervescent granules, but he does dispense specialty products such as Citrocarbonate, Bromo Seltzer and Sal Hepatica.

Granules are dispensed in wide-mouth bottles which permit the entrance of a spoon. Effervescent granules must be packaged in a tight container which excludes air and moisture.

33. ℞
   Citrocarbonate 240

   Sig.: Two teaspoonfuls in glass of water p. c.

34. ℞
   Bassoran granules 200

   Sig.: One or two teaspoonfuls with a large glassful of water b. i. d.

35. ℞
   Senokot 60

   Sig.: Tablespoon h. s. for normal bowel function.

36. ℞
   Siblin . . . . 1 lb.

   Sig.: Two teaspoonfuls in 8 oz. water h. s.

37. ℞
   Bromionyl with barbital 60

   Sig.: Use as directed.

CAPSULES

Capsules are gelatin shells to be filled with an individual dose of powdered and mixed ingredients of a prescription. Capsules can be filled with dry materials, semisolids and liquids that are nonsolvents of gelatin.

Capsules are so familiar a dosage to the physician that it may not occur to him that they are novel to some laymen; yet, nearly every pharmacist of long experience has had empty capsules returned to him for refill. It is neither wise nor necessary for a pharmacist to volunteer advice on administration of every dosage form, but, if he has reason to believe that the customer does not understand the intention of the physician, it is his duty tactfully and inoffensively to make the customer understand. Few persons have difficulty in swallowing a capsule if the capsule is placed on the tongue and swallowed with a drink of water.

On occasion, capsules may be administered rectally or vaginally. When so used, they should be dipped in warm water to facilitate insertion. The physician may desire the contents of a capsule to be dissolved in water to make a solution.

An important function of capsules is to eliminate the taste and the odor of drugs by enclosing the ingredients in an almost tasteless shell which will release the medication in the stomach within 5 minutes.

The flexibility from the viewpoint of the prescriber is restricted only by the bulk of the medication. Even this disadvantage may be overcome easily by administering several capsules when the bulk prescribed is too great to fill a conveniently swallowed capsule.

Capsules cannot be used with substances that react with or dissolve gelatin. Highly soluble drugs administered in capsules form concentrated solutions that irritate the stomach mucosa.

EXTEMPORANEOUS CAPSULES

Hard gelatin capsules are thin shells of gelatin. Each consists of a base and a shorter cap which fits firmly over the base of the capsule. For human consumption 8 sizes are available. The variation in densities of drugs and the wide combinations of drugs used in prescriptions make it impossible to state the capacity of each size in other than approximate terms. The manufacturer attempts to do this by tables printed on the capsule box. As an initial guide for the student, the capacities of capsules in terms of aspirin are given below.

$$
\begin{array}{rl}
000 - & 1,000 \text{ mg.} \\
00 - & 600 \text{ mg.} \\
0 - & 500 \text{ mg.} \\
1 - & 300 \text{ mg.} \\
2 - & 250 \text{ mg.} \\
3 - & 200 \text{ mg.} \\
4 - & 125 \text{ mg.} \\
5 - & 60 \text{ mg.}
\end{array}
$$

Three sizes of veterinary capsules are available. They are Nos. 10, 11 and 12. Their approximate capacities are 30, 15 and 7.5 Gm., respectively.

In addition to the common colorless capsule, there are a variety of colored capsules available. Ordinarily only the pink and the colorless capsule are available to the community pharmacist unless a special order is placed with a capsule manufacturer.

The pink capsules are used to differentiate between two capsule prescriptions for the same person. Colored capsules are used to encapsulate ingredients that would appear unattractive in a colorless capsule. The color and the size of the capsule used should be noted on the prescription to assist in compounding refills.

Capsules are stable under ordinary conditions, but they absorb moisture and soften under high humidity. A dry atmosphere may cause them to become brittle and crack when being filled. In the pharmacy it is advisable to store the empty capsules in glass containers in which they will be protected from dust and extremes of humidity.

Solids for use in capsules are prepared in the manner presented in the discussion of powders. The ingredients are reduced by trituration to about the same particle size and then mixed by geometric dilution.

In selecting the proper size of capsule it may be necessary to weigh one dose and to ascertain by trial the proper size. Since many persons find it difficult to swallow large capsules, the pharmacist selects the smallest capsule that will conveniently hold the prescribed dose. The finished capsule should be filled so that no air spaces are visible within the capsule. When the size has been selected, the required number of capsules should be removed from the container, for their removal singly during the filling process might result in the contamination of the remaining capsules.

In filling capsules, as in all pharmaceutical operations, accuracy and cleanliness must be kept in mind. Each capsules is weighed separately because a capsule is to provide an accurate dose of medication.

The powder to be encapsulated is placed on a paper and pressed down with a spatula until the depth is approximately one third the length of the capsule body. The empty capsule base is held between the thumb and the index finger and is repeatedly pressed vertically into the powder until filled. The cap is fitted over the base and the filled capsule is weighed using an empty capsule of the same size as the tare. An empty capsule may be used as a tare because the empty capsule weighs little compared with the filled capsule; thus only a small error is introduced due to variation in weight of the capsule. If the weight is not accurate, it is adjusted by again pressing more powder into the base or by removing a portion of the contents. Certain powders pack so poorly that the base must be held horizontally and the powder pushed into it by a spatula.

The attraction of gelatin for moisture requires the pharmacist to observe care in handling a capsule. A trace of moisture on the capsule causes a sticky surface to which dry material adheres. The best method of protecting the capsule from moisture and finger prints is to wear finger cots or rubber gloves.

Before compounding in the prescription area, a pharmacist should wash his hands. Clean hands are especially important when the dosage form is manually touched. With open prescription departments, the patron is able to observe the compounding of his prescription. It enhances the public image of the pharmacist when the patient sees the pharmacist washing his hands, wearing finger cots and compounding under sanitary conditions.

Another method by which capsules may be kept free from moisture during compounding is to wash the hands thoroughly, dry them and keep the fingers dry by friction against a towel before each capsule is handled. The towel should be stripped through the clenched fingers until a clearly perceptible heat is felt.

A third method is to use the base of one capsule as a holder for other bases during the filling procedure. This minimizes contact of the fingers with the capsules.

Regardless of how careful the filling operation has been, some traces of material will be found on the outside of the filled capsule. This may be removed by rolling the capsule between the folds of a cloth or by shaking

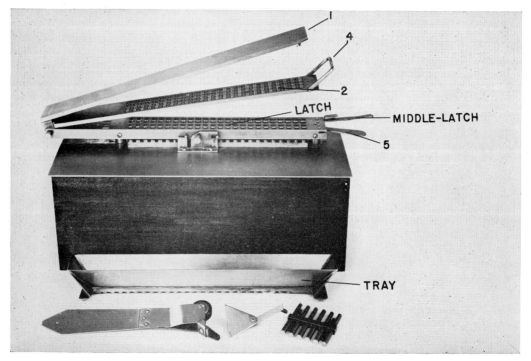

FIG. 3-3.   A hand-operated capsule-filling machine with a capacity of 24 capsules. (Universal Model. Chemi Pharm, 90 W. Broadway, New York, N. Y.)

them in a cloth which has been gathered into the form of a bag.

A few hand operated capsule filling machines have been marketed; one is shown in Figure 3-3. If a large number of capsules are to be made, such a machine saves a considerable amount of time.

Occasional prescriptions are received for viscid or semisolid substances or a combination of dry and liquid substances to be encapsulated. Usually a plastic mass is formed and rolled into a cylinder which is cut into the proper number of segments. The segments should be slightly longer than the capsule so that the ends of the capsule are filled.

Gelatin is not soluble in alcohol, fixed oils and volatile oils. These liquids may be dispensed in hard gelatin capsules. The empty capsule bases are supported by a box in which holes have been punched. A calibrated dropper or pipet is used to deliver the prescribed volume into each capsule base. Care should be taken to ensure that none of the liquid touches the edge of the capsule, since its presence will interfere with proper sealing. As an added precaution to ensure sealing, the capsule chosen should be of such a size that the liquid does not quite fill the base.

In filling capsules with a liquid having a disagreeable odor or taste, particular care must be taken to make certain none of the liquid remains on the outside of the capsule. If the capsules are contaminated in the filling process, they should be washed with alcohol before being dispensed.

When all the bases have been filled, each capsule is sealed by moistening the lower portion of the inside of the cap with water, fitting it over the base, and giving it a half turn. A small applicator or a camel's hair brush dipped in warm water provides a convenient way of moistening the caps; cotton or filter paper should not be used, as they tend to leave lint on the capsule. After the capsules have been sealed, they should be placed on a sheet of paper, where they are allowed to remain for an hour before they are dispensed. This is done to detect poor seals and leakage.

Capsules are dispensed in plastic or glass vials. Vials are more easily portable and protect the capsules better than do paper boxes.

If the vial is of clear glass or plastic, the label may be placed inside the container (where regulations permit), thus preventing it from becoming soiled. A pledget of cotton is placed on top of the capsules to keep them from rattling.

38. ℞

Acetylsalicylic acid	5.0
Phenacetin	3.0
Caffeine	1.0
Codeine phosphate	0.2

M. et Ft. Caps. XX

Sig.: One q. 3 hr.

39. ℞

Cerium oxalate	0.2
Phenobarbital	0.015
Pepsin scales	0.4

Disp. tales #40 capsules

Sig.: One capsule t. i. d. p. c.

40. ℞

| Benzocaine | 0.50 |
| Phenobarbital | 0.05 |

M. ft. D. T. D. # 12 capsules

Sig.: One ut dict.

41. ℞

Codeine phosphate	0.03
Cerium oxalate	0.10
Bismuth subcarbonate	0.20

Ft. tales caps. No. XXX

Sig.: One capsule ½ hr. before meals.

42. ℞

Papaverine hydrochloride	0.06
Aminophyllin	0.10
Sodium phenobarbital	0.15
Nitroglycerin	0.0003

D. T. D. Caps. No. 30

Sig.: One Q. I. D.

43. ℞

Phenobarbital	20
Papaverine hydrochloride	15
Belladonna extract	10

Tales Caps. No. LX

Sig.: One capsule a. c. and h. s.

44. ℞

| Quinine sulfate | 0.6 |
| Calcium lactate q. s. | 10 |

Disp. as placebo. Misce and fill capsules 3 grs.

Dispense #12.

Sig.: One h. s. p. r. n. for sleep.

45. ℞

Desoxyn	2.5 mg.
Thyroid powder	8.0 mg.
Lactose q. s.	

Give 100.

Sig.: One capsule t. i. d. 30 min. a. c.

46. ℞

| Nembutal | 0.050 |
| Phenergan | 0.025 |

Tales Caps. #12

Sig.: One t. i. d. p. r. n. pain.

ELASTIC CAPSULES

Industrially prepared capsules filled with a liquid, a suspension or a powder are known as elastic capsules. Elastic capsules are manufactured by a continuous operation that forms and fills the capsules. Warm, molten gelatin is fed by gravity through a spreader into a metal drum. The gelatin is spread on the rotating drum forming uniform ribbons of gelatin. The ribbons of gelatin converge between rotary dies surmounted by an injection apparatus. The fill is metered under pressure just as the capsule is formed. As the dies continue to rotate, the capsules are sealed and cut from the ribbons.

47. ℞

| Somnos | 0.5 |

Caps. No. 30.

Sig.: One an hour before retiring.

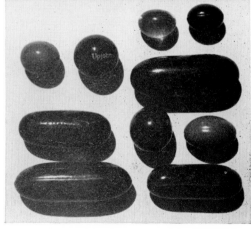

FiG. 3-4. Typical examples of elastic gelatin capsules.

TABLE 3-2. SPECIALTY NAMES OF CAPSULES

SPECIALTY	COMPANY	DESCRIPTION
Capseal	Rocky Mountain Pharmacal	sealed capsule
Cap-So-Loid	Wendt-Bristol	capsule
Clipsule	Lederle	squeezable gelatin capsule convenient for administration to children
Gelseal	Eli Lilly	sealed, elastic gelatin capsule
Hypoglossal	Carnrick Laboratories	buccal or sublingual capsule
Kapseal	Parke, Davis	banded, hard gelatin capsule
Koff-Ball	Lloyd Bros.	chewable gelatin capsule containing liquid medication
Perlette	Philadelphia Laboratories	small elastic capsule
Pulvo-Cap	Pitman-Moore	dry-filled capsule
Pulvule	Eli Lilly	dry-filled, hard gelatin capsule
Radiocap	Abbott Laboratories	hard gelatin capsule containing a radioactive isotope
Spheroid	S. J. Tutag	capsule
Solu-Cap	Sutliff & Case	dry-filled, gelatin capsule

48. ℞

    Multicebrin 100

    Sig.: One with meals.

49. ℞

    Diethylstilbestrol Perles   5   mg.

    Give dozen.

    Sig.: One t. i. d. for 4 days.

50. ℞

    Placidyl 500   mg.

    Caps. No. 30

    Sig.: One h. s.

51. ℞

    Dilantin in oil 0.1

    Dispense 100

    Sig.: One t. i. d.

52. ℞

    Heptuna Plus 100

    Sig.: Two daily.

EFFECT OF PROPERTIES OF DRUGS ON COMPOUNDING TECHNICS

Nearly all substances dispensed in the solid dosage form are dry and stable under ordinary conditions. Compounding and dispensing problems and incompatibilities are encountered less frequently in solid than in liquid preparations; nevertheless, some prescriptions require special compounding procedures and modes of dispensing because of the properties of the drugs.

POTENCY OF THE DRUG

Potent drugs that have doses too small to be weighed on a Class A prescription balance are diluted with an inert powder and an aliquot amount is used. Ordinarily, lactose is used for this purpose. The aliquot method is discussed in Chapter 1. In diluting a potent drug it is advisable to add the drug to some of the diluent in a mortar, after which the remainder of the diluent is added by geometric dilution. By this technic, there is little loss of drug by adhesion to the mortar.

Divided powders weighing less than 250 mg. are inconvenient to administer. If the patient spills a small amount of the powder, the loss is an appreciable part of the intended dose and constitutes a serious underdose of drug. For this reason, lactose is added to drugs of small doses to increase the bulk of the contents of divided powders or cellophane envelopes to a bulk which can be easily handled by the consumer.

53. ℞
    Neostigmine bromide 0.015
    Atropine sulfate 0.0004

D. T. D. Charts. No. XXV

Sig.: One t. i. d. a. c.

A total of 10 mg. of atropine sulfate is required for 25 powders. This is obtained by weighing 1.00 Gm. of a 1:100 trituration of atropine sulfate with lactose. The atropine sulfate and the neostigmine bromide are blended by geometric dilution. To increase the bulk, 195 mg. of lactose is added per powder so that each powder weighs 250 mg.

Potent drugs to be placed in capsules are diluted with lactose to a bulk which is conveniently manipulated by the compounding pharmacist. Some pharmacists find it difficult to handle a No. 5 capsule and prefer to use, by the addition of a diluent, Nos. 3, 2 and 1, which are convenient for both the patient and the pharmacist.

54. ℞
    Papaverine hydrochloride ...... gr. ¼
    Phenobarbital .... gr. ⅓
    Belladonna extract .... gr. ⅛

Give 24 caps.

Sig.: One or two capsules p. r. n.

The total weight of drugs in each capsule is 17/24 gr. This is too small a bulk to be conveniently handled by the pharmacist and will not completely fill a capsule. If the pharmacist adds 2 7/24 gr. of lactose per capsule or 55 gr. for 24 capsules, each capsule will contain 3 gr. which can readily fill a No. 3 capsule.

In some prescriptions, volatile solvents may be used to obtain an even distribution of a potent drug.

55. ℞
    Iodine 0.5
    Boric acid q. s. 30

Sig.: Insufflate as directed.

The iodine is dissolved in a volatile solvent. Alcohol, benzene, chloroform and ether are suitable volatile solvents. The solution of iodine is added gradually to the powdered boric acid in a glass mortar with trituration until the solvent has evaporated. Contact with metal should be avoided. Due to the volatility of the iodine, the powder should be packaged in an airtight glass container with a plastic cap.

INCORPORATION OF LIQUIDS

A small volume of a liquid may be triturated with an equal volume of powder, and the remaining powder added in portions with trituration. With the exception of flavoring oils, the majority of liquids found in extemporaneous prescriptions for solid dosage forms are tinctures or fluidextracts. It is within the province of the pharmacist to replace, without consulting the physician, one of these liquids with an equivalent amount of the corresponding extract.

56. ℞
    Belladonna tincture .... 0.6 ml.
    Acetylsalicylic acid .... 300 mg.

M. Disp. Cap. tales no. x

Sig.: One capsule as directed.

Belladonna tincture contains in each 100 ml. 0.03 Gm. of the alkaloids of belladonna; belladonna extract contains in each 100 Gm. 1.2 Gm. of the alkaloids. The extract is 40 times the strength of the tincture, and the 6 ml. of tincture prescribed may be replaced with 0.15 Gm. of the extract.

If the extract is not available, the liquid may be concentrated to a small volume and lactose added before evaporating to dryness. Lactose acts as an adsorbent on the surface of which the residue precipitates, consequently avoiding a sticky residue when evaporation is complete.

57. ℞
    Hydrastis fluidextract
    Bismuth subnitrate
    Sodium bicarbonate, aa 15

M. et div. in chart. no. x

Sig.: Take 1 powder, mixed with water, after each meal.

The fluidextract must be evaporated, since the amount of dry material prescribed is too great to permit the addition of sufficient inert substance to adsorb the large volume of liquid. The fluidextract is evaporated on a

TABLE 3-3. VAPOR PRESSURE OF SOME
VOLATILE PHARMACEUTICALS

COMPOUND	VAPOR PRESSURE (in mm. of Mercury)	TEMPERATURE (degrees centigrade)
Acetophenone	0.213	25
2-Aminoheptane	5.81	26
Camphor	0.55	23.4
Iodine	0.202	20
Menthol	0.94	28.4
Naphthalene	0.082	25
Paraformaldehyde	10	24
Phenol	1	44.8
Phosphorus, white	0.025	20

water bath, at a temperature not exceeding 70°C., to a syrupy consistency. Lactose is added and the heat continued until a dry powder is formed. This is then intimately blended with the other ingredients of the prescription.

If an extract is not available, a small volume of a liquid may be adsorbed on the other ingredients.

58. ℞
    Calcium carbonate
    Bismuth subcarbonate
    Sodium bicarbonate, aa 15
    Peppermint spirit   8

    M. et div. in chart. no. xxiv

    Sig.: One powder after meals.

There is sufficient dry material to adsorb the peppermint oil which remains after the evaporation of the volatile alcohol.

The technic selected depends on the relative amounts of the liquid present. Evaporation should be used as a last resort, since it is usually attended by a significant loss of material.

VOLATILITY

Volatility is the tendency to enter the vapor phase. Volatility is roughly proportional to the vapor pressure and inversely proportional to the boiling point. To volatilize, a solid must have an appreciable vapor pressure below its melting point.

At a given temperature the vapor pressure of a solid is indicative of its volatility. Only a few solids have a high enough vapor pressure to sublime at atmospheric pressure. Volatilization is immeasurably slow if the vapor pressure of a crystal is low. The rate of volatilization depends not only on vapor pressure but also on temperature and pressure.

The vapor pressure of some solids that are volatile in the region of room temperature are given in Table 3-3. It appears that a solid with a vapor pressure exceeding 0.1 mm. of mercury will vaporize readily.

A dosage form containing volatile substances such as camphor, iodine and menthol should be tightly sealed to minimize loss by vaporization.

Bulk powders, capsules and tablets containing volatile substances are dispensed in airtight glass containers. Divided powders should be double wrapped with an inner paraffin and a bond paper. Protection from loss is increased by use of cellophane envelopes sealed with heat.

59. ℞
    Phenacetin
    Quinine, aa 0.065
    Sodium salicylate 0.10
    Powdered capsicum 0.008
    Peppermint oil 0.20

    M. ft. XII caps. D. T. D.

    Sig.: Ut dict for grippe.

60. ℞
    Chlorobutanol 0.2

    M. et ft. caps. No. 12

    Sig.: One capsule hourly for 3-4 doses.

61. ℞
    Camphor 0.030
    Belladonna extract 0.008
    Quinine sulfate 0.060

    M. et ft. capsules No. 24

    Sig.: One every 2 hours for 4 doses.

Industrially formulated capsules and tablets containing volatile substances are often coated to retard loss of volatile ingredients.

62. ℞
    Rhinitis (Full Strength)

    Give 12 tablets.

    Sig.: Two tablets daily.

HYDRATION

Crystal hydrates that are stable in the air between certain limits of humidity are said to contain water of crystallization.

A mixture of a saturated solution of a salt with the solid has a constant vapor pressure at a given temperature. Diagrammatically, the change of vapor pressure from pure water to pure salt is shown in Figure 3-5 for sodium nitrate.[31]

Point N corresponds to pure anhydrous sodium nitrate with zero vapor pressure. As the salt is dissolved in pure water (W) having a vapor pressure of Y, the vapor pressure of water decreases to X, where the solution is saturated with sodium nitrate corresponding to S.

P represents the vapor pressure of the saturated solution; the ratio of vapor pressure of the solution to pure water is 0.74 at 25°C. If the relative humidity of the air is higher than 0.74—for example, H—the sodium nitrate will attract water and form a saturated solution. After all of the sodium nitrate has dissolved, it will continue to absorb water until the composition of the solution (G) has the same relative vapor pressure as the atmosphere. This phenomenon is deli-quescence and occurs only when the humidity of the air is greater than the vapor pressure of the saturated salt solution.

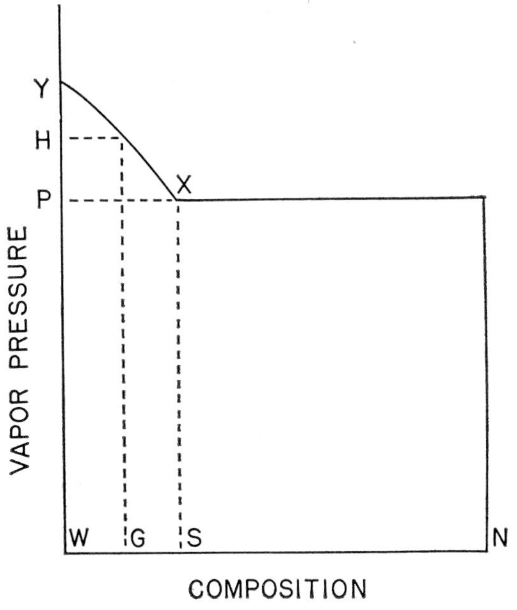

If the relative humidity of the air is less than 0.74, solid sodium nitrate remains unchanged.

Depending on the humidity, a salt hydrate may remain unchanged, deliquesce or give off water. Sodium bromide can exist as the dihydrate and as the anhydrous salt. A saturated solution of sodium bromide has a relative vapor pressure of 0.57 at 25°C. It will deliquesce when the relative humidity of the air is greater than 0.57. The dihydrate has a relative vapor pressure of 0.36 at 25°C. and therefore will give off water when the relative humidity is less than 0.36. This is called efflorescence. Sodium bromide dihydrate is stable only when the relative humidity ranges from 0.36 to 0.57 at 25°C.

The U.S.P. states that borax effloresces in dry air. The vapor pressure-composition curve shown in Figure 3-6 provides a more complete characterization of this substance. A saturated solution of borax has a relative water vapor pressure of 0.99 at 20°C.; for all practical purposes deliquescence does not occur. The relative vapor pressure of borax is 0.39 at 20°C. when it is in equilibrium with the pentahydrate. Therefore, if borax is exposed to air with a relative humidity less than 0.39, it will effloresce to the pentahydrate. The pentahydrate is stable only at relative humidities between 0.39 and 0.25; if the relative humidity becomes less than 0.25, the pentahydrate will effloresce to the anhydrous salt.

FIG. 3-5. Vapor pressure of water in a water–anhydrous salt system at constant temperature.

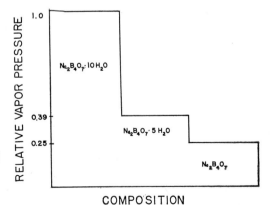

FIG. 3-6. Vapor pressure of water in a water–borax system at 20° C.

Some common crystalline drugs that liberate their water of crystallization in an atmosphere of low humidity and become powdery in appearance are atropine sulfate, scopolamine hydrobromide, terpin hydrate, zinc sulfate and the sulfate and the phosphate of codeine.

Zinc phenolsulfonate effloresces when exposed to the air. If all of the water of hydration were removed from the zinc phenolsulfonate, there would be a loss of 25 per cent of its weight. Efflorescence may alter to a practical extent the dosage of a patient. If cinchonine bisulfate effloresced all of its water of crystallization, there would be a loss of 15 per cent of its weight. Thus, a pharmacist weighing effloresced cinchonine bisulfate instead of hydrated cinchonine bisulfate would be dispensing a 15 per cent greater dose.

A solid containing water of crystallization may lose such water to a greater or less extent on trituration as a result of the heat developed. Furthermore, any occluded water held mechanically in the interior cavities of a crystal will be released as the crystals are reduced to smaller particle size.

Light trituration is recommended with sodium phosphate, sodium sulfate, alums and ferrous sulfate. The best method to ensure a dry powder is to use an equivalent amount of the anhydrous chemical. If the anhydrous chemical is not available, the hydrous form may be dried before mixing.

63. ℞
    Magnesium sulfate
    Sodium sulfate
    Sodium potassium tartrate, aa 15
    Sig.: Heaping teaspoonful in half a cup of hot water night and morning.

On triturating and mixing the three salts a pasty mass is formed. A satisfactory powder could be prepared by using equivalent amounts of the anhydrous form of the salts. The prescription should be dispensed in a tight glass container.

64. ℞
    Sodium salicylate 6.0
    Sodium sulfate 6.0
    Sodium bicarbonate 3.0
    Potassium bitartrate 6.0
    M. ft. Chart. # XX
    Sig.: Take one q. i. d. a. c. & bedtime.

HYGROSCOPICITY

Solids exposed to the atmosphere generally adsorb some water vapor on their surfaces. This is called water of hygroscopicity. It increases with an increase in surface area and humidity.[45,56] The relation between the amount adsorbed and the water vapor pressure is given by an adsorption isotherm. Adsorption is relatively large at small pressures and changes rapidly with vapor pressure change.

A polar molecule such as water is strongly attracted by ions or polar molecules on the surface of a crystal lattice and held firmly by dipole-ion or dipole-dipole interaction, respectively.

Colloidal substances such as cellulose, starch, agar and gelatin adsorb large amounts of water and retain the appearance of dry powders. Such water is called water of imbibition. The water content varies with humidity. As shown in Figure 3-7, potato starch contains 10 per cent of water at a relative humidity of 0.20 and 21 per cent of water at a relative humidity of 0.70. Thus, if the seal is not airtight, the water content changes with the seasons.

Double-wrapped divided powders and sealed cellophane envelopes usually are sufficient to protect hygroscopic substances.

65. ℞
    Sodium bromide
    Sodium salicylate, aa 1.0

    Ft. chart. XXXVI

    Sig.: One q. i. d.

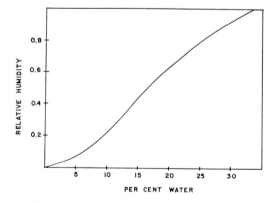

FIG. 3-7. Imbibition of water by potato starch.

66. ℞

| Phenobarbital | 0.03 |
| Ferrous sulfate | 0.30 |

M. ft. D. T. D. #12 caps.

Sig.: Uno daily.

67. ℞

Phenol

Menthol, aa	0.5
Alum	30
Boric acid q. s.	120

Sig.: ʒ i to 1 qt. hot water for douche.

An older method of dispensing hygroscopic powders in a divided powder or a capsule employs the incorporation of an inert substance that preferentially absorbs moisture. Talc, magnesium oxide, magnesium carbonate and starch have been suggested for this purpose. The divided powder is then double wrapped using an inner paraffin paper.

68. ℞

| Ferric ammonium citrate | 0.5 |

Ft. caps. tal. dos. XX

Sig.: One t. i. d.

If the ferric ammonium citrate has been exposed to the air and has absorbed moisture, it will gum up when triturated in the mortar. Dry ferric ammonium citrate may be put into capsules. If the capsules are exposed to humid air, moisture is absorbed within a week. If 60 mg. of magnesium carbonate is added per capsule, the capsule will remain dry after exposure of several weeks to the atmosphere.

The choice of inert ingredient depends on the prescription. Magnesium oxide is alkaline and, in the presence of moisture, will hydrolyze esters. If a clear solution is to be formed, an insoluble absorbent cannot be used.

69. ℞

| Ammonium bromide | 0.1 |
| Tales Chart XII | |

Sig.: Use as directed.

Ammonium bromide absorbs moisture from the air. If magnesium oxide were added, ammonia would be liberated in the presence of moisture. The dry ammonium bromide may be dispensed in the form of a divided powder if double wrapped papers or cellophane envelopes are used.

Deliquescent substances may absorb water from a capsule shell and cause it to crack. Inert absorbents of moisture will aid in maintaining a dry powder, although they are ineffective if the capsules are dispensed in a box. Capsules containing dry deliquescent and hygroscopic drugs dispensed in moisture-tight vials remain stable for long periods of time without the addition of an inert powder.

70. ℞

Sodium citrate	0.12
Calcium iodide	0.06
Guaiacol carbonate	0.03
Aspirin	0.30

Tales caps. No. 12

Sig.: One after each meal.

DEPRESSION OF MELTING POINT

The melting points of certain substances that are solids at room temperature are lowered by contact with certain other substances to the point at which liquefaction occurs. Commonly dispensed drugs exhibiting this phenomenon are acetanilid, aminopyrine, antipyrine, betanaphthol, menthol, thymol, phenol, chloral hydrate and the salicylates.

Any substance that has low intermolecular forces as indicated by low melting point, soft crystalline structure or easy sublimation will probably liquefy when triturated with a chemical of similar nature. Such compounds usually contain aldehydic, ketonic or phenolic groups.

Impurities added to a chemically pure compound will for the most part lower the melting point of that substance. If the melting points of such mixtures are high, the phenomenon offers no problem to the pharmacist. However, many drugs used in medicine have a low melting point, and, when they are mixed intimately with other drugs, the lowered mixed melting point becomes less than room temperature and the mixture liquefies.

Considering atmospheric pressure constant, the particular state that a mixture exists in is primarily a function of temperature and composition. Since pharmaceuticals are prepared to be stable and to be used at room temperature, temperature is not a variable. To the pharmacist the important factor in determining the physical state of a mixture is its composition.

From the phase diagram in Figure 3-8, the physical state of a mixture of camphor and salol can be determined. Point A is the melting point of pure salol. Along the line AO pure salol is separating from the mixture. Point B represents the melting point of pure camphor, and along BO solid camphor is separating. At O both pure salol and pure camphor exist; this is the eutectic point. At room temperature of 25°C., this binary mixture is a liquid when the camphor makes up from 15 to 50 per cent of the mixture.

71. ℞
   Camphor .... 120 mg.
   Salol .... 300 mg.

M. ft. Powder No. 6

Sig.: Use as directed.

Camphor composes 29 per cent of the prescription. At 25°C. the mixture will be a liquid. A salol-camphor prescription containing 75 per cent of camphor will be a dry powder.

Unfortunately, phase diagrams are not available for the multiplicity of combinations found in prescriptions. The physical state depends not only on the proportion of the low melting point ingredients but also on the relative proportion of the higher melting point ingredients. If a liquid is formed, there may be a sufficient quantity of higher melting point material to absorb it effectively. With the almost infinite combinations possible in medicines, it is difficult to make an accurate prediction of the physical state. The practicing pharmacist should recognize probable offenders and compound them as though a liquid would form.

If the amount of liquefying ingredients is small compared with the entire prescription, they may be mixed and the liquids taken up in the pores and on the surface of other ingredients.

72. ℞
   Salicylic acid 5.0
   Menthol 2.0
   Camphor 8.0
   Boric acid 50.0
   Starch 35.0

Sig.: Dust as directed.

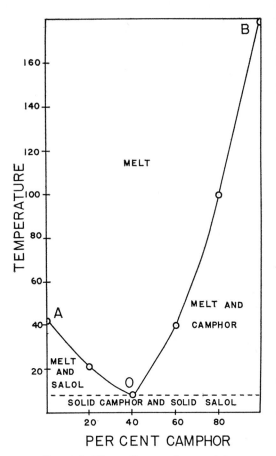

Fig. 3-8. Phase diagram for a salol-camphor mixture.

The camphor, the menthol and the salicylic acid are triturated until liquefaction occurs. The boric acid is added gradually with trituration until the liquid is absorbed. The starch is then added and triturated until the prescription is homogeneous.

If the amount of liquefying substance is large and cannot be absorbed, each of the liquefying drugs is mixed separately with an inert, high melting point protective and then mixed lightly. The inert protective acts as a mechanical barrier or coat to prevent contact between the low melting point substances. Further, if any liquefaction occurs, the liquid is absorbed by the large surface of the protective ingredient.

If the aminopyrine and chloral hydrate are triturated, a liquid is formed. The amount of inert substance required to absorb the liquid would be too bulky for a capsule. Each drug is mixed with an inert absorbent such as kaolin or talc to prevent liquefaction. The chloral hydrate is pulverized and mixed with 150 mg. of kaolin per capsule. The aminopyrine is pulverized and mixed with 300 mg. of kaolin per capsule. The two mixtures are mixed lightly, and the dry powder is filled into No. 00 capsules.

73. ℞
    Chloral hydrate 0.15
    Aminopyrine 0.30

    M. ft. Caps. No. XX

    Sig.: Two on retiring.

74. ℞
    Acid acetylsalicylic 7.5
    Acetophenetidin 4.0

    M. et ft. capsules No. 24

    Sig.: Two capsules t. i. d. a. c.

75. ℞
    Menthol 0.065
    Phenol 0.065
    Zinc oxide 60

    Sig.: Apply ut dict.

76. ℞
    A.S.A. 0.300
    Methenamine 0.050
    Magnesium oxide 0.100
    Caffeine 0.075

    M. caps. D. T. D. #XXX

    Sig.: One p. r. n. headache.

Probably the high melting point and a large specific surface are the primary criteria of a good inert protective. The differences observed between various protectives employed may be largely those of particle size and coating ability. Decreasing the size of an inert protective by one half will reduce by one half the weight of the protective needed to coat the liquefying ingredients.

Kaolin, magnesium oxide and magnesium carbonate are commonly used as inert absorbents.[7,26] Magnesium carbonate is generally the protective of choice, as the oxide may react with other ingredients, carbon dioxide or water to form a hard, insoluble mass.

To avoid liquefaction of a mixture of liquefying substances, an inert, high melting point substance is generally added to surround or coat the drugs, thus preventing them from coming into contact with each other. The amount of inert protective may be rationalized by considering the effect to be only a mechanical coating of the particles.

77. ℞
    Salol
    Aminopyrine, aa 0.2

    M. et fiat caps. D. T. D. No. 50

    Sig.: As directed.

As the melting points of salol and aminopyrine are 43° and 104°C., respectively, one would anticipate possible liquefaction. Assuming spherical particles, trituration in a Wedgwood mortar will reduce the average particle size of the two drugs to a radius of 100 microns. The densities of salol and aminopyrine are approximately 1.0 and 1.1 Gm./cc. respectively. Because of its high melting point (2,800°C.) and its large specific surface area, magnesium oxide is chosen as the inert protective. Magnesium oxide has an average particle size of 10 microns and a density of 1.25 Gm/cc.

1. The area of a single particle of salol is

$$A_1 = 4 \pi R^2 = 4 \pi 10^{-4} \text{ cm}^2.$$

2. The area covered or "shadowed" by a single particle of magnesium oxide is

$$A = \pi R^2 = \pi 10^{-6} \text{ cm}^2.$$

3. The number of particles of magnesium oxide required to coat one particle of salol is

$$\frac{A_1}{A} = \frac{4 \pi 10^{-4}}{\pi 10^{-6}} = 400.$$

4. The weight of a single particle of salol is

$$W_1 = V \rho = \frac{4}{3} \pi R^3 \rho = \frac{4}{3} \pi (10^{-2})^3 = 4.19 \times 10^{-6} \text{ Gm.}$$

5. The total number of particles of salol in the prescription is

$$\frac{10}{W_1} = \frac{10}{4.19 \times 10^{-6}} = 2.4 \times 10^6.$$

6. The number of particles of protective needed to coat all particles of salol is the number of particles of salol multiplied by the number of particles required to coat one particle or

$$2.4 \times 10^6 \times 400 = 9.6 \times 10^8.$$

7. The weight of a single particle of the protective ingredient is

$$W = V \, \rho = \frac{4}{3} \pi \, R^3 \, \rho = 4.19 \, (10^{-3})^3 \, 1.25 =$$
$$5.2 \times 10^{-9} \, Gm.$$

8. The total weight of protective required to coat 10 Gm. of salol is the number of particles of protective multiplied by the weight of a single particle of the protective or

$$5.2 \times 10^{-9} \times 9.6 \times 10^8 = 5 \, Gm.$$

9. Following the same reasoning, it is found that 4.54 Gm. of magnesium oxide is required to coat 10 Gm. of aminopyrine.

10. The total amount of the inert protective necessary to coat the salol and the aminopyrine is 9.5 Gm.

Trial and error have demonstrated that if each of the liquefying substances is diluted with an equal amount of inert absorbent, the result will be a dry powder. The above calculation, based only on mechanical consideration, agrees rather well with the quantity determined by years of experience.

CHEMICAL REACTIVITY

Explosive mixtures usually consist of oxidizing agents and organic compounds. The stronger oxidizing agents used in pharmacy are potassium chlorate, potassium permanganate, sodium peroxide and silver nitrate. The common reducing agents involved in explosions have been charcoal, starch, sugar, tannic acid, sulfur and the sulfides.

With potentially explosive mixtures, trituration is to be avoided. If the powders are to be mixed, they should be triturated separately, and then mixed lightly with a spatula or by tumbling the powders. As a safety measure, it seems obvious that potentially explosive mixtures should not be dispensed. If the physician insists on such a combination, it is advisable, with his consent, to dispense the two ingredients separately.

78. ℞

Potassium chlorate	7.5
Tannic acid	4.0
Sucrose	7.5

M. et ft. chart. 12

Sig.: One p. r. n. gargle in glass of water.

79. ℞

Sulfathiazole	5
Sodium peroxide	15
Boric acid	80

Sig.: Dust on wound t. i. d.

The sodium peroxide will oxidize the sulfathiazole. It should be suggested to the physician that the sodium peroxide be eliminated and a less caustic, nonoxidizing type of antiseptic be dispensed.

Light may provide the energy necessary for a reaction to occur without a change in temperature. Acetazolamide, bismuth salts, cyanocobalamine, many dyes, fumagillin, mercury and silver salts and many other drugs are light sensitive. Photosensitive drugs should be dispensed in amber glass containers.[2] If a suitable amber container is not available the dispensing pharmacist should dispense the prescription in an opaque container and caution the patron that the medication should not be exposed to light.

Some chemicals and drugs such as iodine react directly and rapidly with metal. Care should be observed in the choice of utensils to be used with such drugs. Metal spatulas and metal sieves cannot be used. Other chemicals, such as phenols, undergo reactions catalyzed by trace metal impurities from containers or metal utensils. Plastic caps are used on prescription containers, as they are less reactive than metal caps.

When solid dosage forms are dry, acids and bases or bicarbonates may be mixed without any reaction. If the pharmacist wishes to use this technic, he must begin with dry chemicals, compound in a relatively dry atmosphere and dispense the finished dosage form in a container that seals out moisture.

80. ℞

Pamisyl	0.5
Sodium bicarbonate	0.5

Mix and dispense 50 powders.

Sig.: One powder.

The Pamisyl and the sodium bicarbonate were mixed and the weighed amount of the mixture was packaged in paper envelopes. On dispensing, the powders seemed properly prepared; however, in 3 days the patient returned and complained that some of the envelopes were not as full as the first ones he had taken. Actually, the powders had been accurately weighed. The aminosalicylic acid had reacted with the sodium bicarbonate, in the presence of atmospheric moisture, eliminating water and carbon dioxide with a loss in weight. It could be suggested that the physician use lactose, if the sodium bicarbonate is used as a diluent; however, if the sodium bicarbonate is present to form the soluble sodium aminosalicylate, this would not be acceptable.

81. ℞
    Aminophylline 0.2
    Ascorbic acid 0.1

    M. D. T. D. Caps. No. XXV

    Sig.: One capsule t. i. d.

For several days the capsules appear to be satisfactory, but within a week the powder becomes gummy and brown and possesses an ammoniacal odor. In the presence of moisture, the loosely complexed ethylenediamine reacts with the ascorbic acid. With the consent of the physician, the aminophylline and the ascorbic acid may be dispensed separately or an equivalent weight of anhydrous theophylline may replace the aminophylline.

COMPRESSED TABLETS

A compressed tablet is a unit dosage form prepared by compressing under several hundred kilograms of pressure per square centimeter granulated medicinal substances into a discoid shape by means of dies. A tablet usually has a thickness less than one half of its diameter. Some tablets have distinctive shapes and sizes as a means of associating their identity with a particular company. The physical characteristics of industrially prepared solid dosage forms are so distinctive that the American Medical Association in 1962 published an *Identification Guide for Solid Dosage Forms*. This guide enables one to identify tentatively a tablet, a capsule or a suppository by the use of physical characteristics, such as size, shape, color, markings and coating. The tentative identification is then confirmed by chemical analysis.

In a recent survey it was found that 47.6 per cent of the prescriptions were for compressed tablets. There are several advantages of compressed tablets that make them the most popular dosage form. The obvious advantage of compressed tablets is the convenience of transportation for the manufacturer, the pharmacist and the patient. All pharmaceutical dosage forms are accurate dosage forms, and, usually, the compressed tablet is an accurate dosage in which one tablet represents one dose. A tablet may be scored into halves or quarters, and a uniform tablet assures practical division by the patient into one half or one fourth of the total dose in an intact tablet.

Unpleasant tasting drugs are rendered acceptable by coating the tablets. This may be a sugar coat, a film coat or a press coat. The coating need be designed to protect only during the short time in which the tablet is in contact with the taste buds.

The patient generally finds a tablet the simplest dosage form for self-administration. The intended route of administration determines the size and the shape of the tablet. The maximum size cannot exceed the size of the body passage through which the tablet is to be passed or placed. An oral tablet for an adult should not exceed 7/16 inch in diameter. The bulk of the dose may decide the size of the tablet. When this exceeds 500 mg., most manufacturers divide the therapeutic dose between two tablets, and this becomes the prescribed number of tablets for a therapeutic dose.

The tablet is placed on the tongue and swallowed by drinking a glass of water. Some individuals find it psychologically impossible to swallow a tablet. For such persons and for children, a tablet should first be crushed and moistened with water. The death of a child due to an aspirin tablet becoming lodged in the larynx has been reported.

The pharmaceutical industry has made it still easier to administer tablets by developing the chewable or the soluble oral tablet. The chewable tablet has a base, such as mannitol, which can be chewed or allowed to dissolve in the mouth.

Tablets provide a broad range of drug release. Tablets can be designed for a rapid release of a drug, as illustrated by the many varieties of fast-acting acetylsalicylic acid derivatives that are marketed. Consistent with physiologic function, sustained release tablets provide release of a drug over a period of 8 to 12 hours, maintaining an adequate dosage with the convenience of a single administration.

Our sophisticated society will not accept unappealing medication. A dosage form must be appealing to the patient in order to receive his cooperation in following the dosage regimen established by his physician. Tablets are made elegant by coating, coloring, flavoring, designing appealing shapes and sizes and packaging in attractive containers. The attractiveness of tablets and the possibility that they be mistaken for candy by children makes it necessary that tablets, as well as other medicinals, be kept out of reach of children.

Elegant tablets have been made available to the patient by our pharmaceutical industry at a reasonable cost, because tableting lends itself to mass production methods that increase production while decreasing the cost of labor. An elaborate distribution system makes readily available to the consumer, at low cost, tablets in a wide range of strengths.

Tablets are not only convenient for the pharmacist to store and package, but tablets have few serious disadvantages. Tablet formation is limited by the physical and the chemical properties of a drug. A tablet from an ethical firm implies that the research and developmental pharmacist has corrected or eliminated any problems of stability, incompatibility or other formulation problems prior to marketing the tablet; thus, the community pharmacist, the physician and the patient are not concerned with such problems, except as they may affect therapeutic value.

Although compressed tablets are impractical for the community pharmacist to prepare because of lack of time, equipment, adequate control and advanced training, the pharmacist must have knowledge of the methods of preparation, the factors in their proper disintegration, the correct storage conditions, the types of containers to use, the types of tablets available and their particular advantages and disadvantages. The phar-

macist must be able to converse and advise intelligently about all phases of tablets from production to administration so that he may be of service to the physician and his patient (see Chap. 2).

A pharmacist delivers medication to a consumer with an implied warranty that the purity and the dosage is proper. In extemporaneous prescriptions, the pharmacist exercises great care to make certain each prescription is an accurate dosage form. For obvious reasons, the pharmacist cannot be expected to determine analytically the purity and the accuracy of manufactured products. The pharmacist, acting on faith and the reputation of a firm, accepts label claims of prefabricated products. The pharmacist therefore should buy products from an ethical firm with a good reputation. This is his best assurance that the manufactured product is pure and accurate.

MANUFACTURE OF COMPRESSED TABLETS[29,35,53]

Compressed tablets are manufactured by two methods: dry granulation and wet granulation. To compress a tablet, the ingredients must be free flowing, binding and nonadhesive to the punches and the die. Most substances cannot be compressed directly but must be formed into granules. Granulation is the process by which fine powders are converted to granules with the above characteristics to assure uniform filling and the formation of an easily ejected tablet.

It appears that when the active ingredients are less than 25 per cent of the finished tablet, they may be blended with spray-dried lactose and compressed directly.

WET GRANULATION

Weighing and Mixing the Ingredients. When a production batch of tablets is to be manufactured, the master formula card is reproduced and sent to the chemical and drug supply department. There, the specified weight of each ingredient is weighed and checked. The weighed material is sent to the tablet department where each item is carefully rechecked.

All dry ingredients are in the powdered form so that they will pass through a 60-mesh sieve. The powders are blended by

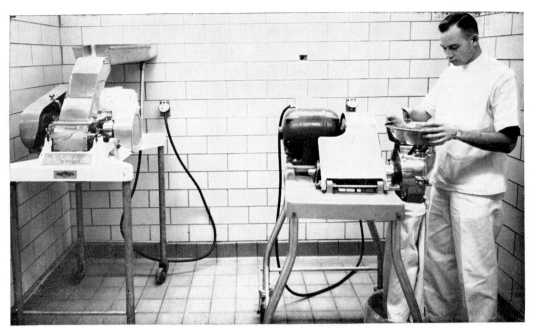

FIG. 3-9.   Reduction of particle size by a small hammer mill. (*Left*) Production size
hammer mill may be used for granulating, pulverizing and dispersing.

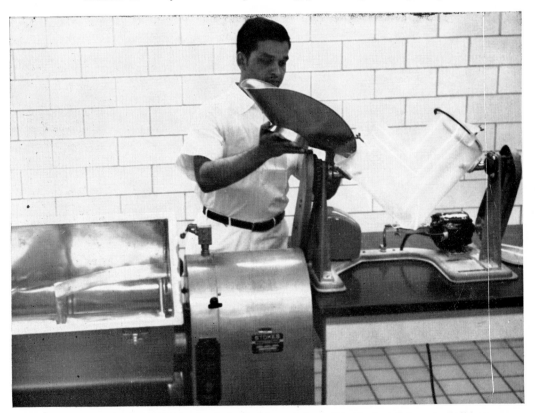

FIG. 3-10.   A plastic V-blender is loaded for mixing. (*Left*) A stainless steel ribbon
blender used for blending the wet granulation.

geometric dilution using V-blenders or other suitable mechanical mixers.

Many of the newer synthetic drugs have a small dose, and it is necessary to increase the bulk of the tablet to a practical and workable size. Common diluents are lactose, sodium chloride, mannitol, calcium carbonate, calcium sulfate and dicalcium phosphate.

Wet Granulating. After the powders are blended, a liquid granulating or binding solution is added to form an adhesive mass which can be granulated. The amount of liquid must be determined empirically for each new formulation, but it is reproducible from batch to batch with a production formula. The liquid is blended thoroughly into the mass with a ribbon blender or other suitable mechanical mixers. When the mass has the proper consistency, it is forced through a wet granulator with a 6-mesh to 10-mesh screen.

The adhesive materials used to bind the powders together into granules are 5 to 10

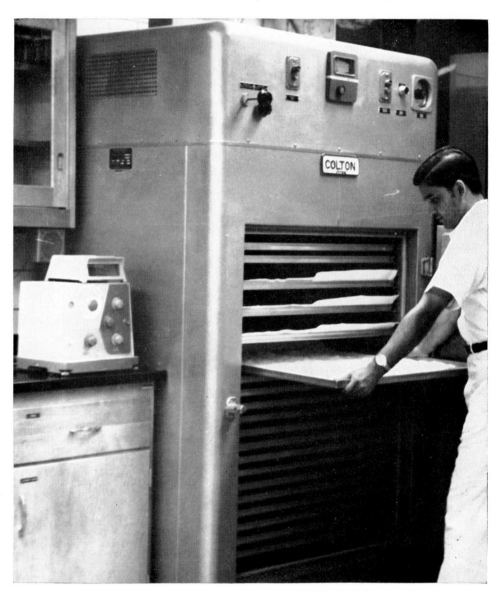

FIG. 3-11.   Oven designed for efficient drying of granulations. (*Left*) Moisture balance for determining the per cent moisture in a granulation.

per cent starch paste, 70 to 85 per cent sucrose solution, 10 to 20 per cent gelatin solution, 10 to 20 per cent acacia mucilage, 25 to 50 per cent glucose solution, 5 to 10 per cent methylcellulose solution, 5 per cent ethylcellulose solution and polyvinylpyrrolidone. Water and alcohol act by means of their solvent effect on the ingredients.

Uniform distribution and the amount of the binder are critical. Insufficient binder leads to poor adhesion, capping and soft tablets. Excessive binder yields a slowly disintegrating and hard tablet; excessive binder makes granulation extremely difficult.

Color may be added to a tablet to convey a characteristic identification, increase patient acceptance or suggest a flavor. Certified dyes are generally distributed throughout the dry mix or dissolved in the binder solution. A 40-mesh granulation is advisable to avoid a mottled tablet.

In a recently developed mixer, the binding solution may be added slowly as a spray. Some formulations will form granules with a minimum of liquid and make it unnecessary to pass the mixture through a wet granulator.

Drying. The wet granulation is spread in a thin layer on trays and dried in an oven at a controlled temperature generally not exceeding 55°C.

Granulating for Compression. The dried granulation is ground to a size appropriate to the size of the finished tablet. For small tablets such as ⅛ inch in diameter, a 30-mesh screen should be used; for tablets up to ⅜ inch a 12-mesh screen should be used. An oscillating granulator has an advantage in that, as soon as a particle is reduced to the proper size, it falls through the screen away from the grinding action and is not further reduced in size. Grinding type granulators and the Fitzpatrick comminutor tend to produce an excess of fine powder.

Many tablets are engraved or embossed with designs on the tablet surface. A 40-mesh granulation is used with engraved or embossed tablets, as coarser particles do not fill as evenly into the engraving on the punch. There is a tendency to compress lettered tablets harder in order to make the letters stand out.

Adding the Lubricant and the Disintegrant. A lubricant is added to ensure uniform feeding of the granules, to prevent sticking to the surface of the punches and the die, to reduce die wall friction and facilitate ejection, and to reduce punch and die wear. Common lubricants are calcium stearate, magnesium stearate, talc, glycine, Sterotex and stearic acid. These must be passed through a 200-mesh sieve to ensure small particle size so that the lubricant will have its proper coating effect. For purely lubricating purposes, more than 1 per cent of a lubricant is not necessary.

Liquid petrolatum has been added or an

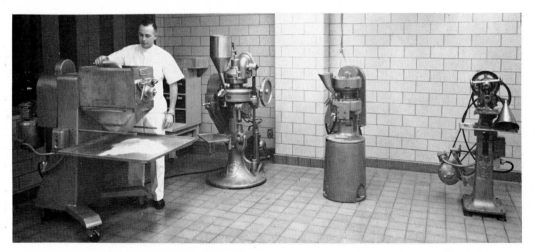

Fig. 3-12. Oscillating granulator being used to reduce the dried granulation to the desired size for compression. The tablet presses in the background are, from left to right, a 22-station rotary, a 4-station induced die feed rotary, and a single punch machine.

ethereal solution sprayed on the granulation. This is not a satisfactory procedure because the hydrophobic coating tends to render the tablet impervious to water and retards disintegration.

A disintegrant is a substance which will rupture the tablet into many small particles soon after administration. The large number of small particles present a greater surface than does an intact tablet and speed solution of the drug. A disintegration time of 15 minutes is satisfactory for most medication.

The most common disintegrant is potato starch. Starch should be dried at 100°C. (see Fig. 3-7) if it is to be used as a disintegrating agent. The high water content of commercial starches may be reduced tenfold by drying; this enhances its disintegrating ability and lessens deterioration of moisture sensitive drugs. In the wet granulation method, some starch is often mixed with the granulation with the hope that it will break apart the individual granules. This seems of doubtful value, as starch imbibes water freely and retains little capacity to act as a disinte-

grant. Other disintegrants are gelatin and numerous algin derivatives.

Compressed tablets of medicaments that dissolve slowly should be designed to disintegrate within a few minutes in water or in the stomach. A tablet must disintegrate within a few hours if it is to have any medicinal effect. A tablet that passes through the gastrointestinal tract is not only useless, but it gives a false clinical picture and may stand in the way of other beneficial treatment.

Tablets composed mostly of soluble materials present no difficulty and generally do not require a disintegrating agent.

Incorporation of an acid and a bicarbonate in a tablet will produce effervescence and disintegrate the tablet. This technic has been used in some saccharin tablets; however, its success has been limited.

Flavor may be added by spraying an alcoholic solution of the flavor onto the dry granules before compression. A more recent technic is to use dry flavors which may be blended at the initial mixing of the ingredients.

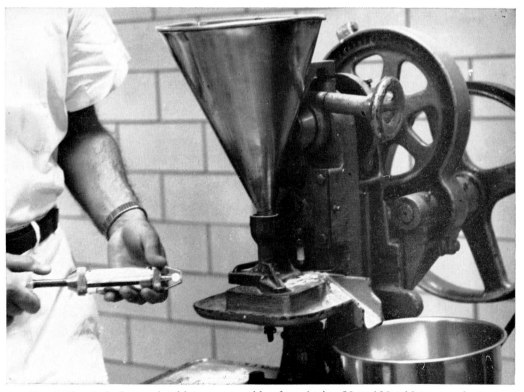

Fig. 3-13. A single punch tablet press capable of producing 80 to 120 tablets per minute. (*Left*) Stokes Hardness Tester is used to determine the hardness of the compressed tablet.

TABLE 3-4. DIFFICULTIES ENCOUNTERED DURING TABLET COMPRESSION

	CAUSE
Capping (splitting off of top after compression)	Excessive pressure Excessive fine powder Insufficient binder Too dry a granulation Worn die or damaged punch face
Improper fill	Damp granulation Machine running too fast Granulation too fine or too coarse
Picking (material sticking to punch face leaving holes in tablet surface)	Unsatisfactory lubricant Damp granulation Static charge Scratched punch face
Mottled tablet	Incomplete mixing
Nondisintegrating tablet	Excessive pressure Excessive binder Excessive lubricant

Compressing. Basically, a single punch tablet machine consists of a die fitted with an upper and a lower punch. With the upper punch out of and above the die and the lower punch at the lowest point of descent within the die, a charge of granulation flows into and fills the die cavity. The upper punch descends, compressing the material as the lower punch remains stationary. The upper punch ascends, followed after a short time by the lower punch, which rises until it is flush with the upper surface of the die. A feed shoe ejects the tablet and fills the die cavity to begin another cycle.

The lower punch is adjusted so that, at its lowest point, the cavity it makes will hold the quantity of granulation necessary to make a complete tablet. At its highest point the lower punch is adjusted flush with the upper surface of the die so that the tablet will be ejected without chipping.

The upper punch is adjusted to control the thickness and the hardness of a tablet. Lowering the upper punch produces a harder and a thinner tablet.

The complexity of the machine, its operation and maintenance are engineering problems. The proper formulation of a stable tablet and the adjustments of the punches are pharmaceutical problems.

The finished tablets are passed along a vibrating wire tray or under an exhaust system to remove any powder. The tablets are then held in quarantine until they have been analyzed and released for bottling by the control department.

For the novice developing a tablet to contain a drug with a small dose, a simple lactose granulation may be used as a basic formulation.

Basic Lactose Granulation

Lactose	350 Gm.
Starch	26
Color	0.25
Magnesium stearate	5
Starch paste, 10%	140 ml.

By geometric dilution, the color is blended with the lactose and the starch. The mixture is moistened with starch paste and the wet mass is passed through a 6-mesh screen. The wet granulation is dried in an oven at 60°C. The dried granulation is passed through a 40-mesh screen. The magnesium stearate is added and the granulation is tumbled for several minutes. The granulation is compressed into tablets with a hardness of 6 Kg.

Neomycin Sulfate Tablet

	Mg. per Tablet
Neomycin sulfate	250
Lactose	100
Starch	100
Acacia	5
Magnesium stearate	5

The neomycin sulfate, the lactose, the starch and the acacia are thoroughly blended. The mixed powders are granulated with methanol containing 10 per cent of water and passed through 6-mesh screen. The wet granulation is placed on paper in trays and dried in an oven. The dried granulation is passed through a 20-mesh screen. Magnesium stearate is blended into the granulation. The granulation is compressed into tablets.

Pediatric Chewable Aspirin Tablet

	Mg. per Tablet
Acetylsalicylic acid (20 mesh)	81
Mannitol	97
Saccharin sodium	1
Acacia	4.5
Starch	11
Talc	8
Magnesium stearate	0.4
Dry flavor	0.6

A mannitol granulation is prepared first. The saccharin sodium and the mannitol are blended. The blend is granulated with 20 per cent acacia mucilage and passed through 8-mesh screen. The mannitol granulation is dried at 45°C. and passed through a 20-mesh screen.

The 20-mesh aspirin is mixed with the dried mannitol granulation. The flavor is added to the starch and mixed thoroughly. The talc and the magnesium stearate are passed through 100-mesh screen and blended with the flavor-starch mixture. This blend is mixed with the mannitol-aspirin mixture. Tablets are compressed to a hardness of 5 Kg. using an 11/32-inch standard concave punch and die set.

PRECOMPRESSION

Wet granulation method is unsuitable for substances injured by heat or for substances that are incompatible with liquid binders. Here the precompression or slugging method is used.

In the slugging process the entire formula is blended and compressed into flat tablets called slugs. Precompression requires a heavy duty rotary tablet machine. The punches and the dies are as much as 1⅜ inch in diameter. Considerable dust results, and the working parts of the machine should be housed and a dust collector attached at the point of com-

pression. These precautions are advisable with all machines.

It is not essential that the slugs be perfectly shaped, as they are ground to the desired granulation size and then compressed into the finished tablet.

Aspirin Tablet, 300 mg.

	Mg. per Tablet
Aspirin granulation containing 10% starch	333.3

The aspirin granulation is compressed into tablets using a 13/32-inch standard concave punch and die set.

Phenobarbital Tablet, 30 mg.

	Mg. per Tablet
Phenobarbital	30
Lactose, spray dried	168
Magnesium stearate	2

The spray dried lactose and the phenobarbital are blended until homogeneous. The magnesium stearate is added to the blend. The blend is compressed into a tablet using a 11/32-inch standard concave punch and die set.

The use of the chilsonator has been suggested to eliminate wet granulation and to speed up and simplify the slugging process. A chilsonator consists of a pair of corded steel rollers scored in a grooving style. The rollers revolve toward each other at a controlled speed. The material to be granulated is fed to these rollers at a controlled rate. The blend is squeezed at a constant pressure varying from one to fifty tons per square inch. The rollers may be heated or chilled as necessary. Any moisture present in the formula is removed by the heat of compression. The compressed granules are discharged in irregular strips of corrugated plaques. These strips are passed through a conventional granulator to secure the proper size granulation from which the finished tablet is compressed.

Other methods have been suggested for preparing granulations. In the pan granulating technic, the blended ingredients are placed in a baffled coating pan and moistened by a spray. When the blend has been adequately moistened, hot air is blown into the pan to dry the granules. The resulting granules approach a spherical shape.

Granulations have been made in V-blenders fitted with spray heads through which the granulating solutions are admitted by trunnion mountings.

Either modification may be connected in such a way that it can be evacuated and dried under a vacuum without transfer of the granulation.

TYPES OF TABLETS

Although all compressed tablets are prepared by the same general procedure, compressed tablets have a wide variety of use. Some common abbreviations for types of tablets are given in Table 3-5. Some specialty names for compressed tablets are given in Table 3-6.

Tablets Used in the Gastrointestinal Tract. Most compressed tablets are swallowed whole with a drink of water. They disintegrate or dissolve in the gastrointestinal tract from which the drug is absorbed in order to exert its therapeutic effect. Some oral tablets are administered by placing the tablet in half a glass of water, stirring and drinking the suspended mixture. These bulk tablets are more or less restricted to antacid products.

82. ℞
    Magnesium and Soda Tablets 100

Sig.: Two in water with meals.

Some pharmaceutical firms have given specialty or trade names to their tablets which are prepared in a distinctive form or shape.

83. ℞
    Digitalis "Tabloid" (Burroughs
    Wellcome) 60

Sig.: One daily.

84. ℞
    Betalin S Diskets (Lilly) 10 mg., No. 100

Sig.: Two daily.

85. ℞
    Coricidin Medilets (Schering) ... 15

Sig.: One t. i. d.

86. ℞
    Dilantin Infatabs (Parke, Davis) .. 100

Sig.: One morning and evening.

TABLE 3-5. ABBREVIATIONS FOR TABLETS

C. T.	compressed tablet
C. C. T.	chocolate colored tablet
C. T. T.	compressed tablet triturate
D. A. T.	delayed action tablet
D. T.	dispensing tablet
E. C. T.	enteric-coated tablet
H. T.	hypodermic tablet
M. C. T.	multiple compressed tablet
R. A. T.	repeat-action tablet
S. C. T.	sugar-coated tablet
T. T.	tablet triturate

87. ℞
    Dexedrine (SKF) 5 mg. 60

Sig.: One t. i. d.

88. ℞
    Empirin Compound with Codeine,
    No. 1 (Burroughs, Wellcome) .. 18

Sig.: One q. 4 hrs.

Chewing tablets or wafers have been available for many years. They are intended to be chewed before swallowing and have been used when the therapeutic dose would make the dosage form too large to swallow.

89. ℞
    Arobon Wafers (Pitman-Moore) .. 12

Sig.: Chew two; then one q. 3 hrs.

90. ℞
    Dical-D Wafers (Abbott) 50

Sig.: Two wafers with each meal.

91. ℞
    Kolantyl Wafers (Merrell) 32

Sig.: Three q. 3 hrs.

The more recent chewing tablet, sometimes called a soluble tablet, has a base of mannitol or glycine and is pleasantly flavored. The soluble chewing tablet will dissolve in the mouth in approximately 1 minute. They may be chewed, sucked or swallowed whole. Chewing tablets are especially adapted for children.

92. ℞
    Deca-Vi-Sol Chewable (Mead John-
    son) 100

Sig.: One tablet daily.

TABLE 3-6. SPECIALTY NAMES OF TABLETS

SPECIALTY	COMPANY	DESCRIPTION
Bitab	National Drug	double strength tablet
Bocap	Bowman Brothers	sugar-coated capsule-shaped tablet
Buccalet	Ciba	curved tablet for buccal or sublingual use
Candisphere	Walker	flavored chewable tablet
Candi-Tab	Merit Pharmacal	flavored chewable tablet
Caplet	Winthrop	elongated tablet
Capsol	Hance Bros.	sugar-coated tablet
Capsotab	Lloyd, Dabney & Westerfield	capsule-shaped tablet
Capsulette	Armour	capsule-shaped tablet
Captab	Bryant	capsule-shaped tablet
Cherro-Chew Tab	Lloyd Bros.	flavored chewable tablet
Chewtab	Jan	flavored chewable tablet
Diplett	Paul E. Elder	flavored pediatric tablet
Discoid	Zemmer	readily soluble, hand-molded tablet
Disket	Eli Lilly	inscribed tablet
Dulcet	Abbott	soluble, flavored, cube-shaped tablet
Duo-Tab	Hiss Pharmacal	two-layered tablet
Filmtab	Abbott	tablet that is coated with a thin film which disintegrates rapidly
Geltab	Stanley Drug	coated tablet
Glosset	Winthrop	sublingual tablet
Hexad	Bowman Bros. Drug	six-sided tablet
Hexette	Bowman Bros. Drug	flavored and colored six-sided tablet
Infatab	Parke, Davis	triangular-shaped, grooved pediatric tablet
Inlay-Tab	Dorsey	flat, capsule-shaped tablet with one drug in shell and others in the inlay
Kote	Vitamix Corporation	coated tablet
Lingual	Key Pharmacal	sublingual tablet
Linguet	Ciba	sublingual tablet
Lingusorb	Ayerst	sublingual tablet
Lozi-Tab	Hoyt	compressed lozenge
Loz-Tablet	Warren-Teed	tablet to be dissolved in the mouth for 5 minutes before swallowing
Mandel	Lederle	flavored chewable tablet
Medilet	Schering	multicolored pediatric tablet
Melet	Pitman-Moore	chewable troche
Membrette	Wyeth	soluble sublingual tablet
Merseal	Merck Sharp & Dohme	film-coated tablet
Mucorette	White	sublingual tablet
Nebutab	Premo	soluble tablet triturate

TABLE 3-6. SPECIALTY NAMES OF TABLETS (*Continued*)

SPECIALTY	COMPANY	DESCRIPTION
Neotrab	Miller	flavored pediatric tablet
Oret	Smith, Miller & Patch	compressed tablet
Ovoid	Winthrop	sugar-coated oval-shaped tablet
Palatab	Central Pharmacal	oblong, scored and flavored pediatric tablet
Pediatab	Phillips-Roxane	flavored tablet
Plastule	Ives	compressed tablet
Pulvoid	Drug Products	compressed tablet
Savoret	Eli Lilly	flavored tablet
Sealet	Premo	coated tablet
Softab	Stuart	soft, soluble tablet
Solvet	Eli Lilly	soluble tablet
Sorbette	Hiss Pharmacal	flavored chewable tablet
Sub-U-Tab	Abbott	sublingual tablet
Tabloid	Burroughs Wellcome	compressed tablet
Tabseal	Rocky Mountain Pharmacal	sealed tablet
Tabule	Neisler	capsule-shaped tablet
Tastitab	Roerig	flavored chewable tablet
Tunglet	Rexall	curved sublingual tablet
Valentab	Moore Kirk	colored and flavored heart-shaped pediatric tablet
Viseal	Biopharma	coated tablet
Zestab	Roche	chewable flavored pediatric tablet

93. ℞
    Viterra Tastitabs (Roerig) 100
    Sig.: One daily.

94. ℞
    Trisulfazine Palatab (Central
      Pharmacal) 30
    Sig.: As directed.

95. ℞
    Unicaps Chewable (Upjohn) 30
    Sig.: 1-2 daily.

Tablets Used in the Oral Cavity. Buccal tablets are small, flat tablets which are placed in the buccal pouch between the cheek and the gums. As the drug is released from the dissolving tablet, the active ingredient is absorbed without passing into the gastrointestinal tract. This is an advantageous route for drugs that would be destroyed by enzymatic action in the gastrointestinal tract. Unfortunately, few drugs are readily absorbed from the oral sulci. Buccal and sublingual administration is limited to glyceryl trinitrate and steroidal hormones.

A starch and lactose base compressed at high forces is used with buccal tablets, as it disintegrates easily in the saliva. No flavor or sweetening agent is added as they would stimulate salivation resulting in undue swallowing and loss of the drug. A well-formulated buccal tablet should dissolve or disintegrate within 30 mintes.

Sublingual tablets are similar to buccal tablets, but the sublingual tablets are placed under the tongue.

96. ℞
    Metandren Linguets (Ciba),
      5 mg. .... No. 25
    Sig.: Place beneath tongue twice daily.

97. ℞

Perandren Buccalets (Ciba),
5 mg. .... No. 30

Sig.: Two daily for 3 days prior to menstruation.

98. ℞

Isuprel Glossets (Winthrop),
10 mg. 50

Sig.: One following attack.

99. ℞

Nitroglycerin H. T. .... 0.3 mg.

Dispense tube of 20.

Sig.: 1-2 tablets sublingually as necessary.

100. ℞

Isordil Sublingual (Ives) 90

Sig.: One q. 4 hrs.

Troches or lozenges are tablets intended to be held in the mouth while they dissolve gradually and maintain the medication in contact with the mouth and the throat for a long period. Troches are used for the local effect of antiseptics, astringents and local anesthetics.

Troches are manufactured by compression or molding. Since troches are intended to dissolve slowly and not to disintegrate, they are formulated somewhat differently from tablets. Troches contain more binder, are compressed harder and have no disintegrating agent added. Granulation and compression are the same as for tablets.

101. ℞

A-C Troches (Abbott) ...... 1 box

Sig.: Dissolve in mouth as needed.

102. ℞

Bradosol Lozenges (Ciba) .. 18

Sig.: Dissolve in mouth as needed.

Tablets Used for Subcutaneous Administration. Pellets or implantation tablets have been developed for subcutaneous implantation of hormones by use of a Kearne implantor or by incision. Generally, the 3.2 x 8 mm. pellets are implanted in the thigh. These sterile pellets serve as a depot which slowly releases the hormone over a prolonged period. Effects are observed for several months after implantation.

Normally no excipients are used in formulating the pellet. The sterile crystalline drug is compressed into the finished pellet under aseptic conditions. Oreton, Percorten acetate and Progynon pellets are available for hospital and clinical use.

Hypodermic tablets are small tablets with opposing flat surfaces which are intended to be dissolved under aseptic conditions just prior to injection. Hypodermic tablets are small so that they readily can be dropped into the barrel of the syringe. They must be capable of dissolving rapidly and completely in water.

Hypodermic tablets may be lightly compressed or molded. Beta-lactose, dextrose and sodium sulfate are used as diluents because of their solubility. Although special precautions are observed in manufacturing the hypodermic tablet, it is doubtful that the solutions prepared from hypodermic tablets are sterile. It probably would be advantageous for the physician to use parenteral solutions sterilized in ampuls.

Atropine sulfate, codeine sulfate, morphine sulfate, nitroglycerin and scopolamine hydrobromide are customarily marketed as hypodermic tablets.

Tablets for Vaginal Use. Tablets compressed into a pear shape for insertion into the vagina are known as inserts. Inserts have a lactose or a sodium bicarbonate base which rapidly releases the drug.

Some tablets are used to make solutions intended to be used as douches. A tablet dissolved in a specified volume of water will make a solution of proper strength of medication for a vaginal douche.

103. ℞

Vioform Inserts (Ciba) 12

Sig.: Insert h. s. after douche.

104. ℞

Neo-Vagisol (Dorsey) 24

Sig.: Insert two high in vagina.

Tablets for Miscellaneous Uses. A few specialized items such as dental cones are used in the mouth. Ilotycin Dental Cones are composed of a sodium bicarbonate and a sodium chloride base. This base will disintegrate and dissolve in the small amount of serum present in approximately ½ hour.

The dental cone is loosely packed in the socket after tooth extraction and contains an antibiotic to prevent local multiplication of bacteria.

Tablets are at times used for convenience in extemporaneous preparations for local use. Tablets such as potassium permanganate tablets and Mercurochrome tablets are used to prepare cleansing and disinfecting solutions. Tablets are available for preparing solutions to be used for chemical sterilization of instruments. One Mercury Bichloride Large Poison Tablet dissolved in a pint of water yields a 1:1,000 solution for disinfectant purposes.

Reagent tablets for diagnostic tests are used by clinics and the patient for self-diagnosis. Acetest reagent tablets are used to test for ketonuria; Hematest reagent tablets are used to detect occult blood; and Ictotest reagent tablets are used to test for urinary bilirubin.

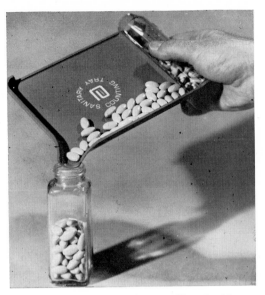

FIG. 3-14. Sanitary capsule, pill and tablet counting tray. (Abbott)

THE DISPENSING OF TABLETS

Tablets should be dispensed in glass or plastic vials or glass bottles. Tablets should not be touched by the hands during packaging procedures. Professional appearance is enhanced by using an Abbott sanitary counting tray which eliminates the fingers touching the tablets or other prefabricated dosages. Not only is handling unsanitary, but moisture from the hands may cause coated tablets to dull and to stick. Cotton should be placed in the vial on top of the tablets.

When a prescription is written for only a few tablets, they may be placed in a cellophane envelope and dispensed in a cardboard box.

Tablets should be stored in tight containers. If the tablets contain a drug that is photosensitive, the tablets must be dispensed in an amber bottle or vial. Exposure to excessive heat, strong light and moisture is to be avoided.

EVALUATION OF SOLID DOSAGE FORMS

Chemical identity and purity of prefabricated solids are implied warranties. Self-analysis and control are left largely to pharmaceutical industry. The pharmaceutical company develops its own assays and specifications for new drugs and dosage forms with the approval of the F.D.A. As chemical analysis by the practicing pharmacist is not feasible, he must rely on the reputation of the manufacturer. There are certain tests which may be carried out in the pharmacy without any elaborate equipment or great expenditure of time. These will help to evaluate some of the desirable characteristics of solid dosage forms.

Accurate Weight. The U.S.P. weight variation tests provide limits for the variation from the observed average in capsules and from the average gross weight for tablets.

To determine the weight variations for hard capsules, 20 intact capsules are weighed and the average gross weight is calculated. The weight of each individual capsule must weigh between 90 and 110 per cent of the average gross weight.

If all capsules do not meet this requirement, the test may be expanded. Then 20 capsules are weighed individually. The contents of the 20 capsules are removed and combined. The weight of the total contents and the average weight are found. Each capsule shell is weighed individually. The net weight of each capsule content is calculated by subtracting the weight of the shell from

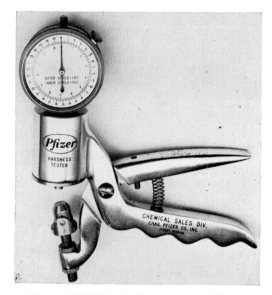

FIG. 3-15. Tablet-hardness tester. (Pfizer)

TABLE 3-7. WEIGHT VARIATION TOLERANCES FOR UNCOATED TABLETS

AVERAGE WEIGHT OF TABLET IN MG.	PERCENTAGE DIFFERENCE
130 or less	10
From 130 through 324	7.5
More than 324	5

the respective gross weight. The difference between the net weight and the average weight should not exceed 10 per cent for more than 2 capsules, and in no case should the difference be greater than 25 per cent.

If more than 2 but less than 7 capsules deviate from the average between 10 and 25 per cent, the net weights of an additional 40 capsules are determined and the average content of the entire 60 capsules is found. To meet specifications not more than 6 of the 60 capsules may exceed 10 per cent of the average, and in no case may the difference exceed 25 per cent.

The weight variation tolerances for uncoated tablets are given in Table 3-7. Twenty tablets are weighed individually. The average weight is calculated. For the tablets to be acceptable, the weights of not more than 2 of the tablets may differ from the average weight by no more than the percentage tabulated and no tablet may differ by more than double the per cent.

Organoleptic Evaluation. The homogeneity of capsule contents and tablets may be judged by visual examination. Speckled powders or tablets indicate improper and incomplete blending of ingredients and heterogeneous distribution of the active medicinals. In scored tablets the drug must be uniformly distributed. If the tablet is divided, the patient will receive that portion of the total active ingredient in the intact tablet only if the entire tablet is homogeneously blended.

The naked eye readily detects lack of uniformity or mottling in a colored tablet. Multiple layered tablets are often laminated into several distinct layers to avoid chemical and physical incompatibilities. Some tablets, such as Naldecon or Coricidin Medilets, are color-speckled tablets. Although these tablets as a whole are not uniform, each layer or granule is homogeneous.

Deterioration of solids may be detected visually or by odor. Aspirin tablets which are improperly formulated, improperly stored or exposed to moisture undergo hydrolysis. On opening a container of such tablets, the odor of acetic acid formed during hydrolysis is quickly discernible. Tablets may fade or darken in color indicating that an unwanted action has occurred.

Hardness. Capsules may be examined for cracks or dents and for brittleness. Tablets that are chipped or cracked are not suitable for dispensing.

The resistance of tablets to mechanical wear is shown in breakage and abrasion, and it is governed by the tensile strength of the compressed tablet. The hardness of a tablet is expressed as that force required to break the tablet. Hardness is used to characterize tablets because it is simple and convenient to measure. Hardness is measured by the Strong Cobb, the Pfizer and the Stokes Hardness Testers. Hardness is expressed in kilograms of force applied. Although the instruments give different hardness values for a set of tablets, it has been found that a constant ratio of hardness results with the Strong Cobb Tester giving results 1.6 times those of the Stokes Tester.

The practicing pharmacist may test tablets by snapping them between his thumb and forefinger. If the tablets do not snap readily,

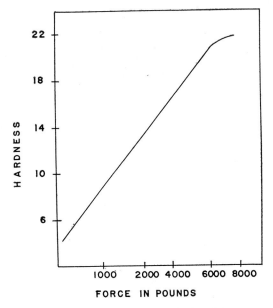

FIG. 3-16. Linear relationship of logarithm of compressional force and hardness of a tablet. (Higuchi, T., Rao, A. N., Busse, L. W., and Swintosky, J. V.: J. Am. Pharm. Ass., *42*:194, 1953)

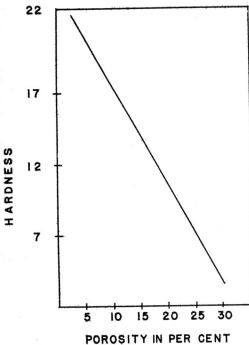

FIG. 3-17. Linear relationship of the hardness and the porosity of a tablet. (Higuchi, T., Rao, A. N., Busse, L. W., and Swintosky, J. V.: J. Am. Pharm. Ass., *42*:194, 1953)

they are too hard and may disintegrate with difficulty. Oral tablets normally have a hardness from 4 to 6; however, sustained release tablets and troches are compressed to at least 10.

As shown in Figures 3-16 and 3-17, hardness is proportional to the logarithm of the force of compression and inversely proportional to the porosity of a tablet. The greater the force of compression used in manufacturing a tablet, the less porous and the harder the tablet will be. Although increasing the hardness makes a more elegant and a less friable tablet, the high force of compression reduces the void space or porosity. With a reduction in porosity, penetration of dissolving or disintegrating fluids into the tablet is diminished, consequently slowing or preventing disintegration of the tablet.

Disintegration. Disintegration time limits are not specified for capsules, since the gelatin shell dissolves rapidly in the gastrointestinal tract. A hard gelatin capsule placed in water at 37°C. should release its contents within 5 minutes.

Factors determining the disintegration of

tablets are the physical and the chemical properties of the granulation, the hardness and the porosity. A tablet is generally formulated with a disintegrating agent, which will cause the tablet to rupture and fall apart in water or gastric fluid.

Disintegration does not imply complete solution of the tablet or the drug. Complete disintegration is that condition in which any tablet residue remaining on the screen of a disintegration apparatus is a soft mass having no palpably firm core. Normally, the disintegration time of a tablet is tested, but the time required for solution of the drug is not expressed.

Most lubricants utilized in tablet production are hydrophobic substances. Excessive lubricant will retard disintegration by preventing the penetration of water into the tablet. A tablet with a great void space will be penetrated by fluid and dissolve or disintegrate more rapidly than a hard, compressed tablet with very low porosity.

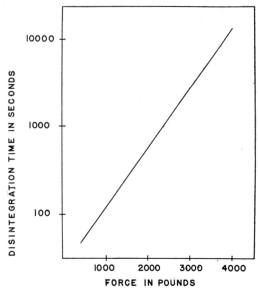

FIG. 3-18. Exponential relationship between disintegration time and the compressional force. (Higuchi, T., Rao, A. N., Busse, L. W., and Swintosky, J. V.: J. Am. Pharm. Ass., *42*:194, 1953)

As shown in Figure 3-18, it has been determined that the logarithm of disintegration time is proportional to the force of compression.

The simplest means of testing the disintegration of a tablet is to drop it in a glass of water. With occasional, gentle agitation the tablet should disintegrate in 15 to 30 minutes.

The *U.S.P.* disintegration apparatus consists of a basket-rack holding 6 open-end glass tubes with a 10-mesh screen on the undersurface. The basket-rack is immersed in a 1-liter beaker containing an appropriate fluid at 37°C. The basket-rack is raised and lowered through a distance of 5 to 6 cm. at the rate of 30 cycles per minute. The volume of fluid used is such that, during the operation, the basket-rack is never less than 2.5 cm. below the surface of the fluid or above the bottom of the beaker.

Each glass tube is supplied with a perforated, grooved disk which is placed on top of the tablet to simulate movement of the gastrointestinal tract.

A tablet is placed in each glass tube and a disk is added. The basket-rack is immersed and moved through the fluid for the time specified in the monograph. At the end of this time, when the basket-rack is lifted, all tablets should have disintegrated completely.

If 1 or 2 tablets did not disintegrate completely, the test is repeated with 12 additional tablets. Not less than 16 of the 18 tablets must disintegrate completely to meet specifications.

Plain coated tablets are tested by first placing a tablet in each glass tube and immersing in water at room temperature for 5 minutes to wash off any soluble external coating. A disk is added to each glass tube, and the apparatus is operated for 30 minutes using artificial gastric fluid at 37°C. After 30 minutes the basket-rack is lifted and the tablets are observed. If the tablets have not completely disintegrated, they are immersed in simulated intestinal fluid and observed. The tablets should disintegrate in the time specified in the monograph. If 1 or 2 tablets fail to disintegrate completely, the procedure is repeated with 12 additional tablets. To meet specifications, not less than 16 of the 18 tablets must disintegrate completely.

Enteric-coated tablets are tested by placing a tablet in each glass tube and immersing in water at room temperature for 5 minutes to wash off any soluble external coating. The apparatus is operated for an hour using simulated gastric fluid. After an hour the basket-rack is lifted and the tablets are observed. No distinctive dissolution or disintegration should be seen. A disk is added to each glass tube. The apparatus is operated in simulated intestinal fluid for a period of time equal to 2 hours plus the time limit specified in the individual monograph. Then the basket-rack is lifted and observed. All of the tablets should have disintegrated completely. If 1 or 2 tablets fail to disintegrate completely, the test is repeated with 12 additional tablets. To meet specifications, not less than 16 of the 18 tablets must disintegrate completely.

Buccal tablets are tested in the same way as uncoated tablets but without disks. The basket-rack is immersed in water for 4 hours. After 4 hours the basket-rack is lifted and the tablets are observed. All tablets should have disintegrated.

The U.S.P. tablet disintegration test does not apply to tablets exceeding 15 mm. in diameter, troches, tablets for hypodermic solution, chewable tablets, repeat action and sustained release tablets.

Hypodermic tablets are tested for solubility. A hypodermic tablet should dissolve completely, producing a clear solution, within 2 minutes when shaken gently in a test tube containing 2.5 ml. of water.

Chapter 2 should be consulted for a discussion of the limitations of such tests in evaluating therapeutic efficacy.

Dissolution. Disintegration time specification is a useful tool for quality control of production, but the disintegration of a tablet does not mean the drug has dissolved. A tablet may pass a disintegration test and yet the drug may be therapeutically unavailable.[12] While the disintegration time of a tablet may influence the rate of drug release to the body, the dissolution rate of the drug from the primary drug particle is fundamentally important, since solution of the drug is essential in order for absorption to occur.[46]

The rate of absorption and consequent physiologic availability of drugs administered orally in compressed tablets is a function of the rate of dissolution in the gastrointestinal fluid. The tablet formulation and

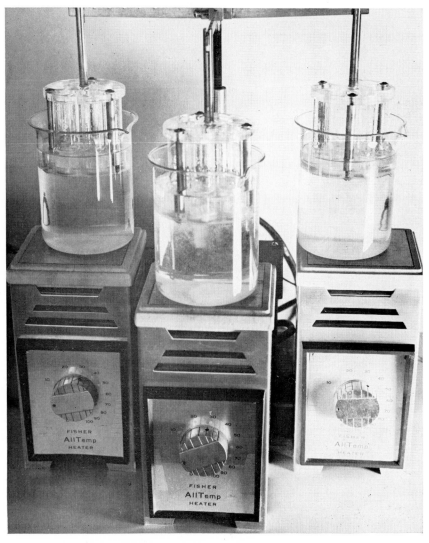

FIG. 3-19. An industrial apparatus for testing tablet disintegration time. (Dorsey Laboratories)

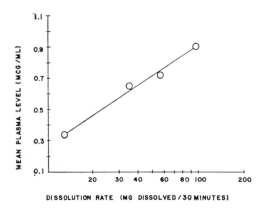

FIG. 3-20. Correlation of dissolution rate and mean griseofulvin plasma level (Katchen, B., and Symchowicz, S.: J. Pharm. Sci., *56*:1108, 1967)

process methods affect the dissolution; therefore, the therapeutic availability of drugs from generically identical tablets may be different.[11,14,22,34,51] There is extreme specificity in the presence or absence of a relationship between dissolution and disintegration time and therapeutic availability.[50]

A correlation between dissolution rate and availability is shown in Figure 3-20 for griseofulvin. The plot shows a linear relationship between the logarithm of the quantity dissolved in simulated intestinal fluid in 30 minutes and the mean plasma level for a 24-hour period after the oral administration of 500 mg. of griseofulvin.[30]

The correlation of in-vitro dissolution rates with blood levels or clinical responses is becoming an accepted technic in product development. Current investigations are attempting to design an in-vitro dissolution test that may be adopted as a standard.

COATING OF SOLIDS

A coating can be applied to a tablet, a pill, a granule or a capsule. A coating may be applied to a solid dosage form to increase the stability if the drug is affected by atmospheric moisture or oxygen, to mask an unpleasant taste, to retard loss of volatile ingredients, to improve the appearance of the solid form or to identify the finished product as being manufactured by a particular pharmaceutical firm. A coating may control the site of action,

as with enteric coating, or it may regulate the release of the drug, as with repeat action products.

105. ℞
Ammonium chloride Enseals . 0.5
Dispense 50.
Sig.: Two tablets every 4 hours.

106. ℞
Ferrous sulfate C. C., 0.2 . . . No. 36
Sig.: One tablet t. i. d. p. c.

107. ℞
Coryza (Bowman) 30
Sig.: One q. 3 hrs. for cold.

108. ℞
Pagitan S. C. Orange . . . . . . No. 50
Sig.: One three times a day.

SUGAR COATING

Commercially, the majority of the coated dosage forms are covered by a sugar coating. The coat is approximately 0.4 to 0.5 mm. in thickness. The maximum weight applied to a tablet by coating is approximately equal to the weight of the uncoated tablet. The amount of material depends on the number of coats required to smooth and color the tablet.

Tablets that are to be coated are compressed with a deep concave punch and die set, producing a tablet approaching a spherical shape. This allows the tablet to be covered more uniformly in the shortest time. Tablets to be coated may be compressed harder than uncoated tablets because they must withstand the additional processing. All dust must be removed from the tablets prior to coating or the tablets will not be uniformly smooth.

Sugar coating requires experience and elaborate equipment which the community pharmacist does not have at his disposal. The industrial equipment consists of motor-driven coating and polishing pans to which an exhaust and a hot air system with a blower is connected. The coating pans are made of stainless steel or copper. Polishing pans are lined with canvas. This lining polishes the tablets as they slide against the fabric. Steam kettles are required to maintain the coating solutions in a pourable state.

Subcoating is effected by the alternate

wetting of the tablet with subcoating solution and application of a coating powder when the tablets are partially dry. This procedure rounds off the sharp edges and builds the tablet to the desired shape. Modified solutions of syrup and gelatin are used as a subcoating solution. Calcium carbonate, starch, sugar and kaolin may be used in the coating powder.

Medium Subcoating Syrup
Acacia 2.25%
Gelatin 2.25
Sucrose 57.25
Distilled water 38.25

Subcoating Powder
Calcium carbonate 35%
Kaolin 16
Talc 25
Sucrose 20
Acacia 4

If a tablet contains a hygroscopic ingredient, a sealing coat is applied so that the water from the solutions applied will not be absorbed by the tablet. Such moisture would eventually penetrate the coating, resulting in discoloration and deterioration of the tablet.

Pharmaceutical glaze or shellac is dissolved in warm alcohol and allowed to stand until solution is complete.

Sealing Coat
Shellac 40%
Alcohol 60

The dust-free tablets are placed in a coating pan. A small amount of shellac solution is applied to the rolling tablets. The operator usually ensures even distribution of the shellac by mixing the rolling tablets with his hand. After 5 minutes of rolling, the cold air is turned on to dry the shellac. After 10 minutes the tablets are dry. A second addition, one half the volume of the first coat, is applied and dried. Two coats usually are adequate for sealing purposes. Excessive coating with shellac will interfere with the disintegration of the tablet.

After the tablet has been sealed, the gelatin syrup at 60°C. is added to the preheated tablets in a rotating coating pan. The tablets are immediately stirred with the hand to distribute the solution. When the gelatin syrup is partially dry (as indicated by the tablets beginning to form a ball), the sub-

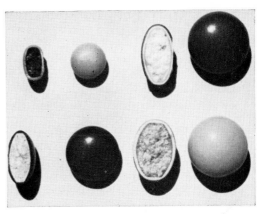

Fig. 3-21. (*Above*) Sugar-coated tablets showing the subcoating, the smoothing and the coloring coats. (*Below*) Enteric-coated tablets.

coating powder is immediately sprinkled into the coating pan until no wet tablets show and the tablets roll freely. An excessive amount of subcoating powder should be avoided.

When the subcoating powder has been taken up by the tablets, the warm air is turned on until the tablets are dry. This requires approximately 15 minutes for small batches.

When the tablets are dry, the warm air is shut off and the coating procedure is repeated until the tablets are nicely shaped and coated. This may require from 5 to 30 coats.

Smoothing is the alternate wetting with a smoothing syrup and drying of the subcoated tablets until they are properly rounded and smooth. Syrups are used as the smoothing solutions.

Smoothing Syrup
Sugar 60%
Distilled water 40

With the tablets rotating in a clean and dust-free pan, the syrup solution at 60°C. is added. After 5 to 10 minutes, when the rotating tablets appear dull and roll freely, warm air is turned on. When the tablets are dry, the process is repeated until the coating is smooth. Drying requires approximately 20 minutes. Five to 25 coats may be necessary to smooth the tablets.

Coloring. With colored tablets, a certified dye is added to the smoothing coat and the depth of color is gradually built up by successive coats. In the initial application, the syrup is colored lightly. After several coats have been applied, several more coats of a more highly colored syrup are applied. Succeeding coats are made darker in color until the last coat has the desired shade. This slow development of color prevents mottling of the coat.

A stock coloring syrup may contain from 0.1 to 0.6 per cent of a certified dye. The first colored syrup may be a 1:15 dilution of the stock coloring syrup; thus, the first colored syrup may have the dye present in 0.005 to 0.04 per cent concentration.

Finishing is the slow, controlled drying of the last syrup coat applied to the tablet. The coating pan is rotated manually with slow drying so that a very smooth finish is formed. When the last syrup is applied, the opening to the coating pan is covered with a cloth. The pan is rotated by hand through one half a revolution every 10 to 15 minutes during a 2-hour period.

Polishing, the final step, is the application of a thin layer of a glossy wax. The wax may be dissolved in warm naphtha or petroleum benzine, and the solution is added to the tablets which are allowed to rotate until the solvent has evaporated. The polishing mixture may be dusted on as a solid which is picked up by the rotating tablets.

Polishing Mixture
Beeswax 90%
Carnauba wax 10

In the sugar coating process considerable time is spent in sealing, rounding and smoothing the tablet and in overcoming the white background during the coloring phase. A suggested modification of this process produces a coating about half as thick and requires half as much time.

The tablets are given 2 coats of acacia, using a gelatin solution as the adhesive. A colorant is added to the gelatin solution so that coloring begins immediately. The tablets are sealed with one coat of a gum or a resin in a suitable solvent. Shellac in alcohol may be used. A pigmented coating suspension is now applied. Generally, 25 coats are adequate to develop the desired color. The tablet is then polished in the conventional way.

FILM COATING

Film coating is the rapid process by which a thin film of coating material is applied or sprayed onto tablets.[38] The process of sugar coating has the disadvantage of being slow and involving much labor, and it greatly increases the weight of the dosage form. Film coating has none of these disadvantages. Film-coated tablets retain their original shape and the thin film permits designs imprinted on the tablet to be seen. The film coat will mask unpleasant taste and protect the tablet from the atmosphere.

There is no significant change in disintegration of a film-coated tablet compared with that of the uncoated tablet. Most film coats will add a luster to a dull uncoated tablet; if required, a film-coated tablet may be polished in the same manner as a sugar coated tablet.

In general, the tablets are given a sealing coat, after which a solution of cellulosic polymers is applied or sprayed on the tablets.[23,58] Hydroxyethylcellulose, sodium carboxymethylcellulose and cellulose acetate phthalate have been used in various combinations with polyethylene glycol and polyvinylpyrrolidone in alcoholic solvents. Zein dispersed in isopropanol by means of the Spans and Tweens has also been used.

109. ℞
    Erythromid Filmtabs 50
    Sig.: Three Q. I. D.

AIR SUSPENSION COATING[19,68]

The Wurster process is an air suspension method for the rapid coating of granules,

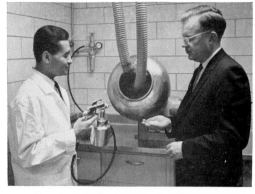

FIG. 3-22. Developmental film coating using a sprayer and 16-inch coating pan fitted with an exhaust and warm air.

powders and tablets. The solids to be coated are fed into a vertical cylinder and supported on a column of air which is being admitted continuously from the bottom of the cylinder in such a volume and at such a pressure that the solids remain suspended. Because of the action of the air stream and the pressure drop at the top of the cylinder, the solids rotate in both horizontal and vertical planes. The coating solution is admitted at a controlled rate. The air coming into the cylinder is heated to provide rapid drying of the coating syrup. Rounding coats on tablets are applied in less than an hour.

The Wurster process may be used to produce granulations. It will granulate rapidly and it needs no separate drying, blending or grinding procedures.

PRESS COATING[67]

Press coating is the process by which a fine, dry granulation is compressed around a core tablet forming what has been called a "tablet within a tablet." Press coating is faster and more economical than the pan coating process, as no sealing or polishing is required. Incompatibilities caused by moisture are avoided, since the press coating process is moisture-free. Press-coated tablets have less weight variation and may be compressed softer than pan-coated tablets. The compression coating process can be used to coat tablets of any shape and size. Press-coated tablets can be engraved or embossed more sharply than can film-coated tablets.

Press-coating machines are of two types. In one type the core is compressed on a standard tablet machine and fed into the compression coater. The second type is basically two rotary machines with a single drive shaft and transfer device so that the compression of the core and the coating is a continuous cycle.

In addition to being used to coat a tablet, the process may be used to prevent contact between incompatible ingredients of the tablet. One of the incompatible drugs is compressed in the core, and the other drug is compressed in the coat or the shell separating the reacting drugs. This technic has also been used with laminated multiple compressed tablets. Each incompatible drug is granulated and compressed separately, forming a

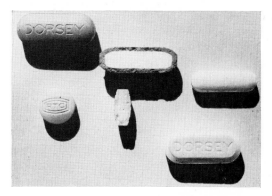

FIG. 3-23. Press-coated tablets and modified press-coated tablets.

finished tablet with two or more layers, each containing one of the incompatible drugs.

Press coating has found wide application in repeat-action and controlled-release medication. In a repeat-action tablet, the core is treated so that it does not disintegrate until 4 to 6 hours have elapsed, while the shell disintegrates rapidly, releasing its drug for the initial dose of the medication.

110. ℞
    Pabirin A C Buffered 50

    Sig.: Two Q. I. D.

111. ℞
    Bonadoxin Tablets 30

    Sig.: One h.s.

112. ℞
    Pyribenzamine-Ephedrine 24

    Sig.: One q. 4 hrs.

ENTERIC COATING

A dosage form is enteric-coated if the coating prevents the disintegration of the tablet in the stomach but permits disintegration in the intestinal tract. Such a coating is needed when a drug is decomposed or inactivated by the pH or the digestive enzymes of the stomach, is irritating to the stomach or is to be placed in the specific area of the intestine.

113. ℞
    Aminosalicylic Acid . . . . . 0.56 Gm.

    Give 60 Enseals.

    Sig.: Six tab. q.i.d.

114. ℞

    Ammonium chloride Emplets   0.5 Gm.

    Give 100

    Sig.: Two t.i.d.

115. ℞

    Diethylstilbestrol E. C. 1 mg.   30

    Sig.: As directed.

Biologic variation affects the release of medication from an enteric-coated dosage form. The emptying time for the stomach may vary from a few minutes to as much as 12 hours. The research and developmental pharmacist uses the average stomach emptying time of 6 hours in formulating an enteric coating. Solid dosage forms remain for a shorter period of time in an empty stomach than in a full stomach. It is generally considered advisable to administer an enteric-coated product 2 hours before meals—the time when the most uniform emptying is observed.

Variation in pH in the regions of the gastrointestinal tract make it preferable that an enteric coat disintegrate independent of pH. More recent enteric coatings are based on the time required for disintegration of the coating when in contact with moisture. One such enteric coating is a mixture of powdered waxes such as carnauba wax or stearic acid and vegetable fibers of agar and elm bark. When the tablets are administered, the vegetable fibers imbibe water, swell and begin the process of disintegration. By varying the ratio of the vegetable fibers to the wax and by varying the thickness of the coating, the time required for disintegration may be controlled.

Gelatin polymerized with formaldehyde, stearic acid, salol, keratin or resins has been used as an enteric coating substance with limited success.

The practicing pharmacist may be called on to coat a capsule, a tablet or a pill with an enteric coating. The traditional salol coat used for extemporaneous enteric coating has been replaced to some extent by one consisting of n-butyl stearate, carnauba wax and stearic acid.[55] All resist the action of the gastric fluid, but, with the exception of carnauba wax, they are hydrolyzed in the intestine.

Forty-five parts of n-butyl stearate, 30 parts of carnauba wax and 25 parts of stearic acid are fused at 75°C. and are maintained at this temperature during the coating process. The capsule is held at one end with tweezers and dipped somewhat more than half its length into the coating mixture. The capsule is withdrawn, its free end is touched to the lip of the dish to remove excess coating mixture, and it is placed on a tile. The operation is repeated until one end of each of the capsules has been coated. Then the coating is completed by grasping the capsule carefully at the coated end and by dipping it in such a fashion that the coats overlap. The cycle should be repeated once to ensure an adequate coating. Although it is possible to coat tablets and pills by this technic, it is difficult to obtain pharmaceutical elegance.

A more recent method of coating with cellulose acetate phthalate may be used to produce acceptable enteric-coated tablets, capsules or pills. Cellulose acetate phthalate has been widely used commercially. The disintegration or dissolution of cellulose acetate phthalate does not require fluids with a high pH but only solutions which will contribute ions to the phthalate carboxyl group and enhance the solubility of cellulose acetate phthalate in aqueous medium. Cellulose acetate phthalate coatings also disintegrate due to the hydrolytic effects of the esterases of the intestinal tract.

Cellulose acetate phthalate may be used extemporaneously.[44] A 10 per cent solution of cellulose acetate phthalate in acetone is placed in a small vial. A capsule is dropped into the solution and removed with tweezers. The capsule is allowed to touch the lip of the vial to catch any excess solution. The capsule is held in the tweezers for a minute, after which it is placed on gauze. In this manner all of the capsules are coated. The cycle is repeated until 3 coats have been applied.

This method has the advantage that no heat is used in the coating process, there is little increase in weight of the dosage form, and tablets may be coated as well as pills and capsules.

MOLDED SOLID DOSAGE FORMS

Tablet triturates are prepared by forcing moistened ingredients into a mold under

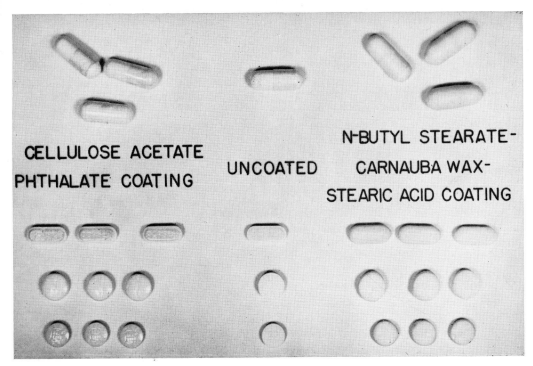

CELLULOSE ACETATE PHTHALATE COATING   UNCOATED   N-BUTYL STEARATE-CARNAUBA WAX-STEARIC ACID COATING

Fig. 3-24. Capsules and tablets enteric-coated with cellulose acetate phthalate or a mixture of n-butyl stearate–carnauba wax–stearic acid. (Parrott, E. L.: J. Am. Pharm. Ass., *NS1*: 158, 1961)

manual pressure. Tablet triturates are flat-faced tablets with a diameter of approximately 5 mm. The diluent used in tablet triturates is lactose or a mixture of lactose and sucrose.

Tablet triturates are administered by placing on the tongue and swallowing with a drink of water. The advantage of tablet triturates is their rapid disintegration and solution. Tablet triturates are fragile and their small size makes them unsuitable for drugs with large doses.

Some tablet triturates are made by compression, but many tablet triturates are still produced by manual molding although the method is costly. The community pharmacist is rarely required to prepare a tablet triturate extemporaneously. The procedure for preparing tablet triturates in the pharmacy will be found in *American Pharmacy*.*

Hypodermic tablets are intended to be dissolved in water, and the solution is to be in-

* Sprowls, J. B.: American Pharmacy. 6th ed. Philadelphia, J. B. Lippincott, 1966.

jected parenterally. Hypodermic tablets are smaller than tablet triturates in order to facilitate placing the hypodermic tablet in the barrel of the syringe. Solution of hypodermic tablets must be rapid and complete. It is doubtful that solutions prepared in this manner are sterile.

Hypodermic tablets are packaged in tubes of 20 tablets. It is preferred that they be dispensed in the original tube in which they are packaged to restrict contamination and to limit the breakage of the fragile tablets.

Tablet triturates are dispensed in a snap-on or screw-cap vial or glass container, using cotton on the bottom and on the top of the tablets to prevent breakage.

116. ℞
  T. T. Saccharin soluble, 1 gr. 100

  Sig.: Use as a sugar substitute.

117. ℞
  T. T. Codeine sulfate, 1 gr. . . . No. 12

  Sig.: One for pain p. r. n.

118. ℞

    H. T. Scopolamine hydrobro-
mide .... 0.32 mg.

Dispense 1 tube.

Sig.: Use as directed.

Pills are oval or spherical solid masses containing drugs to be administered orally. The usual pill weighs from 100 to 300 mg.

Pills have declined in use until it has become a curiosity for a pharmacist to be called on to compound an extemporaneous pill. Although some pills are still produced by pharmaceutical industry, the tablet and the capsule have largely replaced the pill as a dosage form. Pills have no advantages not found in tablets or capsules.

In preparing a pill the powdered ingredients are thoroughly blended. The appropriate excipient is carefully added and the mass is formed by applying considerable pressure with the pestle. When the mass is plastic and cohesive but not sticky, it is removed from the mortar and kneaded with the hands. The correct consistency is reached when the mass tends to peel from the sides of the mortar.

The mass is kneaded in the hands until no cracks show. The mass is then rolled between the palms into a ball. This ball is placed on a pill tile and rolled into a cylinder. The cylinder is cut into the required number of segments.

The cut segments are shaped by rolling one pill at a time in the palm of one hand with the finger of the other.

Since pills are now so little used, it has not been deemed necessary to repeat the details of their production. The procedure for preparing pills will be found in *American Pharmacy*.*

119. ℞

    Alophen pills 15

Sig.: 1-2 h. s.

120. ℞

    Cathartic Compound, Brown,
C. C. .... No. 20

Sig.: Two pills as a laxative.

Lozenges dissolve slowly in the saliva, medicating the throat for a prolonged time.

* Sprowls, J. B.: American Pharmacy. 6th ed. Philadelphia, J. B. Lippincott, 1966.

Those sold over the counter, such as Allenbury's Pastilles and cough drops, are pleasantly flavored to appeal to the sense of taste.

Various types of lozenges, such as troches and pastilles, are prepared by molding masses. Some are prepared similarly to pills with a difference in the final form. Others are manufactured by molding a hot mass which solidifies on cooling.[1] In general, a lozenge consists of the medicinal agent, flavors, sugar and gelatin or a gum.

One candy base is prepared commercially by combining 1,200 lbs. of sugar, 1,000 lbs. of 43° Baume corn syrup and 560 lbs. of water. Warm water is metered into a tank equipped with an agitator. The sugar is added to the water. By means of a steam jacket the sugar solution is heated to 40°C. The corn syrup at the same temperature is metered into the tank. After thorough mixing the mass is pumped into the cookers.

The mass is heated to 115°C. for a short period under atmospheric pressure. The syrup is pumped through a coil, which is surrounded by high pressure steam, and reaches a temperature of 145°C. A vacuum is applied for approximately 10 minutes and water is withdrawn. At this stage, the candy base consists of approximately two thirds sucrose solids, one third corn syrup solids and less than 1 per cent water.

Drugs, color and flavors are thoroughly mixed into the molten mass. As the temperature of the candy will be approximately 90°C., thermolabile drugs cannot be incorporated in a candy base. The mixture is mechanically kneaded and drawn into a thin rope on a spinning machine. The rope is cut and shaped by a die-compressing machine. The lozenges are cooled on moving belts by jets of cool air.

In order to assure stability, troches are packaged in foil or waxed paper to minimize moisture absorption from the atmosphere.

121. ℞

    Cepacol (Merrell) .... 1 box

Sig.: For relief of sore throat.

122. ℞

    Robitussin-DM Cough Calmers 1 pkg.

Sig.: One troche for cough.

123. ℞

Sucrets ....   1 box

Sig.: Dissolve without swallowing.

124. ℞

Synkayvite-C Lozenges 100

Sig.: Two troches t. i. d.

SUSTAINED-RELEASE PHARMACEUTICALS[32,33,54]

Sustained-release medication was introduced into the United States about 1952. At present, sustained-release medication represents about 5 per cent of the total pharmaceutical market. Although 3 major firms produce the majority of the sustained-release medication, there are approximately 50 manufacturers that produce sustained-release products. Some specialty names for capsules and tablets from which the release of the medicinal agents is controlled are given in Table 3-8.

Long-acting oral products have been described by various ambiguous terms. A sustained-release product is one in which a drug is initially made available to the body in an amount sufficient to cause a rapid onset of the desired therapeutic response, after which the level of therapeutic response is maintained at the initial level for a desired number of hours beyond the activity resulting from a conventional dose. A sustained-release product must be formulated so that the rate of release of the drug, after the initial concentration, is equal to the rate at which the drug is eliminated or inactivated. As such a release is difficult to produce, most preparations are prolonged-action products.

A prolonged-action product is one in which a drug is initially made available to the body in an amount sufficient to produce the desired therapeutic response quickly and which then provides for replacement of the disappearing drug at a rate which increases the duration of therapeutic activity compared with that of a single dose.

Repeat-action dosage forms are not prolonged acting products. A repeat-action preparation initially provides a single dose of a drug, and, after several hours, when the therapeutic response of the initial dose has ceased, it provides a second single dose.

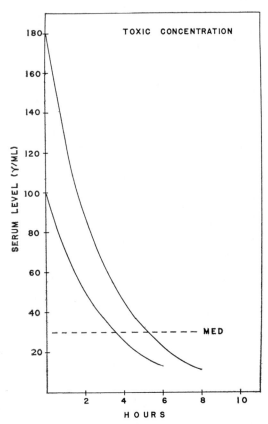

FIG. 3-25. A massive dose results in longer duration of activity, but the serum level rises to a toxic level initially.

By experience, medical science has found that there is a certain amount of a drug which will be required to produce a desired effect in the majority of patients. This dose or serum level is known as the minimum effective dose (M. E. D.). Any dosage which falls below the minimum effective dose does not produce the desired effect.

Ideally, a sustained-release solid dosage form given once daily should provide sufficient drug immediately to produce a rapid, initial therapeutic response and should maintain this level of response for 12 hours on a single administration. Prolonged effect may be achieved by administering massive doses of a drug. This is not an effective method, because, initially, the concentration of the drug greatly exceeds the M. E. D. Any dose that exceeds the M. E. D. is wasted drug, since the desired therapeutic response is ob-

TABLE 3-8. SPECIALTY NAMES FOR CONTROLLED RELEASE DOSAGE FORMS

SPECIALTY	COMPANY	DESCRIPTION
Cenule	Central Pharmacal	time-disintegration capsule
Chroncap	H. R. Cenci Pharmacal	time-disintegration capsule
Chronosule	White	sustained-release capsule
Chronotab	White	sustained-release tablet
Coseal	Hiss Pharmacal	enteric-coated tablet
Cronsule	Louisons Pharmaceuticals	sustained-release capsule
Delay Tab	Southern Drug and Manufacturing	timed-release tablet
Dospan	Merrell	sustained-release tablet
Duracap	Meyer	sustained-release capsule
Dura-Tab	Wynn Pharmacal	sustained-release tablet
Emplet	Parke, Davis	enteric-coated tablet
Encoat	Merrell	enteric-coated tablet
Encore	Premo	repeat action tablet
Enduret	Geigy	sustained-release tablet
Enerel	Premo	enteric-coated tablet
Enkeric	Rorer	enteric-coated tablet
Enpule	Superior Pharmacal	enteric-coated tablet
Enseal	Eli Lilly	time-disintegration, enteric-coated tablet
Entab	Central Pharmacal	enteric-coated tablet
Entell	Buffington	enteric-coated tablet
Enterab	Abbott	enteric-coated tablet
Extentab	Robins	sustained action tablet
Gelet	American Vitamin	enteric-coated tablet
Gradual	Federal Pharmacal	time-disintegration capsule
Gradule	Jan	sustained-release capsule
Gradumet	Abbott	sustained-release tablet
Granucap	S. J. Tutag	time-disintegration capsule
Intervule	Jan	time-disintegration capsule
Juvelet	Dorsey	time-release pediatric tablet
Keensule	Keene Pharmacal	time-disintegration capsule
Longcap	G and G Pharmacal	sustained-release capsule
Lontab	Ciba	sustained-release tablet
Medsule	Medco	timed-release capsule
Medule	Upjohn	timed-release capsule
Palet	Philadelphia	time-disintegration capsule
Plateau Cap	Marion	sustained-release capsule
Prestab	McNeil	sustained-release tablet
Prolong Cap	Gold Leaf Pharmacal	time-disintegration capsule
Prolongsule	Richlyn	time-disintegration capsule

TABLE 3-8. SPECIALTY NAMES FOR CONTROLLED RELEASE DOSAGE FORMS (*Continued*)

SPECIALTY	COMPANY	DESCRIPTION
Repetab	Schering	repeat action tablet
Seal-Ins	Seal-Ins	enteric-coated capsule or tablet
Sequel	Lederle	sustained-release capsule
Singlet	Pitman-Moore	sustained-release tablet
Spansule	Smith, Kline & French	sustained-release capsule
Spacelet	Prime	timed-release tablet
Spancap	Domed	sustained-release capsule
Spantab	Rocky Mountain Pharmacal	time-disintegration tablet
Spascap	Prime	time-disintegration capsule
Stankap	Standex	time-disintegration capsule
Stedytab	Eastern Research	sustained-release tablet
Taysule	Taylor Drug	sustained-release capsule
Tembid	Ives	sustained-release tablet
Tempo-Tablet	Penn Pharmacal	multilayer sustained-release tablet
Tempule	Armour	sustained-release capsule
Ten-Tab	National Drug	sustained-release tablet
Timcap	Vitamix Corp.	time-disintegration capsule
Timecap	Leeds	sustained-release capsule
Timed Cap	Testagar	time-disintegration capsule
Timelet	Rowell	sustained-release tablet
Timeset	Cabot Pharmacal	time-disintegration capsule
Timespan	Roche	sustained-release tablet
Timesule	Arnar Stone	time-disintegration capsule
Timetab	Rocky Mountain Pharmacal	timed-release tablet
Timkap	Betan	time-disintegration capsule
Trisule	Chas. C. Haskell	time-disintegration capsule
Ty-Med	Lemmon Pharmacal	timed-release tablet
Tymcap	Amfre-Grant	time-disintegration capsule
Tymtab	Amfre-Grant	time-disintegration tablet
Unicelle	Hiss Pharmacal	sustained-release pellets

tained at the M. E. D. Massive doses produce a drug concentration that approaches the toxic dose of the drug and markedly increases unwanted side effects.

A soluble drug with a half-life of 2 hours has a M. E. D. serum level of 30 γ/ml. A 250 mg. and a 500 mg. capsule produce a maximum serum level of 100 and 180 γ/ml., respectively. Because the capsule dissolves rapidly and the soluble drug is quickly dis-

solved and absorbed, the time required for release and absorption into the blood stream is small and may be ignored. Assuming a first order elimination from the blood, one can see in Figure 3-25 that by doubling the oral dose the serum level is maintained above the M. E. D. for approximately 2 additional hours.

A conventional capsule, tablet or pill usually is administered 3 or 4 times daily to

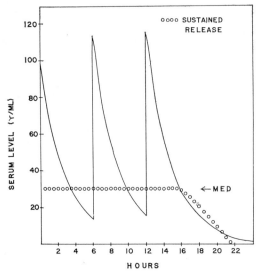

Fig. 3-26. The serum level obtained by the administration of 1 tablet or capsule 3 times a day compared with the serum level obtained from an ideal sustained-release tablet or capsule.

evoke and maintain the desired therapeutic response. Initially each dose will produce a maximum drug concentration far above the M. E. D. As the drug is eliminated and inactivated, the drug concentration falls below the M. E. D. Below this level the therapeutic effect is inadequate until the next dose is administered. Thus multi-doses are wasteful and inadequate.

If a 250 mg. capsule of the soluble drug with a half-life of 2 hours were prescribed to be administered 3 times a day, a patient would probably take a capsule at 8:00 A.M., 2:00 P.M. and 8:00 P.M. and no medication during the night. As shown in Figure 3-26, during the 12 hours immediately after the beginning of administration, the serum level would be adequate approximately 60 per cent of the time. There are 4.7 hours when the serum level falls below the M. E. D. In a 24-hour interval there would be 11.2 hours of adequate serum levels; approximately 50 per cent of the 24-hour period would have therapeutically effective serum concentration.

An ideal sustained-release dosage form will maintain a constant and uniform drug release and concentration as shown in Figure 3-26. With sustained release, the maxima in drug concentration shown with multi-doses

are eliminated with a more economical utilization of the drug and fewer side effects. Sustained release eliminates the fall of drug concentration below the M. E. D. so that the patient is receiving a therapeutically adequate amount of the drug at all times. The elimination of the maxima reduces the total amount of the drug needed to obtain continuity of the desired response. So much drug may be wasted in the maxima that three conventional 50 mg. tablets can be replaced by 100 mg. of the drug in a sustained release form. With the sustained-release form no drug is wasted because the drug concentration does not exceed, and is maintained at, the level of the M. E. D.

In addition to eliminating the peaks and the dips in drug level inevitable with multi-dose administration, sustained release is a convenience to the patient and the nursing staff. With a reduction in the number of doses taken daily, the patient is more cooperative and less likely to forget to take his medication.

For ease of discussion, sustained-release preparations are usually classified according to their method of preparation. From the viewpoint of the physician and the pharmacist who is advising the physician concerning sustained-release products, a classification based on the type of release is most valuable. The type of continuous release from a sustained-release dosage form is release or solution of the drug in a steady, uninterrupted manner from the initial to the final amount of the drug released. An ideal sustained-release product would provide continuous release of its medication. The erosion, the ion-exchange resin and the leaching pharmaceutical technics yield products with this type of release.

Incremental release is that type of release which is not a steady release; rather, the drug is released or dissolved in parts, with a fixed time interval (during which no drug is released) between each part released. The controlled-disintegration type of sustained release provides incremental release.

Methods of Obtaining Sustained Release

Sustained release may be obtained by pharmaceutical, chemical and biologic methods. Medical or biologic means are limited to the immediate use of the physician and are of little significance to the pharmacist.

Controlled Disintegration. The method first used for controlling the release of a drug was the enteric coating. The disintegration of the enteric coating is based on pH of the gastrointestinal tract, chemical and enzymatic action within the gastrointestinal tract, or the time in contact with moisture. The most reliable release is that based on the time in contact with moisture. Although an enteric coating releases the medication in the intestine or after an average time of 6 hours, it is only a controlled and not a sustained-release dosage form.

Repeat-action tablets consist of a tablet within a tablet or a laminated tablet in which the outer shell or a layer disintegrates rapidly, releasing the initial dose for immediate effect. The core is enteric coated with shellac or some resistant coating which protects the core from fluids for approximately 4 hours, after which the core disintegrates releasing a second dose of the medication. The core may be press coated or pan coated with the drug to be released initially.

Repeat-action tablets are also known as delayed-action and timed-release tablets. A repeat-action tablet liberates the drug in an amount that exceeds the immediate need, and the drug level drops sharply after ingestion. The drug level falls below the M. E. D. before the core disintegrates. When the core disintegrates, there is again a drug concentration similar to that from the first dose. Usually, these 2 stages do not overlap, so that there is no therapeutic advantage with repeat-action tablets. The advantage of repeat-action tablets lies in their usefulness to the patient who needs medication during the hours of sleep.

125. ℞
    Triaminic (Dorsey) 12

    Sig.: One swallowed whole in morning.

126. ℞
    Demazin Repetabs (Schering) 24

    Sig.: 2 morning and evening.

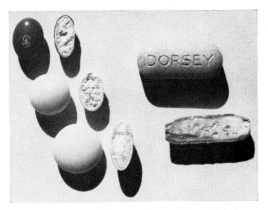

FIG. 3-27. Repeat-action tablets with a pan-coated or a press-coated shell which releases drug for immediate use and a core which does not release any drug for several hours.

127. ℞
    Prestabs Butiserpazide-25
      (McNeil) 30

    Sig.: One daily.

128. ℞
    Bentyl Repeat Action (Merrell) . . 60

    Sig.: One t. i. d.

129. ℞
    Convertin (Ascher) 30

    Sig.: Two with meals.

130. ℞
    Bontril Timed Tablets No. 1
      (Carnrick) 50

    Sig.: One before breakfast.

A plurality of coatings applied to pellets has successfully approached ideal sustained release. Spansule is the best known example of sustained release which depends on different thicknesses of the coating on many pellets to produce various disintegration times.[57,61]

Spansule consists of a capsule containing a large number of pellets coated with various thicknesses of a slowly dispersible substance as well as uncoated pellets or powdered drug to provide initial drug concentration. Each group of the coated pellets, usually 100 per group, contains an equal amount of the drug. The total amount of drug in the sustained form is from 2 to 4 times the dose given in a conventional tablet or capsule.

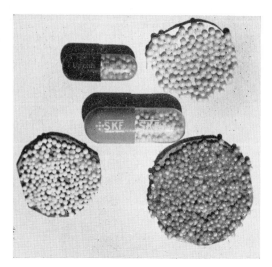

Fig. 3-28 (*Above*) Pellet-type sustained release illustrated by a Module capsule. (*Below*) Left: the immediate-action pellets from a Spansule. Right: the sustained-release pellets from the same capsule.

Any desired release can be obtained by a plurality of coatings but, usually, 3 coated groups are employed. If X represents the thickness of a coating which releases the drug at the end of 9 hours and Y is the number of coated groups, the thickness of the coat for the first group is X/Y, and the thickness of the coat for the second coated group is 2X/Y. In actual production, the coating ranges from 30 to 40 per cent on either side of the median coating. A good approximation may be based on the weight of the coating where X represents the weight of the median coating of the group which disintegrates last.

The nucleus of each pellet is either a 12-mesh to 40-mesh nonpareil or the drug and sucrose made into a pellet. The nonpareils are coated with syrup and the drug, employing conventional pan coating technics. Repeated coats of the drug are added to the nonpareils until by assay the proper weight of drug has been built up on the sugar pellets. These are the uncoated pellets which release the drug for immediate effect.

Three fourths of the uncoated pellets are pan-coated by spraying a warm solution of glyceryl monostearate and beeswax in carbon tetrachloride onto the pellets rotating in a coating pan. Other water-insoluble, indigestible lipids such as paraffin, carnauba wax, bayberry wax or cholesterol may be used to slow disintegration of the coating. Other water-dispersible or digestible substances may be used such as the higher fatty alcohols, stearic acid, diglycol stearate and esters of fatty acids of high molecular weight.

Two thirds of the thinly coated pellets are further coated by the same process. These form the second coated group of pellets covered with a film of intermediate thickness and having an intermediate disintegration time.

Half of the pellets, which are coated with the film having an intermediate disintegration time, are coated further to form a third group of coated pellets which disintegrate at 9 hours.

Each of the 3 groups of coated pellets and the group of uncoated pellets each contains the same weight of the drug. The 4 groups of pellets are blended and encapsulated.

If all of the pellets in each coated group were covered with a uniformly thick coat, the medication would be released after the initial release in 3 discontinuous surges. In actual production, there is some variation of thickness of the coat within each coated group. The variance of thickness within each group permits some pellets to disintegrate sooner than those with the median thickness of that group. The drug so released overlaps the drug remaining from the previous group. Some pellets within a group are slightly thicker than the median thickness and do not disintegrate until later so that the drug released overlaps with the next group. This overlapping between groups provides a smoother and more uniform release which approaches a continuous type of release.

Spansules disintegrate independent of pH with the release mechanism primarily one of moisture vapor pressure permeability of the lipid film. The drug, the composition of the coating and the thickness of the coating determine the rate of moisture permeability.

In addition to promoting a sustained release effect, Spansules provide a more uniform distribution of the drug in the gastrointestinal tract. If a single tablet fails to disintegrate, the benefit of the entire dose is lost. If a few pellets of a Spansule fail to disintegrate, the loss of a small amount of the total drug will not greatly affect the over-all dose.

Fundamentally, Medules function similarly to Spansules. The pellets are of uniform size so that no stratification occurs during the encapsulation process. The release of the medication is dependent on the composition and the thickness of the coating. The coat consists of a styrene-maleic acid copolymer which is pH-sensitive and prevents dissolution in the stomach acid.[60,64]

Shellac coatings may be added in sufficient number to provide delayed disintegration time of nonpareils which have been coated with active ingredients. These pellets are blended with a conventional granulation and compressed into a tablet. Pellets coated with ethyl cellulose are elastic enough so that they can be compressed with a conventional granulation without rupturing the coating during compression.

A sustained-release tablet may be made by compressing a tablet from a blend of a conventional granulation and a sustained-release granulation. The sustained-release granulation consists of the drug coated or granulated with zein, cellulose acetate or ethyl cellulose. Other sustained-release granulations consist of the drug held in a slowly dispersible or digestible matrix of glyceryl esters mixed with fatty acids and alcohols. The waxy ingredients may compose 25 per cent of the delayed-time material.

131. ℞

    Tuss-Ornade Spansule (SKF) 12

    Sig.: One daily.

132. ℞

    Medrol Medules (Upjohn) 60

    Sig.: One in morning and evening.

133. ℞

    Nitroglyn (Key) 50

    Sig.: One before breakfast and h.s.

134. ℞

    Bellergal Spacetabs (Sandoz) 50

    Sig.: One morning and evening.

135. ℞

    Pentritol Tempules (Armour) 45

    Sig.: One A.M. & P.M.

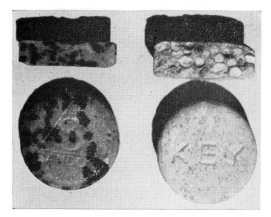

Fig. 3-29. (*Left*) A conventional granulation is compressed with a sustained-release granulation. (*Right*) Sustained-release pellets are compressed within a conventional granulation.

136. ℞

    Timed Amodex Capsules (Testagar) 30

    Sig.: One on arising.

Erosion. In the erosion technic of obtaining sustained release an insoluble tablet is formed which continuously releases the drug due to the uninterrupted surface erosion of the tablet and the solution of the drug. The tablet does not disintegrate and maintains its geometric shape as it passes through the gastrointestinal tract. Because the geometric shape is unchanged while the tablet erodes, there is a continual decrease in the weight of drug released per unit time as the surface area of the tablet is progressively reduced.

The erosion technic is generally used with a press-coated or a pan-coated outer shell which is applied in the conventional manner to the specially formulated core. After administration, the shell disintegrates rapidly, providing an immediate concentration of the drug. The core then begins to erode at a rate determined by the proper blend of a waxy tablet base and the drug. No shellac or enteric materials are used in this method. The drug is suspended in a solid fat or a wax of high molecular weight. As the tablet erodes, the drug is continuously dissolved and is available for absorption.

Industrially, the drug and the melted fats and waxes are blended in a thermostated

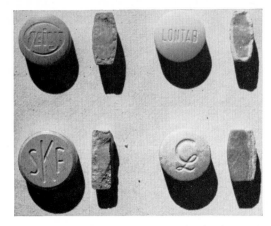

Fig. 3-30. Erosion-type sustained-release tablets. (*Above*) Tablet cores are press coated with a shell to provide immediate drug release. (*Lower right*) The tablet is a laminated tablet with an immediate release and a sustained-release layer.

mixer with milling and sweeping blades to maintain a uniform liquid suspension. The uniform suspension is passed through a steam-jacketed valve onto a cooling drum. The congealed blend is stripped from the drum and ground at low temperature. The resulting granulation is compressed into a tablet and press-coated if desired.

The continuous release of the medication and the elimination of the waste of drug at the maxima obtained with conventional tablets reduce the total drug necessary to maintain a therapeutic response. One Lontab containing 100 mg. of pyribenzamine is therapeutically equivalent to 3 conventional 50 mg. tablets.[59]

Two or 3 separate granulations may be pressed together to form a multiple-layer tablet. One layer contains the drug readily available for immediate use. Another layer —the sustained-release layer—is compressed and formulated so that it will retain its shape during its passage through the gastrointestinal tract. If the layer is cylindrical with a large diameter compared with the height of the layer, the eroding or dissolving surface will remain essentially constant. A constant surface means that the drug will dissolve and be released at a constant rate, more nearly meeting the requirements for an ideal sustained release dosage form.

The erosion or the gradual flaking off of the surface is based on an attrition, and it is independent of pH.

137. ℞
    Preludin Endurets (Geigy) 30

    Sig.: One tablet in midmorning.

138. ℞
    Donnatal Extentabs (Robins) 30

    Sig.: One morning and night.

139. ℞
    Sul-Spantab (SKF) 75

    Sig.: 4 at start; then 2 daily.

140. ℞
    Peritrate Sustained Action
      (Warner-Chilcott) 50

    Sig.: One q. 12 hrs.

141. ℞
    Pen-Vee L-A (Wyeth) 12

    Sig.: Two daily.

142. ℞
    Aminophyllin Dura-Tabs (Wynn) . 18

    Sig.: 1-2 tablets every 12 hrs.

143. ℞
    Novahistine LP (Pitman-
      Moore) 12

    Sig.: One q. 8 hrs.

144. ℞
    Mestinon Timespan (Roche) 25

    Sig.: Two b. i. d.

Leaching is the process by which there is steady dissolution and removal of a drug from an insoluble, intact matrix. One may consider the tablet as an inert sponge with its pores filled with the drug. The intact matrix of Gradumets consists of a copolymer of methyl acrylate and methyl methacrylate which passes unchanged through the gastrointestinal tract and is eliminated in the feces. The Gradumet is produced by compressing a granulation of the drug with the insoluble plastic material.

When the tablet reaches the stomach, some of the drug in the superficial channels is leached out rapidly to provide an immediate therapeutic effect. As the tablet travels along the intestine, the drug is leached out from

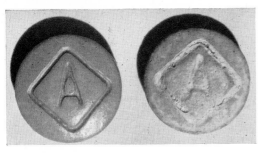

FIG. 3-31. (*Left*) A Gradumet tablet. (*Right*) One which has been exposed to water for 24 hours.

the deeper channels or pores over a prolonged period. The release of the drug is independent of pH and enzyme concentration.

Control of drug release is obtained by varying the porosity and the ratio between the exposed surface of the plastic matrix and the dissolving drug. If the drug is sparingly soluble, a highly soluble substance may be added to facilitate dissolution from the channels. Such a soluble substance is known as a channeling agent.

145. ℞
    Nembutal Gradumets (Abbott) ... 15

    Sig.: One on arising.

Ion Exchange Resin. Ion exchange is the process by which an insoluble resin extracts ions of one kind from solution and exchanges them for ions of another kind originally bonded to the resin.[15] The formation and the dissociation of complexes utilizing organic acids or bases and certain ion exchange resins proceeds at a finite rate. It is claimed that when the ion exchange resin is chosen properly, the rate of dissolution will produce uniform drug release dependent only on the concentration of ions available in the gastrointestinal tract.

The resinate is insoluble and releases the drug by double decomposition in which the drug is exchanged for an ion. Cationic exchange resins are used to replace a specie of cation with another specie of cation. The resins used for sustained release are cationic exchange resins combined with a cationic form of the drug to be released.

The drug is released by an exchange with the cations found in the gastrointestinal fluids.

$$SO_2O \text{ (Drug)} \qquad SO_2ONa$$

$$\bigcirc + NaCl \rightarrow \bigcirc + (Drug)^+Cl^-$$

$$\ldots-CH-CH_2-\ldots \quad \ldots-CH-CH_2-\ldots$$

The rate of release is said to depend only on the total concentration of these cations. Since this concentration is nearly constant throughout the entire gastrointestinal tract, the release is claimed to be predictable, continuous and controlled.

The bead size of the resin affects the rate of release of the adsorbed drug. With a small particle size, the drug is released more rapidly. A 200-mesh bead has a greater surface area per unit weight than a 20-mesh bead. With a greater surface area the drug is eluted or exchanged faster and will not give as prolonged an effect as the larger bead. The degree of cross-linkage of the resin and the quantity of drug removed from the particles during elution affect the rate of release.

Durabond products consist of drugs containing an amine group complexed with tannic acid.[17] This large molecular polyionic complex is claimed to release the drug gradually and uniformly. The complex salts are prepared by reacting an alcoholic solution of the therapeutically active amine with a 20 per cent excess of tannic acid. The reaction mixture is diluted with ice water to complete the precipitation. The precipitated tannate is collected and dried.

The tannate complex is insoluble, but, in the presence of electrolytes and with a lowering of pH, there is an increased release of the amine. The rate of release is often retarded by the addition of polygalacturonic acid.

146. ℞
    Ionamin '30' (Strasenburgh) 30
    Sig.: One 10-14 hrs. before retiring.

147. ℞
    Stimalose Durabond (Irwin-
      Neisler) 50
    Sig.: One daily before breakfast.

CHEMICAL TECHNICS

A biologically active compound may be modified chemically to form an inactive derivative which liberates the parent compound on exposure to enzymatic action in vivo. With such modification, there is at times modified absorption of the drug from the gastrointestinal tract.

To overcome the bitterness of chloramphenicol, the palmitate ester is prepared. The insoluble and tasteless chloramphenicol palmitate is administered to persons who cannot swallow a capsule and to children as a flavored suspension. The palmitate ester has very little antibiotic activity, but it undergoes hydrolysis in the gastrointestinal tract where it is converted into the active alcohol. A somewhat prolonged action results because, as the chloramphenicol palmitate passes along the gastrointestinal tract, there is a continuous hydrolysis and absorption of the active drug until the palmitate remaining is excreted in the feces. A dose of the palmitate equivalent to 500 mg. of chloramphenicol is detectable in the blood for 12 hours.

An active substance may be modified chemically so that its absorption, distribution or metabolism is altered, but the type of response is unchanged. The length of time for which lidocaine exerts its anesthetic effect probably depends on the time required to hydrolyze the amide linkage in the body. If the two methyl radicals in lidocaine are replaced by hydrogen atoms, the resulting compound is rapidly hydrolyzed and exerts its effect for a shorter period. Compared with this compound lidocaine has a more prolonged effect, as the two methyl groups sterically hinder hydrolysis.

MEDICAL TECHNICS

A prolonged effect is obtained by the administration of a second drug which will slow the excretion of the primary drug and prolong its action. Oral penicillin is rapidly excreted by the kidney. The effect of penicillin is prolonged by the administration of probenecid which interferes with the renal excretion of penicillin, so that it is not readily excreted. As penicillin remains in the body longer, its action is extended.

Certain drugs are very lipoid-soluble and are partitioned and deposited in the adipose tissue. The drug deposited in the fat establishes an equilibrium with other body com-

partments and it is gradually released to provide a prolonged effect. Chlorotrianisene is a long-acting estrogen because of this phenomenon.

A prolonged effect may be obtained from the effect of a second drug which modifies a physiologic enzyme system responsible for the inactivation of the primary drug. Acetylcholine is hydrolyzed or inactivated by cholinesterase. Neostigmine combines with and inactivates cholinesterase, thus prolonging the activity of acetylcholine as there is less enzyme available to hydrolyze the acetylcholine.

Medical technics have limited application and are restricted to direct use by the physician. The secondary drug often has undesirable actions in addition to its prolongation effect. At times a massive dose is required to obtain the prolonged effect, and it would involve less risk to the patient to use a conventional dose regimen.

LIMITATIONS OF SUSTAINED RELEASE

Marketed preparations do not release a drug with a constant release per unit time but exhibit a continuously decreasing release with time. The rate of release becomes progressively less than the rate of elimination. Ideally, a sustained-release dosage form should release the drug at a rate equal to the rate of disappearance from the body. The products marketed provide a release of the drug at a rate which appreciably increases the length of activity. They are prolonged-release preparations.

For sustained-release preparations of different mechanism and form, the pattern of release of various drugs is approximated by a first-order equation. For many preparations the rate of release of the drug from the sustained release form is proportional to the amount of drug remaining,

$$-\frac{da}{dt} = ka \qquad (1)$$

or in the integrated form,

$$\log \frac{a}{a_o} = -\frac{kt}{2.3} \qquad (2)$$

where a_o is the total dose of the drug in the product, a is the fraction of the total dose remaining in the sustained-release prepara-

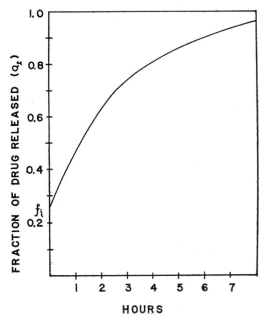

FIG. 3-32. Fraction of the drug released from sustained-release dosage plotted against time. The fraction f_i is released immediately to provide the initial activity. (Wiegand, R. G., and Taylor, J. D.: Drug Standards, *27*:165, 1959)

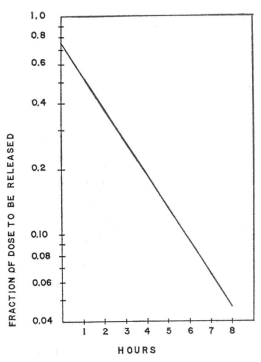

FIG. 3-33. The logarithm of the fraction of drug in the sustained-release solid dosage form is a linear function of time. (Wiegand, R. G., and Taylor, J. D.: Drug Standards, *27*:165, 1959)

tion at time t if a_o is unity, and k is the apparent specific release constant.

With a sustained-release dosage form which releases a fraction of the dose (f_i) immediately and another fraction (f_s) exponentially, the amount of the drug released (a_r) at any time is

$$a_r = a_o f_i + a_o f_s (1 - e^{-kt}) \qquad (3)$$

Obviously, if all of the drug is released, $f_i + f_s = 1$. With the ion-exchange mechanism of sustained release, $f_i + f_s$ is less than 1, indicating that all of the drug is not released.[65]

In promotional literature the release curve is often presented as a plot of the cumulative fraction of the drug released against time as shown in Figure 3-32. Since the amount of drug released at a particular time is of more significance, a better understanding of the drug being released at different times is obtained by a plot of the logarithm of the amount remaining to be released as a function of time as shown in Figure 3-33. With 100 per cent release the intercept on the

ordinate is the logarithm (f_s) and k equals the slope multiplied by 2.303.

Sustained-release products of the leaching and the ion-exchange types release their drug most closely in accord with equation 3. This is to be expected, as the diffusional processes of release from an inert matrix and the ion-exchange mechanism are both first-order processes. With the erosion type tablet, as the surface area decreases the rate of release decreases. Thus, this type of sustained release may be described by equation 3.

Release from a multiple pellet sustained-release product approximates a first order release. This type of preparation probably has the capability of any desired release pattern through the incorporation of pellets with the proper distribution of coating thicknesses. A slight deviation from a first-order pattern is not unexpected, in view of the different form and mechanism of release; however, the release is sufficiently precise to warrant the use of equation 3.

Sustained-release products of all types except the ion-exchange type release part of their drug for immediate use. Since the resinate form releases no drug immediately, the term a_0f_i is zero, and the curve passes through the origin when the cumulative amount of the drug released is plotted as a function of time.

Preparations to be administered occasionally should have a f_i value sufficient to produce a rapid effect. The value depends on the dose incorporated in the preparation and the dose of the specific drug. For products designed for repeated administration, f_i should be as close to zero as possible, since the drug level is not starting from zero after the first administration. This eliminates one source of maxima and troughs in the levels of the drug in the body.

In-vitro experiments have borne out the above relationship which has been correlated with in-vivo urinary excretion patterns of many drugs.

As most drugs are absorbed in the upper intestine to a greater extent than in the lower intestine, the dose or the amount of drug released after 7 or 8 hours should be greater than the drug released at 4 or 5 hours to compensate for the decreased absorption. The opposite release is obtained from most marketed products.

Although sustained-release medication is advantageous, there are limitations in its use. When a precise dose is essential, such as with the digitalis glycosides, sustained release probably should not be used in view of the possibility that physiologic variance may alter the normal release pattern and fail to provide the critical dose required.

Physiologic variance makes it difficult to achieve the ideal pattern of sustained release. This is not a major consideration with a normal individual; however, with persons known to have impaired or erratic gastrointestinal absorption, sustained-release medication should not be used.

Commonly, there is 3 to 4 times the amount of drug in a sustained-dosage form as there is in a conventional one. If the dosage form should be used improperly, such as by chewing an erosion type tablet instead of swallowing the whole tablet, the patient would receive an overdose. For this reason, a drug should not be placed in a sustained-release form unless the margin of safety is substantial.

Pharmaceutically, a drug with a large dose is difficult to develop into a sustained-release form. The bulk resulting from the drug and the excipients which control the release is too great to produce a tablet or a capsule that can be easily swallowed.

Drugs such as digitalis, isopropamide, phenobarbital and sulfamethoxypyridazine have a long biologic half-life and usually require only a single daily dose. With inherently long-acting drugs there is no need for additional treatment to prolong their effect.

Therapeutically, it is not always advantageous to employ sustained-release medication. Sustained-release multivitamins appear to be unnecessary; no beneficial prolonged effect has been demonstrated with riboflavin, ascorbic acid or thiamine. Administration of anticholinergic drugs to persons who are anticholinergic-sensitive may produce side effects, as by altering the gastrointestinal motility and secretions, the absorption of the drug is affected. Cases of angina of effort should not be treated orally with sustained action nitrites. The prolonged effect may obscure the warning signs of pain and lead to overexertion with fatal results.

EVALUATION OF SUSTAINED RELEASE

No single in-vitro test will adequately reflect the availability of a drug from a sustained-release medication. The *U.S.P.* disintegration test does not apply to sustained-release dosage forms, since the amount released per unit time is the critical factor to be evaluated.

In view of the several mechanisms by which sustained release is accomplished, it is doubtful that a single standardized mechanical unit and elution fluid will prove satisfactory. It seems more likely that a mechanical means of testing the release may be developed for each mechanism of release after correlation with clinical release patterns.

In-vitro release tests for sustained-release products are meaningless unless correlated with in-vivo measurements. After the validity of a sustained-release product has been demonstrated by in-vivo testing, in-vitro measurements may be correlated and used for production control.

In-vivo evaluation of sustained release

dosage forms in humans is carried out mainly by determinations of blood level and urine level and by subjective clinical evaluation. The determination of blood levels affords a way of estimating the time of onset and the duration of effect for a drug if the M.E.D. and the maximum blood level concentrations have been determined. Blood levels have been used with prednisolone,[12] penicillin,[43] sulfaethylthiadiazole[48] and caffeine.[4]

Some drugs are used in concentrations so low that they cannot be quantitatively detected in body fluids. Measurement of activity is then a subjective and a somewhat obscure evaluation.

Urinary excretion methods offer a means of measuring the drug absorbed provided that the drug is excreted unchanged or the metabolism of the drug is understood. For such drugs there is a direct relationship between excretion rate and the amount of drug in the blood. Since the clinical response of many drugs parallels their concentration in the blood, a valid relationship exists between the therapeutic effect and the amount excreted in the urine. If a dosage form is found to have prolonged urine levels, it would have prolonged clinical effect. Amphetamine,[13] aspirin,[63] penicillin,[18] sulfaethylthiadiazole,[42] tetracycline,[41] trimeprazine,[25] phenylpropanolamine[24] and riboflavin[66] have been studied by the urinary excretion technic.

Toxicity tests in animals have been used to evaluate ion-exchange resins.[6] To use a toxicity technic, one must have a drug with a relativity high toxicity. In comparing the LD_{50} of the untreated drug with an ion-exchange resinate, the lethal dose is raised and the time until death is longer with the resinate than with the untreated drug. Similar experiments show that the larger beads of the resinate have a higher lethal dose and a longer time until death than small resinate beads. Toxicity studies are valuable in the development of a product; however, they give no indication of the physiologic availability of the drug.

In-vivo roentgenographic technic has been widely used to study the release from encapsulated slow-release pellets. This has proved that there is a wide dispersion of the pellets after 1 hour in the gastrointestinal tract.

Radioactive isotopes have been used as tracers in animal and human studies.[9,16,49] The availability of radioactive drugs has been the restricting factor in the application of this technic.

The final evaluation of sustained-action products must be done by properly designed clinical tests with humans. The actual measurement of drug concentration or activity resulting from a single dose and multiple doses must be compared with that of the sustained-release dosage form.

REFERENCES

1. Adelstein, J., and Frey, R. R.: Art and Science in the Development of Hard Candy Medicinals. Am. Pharm. Ass. Industrial Pharmacy Symposium. Detroit, 1965.
2. Arny, H. V., Taub, A., and Blythe, R. H.: J. Am. Pharm., Ass., 23:672, 1934.
3. Atkinson, R. M., Bedford, C., Child, K. J., and Tomich, E. G.: Antibiot. Chemother., 12:232, 1962.
4. Axelrod, J., and Reichenthal, J.: J. Pharmacol. Exp. Ther., 92:226, 1948.
5. Bauer, G., Rieckmann, P., and Schauman, W.: Arzneimittelforsch., 12:487, 1962.
6. Becker, B. A., and Swift, G.: Toxic. Appl. Pharmacol., 1:42, 1959.
7. Bellafiore, I. J.: J. Am. Pharm. Ass. (Pract.) 14:580, 1953.
8. Binns, T. B., and Dodds, C.. Absorption and Distribution of Drugs. p. 121. Baltimore, Williams and Wilkins, 1964.
9. Bogner, R. L., and Walsh, J. M.: J. Pharm. Sci., 53:617, 1964.
10. Buckwalter, F. H., and Dickinson, H. L.: J. Am. Pharm. Ass. (Sci.), 47:661, 1958.
11. Caminetsky, S.: Canad. Med. Ass. J., 88:950, 1963.
12. Campagna, F. A., Cureton, G., Mirigian, R. A., and Nelson, E.: J. Pharm. Sci., 52:605, 1963.
13. Campbell, J. A., Nelson, E., and Chapman, D. G.: Canad. Med. Ass. J., 81:15, 1959.
14. Carter, A. K.: Canad. Med. Ass. J., 88:98, 1963.
15. Cass, L. J., Fredrick, W. S., and Theodoro, J.: Am. J. Med. Sci., 238:51, 1959.
16. Cavallito, C. J., Chafetz, L., and Miller, L.: J. Pharm. Sci., 52:259, 1963.
17. Cavallito, C. J., and Jewell, R.: J. Am. Pharm. Ass. (Sci.), 47:165, 1958.

18. Chapman, D. G., Shenoy, K. G., and Campbell, J. A.: Canad. Med. Ass. J., *81*:470, 1959.

19. Coletta, V., and Rubin, H.: J. Pharm. Sci., *53*:953, 1964.

20. Dixon, A. S., Scott, J. T., and Harvey-Smith, E. A.: Brit. Med. J., *1*:1425, 1960.

21. Dundon, M. L., and Mack, E.: J. Am. Chem. Soc., *45*:2479, 1923.

22. Frostad, S.: Acta tuberc. scand., *41*:68, 1961.

23. Gross, H. M., and Endicott, C.: Drug Cosmet. Industr., *86*:170, 1960.

24. Heimlich, K. R., MacDonnell, D. R., Flanagan, T. L., and O'Brien, P. D.: J. Pharm. Sci., *50*:232, 1960.

25. Heimlich, K. R., MacDonnell, D. R., Polk, A., and Flanagan, T. L.: J. Pharm. Sci., *50*:213, 1961.

26. Husa, W. J., and Becker, C. H.: J. Am. Pharm. Ass. (Sci.), *29*:78, 1940.

27. Kakemi, K., Arita, T., and Ohashi, S.: J. Pharm. Soc. Japan, *82*:1468, 1962.

28. Kanig, J. L., Lachman, L., and Lieberman, H. A.: Industrial Pharmacy. Chap. 5. Philadelphia, Lea & Febiger, 1970.

29. ———: Industrial Pharmacy. Philadelphia, Lea & Febiger, 1970.

30. Katchen, B., and Symchowicz, S.: J. Pharm. Sci., *56*:1108, 1967.

31. Kolthoff, I. M., and Sandell, E. B.: Textbook of Quantitative Inorganic Analysis. 3rd ed. p. 141. New York, Macmillan, 1952.

32. Lazarus, J., and Cooper, J.: J. Pharm. Pharmacol., *11*:257, 1959.

33. ———: J. Pharm. Sci., *50*:715, 1961.

34. Levy, G., and Hayes, B. A.: New Eng. J. Med., *262*:1053, 1960.

35. Little, A., and Mitchell, K. A.: Tablet Making. 2nd ed. Liverpool, England, Northern Publishing Co., Ltd., 1963.

36. Matsumato, K. K., and Grossman, M. I.: Proc. Soc. Exp. Biol. Med., *102*:517, 1959.

37. Miller, A. B., *et al.*: Physicians' Desk Reference. p. 761. Oradell, N. J., Medical Economics, 1967.

38. Mody, D. S., Scott, M. W., and Lieberman, H. A.: J. Pharm. Sci., *53*:949, 1964.

39. Mullins, J. D., and Macek, T. J.: J. Am. Pharm. Ass. (Sci.), *49*:245, 1960.

40. Nelson, E.: J. Am. Pharm. Ass. (Sci.), *48*:96, 1959.

41. ———: J. Am. Pharm. Ass. (Sci.), *49*: 437, 1960.

42. Nicholson, A. E., Tucker, S. J., and Swin-tosky, J. V.: J. Am. Pharm. Ass. (Sci.), *49*:40, 1960.

43. Ober, S. S., Vincent, H. C., Simon, D. E., and Frederick, K. J.: J. Am. Pharm. Ass. (Sci.), *47*:667, 1958.

44. Parrott, E. L.: J. Am. Pharm. Ass., *NSI*: 158, 1961.

45. ———: Am. J. Pharm. Ed., *30*:470, 1966.

46. Parrott, E. L., Wurster, D. E., and Higuchi, T.: J. Am. Pharm. Ass. (Sci.), *44*: 269, 1955.

47. Reinhold, J. G., Phillips, F. J., Flippin, H. F., and Pollack, L.: Am. J. Med. Sci. *210*:141, 1945.

48. Robinson, M. J., and Swintosky, J. V.: J. Am. Pharm. Ass. (Sci.), *48*:473, 1959.

49. Rosen, E., Ellison, T., Tannenbaum, P., Free, S. M., and Crosley, A. P.: J. Pharm. Sci., *56*:365, 1967.

50. Schroeter, L. C., Tingstad, J. E., Knoechel, E. L., and Wagner, J. G.: J. Pharm. Sci., *51*:865, 1962.

51. Schulert, A. R., and Weiner, R.: J. Pharmacol. Exp. Ther., *110*:451, 1954.

52. Simond, A., Lindquist, K. M., Tendick, F. H., and Rowe, L. W.: J. Am. Pharm. Ass. (Sci.), *39*:52, 1950.

53. Sprowls, J. B.: American Pharmacy. 6th ed. p. 361-366. Philadelphia, J. B. Lippincott, 1966.

54. Stempel, E.: . Am. Pharm. Ass. (Pract.), *20*:334, 393, 1959.

55. Stoklosa, M. J., and Ohmart, L. M.: J. Am. Pharm. Ass. (Pract.), *14*:507, 1953.

56. Strickland, W. A.: J. Pharm. Sci., *51*: 310, 1962.

57. U. S. Patent 2,738,303.

58. U. S. Patent 2,881,085.

59. U. S. Patent 2,887,438.

60. U. S. Patent 2,897,121.

61. U. S. Patent 2,921,883.

62. Vicher, E. E., Snyder, R. K., and Gathercoal, E. N.: J. Am. Pharm. Ass., *26*: 1241, 1937.

63. Vora, M. S., Zimmer, A. J., and Maney, R. V.: J. Pharm. Sci.,*53*:487, 1964.

64. Wagner, J. G., *et al.*: J. Am. Pharm. Ass. (Sci.), *49*:121-139, 1960.

65. Wiegand, R. G., and Taylor, J. D.: Drug Standards, *27*:165, 1959.

66. Wiegand, R. G., Buddenhagen, J. D., and Endicott, C. J.: J. Pharm. Sci., *52*:268, 1963.

67. Windheuser, J., and Cooper, J.: J. Am. Pharm. Ass. (Sci.), *45*:542, 1956.

68. Wood, J. H., and Syarto, J.: J. Pharm. Sci., *53*:877, 1964.

Chapter 4

Solution Dosage Forms

Jere E. Goyan, B.S., Ph.D.,*
and Robert L. Day, Pharm.D.†

A solution may be defined as a homogeneous liquid consisting of at least two components. The student will realize that this definition encompasses a large number of different dosage forms familiar from earlier studies. Thus, we wish to emphasize the similarities between products such as syrups, elixirs and tinctures, rather than their differences.

Solution dosage forms have some important advantages: drugs must dissolve to be absorbed and thereby be effective; many patients (especially children) cannot swallow tablets or capsules, and uniformity of dosage is easily obtainable. However, they do have some disadvantages: they are liable to undergo deterioration and loss of potency; they present many flavoring problems, and many incompatibilities arise due to interactions between dissolved species and to changes in solubility produced by solvent alterations.

In order to mix various dosage forms intelligently the pharmacist must always be aware of the solvents which are used in the original liquids. Thus, changes in alcohol concentration due to mixing an elixir and a syrup will explain the ensuing solubility problems.

The need for several solvents having different properties may be readily understood by consideration of the dissolution process.

SOLUBILITY

THE DISSOLUTION PROCESS‡

In order to discuss solutions, the substance present in largest amount will be designated the solvent, and other substances present in lesser amounts the solutes. The question naturally arises: in which of the three states of matter (gas, liquid or solid) does a dissolved solute exist? The molecules of a dissolved solute do not occupy fixed positions with regard to one another, thereby ruling out the crystalline state. Furthermore, they do not uniformly occupy all volume available in the containing vessel, thus excluding the gaseous state. This leads to the conclusion that a solute dissolved in a liquid is, itself, in the liquid state. Therefore, the dissolution process must contain a step for converting any other state of the solute to the liquid state.

After conversion to the liquid state, the molecules of solute and solvent must be uniformly mixed. This requires a step which consists of overcoming the attractive (cohesive) forces between solute molecules (and between solvent molecules) and replacing them with new forces due to solvent-solute interactions. Such disruption of forces involves work (or energy) changes. This energy rearrangement is known as the interchange energy and may be visualized as follows. Consider two liquids A and B. Assume molecules A and B are similar in size so that a molecule of A will be surrounded by the same number of molecules (m), whether in liquid A or B. Now transfer one molecule of A to liquid B with simultaneous transfer of a molecule of B to liquid A. The work done or interchange energy must then be:

$$\Delta E = -m(2w_{AB} - w_{AA} - w_{BB})\S \quad (1)$$

If this is done with x molecules, the total interchange energy is x times ΔE, the total

* Dean and Professor of Pharmacy and Pharmaceutical Chemistry, University of California.

† Assistant Dean and Lecturer in Pharmacy, University of California.

‡ This treatment is not intended to be a rigorous development of the subject but rather to provide the student with an insight into this very complex field.

§ w_{AA} = work necessary to separate two molecules of A, w_{AB} and w_{BB} similarly.

energy change being designated as the heat of mixing. A negative ΔE corresponds to the release of heat (exothermic process), while a positive ΔE corresponds to absorption of heat (endothermic process). If the difference in attraction is sufficiently great (size differential may also play a part due to changes in m) the two liquids may not be miscible. Cases where the attractions are exactly equal will produce no energy change and will be considered as ideal solutions.

Surprisingly, a good deal of information about a solution may be obtained by studying the vapor above the solution. This may be shown in the following manner.

Consider the saturated vapor above pure liquid A at temperature T. The number of molecules of A returning to the liquid from the vapor phase per second, i.e., the rate of condensation, is proportional to the vapor pressure of A (P^o_A) and the area between the liquid and vapor (S). This may be expressed as:

$$R_C = k_1 P^o_A S \qquad (2)$$

where k_1 is the constant of proportionality. The rate of molecules leaving the liquid by evaporation will be proportional to S.

$$R_E = k_2 S \qquad (3)$$

At equilibrium the rate of condensation must be equal to the rate of evaporation, leading to the following expression for the two constants of proportionality:

$$k_1 = k_2 / P^o_A \qquad (4)$$

Now assume B dissolved in A. In a miscible solution the condensation proportionality constant will be unaffected, since a molecule of A may return at any point on the surface:

$$R_C = k_1 P_A S \qquad (5)$$

where P_A is the pressure of A above the solution. The rate of evaporation of A will depend on the proportion of S which is occupied by A, which, in turn, is dependent on the mole fraction of A, X_A.* This may be expressed as:

$$R_E = k_3 X_A S \qquad (6)$$

* The mole fraction of a solute is the number of moles of the solute divided by the total number of moles in the solution.

Again, at equilibrium $R_E = R_C$, and using equation (4) we obtain:

$$P_A = \frac{k_3}{k_2} P^o_A X_A \qquad (7)$$

In the case of an ideal solution the forces between A-B are equal to those between A-A and B-B, therefore $k_2 = k_3$. This results in the Raoult's Law equation

$$P_A = P^o_A X_A \qquad (8)$$

which may be used to define an ideal solution. If the A-A interactions are stronger than the A-B interactions, $k_2 < k_3$. The vapor pressure of A above the solution will then be greater than that predicted by Raoult's Law. Thus, measurements of the vapor pressure may be used to obtain an understanding of the interactions in the liquid state. It should also be noted that the boiling point of a liquid is a good measure of its cohesive forces. As the cohesive forces increase, k_2 will decrease with no change in k_1 and the boiling point will therefore increase.

The earlier discussion indicates that the solubility of a solid must depend on the energy necessary to melt the solid, usually referred to as the heat of fusion (ΔH_f) and any heat of mixing. The solubility of a gas must depend on the heat of vaporization (ΔH_v) and the heat of mixing. If the interchange energy is zero, an ideal solution exists and some simplifications are possible. The solubility of a gas must decrease with increasing temperature† and the solubility of a solid must increase with increasing temperature.

The equation describing the solubility of a solid which forms an ideal solution, as a function of temperature is the usual van't Hoff type used in describing the effect of temperature on equilibrium.

$$2.3 \log X = \frac{\Delta H_f}{R} \left[\frac{T_m - T}{T T_m} \right] \qquad (9)$$

where R is the gas constant (1.98 calories per degree per mole), T_m is the melting point in degrees Kelvin and X is the mole fraction solubility at temperature T. Note that at the melting point the solid is miscible with the solvent (X approaches 1), as would be expected for an ideal solution. This also pre-

† In order to effect the change in state (gas to liquid) heat must be withdrawn from the gas.

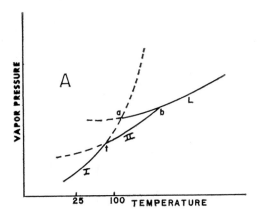 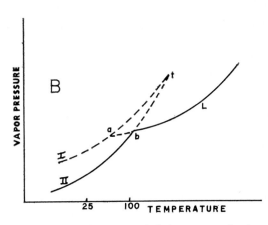

Fig. 4-1. Diagrams of the two polymorphic systems: a = m.p. of polymorph I; b = m.p. of polymorph II; t = transition point. (A) is the enantiotropic system and (B) the monotropic system.

dicts that the lower the melting point of a solid the higher its solubility.* This can be demonstrated by the solubility of fused ring aromatic compounds in benzene (Table 4-1).

TABLE 4-1

Compound	M.P. °C.	Mole Fraction Solubility in Benzene
Naphthalene	80- 81	0.27
Phenanthrene	99-100	0.21
Anthracene	217-218	0.0081

We may also compare a series of closely related substances (Table 4-2), since the interchange energy should be similar for each. The changes in solubility are consequently due to differences in the melting point.

The relationship of melting point and solubility is particularly interesting in the case of polymorphic substances.† Polymorphs are crystal forms of the same substance having different melting points. (The student will recall the different crystal forms of sulfur as an example.) Two distinctly different polymorphic systems are possible. They may be understood most readily by reference to Figure 4-1. The vapor pressures above the crystals and the liquid are plotted vs. the tem-

* The m.p. of a substance decreases as the particle size is reduced below about 2 microns diameter, and the solubility shows a concurrent increase.

† Compare discussion, Chapter 2, page 60.

perature. In part A the transition point (temperature at which both forms have the same vapor pressure) is below the melting point of polymorph I, and the system is enantiotropic. In part B the transition point is above the melting point of polymorph I, and the system is monotropic.

The heat of mixing must be the same for all polymorphs. The solubility will, of course, always be greatest for the polymorph with the highest vapor pressure. Thus, the solubility of a monotropic system follows the rule that the lower melting form will always have the higher solubility. Enantiotropic systems are more complex. Figure 4-1 (*left*) shows that the solubility of polymorph II would be higher at 25°C. but polymorph I would be more soluble at 100°C.

There is currently great interest in the pharmaceutical industry in the investigation

TABLE 4-2

Barbiturate	M.P. °C.	Solubility in Alcohol
Barbital	188-189	1 Gm./14 ml.
Phenobarbital	174-178	1 Gm./10 ml.
Amobarbital	156-158	1 Gm./5 ml.
Pentobarbital	132-133	1 Gm./4 ml.
Secobarbital	95- 96	1 Gm./2 ml.

Sulfonamide	M.P. °C.	Solubility in Water
Sulfadiazine	252-256	1 Gm./13 L.
Sulfamerazine	234-238	1 Gm./5 L.
Sulfapyridine	191-193	1 Gm./3.5 L.
Sulfathiazole	173-175	1 Gm./1.7 L.

TABLE 4-3

COMPOUND	MELTING POINT °C.	SOLUBILITY @ 25°C
Riboflavin		
Polymorph I	291-293	60 mg./liter water
Polymorph II	283	1200 mg./liter water
Methyprednisolone		
Polymorph I	205	9 mg./100 ml. water
Polymorph II	228-237	19.5 mg./100 ml. water
Sulfathiazole		
Form I	174-175	8.15 Gm./100 ml. ethanol
Form II	200-201	14.2 Gm./100 ml. ethanol

of different polymorphs of slightly soluble drugs.[49,79,86] Table 4-3 illustrates both types of polymorphism.

Of course, the consideration of solubility in nonideal systems must take into account the heat of mixing. This may readily be seen by noting that 1 Gm. of phenobarbital is soluble in approximately 800 ml. of water, 700 ml. of benzene, 40 ml. of chloroform, 15 ml. of ether and 10 ml. of ethanol.

The over-all heat effect of the two-step process (fusion and mixing) must be the algebraic sum of the heats of fusion and mixing. This sum may then be used in place of the heat of fusion in equation 9 and a more general equation useful for non-ideal solutions obtained:

$$\log \frac{S_2}{S_1} = \frac{\Delta H}{R}\left[\frac{T_2 - T_1}{T_1 T_2}\right] \quad (10)$$

where S_2 is the molar solubility at T_2, and S_1 at T_1. Therefore, the determination of the solubility at two different temperatures will make it possible to determine ΔH. This equation then may be used to predict solubilities at other temperatures.

Now, it would appear from the previous discussions that the forces between pheno-

barbital molecules are more closely related to those between alcohol molecules than to those between the molecules of any of the other solvents. This is indeed the basis for the rule of thumb that "like dissolves like." It only remains, then, to define what is like what.*

INTERACTION FORCES

All interaction forces are fundamentally electrical in nature. They are the same type of interactions as those responsible for chemical bonding between atoms. However, be-

* The sophisticated reader will note that the entropic contribution to solubility is ignored in this discussion. The maximum contribution due to this term is attained when the solution molecules are mixed in a random (disordered) fashion. Since the solutions with which we deal, in general, are virtually random mixtures, this term has been ignored. The most striking exception to this generalization occurs when hydrocarbons are dissolved in water. It has been shown that hydrocarbons tend to orient the water molecules in their immediate neighborhood, resulting in a more ordered system. Thus the entropy term is unfavorable and the hydrocarbon molecules cluster together. This interaction between hydrocarbon molecules, which occurs in an aqueous medium, has come to be called "hydrophobic bonding," a term which has caused considerable confusion.[50]

TABLE 4-4

INTERACTION	INTERACTION FORCES BETWEEN MOLECULES	INTERACTION ENERGY PROPORTIONAL TO:
Ion-dipole		r^{-2}
Dipole-dipole	(Keesom Forces)	r^{-3}
Ion-induced dipole		r^{-4}
Dipole-induced dipole	(Debye Forces)	r^{-6}
Induced dipole-induced dipole	(London Forces)	r^{-6}

cause of the larger distances over which they are acting they are of considerably smaller magnitude. The electrical nature is quite clear in the case of ions, where the force between them is calculated from Coulomb's Law:

$$f = \frac{q_1 q_2}{Dr^2} \qquad (11)$$

where q is the charge on each ion, D is the dielectric constant of the medium between the ions and r is the distance between the ions. Two other properties of molecules which result in electrical interactions are permanent dipole moments and polarizability. The student will recall that molecules in which the positive and the negative centers do not coincide are known as dipolar molecules. The product of the charges multiplied by the distance between them is known as the dipole moment. Polarizability (usually designated as α) is a measure of the ease with which the average electron distribution in a molecule may be altered by an electric field. This alteration leads to an induced dipole moment in the molecule.

It is now possible to list the various interaction forces usually found in solute-solvent systems (Table 4-4).

The first four cases are easily seen to be electrical interactions and the forces may be predicted with the aid of Coulomb's Law. The last case is more difficult but may be visualized as follows. If we could take an instantaneous snapshot of the electron distribution of a molecule, the molecule would have a dipole moment (averaged over time no dipole exists). This rapidly varying dipole will then induce a dipole in neighboring molecules in phase with itself. These interactions result in an over-all attractive force. Such forces exist between all molecules but are only important when stronger forces are not present to mask them. The polarizability of a molecule is equal to the sum of the polarizabilities of its constituent atoms. London forces will consequently increase with molecular weight. Distance between molecules is also very important, and large flat molecules which may approach each other closely (e.g., benzene) will be more strongly attracted than molecules which are sterically prevented from close association. The sum of the polarizability and the permanent dipole moment may be measured by means of the dielectric constant. The dielectric constant of a liquid may be defined by Coulomb's Law (see equation 11) or as the ratio of the capacitance of a capacitor with the liquid as the dielectric to the capacitance of the same capacitor with air as the dielectric. The permanent and the induced dipoles align themselves oppositely to the applied field, thus decreasing the electric field strength and increasing the capacitance. As the frequency of the applied field is increased the permanent dipole molecules find it increasingly difficult to align themselves in opposition to the applied field. Light may be considered a very high frequency electric field. When light passes through a polarizable liquid its velocity is less than its velocity in air. The relative velocity is defined as the refractive index of the liquid (m). Therefore, the refractive index of a liquid is dependent on the polarizability, increasing as the polarizability increases.*

Several properties of common pharmaceutical solvents are given in Table 4-5.

The contribution of polarizability to the dielectric constant may be shown to be the square of the refractive index. Thus, for substances like benzene the dielectric constant is due almost entirely to polarizability $[(1.5)^2 = 2.25]$ and the molecular interactions are due almost exclusively to London forces. On the other hand, water with its high dielectric constant and low refractive index must consist mainly of dipole-dipole interactions. Water actually contains a special subclass of Keesom forces known as hydrogen bonds. These differ from ordinary Keesom forces in that the small size of the hydrogen atom makes the positive charge more readily available (r will be smaller than in other cases) and thus leads to stronger bonding. Any organic molecule containing N, O or other electronegative atoms will therefore be capable of dipole-dipole interactions. If the electronegative atom is attached to hydrogen, hydrogen bonding will

---

* The actual equation for polarizability is

$$\alpha = 3.96 \times 10^{-25} \left[\frac{m^2 - 1}{m^2 + 2} \right] \frac{\text{M.W.}}{p} \quad \text{Where M.W.}$$

is the molecular weight and p the density of the liquid.

TABLE 4-5

Solvent	B.P. °C.	$\alpha \times 10^{25}$	m(°C.)	D(°C.)
Diethyl ether	35	88	1.35(25)	4.3(20)
Acetone	57	64	1.36(20)	21(25)
Chloroform	61	84	1.44(20)	4.8(20)
Carbon tetrachloride	76	104	1.46(20)	2.2(20)
Ethanol	79	50	1.36(20)	24.3(25)
Benzene	80	100	1.50(20)	2.3(20)
Water	100	14	1.33(20)	78.5(25)
Propylene glycol	189	76	1.43(27)	33.0(25)
Liquid petrolatum	~ 200	> 100	1.48(20)	2-5(20)
Formamide	210	42	1.45(20)	109(20)
Glycerol	290	80	1.47(20)	43(25)

occur. These conditions are quite common in organic medicinals, and, therefore, Keesom forces will play a large role in solubility phenomena of such drugs.

We are now in a position to answer the earlier question: what is like what? The answer is that liquids with similar interaction forces are "like" one another. Water and benzene have similar boiling points and must therefore have approximately equal cohesive forces. However, the cohesive forces in water are primarily of the Keesom type and those in benzene, of the London type. The interaction forces (A-B of our former discussion) will be small (ΔE a large positive number), preventing miscibility of these liquids.

Ion-dipole interactions are particularly interesting, the most important examples being salts in water. The interactions of ions with water dipoles are strong enough to overcome, in many cases, the adverse effect of the high melting point of the salt. However, it must not be assumed that all salts are highly water soluble. In many cases (obvious examples are silver chloride and quinine sulfate), the hydration energy (A-B of our former discussion) is not sufficient to overcome the heat of fusion and solubility is therefore quite low.

However, the formation of a charged species from an uncharged species does lead to an increase in water solubility. Quinine sulfate is considerably more soluble than the free alkaloid, even though it has only slight water solubility. This principle may be used to enhance the water solubility of poorly soluble alcohols. The alcohol is esterified with a dibasic or tribasic acid and the mono ester formed is made into a salt by the addition of sodium hydroxide. The final product is considerably more soluble than the parent molecule and often has good pharmacologic activity. Riboflavin phosphate (water solubility: 100 × riboflavin) is a good example.

An especially important example of salt insolubility occurs when both anion and cation are large organic molecules. In this

TABLE 4-6*

A.D.C.	Solubility Gm./100 ml.	Propylene Glycol	Glycerol	Alcohol	Water qs. ad
71.1	0.22	0	0	15	100
70.4	0.22	20	0	0	100
70.4	0.22	0	10	10	100
65.2	0.22	0	40	0	100
62.3	0.44	0	0	30	100
64.5	0.44	20	0	10	100
63.2	0.44	35	0	0	100
62.6	0.44	0	15	20	100
59.3	0.44	0	40	10	100

* Modified from Krause, G. M., and Cross, J. M.: J. Am. Pharm. Assoc. (Sci.), *40*:137; Peterson, C. F., and Hopponen, R. E.: J. Am. Pharm. Assoc., *42*:540.

case the strong interactions between the ions and the water dipoles are markedly decreased, causing a concurrent decrease in water solubility. This situation commonly occurs when large cation-containing molecules such as benzalkonium chloride and large anion-containing molecules such as sodium fluorescein are mixed in solution leading to precipitation of benzalkonium fluoresceinate. This is a sufficiently general reaction to warrant the "rule of thumb" that large cationic and large anionic molecules should not be used together.[78]

CHANGES OF SOLVENT

Occasionally, it is necessary to change solvents in a pharmaceutical preparation. It has been suggested that the solubility of a substance should be the same in two solvents with the same dielectric constant.[47,84] This can of course be true only if the dielectric constant is due primarily to one type of interaction, e.g., polarizability. This may be illustrated by the solubility of phenobarbital in mixed solvents. Consider the following:

The approximate dielectric constant (A.D.C.) is calculated by neglecting volume changes and using the dielectric constants from Table 4-5. For example, the first value is obtained as follows:

$$A.D.C. = 0.15 \ (21) + 0.85 \ (80) = 71.1$$

If one wishes to predict other solvent combinations it is only necessary to know their dielectric constant and to use ordinary alligation methods.

It is dangerous to push this reasoning too far. For example, in Table 4-6 the solubility increases as the A.D.C. decreases. Thus, it might be expected that the solubility in formamide would be quite small. Actually, the solubility is greater than that in ethanol! This may be rationalized in terms of the balance of high polarizability and dielectric constant of formamide. Phenobarbital has a high polarizability as well as permanent dipoles, thus making formamide a very good solvent.

There has been great interest in attempting to correlate solubility in mixed solvents with dielectric constant and several authors have tested the hypothesis.[41,91] The evidence indicates that a given dielectric constant will produce the greatest solubility for any solvent pair but that the solubility is not equal for different pairs having the same dielectric constant. This again illustrates the difficulty in overlooking the fact that the dielectric constant is composed of more than one factor.

EFFECT OF pH ON SOLUBILITY

The majority of organic medicinal agents are weak acids or bases. Consequently, the solubility of these agents is strongly dependent on the pH of the solution. A qualitative understanding of this phenomenon is obtained by assuming that the charged form of the drug is more water soluble and the uncharged form is therefore the solubility-limiting species. Thus, sodium phenobarbital is freely soluble (1 Gm./ml.) and phenobarbital is only slightly soluble (1 Gm./800 ml.); atropine sulfate is freely soluble (1 Gm./0.4 ml.) and atropine slightly soluble (1 Gm./455 ml.). The two different examples were chosen to illustrate that the charged species may be either the acid form (atropine sulfate) or the base form (sodium phenobarbital) of the medicinal. This type of reasoning is particularly useful in understanding the precipitation seen when a solution of sodium phenobarbital is mixed with an acidic vehicle. It is occasionally desirable to put this qualitative reasoning on a quantitative basis. This is easily accomplished with the aid of the "buffer equation."*

$$pH = pK_A + \log \frac{C_B}{C_A} \qquad (12)$$

where pH = − log hydrogen ion concentration, pK_A = − log acidic dissociation constant, C_B = concentration of the basic species and C_A = concentration of the acidic species. The pH at which any drug will precipitate from solution may be predicted from this equation by insertion of the proper values. The pK_A values and the solubilities are obtained from the literature.† [If only the pK_B (25°C.) values are given, subtract them from 14 to obtain the equivalent pK_A (25°C.).] One then inserts the molar con-

---

* The Henderson-Hasselbach equation; cf. page 62.

† Useful sources are references 133, 134 in the bibliography.

centration of the soluble form reduced by the molar solubility for one concentration term and the molar solubility for the other. This can probably be seen most readily with an illustration.

At what pH would a solution of sodium sulfadiazine (5%) precipitate from solution? Solubility sulfadiazine at 25°C = 1 Gm./ 13 liter. M. W. Sulfadiazine 250, sodium sulfadiazine 272. $pK_A = 6.48$

$$pH = 6.48 + \log \frac{\dfrac{50}{272} - \dfrac{0.077}{250}}{0.077/250}$$

$$= 6.48 + \log \frac{.184}{.308 \times 10^{-3}}$$

$$= 6.48 + 2.00 + 0.78 = 9.26$$

When the solubility of one of the species is low, the validity of the buffer equation should be checked. The exact equation is:

$$pH = pK_A + \log \frac{C_B + H_3O^+ - OH^-}{C_A - H_3O^+ + OH^-} \quad (13)$$

As long as C_A and C_B are at least ten times H_3O^+ or OH^- concentration the simplified version equation 12 is valid. In the example used here, $C_A = 3.08 \times 10^{-4}M$ and $OH^- \cong 0.18 \times 10^{-4}$. Thus the answer is correct. If the approximations are not good, one may obtain a better value by inserting the approximate value and re-solving. This may be illustrated with the previous example.

$$pH = 6.48 + \log \frac{0.184}{.308 \times 10^{-3} + 0.018 \times 10^{-3}}$$

$$= 9.23\ddagger$$

Note that the pH given in this answer is slightly more acidic than the previous one. When the solubility-limiting species is the acid species, any error of this nature will be such that the predicted pH is too high. If the basic species is the solubility-limiting species, the inaccuracy will arise from H_3O^+ not being much smaller than C_B. The predicted pH will therefore be too low. The errors in both cases are such that they give a margin of safety to the predicted pH of precipitation. Therefore, the approximate equation (12)

‡ By a series of such iterations the answer may be obtained to any desired accuracy.

serves the purpose of indicating a pH beyond which precipitation is likely.

Often, the vehicle containing the drug will be hydroalcoholic in nature. The effect of the alcohol will be twofold; it will change the dissociation constant and it will increase the solubility of the less soluble (uncharged) form. The qualitative effect on the dissociation constant can be seen with the aid of Coulomb's Law (equation 11). The introduction of alcohol will lower the over-all dielectric constant and thereby increase the work necessary to separate (dissociate) the ionic species. This means that the equilibrium will always be shifted toward the side containing the fewer charged species. The concurrent increase in the solubility of the uncharged species will be much larger. Thus, the over-all effect will be that the pH of precipitation will be shifted and the solubility at any pH will be increased.

It must always be kept clearly in mind that mixing a weak acid with a weak base will result in neutralization. Thus, if we mix solutions of diphenhydramine hydrochloride and sodium pentobarbital, we may get precipitation of either or both or a salt of the two depending on the relative amounts of each drug used.

Oftentimes exact dissociation constants are not available. In such cases the student may make an "educated guess," depending upon the functional groups of the molecule. For example, aliphatic carboxyl groups have pK_A values of about 4 to 5, etc. Such qualitative information is quite useful in predicting possible incompatibilities between medicinal agents in solution and may be especially valuable in anticipating problems arising when various intravenous solutions are mixed.[16,20,94,98]

SOLUBILIZATION

One other means of effecting solution deserves attention. This process is known as "solubilization" and involves a colloidal solution the particles of which are capable of increasing the ordinary solubility of a compound.[115] This increase in solubility is due to adsorption or incorporation of the solute molecules onto or in the colloidal particle. The colloidal particles usually consist of many molecules of a surfactant arranged so that the nonpolar portions of the surfactant are intermeshed.* The resulting particle is probably in the shape of a sausage, a sphere or a sandwich and is called a micelle. A polarizable non-water-soluble molecule may then be incorporated into the micelle so that its nonpolar portion is in juxtaposition to the nonpolar portion of the micelle.

Most of the properties of solubilized drugs may be understood by assuming that the colloidal surfactant is simply a second invisible phase. Thus, the effect of pH on the solubilization of weak acids may be explained by assuming that the surfactant is a second phase in which the undissociated form is soluble and the dissociated (charged) form is insoluble.[29] In the more general case, one may assume that both forms are soluble but ordinarily the uncharged form is far more soluble (3 to 10 times).[107]

The use of solubilizers in pharmacy dates back to the 19th century. However, their use in internal preparations is relatively recent. The sorbitan esters (Tweens and Spans) have been widely tested and found to be relatively nontoxic. The use of solubilizers has achieved success in vitamin formulations to incorporate the "fat"-soluble vitamins into aqueous preparations. Several studies have shown that vitamin A is more stable and better absorbed in a solubilized aqueous solution than in a true solution in an oil.[18,30] The absorption of iron is also increased by surfactants.[30] However, salicylic acid absorption rate is decreased by solubilization.[69]

Other workers have found that surfactants hasten the color fading of dyes,[111] and can decrease the effectiveness of preserva-

* This interaction is undoubtedly due, in part, to "hydrophobic bonding" (see above).

tives.[24,92,96,115] Therefore, it is necessary that each preparation containing a surfactant be evaluated on an individual basis. Their use in extemporaneous compounding is therefore seriously limited.

STABILITY OF SOLUTIONS

Since no medicinal in solution will last forever, stability is only a relative term. In pharmaceutical practice, most products have sufficient shelf life so that the patient need take no special precautions. However, the student is aware that some products carry expiration dates beyond which they should not be used. Other products require refrigeration and some must be protected from light. In order to understand the need for the preceding precautions let us consider the following experiment.

An organic ester is dissolved in water and the concentration of the drug is determined at time intervals over a period of several days. The concentration may then be plotted as a function of time as shown in Figure 4-2. The slope of this curve at any point may be obtained by determining the slope of the straight line tangent to the curve at the desired point.* For example, the slope at 4 days is computed from the slope of the straight line shown in Figure 4-2 drawn tangent at the 4-day point. The slope of the curve at other times is computed in the same manner. The slope may be determined at several points and the data in Table 4-7 obtained.

* This is done as follows: $m = \dfrac{C_2 - C_1}{t_2 - t_1}$ where C_2 is the concentration at time t_2 and C_1 the concentration at time t_1.

TABLE 4-7

TIME (days)	CONCENTRATION (Gm./100 ml.)	LOG CONCENTRATION	SLOPE	SLOPE/CONCENTRATION
0	6.00	0.778	—	—
4	3.90	0.591	− 0.400	− 0.103
8	2.55	0.407	− 0.280	− 0.110
12	1.65	0.218	− 0.175	− 0.106
16	1.05	0.021	− 0.110	− 0.105
20	0.70			

$$\frac{\Delta C}{\Delta t} = -.106C$$

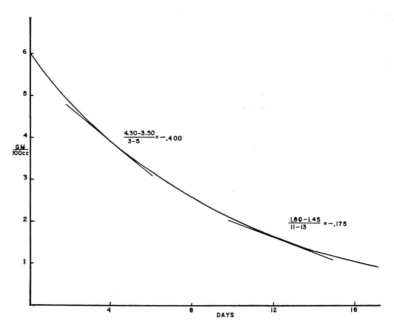

Fig. 4-2. A plot of the concentration of an ester dissolved in water versus time.

Note that the slope divided by the concentration is a constant. This constant will be designated k and the data in Table 4-7 may now be presented in the form of the following equation:

$$\text{slope} = kC = -0.106C \qquad (14)$$

The slope has units of concentration per day and may be expressed as:

$$\text{slope} = \frac{\Delta C}{\Delta t},$$

where ΔC is the change in concentration in the time period Δt. It is thus seen that the slope is the rate of disappearance of the drug from the solution. According to equation 14 this rate is proportional to the concentration of the drug in solution with proportionality constant k.

Now the limit of $\frac{\Delta C}{\Delta t}$ as Δt approaches zero is usually written as dC/dt, leading to the equation:

$$\frac{dC}{dt} = -kC \qquad (15)$$

which upon integration produces the equation as usually written:

$$2.3 \log \frac{C}{C_0} = -kt \qquad (16)$$

predicting that a plot of log C vs. t should be linear with a slope of k/2.3. The data in Table 4-7, plotted in this fashion, are shown in Figure 4-3. In the pharmaceutical literature, it is common to refer to $t_{\frac{1}{2}}$ (the time required for the concentration to be reduced to one half of its original value), rather than k. This value is related to k as follows:

$$2.3 \log \frac{\frac{1}{2} C_0}{C_0} = -k\ t_{\frac{1}{2}}$$

$$\text{or } t_{\frac{1}{2}} = \frac{0.69}{k}$$

Why is the rate of degradation proportional to the concentration in solution?

Assume that in the previous example the drug is disappearing due to the hydrolysis of the ester linkage. It then seems reasonable that the rate of hydrolysis will depend on the number of collisions per second between the water and the drug molecules. (Not every collision will lead to hydrolysis, but a certain fraction of the collisions will do so.) In turn, the number of collisions will depend on the concentration of ester and water molecules. In dilute aqueous solutions the concentration

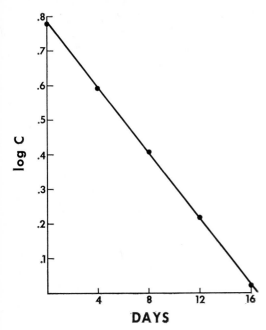

FIG. 4-3. A plot of log ester concentration versus time.

of water will be much greater than the concentration of the ester. The number of collisions per second will therefore depend only on the concentration of drug molecules in the solution, since a small change in drug concentration will have virtually no effect on water concentration. Therefore, the rate of hydrolysis must depend only on the concentration of drug in solution, as seen in equation 14.

This type of rate equation is known as a pseudo first-order reaction. The order of a reaction is the sum of the exponents of all concentration terms on the right-hand side of the equation. The hydrolysis is actually second order:

$$\frac{dC}{dt} = k' \ (C) \ (W) \qquad (17)$$

where W = water concentration. However, the water concentration does not change during the course of the reaction, being in great excess, and may be incorporated with the rate constant k' to produce k and equation 14.

If the amount of water is decreased (e.g., by using propylene glycol in place of water) to the point where the water concentration is comparable with that of the drug, the hydrolysis will depend on both drug and water concentrations. The slope of a plot of concentration of drug versus time would then be divided by the product of drug and water concentration to obtain the rate constant k'.

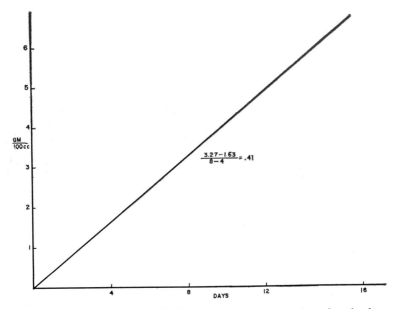

FIG. 4-4. A plot of the alcohol concentration versus time for the hydrolysis of an ester in a saturated solution of the ester.

Another type of behavior would be noted if the saturated drug solution were in contact with excess solid drug. The concentration of drug would now be constant, since the solid would dissolve as rapidly as the drug was hydrolyzed. However, we may determine one of the products of the reactions (e.g., the alcohol) and plot its concentration versus time, as shown in Figure 4-4. This plot may be represented by

$$\frac{dC}{dt} = k'' \qquad (18)$$

or integrating:

$$C = k'' t$$

remembering that the original concentration of the product is zero. This then would be a pseudo zero-order reaction.

Many other types of rate equations are possible, depending on the mechanism of the reaction. Many of the more complex cases may be resolved into parallel or series reactions, each step of which is actually a zero-order or a first-order reaction.

CATALYSIS

A catalyst may be defined as a substance which will greatly increase the rate of the reaction although it does not occur in the stoichiometry.*

Probably the most common catalysts in pharmaceutical solutions are hydronium and hydroxide ions. The hydrolysis of most drugs will be dependent on the relative concentration of such ions. In some reactions other weaker acidic and basic species, e.g., NH_4^+, acetate ion, NH_3, may also be catalysts. Most kinetic studies of drug degradation will therefore include a "pH-rate profile." This is a plot of the log of the rate constant vs. pH. Such a plot will make it possible to predict the pH of maximum stability for a product. For example, the optimum stability range for aqueous solutions of potassium penicillin is found to be pH 6.0 to 6.5.

The effect of pH on hydrolysis may be understood by investigation of the reaction

*Investigation of the rate equation will show that the rate is proportional to the catalyst concentration. Since the catalyst concentration is constant, the concentration may be incorporated into the rate constant.

mechanism (step-by-step pathway) involved.

In acid solution:

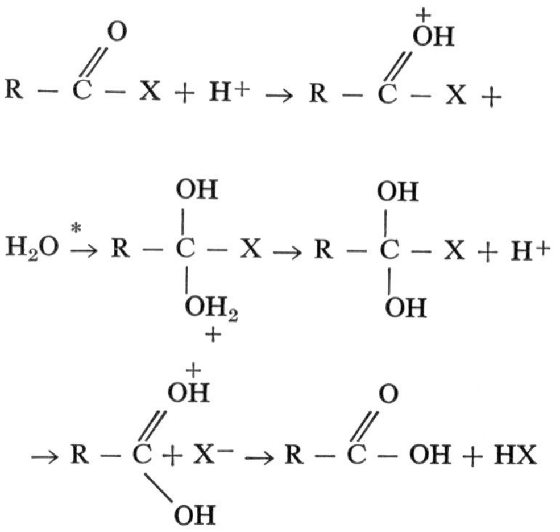

and in alkaline solution

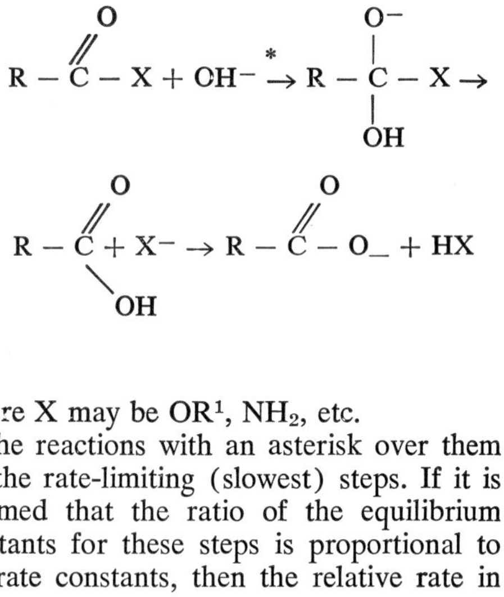

Where X may be OR^1, NH_2, etc.

The reactions with an asterisk over them are the rate-limiting (slowest) steps. If it is assumed that the ratio of the equilibrium constants for these steps is proportional to the rate constants, then the relative rate in acidic and basic media depends on the relative nucleophilic and electrophilic natures of the reactants (OH^-, H_2O, R—C(=O)—X and R—C(=$^+$OH)—X).[54] Usually it is found that the rate constant for base catalysis is much larger (200 to 1,000 times, or more) than the rate constant for acid hydrolysis. The total rate of disappearance may be written:

$$R = k_A(C)(H^+) + k_B(C)(OH^-)$$

At pH 7.0 ($H^+ = OH^-$) the second term will be about 1,000 times the first term. At pH 6.0 the second term will be 10 times larger than the first term *but* the total rate will be only one tenth the rate at pH 7.0. Therefore, it is apparent that most hydrolyzable medicinals will be much more stable at a pH of 5 to 6 than at more basic pH values. Oftentimes the drug will itself change ionic form as the pH changes. For example, in the case of barbital the following equilibrium takes place:

$$B + H_2O = B^- + H_3O^+ \quad (K_A \cong 10^{-8})$$

As you would expect, the rate of degradation varies for the different ionic species interacting. In the above example, the second order rate constant between B^- and OH^- is 1.6×10^4, whereas the rate constant between B^- and OH^- is 5.0×10^1 in agreement with the decrease to be expected from coulombic repulsion between the ions.[43]

Many other catalysts may be encountered. Inorganic heavy metal ions are often indicted, and such unlikely things as sodium phosphate may be catalysts under some conditions.[33]

It is imperative, then, that the degradation

may decrease the hydrolysis rate.[48,66,67] Another method is often used with antibiotics: the drug is packaged in a dry form from which the pharmacist prepares a solution immediately prior to use. Probably the simplest method of stabilization is to decrease the water concentration. Thus, one may prepare a relatively stable aspirin solution by replacing water with alcohol and propylene glycol.[110] It has recently been shown that potassium penicillin G is not inactivated by the presence of alcohol. The problem with penicillin may be circumvented by preparation of water-insoluble salts with large organic cations replacing the potassium ion (cf. the section on solubility). Their low solubility strikingly reduces the degradation rate (equation 18) and makes a suspension which maintains potency in a refrigerator for a year or more.[116] Recent work has shown that dissolving esters in a micellular solution results in considerable stabilization of the ester.[82,83,100,112]

Autoxidation Reactions

Another common stability problem is autoxidation (oxidations involving atmospheric oxygen). Many autoxidations involve free radical mechanisms. The basic scheme for such reactions may be expressed as follows:

A. $RH \xrightarrow[\text{heavy metals}]{\text{light,}} R\cdot$ initiation

B. $R\cdot + O_2 \rightarrow RO_2\cdot$ chain propagation

C. $RO_2\cdot + RH \rightarrow R\cdot + RO_2H$ chain propagation

D. $RO_2\cdot + RO_2\cdot \rightarrow$ products   chain termination

rate of a drug be determined in the final dosage form and not merely in an idealized aqueous solution.

Hydrolytic Degradation

The most important cause of drug decomposition is hydrolysis. This follows, since the majority of organic medicinals are esters or contain other groupings such as substituted amides, lactones, lactams, etc., which are subject to hydrolysis. There are several approaches to this problem.* The addition of agents which form complexes with the drug

* The control of pH has already been discussed.

Many other concurrent reactions may be written but these few will enable us to understand the various approaches to stabilization. The student will readily perceive that the simple kinetic equations which work for other reactions will not be useful here since RH is being destroyed by at least two different reactions, A and C.

The prevention of autoxidation may be attempted by slowing the initiation reaction A. This can be accomplished by use of dark or coated bottles if the photoxidation path is important, and the use of chelating agents such as ethylenediaminetetraacetic acid (Versene) to remove trace ions which are capable of reaction initiation.[126]

Another widely used method is the addition of other easily oxidized substances (inhibitors) which are incapable of chain propagation:

$$RO_2 \cdot + IH \rightarrow I \cdot + RO_2H$$

$$I \cdot \rightarrow prod.$$

Thus, such substances as phenols and amines may be effective antioxidants, since chain propagation requires the structure R-O-O-O which is quite improbable.[122] Often it is necessary to stabilize phenolic and catechol types of drugs (e.g., epinephrine). In this case it is necessary to use a stabilizer which undergoes the initiation step more readily than the drug. The ability of various antioxidants to undergo the initiation step may be compared using oxidation potentials.

Useful antioxidants in oleaginous systems are substances such as α-tocopherol, butyl hydroxyanisole and ascorbyl palmitate.[108] In aqueous systems use may be made of agents such as sodium sulfite, sodium formaldehyde sulfoxylate, sodium bisulfite and ascorbic acid.[31] It is often found that the mixture of two or more antioxidants is synergistic, leading to a much larger increase in stability than predictable from simple additivity.

Hydrogen ion concentration may also have an effect on oxidation rate. In the case of phenolic oxidation the removal of an electron seems to be easier than the extraction of a hydrogen atom:

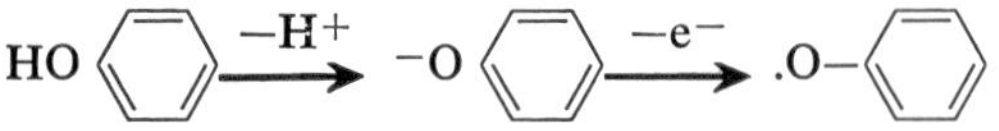

Maintenance of a low pH will prevent ionization, decrease the concentration of species II, and thereby produce significant stabilization of the molecule.[55,102]

The autoxidation of oils in surfactant solutions is quite interesting. Starting with an emulsion of the oil and adding surfactant in steps until a clear solubilized solution is obtained, the oxidation rate at first increases and then decreases greatly when solution is complete. This behavior has been explained by assuming that the initiation step is taking place in the micelle and propagation in the oil phase. Thus, complete solution is equivalent to addition of a chain inhibitor.[15] The effect of solubilization on autoxidation is still an area of controversy and active research.[115]

Effect of Temperature. Most drug degradations increase rapidly with increasing temperature. The quantitative expression of this fact is known as the Arrhenius equation:

$$\log \frac{k_2}{k_1} = \frac{E_A}{2.303 \text{ R}} \left(\frac{T_2 - T_1}{T_1 \times T_2} \right). \quad (19)$$

where k_1 is the rate constant at temperature T_1, k_2 is the rate constant at temperature T_2, and E_A is known as the "activation energy" of the reaction. The increase in rate constant with temperature is rationalized in terms of the increased fraction of molecules having sufficient energy for reaction. Many of the common reactions have "activation energies" of about 12 kilocalories per degree per mole. Solving equation 19 at this value leads to the approximate rule that reaction rate doubles for each 10-degree rise in temperature.

This readily explains the rationale for keeping medications in the refrigerator. The degradation rate will be decreased to approximately ¼ of its degradation rate at room temperature.

Equation 19 is also useful in accelerated stability studies. Thus, one may determine the rate constants at elevated temperatures and using a plot of log k vs. 1/T extrapolated back to room temperature, the rate at room temperature is obtained. Thus, the stability at room temperature may be obtained in a fraction of the time that would be required by ordinary shelf-life studies.

DEGRADATION BY MICRO-ORGANISMS

Although a completely different phenomenon, the growth of micro-organisms in solutions may lead to loss of potency. In many cases (e.g., ophthalmic preparations) the presence of viable organisms in the solutions is undesirable in itself. The most desirable method for avoiding contamination is the use of aseptic technic and sterilization of the solution. This is of utmost importance in the preparation of parenteral and ophthalmic preparations. However, in most ordinary internal and external preparations, the rather tedious and expensive manipulations of aseptic technic are not necessary. The problem

---

* Note the similarity to equation 10.

of contamination may be minimized by the use of suitable antimicrobial or antifungal agents.

The common pharmaceutical solvents alcohol and glycerol are known to possess antimicrobial properties. In addition, the presence of sucrose in high concentration is a useful preservative. Thus, alcohol in concentration of 15 per cent or higher, glycerol at 50 per cent or higher and sucrose solutions of 65 per cent need no other preservatives. When used in combination, the amounts may be less for each ingredient.[11]

It is often desirable to add an antibacterial agent to the solution. Several agents are available for this purpose, the most widely used agents being benzoic acid and the esters of p-hydroxybenzoic acid.

Benzoic acid is a far more effective agent than sodium benzoate;[27] therefore, the preservative action must be strongly dependent on pH. The usual effective concentration of benzoic acid is 0.1 per cent. The concentration of benzoic acid necessary to maintain a free acid concentration of 0.1 per cent in a solution with a pH of 6.0 would be about 6.5 per cent. (p$\bar{K}_A$ of benzoic acid is 4.20.)

Because of this, other agents are needed for nonacidic solutions. This need has been filled by the use of the methyl, ethyl, propyl and butyl esters of p-hydroxybenzoic acid (parabens). The high pK_A of the phenolic hydroxy group (ca. 10) makes their use feasible in almost all pharmaceutical preparations.

These esters differ in their relative activity against various types of micro-organisms. Therefore, use is made of mixtures of parabens as preservatives. The concentration needed is difficult to ascertain, since the recommended concentrations are often higher than the water solubility of the parabens. Solubility data are given in Table 4-8.[88]

TABLE 4-8

PARABEN	WATER	PROPYLENE GLYCOL	ALCOHOL
	Solubility in Gm./100 ml.		
Methyl	0.25	22	52
Ethyl	0.17	25	70
Propyl	0.02	26	95
Butyl	0.02	110	210

In practice a problem arises in the use of parabens because of their very slow rate of dissolution. This may be averted by the use of stock solutions in propylene glycol.

Another problem is likely to arise when parabens are used in solutions containing other molecules with which they may interact through formation of hydrogen bonds.

The interaction with Tween 80 has been thoroughly studied.[92,96] The reaction may be written:

Tween + Paraben = Paraben-Tween

This reaction will follow the law of mass action and may therefore be written:

$$K = \frac{[\text{P-T}]}{[\text{P}][\text{T}]}$$

(Since only the free paraben is antibacterial, it is necessary to add extra paraben to a solution containing such agents.) The total paraben needed is the desired free paraben, P, plus the amount in the complex form, P-T.

Paraben needed $= [\text{P}] + [\text{P-T}] = [\text{P}] + \text{K}[\text{T}][\text{P}]$
$$= \text{P}\,[1 + \text{K}(\text{T})]$$

When P and T are expressed in percentage the value of K for propylparaben is about 0.65 and for methylparaben 4.5. The use of this equation has been shown to predict the required paraben concentration quite accurately.[96]

Since parabens are esters, it is not surprising to find that they degrade relatively rapidly in basic media,[99] $t_{\frac{1}{2}}$ at 70°:

pH	6.0	565 hrs.
	8.0	94 hrs.
	9.0	38 hrs.

It is surprising, however, to find that they are in a few cases degraded by microorganisms.[58] Another possible problem in their use is raised by the occasional reports of allergenic responses to parabens.[109] In spite of the multitude of difficulties, the parabens remain the most widely used and useful of the preservative agents.

The use of preservatives in ophthalmic solutions will be discussed in a later section.

COLORING AND FLAVORING
COLORING

Occasionally the pharmacist encounters a prescription in which coloring will increase patient acceptance. A large number of coal tar colors are available for such use. Probably the easiest approach to the problem is the use of liquid food colors available in grocery stores. Such Food, Drug and Cosmetic dyes are not, in general, as stable as Drug and Cosmetic dyes. However, for use in extemporaneous compounding where long-term stability is not necessary they are quite useful. They consist of solutions of 3 to 4 per cent coloring agent in a propylene glycol–water vehicle. The usual colors are blue, green, yellow and red. Other colors are easily obtained by appropriate mixtures of these.

The dyes are all sodium salts of sulfonic acids. Thus, one would anticipate possible incompatibilities with large cationic molecules such as the salts of alkaloids. However, because of the very low concentration of dye in the final product (ca. $5 \times 10^{-3}\%$) no problem is usually observed. Since sulfonic acids are quite strong, the dyes are not precipitated by ordinary acidic vehicles, although the color may be slightly altered. It is interesting to note that some water soluble F.D.C. dyes have been reacted with large cationic surfactants to obtain oil-soluble dyes.[39]

FLAVORING

It is highly unlikely that anyone would contest the simple statement that the public expects liquid oral medications to be pleasantly flavored and reasonably palatable. In light of this it is sometimes difficult to remember that not too many years ago most liquid products were ghastly tasting preparations— and were even expected to be so. In those days the public had resigned itself to the philosophy that medical treatment *of any type* was unpleasant. Indeed, the greater the discomfort, the more effective it was believed to be. As examples, skin antiseptics (e.g., Iodine tincture) stung when applied to the skin and this was accepted as proof that the product was "working." Ointments, it seemed, *had* to be either tacky, odorous, staining, or grainy before they were qualified to appear in the official compendia. It is evident that liquid oral preparations more than met the public's masochistic expectations. To this day, products such as Aromatic Cascara Sagrada Fluidextract and Elixir of

Iron, Quinine and Strychnine stand out as monumental tributes to mankind's ability to withstand punishment.

In contrast, a modern penicillin preparation provides an excellent yardstick by which to measure the advances in the art-science of flavoring. Potassium penicillin G is a very bitter substance. When a therapeutic dose is dissolved in a teaspoonful of Syrup *U.S.P.*, the assaulted taste buds perceive no sweetness whatsoever. One is aware only that an overwhelmingly bitter viscous liquid has been permitted to enter the oral cavity. Yet there are a large number of oral liquid penicillin preparations on the market, all of which have been flavored and are reasonably palatable. It is because of such remarkable accomplishments as this that the public has become increasingly less tolerant of unpleasant tasting medications. This over-all change in attitude is a tribute to the advances that have been made by the flavoring and pharmaceutical industries.

Flavor Perception

The perception of flavor is actually a composite response to stimuli from many receptor organs which register such characteristics as taste, odor, texture, heat (or cold), pungency or blandness. Usually taste and odor are the predominant contributors. It has been generally accepted that the taste buds can detect only four basic tastes: sweet, sour, bitter, and salty. Taste will therefore be one or a combination of these characteristics (e.g., bitter-sweet, sweet-sour). The sense of smell is at least equally important in flavor perception. A person with a cold often complains that his food is "tasteless" and therefore unappealing. Actually his taste buds are unaffected; it is his sense of smell that has been blocked. It has been suggested[56] that one can detect only seven basic odors: ethereal, camphoraceous, musky, floral, pepperminty, pungent, and putrid. Therefore odor, like taste, is one of or a combination of these characteristics. As an example, almond odor has been described as a mixture of camphoraceous, floral, and pepperminty components.

As mentioned previously, taste and odor are the primary contributors to flavor perception. They become less important when other factors are overwhelming. A person who ingests a teaspoonful of sweetened, orange flavored sand may describe the product as tasting "gritty."

It is obvious that visual responses also play a role in flavor perception and acceptability. If, for example, a strawberry were sculpted into the size and shape of a fly (and colored appropriately) a recipient's eyes would signal his mind with the message, "you are going to eat a fly"—and bias his flavor perception accordingly. Later, somewhat confused, he might admit that the fly tasted a little like a strawberry, but there is little hope that he would describe the encounter as delicious, or request another. Occasionally the manufacturers of pharmaceuticals use a visual distraction as a flavoring technic. One commonly prescribed antihistamine is peach flavored, but colored blue. Another has a cola flavor, yet is colored orange. While the brain is attempting to decide what a blue peach or orange cola is, the bitter drug has been swallowed.

Flavoring Considerations

The process whereby a particular flavor is eventually selected for a particular drug is composed of many steps. For this reason a pharmacist can be thankful that he is seldom called upon to solve a flavoring problem. When he is, he will probably try cherry, mint, lemon, or orange flavors because these are readily available and have been reported to be useful for the majority of extemporaneous flavoring problems.[124] A pharmaceutical manufacturer cannot rely solely on the aforementioned flavors, nor can he approach the problem casually. Since the financial success of his product depends ultimately upon patient acceptance as well as therapeutic merit, he devotes a great deal of talent and money to the developing of an ideally flavored product.

Although every manufacturer has developed his own approaches to flavoring, in general one of the first steps is the determination of the taste characteristics (bitter, sour, aftertaste, etc.) of the drug to be masked. If these characteristics are extreme in nature, he may attempt to synthesize a less water-soluble derivative of the drug. If successful, the eventual product will be a suspension. In any event, after the taste characteristics have been determined, he may apply some general guidelines[19,61,64,76]: sour or salty drugs are sometimes masked by citrus flavors (orange, pineapple, etc.), bitter drugs are sometimes more palatable in chocolate, mint, or raspberry flavors. He may also use a flavor guide published by a flavor manufacturer[95] for additional recommendations.

It is important to note that the dosing regimen of a product must be taken into consideration when selecting test flavors. If a product is to be taken many times a day, certain flavors are rejected becaused the patient rapidly tires of them. A strawberry flavored antacid would not be expected to be popular, whereas peppermint appears to be quite acceptable for multiple daily dosing. Another factor to be considered is the average age of the population who will be taking the drug. Children readily accept very sweet recognizable flavors (cola, orange, fruit, etc.) while adults may reject these, preferring less sweetened products. Elderly patients may prefer mint, wine, or liquor flavors. On occasion a manufacturer blends flavors to achieve a "non-descript" flavor,[125] a technic used for flavoring many penicillin preparations.

Sooner or later, a series of test preparations are submitted to a tasting panel, whose preferences are then statistically analyzed. Table 4-9 reproduced from a survey published in 1963[124] gives some idea of the frequency with which various flavors appear in certain classes of drugs.

Stability

Throughout the total process of flavor design, a manufacturer must be concerned about the stability of his final product. As

TABLE 4-9*

Flavor	Antibiotics	Vitamins	Cough Preparations
Cherry	19%	21%	30%
Orange	17%	21%	–
Fruit	21%	19%	–
Raspberry	–	–	22%
All others	43%	39%	48%

* Wesley, F.: J. Am. Pharm. Ass., NS3:208, 1963.

indicated in previous sections of this chapter, drugs that are in solution are considerably more susceptible to chemical degradation than are drugs in solid form (powder, suspension, etc.) In a flavored product there is also the possibility that the flavoring ingredients will interact or affect the stability of the active drug. The manufacturer therefore attempts to design his product to meet useful shelf-life specifications as well as patient acceptance. Occasionally these two demands are incompatible, and specialized oral dosage forms must be designed. As an example, potassium penicillin G is most acceptable, but least stable, in an acid-buffered citrus flavor blend. To overcome this difficulty, this product is packaged in dry powder form, to which the pharmacist adds water prior to dispensing (see "encapsulated flavors").

Flavors—Natural vs. Synthetic

It has been estimated[108] that more than 1,100 different flavoring substances are currently available to the food and pharmaceutical industries. Seven hundred fifty of these are totally synthetic. Recently the trend in the flavoring industry has been to replace many of the natural flavors with synthetic substitutes or equivalents. This has been prompted by the many disadvantages of natural flavors: they are expensive; the supply is limited, to some extent dependent upon growing seasons; they are non-uniform in composition, and they are unstable. For these reasons synthetic flavoring ingredients have been incorporated into a wide variety of food and pharmaceutical products. Daily, the average American is unknowingly exposed to a barrage of synthetically flavored products, starting with his glass of orange juice in the morning and ending with the brushing of his teeth at night. The student is advised to scan the flavor advertisements that appear in various periodicals.[1,26] He will discover that items such as tomato, cantaloupe, chicken, coffee, and watermelon have succumbed to the skill of the synthetic chemist. Further exposure to the wide variety of available flavors may be found in a catalog requested from one of the major flavor manufacturers.[34,35,37,72,89]

Flavor Types

Once a specific flavor has been selected for a product, depending upon the particular requirements of the situation, a flavoring pharmacist selects one of the several types of flavoring ingredients that are available:

Volatile Oils. A volatile oil is the most concentrated form of flavoring ingredient available, having the ability to flavor many thousand times its own weight of a product. It may be prepared by expression, distillation, or solvent fractionization of a natural product, or synthetically. Since it is an oil and is water insoluble, special technics must be used when it is incorporated into a product (e.g., incorporation into ethyl alcohol, propylene glycol, use of a filter aid such as talc). It is usually colorless and food colors must be added for a natural effect. Ordinarily it cannot be used to flavor dry-mix products, since it may cause "caking" of the powders or interact with the active ingredients.

Encapsulated Flavors. An encapsulated flavor is a specialized flavor form that is available as a free flowing powder and is commonly used in dry-mix preparations (e.g., potassium penicillin G). The flavor powder is prepared by simultaneously spray-drying a volatile oil with a hydrocolloid solution (such as acacia). The resultant dry particle is embedded with the volatile oil which becomes less susceptible to evaporation, oxidation, or interaction with subsequently added ingredients. An encapsulated flavor is somewhat less concentrated than a volatile oil; however, it offers the advantage that the flavor is rapidly dissolved in water (because of the available surface area). As with volatile oils, food colors must be added to obtain a natural effect.

Finished Flavors. A finished flavor contains a volatile oil (or natural product concentrate) suitable coloring agents, and is water soluble. It is a "ready-for-use" flavor. In certain cases (orange, lemon, etc.) this type of flavor will also contain a synthetic "clouding" agent to mimic the haze of a natural product. This type flavor is considerably less concentrated than a volatile oil although one part will flavor somewhere between 100 to 500 parts of a final product.

Sweetening Agents

Although sucrose can be considered to be a classic sweetening agent for pharmaceuticals and is still fairly popular, there has been a tendency at the industrial level to blend it, or replace it entirely, with synthetic sweetening agents. This has been prompted by the fact that, on a weight basis, sucrose is an inefficient sweetening agent. Secondly, sucrose syrups are susceptible to microbial attack and chemical degradation. Furthermore, sucrose tends to crystallize around the lip of a bottle containing a sucrose liquid and can cause cap-locking,[123] so that the bottle cap becomes difficult or impossible to remove. Most of these shortcomings are overcome by the use of the synthetic sweetening agents, which (with the exception of sorbitol) have the added advantage of being less costly.

Sorbitol. Sorbitol is a white crystalline material reported to be approximately one half as sweet as sucrose on a weight basis. It readily dissolves in water and is occasionally used in lozenges because as it goes into solution it creates a pleasant cooling sensation. In large doses it acts as a laxative and when eventually absorbed from the gastrointestinal tract it is about 98 per cent metabolized. Because this material is hygroscopic it is commonly used as a humectant in cosmetic or pharmaceutical lotions and creams.

Saccharin Sodium. Saccharin sodium readily dissolves in water and is reported to be 300 to 550 times sweeter than sucrose of equal weight (depending upon its use). Many persons complain of a bitter metallic aftertaste. Aqueous solutions are relatively stable at room temperature, but heating (especially in the presence of an acid) will cause hydrolysis to sulfonamidobenzoic acid —a harmless but bitter substance. Saccharin is excreted unmetabolized less than 24 hours after ingestion.

PACKAGING

The student is familiar from his laboratory studies with the ordinary glass bottles used for packaging liquids. The need for brown bottles which absorb the highly energetic blue wavelengths should be apparent from the earlier discussion of autoxidation. The green dropper bottles often used will transmit ultraviolet radiation and are therefore no improvement over clear bottles.

The past few years have seen the introduction of plastic containers for liquids. They have certain advantages in terms of breakage and opacity. However, their ability to adsorb preservatives and drugs and allow free passage of gases militates against their usage in several systems.[8,62,73] Their use for any product must be tested on an individual basis, and it will probably be several years before they may be used widely in prescription practice.

SPECIAL SOLUTIONS

Although the general principles developed earlier are applicable to all solutions, some dosage forms require special technics.

OPHTHALMIC SOLUTIONS

It is generally agreed that ophthalmic solutions should be sterile, should contain a preservative and should have an osmotic pressure and pH similar to that of normal lacrimal fluid. Each of these requirements will be discussed separately.

Sterility

If one considers the limitations of the defense mechanisms of the eye, it becomes self-evident that ophthalmic preparations should be sterile. Tears—unlike blood—do not contain antibodies or the mechanisms for producing them. Therefore the primary defense mechanisms against eye infection are the simple washing action of tearing, and an enzyme found in tears (lysozyme) which has the ability to hydrolyze the polysaccharide coat of *some* microorganisms. Of those organisms unaffected by lysozyme, the one most capable of causing eye damage is *Pseudomonas aeruginosa (Bacillus pyocyaneus)*. The seriousness of an infection caused by this organism is brought home by an examination of the clinical literature which abounds with such terms as enucleation of the eye and corneal transplants.[13,14,21] It is important to note that this is not a rare organism: it may be found in the intestinal tract or on the normal skin of man and may even be an airborne contaminant. Thus contamination of ophthalmic solutions (commercial or compounded) is not surprising if they are not handled properly.

FDA Requirements. Because of the potential problems arising from contaminated eye preparations, the FDA ruled in 1953 that any commercially prepared ophthalmic preparation must be sterile or it would be considered to be misbranded and adulterated. In 1963 the FDA further recommended that the labels of ophthalmic preparations bear the following caution, "Do not touch dropper tip (or other dispensing tip) to any surface since this may contaminate the solution." Since a pharmacist in his usual dispensing technic removes this label, it is imperative that he reproduce the caution, or verbally transmit it to the patient.

Although the 1953 FDA ruling applied only to the commercial manufacturers of ophthalmic preparations, the moral and ethical implications to the community pharmacist are clear: *any* compounded ophthalmic solution should be sterile. If a pharmacist lacks equipment to prepare a sterile solution, he is ethically bound to dispense a commercial preparation if available.

It is important to note that sterility is not accomplished by a partial approach. The use of distilled water, or sterile distilled water, with a nonsterile chemical and a sterile or nonsterile container accomplishes absolutely nothing. Using a sterile chemical, sterile distilled water, a sterile container *and* mixing the ingredients together in a nonsterile measuring device is equally self-defeating. In other words, there is no such thing as a partially sterile solution. Tap water should *never* be used in manufacturing ophthalmic preparations. Aside from containing minerals which may catalyze the degradation of the active ingredients, water from faucets equipped with aerators is highly contaminated with microorganisms (including Pseudomonas).[127]

The problems mentioned above are dramatically illustrated in a recent article by MacDonald *et al.* (Am. J. Ophthal. *68*:1099, 1969): Pilocarpine solution, one per cent, was prepared extemporaneously by 66 pharmacists. Fifty-two of the 66 pharmacy-prepared solutions were found to be contaminated with bacteria and/or fungi! In contrast, only one of the 34 samples from pharmaceutical companies was found to be contaminated.

Technics. In order to ensure sterility of the final product, the solution should be prepared under aseptic conditions (sterile hood, laminar air flow hood, etc.). The ready availability of inexpensive household pressure cookers makes possible the sterilization of the utensils used in preparing ophthalmic solutions, the dropper bottles, or in some cases the prepared solution in the dropper bottle. When the active ingredient cannot stand autoclaving temperatures, solutions may be rendered sterile by filtration technics. One approach is the use of a glass chamber which houses a Selas bacterial filtration unit[90] that filters the solution by means of vacuum aspiration into a previously sterilized dropper bottle. A less cumbersome approach was made possible by the development of the Millipore filter.* When this filter is used in combination with a large syringe (10-30 ml.) and a Swinny adapter (and possibly a Cornwall 3-valve multifilling adapter), all bacteria can be removed from a solution.[57] The presterilized Swinnex disposable unit* makes this system even more desirable, since, aside from a syringe, no permanent equipment is necessary. Another disposable presterilized filtration unit[45] comes complete with a syringe, filtration unit and plastic dropper bottle, and reduces the total sterilization process to a few simple steps.

Utilizing such technics as those mentioned above, it is possible for the original prescription to leave the pharmacy in a sterile condition. However, the pharmacist's responsibility does not end here.

Preservatives

Attention to the future conditions of use of the final product is also important. If the solution is to be used in a physician's office or a clinic, the possibility of inoculation of pathogens into the solution becomes great.[71] For example, an epidemic of Pseudomonas infection in a Rotterdam hospital, a few years ago, revealed that a large number of eyedrops in clinical use were infected.

---

* Information is available from the Millipore Co., Bedford, Mass.

Further study of the solutions in use in the consulting rooms of 12 eye surgeons in Rotterdam showed contamination in at least one preparation in each of 9 of the 12 rooms examined.[38] Thus, it is necessary that ophthalmic solutions for such use be "self-sterilizing." Solutions for home use are much less liable to such "cross infections," but it seems reasonable to use a preservative for this type of preparation also. A third general type of eye medication is more likely to be seen only in hospital pharmacies. Preparations for use in traumatized eyes or during surgery should be compounded for the use of only one patient. This preparation will only be used once, and therefore preservatives should be omitted.[87,113]

The problem arises as to what preservative should be used. This is a particularly knotty problem which has puzzled investigators for several years. The literature is conflicting and confusing and the popularity of various agents rises and falls with alarming rapidity.

It seems unlikely that much can be gained by reiteration of the history of such preservatives. Therefore, only a few examples which are presently accepted will be discussed.

The quaternary ammonium compounds, especially benzalkonium chloride, have become accepted as excellent broad-spectrum preservatives effective against both gram-positive and gram-negative organisms.[68] However, there has been a question raised as to their effectiveness against certain strains of Pseudomonas.[105] It has been suggested that the addition of 0.01 to 0.1 per cent of disodium ethylenediaminetetraacetate will make such resistant organisms susceptible to the usual 1:10,000 benzalkonium chloride solutions.[70,87] Dale and co-workers suggested that a mixture of benzalkonium chloride (0.02%) and neomycin sulfate (0.5%) might be an excellent combination.[21,22] Another possibility is benzalkonium chloride (0.01%) and polymyxin B 1,000 units/cc. The use of polymyxin B has been questioned, since it is one of the few drugs useful against clinical infections of Pseudomonas. However, development of a new antibiotic useful against Pseudomonas infections seems to reduce the validity of this argument.[97] Note that the need for benzalkonium chloride is due to the narrow spectrum of the suggested antibiotics.

The quaternary ammonium preservatives have some incompatibilities which must be taken into account with their use. They have been reported to be incompatible with 5 per cent (but not 2%) boric acid, nitrates, salicylates and fluorescein. In the case of nitrates and salicylates where the cation is the pharmacologically active agent, the best method is to change to the chloride or another salt which would be compatible with quaternaries. One other effect of the addition of benzalkonium chloride should be noted. The surface tension reduction will decrease the drop size of the solution with concurrent reduction in dosage per drop. (The drop is reduced from 0.05 cc./drop to about 0.03/drop in a 0.01% solution.)

Chlorobutanol has been strongly recommended in the past.[119] However, it has some distinct disadvantages. It is difficult to effect solution of the 0.5 per cent concentration required and it is rapidly destroyed by autoclaving or in basic solution. It is also incompatible with silver nitrate and sodium salts of sulfa drugs.[40]

The organic mercurials such as phenylmercuric nitrate have been used for several years as preservative agents.[53] Unfortunately, organic mercurial agents are much slower acting than other agents and tend to be sensitizing when used over long periods of time. Phenylmercuric nitrate is also incompatible with halides, which further detracts from its usefulness. It may be used with salicylate and nitrate salts in place of quaternaries. Thimerosal has been recommended for ophthalmic use in combination with polymyxin B. It worked well at the pH tested by the authors (6.8) but could not be used at more acidic pH values because of precipitation of the free acid form of thimerosal.[59]

Since fluoroscein has been mentioned, it is perhaps appropriate to discuss a problem associated with its use. Fluorescein solutions are used by all practitioners in fitting contact lenses and by physicians in delineating corneal lesions such as may occur as a result of trauma, chemical burns, or erosive pathologic processes of any kind.[65] However, fluorescein solutions are a notorious source of Pseudomonas infections,[101] and the U.S.P. suggests that only single dose preparations should be used.[121] The message here is clear and direct: no pharmacist should prepare fluorescein solutions for use in the eye. Instead he should recommend presterilized unit-dose preparations.

Osmotic Pressure

It was not many years ago that a great deal of energy was expended in the effort to assure the correct osmotic pressure of ophthalmic solutions. Later, it was possible to read in an Italian pharmaceutical journal a quotation from a Swiss pharmaceutical journal, which originated in an American pharmaceutical journal, that assures us that osmotic pressure is relatively unimportant![104] This viewpoint is based on the fact that the eye is insensitive to a rather large range of osmotic pressure. This concept has been challenged on the grounds that although pain may not be elicited, tearing may result, and, thus, medications may be washed out of the eye.[120] Therefore, it seems that the safest method is to adjust the osmotic pressure of solutions for use in the eye to a practical range.

The student will recall the earlier discussion of Raoult's Law. This law states that the vapor pressure above a liquid is proportional to the mole fraction of the liquid in the solution. Thus, as the mole fraction of solute is increased the mole fraction of solvent will decrease (sum of all mole fractions must equal one) and the vapor pressure of the solvent must necessarily decrease. Let us now visualize an aqueous solution and pure water separated by a membrane which will allow water molecules to pass freely but will not allow the passage of solute molecules (Fig. 4-5). Since the vapor pressure of the water is greater than the vapor pressure of the solution, water will pass through the membrane into the solution. In order to prevent this transfer we may increase the pressure on compartment B (F_B) with the piston until the volume of water in B no longer increases with time. Thus, we have increased the vapor pressure of the solution until it is equal to the vapor pressure of the pure water. Osmotic pressure π is defined as the difference in pressure necessary to prevent passage of solvent in one direction, i.e.,

$$\pi = F_B - F_A$$

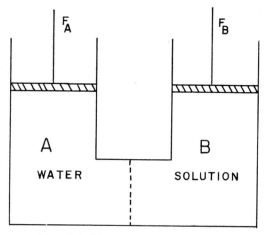

FIG. 4-5. Water (A) and an aqueous solution (B) separated by a semipermeable membrane with impervious pistons exerting pressures F_A and F_B, respectively, above each compartment.

It may appear that the osmotic pressure should be a rather small force, since the vapor pressure differences are quite small for dilute aqueous solutions vs. water. This is far from true, osmotic pressures often being as high as several atmospheres of pressure! The explanation for this lies in the fact that large increases in applied pressure must be exerted in order to produce small increases in vapor pressure. The equation relating the two pressures is:

$$F = \frac{2.3RT}{\overline{V}} \cdot \log \frac{P}{P^*},$$

where R and T have their usual meanings, $\overline{V}$ is the volume per mole of liquid (e.g., 18 ml./mole for water), P^* is the vapor pressure when F (applied pressure) is zero and P is the vapor pressure for a given value of F. From this definition we may derive a relationship for predicting π for various concentrations of solute:

$$\pi = F_B - F_A = \frac{2.3RT}{\overline{V}} \log \frac{P_B}{P^*_B} - \frac{2.3RT}{\overline{V}} \log \frac{P_A}{P^*_A}$$

Now, $P_A = P_B$ (vapor pressure of water and solution are equal), $P_A^* = P_w^\circ$ where P_w° is the vapor pressure of pure water, and $P_B^* = P_w^\circ X_W = P_w^\circ [1 - X_s]$ where X_W is the mole fraction of water and X_s is the mole fraction of solute in the solution.

Thus,

$$\pi = \frac{2.3RT}{\overline{V}} \log \frac{P_B \, P^*_A}{P^*_B \, P_A} = \frac{2.3RT}{\overline{V}} \log$$

$$\frac{P_W^{\circ}}{P_W^{\circ} [1 - X_s]} = -\frac{2.3RT}{\overline{V}} \log [1 - X_s].$$

For dilute solutions, $[1 - X_s]$ approaches one and $2.3 \log [1 - X_s]$ is approximately equal to $-X_s$. (The student may verify this by checking the equality for small values of X_s.)
Therefore:

$$\pi = +\frac{RT}{\overline{V}} X_s$$

By definition,

$$X_s = \frac{\text{moles solute (m)}}{\text{moles water + moles solute}},$$

and for dilute solutions, where the moles of solute are much smaller than the moles of water,

$$X_s = \frac{\text{moles solute (m)}}{\text{moles water}}.$$

The moles of water multiplied by the volume per mole gives the volume of water (V). Thus,

$$\pi = \frac{m}{V} RT = 0.082 \, MT \qquad (20)$$

where M is the molarity of the solute. We may predict the osmotic pressure of a 5 per cent glucose solution (which has the same osmotic pressure as lacrimal fluid) at 25°C. as follows:

$$\pi = 0.082 \times \frac{50}{180} \times 298$$

$$= 6.8 \text{ atmospheres} = 100 \text{ lb./in.}^2$$

The vapor pressure differential ($P_W^{\circ} - P$) producing this osmotic pressure may be estimated with the aid of Raoult's Law to be only 2.78×10^{-2} mm. of mercury or 5.6×10^{-4} lb./in.^{2}

The effect of 100 lb./in.^{2} on a semipermeable membrane such as the cornea of the eye is easily understood. Such pressures would never actually be obtained with ophthalmic medication, since the pressure differential would have to be generated by movement of water molecules across the cornea.

The stimulus will, of course, induce lacrimal secretion which rapidly dilutes and washes out the offending liquid.

Incorrect answers are obtained if one attempts to use equation 20 for predicting the osmotic pressure of electrolytes. This may be explained by assuming that the molecules dissociate into g particles. The mole fraction of solute X_s will then be multiplied by g:

$$X_s = \frac{(g)(m)}{\text{moles water}}$$

For example, with potassium chloride, the number of moles both of potassium and of chloride ions are equal to the number of moles of potassium chloride added and the total number of moles of solute is therefore doubled by dissociation. Of course, dissociation is never complete and the factor g is always less than the theoretic number of particles possible. It is therefore necessary to determine the factor experimentally. The experimental correction factor is usually designated as i. Equation 20 then becomes:

$$\pi = 0.082 \, i \, MT.^* \qquad (21)$$

Fortunately, it is not necessary to obtain i values for all salts encountered, since the variation between salts of similar types (e.g., NaCl and KCl, or $MgSO_4$ and $CaSO_4$) is negligible. They also vary somewhat with concentration but this effect is also unimportant for practical compounding. A listing of i values is given in Table 4-10.

Two solutions which have the same osmotic pressure are defined as iso-osmotic. The term isotonic is more widely used in pharmacy. This term is defined in terms of an actual cell membrane. For example, a solution in which a red blood cell neither swells nor shrinks will be isotonic with the red blood cell contents. The term is often loosely used and the possibility that one of the solutes penetrates the membrane should not be overlooked. When penetration occurs, the solution may be iso-osmotic but not isotonic.[46] Lacrimal fluid (and blood plasma) has been found to be isotonic with 0.9 per cent sodium chloride.[51] Most practical

* Knowing i and π (6.8 atmospheres) it therefore is possible to determine the molarity of any substance necessary to prepare an iso-osmotic solution.

TABLE 4-10. AVERAGE i VALUES FOR VARIOUS IONIC TYPES†

TYPE	i VALUE	EXAMPLES
Nonelectrolytes	1.0	Sucrose, dextrose, glycerin
Weak electrolytes	1.1	Phenobarbital, boric acid
Uni-univalent electrolytes	1.8	Sodium chloride, procaine HCl, sodium phenobarbital
Uni-divalent electrolytes	2.3	Atropine sulfate, calcium sulfate
Di-univalent electrolytes	2.6	Calcium chloride
Di-divalent electrolytes	1.1	Zinc sulfate, calcium sulfate
Uni-trivalent electrolytes	2.8	Sodium citrate
Tri-univalent electrolytes	3.2	Ferric chloride
Tetraborate electrolytes	4.1	Sodium borate

† Modified from Wells, J. M.: Am. Pharm. Ass. [Pract.] 5:99, 1944.

methods of preparing isotonic solutions use this concentration as a guide.[42,75] Thus, in the sodium chloride equivalent method the concentration of each ingredient is changed (mentally) into the equivalent amount of sodium chloride and additional sodium chloride sufficient to make the final percentage 0.9 is added. The sodium chloride equivalent E is found in the following fashion:

$$(\text{Osmotic pressure of NaCl}) = \pi_1 = 0.082 \times 1.82 \times \frac{58.5}{\text{wt. NaCl}} \times 298 = 0.76 \times \text{wt. NaCl}$$
$$= .76\ E$$

Osmotic pressure of one weight unit of solute

$$= \pi_2 = 0.082 \times i \times \frac{1}{\text{M.W.}} \times 298 = 24.5\ i/\text{M.W.}$$

Therefore

$$E = \frac{24.5}{0.76}\ \frac{i}{\text{M.W.}} = 32 \times \frac{i}{\text{M.W.}} \quad (22)$$

Now, E is the number of weight units of sodium chloride equivalent to one weight unit of the other solute, therefore the two π may be set equal and solved for E.

Knowing the value of i and the molecular weight of any given drug makes it possible to obtain the required value of E. E will have any weight units as desired. Thus, it is the number of grains equal to 1 grain of the ingredient, or, equally well, the number of Gm. equal to 1 Gm. of the ingredient. A listing of useful E values is given in Table 4-11. (Note that many of these values are experimental and may differ slightly from values calculated with the aid of equation 22.)

The use of these values may be illustrated by prescription examples:

1. ℞
   Procaine HCl 2%
   Mft isotonic solution .... fℨii

Since the prescription is in the apothecary system, we shall assume that 18 gr. of procaine HCl are used. E = 0.18. Therefore, a solution with an osmotically equivalent amount of sodium chloride would contain 3.2 gr. of sodium chloride. Two ounces of an 0.9 per cent solution would contain 8 gr. of sodium chloride. Therefore, we need an additional 4.8 gr. of sodium chloride to render the prescription isotonic.

2. ℞
   Eserine salicylate 0.5%
   Pilocarpine nitrate 1.0%
   Sodium sulfite 0.1%
   Mft Isotonic solution .... 30 cc.

This prescription is written in the metric system and will be manipulated in that system.

   0.15 × 0.14 = 0.02 Gm. NaCl
   0.30 × 0.21 = 0.06 Gm. NaCl
   0.03 × 0.57 = 0.02 Gm. NaCl
   ————————
   0.10 Gm. NaCl total
   0.9% NaCl = 0.27 Gm.

Therefore, 0.17 Gm. additional NaCl is needed.

TABLE 4-11. SODIUM CHLORIDE EQUIVALENTS FOR SOME COMMON DRUGS

Acriflavine	0.10	Caffeine and sodium benzoate U.S.P.	0.26
Adeniphene HCl	0.22	Caffeine and sodium salicylate	0.21
Adenosine 5 monophosphate	0.41	Calcium aminosalicylate N.F.	0.27
Adrenalone HCl	0.27	Calcium chloride U.S.P.	0.51
Alcohol U.S.P.	0.65	Calcium chloride ($6H_2O$)	0.35
Alcohol, dehydrated N.F.	0.70	Calcium chloride, anhydrous	0.68
Alum (potassium) N.F.	0.18	Calcium disodium edetate U.S.P.	0.21
Aminacrine HCl	0.17	Calcium gluconate U.S.P.	0.16
Aminocaproic acid	0.26	Calcium lactate N.F.	0.23
Aminophylline U.S.P.	0.17	Calcium levulinate	0.27
Amiodoxyl benzoate	0.20	Calcium pantothenate U.S.P.	0.18
Amitriptyline HCl	0.18	Carbachol U.S.P.	0.36
Ammonium carbonate N.F.	0.70	Cetyltrimethyl ammonium bromide	0.09
Ammonium chloride U.S.P.	1.12	Chiniofon	0.13
Ammonuim lactate	0.33	Chloramine-T	0.23
Ammonium nitrate	0.69	Chlorcyclizine HCl U.S.P.	0.17
Ammonium phosphate dibasic	0.55	Chloramphenicol sodium succinate U.S.P.	0.14
Ammonium sulfate	0.55	Chlordiazepoxide HCl N.F.	0.22
Amobarbital sodium U.S.P.	0.25	Chlorobutanol (hydrated) U.S.P.	0.24
Amphetamine phosphate N.F.	0.34	Chlorpheniramine maleate U.S.P.	0.17
Amphetamine sulfate N.F.	0.22	Chlorpromazine HCl U.S.P.	0.10
Amprotropine phosphate	0.18	Chlortetracycline sulfate	0.13
Amydricaine HCl	0.24	Citric acid U.S.P.	0.18
Amydricaine nitrate	0.19	Cocaine HCl U.S.P.	0.16
Amylcaine HCl	0.22	Codeine HCl	0.15
Antazoline HCl	0.23	Codeine phosphate U.S.P.	0.14
Antazoline phosphate N.F.	0.20	Cupric sulfate N.F.	0.18
Antimony potassium tartrate U.S.P.	0.18	Cupric sulfate, anhydrous	0.27
Antipyrine N.F.	0.17	Cyclizine HCl U.S.P.	0.20
Apomorphine HCl N.F.	0.14	Cyclomethycaine sulfate	0.13
Arecoline HBr N.F.	0.27	Cyclopentamine HCl N.F.	0.36
Arsenic trioxide N.F.	0.30	Cyclopentolate HCl U.S.P.	0.20
Ascorbic acid U.S.P.	0.18	Cyclophosphamide N.F.	0.10
Atropine methyl nitrate	0.18		
Atropine sulfate U.S.P.	0.13	Decamethonium bromide	0.25
Aurothioglucose U.S.P.	0.03	Demecarium bromide	0.12
		Dexamethasone sodium phosphate N.F.	0.17
Bacitracin U.S.P.	0.05	Dextroamphetamine HCl	0.34
Barbital sodium	0.30	Dextroamphetamine phosphate N.F.	0.25
Benoxinate HCl	0.18	Dextrose U.S.P.	0.16
Benzalkonium Chloride U.S.P.	0.16	Dextrose, anhydrous	0.18
Benzethonium chloride U.S.P.	0.16	Dibucaine HCl U.S.P.	0.13
Benzethonium chloride N.F.	0.05	Dibutoline sulfate	0.16
Benzpyrinium bromide N.F.	0.20	Dichlorophenarsine HCl	0.55
Benztropine mesylate N.F.	0.21	Dicyclomine HCl	0.18
Benzyl alcohol N.F.	0.17	Diethylcarbamazine citrate U.S.P.	0.14
Bethanechol chloride U.S.P.	0.39	Dihydrocodeinone enolacetate HCl	0.14
Bismuth potassium tartrate	0.09	Diphenhydramine HCl U.S.P.	0.28
Bismuth sodium tartrate	0.13	Diphemanil methylsulfate	0.15
Boric acid U.S.P.	0.50	Dihydrostreptomycin sulfate	0.06
Bromodiphephydramine HCl	0.17	Dimethindene maleate	0.12
Brompheniramine maleate N.F.	0.09	Diperodon HCl	0.14
Butacaine sulfate	0.20	Dipyrone	0.19
Butethamine formate	0.26	Disodium edetate U.S.P.	0.23
Butethamine HCl N.F.	0.25	Dycoline HCl	0.24
		Dyphylline	0.12
Caffeine U.S.P.	0.08		

TABLE 4-11. SODIUM CHLORIDE EQUIVALENTS FOR SOME COMMON DRUGS (*Continued*)

Drug	NaCl Eq.	Drug	NaCl Eq.
Edrophonium chloride U.S.P.	0.31	Imipramine HCl N.F.	0.20
Emetine HCl U.S.P.	0.10	Intracaine HCl	0.23
Ephedrine HCl N.F.	0.30	Iodophthalein sodium	0.17
Ephedrine lactate	0.26	Iodopyracet N.F.	0.11
Ephedrine sulfate U.S.P.	0.23	Iodopyracet diethylamine	0.12
Epinephrine bitartrate U.S.P.	0.18	Isoniazid U.S.P.	0.25
Epinephrine HCl	0.29	Kanamycin sulfate U.S.P.	0.07
Ergonovine maleate U.S.P.	0.16		
Erythromycin glucoheptonate U.S.P.	0.07	Lactic acid U.S.P.	0.41
Erythromycin lactobionate U.S.P.	0.07	Lactose U.S.P.	0.07
Ethaverine HCl	0.12	Lidocaine HCl U.S.P.	0.22
Ethylenediamine U.S.P.	0.44	Lobeline HCl	0.16
Ethylhydrocupreine HCl	0.17		
Ethylmorphine HCl N.F.	0.16	Magnesium chloride	0.45
Ethylnorepinephrine HCl	0.32	Magnesium sulfate U.S.P.	0.17
Evans Blue U.S.P.	0.06	Mannitol N.F.	0.17
		Maphenide HCl	0.27
Ferric ammonium citrate, Green	0.17	Menadione-diphosphate	0.25
Ferric cacodylate	0.09	Menadione sodium bisulfite	0.20
Ferrous gluconate	0.15	Meperidine HCl	0.22
Ferrous lactate	0.21	Mephenesin N.F.	0.19
Fluorescein sodium U.S.P.	0.31	Mephentermine sulfate N.F.	0.22
D-Fructose	0.18	Mepivacaine HCl N.F.	0.21
Furtrethonium iodide	0.24	Merbromin N.F.	0.14
		Mercaptomerin sodium U.S.P.	0.18
Galactose	0.18	Mercuric cyanide	0.15
Gallamine triethiodide N.F.	0.08	Mercurophylline N.F.	0.13
Glucosulfone sodium U.S.P.	0.16	Mercury bichloride N.F.	0.13
D-Glucuronic acid	0.20	Mersalyl U.S.P.	0.12
L-Glutamic acid	0.25	Metaraminol bitartrate U.S.P.	0.20
Glycerin U.S.P.	0.35	Methacholine bromide N.F.	0.28
Guanidine HCl	0.65	Methacholine chloride N.F.	0.32
		Methantheline bromide N.F.	0.15
Heparin sodium U.S.P.	0.08	Methadone HCl U.S.P.	0.18
Hexafluorenium bromide	0.11	Methapyrilene HCl N.F.	0.19
Hexamethonium bromide	0.22	Methamphetamine HCl U.S.P.	0.37
Hexamethonium chloride	0.27	Methdilazine HCl	0.10
Hexamethonium tartrate	0.16	Methenamine N.F.	0.23
Hexobarbital sodium N.F.	0.26	Methionine N.F.	0.28
Hexylcaine HCl	0.26	Methitural sodium	0.25
Hippuran®	0.16	Methoxamine HCl U.S.P.	0.26
Histalog®	0.51	Methoxyphenamine HCl	0.26
Histamine DiHCl	0.40	p-Methylaminoethanol-phenol tartrate	0.17
Histamine phosphate U.S.P.	0.25	Methylatropine bromide	0.14
Histidine monohydrochloride	0.29	Methyldopate HCl	0.21
Holocaine HCl	0.20	N-Methylglucamine	0.20
Homatropine HBr U.S.P.	0.17	Methylphenidate HCl N.F.	0.22
Homatropine methylbromide U.S.P.	0.19	Monoethanolamine N.F.	0.53
Hyaluronidase N.F.	0.01	Morphine HCl	0.15
Hydralazine HCl N.F.	0.37	Morphine nitrate	0.19
Hydrastine HCl	0.15	Morphine sulfate U.S.P.	0.14
Hydromorphone N.F.	0.22		
Hydroxyamphetamine HBr U.S.P.	0.26	Nalorphine HCl U.S.P.	0.21
Hydroxyquinoline sulfate	0.21	Naphazoline HCl N.F.	0.27
Hydroxystilbamidine isethionate U.S.P.	0.16	Narcotine HCl N.F.	0.10
Hyoscyamine HBr U.S.P.	0.19	Neoarsphenamine	0.40
Hyoscyamine sulfate N.F.	0.14	Neomycin sulfate U.S.P.	0.11

TABLE 4-11. SODIUM CHLORIDE EQUIVALENTS FOR SOME COMMON DRUGS (*Continued*)

Neostigmine bromide U.S.P.	0.22	Propiomazine HCl	0.15
Neostigmine methylsulfate U.S.P.	0.20	Propoxycaine HCl	0.19
Niacinamide U.S.P.	0.26	Propylene glycol U.S.P.	0.45
Nicotinic acid N.F.	0.25	Pyrathiazine HCl	0.17
Nikethamide U.S.P.	0.18	Pyridoxine HCl U.S.P.	0.37
		Pyrilamine maleate N.F.	0.18
Oxophenarsine HCl U.S.P.	0.24		
Oxycodone	0.14	Quinacrine HCl U.S.P.	0.18
Oxyquinoline sulfate	0.21	Quinacrine methanesulfonate	0.11
Oxytetracycline HCl U.S.P.	0.13	Quinidine gluconate U.S.P.	0.12
		Quinidine sulfate U.S.P.	0.10
Panthesin	0.18	Quinine bisulfate	0.09
d-Pantothenyl alcohol	0.18	Quinine dihydrochloride	0.23
Papaverine HCl N.F.	0.10	Quinine hydrochloride	0.14
Pargyline HCl	0.29	Quinie and urea hydrochloride U.S.P.	0.23
Penicillin G potassium U.S.P.	0.18		
Penicillin G sodium U.S.P.	0.18	Racephedrine HCl N.F.	0.31
Pentobarbital sodium U.S.P.	0.25	Resorcinol U.S.P.	0.28
Pentolinium tartrate	0.17	Scopolamine HBr U.S.P.	0.12
Pentylenetetrazol N.F.	0.22	Scopolamine methylnitrate	0.16
Phenarsone sulfoxylate	0.33	Secobarbital sodium U.S.P.	0.24
Phenindamine tartrate N.F.	0.17	Silver nitrate U.S.P.	0.33
Pheniramine maleate N.F.	0.16	Mild silver protein N.F.	0.17
Phenobarbital sodium U.S.P.	0.24	Strong silver protein	0.08
Phenol U.S.P.	0.35	Sodium acetate, anhydrous	0.77
Phentolamine mesylate U.S.P.	0.17	Sodium acetate N.F.	0.46
Phenylephrine HCl U.S.P.	0.32	Sodium acetazolamide U.S.P.	0.23
Phenylephrine tartrate	0.19	Sodium aminosalicylate U.S.P.	0.29
Phenylpropanolamine HCl	0.38	Sodium antimonyl tartrate	0.13
Phenylpropylmethylamine	0.38	Sodium arsenate, dibasic	0.25
Physostigmine salicylate U.S.P.	0.16	Sodium ascorbate U.S.P.	0.33
Physostigmine sulfate	0.13	Sodium benzoate U.S.P.	0.40
Pilocarpine HCl U.S.P.	0.24	Sodium bicarbonate U.S.P.	0.65
Pilocarpine nitrate U.S.P.	0.23	Sodium biphosphate, anhydrous	0.46
Piperocaine HCl U.S.P.	0.21	Sodium biphosphate U.S.P.	0.40
Piridocaine HCl	0.24	Sodium biphosphate ($2H_2O$)	0.36
Plaquenil® phosphate	0.18	Sodium bismuth thioglycollate	0.19
Polymyxin B sulfate U.S.P.	0.09	Sodium bisulfite U.S.P.	0.61
Polysorbate 80 U.S.P.	0.02	Sodium borate U.S.P.	0.42
Potassium acetate N.F.	0.59	Sodium bromide N.F.	0.57
Potassium chlorate N.F.	0.49	Sodium cacodylate N.F.	0.32
Potassium chloride U.S.P.	0.76	Sodium carbonate, anhyd.	0.70
Potassium iodide U.S.P.	0.34	Sodium carbonate, monohydrated U.S.P.	0.60
Potassium nitrate	0.56	Sodium chloride U.S.P.	1.00
Potassium permanganate U.S.P.	0.39	Sodium citrate U.S.P.	0.31
Potassium phosphate N.F.	0.46	Sodium colistimethate U.S.P.	0.15
Potassium phosphate, monobasic	0.44	Sodium folate	0.12
Potassium sulfate	0.44	Sodium hypophosphite	0.61
Pralidoxime chloride	0.32	Sodium iodide U.S.P.	0.39
Pramoxine HCl	0.18	Sodium lactate	0.55
Probarbital calcium	0.25	Sodium lauryl sulfate U.S.P.	0.08
Probarbital sodium	0.32	Sodium metabisulfite	0.67
Procainamide HCl U.S.P.	0.22	Sodium nafcillin	0.14
Procaine HCl U.S.P.	0.21	Sodium nitrate	0.68
Prochlorperazine edisylate U.S.P.	0.06	Sodium nitrite U.S.P.	0.84
Promazine HCl N.F.	0.13	Sodium oxacillin U.S.P.	0.17
Promethazine HCl U.S.P.	0.18	Sodium phenylbutazone	0.18

TABLE 4-11. SODIUM CHLORIDE EQUIVALENTS FOR SOME COMMON DRUGS (*Continued*)

Sodium phosphate exsiccated, N.F.	0.53	Tetraethylammonium chloride	0.34
Sodium phosphate N.F.	0.29	Tetrahydrozoline HCl	0.28
Sodium phosphate, dibasic (2H$_2$O)	0.42	Theophylline N.F.	0.10
Sodium phosphate, dibasic (12H$_2$O)	0.22	Theophylline sodium glycinate N.F.	0.31
Sodium propionate N.F.	0.61	Thiamine HCl U.S.P.	0.25
Sodium riboflavin phosphate	0.08	Thiethylperazine maleate	0.09
Sodium ricinoleate	0.10	Thiopental sodium U.S.P.	0.27
Sodium salicylate U.S.P.	0.36	Thioproprazate Di HCl	0.16
Sodium sulfate N.F.	0.26	Thioridazine HCl	0.05
Sodium sulfate, anhydrous	0.58	Tolazoline HCl	0.34
Exsiccated sodium sulfite N.F.	0.65	Trasentine® HCl	0.22
Sodium sulfobromophthalein U.S.P.	0.06	Tribromoethanol U.S.P.	0.05
Sodium suramin	0.10	Trifluoperazine Di HCl	0.18
Sodium thiosulfate N.F.	0.31	Trimeprazine tartrate	0.06
Sorbitol (½ H$_2$O)	0.16	Trimethadione U.S.P.	0.23
Stibamine glucoside	0.14	Trimethaphan camphorsulfonate	0.10
Stibophen U.S.P.	0.18	Trimethobenzamide HCl N.F.	0.10
Streptomycin calcium chloride complex	0.20	Triplennamine HCl U.S.P.	0.30
Streptomycin HCl	0.17	Tropacocaine HCl	0.25
Streptomycin sulfate U.S.P.	0.07	Tropicamide	0.09
Strychnine HCl	0.18	Tryparsamide U.S.P.	0.20
Strychnine nitrate	0.12	Tuaminoheptane sulfate N.F.	0.27
Sucrose U.S.P.	0.08	Tubocurarine chloride U.S.P.	0.13
Succinylcholine chloride U.S.P.	0.20	Urea U.S.P.	0.59
Sulfacetamide Sodium U.S.P.	0.23	Urethan	0.31
Sulfadiazine Sodium U.S.P.	0.24		
Sulfamerazine Sodium U.S.P.	0.23	Valethamate bromide	0.15
Sulfapyridine sodium	0.23	Vancomycin HCl U.S.P.	0.05
Sulfathiazole sodium	0.22	Vinbarbital sodium	0.26
Sulfisoxazole diethanolamine	0.18	Viomycin sulfate	0.08
Sympocaine® HCl	0.18	Warfarin sodium U.S.P.	0.17
Synkamin® HCl	0.32		
Synthenate® tartrate	0.19	Xylometazoline HCl	0.21
Tannic acid N.F.	0.03	Zinc chloride U.S.P.	0.61
Tartaric acid N.F.	0.25	Zinc phenolsulfonate	0.18
Tetracaine HCl U.S.P.	0.18	Zinc sulfanilate	0.21
Tetracycline HCl U.S.P.	0.14	Zinc sulfate U.S.P.	0.15
Tetraethylammonium bromide	0.33	Zinc sulfate, dried	0.23

Adapted from Hammarlund, E. R., and Pederson-Bjergaard, K.: J. Am. Pharm. Ass. (Sci.) *47*:107, 1958 and Hammarlund, E. R., Deming, J. G., and Pederson-Bjergaard, K.: J. Pharm. Sci. *54*:160, 1965.

3. ℞

Ephedrine sulfate 3%
                                          30|

Mft Isotonic solution
    $0.9 \times 0.23 = 0.21$

The closeness of the answer raises the question of whether it is really necessary to add the other 60 mg. of sodium chloride. Several studies have shown that the eye does not perceive differences if the solution is equivalent to 0.5 to 2.0 per cent sodium

chloride.[104,113] Most authors have recommended the use of 0.7 to 1.5 per cent NaCl as the practical concentration range. Therefore, it would be reasonable to omit the addition of any further sodium chloride to this prescription or any other which falls in the above range.

4. ℞

Sodium sulfacetamide . . . .   30 |
Sodium bisulfite | 1
Water q.s. ad 100

Let us assume that the E value for sodium sulfacetamide is not given in the Table and it will therefore be necessary to estimate it as follows:

$$E = \frac{32 \times 1.82}{254} = 0.23$$

$$30 \times 0.23 = 6.9$$

Without further calculation, this prescription is obviously hypertonic. Since there is no source of negative sodium chloride, it will be necessary to compound this prescription as written with no additional salts.

Most ophthalmic solutions are buffered as well as adjusted for tonicity, and the adjustment of buffered collyria will be discussed in the next section.

Hydrogen Ion Concentration. The normal pH of lacrimal fluid was the subject of debate for many years but is now known to be approximately the same as that of blood, 7.4.[52] Thus, it might seem reasonable to buffer all ophthalmic preparations to this value. However, other factors must be considered.[51] For example, the solubility and the stability of most ophthalmic drugs are strongly dependent on pH. The solubility of weak acids (e.g., atropine sulfate, pilocarpine nitrate) will decrease as the pH increases, and the solubility of weak bases (e.g., sodium fluorescein, sodium sulfadiazine) will decrease as the pH decreases. Many ophthalmic drugs are amides and esters which are liable to hydrolytic degradation. The use of pressure cookers for sterilization greatly magnifies the stability problem. If the "rule of thumb" that the reaction rate doubles for each 10 degree rise in temperature is used, the rate at 121°C. will be approximately 2^{10} times as rapid (as at room temperature)! Fifteen minutes at 121°C. will therefore be equivalent to approximately 10 days at room temperature. (The heating and the cooling times will also increase the degradation.) As mentioned earlier (cf. section on stability) such drugs are more stable in slightly acidic solution. Solutions with a pH greater than 5.0 should probably be sterilized by filtration.

The effect of pH on therapeutic activity in the eye is debatable. Most authors believe that penetration of biologic membranes such as the cornea is accomplished by the uncharged species of a drug.[114] Therefore, it would be expected that weak acids are more effective at lower pH values and weak bases at higher pH values.

This particular argument becomes academic if the buffer capacity of lacrimal fluid is great enough to bring the pH of instilled solutions back to pH 7.4 immediately. If this were true, the pH of the applied solution would have no effect on pharmacologic activity. Some workers have obtained results which indicate that this is true.[36,103] One publication disputes these results. Tolazoline hydrochloride was found to be ineffective at a pH of 5.30, although quite effective at pH values greater than 6.05. The author explains his results with an experiment with artificial tears. He shows that artificial lacrimal fluid required ½ to 1 hour to neutralize added drug. The student should note that this is a rate phenomenon—the buffer capacity is adequate, but the return of pH to normal is slow.[32]

Many authors consider a nonbuffered solution of pH 5.00 (e.g., 2% boric acid) to be well tolerated.[74] However, others claim that any pH less than 6.2 is distinctly irritating and leads to tearing.[32,120]

These remarks should alert the student to the controversy surrounding the concept of buffered ophthalmic solutions. Although many different buffer systems have been suggested, the two which have been widely accepted are: 2 per cent boric acid. pH $\cong$ 5 (it is, of course, not actually a buffer but it is usually so named) and the Hind-Goyan buffer pH 6.8.[51]

Sodium acid phosphate (anhydrous)	4.00 Gm.
Disodium phosphate (anhydrous)	4.73 Gm.
Sodium chloride	4.30 Gm.
Distilled water, q.s.ad	1,000 ml.

Each solution should contain a preservative and, where necessary (e.g., epinephrine, eserine), an antioxidant such as 0.2 per cent sodium bisulfite. The E values for buffer solutions must always be considered when they are used in compounding. The E values for the two buffer solutions above are:

$$E \text{ (Boric acid)} = 0.47 \qquad 2 \times .47 = 0.94 \text{ Gm.}/100 \text{ ml.}$$

$$
\begin{aligned}
E \text{ (NaH}_2\text{PO}_4\text{)} &= 0.46 & 4 \times .46 &= 1.84 \\
E \text{ (Na}_2\text{HPO}_4\text{)} &= 0.53 & 4.73 \times .53 &= 2.50 \\
E \text{ (NaCl)} &= 1.0 & &\underline{4.30} \\
& & &\overline{8.64} \text{ Gm.}/1{,}000 \text{ ml.}
\end{aligned}
$$

Both of these formulations therefore are in the isotonic range without added medicinal agent. This is quite useful, since the large majority of drugs are used in such low concentration that their addition will still leave the final product within the isotonic range with further adjustment unnecessary. Excellent general directions for the preparation of ophthalmic prescriptions may be found in *N.F. XII.*[87]

Viscosity Adjustment. The use of 0.33 per cent (4,000 c.p.s.) methylcellulose with 1:50,000 benzalkonium chloride has been recommended as a tear substitute.[80] Methylcellulose in 1 per cent concentration may be used to increase the viscosity of an ophthalmic solution in order to delay the rapid washing away of the solution.[10,85]

PARENTERAL PRODUCTS

Until recently, the average pharmacist only occasionally encountered parenteral products (or injectables). Unless he practiced in a hospital pharmacy or in a pharmacy which specialized in medical supplies, exposure to this particular dosage form was limited to an occasional prescription, or a request for insulin. This is changing, however, and will continue to change in the future. Partially in response to external pressures (government) and partially in response to evolving concepts in pharmaceutical practice, the pharmacist of today is directing an ever increasing amount of attention to total health care systems. As a result, hospital pharmacy practice is expanding, and more and more pharmacists are taking up practice in community medical center pharmacies. Some are experimenting in group-clinic practice. Others, while practicing in traditional community pharmacies, are serving as consultants to nursing homes and extended care facilities. With each of these evolving modes of practice has come the need for an increased knowledge of parenteral products.

We are told that the term "parenteral" comes from a fusion of two Greek words (para, enteron) and means "besides the intestine." While this description excludes only the oral and rectal route, in actual use this term has come to mean any product that is injected directly into a fluid system of the body (blood, lymph, intra- or extracellular liquids). Because a parenteral product is injected directly in body fluids and bypasses many of the body's protective mechanisms, it must meet rigid sterility and pyrogen specifications. This requires specialized equipment and manufacturing facilities. Furthermore, the product should be designed to meet certain pH and isotonicity requirements so as to minimize discomfort upon administration. The problems inherent in parenteral drug manufacturing are such that very few pharmacists attempt to manufacture these products. They have left this task to the large pharmaceutical manufacturers. Instead, the pharmacist has turned his attention to the problems that can arise after such a product comes into his hands. Much of this knowledge is general in nature and much of it can be learned only by experience.

There is little doubt that, from the patient's point of view, a parenteral product is one of the least desirable dosage forms. This is based upon a general fear of pain from a needle, the anticipation of which is far worse than the actual event. For this and other reasons a parenteral product is usually reserved for those situations in which the other dosage routes (oral, topical, etc.) are either medically undesirable, or ineffective—for example, when:

1. The required drug is poorly absorbed from the gastrointestinal tract, or rapidly degraded in the stomach or intestine and is therefore available *only* in injectable form (e.g., Insulin, Adrenocorticotropic Hormone ACTH).

2. The oral or rectal route is contraindicated because of damage or surgery to the esophagus or gastrointestinal tract.

3. The patient is unconscious, nauseated, or uncooperative.

4. Immediate blood levels of the drug are required (emergency situations).

5. The drug cannot be expected to reach the required site (brain, spinal column, etc.) *via* other dosage routes.

There are various specific sites for the injection of parenteral products. Some of the more common are:

Intravenous (I.V.)—injected directly into a vein (An I.V. product is usually a solution, rarely a fine emulsion, but *never* a suspension of solids)

Intramuscular (I.M.) — injected into a skeletal muscle (usually in the deltoid or gluteal regions)

Subcutaneous (S.C.)—injected into the tissue directly below the skin

Intradermal (I.D.) — injected into the skin layer

Intraspinal—injected into the spinal column

Physical Classifications. Injectables are available in many physical forms. The particular form is dictated, to some extent, by the stability of the drug, its solubility and dissolution characteristics, the desired time for onset of action, and the site of administration. In general, parenteral products will fall into one of the five following physical classifications:

1. Solutions—in water or oil (e.g., sodium bicarbonate soln.; estrone in oil (Theelin in oil))

2. Dry soluble powders to which a solvent will be added prior to administration (e.g., aqueous penicillin G)

3. Dry insoluble powders to which a liquid will be added prior to administration (e.g., Triamcinolone Diacetate Suspension)

4. Suspensions, ready for injection (e.g., Cortisone Acetate)

5. Emulsions (e.g., Lipomul I.V.)

Containers. Parenteral products are available in many different containers, each designed for a specific purpose. An *ampul,* for example, is a single-dose slender glass container with a pinch-neck which is broken off at the time of use. Available in sizes ranging from 0.5 to 1,000 milliliters, an ampul for obvious reasons cannot be stored once it has been opened. Other single-dose containers are disposable pre-loaded syringes (ready to be used) and large round bottles with rubberlike stoppers containing 500 to 1,000 milliliters of intravenous liquids (dextrose, etc.).

The multidose vial, which as the name implies, is designed for multiple withdrawal of the contents, is another kind of container with a rubberlike stopper for parenteral products. At the time of use, a syringe with a needle is used to inject a volume of air equal to the volume of liquid to be withdrawn. This prevents the formation of a vacuum which could eventually aspirate contaminating material from outside of the vial. Because of stability problems and possible contamination from multiple use, the *U.S.P.* limits the size of multidose vial to 30 milliliters and further requires that the solution contain an antimicrobial preservative (a specification not demanded of single-use products).

A problem associated with rubberlike stoppers is "coring." [17] Such a "core" can be either a round plug produced by the passage of the hollow syringe needle through the stopper, or a jagged piece of stopper material which breaks off when a needle passes by or across a hole made by a previous withdrawal. This material collects in the vial, and may eventually be drawn up into a syringe and injected into a patient. To avert the possibility of inducing a foreign body reaction, or causing blockage of blood capillaries, the user of a multidose vial should carefuly inspect the vial, if it has been used previously, and should always take care to insert the needle in a section of the stopper through which a needle has not previously passed.

Storage. As a regular procedure, a pharmacist should establish the habit of scanning the labels of parenteral products for storage information. Some products, because of relative instabilities, must be stored in a refrigerator, whereas others may be safely stored at room temperature. Every product should be carefully inspected for an expiration date (the date on which the concentration of the active ingredient may be expected to fall below some predetermined percentage of the labeled concentration).

Incompatibilities of Parenteral Admix-

tures. A common practice, especially associated with institutional settings, is the mixing of two or more parenteral products together for simultaneous injection. This may be done in a syringe, or in a single or multidose container. One survey,[16] performed in an institution, reveals the extent of the mixing of parenteral products. Of the 1,565 injections received by 264 patients, 60 per cent were mixtures containing one additive, 20 per cent contained two additives, and 6 per cent contained three additives. In another study[77] it was found that 30 per cent of the preparations injected contained one additive ingredient, 24 per cent contained two additives, 14 per cent contained three additives, 18 per cent contained four additives, and 14 per cent contained five or more additives. The reasons for mixing parenteral products are obvious, since it is convenient to add all the ingredients into one container so that only one, rather than a multiple number of skin punctures, need be made. Such a practice, however, raises myriad potential problems and has drawn a great amount of attention in the last several years. The first of these problems is *therapeutic incompatibility,* a term which may be defined as undesirable biologic interactions between two or more ingredients leading to potentiation or diminution of the effectiveness of one or more of the ingredients, or the production of toxic reaction (see Chap. 11). A second problem is that one parenteral product may be physically or chemically incompatible with another. As the number of additives increases, the probability of an incompatibility increases as well.

The differences between physical and chemical incompatibilities are often difficult to define; therefore we shall outline the possible effects of mixing one or more parenterals together, rather than attempt to define one as a physical, another as a chemical incompatibility. When parenterals are mixed together, one or more of the following results are possible:

I. The mixture is compatible.
II. There is a change in pH.
   A. One or more drugs are forced out of solution (visible).
   B. One or more drugs are rapidly degraded.
   1. A precipitate forms (visible).
   2. There is a color change (visible).
   3. There is no observable change (invisible).
III. One or more drugs react with or inactivate another (complexation, etc.).
   A. A precipitate forms (visible).
   B. There is a color change (visible).
   C. There is no observable change (invisible).

Under usual circumstances a mixed product exhibiting a color change or a precipitate is evidence of an incompatibility, and the mixture should not be administered. At best, the components of the mixture should be administered separately, and preferably at different injection sites.

The nonvisible incompatibilities (suggested above) are of great concern. They are not necessarily predictable and in many cases have not been discovered until it was observed that therapeutic activity was either absent or decreased. As specific examples, it has been reported[25] that tetracycline, oxytetracycline and chlortetracycline lose their biologic activity when mixed with vitamin B complex injectables. Elsewhere it has been reported[60] that (because of pH change) penicillin G potassium in a 5 per cent dextrose solution is inactivated by the addition of tetracycline hydrochloride injection. In neither case was the interaction visible or apparent. The list of incompatible parenteral products is quite large, and grows daily. To help solve this problem several manufacturers have published compatibility charts[3,5] and others have been published by pharmacists.[2,4,12,28,44,63,81,93,106] The majority of these charts suffer from many shortcomings: few concern themselves with the addition of more than one additive; most cite only visible incompatibilities and ignore nonvisible and therapeutic incompatibilities. Those charts published by a manufacturer usually involve only those products of that manufacturer thus ignoring possible incompatibilities with products from other manufacturers. Also, manufacturers change the formulation of their parenterals from time to time, thus making obsolete much of the charted information.

Whenever a pharmacist is called upon to

prepare a mixture of two or more parenterals (admixtures) he should fully keep in mind the physico-chemical principles cited previously in this chapter. Secondly, he should keep himself fully informed by regularly scanning those journals which publish incompatibility information.

As a final point, a safe but occasionally difficult rule to follow clinically is, "When in doubt, don't mix."

Technics of Mixing Parenteral Products. When several parenteral products are mixed together, at least one of the preparations is removed from its sterile container and introduced into another. Although the transferring device is sterile (frequently a syringe), there is a short period during which the ingredients or the transferring device is exposed to the atmosphere. Since a cubic foot of air contains anywhere between 35,900 to 1,325,000 suspended particles[7] some of which are bacterial, special precautions must be taken to prevent contamination. Therefore a pharmacist who prepares parenteral mixtures should attempt to perform these functions in an environment that minimizes the possibility of bacterial contamination. The simplest approach is the use of a hood, which is little more than a draft-free box, that has been previously scrubbed with a disinfectant and/or is bathed in ultraviolet light when not in use. Unfortunately, this device is open at one end, and the pharmacist's movements can create air currents which pull in contaminated air from the outside. Another approach is the use of a sealed chamber, manipulative access to which is through a pair of extra-long gloves. The use of a device such as this is cumbersome and time consuming. A more recent development is an open-ended hood with a positive pressure of bacteriologically filtered air. However, since the air tends to swirl around the inside of the hood, it is still possible for contaminated external air to be pulled inside. Most of the aforementioned shortcomings have been overcome by a device called a laminar air flow hood (Fig. 4-6). This is also a positive pressure device whose air supply is forced through a HEPA (high efficiency particulate air) filter and is 99.99 per cent bacteria free. As the air leaves the filter, special corrugated separators direct it into

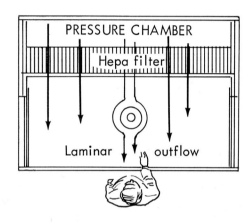

FIG. 4-6. (*Top*) Cross section of laminar flow through HEPA filter. (*Bottom*) Top view of laminar flow through HEPA filter. (Abbott Laboratories, North Chicago, Ill.)

parallel (laminar) streams. Air structured in this manner is free from eddy currents and swirls and presents a sterile, solid front to the external environment. This solid front acts as a continuous broom and sweeps away any bacteria introduced by the operator. For this reason, laminar air flow hoods do not require the use of an ultraviolet light when not in use, since merely turning the device on and allowing it to run for 20 minutes or so effectively removes suspended bacteria.

Since laminar air flow hoods are relatively inexpensive and certainly less bothersome than the maintenance of sterile rooms and hoods, it seems likely that their popularity will increase. At present these devices are manufactured by more than thirty firms, and the student is referred to a series of articles[6,28] that list these sources and review the present state of the art.

It is distressing to note that parenteral mixtures which have been prepared with scrupulous sterile technic are not uncommonly stored for minutes or hours on medication carts, in medication rooms, in hallways or on desk tops fully exposed to the unsterile environment of the air. Storage in this haphazard manner defeats the whole purpose of sterile technic, since the container (and especially the stopper) is easily contaminated with bacteria. Therefore the pharmacist's involvement must extend to the point of administration. Not only must he ascertain that storage conditions are such as to prevent eventual contamination of his product; he also must thoroughly understand the nursing technics used in its administration.

Pharmaceutical Solutions

The student will find it instructive to read the package inserts found in modern proprietaries. A few sample formulations are given in the following. The student should study them and attempt to understand the need for each of the nontherapeutic agents.

Aldomet* Injection

Methyldopa hydrochloride	250 mg.
Citric acid (anhydrous)	25.0 mg.
Sodium bisulfite	16.0 mg.
Disodium edetate	2.5 mg.
Monothioglycerol	10.0 mg.
Sodium hydroxide to adjust pH	
Methylparaben	0.15%
Propylparaben	0.02%
Water q.s. ad	5.0 ml.

Compazine* Injection

Prochlorperazine ethanedisulfonate	5 mg.
Sodium sulfite	1 mg.
Sodium bisulfite	1 mg.
Sodium phosphate	8 mg.
Sodium biphosphate	12 mg.
Water	q.s.ad 1 ml.

* Trade mark.

Digitalline Nativelle*

Chief Glycoside of *Digitalis purpurea*	0.2 mg./ml.
P.E.G.—300	28.6%
Glycerine	43.8%
Benzyl alcohol	4.0%
Ethanol	5.0%
Water for injection	18.6%
Amber Ampules	

Elavil* Injection

Amitriptyline HCl	10 mg.
Dextrose	44 mg.
Methylparaben	1.5 mg.
Propylparaben	0.2 mg.
Water for injection	q.s.ad 1 ml.

Epitrate* "Ophthalmic"

l-Epinephrine bitartrate	2 %
Chlorobutanol	0.5%
Methylaminoacetopyrocatechol HCl	
Sodium bisulfite	
Sodium chloride	
Dioctyl sodium sulfosuccinate	
Sodium EDTA	

Fluorouracil Injection

5-Fluorouracil	500 mg.
Sodium hydroxide to adjust pH to approximately 9.0	
Water q.s. ad	10 ml.

Hydrocortone* Phosphate Injection

Hydrocortisone-21-phosphate, disodium salt	50 mg.
Creatinine	8 mg.
Sodium citrate	10 mg.
Sodium bisulfite	3.2 mg.
Phenol	5 mg.
Sodium hydroxide to adjust pH	
Water	q.s.ad 1 ml.

Neo-Synephrine* Injection

Phenylephrine HCl	10 mg.
Sodium bisulfite	2 mg.
Citrate buffer	q.s.ad 1 ml.
Sodium chloride	

Phenergan* Injection

Promethazine hydrochloride	25 mg.
Sodium formaldehyde sulfoxylate	0.75 mg.
Disodium edetate	0.1 mg.
Sodium metabisulfite	0.25 mg.
Calcium chloride	0.04 mg.
Phenol	5 mg.
Sodium acetate buffer	q.s.ad 1 ml.

* Trade mark

Serpasil* Injection

Reserpine	2.5 mg.
Adipic acid	10 mg.
Dimethylacetamide	0.1 ml.
Sodium EDTA	0.1 mg.
Benzyl alcohol	.01 ml.
P.E.G. 300	.05 ml.
Ascorbic acid	0.5 mg.
Sodium sulfite	0.1 mg.
Water for injection	q.s.ad 1 ml.
(packaged in dark bottle)	

Sparine* Injection

Promazine HCl	.25 mg.
Sodium formaldehyde	
sulfoxylate	0.75 mg.
Sodium metabisulfite	0.25 mg.
Sodium EDTA	0.099 mg.
Calcium chloride	0.039
Sodium acetate buffer	q.s.ad 1 ml.

Solu-Cortef* Injection
(when mixed)

Hydrocortisone sodium	
succinate (equivalent to	
100 mg. hydrocortisone)	
Sodium biphosphate	0.8 mg.
Sodium phosphate	8.73 mg.
Chlorobutanol	10 mg.
Water q.s. ad	2.0 ml.

Tigan* Injection

Trimethobenzamide	
hydrochloride	100 mg.
Phenol	0.45%
Sodium citrate	0.5 mg.
Citric acid	0.2 mg.
Sodium hydroxide to adjust	
pH to approximately 5.0	
Water q.s. ad	1 ml.

Tussar* Syrup

d-Methorphan hydrobromide	60 mg.
Pheniramine maleate	45 mg.
Phenylpropanolamine HCl	30 mg.
Sodium citrate	780 mg.
Citric acid	120 mg.
Chloroform	90 mg.
Methylparaben	30 mg.
Vehicle q.s. ad	30 ml.

Tyzine* Nasal Solution

Tetrahydrozoline HCl	1 mg.
Benzalkonium chloride	0.02%
Disodium EDTA	0.1%
Certified color	q.s.
Sodium chloride and sodium	
citrate	
Adjust to optimum pH with	
HCl	q.s.ad 1 ml.

* Trade mark

Xylocaine* Injection 2%

Lidocaine hydrochloride	20 mg.
Sodium chloride	6 mg.
Methylparaben	1 mg.
Sodium hydroxide to adjust pH	
Water q.s. to	1 ml.

The student should be aware that texts can only distill the results of many years of research and study. In order to truly appreciate the problems involved and to understand more fully the subjects discussed, he will find reading some of the original references rewarding.

REFERENCES

1. American Perfumer and Cosmetics, 800 N. Court St., Pontiac, Ill.
2. Anon.: Incompatibilities of Parenteral Products. The University of Iowa, College of Pharmacy, Iowa City, Iowa, Jan. 1964.
3. Anon.: Compatibiiity Guide — Physical Compatibility of Intravenous Solutions with Various Antibiotics and Additives. Cutter Labs., Berkeley, Calif., May 1964.
4. Anon.: Pharmacy Department Intravenous Additive Incompatibilities. National Institutes of Health, Clinical Center, Pharmacy Department, Bethesda, Maryland, March 1967.
5. Anon.: Physical Compatibility of Parenteral Admixtures. Abbott Laboratories, N. Chicago, May 1967.
6. Anon.: Hospital Pharmacy, 3:3, 1968.
7. Baker, A. K.: Bull. Parenteral Drug Ass., 14(1):8, 1960.
8. Beal, H. M., et al.: J. Pharm. Sci., 56: 1310, 1967.
9. Beck, K. M.: Food Technology, 11:156, 1957.
10. Bergy, G. A.: J. Am. Prof. Pharm., 18: 340, 1952.
11. Block, S. S.: Industrial Preservatives. In: Reddish, G F.: Antiseptics, Disinfectants, Fungicides and Sterilization. ed. 2. p. 733. Philadelphia, Lea & Febiger, 1957.
12. Bogash, R. C.: Bull. Am. Soc. Hosp. Pharm., 12:445, 1955.
13. Brown, M. R. W.: Proc. Roy. Soc. Med., 60:354, 1967.
14. Brown, M. R. W., and Norton, D. A.: J. Soc. Cos. Chem., 16:369, 1965.
15. Carless, J. E., and Nixon, J. R.: J. Pharm. Pharmacol., 12:348, 1960.

* Trade mark

16. Carlin, H., and Perkins, A. J.: Am. J. Hosp. Pharm., 25:271, 1968.

17. Charlebois, P. A.: Can. Anaes. Soc. J., 13:585, 1966.

18. Coles, C. L. J., and Thomas, D. F. W.: J. Pharm. Pharmacol., 4:898, 1952.

19. Cook, M. K.: Drug Cosm. Ind., 81:750, 1957.

20. Cooper, J., and Lachman, L.: J. Am. Pharm. Ass., NS4:118, 1964.

21. Dale, J. K., Nook, M. A., and Barbiers, A. R.: J. Am. Pharm. Ass. [Pract.], 20:32, 1959.

22. Dale, J. K., and Rundman, S. J.: J. Am. Pharm. Ass., 18:421, 1957.

23. Davies, W. L., and Lamy, Peter P.: Hospital Pharmacy, 3:7, 1968.

24. Deluca, P. P., and Kostenbauder, H. B.: J. Am. Pharm. Ass. [Sci.], 40:430, 1960.

25. Dony-Crotteux, J.: J. Pharm. Belg., 12:179, 1957.

26. Drug and Cosmetic Industry, 101 West 31st St., New York, 10001.

27. Dunn, C. G.: Food Preservatives. In: Reddish, G. F.: Antiseptics, Disinfectants, Fungicides and Sterilization. ed. 2. p. 677. Philadelphia, Lea & Febiger, 1957.

28. Dunworth, R. D., and Kenna, F. R.: Am. J. Hosp. Pharm., 22:190, 1965.

29. Dyer, D. L.: J. Colloid Sci., 14:640, 1959.

30. Eickholt, T. H., and White, W. F.: Drug Standards, 28:154, 1960.

31. Engelhardt, R. J., Schell, F. M., and Lichtin, J. L.: J. Am. Pharm. Ass., NS8:198, 1968.

32. Etter, J. C.: Pharm. acta helv., 36:238, 1961.

33. Finholt, P., Jürgensen, G., and Kristiansen, H.: J. Pharm. Sci., 54:387, 1965.

34. Firmenich Inc., 250 West 18th St., New York 10011.

35. Florasynth Labs. Inc., 900 Van Nest Ave., New York 10001.

36. Floyd, G., Kronfeld, P. C., and McDonald, J. E.: J. Am. Pharm. Ass. [Sci.], 42:333, 1953.

37. Fritzsche Bros. Inc., Port Authority Bldg., 76 Ninth Ave., New York 10011.

38. Goettsch, F. J. B.: Ophthalmologica, 132:167, 1956.

39. Goldemberg, R. L., O'Leary, S., and Ziskin, N. A.: Proc. Sci. Sect. Toilet Goods Ass., 36:16, 1961.

40. Goldstein, S. W.: J. Am. Pharm. Ass. [Pract.],14:498, 1953.

41. Gorman, W. G., Hall, G. D.: J. Pharm. Sci., 53:1017, 1964.

42. Goyan, F. M., Enright, J. M., and Wells, J. M.: J. Am. Pharm. Ass. [Sci.], 33:74, 1944.

43. Goyan, J. E., Shaikh, Z. I., and Autian, J.: J. Pharm. Sci., 49:627, 1960.

44. Grant, H. R.: Hosp. Pharmacist, 15:67, 1962.

45. Hammarlund, E. R.: J. Am. Pharm. Ass., NS4:542, 1964.

46. Hammarlund, E. R., and Pederson-Bjergaard, K.: J. Am. Pharm. Ass. [Sci.], 50:24, 1961.

47. Higuchi, T.: Solubility. In: Lyman, R.: Pharmaceutical Compounding and Dispensing. p. 167. Philadelphia, J. B. Lippincott, 1949.

48. Higuchi, T., and Lachman, L.: J. Am. Pharm. Ass. [Sci.], 44:521, 1955.

49. Higuchi, W. I., Lau, P. K., Higuchi, T., and Shell, J. W.: J. Pharm. Sci., 52:150, 1963.

50. Hildebrand, J. H.: J. Phys. Chem., 72:1841, 1968.

51. Hind, H. W., and Goyan, F. M.: J. Am. Pharm. Ass. [Sci.], 36:33, 1947.

52. ————: J. Am. Pharm. Ass. [Sci.], 38:477, 1949.

53. Hind, H. W., and Szekely, I. J.: J. Am. Pharm. Ass. [Pract.], 14:644, 1953.

54. Hine, J., and Bayer, R. P.: J. Am. Chem. Soc., 84:1989, 1962.

55. Horner, L.: Autoxidation of various organic substances. In: Lundberg, W. O.: Autoxidation and Antioxidants. p. 205. New York, Interscience, 1961.

56. Hornstein, I., Teranishi, R.: Chem. and Eng. News, 45:93, 1967.

57. Hugill, P. R., Osheroff, B. J., and Skolaut, M. W.: Am. J. Hosp. Pharm., 17:525, 1960.

58. Hugo, W. B.: Scientific and Technical Symposia, 112th Annual Meeting of the American Pharmaceutical Association. p. C 111, 1965.

59. Iannarone, M., and Eisen, J.: N. J. J. Pharm. June, p. 24, 1961.

60. Im, S., and Latiolais, C. J.: Amer. J. Hosp. Pharm., 23:333, 1966.

60. Janovsky, H. L.: Drug Cosm. Ind., 86:335, 1960.

62. Kim, H. K., and Autian, J.: J. Am. Pharm. Ass [Sci.], 49:227, 1960.

63. Kirkland, W. D., et al.: Am. J. Hosp. Pharm., 18:694, 1961.

64. Konigsbacher, K. S.: Drug Cosm. Ind., 85:168, 1959.

65. Krezanoski, J. Z., Hind, H. W., and Szekely, I. V.: J. Am. Pharm. Ass., NS2:417, 1962.

66. Lachman, L., and Higuchi, T.: J. Am. Pharm. Ass. [Sci.], 46:32, 1957.

67. Lachman, L., Ravin, L. J., and Higuchi, T.: J. Am. Pharm. Ass. [Sci.], 45:290, 1956.

68. Lawrence, C. A.: J. Am. Pharm. Ass. [Sci.], 44:457, 1955.

69. Levy, G., and Reuning, R. H.: J. Pharm. Sci., 53:1471, 1964.

70. MacGregor, D. R., and Elliker, P. R.: Canad. J. Microbiol., 4:499, 1958.

71. McPherson, S. D., Jr., and Wood, R. M.: Am. J. Ophthal., 32:673, 1949.

72. Magnus, Mabee, Reynard, 16 Besbrosses St., New York 10013.

73. Marcus, E., Kim, H. K., and Autian, J.: J. Am. Pharm. Ass. [Sci.], 49, 457, 1959.

74. Martin, F. M., Jr., and Mims, J. L.: Arch. Ophthal. (Par.), 44:561, 1950.

75. Meer, T.: SKF Selected Pharmaceutical Research Reference, Manuscript No. 4 (1957), SKF Laboratories, Philadelphia, Pa.

76. Mellen, M., and Seltzer, L. A.: J. Am. Pharm. Ass. [Sci.], 25:759, 1936.

77. Meyers, E. L. A.: Bull. Parenteral Drug Ass., 20:1, 1966.

78. Miller, O. H.: J. Am. Pharm. Ass. [Pract.],13:657, 1952.

79. Milosovich, G.: J. Pharm. Sci., 53:484, 1964.

80. Mims, J. L.: Arch. Ophthal. (Par.), 46:664, 1951.

81. Misgen, R.: Am. J. Hosp. Pharm., 22: 92, 1965.

82. Mitchell, A. G.: J. Pharm. Pharmacol., 14:175, 1962.

83. Mitchell, A. G., and Broadhead, J. F., J. Pharm. Sci., 56:1261, 1967.

84. Moore, W. E.: J. Am. Pharm. Ass. [Sci.], 47:855, 1958.

85. Mueller, W. H., and Deardorff, D. L.: J. Am. Pharm. Ass. [Sci.], 45:334, 1956.

86. Mullins, J. D., and Macek, T. J.: J. Am. Pharm. Ass. [Sci.], 49:245, 1960.

87. National Formulary: ed. 12. p. 481. 1965.

88. Neidig, C. P., and Burrell, H.: Drug Cosm. Ind., 54:408, 1944.

89. Orbis Products Corporation, 601 West 26th St., New York 10001.

90. Parrott, E. L., Wurster, D. E., and Busse, L. W.: J. Am. Pharm. Ass. [Pract.], 19: 645, 1953.

91. Paruta, A. N., Sciarrone, B. J., and Lordi, N. G.: J. Pharm. Sci., 53:1349, 1964.

92. Patel, N. K., and Kostenbauder, H. B.: J. Am. Pharm. Ass. [Sci.], 47:289, 1958.

93. Patel, J. A., and Phillips, G. L.: Am. J. Hosp. Pharm., 23:409, 1966.

94. Pelisser, N. A., and Burgee, S. L.: Hospital Pharmacy, 3:15, 1968.

95. Pharmaceutical Flavoring Guide. Fritzsche Bros., N. Y., N. Y.

96. Pisano, F. D., and Kostenbauder, H. B.: J. Am. Pharm. Ass. [Sci.], 48:310, 1959.

97. Pryor, J. G., Apt, L., and Leopold, I. H.: Arch. Ophthal. (Chicago) 67:612, 1962.

98. Putney, B.: J. Am. Pharm. Ass., NS6: 643, 1966.

99. Raval, N. N., and Parrott, E. L.: J. Pharm. Sci., 56:274, 1967.

100. Riegelman, S.: J. Am. Pharm. Ass. [Sci.], 49:339, 1960.

101. Riegelman, S., et al.: J. Am. Pharm. Ass. [Sci.], 45:93, 1956.

102. Riegelman, S., and Fischer, E. Z.: J. Pharm. Sci., 51:210, 1962.

103. Riegelman, S., and Vaughan, D. G., Jr.: J. Am. Pharm. Ass. [Pract.], 19:474, 1958.

104. Riegelman, S., Vaughan, D. G., Jr., and Okumoto, M.: J. Am. Pharm. Ass. [Pract.], 16:742, 1955.

105. ———: J. Am. Pharm. Ass. [Pract.], 45:94, 1956

106. Riffkin, C.: Am. J. Hosp. Pharm., 20: 19, 1963.

107. Rippie, E. G., Lamb, D. J., and Romig, P. W.: J. Pharm. Sci., 53:1346, 1964.

108. Sanders, H. J.: Chem. and Eng. News, 44:108, 1966.

109. Schorr, W. P., and Mohajerin, A. H.: Arch. Dermatol., 93:721, 1966.

110. Schwarz, T. W., Shvemar, N. G., and Renaldi, R. G.: J. Am. Pharm. Ass. [Pract.], 19:40, 1958.

111. Scott, M. F., Goudie, A. J., and Huetteman, A. J.: J. Am. Pharm. Ass. [Sci.], 49:467, 1960.

112. Sheth, P. B., and Parrott, E. L.: J. Pharm. Sci., 56:983, 1967.

113. Soehring, K., Klingmuller, O., and Neuwald, F.: Arzneimittel-Forsch., 9:349, 1959.

114. Swan, K. C., and White, N. G.: Am. J. Ophthal., 25:1043, 1942.

115. Swarbrick, J.: J. Pharm. Sci., 54:1229, 1965.

116. Swintosky, J. V., et al.: J. Am. Pharm. Ass. [Sci.], 45:37, 1956.

117. Talmage, J. M., Chafetz, L., and Elefant, M.: J. Pharm. Sci., 57:1073, 1968.
118. Technical Bulletin No. 355, Abbott Laboratories, Chemical Marketing Division, North Chicago, Ill.
119. Theodore, F. H., and Feinstein, R. R.: J.A.M.A., 152:1631, 1953.
120. Tozer, G. A.: J. Am. Prof. Pharm., 25: 30, 1959.
121. United States Pharmacopeia. ed. 17. p. 792, 1965.
122. Uri, N.: Mechanism of Antioxidation. In: Lundberg, W. O.: Autoxidation and Antioxidants. p. 1660, New York, Interscience, 1961.
123. Ward, D. R., Lathrop, L. B., and Lynch, M. J.: Drug Cosm. Ind., 98:48, 1966.
124. Wesley, F.: J. Am. Pharm. Ass., NS3: 208, 1963.
125. ———: Drug Cosm. Ind., 98:37, 1966.
126. West, G. B., and Whittet, T. D.: J. Pharm. Pharmacol. Trans., 113 T, 1960.
127. Wilson, M. G., Nelson, R. C., and Boak, R. A.: J.A.M.A., 175:1146, 1961.

GENERAL REFERENCES

Solubility

128. Hildebrand, J. H., and Scott, R. L.: Regular Solutions. Englewood Cliffs, N. J., Prentice-Hall, Inc., 1962.

Stability

129. Schou, S. A.: Am. J. Hosp. Pharm., 17: 5, 1960.
130. Schou, S. A.: Ibid., 17:153, 1960.
131. Parrott, E. L.: J. Am. Pharm. Ass. NS6: 73, 1966.

Flavoring

132. Crocker, E. C.: Flavor. New York, McGraw-Hill, 1945.

Physical Pharmacy

133. Martin, A. N.: Physical Pharmacy, ed. 2. Philadelphia, Lea & Febiger, 1970.

Physical Constants

134. The Merck Index, ed. 8. Rahway, N. J., Merck & Co., 1968.

Chapter 5

Liquid Dosage Forms Containing Insoluble Matter

Theodore R. Bates, Ph.D.*

A significant number of therapeutic agents because of their complex organic nature are relatively insoluble in aqueous media as well as in the limited number of nonaqueous, nontoxic liquid vehicles commonly available to the practicing pharmacist. The need to deliver these drugs to the patient in physicochemically stable, biologically available and pharmaceutically elegant form has given rise to the utilization of the two types of dosage forms to be discussed in this chapter—solid-in-liquid dispersions (suspensions) and liquid-in-liquid dispersions (emulsions). Both dosage forms have found widespread use for drugs which are intended for oral and parenteral administration and external application.

A pharmaceutical suspension may be defined as a coarse dispersion in which finely divided insoluble solid (drug) particles, usually greater than 0.1 micron in diameter, are dispersed in a liquid medium (aqueous or oleaginous). The solid particles are maintained in the dispersed state by the addition of a dispersing or suspending agent to the system. Lotions, magmas, mixtures and gels are pharmaceutical products which conform to this general definition, but differ essentially as to the particle size of the dispersed phase. This class of preparations may be considered to include both powders in the dry form to be placed in suspension at the time of dispensing and medicinal substances suspended in liquid vehicles with or without suspending and flavoring agents.

An emulsion or liquid-in-liquid dispersion is a preparation consisting of two immiscible liquids, usually water and oil, one of which is dispersed as small globules in the other. If oil is the dispersed phase and water the external phase the emuslion is of the oil-in-water (o/w) type. The reverse is true in the case of a water-in-oil (w/o) emulsion. Emulsions of the former type are usually employed for medicinal agents intended for oral administration, whereas both types are used for externally applied products. The dispersed phase globules of an emulsion range from about 0.1 to 10 microns and are sometimes as small as 0.01 micron or as large as 50 to 100 microns.

The problems encountered by the dispensing or manufacturing pharmacist in the formulation of both suspensions and emulsions are intimately associated with the inherent thermodynamic instability of these types of dosage forms. The effect of gravity in causing the sedimentation of the dispersed solid phase of suspensions and the separation of phases in emulsions must be overcome if the patient is to be provided with a uniform dose of the medicament contained therein.

Since compounding equipment and stabilizing agents are similar or identical for both classes of preparations, both are discussed in this chapter rather than following the traditional method of considering suspensions and emulsions separately.

* Associate Professor of Pharmacy, School of Pharmacy, University of Connecticut.

PROPERTIES OF LIQUID DOSAGE FORMS CONTAINING INSOLUBLE MATTER

Until recently, the major concern regarding an acceptable suspension or emulsion was its ability to remain dispersed long enough to provide a uniform dose when taken orally, injected or applied to the skin. External suspensions necessarily required as small a particle size as possible to eliminate grittiness when applied to the skin surface.

Particles settling under the force of gravity are considered to follow Stoke's equation:

$$V = \frac{d^2(p - p_0)g}{18\eta_0}$$

where V is the settling rate, d is the mean diameter of the particles, p is the density of the particles, p_0 is the density of the dispersion medium, g is the acceleration due to gravity and η_0 is the viscosity of the dispersion medium. The applicability of Stoke's equation is limited to the following conditions: (1) The dispersion medium is of infinitely large volume compared with the dispersed phase; (2) the dispersed phase consists of smooth and rigid true spheres; (3) the particles are independent and not flocculated; (4) the particle velocity is small; (5) there is no slip between particle and liquid; (6) the particle is large enough to be unaffected by the kinetic motion of the suspending liquid and (7) electrical effects between particles and the liquid are negligible.

It is immediately apparent that pharmaceutical suspensions and emulsions, because of the high concentration of the dispersed phase, do not meet the above criteria. Higuchi[15] has modified the approach to creaming and settling by treating the suspension and the emulsion as systems of fluid flow through a packed bed.

Heterogeneous dispersions are stabilized by treatment of two factors of Stoke's equation—particle diameter (d) and the viscosity of the dispersion medium (η_0). An attempt is made to retard settling or creaming by reduction of the particle size of the dispersed phase to the smallest diameter feasible within limits of the equipment available and by increasing the viscosity of the dispersion medium by the addition of various hydrocolloids and other agents. The problem is compounded by the fact that very small particles possess a great deal of energy. In a system of high concentration of dispersed phase this results in considerable particle-particle interaction in an attempt to reduce the surface free energy, lowering the total surface by particle agglomeration.

Martin[23] considers another approach to the stabilization of suspensions, in addition to the use of protective colloids, i.e., the application of surfactants to reduce the interfacial tension between the particle and the liquid. He also discusses the use of dispersing or deflocculating agents. Examples of the latter are the Darvans (R. T. Vanderbilt Co.), Daxads (Dewey and Almay) and the Marasperses (Marathon Corp.). The Daxads and the Darvans are polymerized organic salts of the alkyl aryl type represented by the following formula:

$$Na^+ \; {}^-O_3S \cdot CH_2 \cdot Aryl \cdot SO_3{}^- \; Na^+$$

The Marasperses are calcium and sodium lignosulfonates. Deflocculating agents are not classified as true surfactants and do not greatly lower surface tension. They seem to be absorbed on the surface of the particle through polar forces, greatly increasing the negative charge on the particle and resulting in particle-particle repulsion.

CAKING VS. FLOCCULATION

If particles immersed in a liquid are not in true solution, usually the thermodynamic considerations favor aggregation. Lowering the interfacial tension will tend to significantly reduce, but not completely eliminate, the associated free energy change. It is, however, possible to reduce the rate of aggregation by surrounding the particles with an electrically charged or uncharged barrier. Since most solid-in-liquid dispersions do not remain evenly dispersed for long periods of time, consideration must be given to the eventual result of the settling of particles in a suspension. The suspension must be prepared in such a manner that the solids are redistributed with ease by shaking so that the patient is able to obtain a uniform dose of the medicament.

When two or more particles in a suspended state make contact the end result is either *caking* or *flocculation*. Haines and

Martin[11,12,13] and Hiestand[14] classify particle-particle interactions in two ways: physical and/or chemical reactions forming strong bonds between particles resulting in *caking* and weakly bonded reactions of the van der Waals type leading to *flocculation*. Studies conducted by Haines and Martin[11,12,13] of the caking in pharmaceutical suspensions indicated that a suspension in a state of fine deflocculated particles leads to caking. In some cases, commonly used suspending agents and electrolytes exaggerate caking.

Caked suspensions, because of the close-packed structure of the settled particles, usually possess low sedimentation volumes (i.e., the ratio of the ultimate settled height or volume of solids after sedimentation to the total height or volume of the original suspension before settling). These types of suspensions are quite difficult to resuspend. In flocculated suspensions, the loosely packed, porous structure of the settled particles results in a large sedimentation volume. The relatively weak particle-particle interaction in a flocculated system allows ease of redispersion of the settled particles. Overbeek,[27] considering the influence of particle size on the effectiveness of shaking in redispersing a coarse suspension, states:

Qualitatively this easy repeptization can be explained in the following way: By agitation a shearing motion of the liquid is excited. This causes a force trying to tear two neighboring particles apart, which force is proportional to the radius of the particles (Stokes' Law) and to the distance between their centres (difference in the velocity of the liquid). So the separating force is proportional to the square of the radius of the particles. On the other hand, the attractive force is, at best, proportional to the first power of the radius of the particles (London force for spherical particles), and if the particles are not very regularly formed, the attractive force will soon be independent of the overall dimensions. . . . It may be remarked here that although a flocculated suspension is easily repeptized it is very difficult to redisperse the compact sediment of a stable suspension . . . the sediment is so compact that the particles can only be attacked by hydrodynamic motions layer by layer which evidently is a very slow process.

The compact sediment mentioned by Overbeek refers to that which is formed when the particles of a colloidally stable, but pharmaceutically unstable, deflocculated suspension settle.

The problem confronting the dispensing or manufacturing pharmacist is to control the flocculation in a manner that will provide the desired characteristics in the vehicle when using particle sizes chosen on therapeutic criteria. Haines and Martin[11,12,13] suggest that controlled flocculation, rather than deflocculation, will prevent caking in some pharmaceuticals. The study recommended the use of a nontoxic flocculating agent, together with a viscosity-increasing agent, to stabilize and flocculate suspensions. Hiestand[14] considers various methods of providing a condition of controlled flocculation.

A classic example of clay formation is shown by a mixture of hydrated magnesium oxide and sodium bicarbonate in an aqueous suspension. Magnesium carbonate crystals slowly form and fuse to a compact mass, which will not resuspend. Replacing the magnesium oxide by magnesium carbonate in the original compounding prevents this formation.

PARTICLE SIZE IN RELATION TO PHARMACOLOGIC ACTION

Drugs must be in solution before they can be absorbed across the gastrointestinal mucosa. In the case of dosage forms that contain water insoluble drugs the rate and/or extent of gastrointestinal absorption or absorption from another site in the body is usually dissolution-rate limited. According to the Noyes-Whitney relationship, which governs the rate of dissolution of pharmaceuticals, if the surface area of the dissolving drug exposed to the fluids of the gastrointestinal tract is increased by means of particle size reduction then the rate of solution is generally increased and hence the rate and/or extent of absorption (see Chapter 2).

Numerous investigations have substantiated the observations made by Reinhold et al.[29], in a study of the effect of particle size on the blood levels of sulfadiazine following the oral administration of suspension dosage forms to human subjects. The maximum blood levels of sulfadiazine following the administration of a suspension containing microcrystalline drug particles (1 to 3 micron particle size) were approximately 40 per cent higher and occurred two hours earlier than with the suspension containing coarser sulfadiazine particles (U.S.P.). Not only was the rate of absorption increased by particle size reduction, but there was a 20 per cent increase in the extent of absorption. Greengard and Wooley[8] evaluated the effect of administering sulfur in a colloidal form and also in the form of a 100-mesh powder. It was reported that the colloidal form was absorbed at a rate three to four times faster than that of the powder form of the drug.

Several authors[7,18,19,21,34] have reported that better absorption of drugs from ointment bases consistently occurs on reduction in size of the particulate matter dispersed in the base.

Investigators, cognizant of the importance of fine particles, have devised improved methods for obtaining these materials. Essentially, the processes can be classified into two broad categories. The first involves methods based on a reduction in size of a preformed crystal, powder or agglomerate. The second entails a condensation or an agglomeration of smaller discrete units to form particles of specific size. The first method is used more often at present for producing particles of low micron size, but, because of many difficulties inherent to this process, condensation methods are being investigated.

The reduction processes can be subdivided in the following manner: (a) those procedures in which the solid to be treated is dispersed in a liquid medium and acted on in that medium, and (b) those methods in which the materials are processed in the dry form.

Most equipment for dry pulverization of substances to provide particles in the micron range operates on procedures that are quite similar. The material to be pulverized is exposed to streams of high-velocity air. The solids are carried into the violent turbulence by sonic or supersonic velocity streams. In this turbulent environment the particles collide with one another and with the walls of the chamber to yield low-micron particles.

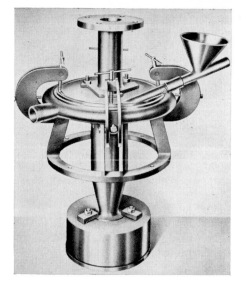

Fig 5-1. Sturtevant micronizer.

The Sturtevant Micronizer* is an example of equipment of this type (Fig. 5-1).

The wet or the suspended solid procedure is the method most often used in prescription practice to prepare suspensions. Since prescription laboratory equipment is available for this purpose, it will be discussed under solid-in-liquid dispersions (p. 205).

Another approach to the production of particles of low micron size has been through controlled crystallization. Crystallization is essentially a two-phase operation which is initiated by the formation of nuclei or grains and is concluded with subsequent growth of nuclei to macro size. By taking a supersaturated solution and causing rapid crystallization during high-speed stirring and a sudden drop in temperature small particles in the range of 5 microns and below can be produced. These fine crystals can be resuspended for oral, topical and parenteral administration. Investigation by Atkinson et al.[1] and Kraml et al.[17] on the effect of griseofulvin particle size on blood levels in man has resulted in a halving of the oral dose of griseofulvin by control of particle size below 5 microns.

Changes in the crystal form of drugs present in oral and parenteral suspensions may occur during their preparation, with

* Sturtevant Mill Company, Boston 22, Mass.

time or with changes in storage temperature. The increase in biological availability or absorption rate of the drug, produced by particle size reduction, can be significantly altered if crystal form changes occur in the finished suspension. The influence of complexation, crystal form and viscosity on the onset and intensity of the pharmacologic response produced by drugs contained in suspension dosage forms is discussed in Chapter 2.

SOLID-IN-LIQUID DISPERSIONS (SUSPENSIONS)

In the preparation of suspensions in prescription practice the pharmacist is somewhat limited in the modifications which he can make to produce a stable and elegant product, being confined by the manner in which the prescription is written. However, there are two methods which he can use for suspension stabilization: (a) reduction of the size of the dispersed particle either by breaking up aggregates or reducing individual particles to a finer state of subdivision, and (b) increasing the viscosity of the dispersion medium by the use of suspending agents.

Equipment for Particle Size Reduction. Small-scale equipment is now available to the pharmacist in increasing quantities. Apparatus for the production of the shearing force necessary for breaking up aggregates

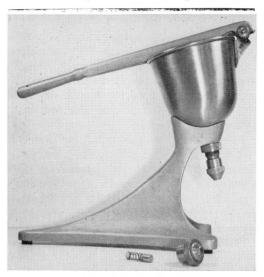

FIG. 5-2. Hand homogenizer.

Blendor Head

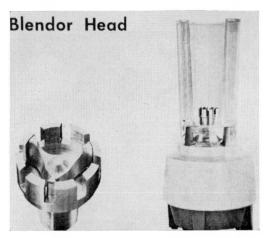

FIG. 5-3. Waring Blendor with polytron assembly.

of particles was once confined to the mortar and pestle. Most of the equipment available is equally applicable to the stabilization of emulsions by particle size reduction.

One useful compounding tool is the hand homogenizer (Fig. 5-2), consisting of a piston which forces the liquid through an orifice closed by a brass pin held in place by a spring. The pressure exerted by hand-pumping the piston causes the aperture to open and allow the liquid to pass. Considerable shearing action results in the deagglomeration of solids and the reduction of globule size in emulsions.

The general household use of the blender (Waring Blendor, Osterizer, etc.) for food preparation has resulted in a general reduction in the cost, and the prescription department has gained a mixing unit of high efficiency for the dispersing of solid aggregates and the reduction of globule size. In addition, the Waring Blendor has a homogenizing attachment ideal for prescription use. The Polytron Assembly* (Fig. 5-3) consists of a 3-bladed rotor running within an 8-slotted stator. Operating as a centrifugal pump, the rotor blades drive material at high speed against the shearing edges of the stator slots. The large number of shearing faces accelerates particle size reduction for fast dispersing and homogenizing. The unit possesses the advantage of high shear and low capacity, permitting its use in prescription practice.

* Will Scientific Inc., Rochester 9, N. Y.

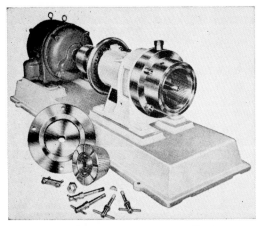

Fig. 5-4. Charlotte ND-1 Sanitary model colloid mill with rotor removed to show rotor-stator arrangement.

Certain of the colloid mills available can be used for stabilization of suspensions and emulsions in quantities small enough for prescription compounding. The Charlotte ND-1* mill with a capacity of 1 to 35 gallons per hour (Fig. 5-4) is an example of this type. The disadvantage of a colloid mill lies in its rather high cost for a prescription department.

The ball and pebble mill may be used for particle size reduction of solid-in-liquid dispersions. However, the time required for processing of the suspension may often eliminate its use in extemporaneous prescription compounding.

Suspensions Without Suspending Agents. Some solid-in-liquid dispersions may be written for and prepared without a suspending agent, depending on the density of the dispersed particles, their tendency to flocculate or cake and how well they are wetted by the dispersion medium. The following prescriptions are written examples of this type:

1. ℞

Liquor carbonis detergens	1.0 ml.
Zinc oxide	18.0 Gm.
Starch	18.0 Gm.
Glycerin	28.0 ml.
Lime water q.s. ad	90.0 ml.

M. Ft. lotion.

Sig.: Apply h.s.

* Chemicolloid Laboratories Inc., Garden City Park, N. Y.

2. ℞

Resorcinol	1.80
Sodium biborate	0.82
Starch	3.75
Calamine	3.75
Alcohol 70% ad	60.00

M.

Sig.: Apply to acne q.d.

3. ℞

Magnesium sulfate	℥ i
Light magnesium carbonate	℥ iss
Aq. menth. pip. q.s. ad	℥ iv

M. ft. susp.

Sig.: ℥ i h.s.

4. ℞

Magnesium trisilicate	2.4 Gm.
Light magnesium carbonate	2.4 Gm.
Sodium bicarbonate	2.4 Gm.
Belladonna tincture	3.0 ml.
Peppermint water ad	60.0 ml.

M. ft. mistura.

Sig.: ℥ ii ½ hr. p.c.

5. ℞

Zinc sulfate	40%
Potassa sulfurata	22%
Glycerin	3%
Stronger rose water	3%
Purified water q.s.	

M. ft. tal. lot. 90.0.

Sig.: Apply to face b.i.d.

This is a concentrated White Lotion (Lotio Alba). Dissolve the zinc sulfate in enough water to make 54 ml. and the sulfurated potash in enough water to make 30 ml. Filter each and slowly add the sulfurated potash solution to the zinc sulfate solution with constant trituration in a mortar. Add the glycerin and the water and mix well. Dispense in a wide-mouth bottle.

In most cases of this type, improvement may be made by the addition of a suspending agent to increase the viscosity of the preparation, and the physician may be contacted for such changes. Hand homogenization or treatment in a blender will further increase the elegance of the product.

Stabilization by Increasing the Viscosity of the Dispersion Medium. In addition to deagglomeration of solids and reduction of particle size to prevent settling of a suspension, certain viscosity-increasing agents are available for compounding use. Since this represents the easiest approach to suspension stabilization, it is the one most often used.

The requirements for an agent of this type are: (a) that it have no therapeutic action itself in the concentration used; (b) that it be relatively chemically inert over a wide pH range; (c) that it form a viscous dispersion in low concentration; (d) that it not change in viscosity over a period of storage, and (e) that it either be soluble in water or swell in it.

This group of suspending agents is classified as protective colloids, capable of forming a film around the dispersed particle and/or imparting high viscosity to the dispersion medium. In addition to retarding flocculation of the dispersed particles, protective colloids reduce the sedimentation rate by increasing the viscosity of the dispersion medium.

Rheologic Properties of Solid-in-Liquid Dispersions. With the exception of suspensions in which there is a very large percentage of dispersed phase compared with dispersion medium, the flow properties may be considered essentially those of the agent used to increase the viscosity of the system. Proper selection of a suspending agent or a mixture of suspending agents, according to the flow properties of their aqueous dispersions, will simplify the production of an acceptable suspension.

Viscosity-increasing agents, with the exception of newtonian materials such as glycerin, sucrose solutions, etc., are classified as non-newtonian substances, i.e., those materials which do not follow Newton's equation of flow. Figure 5-5 shows the flow characteristics of various materials.

A newtonian liquid (Fig. 5-5, A) flows when acted on by any force, the rate of shear being directly proportional to the shearing stress, as shown by the straight line extending to the origin. Non-newtonian substances exhibit flow that has been classified into several types; plastic flow, thixotropic flow, pseudoplastic flow and dilatant flow.

A liquid that exhibits plastic flow (Fig. 5-5, B) does not flow until the applied shearing stress exceeds a minimum value. This minimum shearing stress is designated as the yield value.

Plastic flow is frequently associated with an internal structure which is temporarily destroyed by stirring or shaking, but reforms on standing. A substance that exhibits this flow pattern is said to be thixotropic (Fig. 5-5, C) and the property is designated as

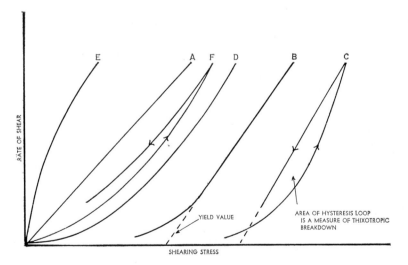

Fig. 5-5. Characteristic flow curves of various substances. (A) Newtonian substance. (B) Plastic substance. (C) Thixotropic substance. (D) Pseudoplastic substance. (E) Dilatant substance. (F) Pseudoplastic substance with thixotrophy. (Martin, A. N.: Physical Pharmacy, Philadelphia, Lea & Febiger)

thixotropy. The clays bentonite, hectorite and Veegum* are thixotropic substances. These substances form a gel structure on standing but become liquid on shaking; thus, they have many applications in suspension stabilization.

Most of the natural and the synthetic hydrocolloids exhibit pseudoplastic flow (Fig. 5-5,D); these include tragacanth, methylcellulose, sodium carboxymethylcellulose, the algins and Carbopol 934.† A substance which shows this property flows more readily as it is sheared and begins to flow at low shearing stress, but no part of the curve exhibits linearity. As a result, the viscosity of pseudoplastic materials can be expressed adequately only by a plot of the entire consistency curve.

Dilatant flow is exhibited by suspensions with high concentrations of solids, such as paints, inks, pastes, etc. These substances show increased resistance to flow with increased shearing stress (Fig. 5-5, E).

Figure 5-5 illustrates ideal flow patterns of non-newtonian substances. This would seldom be shown in actual substances. For example, some pseudoplastic materials do show thixotropy due to breakdown of structure with shear (Fig. 5-5, F).

Classification of Dispersion Stabilizers. Protective colloids are classified in several ways, one of which is their general division into similar chemical classifications, as follows:

1. Natural plant and animal hydrocolloids
   A. Plant derivatives
   B. Animal derivatives
2. Modified plant derivatives
3. Clays
4. Synthetic hydrocolloids

PLANT HYDROCOLLOIDS

Acacia is the dried gummy exudation of *Acacia senegal* and various other acacia trees throughout the world. It is often designated in commerce as "gum arabic." It is a mixture of the calcium, the magnesium and the potassium salts of arabic acid. As with other natural hydrocolloids, the viscosity of acacia solutions is affected by the age of the tree

* R. T. Vanderbilt Co., New York 17, N. Y.
† B. F. Goodrich Chemical Co., Cleveland 15, Ohio.

from which the gum is collected, amount of rainfall, storage conditions, pH, addition of salts, etc. Acacia solutions retain their viscosity through a pH range of 4 to 10. Because of the low viscosity of acacia dispersions, they are less used as suspension stabilizers than are some of the other plant hydrocolloids. However, acacia is used as an emulsifying agent and will be discussed further under emulsions. The following prescriptions illustrate the use of acacia as a suspension stabilizer.

6. ℞
   Heavy magnesium oxide ..... ℨ ii
   Magnesium sulfate .... ℨ vii
   Glycerin .... ℥ i
   Acacia mucilage .... ℥ i
   Peppermint water ad .... ℥ iii
   M.

   Sig.: ℥ ss t.i.d.

7. ℞
   Precipitated sulfur .... 4.8 Gm.
   Camphor .... 0.4 Gm.
   Acacia, fine powder .... 2.4 Gm.
   Lime water .... 60.0 ml.
   Aqua Rosae q.s. ad .... 120.0 ml.
   M. ft. lotion.

   Sig.: Apply to affected area q. 4 hr.

Tragacanth is the dried exudation of *Astragalus gummifer* and other species of *Astragalus*. The gum consists of 60 to 70 per cent of bassorin and 30 to 40 per cent of tragacanthin. In water, bassorin swells to form a gel and tragacanthin a colloidal dispersion. Tragacanth owes its effectiveness to its capacity to hydrate to form a viscous dispersion when placed in water. Although tragacanth hydrates very slowly, its rate may be increased by the shearing action of repeated hand homogenization of the dispersion. Tragacanth dispersions exhibit maximum viscosity at a pH of 5, showing a rapid drop in storage in a range below pH 4.5 and above pH 6.[31]

8. ℞
   Camphor spirit 6.0
   Alcohol 6.0
   Precipitated sulfur 3.6
   Tragacanth, fine powder 0.9
   Purified water ad 60.0
   M.

   Sig.: Apply to face night and morning.

Mix the precipitated sulfur with the tragacanth and gradually add about 40 ml. of water with constant trituration. Mix the camphor spirit and the alcohol and add this mixture to the sulfur suspension. Add enough purified water to make 60 ml.

The following prescription illustrates the use of tragacanth as a viscosity-increasing agent and a film former in a podiatric preparation:

9. ℞

Camphor	. . . .	gr. vii
Menthol	. . . .	gr. xiv
Tragacanth	. . . .	℥ ss
Glycerin	. . . .	℥ iss
Alcohol	. . . .	℥ iss
Amaranth solution 1%	. . . .	♏ xii
Purified water ad	. . . .	℥ iii

M. ft. lotion.

Sig.: Apply to feet q. 4 hr. ut. dict.

Dissolve the camphor and menthol in the alcohol. Triturate the glycerin with the tragacanth to a smooth paste. Add the alcohol solution, the amaranth solution and the purified water in divided portions to make the final volume.

Algins. The term designates the water-soluble derivatives of alginic acid, obtained by extraction from species of kelp. Alginic acid is a linear polymer of anhydro-β-D-mannuronic acid. The most important derivatives are the sodium, the potassium and the ammonium salts and the propylene glycol ester. Careful control of manufacturing conditions has made available a series of products ranging from low to high viscosity. Since the alginic acid salts are anionic in character, they show their greatest viscosity stability at pH 5 and above. When propylene glycol* alginate was made available, the range of usefulness was extended to pH ranges below pH 5.

Sodium alginate, the derivative most frequently used, is soluble in water and insoluble in alcohol. Low concentrations of alcohol produce higher initial viscosity values than does water alone, while higher concentrations (30 to 40%) precipitate sodium alginate from aqueous dispersions.[6]

Other natural plant hydrocolloids are used

* Kelcoloid S, Kelco Company, San Diego, Calif.

to a lesser extent than are acacia, tragacanth and the algins and are not encountered normally in prescription practice. Karaya, the dried exudation of *Sterculia urens,* is used to a great extent in the food industry and to a lesser extent in pharmaceuticals. Its main application is as a bulk laxative. Locust bean gum and guar gum—very similar in properties—are used to some extent in pharmaceuticals. Carrageenin, the dried extract of certain species of seaweed, is also used to a limited extent as a suspending agent and a stabilizer of emulsions.

10. ℞

Zinc oxide	3.6 Gm.
Starch	3.6 Gm.
Glycerin	3.0 ml.
Sodium alginate, med. viscosity	0.6 Gm.
Liq. calc. hydrox.	30.0 ml.
Aq. Ros. q.s. ad	60.0 ml.

M. ft.

Sig.: Apply as directed.

Triturate the sodium alginate, the starch and the zinc oxide together with the glycerin to form a paste. Gradually add the lime water and, finally, the rose water to volume.

Preservation of Natural Hydrocolloid Dispersions. The natural hydrocolloids are very subject to decomposition due to micro-organisms. Thus, when they are used as suspending or emulsifying agents, certain of the preservatives must be used. Among the acceptable ones are phenylmercuric nitrate 1:50,000, thimerosal 1:50,000, sodium benzoate 1.5 per cent and a combination of methylparaben 0.2 per cent and propylparaben 0.02 per cent.

ANIMAL HYDROCOLLOIDS

The hydrocolloids derived from animal sources, i.e., gelatin, egg yolk and casein, are used principally as primary emulsifiers or stabilizers in emulsification and will be discussed in this chapter under emulsions.

MODIFIED PLANT DERIVATIVES
(CELLULOSE DERIVATIVES)

The cellulose derivatives have become important as viscosity-increasing agents because they possess certain properties that the natural hydrocolloids do not share. The synthetic cellulose derivatives are produced under chemical control of raw materials and reaction product; thus, reproducible results in usage are more likely, in contrast to natural gums whose quality is subject to the vagaries of nature. Furthermore, they are free from insoluble substances and other matter (inorganic salts, etc.), resulting in a clearer dispersion.

Methylcellulose. By treatment of cellulose with alkyl halides such as methyl chloride a series of cellulose ethers may be obtained— the methylcelluloses.* Although they are available in viscosity types from 15 centipoises to 4,000 centipoises (the absolute viscosity of 2% aqueous dispersions at 20° C.), two viscosity types—1,500 centipoise and 4,000 centipoise—are most often used in pharmaceuticals. Methocel HG is the designation for a mixed methyl and hydroxypropyl ether of cellulose. Methylcellulose is soluble in cold water and insoluble in most of the common organic solvents. Methylcellulose differs from most hydrocolloids in that its dispersions gel on heating, while those of other hydrocolloids gel on cooling. As the temperature approaches 50° C., the gel point of the methylcelluloses, the outer layers of water molecules which are attached to the methylcellulose molecule break away. When enough of the attached water molecules are lost from the polymer chain, the solution is transformed into a gel. This phenomenon is reversible on cooling. Methocel HG has a gel point 10 to 15° C. higher than Methocel.

Dispersion of methylcellulose presents something of a problem, and, as a result, it is very often used in the form of a mucilage in prescription compounding. However, there are three ways in which it can be handled. One method is, first, to mix the methylcellulose thoroughly with one third of the required amount of water as hot water (80-90° C.), then, to add the remainder of the water as cold water. The second method is to mix the methylcellulose with a small amount of alcohol or glycerin before adding the cold water, to prevent lumping. If methylcellulose is to be used in a formulation containing other dry ingredients, it may be

* Methocel, Dow Chemical Company, Midland, Michigan.

blended with these ingredients prior to mixing with water.

11. ℞

Coal tar solution	3.0
Glycerin	1.5
Aqua Hamamelidis ad	30.0

M.

Sig.: Pat on abraded area and allow to dry.

When 10 ml. of a 2 per cent Methocel HG dispersion is thoroughly mixed with the coal tar solution and the other ingredients added gradually, a stable dispersion results.

12. ℞

Phenacetin	℥ iss
Glycerin	℥ i
Methylcellulose, 400 cps., 3% sol.	℥ vii
Aromatic elixir ad	℥ iii

M. ft. Mist.

Sig.: ℥ i q. 4 hr. for pain.

Triturate the phenacetin with the glycerin, add the methylcellulose dispersion and mix. Gradually add the aromatic elixir to volume.

Sodium carboxymethylcellulose is prepared by treating highly purified cellulose with alkali and subsequent reaction with sodium monochloroacetate. It is a fibrous or granular powder, light cream to white in color, and is readily soluble in hot or cold water. As opposed to methylcellulose, the viscosity of sodium carboxymethylcellulose (carboxymethylcellulose, C.M.C.) decreases with increasing temperature. Its dispersions fall within the pH range of 6.5 to 8.

Carboxymethylcellulose has a good tolerance to ethanol, with up to 40 per cent of ethanol permissible in low concentration dispersions. If it is mixed with mineral acids, the free acid of carboxymethylcellulose is formed; and precipitation results when a critical excess of the acid has been produced.

Carboxymethylcellulose is available in three viscosity grades: low viscosity—25 to 50 cps. in 2 per cent dispersion; medium viscosity—400 to 600 cps. in 2 per cent dispersion; and high viscosity—approximately 1,500 cps. in 1 per cent dispersion.

13. ℞

Barium sulfate	350.0 Gm.
CMC 70, Prem. Grade, low viscosity	20.0 Gm.
Dioctyl sodium sulfosuccinate sol. 1%	160.0 ml.
Flavor	5.0 ml.
Saccharin sodium	0.5 Gm.
Sorbitol solution 70%	150.0 ml.
Purified water to make	1,000.0 ml.

M.

14. ℞

Sulfadiazine	6.00 Gm.
Sulfamerazine	6.00 Gm.
Sodium lactate	36.00 ml.
Saccharin sodium	0.70 Gm.
Tr. lemon peel	3.60 ml.
CMC med. visc. sol. 1% q.s. ad	120.00 ml.

M.

Sig.: 5.0 q. 4 hr.

Powder the sulfadiazine and the sulfamerazine in a mortar, add the sodium lactate, the saccharin sodium and the CMC solution with constant trituration.

Microcrystalline cellulose,* which is prepared by severe acid hydrolysis of cellulose, can be dispersed in water to form high viscosity thixotropic dispersions that are stable over long periods. Early investigation[20] indicated that microcrystalline cellulose has excellent capability as a suspending agent.

CLAYS

The clay minerals of the montmorillonite structure have long been used as stabilizing agents for suspensions, due to their ability to form thixotropic dispersions of high viscosity. The suspending properties of these clays are due chiefly to their singular latticelike crystalline structure. The three clays most often used are bentonite, hectorite and Veegum.*

Bentonite (*U.S.P. XVII*) is described as a native, colloidal hydrated aluminum silicate, pale buff or cream colored, free from grit, with a slightly earthy taste. The best grades of bentonite usually swell in water to 15 times their dry volume, forming a thixotropic dispersion in low concentrations. As a suspending agent, a 2 to 5 per cent dispersion of bentonite is used. Bentonite is anionic in character and is markedly influenced by pH, showing maximum viscosity in the alkaline range. In addition, incompatibilities may be expected with cationic substances such as benzalkonium chloride, gentian violet, thiamine hydrochloride, etc.

Electrolytes change the character of bentonite dispersions in many respects, depending on the kind of electrolyte, the concentration of bentonite and the concentration of electrolyte relative to bentonite. Monovalent ions have the least effect, and trivalent the greatest effect. An excess of either cations or anions results in coalescence and flocculation of bentonite particles.

15. ℞

Menthol	0.23
Phenol	0.45
Liq. carb. det.	9.00
Talc	18.00
Glycerin	13.50
Bentonite	3.60
Purified water ad	90.00

M.

Sig.: Apply t.i.d.

Mix the powders with the glycerin in a mortar, dissolve the menthol and the phenol in the coal tar solution and add to the glycerin paste; gradually add the water with constant trituration to volume.

16. ℞

Zinc oxide	12 Gm.
Talc	12 Gm.
Glycerin	12 ml.
Alcohol	8 ml.
Magma bentonite	48 ml.
Purified water ad.	120 ml.

M.

Sig.: Leiner's Lotion.

Triturate zinc oxide, talc, glycerin and alcohol together; gradually add the bentonite magma with constant trituration and, finally, the purified water to volume.

Hectorite,† a member of the montmorillonite group of clays, is closely related to bentonite. As a result, its behavior is very

---

* Avicel, American Viscose Corporation, Marcus Hook, Pa.

* Veegum F and Veegum HV, R. T. Vanderbilt Co., New York 17, N. Y.

† Available as Macaloid, Inerto Company, 1489 Folsom St., San Francisco, Calif.

similar and it may be used in the same manner. Certain properties, especially its greater rate of hydration and its white color, give it some advantages over bentonite.

Veegum may be considered to be a highly purified form of bentonite. The purification procedure removes silica, grit, nonhydrating materials, etc. Veegum is supplied in the form of white flakes (Veegum HV), which swell on hydration as does bentonite. Its behavior as to pH changes, alcohol and electrolytes closely follows that of bentonite. Veegum dispersions are thixotropic as are those of bentonite. Veegum is generally used in concentrations of 1.5 to 2 per cent.

17. ℞
    Prepared chalk . . . .   3.6   Gm.
    Saccharin sodium . . . .   0.018 Gm.
    Veegum HV magma 3% . .   30.0   ml.
    Cinnamon water . . . .   24.0   ml.
    Purified water ad. . . . .   60.0   ml.

    M.

    Sig.: Chalk Mixture. 15 ml. a.c.

Mix the Veegum magma with the cinnamon water, and add enough of this mixture to the saccharin sodium and the prepared chalk in a mortar to form a smooth paste. Gradually incorporate the remainder of the diluted magma and, finally, enough purified water to make 60 ml.

All of the clay dispersions may be prepared in the same manner. However, it must be remembered that bentonite takes a longer period of time to hydrate and will take as much as 24 hours to reach its maximum viscosity. When the dry powder is used, the clay is triturated with the insoluble substances in a mortar and the vehicle is added a little at a time until the final volume is reached. When a magma of the clay is used, it is usually in the concentration of 2 to 5 per cent. Bentonite magma is prepared by sprinkling the powder on hot purified water and allowing to stand for 24 hours with occasional stirring. Magmas of all the clays may also be prepared by adding the clay to hot purified water with rapid stirring, as in a blender.

Since the clays will support growth of micro-organisms under certain conditions, a preservative is generally considered desirable, i.e., a methylparaben (0.2%)-propyl-paraben (0.02%) combination or sodium benzoate 0.1 per cent.

SYNTHETIC HYDROCOLLOIDS

In the attempt to overcome some of the disadvantages of natural products, especially the lack of purity and uniformity of hydrocolloids of plant origin, many synthetic polymers have been prepared. Of these a carboxy vinyl polymer* of high molecular weight has had the most extensive use. Supplied as a white powder in the acid form, it is neutralized with alkali and exhibits its greatest viscosity at a pH range of 5 to 10. Carbopol 934 may be used in both internal and external preparations. The following kaolin-pectin prescription shows an example of the use of Carbopol 934 as a suspending agent.

18. ℞
    Kaolin 11.66
    Pectin 0.26
    Carbopol 934 . . . .   0.18
    Sucaryl sodium 0.60
    Peppermint oil 0.35
    Methyl salicylate 0.35
    Sodium carbonate to neutralize
    Distilled water ad 60.00

    M.

It must be remembered in the use of Carbopol that its neutralized gels tend to undergo oxidative degradation when exposed to light. Schwarz and Levy[30] reported this loss of viscosity and attributed it to the presence of trace metals. Therefore, when Carbopol is used as a suspending agent, the suspensions should be protected from light or contain antioxidants or EDTA to complex trace metal ions.

Carbopol is also quite sensitive to small amounts of electrolytes, showing a marked decrease in viscosity in its neutralized aqueous dispersion. Preservatives which are ionic, such as benzoic acid, sodium benzoate, etc., can cause the decrease in viscosity.

IONIC BEHAVIOR OF HYDROCOLLOIDS

In employing viscosity-increasing agents, the chemical reactivity of these substances should be taken into account. Most of the suspending agents used are anionic in nature

* B. F. Goodrich Chemical Co., Cleveland 15, Ohio.

(acacia, tragacanth, sodium alginate, karaya, carrageenin, sodium carboxymethylcellulose, Carbopol 934, bentonite, hectorite and Veegum). Methylcellulose, microcrystalline cellulose and propylene glycol alginate are nonionic. Nakashima and Miller,[24] in a study of ionic incompatibilities of suspending agents, showed that the use of some anionic suspending agents resulted in the precipitation of organic cationic substances such as thiamine hydrochloride, neomycin sulfate, benzalkonium chloride, etc., with the resulting possibility of inactivation of the substance. This was especially evident with the clays and indicates the need for care in selection of a viscosity-increasing agent to be combined with cationic substances.

Preparation of Suspensions

Figure 5-6 shows the steps involved in preparing and stabilizing a pharmaceutical suspension.[25] The first step involves increasing the wettability of the micronized hydrophobic solid particles by the dispersion medium, which may be accomplished by the addition of a wetting agent to the system. Glycerin, U.S.P. alcohol or suitable nontoxic surface active agents are commonly employed for the purpose of facilitating the initial dispersion of powders in aqueous

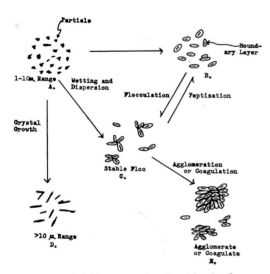

Fig. 5-6. Processes involved in the formation of pharmaceutical suspensions. (Nash, R. A.: Drug and Cosmetic Industry, *97* (6):843, 1965)

media. The particles in the deflocculated state (B) are of a relatively small particle size; they usually carry an electrical charge and, because of repulsive forces existing between like charged particles, have less of a tendency to settle. However, a deflocculated suspension is pharmaceutically unstable, and, once the particles of such a suspension settle to the bottom of the container, they form a compact mass or cake which is difficult to resuspend. To meet this problem appropriate methods are employed to partially flocculate (C) the deflocculated suspension so as to prevent the formation of a caked suspension (E). Care must be exercised to avoid the addition of too much flocculating agent (e.g., electrolytes, surface active agents or hydrocolloids), since it is possible to bypass the flocculated state and produce a deflocculated suspension (E) by reversing the charge on the dispersed particles. The degree of flocculation can be monitored microscopically.

The suspending agent used in the preparation of pharmaceutical suspensions may act as a protective colloid to keep the particles from caking, as a flocculating agent to produce the desired degree of flocculation, or to provide a *structured vehicle*[14] to support the flocs while not preventing flow when the mixture is agitated and poured from the container.

It should be borne in mind that although the vehicle in most pharmaceutical suspensions is aqueous there are some products in which the vehicle is oleaginous in nature. These nonaqueous suspensions present additional stability problems. The nature of the electrical barrier surrounding the dispersed phase particles, which aids in stabilizing some aqueous suspensions, is usually significantly altered in the presence of a solvent of low dielectric. The low dielectric constant of oleaginous solvents tends to reduce the potential energy that must be overcome to bring two suspended particles together. As a result, such suspensions are not well protected against excessive flocculation by the electrical double layer surrounding the particles.

Micronized suspensions intended for parenteral administration via the intramuscular route must be prepared from sterile ingre-

Surfactants

Pluronic F-68
Polysorbate 80, U.S.P. (Tween 80†)
Polyoxyethylene sorbitan monolaurate
Emulphor EL-620
Sorbitan trioleate (Span 85†)
Lecithin

Hydrocolloids

Sodium carboxymethylcellulose
Polyvinylpyrrolidone
Gelatin (nonantigenic)
Methylcellulose

Solvents

Water for injection
Sodium chloride injection
Ringer's injection
Dextrose and sodium chloride injection
Lactated Ringer's injection
Fixed oils (*Note:* must meet U.S.P. require-
    ments)
Polyethylene glycol
    300   Used as a portion of
Propylene glycol   an aqueous vehicle
Sorbitol

Others

Aluminum monostearate
Silicone Antifoam

* Adapted from Macek, T. J.: J. Pharm. Sci.,
52:694, 1963.
† Trademark.

dients under aseptic conditions. The agents
used in their preparation and stabilization
should meet at least four principle criteria,
as outlined by Macek.[22] They should be:

1. Nontoxic, nonpyrogenic, nonantigenic,
nonirritating, nonhemolytic and of the highest purity.

2. Potent dispersants and/or stabilizers
so that only small amounts are required.

3. Stable, especially upon prolonged storage and preferably under the conditions of
higher temperatures which one would like
to employ for positive sterilization.

4. Approved by the federal Food and
Drug Administration for parenteral use.
The *United States Pharmacopeia XVII* and
the *National Formulary XII* set forth additional standards for ingredients used in the

preparation of parenteral dosage forms, and
should be consulted before preparing parenteral suspensions.

Table 5-1 is a partial listing of agents
commonly employed in parenteral suspensions. The finished sterile suspension should
possess good stability, resuspendability, and
syringeability (i.e., the ability of the suspension to pass through a hypodermic
needle). The last-named property is dependent on the viscosity and density of the
vehicle and, to a lesser extent, on the particle size and concentration of the suspended
drug.*

LIQUID-IN-LIQUID DISPERSIONS (EMULSIONS)

The pharmacist encounters the emulsion
system in his dispensing practice more often
than he may realize and should be thoroughly
familiar with emulsion technology. He probably will be concerned less with emulsions
to be taken internally than with external oil-
in-water or water-in-oil lotions used both for
their emollient action and as viscous liquid
carriers for insoluble medicinal agents.

It is assumed that the student is thoroughly familiar with the theories of emulsification and the terminology of this class of
pharmaceuticals. However, it may be wise to
review some of the features of an emulsion
system. Although an emulsion may be considered as a two-phase system consisting of
two immiscible liquids, one of which is dispersed throughout the other in the form of
globules, from a practical standpoint a third
component—the emulsifying agent—must be
added to stabilize the heterogeneous dispersion. This third substance orients itself at the
interface, thereby acting as a bridge between
the immiscible liquid pair. It reduces the
interfacial tension between the two and forms
a film around the dispersed globule, preventing or retarding coalescence of the internal
phase. Emulsion technology, as far as the
pharmacist is concerned, involves a knowledge of the types of emulsions which he will
encounter, plus an awareness of the myriad
of emulsifying agents which he has at his dis-

* References 2, 3 and 22 should be consulted
for a more detailed discussion of parenteral suspensions.

posal for producing satisfactory oil-in-water and water-in-oil emulsions.

The pharmacist must realize that the stability of an emulsion may be improved if (a) the particle size of the internal phase is decreased as far as possible; (b) the optimum ratio of oil to water is used, and (c) the viscosity of the system is increased.

Globule Size. As the globules of the internal phase are reduced to a size approaching the colloidal range (under 5 microns), they are influenced by brownian motion; this helps to keep the globules in a uniform dispersion. This is accomplished by shearing action resulting from efficient and prolonged trituration in a mortar, the passing of the emulsion through a hand homogenizer or a colloid mill or mixing it in a blender.

Phase-Volume Ratio. The volume of the internal phase compared with that of the external phase (phase-volume ratio) will influence the characteristics of an emulsion. Generally speaking, the most stable emulsions have an internal phase occupying between 40 and 60 per cent of the emulsion. As the percentage of internal phase increases the viscosity of the emulsion rises due to the packing of the globules of the internal phase, preventing free movement in the external phase. When the concentration of the internal phase approaches 80 per cent, there is mechanical crowding to such an extent that the emulsion usually has the consistency of a paste.

Viscosity. The pharmacist is limited in the changes which he can make in the phase-volume ratio of an emulsion; however, he may increase stability by adding certain ingredients to increase the viscosity of the external phase. To raise the viscosity of the external phase of an oil-in-water emulsion he must add a substance which is soluble in or miscible with water and, also, has the capacity to increase viscosity. The polyethylene glycols, cellulose ethers, natural and synthetic gums and clays have been used successfully as viscosity-increasing agents. If the pharmacist wishes to raise the external phase viscosity of a water-in-oil emulsion, he must add to the system a substance which is soluble in or miscible with the oil phase and will increase its viscosity. Among the substances which have been used for accomplishing this

in water-in-oil emulsions are viscous oils, waxes, fatty alcohols and fatty acids.

Classification of Emulsifying Agents. Emulsifying agents may be classified into three main groups:

1. Natural emulsifying agents
   A. Those from vegetable sources
      a. Carbohydrates such as acacia, tragacanth, chondrus and pectin
      b. Those derived from cellulose
   B. Those from animal sources
      a. Gelatin, egg yolk and casein
      b. Wool fat and cholesterol
2. Finely divided solids
3. Synthetic emulsifying agents
   A. Anionic
   B. Cationic
   C. Nonionic

NATURAL EMULSIFYING AGENTS FROM VEGETABLE SOURCES

The natural emulsifying agents from vegetable sources all have some of the same features, as they are all carbohydrate derivatives, glycoside-like and anionic in nature; all produce oil-in-water emulsions under normal circumstances and are sensitive to high concentrations of alcohol or salts. They are differentiated by the way in which they act as emulsifiers. Those which reduce interfacial tension and form a tough mechanical film around the dispersed phase are considered to be "true" emulsifiers; those which function by increasing viscosity to the extent of preventing creaming and coalescence are considered "quasi" emulsifiers.

Acacia was discussed under suspending agents previously in the chapter. In general, it yields good, stable and palatable emulsions of low viscosity. Other gums, such as tragacanth, agar or pectin, are often added in small quantities to increase the viscosity of the system.

Acacia emulsions may be made by the wet gum (English), the dry gum (Continental) or the bottle method (with volatile oils). (See p. 224.) The ratio of gum to oil varies from 1 part of acacia to 2 parts of volatile oil to 4 parts of fixed oil. The following prescription illustrates the use of acacia as an emulsifying agent.

19. ℞
Kaolin .... 10.8 Gm.
Aluminum hydroxide .... 0.5 Gm.
Mineral oil .... 18.0 ml.
Acacia .... 4.5 Gm.
Peppermint water ad. ...... 90.0 ml.

M. ft. emulsion.

Sig.: One tablespoonful q.d.

Triturate the liquid petrolatum with the acacia. Add 9 ml. of peppermint water and form a primary emulsion. Mix the kaolin and the aluminum hydroxide with the remainder of the peppermint water and add slowly to the nucleus.

20. ℞
Ol. ricini .... 31.5 ml.
Acacia, in fine powd. .... 8.1 Gm.
Tr. vanilla .... 2.3 ml.
Syrup .... 18.0 ml.
Dist. water ad .... 90.0 ml.

M. ft. emulsion.

Sig.: Three tablespoonfuls at bedtime.

Triturate the acacia with the oil. Add 16 ml. of water all at once and form an emulsion. Incorporate the syrup, the tincture and the remainder of the water in small amounts with trituration.

Tragacanth emulsions may be made by either the wet gum or the dry gum method, keeping in mind that 0.1 Gm. of tragacanth is required where 1 Gm. of acacia was used. When the wet gum method is used, a mucilage is made of 1 part of gum to 20 parts of water. Tragacanth emulsions are stable but tend to be coarser than those made from acacia. Passing through a hand homogenizer materially improves their particle size and appearance. The following liniment uses tragacanth as the emulsifier:

21. ℞
Liquid petrolatum 18.00
Bergamot oil .... .30
Lavender oil .... .30
Sodium benzoate .... .48
Tragacanth 1.80
Distilled water ad 120.00

M. ft. emulsion.

Triturate the liquid petrolatum with the tragacanth until smooth, add 38 ml. of water all at once and make an emulsion. Dissolve the preservative in 12 ml. of water and add gradually. Add the oils and enough distilled water to make 120 ml. This emulsion demands a larger amount of tragacanth than normal because the low percentage of liquid petrolatum increases the viscosity requirement.

Agar is employed to some extent as an auxiliary emulsifier in liquid petrolatum emulsions. To increase viscosity it is used in the amount of 1 per cent of the total volume of the emulsion. The general procedure is to prepare an emulsion with acacia, water and oil and then add a 2 per cent agar mucilage to this emulsion.

Chondrus. In itself, Chondrus is not very adaptable to prescription use because of the difficulty in preparing the mucilage from the plant. However, its refined dried extract, carrageenin, is available under the names of Sea Kem* and Kraystay† in a variety of types, depending on their ultimate use. These substances are rather sensitive to electrolytes and hydrolyze at low pH values. They will tolerate up to 20 per cent of alcohol before gelling.

Pectin is often used alone or in combination with acacia as an emulsifier. When employed alone, 0.1 Gm. of pectin is used to replace 1 Gm. of acacia in the emulsion. When used to increase the viscosity of acacia emulsions, a concentration of approximately 1 per cent of the final emulsion volume is employed.

22. ℞
Liquid petrolatum 50.0
Pectin 1.0
Syrup 10.0
Methyl salicylate 0.4
Purified water ad 100.0

M. ft. emulsion.

Mix the pectin and half of the liquid petrolatum in a mortar, add 25 ml. of purified water all at once and triturate until an emulsion is formed. Allow to stand for 10 minutes and continue trituration until white and creamy. Add slowly, with trituration, the remainder of the liquid petrolatum, the syrup, the methyl salicylate and the rest of the purified water.

* Sea Plant Corporation, New Bedford, Mass.
† Phenix Foods Company, Chicago 90, Ill.

Algins. Sodium alginate, discussed earlier in the chapter, is classed with tragacanth and pectin as one of the substances which emulsifies principally by increasing the viscosity of the mixture. Satisfactory emulsions may be obtained with 50 per cent of oil with the use of about 1 per cent of sodium alginate, medium viscosity. Propylene glycol alginate* may be used in prescriptions of the following type:

23. ℞
Paraldehyde 15.0
Syr. Pruni virginianae 75.0
Kelcoloid S 0.6

M. ft. emulsion.

Sig.: 15.0 ml. h.s.

Form a mucilage with about 15 ml. of the wild cherry syrup and the propylene glycol alginate and gradually add the paraldehyde in increasing amounts, with constant trituration, until emulsification is complete; then add the remainder of the wild cherry syrup.

Other Emulsifiers. At various times substances such as honey, malt extract, licorice extract, etc., have been used as emulsifying agents. Since they are little used, they will not be discussed here.

NATURAL EMULSIFIERS DERIVED FROM CELLULOSE

The modified celluloses are generally thought of as agents for the suspending of solids but may be used successfully in many emulsion formulations. They possess the advantages over the natural gums of higher purity and less sensitivity to changes in environment: pH, concentration of electrolytes and the presence of mold or bacterial organisms.

Methylcellulose has been described in some detail under suspensions. It may be used both as a primary emulsifying agent and as an auxiliary emulsifier to increase the viscosity of emulsions. Excellent emulsions can be obtained with mineral oil and cod liver oil, using methylcellulose as the primary emulsifier.[26] A dispersion of the methylcellulose is made, placed in a mortar and the oil added in small amounts with constant trituration.

* Kelcoloid S, Kelco Company, San Diego, Calif.

24. ℞
Castor oil . . . . ℥ i
Methocel HG 2% Sol. . . . . ℥ i
Vanilla Tr. . . . . ♏ xx

M. ft. emulsion.

Sig.: ℥ ss h.s.

Make a 2 per cent Methocel HG† dispersion, place in a mortar and gradually add the oil, with constant trituration, to form an emulsion. Add the flavor.

Sodium Carboxymethylcellulose (CMC) may also be used as a primary emulsifier but is generally used with other emulsifiers to increase viscosity.

EMULSIFYING AGENTS FROM ANIMAL SOURCES

Egg yolk, egg albumin, casein and condensed milk have been used occasionally as emulsifying agents in pharmaceuticals. However, gelatin remains the one which is used frequently in the production of oil-in-water emulsions, especially with mineral oil.

Gelatin. The *U.S.P.* distinguishes two types of gelatin: "Gelatin derived from an acid-treated precursor is known as Type A (Pharmagel A) and exhibits an isoelectric point between pH 7 and 9, while gelatin derived from an alkali-treated precursor is known as Type B (Pharmagel B) and has an isoelectric point between pH 4.7 and 5."

Pharmagel A is generally used in an acid solution in the range of pH of 3 to 3.5. At this pH it is positively charged and is incompatible with negatively charged hydrocolloids such as acacia, tragacanth or agar. Pharmagel B is used in a pH range above its isoelectric point. In this range, it is negatively charged and is compatible with the negatively charged hydrocolloids.

When gelatin is used as an emulsifier, it is impossible to make a satisfactory emulsion with mortar and pestle. Homogenization or treatment with a colloid mill is necessary. In prescription practice the hand homogenizer has proved to be quite satisfactory.

Gelatin may be used in a low concentration—in the area of 1 per cent—of the total emulsion volume. The procedure consists of adding most of the water in the formula to

† Dow Chemical Company, Midland, Mich.

the gelatin, heating to 98-100° C. and stirring until the gelatin is dissolved. When cool, the gelatin solution, the oil and the other ingredients are mixed roughly and passed through a hand homogenizer several times.

25. ℞
Pharmagel A	1.20	Gm.
Tartaric acid	70	mg.
Syrup	12	ml.
Vanillin	5	mg.
Alcohol	7.2	ml.
Liquid petrolatum	60	ml.
Purified water ad	120	ml.

M. ft. emulsion.

Sig.: ℥ ss h.s.

Add the Pharmagel A and the tartaric acid (to bring pH to acid range) to 36 ml. of water. Heat at boiling for 5 to 10 minutes until all of the gelatin dissolves. Cool to 50° C., add liquid petrolatum, syrup, flavor, alcohol and enough purified water to make 120 ml. Pass through the hand homogenizer several times.

All of the previous substances discussed as emulsifying agents have certain things in common: all normally are soluble or dispersible in water and are oil-in-water emulsifiers. In addition, if emulsions are to be stored for any period of time, preservatives must be added. The ones most used are sodium benzoate, benzoic acid, alcohol and the parabens.

Wool Fat and Cholesterol. Wool fat and its main active ingredient are used more often as water-in-oil emulsifiers in ointments and creams or emollients. When they are used in liquid preparations of the lotion type, they are generally auxiliary emulsifiers.

Finely Divided Solids

Many finely divided solids, especially those which are highly hydrated in dispersion, will form very stable emulsions, usually of the oil-in-water type. Examples of compounds of this type which will orient at the interface between oil and water are bentonite and the other clays, magnesium hydroxide, aluminum hydroxide and magnesium trisilicate. Sometimes the emulsion may be prepared by agitating the magma of the compound with the oil in a bottle. Usually, the magma is placed in a mortar and the oil added in small amounts with constant trituration. Hand homogenization or treatment in a blender greatly improves this type of emulsion. The following prescriptions are examples:

26. ℞
Liquid petrolatum	℥ ii
F.E. cascara	℥ i
Magma magnesia ad	℥ iv

M. ft. emulsion.

Sig.: ℥ ss h.s.

Place the magma magnesia in a mortar. Add the liquid petrolatum, with constant trituration, in small amounts until all has been emulsified. Add the fluidextract. Mix. If necessary, pass through a hand homogenizer.

27. ℞
Cottonseed oil	30.0
Oleic acid	0.6
Aluminum hydroxide gel	15.0
Purified water ad	60.0

M. ft. emulsion.

Place the aluminum hydroxide gel in a mortar, gradually add a mixture of the oil and the oleic acid with constant trituration until completely emulsified. Add the purified water to volume. Hand-homogenize if necessary.

28. ℞
Camphor	0.3
Menthol	0.3
Phenol	0.6
Olive oil	24.0
Bentonite magma ad	60.0

M.

Sig.: Apply to itching area.

Triturate the three eutectic substances together and add the olive oil. Place the bentonite magma (35 ml.) in a Wedgwood mortar and gradually add the oil solution in small amounts, with constant trituration, until completely emulsified. Hand-homogenization greatly improves this preparation.

Synthetic Emulsifying Agents

A few of the substances that belong to a large group classified as surface-active agents or surfactants have emulsification also as one of their applications. The usual method for grouping these compounds is according to their behavior in solution. Most of the surfactants ionize in water, and either the anion or the cation is responsible for the surface-active properties. If the anion is the surface-active portion of the molecule, it is termed an *anionic* surfactant. If the cation is the surface-active portion of the molecule, it is called a *cationic* surfactant. If it is a molecule which possesses surface-active properties but does not ionize, it falls into the classification of *nonionic* surfactants. In the following sections those compounds which are used principally as emulsifying agents will be discussed.

Anionic Emulsifying Agents

In this group appear three important types: soaps, sulfated compounds and sulfonated compounds. All have one characteristic in common—their incompatibility with acids, cationic surfactants and cations which will react with the anion to form an insoluble compound.

Soaps may be considered as the reaction products of fatty acids above C_{14} with alkaline substances, i.e., KOH, NaOH, NH_4OH, $Ca(OH)_2$, $Zn(OH)_2$, $Mg(OH)_2$ or an organic amine such as triethanolamine. When they are used as emulsifying agents, the reaction forming the soap usually takes place during the preparation of the emulsion.

ALKALI SOAPS (MONOVALENT). These substances produce oil-in-water emulsions, impart alkalinity to the finished preparation (pH 9 to 10) and are seldom used in internal preparations because of their bitter taste and laxative action. In the presence of excessive amounts of multivalent cations such as calcium ions an insoluble soap is precipitated. In an acid medium the alkali soaps form the free fatty acids. Since the free fatty acids are feeble emulsifying agents, this usually results in breaking of the emulsion. The following formula is a lotion type utilizing an alkali soap as the emulsifier.

29. ℞

Stearic acid	3.5 Gm.
Glycerin	8.0 Gm.
Potassium hydroxide	0.2 Gm.
Alcohol	8.0 Gm.
Lanolin	2.0 Gm.
Purified water	78.3 Gm.

The procedure used in compounding this is a standard one for emulsions of this type. The water-soluble substances—in this case the glycerin, potassium hydroxide, alcohol and water—are heated together to about 70° C. The fat-soluble ingredients—lanolin and stearic acid—are heated to the same temperature, the two solutions are mixed and allowed to cool to room temperature with stirring.

This type of lotion base is used less often than others because of its alkalinity and tendency toward skin irritation and sensitization.

METALLIC SOAPS (DIVALENT). This group results from the reaction of fatty acids (whether alone or as a component of a fixed oil) with zinc hydroxide, magnesium hydroxide or calcium hydroxide. Neither the zinc soap (zinc stearate) nor the magnesium soap (magnesium stearate) is used as an emulsifier. However, the calcium soap is one of the emulsifiers most used in dermatologic practice.

Calcium oleate produces water-in-oil emulsions, imparts alkalinity to the finished emulsion and is limited to external use because of the characteristic taste of soaps. It is sensitive to an acid medium which liberates the free fatty acid but has a higher acid tolerance than the alkali soaps.

Emulsions using a calcium soap as the emulsifying agent are prepared by mixing calcium hydroxide solution with a fixed oil in equal portions or with the oil in excess. If the acid value of the oil is too low, the addition of a small amount of oleic acid often will produce a satisfactory emulsion. This emulsion base may be used as a vehicle for insoluble solids. The following are lotion-type dermatologic prescriptions of record:

30. ℞

Pulv. calamine	3.
Zinc oxide	2.
Olive oil	
Lime water, aa	30.

M.

Sig.: Apply locally b.i.d. et h.s.

Shake the lime water and the olive oil in a 2-fl. oz. bottle until a creamy emulsion results. Place the powders in a mortar and add the prepared w/o emulsion with trituration.

31. ℞

Pulv. calamine
Zinc oxide, aa .... 6.
Sol. calc. hydrox. .... 25.
Olive oil .... 9.
Purified water ad .... 50.

M.

Sig.: Locally ut dict.

Since the volume of lime water exceeds that of the oil (which will be the external phase), first mix the full amount of olive oil with an equal volume (9 ml.) of lime water. Agitate until the emulsion forms. Place the powders in a mortar; add the remainder of the lime water and 16 ml. of distilled water, then the w/o emulsion. Mix thoroughly.

SOAPS OF ORGANIC AMINES. Several of the organic amines have been used to form soaps; however, triethanolamine is the one used in many lotion bases. When reacted with stearic or oleic acid, the soap that is formed acts as an excellent oil-in-water emulsifier. It produces a slightly alkaline emulsion, in the range of pH 7.5 to 8. Like other soaps, it is incompatible with acidic substances and acidic solutions. The procedure for preparing emulsions containing triethanolamine soaps is the same as that for the alkali soaps.

32. ℞

Menthol .... 0.04 Gm.
Stearic acid .... 2.40 Gm.
Cetyl alcohol .... 1.20 Gm.
Wool fat .... 0.80 Gm.
Liquid petrolatum .... 4.00 ml.
Triethanolamine .... 1.20 ml.
Water .... 88.00 ml.
Perfume q.s.

M. et Sig.: Back Rub Lotion (Peter Bent Brigham Hospital).

Heat the menthol, the stearic acid, the cetyl alcohol, the wool fat and the liquid petrolatum to 70° C. Dissolve the triethanolamine in the water and heat to 70° C. Mix the two solutions. Stir until cool.

33. ℞

Hydrous wool fat .... 20.0 Gm.
Stearic acid .... 2.0 Gm.
Light liquid petrolatum .... 10.0 ml.
Triethanolamine .... 0.8 ml.
Rose water q.s. ad .... 100.0 ml.

M. ft. lotion.

Sig.: Lanolin Lotion.

Heat the wool fat, the stearic acid and the light liquid petrolatum to 70° C. Dissolve the triethanolamine in the rose water and heat to 70° C. Mix the two solutions. Stir until cool.

It is interesting to note that triethanolamine soaps have an HLB value in the range of 12, which explains why they have been used so successfully as emulsifiers for liquid petrolatum (required HLB is about 12). (For discussion of HLB see p. 221 and Table 5-2.)

Sulfated Compounds. Many surfactants of the sulfated group are available. They are produced by sulfating a long-chain alcohol and making the alkali or amine salt. Sodium lauryl sulfate, composed of a mixture of sulfated alcohols with lauryl alcohol the principal one, has been used in pharmaceuticals for a number of years as an oil-in-water emulsifier. It has the advantage over soaps of being less sensitive to acids and compatible with calcium salts, since calcium lauryl sulfate is not water-insoluble. When used by itself, so-

TABLE 5-2. "REQUIRED HLB" VALUES FOR
O/W EMULSIONS OF COMMON
INGREDIENTS*

Acid, stearic	15-18
Alcohol, cetyl	13-16
Alcohol, stearyl	13-16
Isopropyl esters	9-13
Lanolin, anhydrous	10-12
Oils	
Vegetable	6-10
Mineral	10-12
Petrolatum	7-11
Waxes	
Beeswax	8-12
Microcrystalline	9-12
Paraffin	8-11

* The Required HLB of any material is likely to vary slightly with the source of the material, the concentration desired, and the method of preparation, and should be verified against your own ingredients at your own desired concentration and with your own manufacturing technic.

Materials that are surface active, such as fatty acids, fatty alcohols, etc., when used at high concentrations, will likely require a higher HLB.

The Required HLB for making W/O emulsions of any material will lie in the range of 3 to 8; for solubilization in water, in the range of 10 to 18.

From Guide to the Use of Atlas Sorbitol and Surfactants in cosmetics, Atlas Chemical Industries, Inc., Wilmington, Del., 1962.

dium lauryl sulfate forms emulsions of rather poor stability. Therefore, it is employed with stabilizers such as cetyl or stearyl alcohol. Sodium lauryl sulfate has been avoided by dermatologists, who consider it a primary irritant to the skin. The following formula includes sodium lauryl sulfate as the emulsifier.

34. ℞
Cetyl alcohol .... 2.4 Gm.
Light liq. petrolatum ...... 19.2 ml.
Sodium lauryl sulfate ..... 0.6 Gm.
Purified water ad .... 120.0 ml.

M. ft. emulsion.

Heat the cetyl alcohol and light liquid petrolatum to 70° C., dissolve the sodium lauryl sulfate in the water and heat to the same temperature. Mix and stir until cool. This may be used as a stock lotion base.

Sulfonated Compounds. Dioctyl sodium sulfosuccinate* is the major representative of this group of sulfonated surfactants. It is used both as a wetting agent and as an emulsifier in pharmaceuticals.

Cationic Emulsifying Agents

The cationic surfactants may be used as oil-in-water emulsifiers. However, because of their superior bacteriostatic properties they are seldom used as emulsifying agents. Benzalkonium chloride is representative of this group of compounds.

Nonionic Emulsifying Agents

The nonionic surfactants used in pharmaceuticals are complex esters, ethers or ester-ethers of alcohols. They possess the advantage over anionic and cationic agents of stability over a wide range of pH. Most nonionics can be made by taking practically any hydrophobic compound which has in its structure a carboxy, hydroxy, amido or amino group with free hydrogen attached to the nitrogen and reacting it with ethylene oxide. Furthermore, the properties of each compound can be changed considerably simply by changing the molar portion of ethylene oxide, that is, by changing the length of the polyoxyethylene chain. Most of the nonionics

* Aerosol OT, American Cyanamide Company, New York 20, N. Y.

are viscous liquids or soft pastes. The ethylene oxide type accounts for 80 to 90 per cent of all nonionics used.

The HLB System. With the development of the nonionic emulsifiers a great amount of interest was taken in more exact methods of determining whether an emulsion remained stable or not and whether the proper amount and type of emulsifier was being used. Griffin[9,10] assigned to the respective components of emulsion systems a value indicating their relatively lipophilic (nonpolar) or hydrophilic (polar) characters. This value represents the ratio between the lipophilic portion of the molecule and the hydrophilic portion and is called the hydrophile-lipophile balance (HLB).

Each emulsifier and major component of an emulsion was assigned an HLB value of from 1 to 20. Although higher values are known, most surfactants fall below 20. The higher the HLB value of an emulsifier the more the polar portion predominates, and the lower the value the more the nonpolar portion predominates. It has been found that water-in-oil emulsions are formed when the emulsifiers are in the range of HLB 3 to 6, while oil-in-water emulsions are formed from HLB 8 to 18. Substances with low HLB values are predominantly oil-soluble while those with high HLB values are predominantly soluble or miscible in water.

USE OF THE HLB SYSTEM. The HLB value of the oil phase of an emulsion, i.e., oils, waxes, etc., must first be considered to determine what will be the matching HLB of the emulsifier or emulsifier blend required to produce a stable emulsion. Many of the substances in the oil phase have already been assigned HLB values and may be determined from available tables. Table 5-2 lists some of the "Required HLB" values of common ingredients of emulsion formulae.

As an example of the use of the HLB system the following formula is given.†

Liquid petrolatum	35%
Wool fat	1%
Cetyl alcohol	1%
Emulsifier	7%
Water	56%

† See footnote to Table 5-2.

TABLE 5-3. HLB VALUES OF SOME SELECTED EMULSIFYING AGENTS

CHEMICAL OR GENERIC NAME	TRADE NAME	HLB
Sorbitan Trioleate	Span or Arlacel 85*	1.8
Sorbitan Tristearate	Span 65*	2.1
Sorbitan Sesquioleate	Arlacel 83*	3.7
Glyceryl Monostearate		3.8
Sorbitan Mono-oleate	Span or Arlacel 80*	4.3
Sorbitan Monostearate	Span or Arlacel 60*	4.7
Glyceryl Monostearate (Self-emulsifying)	Aldo 28†	5.5
Sorbitan Monopalmitate	Span or Arlacel 40*	6.7
Acacia		8.0
Sorbitan Monolaurate	Span or Arlacel 20*	8.6
Gelatin		9.8
Polyoxyethylene Sorbitan Trioleate	Tween 85*	11.0
Polyethylene Glycol 400 Monostearate		11.6
Triethanolamine Oleate		12.0
Polyoxyethylene Sorbitan Monostearate	Tween 60*	14.9
Polyoxyethylene Sorbitan Mono-oleate	Tween 80*	15.0
Polyoxyethylene Sorbitan Monopalmitate	Tween 40*	15.6
Polyoxyethylene Sorbitan Monolaurate	Tween 20*	16.7
Sodium Oleate		18.0
Sodium Lauryl Sulfate		above 20.0

* Atlas Chemical Company, Wilmington 99, Delaware.
† Glyco Chemicals Corp., New York 1, N. Y.

and an o/w lotion vehicle is desired. The percentage composition of the oil phase is $35\% + 1\% + 1\% = 37\%$ and its required HLB for o/w emulsification can be calculated as follows:

Required HLB

Liquid Petrolatum $= \dfrac{35}{37} = 94.6\% \times 12 = 11.4$

Wool Fat $= \dfrac{1}{37} = 2.7\% \times 10 = 0.3$

Cetyl Alcohol $= \dfrac{1}{37} = 2.7\% \times 15 = 0.4$

Estimated required HLB of emulsifier 12.1

Therefore, an emulsifier or a combination having an HLB range of 11 to 13 probably will be satisfactory.

Table 5-3 shows some of the HLB values of some emulsifying agents.

There are many other surfactants for which the HLB values have been determined. Once the required HLB value of the oil phase has been determined, an emulsifier or a blend of emulsifiers may be selected of approximately that HLB. For Atlas emulsifiers charts are available giving HLB values of various blends.

In the formula given with Table 5-2, with a required HLB value of 12.1, a single emulsifier such as polyethylene glycol 400 monostearate might prove satisfactory. More often a blend of two emulsifiers of similar structure, one with a high HLB value and the other with a low HLB value, is chosen. If, in the above case, Tween 80 (HLB–15) and Arlacel 80 (HLB–4.3) were selected, the proportion of each could be determined by alligation. This would give 78 parts of Tween 80 to 29 parts of Arlacel 80, or 5 per cent of Tween 80 and 2 per cent of Arlacel 80.

There are many nonionic emulsifiers available, but the pharmacist will find that he encounters a relatively low number in emulsion compounding.

Glycol esters consist of reaction products when a glycol (glycerin, propylene glycol, diethylene glycol, polyethylene glycol, etc.) reacts with a fatty acid—usually, stearic acid. With the exception of the polyethylene glycol stearates, they are rather poor emulsifying agents when used alone. If a small amount of an anionic surfactant such as sodium stearate or sodium lauryl sulfate is added, they become efficient oil-in-water emulsifiers. Two of the group are used in pharmaceuticals: glyceryl monostearate, self-emulsifying, and polyethylene glycol 400 monostearate.

GLYCERYL MONOSTEARATE S. E. This mixture serves as an emulsifier in many pharmaceutical and cosmetic emulsions. Because it depends for its emulsifying efficiency on the blend of nonionic-anionic emulsifiers, it has the incompatibilities of the anionics, i.e., sensitivity to an environment of low pH. When used in liquid preparations, glyceryl monostearate S. E. is present as a co-emulsifier along with amine soaps, etc. An acid-stable self-emulsifying glyceryl monostearate containing a small amount of a nonionic emulsifying agent of high HLB is available as Arlacel 165* for use in lotion formulas containing acidic salts.[33]

35. ℞
Cetyl alcohol	5%
Arlacel 165	5%
Sorbitol solution	5%
Water	85%
Preservative q.s.	

M. ft. lotion base 120 ml.

Heat the cetyl alcohol and the Arlacel 165 to 70° C.; heat the sorbitol solution and the water to the same temperature. Mix and stir until cool.

POLYETHYLENE GLYCOL 400 MONOSTEARATE. The polyethylene glycol esters may be used not only as nonionic emulsifiers but also as suspending agents. They are found in many cosmetic lotions in conjunction with anionic emulsifiers such as triethanolamine stearate.[28]

36. Cleansing Lotion
1. Stearic acid		2.0 Gm.
2. Liquid petrolatum		15.0 ml.
3. Isopropyl myristate		2.0 ml.
4. Polyethylene glycol 400 monostearate		10.0 Gm.
5. Lanolin		5.0 Gm.
6. White wax		8.0 Gm.
7. Propylene glycol		5.0 ml.
8. Triethanolamine		1.0 ml.
9. Preservative		0.1 Gm.
10. Purified water q.s. ad		100.0 ml.

* Atlas Chemical Company, Wilmington 99, Delaware.

Mix and heat ingredients 1 through 6 to 70 to 75° C.; dissolve 7, 8 and 9 in the water and heat to the same temperature. Add the aqueous solution to the oil solution and stir uniformly to room temperature.

Sorbitan Esters. Although there are many nonionic emulsifiers available which are satisfactory for use in pharmaceuticals, the Tweens* and the Spans* have had the most application.

The Spans and the Arlacels are prepared by esterification of sorbitan with various fatty acids. Table 5-3 shows their chemical composition. The Arlacels are a highly purified grade of the Spans, intended for pharmaceutical and cosmetic use.

The Tweens are derived from Spans by treatment of the nonesterified hydroxy groups with ethylene oxide to form polyoxyethylene side chains. Chain length can be controlled to give surfactants of varying polarities. Tween 80 is official in U.S.P. XVII as Polysorbate 80.

37. ℞
Zinc oxide	12.0 Gm.
Talc	12.0 Gm.
Lanolin	12.0 Gm.
Peanut oil	48.0 ml.
Alum acetate sol.	2.4 ml.
Polysorbate 80	2.4 ml.
Purified water ad	120.0 ml.

M.

Sig.: Burow's Emulsion.

Heat the lanolin, the peanut oil and the polysorbate 80 to 60° C. Mix well and cool to room temperature. Mix with the zinc oxide and the talc in a mortar. Add the aluminum acetate solution followed by the water with constant trituration.[16]

38. ℞
Castor oil	45.0 ml.
Span 80	6.3 ml.
Tween 80 (0.67% sol.)	38.7 ml.
To make	90.0 ml.

M. Sig.: Castor Oil Emulsion.

Mix the Span 80 and the castor oil. Place the Tween 80 solution in a mortar and add the Span-castor oil mixture in small proportions with constant trituration.[20]

* Atlas Chemical Company, Wilmington 99, Delaware.

GENERAL PREPARATION OF EMULSIONS

The pharmacist must be able to prepare emulsions extemporaneously using the mortar and pestle, together with whatever other small-scale equipment he may have at his disposal. In general, when working with the gums, he uses one of three methods of preparation.

Dry Gum Method (Continental Method). This method involves the preparation of a concentrated emulsion or nucleus of oil, acacia and water by the following procedure. The acacia and the oil are placed in a dry Wedgwood or porcelain mortar, in the ratio of 4 parts by volume of fixed oil to 1 part by weight of acacia. When the acacia is thoroughly distributed throughout the oil, 2 parts by volume of water are added all at once, followed by rapid trituration until the emulsion is formed. This nucleus is triturated for at least 5 minutes, then the additional ingredients are added. Water-soluble ingredients should be dissolved in water and added to the nucleus in small amounts with constant trituration. Insoluble substances should be finely powdered and triturated with the nucleus. Alcohol should be diluted with water and added in small quantities. Oil-soluble substances are dissolved in the oil before the nucleus is made. Finally, the emulsion is transferred to a graduate and brought to volume with water.

When tragacanth or pectin are used in place of acacia $\frac{1}{10}$ the amount of each is required. The ratio for forming the nucleus becomes 4:2:0.1 instead of 4:2:1. With linseed oil or liquid petrolatum the ratio of oil to acacia is often a 3:1 ratio, making the primary emulsion or nucleus a 3:2:1 ratio.

Wet Gum Method (English or American Method). This procedure involves the preparation of a mucilage of acacia with water, usually in the same ratio as is used in the dry gum method. A smooth mucilage is made by triturating 1 part by weight of acacia to 2 parts by volume of water. If tragacanth or pectin is used, the ratio of gum to water becomes 1 to 20. If the gum is a fine powder, it may be wetted with a small amount of glycerin or alcohol to prevent lumping when the water is added.

After the mucilage is made, the oil is added in small increments with constant trituration until all is emulsified. The nucleus is now triturated for 5 minutes and diluted as described under the dry gum method. If, during the addition of the oil to the mucilage, the viscosity of the emulsion becomes too high, small amounts of water may be added to return to the original viscosity.

Bottle Method. The bottle method is merely a variation of the dry gum method, used with volatile oils. One part by weight of acacia is thoroughly mixed with 2 or 3 parts by volume of volatile oil by shaking in a bottle. Two parts by volume of water are added all at once and the shaking continued until the emulsion is formed. Other ingredients and the remainder of the water are added in small quantities with constant shaking.

MICROEMULSIONS

The pharmaceutical emulsions described thus far are termed *macro*-emulsions in that the particle size of the dispersed phase globules are seldom smaller than 0.5 micron in diameter. However, under proper conditions it is possible to prepare an emulsion system in which the diameter of the dispersed phase globules are in the range of 100 to 600 Å.[29a] Such an emulsion is referred to as a *micro*-emulsion.* These emulsions differ from macro-emulsions in that (1) they are thermodynamically stable, since a metastable, negative interfacial free energy (tension) exists between the two immiscible phases of the emulsion; (2) they are usually transparent, owing to the fact that the globule diameter of the internal phase is less than $\frac{1}{4}$ the wavelength of light, and (3) they are formed spontaneously without the necessity for homogenization.

In order to produce a micro-emulsion it is necessary to employ a high concentration (usually 10 to 40%) of emulsifiers so as to reduce the interfacial tension of the system to below zero.[26a] At present, this requirement has limited the pharmaceutical use of this type of emulsion because of the potential internal and/or external toxicity of high concentrations of emulsifiers. They have found some use in cosmetic preparations (e.g., clear hair dressings).

*Reference 26a should be consulted for a more detailed discussion of micro-emulsions.

ABSORPTION OF DRUGS FROM EMULSION DOSAGE FORMS

The gastrointestinal absorption characteristics of drugs from an emulsion dosage form have received scant attention in the literature, as compared to those of other types of dosage forms. An emulsion of the oil-in-water type is the one most appropriate for oral administration, and the in-vivo release of a lipid-soluble drug from such a vehicle depends primarily on the oil:water partition coefficient of the drug, the globule size and nature of the internal phase and, possibly, the nature and concentration of emulsifier employed in its preparation.

Wagner and co-workers[34b] studied the effect of dosage form on the serum levels of the lipid-soluble nonsteroidal anti-inflammatory agent indoxole, following its oral administration to human subjects. The emulsion dosage form, in which the drug was dissolved in the internal oleaginous phase, not only produced a significantly higher apparent serum concentration of drug, but also was apparently more completely available to the body as compared to the drug administered in an aqueous suspension or hard filled gelatin capsule. Similar results have been reported for emulsion systems containing sulfa drugs,[6a,10a,17a,23a,31a] and there is some indication that sustained plasma levels were also achieved.[6a,31a] A recent patent by Vogenthaler[34a] claims that the efficacy and the duration of therapeutic activity of water-soluble drugs are increased when the drugs are orally administered in a *special* emulsion as compared to either aqueous or lipid vehicles or a lipid-aqueous emulsion compounded in the conventional manner. The special emulsion referred to in the patent differs from the conventional emulsion in the method of preparation and in the fact that the former emulsion contains drug in both phases, whereas the conventional emulsion contains drug only in the oleaginous phase.

Although the exact mechanism by which the emulsion dosage form produces these desirable biologic effects has not been elucidated, it has been suggested, at least in the case of indoxole,[34b] that both the drug and the oil phase of the emulsion enter into the enterohepatic circulatory system, which increases the possibility for intestinal reabsorption of the drug.

Once suitably investigated, the emulsion dosage form may well prove to be an important vehicle for the oral delivery of certain pharmacologically important drugs.

PRESERVATION OF LIQUID DOSAGE FORMS CONTAINING INSOLUBLE MATTER

Molds, yeasts and bacteria find the aqueous phase of suspensions and emulsions a fine medium for growth. For this reason preservatives must be added to both solid-in-liquid and liquid-in-liquid dispersions which are to be stored for more than a few days.

Benzoic acid (0.1 to 0.2%), sodium benzoate (0.1 to 0.2%), alcohol (5 to 10%), phenylmercuric nitrate and acetate (1:10,000 to 1:25,000), phenol (0.5%), cresol (0.5%), chlorobutanol (0.5%), sorbic acid (0.2%) and the cationic quaternary ammonium compounds (1:10,000 to 1:50,000) have been used as antibacterial preservatives with varying degrees of success.

The most popular preservatives, because they are active against bacteria, yeasts and molds, have been the parahydroxybenzoic acid esters: butylparahydroxybenzoate (butylparaben 0.02%), methylparahydroxybenzoate (methylparaben) and propylparahydroxybenzoate (propylparaben). A combination of methylparaben 0.2 per cent and propylparaben 0.02 per cent seems to be the mixture of choice.

In the use of preservatives, consideration must be given to the possibility of a reaction occurring between the substance used as a preservative and the suspending agent or the emulsifier that may inactivate the preservative. The result may be the formation of an inactive complex or an ionic reaction.

It has been shown[32] that complex formation takes place between methylcellulose and the parahydroxybenzoic acid esters. Barr and Tice[4] reported the growth of micro-organisms in the presence of surfactants containing polyether groups. A large number of nonionic surfactants used in pharmaceuticals belong to this class. These substances also tend to form complexes. The investigators reported that sorbic acid 0.2 per cent proved to be a satisfactory preservative.

With the use of polymeric substances—natural and synthetic—as suspending and emulsifying agents, care must be taken to select a preservative for a particular system to avoid possible inactivation of the preservative.

PACKAGING, DISPENSING AND STORAGE OF LIQUID DOSAGE FORMS CONTAINING INSOLUBLE MATTER

All suspensions and emulsions are heterogeneous and should be dispensed with a "shake well" label. They should be stored in a manner to prevent freezing or exposure to high temperature. If they are not sensitive to light, they may be dispensed in clear glass. When suspensions and emulsions are viscous, wide-mouth bottles should be used. It is often advantageous to package dermatologic prescriptions in polyethylene squeeze bottles.

REFERENCES

1. Atkinson, R. M., Bedford, C., Child, K. J., and Tomich, E. G.: Antibiotics and Chemotherapy 12:232, 1962.
2. Avis, K. E.: Remington's Pharmaceutical Sciencies. ed. 13. p. 498. Mack, Easton, Pa., 1965.
3. Ballard, B. E., and Nelson, E.: Remington's Pharmaceutical Sciences. ed. 13. p. 627. Mack, Easton, Pa., 1965.
4. Barr, M., and Tice, L. F.: J. Am. Pharm. Assoc. (Sci.), 46:442, 445, 1957.
5. Battista, O. A., and Smith, P. A.: Ind. and Eng. Chem., 54:20, 1962.
6. Bollinger, von Marie, and Munzel, K.: Pharm. acta helv., 34:79, 1959.
6a. Daeschner, C. W., Bell, W. R., Stivrins, P. C., Yow, E. M., and Townsend, E.: A.M.A. Arch. Dis. Child., 93:370, 1957.
7. Fleming, W., and Wolf, M.: Am. J. Syphilis, Gonorrhea and Venereal Dis., 30:47, 1946.
8. Greengard, R. and Wooley, J. G.: J. Biol. Chem., 132:83, 1940.
9. Griffin, W. C.: J. Soc. Cos. Chem., 1:311, 1949.
10. ———: J. Soc. Cos. Chem., 5:1, 1954.
10a. Hagler, S., Kaufman, A., Kaiser, E., Lillien, M., and McClain, H.: J. Pediat., 50:16, 1957.
11. Haines, B. A., Jr., and Martin, A. N.: J. Pharm. Sci. 50:228, 1961.
12. ———: J. Pharm. Sci. 50:753, 1961.
13. ———: J. Pharm. Sci. 50:756, 1961.
14. Hiestand, E. N.: J. Pharm. Sci., 53:1, 1964.
15. Higuchi, T.: J. Am. Pharm. Assoc. (Sci.), 48:657, 1958.
16. Hospital Formulary, Hamilton, Illinois, The Hamilton Press, 1959.
17. Kraml, M., Dubuc, J., and Gaudry, R.: Antibiotics and Chemotherapy, 12:239, 1962.
17a. Krugman, S.: Ann. N. Y. Acad. Sci., 69:399, 1957.
18. Lafferty, G., and Gross, H.: J. Am. Pharm. Assoc. (Sci.), 44:212, 1955.
19. Laug, P., Vos, E., and Kunze, F.: J. Pharmacol. Exp. Ther., 89:52, 1947.
20. Lichtin, J. L., and Lichtin, A.: J. Am. Pharm. Assoc. (Pract.), 14:295, 1953.
21. MacDonald, L., and Himmlick, R. J.: J. Am. Pharm. Assoc. (Sci.), 37:368, 1948.
22. Macek, T. J.: J. Pharm. Sci., 52:694, 1963.
23. Martin, A. N.: Physical Pharmacy. Lea & Febiger, Philadelphia, 1960.
23a. May, C. N., and Hassler, W. H.: Bull. Am. Soc. Hosp. Pharmacists, 14:419, 1957.
24. Nakashima, J. Y., and Miller, O. H.: J. Am. Pharm. Assoc. (Pract.), 16:496, 1955.
25. Nash, R. A.: Drug and Cos. Ind., 97(6):843, 1965.
26. Osborne, G. E., and DeKay, H. G.: J. Am. Pharm. Assoc. (Pract.), 2:420, 1941.
26a. Osipow, L. I.: Surface Chemistry, Theory and Industrial Applications. pp. 337-341. New York, Reinhold, 1962.
27. Overbeek, J. Th. G.: Colloid Science. vol. 1. p. 1331. New York, Elsevier, 1952.
28. Polyglycol Esters, Kessler Chemical Company, Philadelphia.
29. Reinhold, J. G., Phillips, F. J., Flippin, H. F., and Pollack, L.: Am. J. Med. Sci., 210:141, 1945.
29a. Schulman, J. H., and Montagne, J. B.: Ann. N.Y. Acad. Sci., 92:366, 1961.
30. Schwarz, T. W., and Levy, G.: J. Am. Pharm. Assoc. (Sci.), 47:442, 1958.
31. Schwarz, T. W., Levy, G., and Kawagoe, H. H.: J. Am. Pharm. Assoc. (Sci.), 47:695, 1958.
31a. Svenson, S. E., et al.: Antibiot. Med., 2:148, 1956.
32. Tillman, W. J., and Kuramoto, R.: J. Am. Pharm. Assoc. (Sci.), 46:211, 1957.

33. Typical Pharmaceutical Formulations for Topical Application, Atlas Chemical Company, Wilmington, Delaware, 1960.

34. Vicher, E., Snyder, R., and Gathercoal, E. J.: J. Am. Pharm. Assoc. (Sci.), *26*: 1241, 1937.

34a. Vogenthaler, C. A.: U.S. Patent No. 3,238,103, 1966.

34b. Wagner, J. G., Gerard, E. S., and Kaiser, D. G.: Clin. Pharmacol. Therap., *7*:610, 1966.

Chapter 6

Semisolid Dosage Forms

Seymour Blaug, Ph.D.*

The terms salve, ointment and cream indicate preparations that have in common the property of being semisolids which are spread easily on the skin. While these terms are sometimes used interchangeably, they are at other times used to represent gradations in viscosity, the salve being considered most viscous, the ointment less and the cream least.

Semisolid dosage forms include primarily those preparations to be applied to cutaneous tissue, such as ointments, cerates, creams, jellies, pastes, plasters and poultices.

A dermatologic prescription is usually applied to highly sensitive, diseased or denuded areas, and the application of such a prescription requires the patient's cooperation. Therefore, such preparations should be easily applied and should be prepared so that the completed product is not grainy to the touch.

Ointments constitute one of the oldest forms of dermatologic therapy. Zopf[95] gives a brief history of the development of the modern ointment.

It is interesting to note that in the 1968 National Prescription Audit conducted by R. A. Gosselin and Company, dermatologics rank second (oral medications are first) in frequency prescribed, based on the volume of new prescriptions reported. Ten other dosage forms—ophthalmics, parenterals, etc.—are ranked below dermatologic medications.

An ointment has been defined as a "fatty preparation of such consistency as to be easily applied to the skin with rubbing." Our present concept of an ointment is much broader: ointments are soft, semisolid preparations intended for application to cutaneous tissue

* Professor of Pharmacy, College of Pharmacy, The University of Iowa.

with or without inunction. They may be entirely free of oleaginous materials. Because of their physical properties they are used in dermatologic therapy for three purposes: (1) as lubricating agents (emollients); (2) as vehicles in which to incorporate drugs required to treat skin disorders; and (3) as protective coverings to prevent contact of the skin surface with chemicals, aqueous solutions and some organic solvents.

There are several factors which influence the selection of the type of preparation to be used topically. Among these factors are the diagnosis, the effect desired, the condition of the patient and the area or areas to be treated. The selection of base for the extemporaneous preparation of an ointment is the privilege of the physician. However, it is the responsibility of the pharmacist to prepare products that are pharmaceutically correct. In exercising this responsibility the pharmacist may generally make minor changes necessary for the preparation of a superior product. This may involve the use of small amounts of inert materials as levigating and/or solubilizing agents. However, the pharmacist must be certain that the levigating or solubilizing agent does not interact or interfere with the active ingredient and is not considered to be a sensitizing agent. For example, some physicians may consider lanolin, used occasionally as a levigating agent or for its hydrophilic value, as a skin sensitizer. Blaug et al.[11,12,18] have shown that many agents used as solubilizers or as dispersing agents interact with preservatives and active ingredients commonly used in semisolid dosage forms.

It is most important that the pharmacist consult with the physician before changing the type of base or the form of an active constituent in a dermatologic prescription. Alteration from an oleaginous base to an emulsion base may effect the absorption and percutaneous action of the active ingredient necessitating either an increase or decrease in concentration of the therapeutic agent.

EFFECTS OF LOCALLY APPLIED DRUGS

Topical medication is prescribed to produce a specific beneficial effect. The principal effects of most substances applied to the skin are indicated by their generic names.

Antipruritic agents relieve itching in various ways. Commonly used agents and strengths include menthol 0.25 per cent, phenol 0.5 per cent, camphor 2 per cent and coal tar 2 to 10 per cent.

Keratoplastic agents tend to increase the thickness of the horny layer. Salicylic acid 1 to 2 per cent is an example of a keratoplastic agent, whereas stronger strengths of salicylic acid are keratolytic.

Keratolytic agents remove or soften the horny layer. Commonly used agents of this type include salicylic acid 4 to 10 per cent, resorcinol 2 to 4 per cent and sulfur 4 to 10 per cent. A strong destructive agent is trichloracetic acid, full strength.

Antieczematous agents remove oozing and vesicular excretions by various actions. Some may act as protectives, keratolytics and antipruritics. The common antieczematous agents include 2 per cent boric acid solution packs or soaks, coal tar solution 2 to 5 per cent and hydrocortisone and derivatives 0.5 to 1 per cent incorporated in lotions and ointments.

Antiparasitics destroy or inhibit living infestations. Agents of this type include benzyl benzoate 10 to 30 per cent emulsion or lotion, sulfur ointments, n-ethyl-o-crotonotoluidine 10 per cent (Eurax Cream)[*] and gamma benzene hexachloride 1 per cent (Kwell Ointment)[†].

Antibacterial and Antifungal Agents destroy or inhibit bacteria and fungi. Commonly used agents include iodochlorhydroxyquin 3 per cent (Vioform Cream and Oint-

ment)[‡] and antibiotics such as bacitracin 500 units/Gm., tetracycline hydrochloride ointment 3 per cent, and Chloromycetin Cream.[§] Antifungal agents include Benzoic and Salicylic Acid Ointment, undecylenic acid and zinc undecylenate in various bases, tolnaftate cream 1 percent (Tinactin Cream)[||] and nystatin cream 100,000 units/Gm. (Mycostatin Cream).[#]

Antiseborrheics are agents that alleviate seborrhea (excessive discharge of sebum from the glands) by various actions, i.e., antipruritics. Examples are ammoniated mercury 2 to 10 per cent, coal tar 1 to 5 per cent, ichthammol 4 to 10 per cent, resorcinol and sulfur ointments, salicylic acid ointments.

Emollients are agents that soften the skin surface. Mineral oil, white petrolatum, cold creams and w/o emulsion bases are examples of such agents. However, recent investigations by Blank[4] with callus tissue have revealed that the water content of the stratum corneum is probably the prime factor in determining its softness and flexibility. In living skin, moisture is continuously reaching the stratum corneum (outermost layer of the epidermis) and being evaporated off the surface of the skin as "insensible perspiration."[77] One source of this moisture supply is the tiny orifices of the eccrine glands (small sweat glands opening directly onto the skin surface). The second source is through the transepidermal transport of moisture but its source is still the subject of discussion.[77] Mali[53] demonstrated the existence of a barrier membrane lying just below the stratum corneum which limits the amount of transepidermal moisture which can reach the outer layer of the skin, thus confirming earlier studies of Blank.[5] This moisture reaching the stratum corneum is in the main evaporated into the atmosphere but a small percentage is retained in the stratum corneum, accounting for its softness and flexibility. It has been demonstrated[10,30] that there is present in the stratum corneum a water-extractable nitrogenous material capable of binding up to 3 times its weight in water. Should there be a

[*] Geigy Chemical Corporation, Yonkers, New York.
[†] Reed and Carnrick, Kenilworth, New Jersey.
[‡] Ciba Pharmaceutical Products, Inc., Summit, New Jersey.
[§] Parke Davis and Co., Detroit, Michigan.
[||] Schering Corporation, Bloomfield, N. J.
[#] E. R. Squibb and Sons, N. Y.

deficiency of water-binding material in the stratum corneum, a dry skin condition may result.

Excessive moisture loss can occur when the water vapor pressure in the surrounding atmosphere is extremely low, such as exists under low relative humidity conditions especially on cold, windy days.

Blank[4] and Peck[68] have shown that oleaginous materials such as mineral oil and lanolin per se do not soften dead, dried and callus tissue. However, the action of these materials may be different on living skin.[6]

Oleaginous materials may act as skin softeners by retarding moisture evaporation from the surface of the skin by forming an occlusive film which retards moisture evaporation. Materials that absorb moisture from the air and add such moisture to the stratum corneum or materials that retard moisture loss from the skin by virtue of their emulsifying ability may be classified as moisturizing agents in that they aid in increasing moisture content and hence the softness of the skin.

Protectives are agents that protect the skin against moisture, air and chemicals. Petrolatum, zinc oxide ointment, starch ointment and silicone ointments and lotions frequently are so employed. Water-removable emulsion bases do not protect the skin very well against aqueous solutions. However, sunscreening agents that filter out ultraviolet rays may be incorporated in various types of dermatologic vehicles. The protective agent in this case would be the active ingredient, not the base.

CLASSIFICATION OF OINTMENTS

Ointments are usually classified according to their composition and/or their therapeutic action, based on their degree of penetration on application to the skin.

Based on composition, ointments can be classified as follows:

1. Oleaginous or Hydrocarbon Base-
    Petrolatum, fixed oils of vegetable origin, mixtures of petrolatum with wax or other stiffening agents, oils of animal origin, such as lard and silicones
    A. Anhydrous
    B. Nonhydrophilic
    C. Insoluble in water
    D. Not water removable

2. Absorption Base
    Hydrophilic bases such as Anhydrous Lanolin and Hydrophilic Petrolatum
    A. Anhydrous
    B. Hydrophilic
    C. Insoluble in water
    D. Not water removable
    Hydrous (Emulsion Base, w/o)—Lanolin, Rose Water Ointment, Cold Cream
    A. Hydrous
    B. Hydrophilic
    C. Insoluble in water
    D. Not water removable
    E. Water-in-oil emulsion

3. Emulsion Base (o/w)
    Hydrophilic Ointment, vanishing creams
    A. Hydrous
    B. Hydrophilic
    C. Insoluble in water
    D. Water removable
    E. Oil-in-water emulsion

4. Water Soluble Base
    Polyethylene Glycol Ointment
    A. Anhydrous
    B. Hydrophilic
    C. Water soluble
    D. Water removable
    E. Greaseless

Goodman[32] classified ointments according to their degree of penetration on application to the skin as:

1. Epidermatic ointments, or those which demonstrate little or no power of penetration into the skin. This group includes the oleaginous and the hydrocarbon bases.

2. Endodermatic ointments, or those which possess some power of penetration into the skin. Lard, lanolin and vegetable oils are included in this group.

3. Diadermatic ointments, or those which penetrate the skin permitting or encouraging systemic absorption of active constituents incorporated in the base. Emulsion type and water-soluble bases belong to this class. This classification is not sound because absorption can occur from any ointment base depending on the solubility of the medicant, the extent of hydration and the condition of the skin (cut, abraded, eczematous etc.).

Lane and Blank[45] have classified ointments and dermatologic vehicles according to physical differences between the vehicles, i.e., aqueous vehicles, e.g., water, aqueous lotions; vehicles which act as oils, e.g., petrolatum, wool fat, pastes; vehicles which act as powders, e.g., starch, talc; vehicles which act as organic solvents, e.g., alcohol, ether, acetone.

GENERAL INDICATIONS FOR OINTMENT BASES

It is not possible to list completely the specific vehicle in which to incorporate a particular drug for the best treatment of a given disorder. However, the pharmacist should be able to recommend to the general practitioner or the dermatologist the type of base that can be used to produce a stable antibiotic ointment, or that can be used as a skin lubricant or as a vehicle to be used on the scalp. He should also have a general knowledge of the factors that promote the absorption of drugs from ointments and other semisolid dosage forms. Generally, the o/w emulsion bases or water-soluble bases are indicated when vehicles which are water removable and not greasy to the touch are desired. As vehicles for medication to be applied to the scalp, they are most suitable because they can be easily washed out of the hair. They may be preferred for cosmetic reasons.

Water-in-oil emulsion bases form relatively occlusive oil films on the skin surface. They are little affected by atmospheric conditions and exchange water vapor slowly. They are not very miscible with sweat. Consequently, they promote the accumulation of sweat at the skin-vehicle interface producing hydration of the skin surface. Hence, water-in-oil emulsions are used to provide lubrication and are especially indicated when the skin is dry. Oleaginous vehicles differ from water-in-oil emulsions in the occlusiveness of the film formed on the skin surface.

Oleaginous vehicles are also indicated when skin lubrication and hydration are desired, since, like water-in-oil emulsions, they form occlusive oil films on the skin surface. They differ from water-in-oil emulsions only in the exaggeration of this occlusive character.

For most antibiotics, inert oleaginous or anhydrous w/o emulsion bases offer greater stability than o/w emulsion bases or the water miscible, hygroscopic bases.

The nonvolatile water-miscible vehicles such as Polyethylene Glycol Ointment are freely miscible with sweat. They will not soften dry skin, since they do not retard the evaporation of sweat; hence, they maintain the least hydration at the skin-vehicle interface. This is especially true when the relative humidity is low. However, such vehicles are useful when water removability is desired, such as for application to hairy regions.

EFFECTS OF VEHICLES ON THE SKIN

Hydration of the Skin. A large percentage of topical preparations are used solely for their physical effect on the skin surface, such as the control of hydration. Other topical preparations are used as vehicles, and their primary function is to deliver an incorporated medicament to a certain area of the skin. Before discussing the effect of the vehicle on drug diffusion and penetration, let us consider the role of the vehicle or base on the degree of hydration induced in the stratum corneum.

The stratum corneum or horny layer of the epidermis is the outermost layer of the skin. It is made up of stratified layers of dead keratinized cells that are constantly being shed. The chemical protein in these cells, keratin, is hygroscopic and softens when it contains sufficient water. This water diffuses from inner layers of the skin and may be taken up from the atmosphere under certain conditions. Monash and Blank[60] and Monash[59] have demonstrated that the inner two thirds of the stratum corneum constitutes the main barrier to water loss, and that the outer one half to two thirds of the stratum corneum is the main barrier to percutaneous penetration. The thickness of this outer keratin area differs in different parts of the body according to the degree of protection required, being thickest on the palms of the hands and the soles of the feet. Hence, penetration may proceed at a slower rate through skin areas with a thicker layer of outer keratin, being drastically reduced through the palms and the soles. On the other hand, the outer keratin area is exceptionally thin on the face, a point to be remembered in considering the possible penetration of cosmetic materials.

The degree of hydration induced in the stratum corneum is one of the more important characteristics of a vehicle or other topical preparation. As the permeability to water vapor of the ointment or the lotion film on the skin increases, there is a corresponding decrease in the degree of equilibrium hydration induced in the stratum corneum.

Oleaginous vehicles are the most occlusive and induce the greatest hydration of the stratum corneum through sweat accumulation. Oleaginous vehicles containing a lipophilic surfactant, such as anhydrous water-in-oil emulsion vehicles, are somewhat less occlusive.

Oil-in-water emulsions probably show the greatest variation in permeability to water vapor. This is due to the greater variety of ingredients in such formulations. Shelmire[80] has shown that a basic formula (oil, surfactant and water) for an oil-in-water emulsion vehicle will not produce a film of maximum water-retaining capacity unless a fourth substance is added, usually one of the long-chain saturated alcohols, esters or acids. As the outer phase of an oil-in-water emulsion evaporates from the skin the emulsion tends to invert, leaving a continuous oil film containing other dissolved or suspended substances. The long-chain alcohols, esters and acids dissolved or suspended in the oil probably increase the viscosity and the cohesion of the oil film, thus inhibiting the evaporation of water from the skin surface.

Powers and Fox[73] studied the effect of representative fatty materials, humectants and emulsifiers on rate of moisture loss from the skin. The materials which retarded moisture loss from the skin most effectively were primarily the water-insoluble non-surface-active fatty or oily compounds. This type of compound forms a semiocclusive barrier on the surface of the skin, thus retarding the rate of water evaporation.

Surfactants used in oil-in-water emulsions had little effect in influencing the rate of moisture loss from the skin.

Glycerin and propylene glycol, used in many emulsion formulations, consistently increased the amount of moisture lost to a dry atmosphere. Although these humectants will decrease the rate of water loss from the vehicle itself and prevent crust formation, they will actually increase the rate of water loss from the stratum corneum. Certain of the water-soluble polyoxyethylene esters and ethers also did this. Humectants and polyoxyethylene esters and ethers may accelerate water loss by drawing moisture from within the skin to the surface under dry or low humidity conditions. They may also interfere with the rigidity of the final oil film on the skin and probably interfere with inversion of an oil-in-water emulsion.

Water-soluble vehicles such as Polyethylene Glycol Ointment do not wet the skin and do not retard the evaporation of water from the stratum corneum; hence, they produce the least change in hydration from the time of application until equilibrium.

In summary, water-containing vehicles wet the skin initially, but the degree of hydration decreases as the aqueous phase evaporates. Although oleaginous vehicles do not wet the skin initially, they do produce a steady increase in hydration as moisture is prevented from evaporating by the occlusive oil film.

GENERAL FACTORS AFFECTING PERCUTANEOUS ABSORPTION

Percutaneous Absorption. Any discussion of semisolid dosage forms must start with a consideration of how drugs penetrate the skin. In order to determine how drugs penetrate the skin one must examine: (1) the functions and physiology of the skin, and (2) factors influencing penetration of the skin.

FUNCTIONS AND PHYSIOLOGY OF THE SKIN. One can divide the functions into those related to the skin as a protective covering for the body and those related to the skin as a barrier to topically applied medicated applications.

Wells and Lubowe[93] and Tregear[91] have reviewed the physical functions of the skin. Among the functions performed by the skin are respiration and heat regulation, sebum and sweat production, acting as a barrier to allergens, irritants and bacteria, and regulating water balance of the body through perspiration.

The skin is a complex organ that is estimated to have, in the average man, a total surface area of 18 square feet. According to Lubowe,[48] each square inch of skin is liber-

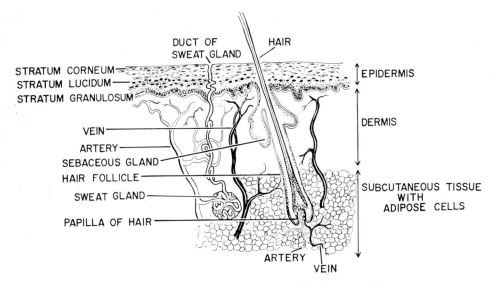

FIG. 6-1. Vertical section of human skin (schematic).

ally endowed with nerves, sweat glands, blood vessels, sensory apparatuses for heat and cold, sensory cells, sebaceous glands, hairs, muscles and cells, nerve endings to record pain, and pressure apparatuses for the sense of touch.

The structure of adult human skin is very complex. It can be conveniently classified into three layers: (1) the epidermis (cuticle), (2) the dermis (corium or true skin), and (3) the subcutaneous tissue (hypoderm).

The third layer is often considered as a part of the dermis and consists of subcutaneous fibrous tissue and adipose cells. A vertical section of the skin is shown schematically in Figure 6-1.

Because the epidermis is the external or outer surface of the skin it is the site of application of cosmetics and medicated topical preparations and, hence, is of particular interest to pharmacists and dermatologists. The epidermis varies in thickness from about 1 mm. on the palms of the hands and soles of the feet to about 0.1 mm. or less on parts of the face and body. It is covered with a surface film composed of emulsified lipids. The film is discontinuous and offers little resistance to penetrating molecules.[33]

Histologists classify the epidermis into five layers:

1. Stratum corneum, or horny layer.

2. Stratum lucidum, sometimes called the "barrier layer."
3. Stratum granulosum, or granular layer.
4. Stratum malpighii, the prickle cell layer.
5. Stratum germinativum, the basal cell layer.

It should be remembered that these subdivisions represent changes in cell structure as one moves toward the surface rather than distinct separate layers. The layers merge into one another almost imperceptibly.

The stratum corneum, or horny layer, consists of several layers of flattened cells composed of keratin. This layer is thickest on the soles of the feet and palms of the hands (0.6 to 0.8 mm.) and is exceptionally thin on the face.

The horny layer is a tough and relatively insensitive layer that is continuously being shed and being replaced. "Dead" cells, which are constantly being shed, are replaced by the cornification of other cells that are evolved from the germinal, or basal, layer and proliferated or pushed up from below. The chemical composition of stratum corneum is protein, 85% (approximately 15% water soluble, 65% keratin or cytoplasmic protein and 5% membrane protein); lipid, 7-9% (C_{16}-C_{18} saturated and unsaturated free acids and esters, tri-glycerides and cholesterol and related sterols); other, 6-8% (mucopolysac- charides, carbohydrate, mucins, lipo amino acids, etc.).

The lipid film covering the stratum corneum usually has a pH of 4.5 to 6.5, according to the region tested, with the pH in females usually being slightly higher (less acid) than in males.[61] Drastic alteration of the pH of this so-called "acid mantle" may lower the ability of the skin to resist bacterial attack. Jacobi and Heinrich[38] refer to the acid mantle of the skin as the first line of the body's defense against external influences.

Peck et al.[67,69] pointed out that acidity per se does not make the acid mantle a bar- rier to bacterial and fungal attack. The bac- teriostatic character of the acid mantle is probably associated with the type of acids found in the acid mantle of the skin, as well as the buffer capacity of the acid mantle. Pers- piration and sebum have fungistatic and bac- teriostatic properties associated with their lower fatty acids and long chain unsaturated fatty acids. The buffering capacity of the skin is probably associated with the presence of free amino acids, protein debris, fatty acids, lactic acid, and bicarbonates and lactates.

Because the horny layer is composed largely of keratin, a protein that absorbs large quantities of water and other polar com- pounds, it may become a reservoir for pene- trating agents, thereby maintaining a maxi- mum concentration gradient just above the stratum lucidum. Penetrants such as ions and dyes may be bound by the stratum corneum thus hindering their penetration beyond the orifices of the hair follicles.[7,33]

The capacity of epidermal keratin to ab- sorb water may affect penetration in another way. When the horny layer is well hydrated, hydrophilic and hydrophobic compounds can penetrate to the stratum lucidum more read- ily. Thus, the percutaneous absorption of some compounds may be increased by phar- maceutical formulations that produce an oc- clusive film on the skin surface. Covering the skin with an occlusive dressing, such as wrapping with a plastic film, is likely to pro- duce a higher degree of occlusion than can be obtained with ointments. The effect of oc- clusion is related to better hydration of the stratum corneum and to an increase in the surface temperature of the skin. McKenzie

and Stoughton[52] have shown that the minimal effective concentration of topically applied corticosteroids is markedly reduced when the site of application is occluded.

The outer layers of flattened keratinized cells in the stratum corneum are thought by some to be less densely packed than those ad- jacent to the underlying granular layer. This led to the designation of the region between the stratum corneum and the granular layer (the stratum lucidum) as a "barrier zone." This zone, which is several microns thick, is reported to act as a barrier to the transfer of water across the skin.[5,78] The "barrier zone" reportedly[92] prevents the penetration of mole- cules having molecular weights greater than 200 or 300. The existence of a "barrier zone" has not been proved conclusively, and most theories pertaining to percutaneous absorp- tion consider the entire stratum corneum as a compactly packed layer (10 to 50 microns thick) that acts as the major barrier to pene- tration. After penetrating the stratum cor- neum the penetrant is exposed to the 200- micron-thick layer of living tissue, the dermis, which can be a formidable barrier for non- polar molecules because of its aqueous char- acteristics. Therefore, molecules that pene- trate the stratum corneum either are bound in the lower epidermis or the dermis, or are carried away by the tissue fluids in the dermis to the blood vessels and lymphatics.[33]

Tregear[9] believes that the evidence to sup- port the existence of a barrier zone at the base of the stratum corneum is not conclusive, because, if such a layer is present, one would expect a more critical change of permeability with stripping of the outer layers of the skin and a definite relation of penetrant solubility to permeability.

Kligman[41] has proposed that the entire horny layer is involved in barrier function. This view is receiving acceptance by other investigators and has been re-emphasized by Scheuplein.[79] Matoltsy et al.[56] offer evidence suggesting that the plasma membrane pro- teins of the horny cells may also take part in barrier function.

The innermost layer of the epidermis—the stratum germinativum, or basal cell layer— is the reproductive layer. In this layer the cells are constantly undergoing mitosis, the daughter cells gradually progressing toward the skin surface. As such cells migrate, they change in shape and composition until they become the horny cells of the stratum corneum.

The dermis, or true skin, differs morphologically from the epidermis. The dermis consists of dense fibrous tissue together with blood and lymph vessels, hair follicles, sebaceous and sweat glands, and muscle and nerve fibers. As an aqueous layer, it probably acts as a barrier to the passage of nonpolar molecules.

POSSIBLE AVENUES OF PENETRATION. Griesemer[33] describes the possible avenues of penetration into and through the unbroken skin as: (1) between the cells of the stratum corneum, (2) through the walls of the hair follicles, (3) through the sweat glands, (4) through the sebaceous glands, and (5) through the cells of the stratum corneum.

Tregear[89] concludes that the route of entry of substances into and through the skin is the epidermis itself, the penetrant moving between the cells and possibly through them rather than through the accessory structures, i.e., hair follicles and sweat glands. He regards the resistance to this entry as a property of the keratinized cell matrix of the epidermis, uncomplicated by "active processes." The removal of keratinized cells from human skin by repeatedly stripping the skin with adhesive tape has been shown to make the skin more permeable than normal skin to water,[5] local anesthetics[59] and endogenous ions.[46] Each stripping either removes some of the impermeable material and/or disturbs it at a lower level. As the last few layers of stratified cells are removed by successive strippings, the permeability of the remaining skin is greatly increased. This increase may be due to the reduction in the thickness of the remaining skin, and/or it may indicate that the lower layers of the stratum corneum removed by stripping are the least permeable of the layers removed. According to Marzulli,[55] the membranes removed by stripping sometimes have an impermeability as great, or nearly as great, as that of the whole skin.

FACTORS INFLUENCING PENETRATION. The following factors must be considered in any discussion of percutaneous absorption: (1) skin condition, (2) solubility of penetrant, (3) concentration of penetrant, (4) skin hydration, (5) the vehicle, (6) solvents, and (7) other factors.

Skin Condition. Damage to the skin, such as that caused by scratches, blisters, cuts etc., and skin modifying processes, such as eczema and hyperemia, are known to affect permeability—i.e., there is a marked increase in the penetration of drugs following such trauma.[8,33] Treatment of the skin with keratolytics or with organic solvents such as acetone, alcohol or hexane may increase the permeability of the epidermis to water, the effect varying with the keratolytic agent used and the length of time the epidermis is exposed to the organic solvent.[65,91]

Solubility of Penetrant. The solubility characteristics of a penetrant are probably of more importance than molecular size in determining its ability to penetrate the skin, although molecular size does play some part in determining the rate of penetration of a substance through the skin. Molecules as small as helium pass through the skin very rapidly, whereas large molecules such as human serum albumin pass through the skin very slowly.[43,90] According to Tregear,[91] within a narrow range of molecular size there is no correlation between size and penetration rate.

Treherne,[92] using excised human skin, related the permeability constants of a series of compounds to their ether/water partition coefficients. He suggested that skin penetration might be favored by a partition coefficient of one or nearly one. Higuchi[35] also pointed out the importance to percutaneous absorption of such factors as the distribution coefficient of the penetrant between the vehicle and the barrier of the skin, and the solubility of the penetrant in the vehicle.

Using a vasoconstrictor assay, McKenzie and Aitkinson[51] studied the topical activity of betamethasone and 23 esters of betamethasone. The results of their study can be related to the lipid/water partition coefficients of the esters—i.e., activity decreased as the esters became more lipid-soluble and less water-soluble. Similarly, activity decreased when the esters were more soluble in water and less soluble in lipids.

Concentration of Penetrant. Shelmire[81] found that the major factors affecting the total penetration from medicated applications are skin hydration, concentration of the penetrant and its state of solution in the vehicle, and contact time of the medicated preparation on the skin.

According to Higuchi,[35] for all penetrants the rate of penetration is controlled by the lack of permeability of the skin. If one assumes that the vehicle containing the penetrant does not appreciably affect the skin, then the rate of percutaneous penetration is maximum for penetrants possessing the highest possible thermodynamic potential. If the thermodynamic activity of the penetrant in different vehicles were maintained constant, then the rate of percutaneous penetration from the different vehicles would be approximately constant. However, the thermodynamic activity of the penetrant in a vehicle is not constant. It varies with the solvent properties of the vehicle for the penetrant and the concentration of the penetrant. Thus, all vehicles containing the penetrant in suspension (system has solid drug in equilibrium with that in true solution) do not produce the same rate of penetration because, although at saturation the escaping tendency for a molecule becomes fixed, the total number of molecules in solution varies with the solvent properties of the vehicles for the penetrant. The total number of molecules in solution is an important factor because the flux in a given direction through a membrane (the skin) depends on the concentration (strictly speaking, the activity) in the phase of origin (the vehicle). The activity increases up to saturation of the vehicle. Activity is the im-

portant factor rather than any absolute concentration, and therefore, for a given concentration of the penetrant, vehicles that have a lower affinity for the penetrant normally produce faster penetration when the solubility is exceeded in all vehicles. Reduction of particle size of the suspended penetrant improves its penetration.[3]

Higuchi[35] points out that large concentration gradients may develop in the ointment phase (the rate-controlling step is in the applied phase rather than in the skin barrier), such as develop in cases involving absorption by injured skin or where highly insoluble penetrants are suspended in ointment bases. In his mathematical treatment of the latter instances, Higuchi shows that the rate of release of penetrants from such suspension type ointments can be regulated by controlling the penetrant concentration, the solubility of the penetrant (if a partly aqueous base is used, the solubility can be varied by changing the effective pH of the vehicle for insoluble acidic and basic drugs), and the diffusion constant of the penetrant in the vehicle (a decrease in the viscosity of the vehicle should yield an increased diffusion coefficient for the drug).

Skin Hydration. Higuchi[35] states that because water is particularly well absorbed by protein and protein degradation products contained in the outer skin, the transfer properties of the several layers are probably strongly influenced by the presence of water. Using glyceryl monostearate as the penetrant and artificial membranes as barriers, Higuchi

TABLE 6-1. EXPERIMENTAL EXCRETION RATES AND OTHER PHYSICAL CONSTANTS OF THE TEST PENETRANTS*

No.		GLYCOL SALICYLATE	METHYL SALICYLATE	ETHYL SALICYLATE
1.	Hydrous system rate (moles/100 cm²/hr.) calculated as the salicylate ester	11.7	8.6	2.9
2.	Anhydrous system rate (moles/100 cm²/hr.) calculated as the salicylate ester	1.3	2.7	1.5
3.	$\dfrac{\text{Rate hydrous system}}{\text{Rate anhydrous system}}$	9.0	3.2	2.0
4.	Per cent water solubility	1.27	0.08	0.03
5.	Distribution coefficient (olive oil/water)	7.7	343	1,170
6.	Relative distribution coefficient (glycol salicylate 1)	1	45	152

*From J. Pharm. Sci. *50*:291 (1961).

demonstrated the relationship between permeability and relative humidity. At low humidities permeability was relatively insensitive to relative humidity whereas, at relative humidities near 100 per cent, the rate of penetration was very dependent on water activity. He attributed this to imbibition of water by the barrier phase exposed to saturated water vapor and consequent changes in both the diffusion coefficient and activity coefficient of the penetrant.

Shelmire[80,81] concludes that the two important factors in determining the rate of diffusion of penetrant from the vehicle to the skin surface are the degree of hydration at the skin-vehicle interface, and the miscibility of the vehicle with the skin secretions.

Using an absorption cell attached to the forearm of human subjects, Wurster and Kramer[94] studied the absorption of three salicylate esters under hydrous and anhydrous skin conditions. As shown in Table 6-1, the absorption rates for the three drugs can be related to their distribution coefficients and their per cent solubility in water. As the distribution coefficient decreased, the absorption rate increased under hydrous conditions. The rates shown in Nos. 1 and 2 are for 100 sq. cm. of skin surface. Wurster and Kramer[94] demonstrated that the excretion rate is directly proportional to the area of skin surface through which the salicylate diffuses. No. 3 expresses the ratio of the rate in the hydrous system to the rate in the anhydrous system. The ratio shows the increase in rate produced by hydration. This ratio decreases with the decreasing solubility of the salicylate. Urinary salicylate was determined at various time intervals and plotted against time. Figures 6-2 to 6-4 show that for the three salicylates studied the absorption was greater when a hydrous skin condition was maintained.

The Vehicle. Medical and pharmaceutical literature is replete with conflicting reports on the importance of the vehicle in the percutaneous absorption of penetrants. Barr,[1] in his review article on percutaneous absorption, discusses some of these conflicting reports. One should bear in mind that many percutaneous absorption studies are carried out in animals whose skin permeability may differ considerably from that of man. For example, although the hair follicles are not considered an important route of entry for penetrants in man, most mammals have many more hairs per square centimeter of skin than does man. Therefore, in man the invaginated area of stratified epithelium within the hair follicles is small relative to that on the skin. A similar calculation for rabbit or horse skin indicates that much more epithelium lines the hair follicles than covers the surface of the skin. Thus, in certain mammals, the potential for penetration through the hair follicles is very large. In fact, the permeability of rodent skin to many diverse substances is three to five times that of human skin.[91] Furthermore, many of the studies conducted using human skin are valid only for a particular penetrant—e.g., salicylic acid[64,85] and radioactive iodine or potassium iodide.[16,58]

Solvents. Higuchi[35] states that application of most solvents appears to cause marked alteration in the resistance of the skin barrier toward penetration. According to Rothman,[77] the absorption of water-soluble and lipid-soluble substances is encouraged by organic solvents that dissolve skin lipids. Whether this is due to the effect of such treatment on the follicular openings or modification of the tissue layers in the epidermis has not been established. More polar solvents such as propylene glycol have been found, in some investigations, to enhance penetration,[26,50] whereas in others it has been found to retard penetration or to have no effect.[29] This may be due to the concentration of propylene glycol used in the vehicle and the solubility of the penetrant in the propylene glycol. The thermodynamic activity of a penetrant will increase up to saturation of the vehicle hence one would expect its release rate to be highest at a propylene glycol concentration required to just saturate the vehicle with the penetrant. Poulsen *et al.*[72] studied the effect of propylene glycol concentration on the in-vitro release of fluocinolone acetonide and its acetate ester. Their results showed that maximum release for a given concentration of steroid was obtained from vehicles containing approximately the minimum amount of propylene glycol necessary to dissolve the steroid completely. A decrease in steroid release resulted when excess propylene glycol was present owing to increased affinity of the vehicle for the steroid. When the amount of

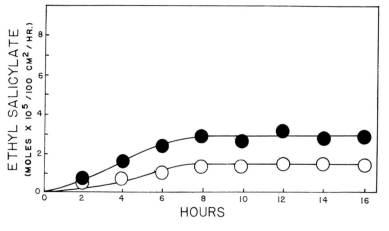

Fig. 6-2. Urinary excretion data showing the influence of moisture on the percutaneous absorption rate of ethyl salicylate. ● Hydrous system; ○ Anhydrous system.

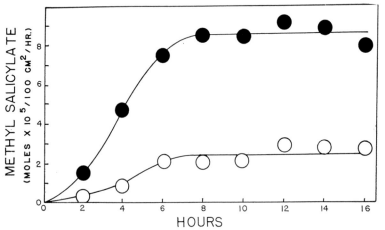

Fig. 6-3. Urinary excretion data showing the influence of moisture on the percutaneous absorption rate of methyl salicylate. ● Hydrous system; ○ Anhydrous system.

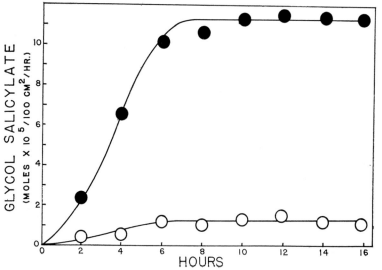

Fig. 6-4. Urinary excretion data showing the influence of moisture on the percutaneous absorption rate of glycol salicylate. ● Hydrous system; ○ Anhydrous system.

propylene glycol present was insufficient to dissolve all the steroid, then diffusion into the receptor phase (analogous to the skin in vivo) became dissolution-rate-limited and the release rate was reduced.

The enhancement of percutaneous absorption of various compounds by dimethylsulfoxide has been reported. Stoughton[84] reported an increase in the penetration of hydrocortisone and triamcinolone acetonide from an alcoholic solution containing 40 per cent of dimethylsulfoxide. Kligman[42] studied the percutaneous absorption of a large number of different types of compounds in different concentrations of dimethylsulfoxide and other solvents. In most cases he found absorption greatly enhanced from solutions containing dimethylsulfoxide. Collon and Winek[21] reported that a dimethylsulfoxide vehicle increased the penetration of sodium and zinc pyridinethione (antifungal and antibacterial agents) when applied to rabbit skin. The ability of dimethylsulfoxide to promote skin penetration may be due to its strong affinity for both polar and nonpolar materials.

Other Factors. The site of application and length of time such application remains in contact are factors that influence the percutaneous absorption of penetrants. Drugs that penetrate the stratum corneum do so most readily where the outer keratic layer is thin. According to Shelmire,[82] the rate of absorption is directly proportional to the thickness of the skin barrier and the extent of absorption is directly proportional to the area of skin covered by the ointment.

Although, in vitro, palmar skin is more permeable to water than is trunk skin,[53] iodine penetrates palmar skin at only one third of the rate it penetrates forearm skin in vivo.[87] Using tri-n-butyl phosphate, Marzulli[55] showed that, in vitro, plantar skin was penetrated much more slowly than skin from other regions. He also showed that postauricular and scrotal skin were the most permeable to tri-n-butyl phosphate. Blank *et al.*[9] compared the permeability of scrotal and abdominal skin to hydrogen sulfide, salicylic acid and water vapor. They showed that excised scrotal skin was more permeable than abdominal skin to these substances.

In general, the quantity of drug absorbed is proportional to the time the vehicle is in contact with the skin. However, this may be affected by secondary changes of drug concentration due to changes in degree of skin hydration and evaporation of water from an emulsion vehicle. Malkinson[54] demonstrated that rate of penetration of a medicament decreases with time as the tissues become saturated with the drug.

OLEAGINOUS BASES

Oleaginous bases include lard, vegetable oils (usually used as components of vehicles) and hydrocarbons such as petrolatum, liquid petrolatum, paraffin and jelled mineral oil. Also included in this group of semisolid preparations are bases consisting of or containing silicones, used primarily as protectives.

Lard. The purified internal fat of the abdomen of the hog was employed extensively in the past as a vehicle or as a component of vehicles. It is soft and greasy and, like other vehicles in this category, it forms an occlusive film when applied topically. Lard will absorb approximately 15 per cent of its weight of water. Stiffening agents such as spermaceti or beeswax can be incorporated to improve its physical properties. Lard has largely been replaced by benzoinated lard prepared by the addition of 1 per cent Siam benzoin. This preparation has better keeping qualities than lard because of the balsamic acids (primarily benzoic acid) and coniferyl benzoate contained in the Siam benzoin. These constituents serve as antioxidants and preservatives. Lard is rarely used as a component of topical preparations in modern dermatologic practice.

Vegetable Oils. Olive, cottonseed persic, sesame and other oils are seldom employed as vehicles. However, they are frequently employed in semisolid preparations as softening agents for preparations containing waxes or for their emollient effect. They are often employed in emulsion lotions and emulsion type ointment bases.

Petrolatum (Petroleum Jelly). Petrolatum *N.F.* is a tasteless, odorless, unctuous mass obtained from petroleum. It varies in color from yellow to light amber. White Petrolatum *U.S.P.* is petrolatum wholly or nearly decolorized. It is preferred when a white or a translucent ointment is desired. Both petro-latums consist of microcrystalline, solid hy-drocarbons suspended in liquid and semi-solid hydrocarbons.

Petrolatums are employed extensively as components of many emulsion bases, either oil-in-water or water-in-oil types. They are also used as occlusive, emollient, protective coverings for the skin. Steigleder and Raab[83] studied a variety of semisolid bases with re-spect to their protective action on the skin surface against contact with water. White petrolatum showed the best protective action. Addition of silicone did not enhance the protective qualities of the base. Data indi-cated that ointments have a prolonged influ-ence on the skin surface, even when pro-tection against water was no longer complete.

Petrolatum bases are greasy and difficult to remove from the skin. Also, they are in-capable of absorbing aqueous solutions (5 to 10% of water can be incorporated by trituration). However, this can be remedied by incorporating 15 per cent of anhydrous lanolin with petrolatum; this mixture will ab-sorb up to 50 per cent of water.

The major advantage of hydrocarbon oint-ments over oleaginous bases prepared from animal fats and vegetable oils is that they do not rancidify. Cold Cream *U.S.P.* possesses this advantage over the Rose Water Oint-ment prepared from a vegetable oil.

1. ℞

Iodine	0.3
Petrolatum q.s.	30.0

Sig.: Apply at bedtime.

Dissolve the iodine in a small amount of water containing 0.3 Gm. of potassium iodide. Incorporate the solution in 10 Gm. of anhy-drous lanolin and then incorporate the petro-latum.

2. ℞

Starch	20.0
Zinc oxide	10.0
Petrolatum q.s.	60.0

Sig.: Protective ointment. Apply as di-rected.

Incorporate the starch and the zinc oxide by levigating with the petrolatum. A portion of the petrolatum can be melted and used as the levigating agent. Incorporate the remaining petrolatum.

3. ℞

Peru balsam	5.0
Sulfur	5.0
Salicylic acid	3.0
Petrolatum q.s.	30.0

Sig.: Apply locally as directed.

Levigate the sulfur and the salicylic acid with a small portion of the petrolatum. Mix the Peru balsam with an equal weight of castor oil and incorporate with the concentrate, then add the remainder of the base and mix well.

Prescription 1 demonstrates the incorpora-tion of a water-soluble medicament in pet-rolatum. Medicaments such as iodine, mer-bromin, etc., should not be incorporated by trituration. They must be dissolved in water prior to incorporation in the base. Prescrip-tion 2 is a stiff, protective type of ointment. If a levigating agent such as liquid petrolatum is used, the preparation becomes too soft. In general, the vehicle itself should be used as the levigating agent in most ointment pre-scriptions. The use of auxiliary agents such as liquid petrolatum results in undue soften-ing of the preparation. Prescription 3 illus-trates the use of a special levigating agent, castor oil. It is used to prevent the "bleeding" or separation of Peru balsam from the oleaginous vehicle since Peru balsam is only slightly soluble in most oleaginous vehicles. Ichthammol also can be readily incorporated in petrolatum by first triturating it with an equal weight of castor oil. Castor oil acts as a solubilizing agent for some of the more polar constituents in Peru balsam and ich-thammol such as resin acids and salts of sulfo-ichthyolic acid. Ichthammol Ointment *N.F.* employs anhydrous lanolin as the levigating agent. However, Peru balsam and ichtham-mol can be incorporated directly in emulsion bases such as Hydrophilic Ointment *U.S.P.* to produce a stable product.

Anhydrous petrolatum bases are also em-ployed extensively when antibiotics such as penicillin, the tetracyclines, chloramphenicol and bacitracin are to be prepared in a semi-solid dosage form. Extensive hydrolysis occurs if these antibiotics are incorporated in water-containing emulsion bases or in water-soluble bases such as Polyethylene Glycol Ointment *U.S.P.* If it is desired to in-corporate these antibiotics in emulsion type or water-soluble bases, the ointments should be refrigerated. Neomycin, tyrothrycin and polymyxin B are stable at room temperature in all types of ointment bases.

White Ointment, *U.S.P.* and **Yellow Ointment,** *N.F.* These hydrocarbon bases consist, respectively, of white and yellow petrolatum, stiffened (respectively) with white and yellow wax. Both serve as emollient vehicles for other ointments. Both the White and the Yellow Ointments are known as Simple Ointment. White Ointment should be employed to prepare white ointments and Yellow Ointment should be used to prepare colored ointments when Simple Ointment is prescribed. Variations are permitted in the amounts of petrolatum and wax, to maintain a suitable consistency at extreme climatic conditions.

4. ℞
   Bismuth subnitrate 30.0
   White wax 10.0
   White petrolatum 60.0

   Sig.: Apply as directed.

Melt the wax and the petrolatum on a water bath. Use a portion of the melted base to levigate the bismuth subnitrate. Stir the remaining base until congealed and incorporate the well triturated bismuth subnitrate. A very stiff preparation results.

5. ℞
   Zinc sulfate
   Sulfurated potash
   Calamine .... $\overline{aa}$ 4.0
   Anhydrous lanolin
   Petrolatum q.s. 60.0

   Sig.: Apply to skin.

Prepare white lotion. Filter off the water and incorporate the residue in the wool fat. Levigate the calamine on a slab with a small amount of petrolatum. Incorporate the calamine and the white lotion residue in the remaining petrolatum.

6. ℞
   Iodine 1.0
   Potassium iodide 1.0
   Yellow ointment q.s. 30.0

   Sig.: Apply as directed.

Dissolve the potassium iodide in a small quantity of water. Dissolve the iodine in this solution. Incorporate the iodine solution in 5 Gm. of anhydrous lanolin and incorporate sufficient yellow ointment to make 30 Gm.

Plastibase* (Jelene) consists largely of mineral oils jelled with high molecular weight hydrocarbon waxes. The liquid phase is mobile and is retained in what is believed to be a matrix of submicroscopic interstices.

An unique feature of Plastibase is its unusual temperature-viscosity relationship. It melts at 90 to 91° C. and maintains its ointmentlike consistency over a wide temperature range (—15° to 60°).

In-vitro studies[31,40] indicate that Plastibase permits a greater release of an incorporated medicament than does petrolatum. This is associated with the mobility of the oil phase, permitting a drug to diffuse into the surrounding media.

Menthol, salicylates and camphor are dissolved by Plastibase, producing ointments that are too soft. This is probably due to interaction with the high molecular weight waxes used to gel the mineral oil. Coal tar, when incorporated in Plastibase, also produces a very soft ointment. Prescriptions using Plastibase as the vehicle cannot be prepared by fusion because it is difficult to cool the resulting mixture to a smooth consistency.[31] In preparing Plastibase commercially, a shock cooling procedure (very rapid cooling to a low temperature) is used.

Silicones cannot be considered as hydrocarbon materials, since their basic structure is not carbon but an alternate chain of silicon and oxygen atoms, i.e., –Si–O–Si–O. They are included in the oleaginous group of ointments because they are oily fluids or greasy semisolids similar in appearance to and possessing some of the physical properties of liquid petrolatum and petrolatum such as inertness and immiscibility with water.

Physically, silicones vary from low viscosity fluids through high viscosity liquids and semisolids to solids, depending on the substituent organic groups attached to the silicon and the degree of cross-linking of the polymer.

Silicone fluids are used extensively in semisolid preparations to provide a protective barrier against common skin irritants. The fluids are odorless, tasteless, relatively inert chemically and physiologically[76] and water repellent.

* Trade name of E. R. Squibb & Sons, New York, N. Y.

Dimethicone, a water-repellent silicone fluid consisting of dimethylsiloxane polymers, is used in the form of an ointment containing 30 per cent silicone in a petrolatum base. Dimethylsiloxane polymers are commercially available as D.C. 200 (Dow Corning) fluids of various viscosities. Usually, the 1,000-cts. fluid is used in protective ointments.

$$CH_3-\underset{\underset{CH_3}{|}}{\overset{\overset{CH_3}{|}}{Si}}-O-\left[\underset{\underset{CH_3}{|}}{\overset{\overset{CH_3}{|}}{Si}}-O\right]_n \underset{\underset{CH_3}{|}}{\overset{\overset{CH_3}{|}}{-Si}}-CH_3$$

Dimethicone

Alcohol-soluble silicones are used in protective formulations, suntan lotions, hair sprays and shave lotions. The alcohol-soluble silicones are methylphenylpolysiloxanes, which possess the typical characteristics of dimethylsiloxanes except for solubility in 95 per cent alcohol.[66] Dow Corning* 555 fluid is a commercially available alcohol-soluble silicone.

A series of organosilicone copolymers with unique solubility characteristics are available as L-520, L-521 and L-522 fluids.[†] L-520 and L-521 are soluble in water and dilute alcohol solutions.

In addition to the incorporating of silicone fluids in petrolatum, these can be emulsified in oil-in-water or water-in-oil type of emulsions, in much the same manner as mineral oil. Plein and Plein[70] have prepared silicone-containing ointments such as silicone cold cream, silicone hydrophilic ointment, etc.

Vanisil Silicone Ointment[71]

7. ℞
Stearic acid (Pearlstearic) 10.0
Synthetic Japan Wax 2.0
D.C. 200, 1000 cts. Silicone Fluid 20.0
Potassium hydroxide 0.5
Methylparaben 0.025
Propylparaben 0.015
Distilled water 67.5

Warm the aqueous mixture of the potassium hydroxide and the parabens to 75° and slowly add it to the warmed stearic acid, Japan wax, D.C. 200 mixture. Stir until the ointment congeals.

* Dow Corning Corporation, Midland, Michigan.
† Union Carbide Corporation, Silicones Division, New York, N. Y.

Steigleder and Raab[83] studied the protective action of a petrolatum ointment containing 25 per cent silicone and a neutral, petrolatum-free ointment containing 25 per cent silicone. These were compared with the protective action afforded the skin surface against contact with water by petrolatum, Hydrophilic Petrolatum *U.S.P.,* Hydrophilic Ointment *U.S.P.,* Zinc Ointment *U.S.P.* and Olive Oil *U.S.P.* White petrolatum showed the best protective effect.

SPECIALTIES CONTAINING SILICONES AND SILICATES

Covicone (Abbott)—a plasticized combination of dimethylpolysiloxane, nitrocellulose and castor oil in a vanishing cream base, used to protect the skin from occupational dermatoses and skin contact allergies

Domicone (Dome)—Acid Mantle Cream (a buffered solution of aluminum acetate in an oil-in-water type of emulsion base) containing 20 per cent silicone

Silicote (Arnar-Stone)—a specially refined petrolatum base containing 30 per cent silicone

Kerodex Barrier Creams (Ayerst)—available as water-repellent and water-soluble preparations containing magnesium silicate, diatomaceous silica, zinc oxide, zinc stearate and kaolin

ABSORPTION BASES

The term absorption as used in the above title does not refer to the therapeutic efficacy of bases when applied to the skin but to their hydrophilic or water-absorbing properties. This class of bases may be divided into two groups, one group consisting of anhydrous bases which permit the incorporation of aqueous solutions with the formation of a water-in-oil emulsion, i.e., Hydrophilic Petrolatum *U.S.P.,* Anhydrous Lanolin *U.S.P.* The second group consists of hydrous water-in-oil emulsions, which permit the incorporation of additional quantities of aqueous solutions, i.e., Lanolin *U.S.P.,* Rose Water Ointment *N.F.* and Cold Cream *U.S.P.*

Hydrophilic Petrolatum *U.S.P.* This base enables the pharmacist to incorporate water or a solution of medicinal substances in water resulting in the formation of a water-in-oil emulsion. The original formula for hydrophilic petrolatum contained cholesterol and anhydrous lanolin. Anhydrous lanolin has since been deleted and the cholesterol content increased from 1 to 3 per cent, enabling the incorporation of large quantities of aqueous solutions.

8. ℞
   Aluminum acetate solution 10.0
   Hydrophilic petrolatum q.s. 100.0
   Sig.: Apply as directed.
   University of Iowa Absorption Base
9. ℞
   Cholesterol 30.0
   Cottonseed oil 30.0
   White petrolatum 940.0

Heat the white petrolatum and the cottonseed oil to 145° C. Remove from the heat, add the cholesterol and stir until congealed.

Anhydrous Lanolin *U.S.P.* **(Wool Fat).** Anhydrous lanolin is the purified, anhydrous, fatlike substance from the wool of sheep. It contains the sterols cholesterol and oxycholesterol as well as triterpene and aliphatic alcohols. Although called a fat, wool fat is more accurately classified chemically as a wax. The emulsifying and the emollient actions of lanolin are thought to be due to the alcohols which are found in the unsaponifiable fraction when lanolin is treated with alkali.[88] Wool wax alcohols constitute about 50 per cent of this fraction which consists of approximately 30 per cent of cholesterol, 25 per cent of lanosterol, 3 per cent of cholestanol, 2 per cent of agnosterol and 40 per cent of various other alcohols. Anhydrous lanolin is capable of taking up about twice its weight of water. It is too sticky and tenacious to be used by itself but mixes readily with other oleaginous materials to increase the hydrophilic property of the base. Lanolin *U.S.P.* contains 25 to 30 per cent of water.

10. ℞
    Burow's solution 5.0
    Zinc oxide 5.0
    Boric acid ointment 10.0
    Lanolin 5.0
    White petrolatum q.s. 60.0

The British Pharmacopoeia contains a monograph for an absorption base under the name Wool Alcohols Ointment.

Wool Alcohols Ointment B.P.

11. ℞
    Wool alcohols 60.0
    Hard paraffin 240.0
    White or yellow soft paraffin 100.0
    Liquid paraffin . . . .   600.
Melt together and stir until congealed.

Wool Alcohols is a crude mixture of sterol and triterpene alcohols prepared by hydrolyzing wool fat with alkali and separating the fraction containing cholesterol and other alcohols. The preparation is claimed to be much less odoriferous than lanolin.

Lanolin can be converted by means of various physical and chemical procedures into functional derivatives for use in pharmaceutical and cosmetic formulations. Conrad and Maso[22] discuss some of the lanolin derivatives and give representative formulations that illustrate their many uses—for example, as emulsifiers, moisturizers and emollients, for slip and lubricity, as dispersing and solubilizing agents, etc. Two of the better known lanolin derivatives are acetylated lanolin and ethoxylated lanolin.* These lanolin derivatives are prepared by controlled acetylation and ethoxylation of the hydroxyl groups of lanolin hydroxyesters. As a result of chemical modification, acetylated lanolin is considered hypoallergenic.[27] Ethoxylated lanolin is a water-soluble lanolin that is a convenient source of whole lanolin for aqueous, alcoholic and emulsified topical preparations. In addition, it is a nonionic oil-in-water emulsifier.

Products referred to as "Liquid Lanolin," "Lanolin Oil," or "Dewaxed Lanolin" are true liquid lanolins prepared by the fractional crystallization or molecular distillation of solid lanolin. Liquid lanolin is a water-in-oil emulsifier with improved solubility in mineral oil and other organic solvents. Descriptions of liquid lanolin and suggested formulas containing liquid lanolin were published by Clark[19] and by Lower and Cressey.[47]

Although some dermatologists consider lanolin a sensitizing agent, a review[63] of the medical literature yields a total of about 100 cases of lanolin sensitization reported over a period of 30 years. Considering the widespread use of lanolin in cosmetics and pharmaceuticals, this is an extremely low incidence of sensitization and indicates that lanolin is not a potent sensitizer. However, Hjorth and Trolle-Lassen[37] made a detailed study of lanolin sensitivity and reported that the incidence of sensitivity to lanolin among patients with eczema is quite impressive. Sulzberger *et al.*[86] patch tested 19 patients

* Modulan and Solulan 75, American Cholesterol Products, Inc., Edison, N. J.

TABLE 6-2. WATER NUMBER OF FATTY ALCOHOL, ANHYDROUS LANOLIN AND
PETROLATUM MIXTURE

FATTY ALCOHOL	ANHYDROUS LANOLIN	PETROLATUM	WATER NUMBER	
			WHITE PETROLATUM	YELLOW PETROLATUM
Cetyl alcohol, 4%	10%	86%	104.1	108.3
Stearyl alcohol, 6%	10%	84%	118.2	114.5

sensitive to lanolin with components and derivatives of lanolin and concluded that the allergen was in the aliphatic fraction of the alcoholic component.

Rose Water Ointment N.F. (Cold Cream). This preparation was originated by Galen and was known for centuries as Ceratum Refrigerans. Cold cream prepared with expressed almond or persic oil is readily absorbed by the skin and produces a sensation of coolness. The emulsifier in rose water ointment and in cold cream is the sodium salt of hexacosanoic acid (cerotic acid), $C_{25}H_{51}COOH$, found in the white wax. Cold cream is used as an emollient ointment or as a vehicle for medicaments. It belongs to the group 2 type of absorption bases, the hydrous water-in-oil emulsions.

Cold Cream U.S.P. (Petrolatum Rose Water Ointment). This preparation differs from Rose Water Ointment N.F. in the replacement of the expressed almond or persic oil by an equal weight of liquid petrolatum. This produces an ointment which is not subject to rancidity. However, petrolatum rose water ointment is nonabsorbent and remains greasy to the touch, producing less cooling sensation than Rose Water Ointment. The petrolatum-containing ointment is used primarily as an emollient and a cleansing cream (used to remove makeup and grease paints). It is very similar to the commercially available cleansing cream or theatrical cream.

WATER NUMBER

Most oleaginous bases can become absorption bases by the addition of an ingredient or ingredients that increase the water number of the oleaginous base. Casparis and Meyer[17] defined the water number as the largest amount of water (in Gm.) that 100 Gm. of an ointment base or fat will hold at normal temperature (20°). They also described a titration method for determining the water number of an ointment base. A more sensitive method utilizes the Karl Fisher reagent and an instrument such as the aquameter. Halpern and Zopf[34] investigated the hydrophilic properties of the saturated fatty alcohols from C_{10} to C_{18}. Casparis and Meyer reported the water number of petrolatum as 9.3 to 15.6 and lard as 7.5. They found that 4 per cent cetyl alcohol increased the water number of petrolatum to between 38.8 and 51.5, while 3 per cent cetyl alcohol increased the water number of lard to 244.9. There appears to be a definite relationship between concentration of fatty alcohol and the water number of the vehicle. Stearyl alcohol was found to produce the greatest potentiation of the water number of petrolatum, although cetyl alcohol had the lowest optimum concentration, i.e., in white petrolatum 5 per cent cetyl alcohol raised the water number to 38, whereas 7 per cent stearyl alcohol raised it to 42.

As shown in Table 6-2, combinations of cetyl or stearyl alcohol and wool fat increased the water number of petrolatum more than either cetyl or stearyl alcohol alone.

Since the water number indicates the maximum amount of water that the base will hold, it is advisable to add water in quantities of 10 to 15 per cent less than is indicated by the water number. This will preclude the possibility of water bleeding from the base because of temperature variations.

12. ℞
White wax 7.0
Sodium borate 0.5
Precipitated sulfur 5.0
Rose water 18.0
Liquid petrolatum q.s. 60.0
Sig.: Apply to skin twice daily.

Melt the wax on a water bath with the liquid petrolatum. Dissolve the sodium borate in the rose water, warm to about 65° and gradually add the warm solution to the melted mixture. Stir until congealed. Use a portion of the base to levigate the sulfur, incorporate the remaining base.

SPECIALTY ABSORPTION BASES (ANHYDROUS AND HYDROUS)

Almatone (Almay)—a hypoallergenic ointment containing lanolin derivatives with spermaceti and petrolatum

Aquaphor (Duke)—absorption base containing 6 parts of woolwax alcohols and 94 parts of aliphatic hydrocarbons

Hydrotex (Texas Pharmacal)—a neutral, oleaginous absorption base consisting of sorbitan sesquioleate, white wax and blended petrolatums

Lanolor (Squibb)—lanolin, purified and deodorized

Nivea Cream (Duke)—an emulsion of neutral aliphatic hydrocarbons in water with woolwax alcohols

Polysorb (Fougera)—a wax-petrolatum mixture containing sorbitan sesquioleate as the emulsifying agent

EMULSION BASES

The outstanding characteristic of this group of semisolid bases is water removability. Since these bases are oil-in-water emulsions, they are diluted readily by the external phase and, hence, are readily removed from the skin or clothing. Although these bases are also termed hydrophilic bases (Hydrophilic Ointment *U.S.P.*) they will not take up more than 30 to 50 per cent of their weight in water without losing their ointment consistency.

Emulsion bases are not as occlusive as oleaginous bases or anhydrous and hydrous absorption bases. However, they are cosmetically appealing and are useful when a medicament is to be applied to a hairy region such as the scalp. Many cosmetic preparations such as vanishing creams, foundation creams, etc., are o/w emulsion preparations. They do not leave a greasy residue when applied to the face.

In addition to oil and water, an emulsion base may contain high molecular weight fatty alcohols such as cetyl and/or stearyl alcohol. These alcohols improve the stability of the base by increasing its consistency and also enhance the water-holding ability of the base. Most emulsion bases, because of their external aqueous phase, also contain a humectant such as glycerin, propylene glycol or sorbitol. These substances reduce water loss through evaporation and may assist in obtaining a more intimate dispersion of oils, grease, etc., in water.

The choice of emulsifier is important, since solubility of the emulsifying agent is a determining factor in the type of emulsion produced. In general, an agent that is soluble in water or more readily wetted by water than by oil will form an o/w emulsion.

One should not overlook the fact that this generalization has many exceptions. Oil-in-water emulsions can be prepared using emulsifying agents that are lipophilic, even when the oil phase represents 60 to 70 per cent of the total emulsion volume. Davies[25] and Riegelman[74] point out the importance of viscosity, coalescence rate of dispersed oil and water droplets, phase-volume ratio of oil and water and the concentration of surfactant in determining the type of emulsion that forms.

Emulsifying agents include monovalent soaps, amine soaps, sulfated fatty alcohols, polyglycol esters, quaternary ammonium compounds and many nonionic polyoxyethylene derivatives. Ionic agents such as soaps, sulfated fatty alcohols and quaternary compounds are sensitive to the presence of other ions and to changes in pH. Thus, anionic emulsifying agents such as soaps may be ineffective in formulations containing buffer salts or cationic materials, and cationic agents such as the quaternary compounds are ineffective in the presence of anionic materials such as soap. Ointments prepared with anionic agents are not stable at pH's much below 5 to 6. On the other hand, nonionic agents do not ionize, hence are compatible with electrolytes and ionic emulsifying agents. In general, nonionic agents are less irritating than anionic agents, which are less irritating than cationic agents.

The British Pharmacopoeia[15] contains a monograph for an emulsifying wax that is a mixture of two compounds that combine to form a stable complex. Emulsifying waxes are used to formulate anhydrous ointments capable of admixture with considerable quantities of water or aqueous solutions to form stable oil-in-water emulsions.

Emulsifying Wax B. P.

Sodium lauryl sulfate 10.0
Cetostearyl alcohol 90.0
Emulsifying Ointment B. P.
Emulsifying wax 30.0
Liquid paraffin 20.0
White soft paraffin 50.0

Emulsifying ointment is used to prepare Aqueous Cream B. P., which contains about 70 per cent water.

Although there are no official emulsion bases prepared with a cationic emulsifying agent, the British Pharmaceutical Codex[13] includes a cationic equivalent of Emulsifying Wax B. P.

Cetrimide Emulsifying Wax

Cetrimide* 10.0
Cetostearyl alcohol 90.0

Cetrimide emulsifying wax is used in the preparation of cetrimide emulsifying ointment, which in turn is used to prepare cream of cetrimide. These vehicles can be used for the incorporation of cationic and nonionic medicaments.

The British Pharmaceutical Codex[13] also contains a monograph for cetomacrogol emulsifying wax, a nonionic emulsifying wax prepared with a condensate of cetyl or cetostearyl alcohol with ethylene oxide.

Nonionic emulsifying agents are widely used in cosmetic and dermatologic formulations. One must keep in mind that preservatives and medicaments may interact with the nonionic emulsifying agent in such formulations. Blaug et al.[11,12,17] have shown that many commonly used nonionic surfactants interact with preservatives and active ingredients used in semisolid dosage forms. For example, Hydrophilic Ointment U.S.P. XV contained polyoxyl 40 stearate (Myrj 52),† a nonionic surfactant, as the emulsifying agent. However, it was noted that medicaments containing an acidic hydrogen such as benzoic and salicylic acids, phenol, etc., produced a marked softening of the base. For this reason the U.S.P. XIV formula containing sodium lauryl sulfate, an anionic agent, was readopted in U.S.P. XVI.

* Chiefly tetradecyltrimethylammonium bromide.
† Atlas Chemical Industries, Inc., Wilmington, Delaware.

13. ℞
Bacitracin 500 units/Gm.
Stearyl alcohol 15.0
White wax 1.0
Glycerin 5.0
Myrj 52 .... 5.0
Water 74.0
Sig: Apply to infected area three times daily.

Prepared as above, the preparation becomes very soft due to interaction between the Myrj 52 and constituents in Bacitracin. Replace the Myrj with 2.0 Gm. of sodium lauryl sulfate. Melt the stearyl alcohol and the wax on a water bath and heat to about 65°. Dissolve the sodium lauryl sulfate and the propylene glycol in the water and heat to about 65°. Slowly add the oil phase to the water phase with stirring. Stir until the preparation congeals. Levigate the bacitracin with a small amount of the base, then incorporate the remaining base. Preparation must be refrigerated. For greatest stability bacitracin should be incorporated in an anhydrous base.

14. ℞
Salicylic acid 0.6
L.C.D. 3.0
Zinc oxide 3.0
Starch 3.0
Water-removable base q.s. 30.0
Sig.: Apply as directed.

Dissolve the salicylic acid in the L.C.D. and incorporate in hydrophilic ointment. Levigate the zinc oxide and the starch with a portion of the hydrophilic ointment. Incorporate in the remaining base.

15. ℞
Salicylic acid 0.6
Sulfur 0.6
Neobase q.s. 30.0
Sig.: Apply to scalp.

16. ℞
Coal tar 2.0
Zinc oxide 5.0
Polysorbate 80 .... 0.5
Petrolatum q.s. 60.0
Sig.: Apply to arm daily.

Mix the coal tar with the polysorbate 80. Levigate the zinc oxide with a small portion of petrolatum and incorporate the coal tar and the zinc oxide in the remaining petrolatum. The polysorbate 80 serves a dual purpose. It functions as a dispersing agent and also aids in the removal of the ointment from the skin.

17. ℞

Salicylic acid	0.6
Undecylenic acid	1.0
Hydrophilic base q.s.	60.0

Sig.: Apply between toes once daily.

18. ℞

Ammoniated mercury	22%
Liquid petrolatum	20%
Stearic acid	8%
Cetyl alcohol	2%
Triethanolamine	1%
Distilled water q.s.	60.0

Sig.: Apply locally p.r.n.

The emulsifier, triethanolamine stearate, is prepared in situ. Melt the cetyl alcohol and the stearic acid on a water bath. Add the liquid petrolatum and warm to 70°. Disperse the triethanolamine in the water, heat to 70° then add to the melted oil phase with stirring. Stir till congealed. Use a portion of the base to levigate the ammoniated mercury then incorporate the remaining base.

19. ℞

Sulfur	2.0
Phenol	0.5
Cetyl alcohol	8.0
White wax	0.5
Propylene glycol	5.0
Sodium lauryl sulfate	1.0
Distilled water q.s.	60.0

Sig.: Apply to scalp as directed.

SPECIALTY EMULSION BASES (O/W)

Almay Emulsion Base (Almay)—a hypoallergenic greaseless o/w base

Cetaphil (Texas Pharmacal)—a water removable greaseless base free from any fatty material. It contains cetyl alcohol, stearyl alcohol, propylene glycol, sodium lauryl sulfate and water.

Dermabase (Borden Pharm.)—a hypoallergenic greaseless emulsion base

Dermovan (Texas Pharmacal)—an acid-pH vanishing cream type of base, compatible with acid-reacting medicaments. The base consists of glyceryl monostearate (acid-emulsifying), spermaceti, mineral oil, glycerin and water

Multibase (Ar-Ex)—a hydrophilic, nondehydrating vanishing cream type base

Neobase (Burroughs Wellcome)—liquid petrolatum, polyhydric alcohol esters, propylene glycol and water to form an o/w emulsion base

Phorsix (Texas Pharmacal)—an o/w emulsion base made with nonionic emulsifiers. The base is adjusted to a pH of 4.6

Unibase (Parke, Davis)—nongreasy base

consisting of higher fatty alcohols, petrolatum, glycerin, water and an emulsifying agent. It has a pH approximating that of the skin. Unibase will absorb 30 per cent of its own weight of water

Velvachol (Texas Pharmacal)—a hydrophilic emulsion base compatible with acids, bases, strong electrolytes and many other medicaments. The base contains cholesterin, sodium lauryl sulfate, cetyl alcohol, stearyl alcohol, petrolatum, liquid petrolatum and water.

WATER-SOLUBLE BASES

This group of so-called greaseless ointment bases is comprised of water soluble ingredients, the polyethylene glycol polymers known as Carbowax* compounds. Polyethylene Glycol Ointment *U.S.P.* is the only pharmacopoeial preparation in this group. Nitrofurozone soluble Dressing *N.F.* is a medicated polyethylene glycol semisolid preparation.

The polyethylene glycols of interest in ointment formulation are those that vary in molecular weight from 1,000 to 6,000. Consistency of these compounds varies from a soft petrolatumlike semisolid to hard, waxy solids, the consistency increasing with molecular weight. The outstanding feature of these compounds is water solubility. Patch tests have shown the polyethylene glycols to be innocuous and no more irritating than lanolin or petrolatum when applied to the skin.[49]

Polyethylene glycol 1500, a soft petrolatumlike semisolid, can be used as a vehicle for the topical application of medicaments. However, the higher molecular weight polyethylene glycols are usually blended with the low molecular weight (200-600) liquid polyethylene glycols for ointment formulation. For example, Polyethylene Glycol Ointment *U.S.P.* is a blend of PEG 4000 and polyethylene glycol 400. The base for Nitrofurozone Soluble Dressing *N.F.* consists of a blend of polyethylene glycols 300, 1,540 and 4,000.

Polyethylene Glycol Ointment *U.S.P.* possesses many desirable properties. It washes off readily with water, it is not greasy, it shows no physical changes on aging and it permits ready dispersion of water-soluble me-

* Union Carbide Chemicals Co., New York, N. Y.

dicaments. However, the solubility of this base precludes the addition of aqueous solutions much in excess of 5 per cent of the total formula. Inclusion of 5 per cent stearyl or cetyl alcohol in the formula increases the water number of the ointment, allowing the inclusion of 20 per cent of water.

20. ℞
Burow's solution 5.0
Polyethylene glycol ointment q.s... 30.0
Sig.: Apply to irritated area three times daily.

The water solubility of polyethylene glycol ointment precludes the inclusion of the Burow's solution. Replace 2 Gm. of the ointment base with cetyl alcohol. Melt the cetyl alcohol and the polyethylene glycol ointment on a water bath. Add the Burow's solution and stir until congealed.

Medicaments such as benzoic and salicylic acids, phenol and tannic acid have a solubilizing effect on ointment bases containing the high molecular weight PEG compounds. This may result in an undue softening of the base. These medicaments have been shown to interact with the high molecular weight polyethylene glycols, the complexes formed having different solubility characteristics from those of the parent compounds.[36]

In-vitro studies[20,57] have shown that medicaments diffuse readily from PEG bases. However, Shelmire[80] has shown that, although diffusion of a medicament to the skin surface from a polyethylene glycol vehicle is high, little percutaneous absorption occurred. Michelfelder and Peck[57a] also found that a polyethylene glycol vehicle is not a suitable vehicle for a water soluble drug, if one desires percutaneous absorption.

Polyethylene Glycol Ointment can be used as a base for insoluble medicaments as well as for water and water-soluble medicaments.

℞
Sulfur 1.0
PEG Ointment q.s. 30.0
Sig: Apply to scalp h.s.

Levigate the finely powdered sulfur with a small portion of the base and gradually add the remainder of the base with thorough trituration. Polyethylene glycols have been used to prepare water-removable emulsion bases to which varying quantities of water can be added. Landon and Zopf[44] developed the following PEG emulsified base:

21. ℞
PEG 4000 .... 20.0
Stearyl alcohol 34.0
Glycerin 30.0
Sodium lauryl sulfate 1.0
Purified water 15.0

Heat the PEG, the stearyl alcohol and the glycerin on a water bath to 75° C. Add, with stirring, to the water previously heated to 75° C. and containing the sodium lauryl sulfate. Stir until the base congeals.

PEG emulsified bases are not truly water-soluble. The PEG has an adjuvant action as an emulsifier and improves the water removability factor of the base. In addition, larger quantities of aqueous solutions can be added to such bases than can be added to polyethylene glycol vehicles.

Polyethylene glycol vehicles form non-occlusive films on the skin. The residual film from such bases can and will take up water which has diffused through the skin or come from the sweat glands, permitting the loss of such water to the environment. Since polyethylene glycol vehicles do not maintain hydration of the skin surface, it is understandable why water soluble medicaments are not transferred readily to the skin surface.

Often included in the group of water-soluble bases are semisolid bases that are not soluble in water but swell with water. Such bases are hydrous and usually contain an emulsifying agent. Included in this group are preparations produced through the use of bentonite, Veegum,* gelatin and cellulose derivatives. Guth et al.[2,24] prepared bentonite ointment bases in which various antibacterial agents were incorporated. These ointments showed high in-vitro activity.

22. ℞
Bentonite 20.0
Sodium lauryl sulfate 0.5
Glycerin 10.0
Purified water 69.5

Sprinkle the bentonite on the liquid portion of the base and stir at a slow rate of speed in a mechanical mixer until a homogeneous preparation results.

* R. T. Vanderbilt Company, Inc., New York, New York.

Universal Ointment Base*

23. ℞

Veegum	10.0
Sodium lauryl sulfate	0.1
Methylparaben	0.1
Glycerin	10.0
Tween 80	1.0
Purified water	78.8

Add the Veegum to the water slowly, agitating continually until smooth. Add the other ingredients, stir until smooth.

Massachusetts General Hospital Ointment Base[62]

24. ℞

Polyethylene glycol 200 mono-stearate	15.0
Veegum	5.0
Polysorbate 80	1.0
Methylparaben	0.1
Purified water	78.9

These bases are not greasy, spread readily without rubbing and form a protective film; yet, they can be easily removed from the skin with water. They do not alleviate dryness as well as does petrolatum because they are not occlusive. The residual film left on the skin by these bases will take up water which has diffused through the skin or come from the sweat glands; hence, they are vehicles of choice when an ointment is to be applied to a moist lesion.

OPHTHALMIC OINTMENTS

Special precautions must be taken in the preparation of an ophthalmic ointment. The active ingredient is added to the ointment base, either as a finely powdered chemical or as a solution. Where possible, the active ingredient should be sterile, as should a solution of the active ingredient. Not all of the drugs prescribed in ophthalmic ointments are available as sterile chemicals. If available, ampuls or vials of the dry parenteral powder should be used. However, although capsules, tablets or the bulk chemicals may not be sterile, they usually do not support bacterial growth within the lattice structure of the dry material; hence, they can usually be used where the sterile powder is not available.

Powders or tablets should be triturated and

*R. T. Vanderbilt Company, Inc., New York, New York.

incorporated in the ointment base aseptically. This can be accomplished by using sterile utensils. The mortar and the pestle, graduates, spatulas, etc., can be sterilized by autoclaving (a pressure cooker can be used). If an ointment slab is used, it can be washed with an antiseptic solution (preferably by an antiseptic dissolved in 70% alcohol). These precautions are necessary to prevent contaminants from infecting the eye, particularly an eye which is already injured. Riegelman and Vaughn[75] use the term "injured eye" to indicate one in which the corneal epithelium has been damaged. An intact epithelial layer acts as an effective barrier to organisms which might otherwise invade the cornea. Hence, sterility is probably of greater importance when the ointment is to be applied to an injured eye than when it is to be applied to an intact eye (i.e., one in which corneal epithelium has not been damaged).

Most ophthalmic ointments are prepared with a petrolatum base, a petrolatum-mineral oil base or a petrolatum-lanolin base. A petrolatum-lanolin base is sometimes used when an aqueous solution of the active ingredient is to be incorporated in an ophthalmic ointment. Whatever type of base is used, it must be nonirritating to the eye and should permit diffusion of the active ingredient from the base to the secretions of the eye. Although absorption bases, o/w emulsion bases and water soluble bases can be employed for ophthalmic drugs, they may be irritating. The irritation is probably due to the surface-active agent in the base. At the same time, the surface-active agent may increase the availability of the drug in the eye.

The British Pharmaceutical Codex[14] gives a formula for the preparation of a sterile ophthalmic ointment base.

Ophthalmic Ointment

Yellow soft paraffin	80.0
Liquid paraffin	10.0
Anhydrous lanolin	10.0

Heat together the anhydrous lanolin, the yellow soft paraffin and the liquid paraffin, filter while hot through a coarse filter paper in a heated funnel, and sterilize by heating for a sufficient time to ensure that the entire base is maintained at a temperature not lower than 160° for not less than 1 hour. Allow to cool before incorporating the medicament.

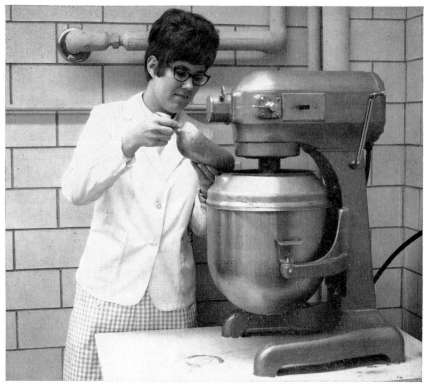

FIG. 6-5. Mixing is an essential part of ointment manufacture. The active ingredient is being added to the ointment in a Hobart Mixer. (Industrial Pharmacy Laboratory, University of Iowa, College of Pharmacy)

Petrolatum or a petrolatum-mineral oil base may be heat-sterilized in a hot-air oven at 175° C. for 2 hours. After the active ingredient is aseptically incorporated in the sterile vehicle, the ointment should be transferred into sterile ophthalmic-tipped tubes. The tubes can be sterilized by storage in 70 per cent alcohol for 24 hours prior to use. The use of tubes reduces the possibility of contaminating the ointment.

PREPARATION OF OINTMENTS

Mechanical Incorporation. Whether an ointment is applied to an irritated area of the skin or to intact skin, it should be homogeneous, smooth and free from granular or gritty particles. The usual technic used by the pharmacist to prepare such an ointment involves mechanical incorporation of the active ingredient in the ointment base on an ointment slab with a spatula. A mortar and a pestle are often used to incorporate liquids

in an ointment base. The mortar and pestle are probably not as efficient as the ointment slab and the spatula for incorporating insoluble powders in an ointment base because of the small surface area levigated at any one time.

Mechanical incorporation of a medicament on an ointment slab requires a ground glass plate and two stainless steel spatulas. Hard rubber spatulas or wooden tongue depressors should be used when danger of chemical reaction between the steel spatula and certain medicaments, i.e., iodine, tannic acid, salicylic acid, mercuric salts, etc., exists.

Before incorporating insoluble medicaments in an ointment base, the medicaments must be reduced to an impalpable powder. This can be accomplished on a slab by levigating the medicament with a small portion of the base to form a smooth nucleus. The nucleus is then incorporated with the remaining base. If very small amounts of medicaments are to be incorporated, a small amount

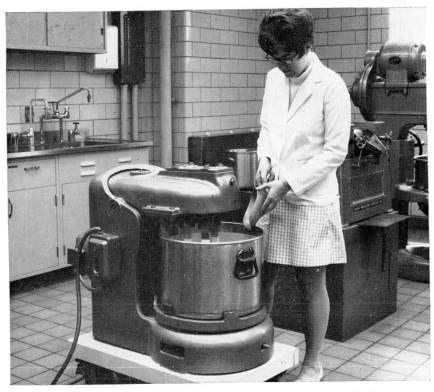

FIG. 6-6. The adding of active ingredient to ointment in a J. H. Day change can mixer. (Industrial Pharmacy Laboratory, University of Iowa, College of Pharmacy)

of mineral oil or a vegetable oil can be used as a levigating agent. However, the use of levigating agents (other than the base itself) usually results in a marked softening of the finished product. The details of preparing an ointment by mechanical incorporation are thoroughly understood. However, some medicinal substances require special technics on the part of the pharmacist in order to prepare a very smooth homogeneous product.

Alkaloids can easily be incorporated in ointment vehicles if used in the salt form. The alkaloidal salt should be dissolved in the smallest quantity of water possible. The aqueous solution can be incorporated directly in absorption bases, emulsion bases and water-soluble bases. If an oleaginous base is prescribed, the aqueous solution can be incorporated with a small quantity of anhydrous lanolin before incorporating in the oleaginous base. See ℞ Nos. 1 and 10.

Coal tar can be incorporated readily in oleaginous bases and pastes by first dispers-

ing the tar with Polysorbate 80 *U.S.P.*, a non-ionic surfactant. The dispersed coal tar is then incorporated in the base. One per cent of coal tar can be dispersed with 0.5 per cent of polysorbate 80. Coal Tar Ointment *U.S.P.* is an example of such a preparation. Coal tar usually can be incorporated in emulsion bases such as Hydrophilic Ointment *U.S.P.* by simple trituration.

Viscid materials such as ichthammol and Peruvian balsam are only slightly soluble in most oleaginous bases and, frequently, after incorporation in such bases, the ichthammol or the Peruvian balsam "bleeds" or separates from the base. Both materials can be incorporated in an oleaginous base by first dispersing them in an equal weight of castor oil. (See ℞ No. 3.) Peruvian balsam and ichthammol can be incorporated in emulsion bases such as Hydrophilic Ointment *U.S.P.* with a minimum amount of trituration.

Fusion. Ointments containing hard, waxy ingredients such as wax, spermaceti, paraffin,

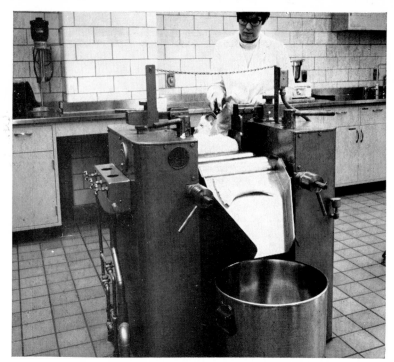

FIG. 6-7. A Kent three-roller mill used in the large-scale production of ointments. (Industrial Pharmacy Laboratory, University of Iowa, College of Pharmacy)

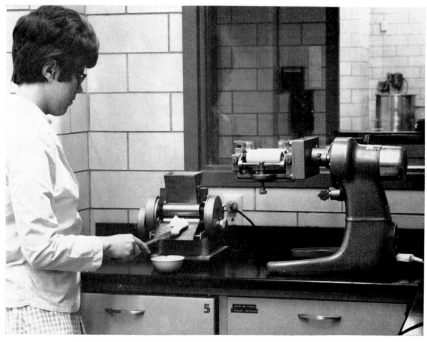

FIG. 6-8. Three-roller mills used for milling small batches of ointment. (*Left*) ASRA ointment mill. (*Right*) Erweka three-roller mill with detachable motor unit for all-purpose use. (Industrial Pharmacy Laboratory, University of Iowa, College of Pharmacy)

polyethylene glycols, high molecular weight fatty alcohols, etc., plus soft materials such as petrolatum and/or glycols, surfactants, water, etc., are prepared by the fusion process. This process also can be used to incorporate medicaments that are readily soluble in the melted base or to incorporate aqueous solutions in water-soluble bases.

In the fusion process, the ingredient with the highest melting point is placed in a beaker or evaporating dish and melted on a water bath. The other ingredients are added in order of decreasing melting points until the soft oleaginous materials have all been thoroughly incorporated. The base must be stirred until it congeals to prevent the separation of large particles of the ingredients with higher melting points. An active ingredient that is soluble in the base can be added to the warm base just before it congeals. Perfume oils and other volatile materials should be added after the base has cooled to about 35 to 40° C. An active ingredient which is insoluble in the base should not be sprinkled on the melted base. Instead, the medicament should be levigated with a small portion of the melted base. When the remaining base has congealed it can be incorporated with the levigated mass.

Emulsion bases are usually prepared by fusion. Waxes, fatty alcohols, lanolin and any oleaginous materials are melted in a suitable vessel. The emulsifying agent is dispersed in the water, previously heated to approximately the same temperature as the oleaginous phase. Any water-soluble ingredients, such as preservatives, and humectants such as glycerin or propylene glycol are dissolved in the water. The aqueous phase is added to the oleaginous phase with stirring and the mixture is stirred until the base is congealed.

25. ℞

Bismuth subnitrate	15.0
White wax	10.0
Paraffin	5.0
Petrolatum	70.0

Sig.: Apply as directed.

Melt the wax, the paraffin and the petrolatum on a water base. Use a portion of the melted base to levigate the bismuth subnitrate on an ointment slab. Stir the remaining base until it congeals, then combine with the levigated mixture.

26. ℞

Burow's solution	5.0
Polyethylene glycol 400	20.0
Polyethylene glycol 4,000	35.0

Sig.: Apply to irritated area daily.

Melt the p.e.g. 4,000 on a water bath. Add the p.e.g. 400 and stir. Add the Burow's solution before the mixture congeals and stir until the ointment congeals.

27. ℞

Sulfur	2.0
Cetyl alcohol	8.0
White wax	0.7
Propylene glycol	5.0
Sodium lauryl sulfate	1.0
Purified water q.s.	60.0

Sig.: Apply to scalp as directed.

Melt the white wax and the cetyl alcohol on a water bath. Disperse the sodium lauryl sulfate in the water previously heated to approximately the same temperature as the cetyl alcohol-wax phase and add to the wax phase with stirring. Stir until congealed. Levigate the sulfur with the propylene glycol, then combine with the congealed base.

PACKAGING, STORAGE AND LABELING OF OINTMENTS

Packaging. Ointments are usually dispensed in either ointment jars or tubes, jars being used most frequently by the community pharmacist. Ointment jars are available in brown, green or opaque white glass.

Ointments prepared by mechanical incorporation should be packed in jars uniformly, to avoid air pockets. A spatula can be used to fill the jar which should be tapped against the palm of the hand during filling to ensure that the air pockets are filled by the ointment. The container size should be such that the ointment fills the container but does not contact the lid liner. After the jar has been filled, the spatula should be used to smooth the surface of the ointment and give the product a finished appearance.

Ointments prepared by fusion can usually be packed while the ointment is still warm and fluid enough to be poured directly into the jar. It is usually unnecessary to smooth the surface of ointments packed in this manner.

The use of collapsible tin tubes avoids the possibility of ointment contamination through use. Furthermore, a collapsible tube presents

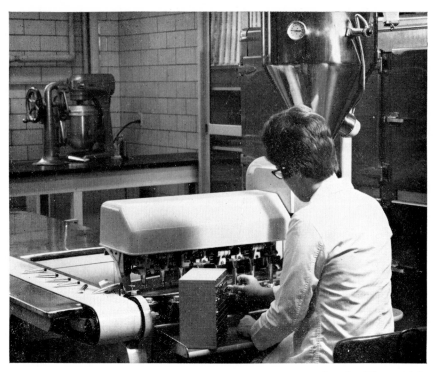

FIG. 6-9. Ointment tubes being fed into an Arenco automatic tube filler, which air-cleans and vacuums each tube before filling it with a measured amount of ointment. (Industrial Pharmacy Laboratory, University of Iowa, College of Pharmacy)

a minimum of ointment surface to the action of air and light. Collapsible tin tubes are available with special tips for application of ointments to the eye, the nose, the rectum or the vagina.

Ointment tubes are easily filled by placing the ointment on a powder paper longer than the tube. Shape the ointment to form a cylinder shorter than the container. Roll the cylinder with the paper to form a tube having a diameter smaller than that of the collapsible tube. Slip the tube into the container then flatten about ⅛ inch of the open end of the tin tube with a spatula. Holding the flattened edges of the tube together with the spatula, grasp the protruding paper and slowly withdraw it from the container. This leaves the ointment inside the collapsible tube. Make two ⅛-inch folds at the flattened end of the tube to prevent any ointment from being extruded. The cap end of the tube should be open during the process of filling and closing.

Storage. Ointments should be stored in a cool place, primarily to prevent the base from liquefying. If the base should liquefy, insoluble medicaments may settle to the bottom of the container. Emulsion bases may separate into two phases if allowed to soften or liquefy. Water-containing ointments should not be unduly exposed to the air, since evaporation of water may change the physical characteristics of the ointment.

When dispensing an ointment from a stock container, scrape the ointment from the surface. Digging into the ointment exposes a greater surface area, increasing the possibility of rancidity, water loss and mold growth.

Labeling. Special strip-form labels, which encircle the ointment jar or tube, are available. Labels should be covered with cellophane tape to prevent soiling.

Labels are somewhat difficult to attach to collapsible tin tubes. Coat the area of the tube to be labeled with benzoin tincture. Permit the tincture to dry and then apply the strip-form label. Labels should be attached

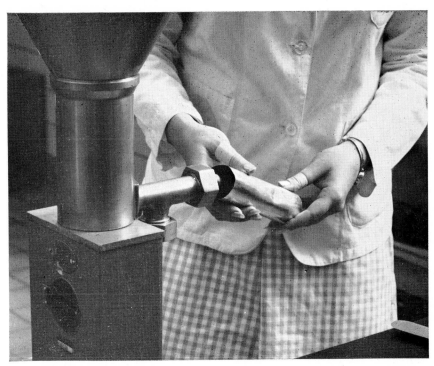

FIG. 6-10. Ointment tube being filled with a foot-operated Anderson paste and cream filler. (Industrial Pharmacy Laboratory, University of Iowa, College of Pharmacy)

near the top of the tube to prevent destruction and soiling while the ointment is being used.

OTHER TOPICAL PREPARATIONS

This section includes topical preparations which do not fit easily into the classification of ointments previously outlined. Included in this group are cerates, creams, pastes, plasters and poultices. These preparations differ in consistency from ointments and are usually medicated. Some, i.e., cerates, plasters and poultices, are spread on cloth before applying to the skin.

Cerates are ointmentlike preparations with a consistency between those of ointments and of plasters. As the name implies, true cerates always contain wax (cera). However, spermaceti, paraffin, suet or rosin have been employed as stiffening agents in cerates. Cerates are mainly of historical interest.

Cerates are used by spreading at ordinary temperatures on cloth and applying to the skin. They should not be soft enough to liquefy when applied to the skin. Cerates are usually prepared with lard, oil or petrolatum and a sufficient quantity of high melting wax to give the proper consistency. Because of the high melting ingredient, cerates are prepared by fusion. Five cerates were official in *N.F. VIII*: Simple Cerate, Rosin Cerate, Compound Rosin Cerate, Cantharides Cerate and Lead Subacetate Cerate.

Cerates are seldom prescribed in modern dermatologic practice. They formerly were used as dressings and protectives for inflamed and ulcerative areas of the skin.

Creams are usually thought of as a soft cosmetic type of preparation, i.e., vanishing creams, hand creams, face creams, etc. Pharmaceutically, medicated creams are semisolid or thick liquid emulsions containing medicaments dissolved or suspended in the emulsion and intended for external application. In general, creams belong to the oil-in-water emulsion classification of ointments. However, many preparations are referred to as creams because of consistency and appearance without regard to the type of base used.

In the British Pharmacopoeia creams are medicated liquid emulsions consisting of a mixture of lanolin, olive oil or other fixed oil and lime water. These preparations are water-in-oil emulsions similar to lime liniment and calamine liniment. The *B.P.* also uses the term cream as a synonym for several ointments and pastes.

In addition to Cold Cream, *U.S.P. XVIII* contains monographs for Gamma Benzene Hexachloride Cream, Gentamicin Sulfate Cream, Hydrocortisone Cream, Iodochlorhydroxyquin Cream, Tolnaftate Cream and Triamcinolone Cream. Most proprietary medicated creams are prepared with water-soluble or water-removable bases.

Pastes encompass two classes of ointment-like preparations for external use—the fatty pastes such as zinc oxide paste and the non-greasy pastes containing glycerin with pectin, gelatin, tragacanth, etc. Pastes are usually stiffer and less greasy than ointments due to a high proportion of powdered ingredients such as starch, zinc oxide and calcium carbonate in the base. Powders may be present to the extent of 50 per cent, e.g., Zinc Oxide Paste *U.S.P.* which contains 25 per cent zinc oxide and 25 per cent starch in white petrolatum.

Pastes are less greasy and more absorptive than ointments because of their high proportion of powdered medicaments having an affinity for water. Therefore, they are preferred for acute lesions having a tendency toward oozing, crusting or vesiculation. Such pastes are less penetrating and less macerating than ointments and tend to absorb the serous exudate. Medicaments incorporated in pastes are absorbed less readily than from ointments and, therefore, have a more superficial action.

In addition to powders, fatty pastes are composed of liquid petrolatum, petrolatum or fatty materials such as lanolin, benzoinated lard, etc. There are two official fatty pastes: Zinc Oxide Paste *U.S.P.* (Lassar's Plain Zinc Paste) and Zinc Oxide Paste with Salicylic Acid *N.F.* (Lassar's Zinc Paste with Salicylic Acid).

28. ℞
    Zinc oxide 25
    Starch 25
    Calamine 5
    Petrolatum q.s. 100
    Sig.: Apply as directed.

Triturate the calamine with the zinc oxide and the starch and incorporate the powders in the petrolatum. A portion of the petrolatum can be melted and used to triturate the powders. Liquid petrolatum should not be used as a levigating agent, since the amount required would result in softening of the product.

29. ℞
    Sulfur 1.0
    Salicylic acid 1.0
    Lassar's paste q.s. 30.0
    Sig.: Apply twice daily and h.s.

Levigate the sulfur and the salicylic acid with a small amount of the base or with a very small quantity of liquid petrolatum. Incorporate the remaining base. Since the amount of medicament contained in this prescription is small, a levigating agent such as liquid petrolatum can be used.

30. ℞
    Ichthammol 1.0
    Starch 25.0
    Zinc oxide paste q.s. 60.0
    Sig.: Apply at night.

The second class of pastes, made with glycerin and gelatin or pectin, are useful when fatty bases are undesirable, i.e., for application to wet surfaces. The nongreasy pastes are advantageous when applied to moist surfaces because of their miscibility with water.

Fantus and Dyniewicz[28] introduced pectin and tragacanth pastes for the treatment of bedsores and ulcers. The preparation of these pastes and other nongreasy pastes differs from the preparation of fatty pastes, since the basic ingredient of the paste—pectin, tragacanth, etc.—must hydrate. In general, the pastes can be prepared by first wetting the hydrocolloid with a small amount of glycerin and then adding a sufficient quantity of hot water.

31. ℞
    Pectin 5.0
    Glycerin 10.0
    Ringer's solution q.s. 60.0
    Sig.: Pectin paste.

Mix the pectin with the glycerin. Then, while stirring, add the Ringer's solution previously heated to 100°. Continue stirring to make a smooth paste.

Glycerogelatin pastes are prepared by allowing the gelatin to hydrate in hot water and then adding the powdered medicaments which previously have been rubbed to a smooth paste with the glycerin. Glycerogelatin pastes soften at body temperature and may be applied after they have been softened by warming. Zinc Gelatin *U.S.P.* is a firm glycerogelatin paste. It is used by placing the jar in hot water to melt the paste, which is then applied to the skin with a brush. The paste congeals on the skin, forming a protective film.

32. ℞
Zinc oxide	20.0
Calamine	20.0
Gelatin	10.0
Glycerin	10.0
Purified water q.s.	100.0

Sig.: Apply to itching area.

Add the gelatin to the water with stirring, then heat on a water bath until the gelatin dissolves. Add the zinc oxide and calamine, previously triturated with the glycerin. Stir until a smooth paste results.

Nongreasy, water-dispersible pastes must be stored in tightly closed containers to prevent the loss of water. On standing for several months, pectin pastes may liquefy. The liquefaction may be due to enzymatic hydrolysis of the pectin caused by mold growth. The parabens or benzoic acid should be employed to prevent mold growth.

Plasters are solid or semisolid adhesive masses spread on cotton, felt, linen or muslin and intended for topical application to various parts of the body.

The older type of plaster, prepared by reacting litharge and oil, was known as diachylon plaster (Lead Oleate Plaster *N.F. IX*). This type of plaster required the application of heat in order to spread and apply the plaster to the skin. Plasters are now prepared with a base of India rubber or with mixtures of vinyl resin, plasticizers and other chemical additives. These plasters are adhesive at body temperature and, hence, can be applied readily without heating. Furthermore, the newer adhesive plasters possess a lower incidence of irritation and sensitization than the older plasters which contained such ingredients as rosin and pitch. Plasters in general may be somewhat irritant, partly because they prevent evaporation from the skin and partly because of the small quantities of volatile oils contained in the resins from which plasters are often prepared.

Years ago, the pharmacist prepared plasters extemporaneously. With the introduction of machine-made plasters, the hand-spread plasters became obsolete. However, the pharmacist should instruct the patient purchasing a plaster as to the method of applying. The part to which the plaster is applied must be dry and clean to ensure close contact between the skin and plaster.

The plaster serves two purposes: (1) it affords protection and mechanical support and (2) it may be medicated, in which case it brings medication into close contact with the skin surface. The demand for medicated plasters is limited to those containing salicyclic acid and mustard. One plaster is official in the *U.S.P.*: Salicylic Acid Plaster, and none are official in the *N.F.*

Poultices or cataplasms are soft preparations applied to the skin while hot in order to reduce inflammation or, in some cases, to act as counterirritants. They apply moist heat to the body areas and theoretically draw infectious materials from body tissues. The drawing action is ascribed to the hygroscopic nature of the ingredients used as the poultice base, i.e., kaolin, flaxseed and other mucilaginous substances. The last official poultice was Kaolin Cataplasm *N.F. IX*. It contained kaolin, boric acid, thymol, methyl salicylate, peppermint oil and glycerin and was used as a warming poultice for deep-seated inflammations.

REFERENCES

1. Barr, M.: J. Pharm. Sci. *51*:395, 1962.
2. Barr, M., and Guth, E. P.: J. Am. Pharm. Ass. [Sci.] *40*:13, 1957.
3. Barrett, C. W., Hadgraft, J. W., Caron, G. A., and Sarkany, I.: Brit. J. Derm *77*:576, 1965.
4. Blank, I. H.: Invest. Derm. *18*:433, 1952.
5. ———: J. Invest. Derm. *21*:259, 1953.
6. ———: Proc. Sci. Sec. Toilet Goods Ass. *23*:19, 1955.
7. Blank, I. H., and Gould, E.: J. Invest. Derm. *33*:327, 1959.
8. Blank, I. H., Griesemer, R. D., and Gould, E.: J. Invest. Dermatol. *30*:187, 1958.

9. Blank, I. H., Smith, J. G., and Fischer, R. W.: J. Invest. Dermatol. *36*:337, 1961.

10. Blank, I. H., and Shappirio, E. B.: J. Invest. Derm. *25*:391, 1955.

11. Blaug, S. M., and Ahsan, S. S.: Drug Stand. *28*:95,1960.

12. ———: J. Am. Pharm. Ass. [Sci.] *50*:441, 1961.

13. *British Pharmaceutical Codex.* The Pharmaceutical Press, London, 1968, p. 1031.

14. *British Pharmaceutical Codex.* The Pharmaceutical Press, London, 1968, p. 1092.

15. *British Pharmacopoeia,* The Pharmaceutical Press, London, 1968, p. 373.

16. Canals, E., and Gidon, M.: J. Pharm. Chim. *2*:102, 1925.

17. Casparis, P., and Myer, E. W.: Pharm. acta helv. *10*:163, 1935.

18. Chakravarty, D., Lach, J. L., and Blaug, S. M.: Drug Stand. *25*:137, 1957.

19. Clark, E. W.: Am. Perf. Cosmet. *77*:89, 1962.

20. Clark, W. G.: Am. J. Med. Sci. *212*:523, 1946.

21. Collom, W. D., and Winek, C. L.: J. Pharm. Sci., *56*:1673, 1967.

22. Conrad, L. I., and Maso, H. F.: Am. Perf. Cosmet. *77*:97, 1962.

23. Cyr, G. N., Skauen, D. M., Christian, J. E., and Lee, C. O.: Am. Pharm. Ass. [Sci.] *38*:615, 1949.

24. Darlington, R. C., and Guth, E. P.: J. Am. Pharm. Ass. [Pract.] *11*:82, 1950.

25. Davies, J. T.: J. Soc. Cosmet. Chem. *12*: 193, 1961.

26. Dillaha, C. J., Jansen, G. T., and Honeycutt, M. W.: Progr. Derm., Quart. Bull. Dermatol. Foundation, New York, 1966.

27. Everall, J., and Truter, E. V.: J. Invest. Derm. *22*:493, 1954.

28. Fantus, B., and Dyniewicz, H.: J. Am. Pharm. Ass. [Sci.] *28*:548, 1939.

29. Feldman, R. J., and Maibach, H. I.: Arch. Derm. *94*:649, 1966.

30. Flesch, P., and Esoda, E. C. J.: J. Invest. Derm. *28*:5, 1957.

31. Foster, W., Wurster, D. E., Higuchi, T., and Busse, L. W.: J. Am. Pharm. Ass. [Sci.] *40*:123, 1951.

32. Goodman, H.: J. Am. Pharm. Ass. [Pract.] *3*:7, 1942.

33. Griesemer, R. D.: J. Soc. Cosmet. Chem. *11*:79, 1960.

34. Halpern, A., and Zopf, L. C.: J. Am. Pharm. Ass. [Sci.] *36*:101, 1947.

35. Higuchi, T.: J. Soc. Cosmet. Chem. *11*: 85, 1960.

36. Higuchi, T., and Lach, J. L.: J. Am. Pharm. Ass. [Sci.] *43*:465, 1954.

37. Hjorth, N., and Trolle-Lassen, C.: Trans. St. John's Hosp. Derm. Soc., London *49*: 127, 1963.

38. Jacobi, O., and Heinrich, H.: Proc. Sci. Sect. Toilet Goods Ass. No. 21, 1954.

39. Johnston, G. W., and Lee, C. O.: J. Am. Pharm. Ass. [Sci.] *32*:278, 1943.

40. Jones, E. R., and Lewicki, B.: J. Am. Pharm. Ass. [Sci.] *40*:509, 1951.

41. Kligman, A. M.: *The Epidermis.* Academic Press, New York, 1964, p. 387.

42. ———: J. Am. Med. Ass. *193*:140, 1965.

43. Klocke, R. A., Gurtner, G. H., and Farhi, L. E.: J. Appl. Physiol. *18*:311, 1963.

44. Landon, F. W., and Zopf, L. C.: J. Am. Pharm. Ass. [Pract.] *4*:251, 1943.

45. ———: Am. Prof. Pharm. *13*:357, 1947.

46. Lawler, J. C., Davis, J. C., and Griffiths, E. C.: J. Invest. Derm. *34*:301, 1960.

47. Lower, E. S., and Cressey, S.: Drug Cosmet. Ind. *81*:450, 1957.

48. Lubowe, I. I.: *New Hope for Your Skin.* Dutton and Co., New York, 1963.

49. McClelland, C. P., and Bateman, R. L.: J. Am. Pharm. Ass. [Pract.] *10*:30, 1949.

50. MacKee, G. M., Sulzberger, M. B., Herrmann, F., and Baer, R. J.: J. Invest. Derm. *6*:43, 1945.

51. McKenzie, A. W., and Aitkinson, R. M.: Arch. Derm. *89*:741, 1964.

52. McKenzie, A. W., and Stoughton, R. B.: Arch. Derm. *86*:608, 1962.

53. Mali, J. W. H.: J. Invest. Derm. *27*:451, 1956.

54. Malkinson, F. D.: J. Invest. Derm. *31*:19, 1958.

55. Marzulli, F. N.: J. Invest. Derm. *37*:387, 1962.

56. Matoltsy, A. G., Downes, A. M., and Sweeney, T. M.: J. Invest. Derm. *50*: 19, 1968.

57. Meyers, D. B., Nadkarni, M. V., and Zopf, L. C.: J. Am. Pharm. Ass. [Pract.] *32*:231, 1949.

57a. Michelfelder, T. J., and Peck, S. M.: J. Invest. Derm. *19*:237, 1952.

58. Miller, O. B., and Selle, W. A.: J. Invest. Derm. *12*:19, 1949.

59. Monash, S.: J. Invest. Derm. *29*:367, 1957.

60. Monash, S., and Blank, H.: A.M.A. Arch. Derm. *78*:710, 1958.

61. Montagna, W.: *The Structure and Function of the Skin.* Academic Press, New York, 1962.

62. Murphy, J. T. (ed.): Formulary of the Massachusetts General Hospital and The Massachusetts Eye and Ear Infirmary, pp. 91, 92, 94, 95, 1951.
63. Newcomb, E. A.: J. Soc. Cosmet. Chem. *17*:149, 1966.
64. Nogami, H., Hasegawa, J., and Hanano, M.: Pharm. Bull. Tokyo *4*:347, 1956.
65. Onken, H. D., and Moyer, C. A.: Arch. Dermatol. *87*:584, 1963.
66. Pail, D., and Todd, C. W.: Am. Perf. Cosmet. *77*:162, 1962.
67. Peck, S. M.: Proc. Sci. Sect., Toilet Goods Ass. *18*:33, 1952.
68. Peck, S. M., and Glick, A. W.: J. Soc. Cos. Chem. *7*:530, 1955.
69. Peck, S. M., Rosenfeld, H., Leifer, W., and Bierman, W.: Arch. Derm. *39*:126, 1939.
70. Plein, J. B., and Plein, E. M.: J. Am. Pharm. Ass. [Sci.] *42*:79, 1953.
71. ———: Bull. Am. Soc. Hosp. Pharm. *13*:38, 1956.
72. Poulsen, B. J., Young, E., Coquilla, V., and Katz, M.: J. Pharm. Sci. *57*:928, 1968.
73. Powers, D. H., and Fox, C.: Drug Cosmet. Ind. *82*:32, 1958.
74. Riegelman, S.: Am. Perf. Cosmet. *77*:31, 1962.
75. Riegelman, S., and Vaughn, D. G., Jr.: J. Am. Pharm. Ass. [Pract.] *19*:474, 1958.
76. Rochow, E. G.: *Chemistry of the Silicones,* ed. 2. New York, Wiley, 1951.
77. Rothman, S.: *Physiology and Biochemistry of the Skin.* University of Chicago Press, Chicago, Illinois, 1954.
78. ———: J. Lab. Clin. Med. *28*:1305, 1943.
79. Scheuplein, R. J.: J. Invest. Derm. *45*:334, 1965.
80. Shelmire, J. B.: J. Invest. Derm. *26*:105, 1956.
81. ———: Arch. Derm. *78*:191, 1958.
82. ———: A.M.A. Arch. Derm. *82*:24, 1960.
83. Steigleder, G. K., and Raab, W. P.: J. Invest. Derm. *38*:129, 1962.
84. Stoughton, R. B.: Arch. Derm. *91*:657, 1965.
85. Strakesch, E. A.: Arch. Derm. Syphilol. *47*:16, 1943.
86. Sulzberger, M. B., Warshaw, T., and Herrmann, F.: J. Invest. Derm. *20*:33, 1953.
87. Tas, H., and Feige, Y.: J. Invest. Derm. *30*:193, 1958.
88. Tiedt, J., and Truter, E. V.: Chem. Ind., London *403*, 1952.
89. Tregear, R. T.: J. Soc. Cosmet. Chem. *13*:145, 1962.
90. ———: J. Invest. Derm. *46*:24, 1966.
91. ———: *Physical Functions of Skin.* Academic Press, London and New York, 1966.
92. Treherne, J. E.: J. Physiol. *133*:171, 1956.
93. Wells, F. V., and Lubowe, I. I.: *Cosmetics and the Skin.* Reinhold Publishing Company, New York, 1964.
94. Wurster, D. E., and Kramer, S. F.: J. Pharm. Sci. *50*:288, 1961.
95. Zopf, L. C.: *In* Sprowls, J. B., and Beal, H. M. (eds.): American Pharmacy, ed. 5, p. 315, Philadelphia, J. B. Lippincott, 1960.

Chapter 7

Suppositories

Charles F. Peterson, Ph.D.*

Suppositories are solid, shaped unit dosage forms for the application of medication to the rectum, the vaginal cavity or the urethral tract. Certain manufacturers refer to the last two dosage forms as "inserts," particularly when made by compression as a specially shaped tablet. These melt or dissolve in the secretions of the cavity and usually release the medication over a prolonged period. The suppository, a solid dosage form, is conveniently inserted within the cavity and after a short time becomes a semi-fluid, having ointment-like consistency. Similarly there are a number of ointments and creams which are applied to the rectal or the vaginal cavity (usually with a special device). Therefore, the concepts of ointment formulation are used in suppository formulation and should be kept in mind for rational use of rectal and vaginal medications.

The use of suppositories has been traced to the time of the ancient Egyptians and Greeks.[14] Hippocrates recorded the use of herb and soap mixtures which were inserted rectally to stimulate the defecation reflex. This use of suppositories appears in many early writings. Systemic absorption of drugs did not appear to be important to these ancients, although some mixtures containing potent drugs such as mandrake and poppy seeds were mentioned. Perhaps the lack of a suitable base and, consequently, of availability of the active drug kept this dosage form from dependable use.

In the late 18th century, cocoa butter became available and Antoine Baumé recognized and promoted its usefulness as a suppository base in Europe. In 1852, A. B.

Taylor suggested the use of cocoa butter as a suppository base to American pharmacists.[30] It was recognized as Theobroma Oil in *U.S.P. V.* and its use and the employment of suppositories gradually increased.

Suppositories are classified by the site to which they are to be applied and whether the medication is intended for local or systemic effects. The size and the shape of the suppository are such that they facilitate insertion into the body opening. Some manufacturers of "inserts" furnish an apparatus designed to place the "insert" high in the vaginal tract and beyond the reach of the fingers. This type of preparation will be considered to be a special category of suppositories, since, in general, suppositories are placed with the fingers into the intended opening. The pharmacist should make sure that the patient understands the correct application of the dosage form dispensed to the patient.

When used without qualification, the term suppository usually signifies the dosage form intended for rectal insertion. The *U.S.P.* describes rectal suppositories for adults as usually weighing about 2 Gm. each and having a tapered shape.[32] The most popular shapes appear in Figure 7-1. Of these shapes, the one preferred by many is the modified torpedo. On insertion of the blunt head, the pressure exerted on the suppository by the external anal sphincter is translated into movement which forces the suppository into the rectum. The modified torpedo is formed most satisfactorily by molding as in the fusion process. In hand rolling, the cylindrical shape is more easily attained. The largest diameter should be about 13 mm., usually tapered to about

* Professor of Pharmacy, Temple University, Philadelphia, Pa.

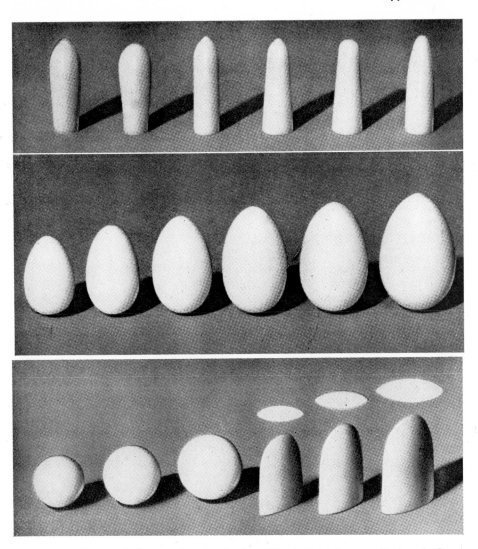

FIG. 7-1. Sizes and shapes of suppositories. (*Top*) Rectal suppositories, 1 Gm.: torpedo; cylindrical; tapered. (*Center*) Vaginal ovals. (*Bottom*) Vaginal balls and pessaries, with cross section. (From Chemical and Pharmaceutical Co., Inc., 260 West Broadway, New York, N. Y.)

7 mm., and the length about 25 to 35 mm. For the small child, the diameter and the length is less, with reduction of weight to about 1 Gm.

Vaginal suppositories are more varied in shape and usually have globular, ovoid or modified conical shapes. They are described as weighing about 5 Gm., but, examination of the majority of commercial vaginal suppositories has shown that many weigh between 3 and 4 Gm. and some weigh as much as 8 Gm. The vaginal suppository is used primarily for local effects, although it should be kept in mind that the mucous epithelial surface in the vaginal tract is well supplied with circulation so that medication may be absorbed and have systemic effects.

Urethral suppositories (which may be called "inserts") are the form least used. These are slender rods, 3 to 6 mm. in diameter, preferably somewhat flexible, yet firm enough for insertion. For the male urethra these are 100 to 150 mm. long and for the female 60 to 75 mm.

MEDICATION BY SUPPOSITORY AND RELATED DOSAGE METHODS

Suppositories and the related dosage methods, such as ointments, enemas and vaginal douches, are classified as special topical applications either to the vaginal tract or to the rectum. Most of these medications are intended to produce only local action; systemic drug absorption is intentional only by the rectal route.

Medications introduced into the vaginal tract are intended almost invariably for local action such as anti-infective, spermatocidal or cleansing. Systemic action of drugs placed in the vagina has been observed,[19a] usually as an unwanted effect. The usual intent of vaginal medication is that the drug be well diluted with the inert vehicle and remain where placed for a relatively long period as a nonirritating preparation without any systemic effects.

Local rectal medication may have one of two contrasting therapeutic effects: (1) the soothing effect of a local anesthetic or an anti-infective such as the preparations used for hemorrhoidal treatment, or (2) the effect of the evacuant suppositories and the cleansing enemas that are used to stimulate the defecation reflex and to empty the rectum and lower colon.

SYSTEMIC DOSAGE BY RECTAL SUPPOSITORY

An important use of rectal medication is the administration of drugs for their systemic effects when other routes are unavailable, e.g., rectal administration of an antiemetic when the patient is unable to retain the drug in oral dosage form, because of cyclic vomiting. Or, if the drug is one that may interfere with the gastrointestinal enzymes (or vice-versa) if administered orally, the rectal route may be preferred. With some drugs, this route is as effective as parenteral administration. Furthermore, the rate at which the drug is made available for absorption may be controlled by compounding with an appropriate vehicle.

The implications of the choice of vehicle for the drug and the possibility of a rapid or prolonged duration of action are considered in terms of the rectum as the site of application. The suppository is the usual dosage form for this application; however, the physician should also consider the rectal retention enema, by means of which the drug solution is placed into the lower colon immediately within the inner sphincter.

It has been pointed out that the physician should determine the state of rectal functioning and the sensitivity of the patient for whom rectal administration is contemplated.

The function of the normal rectum is expulsion rather than retention, but there are individuals whose lower bowel is quite insensitive and habitually contains fecal matter. . . . On the other hand, there are those whose rectums are exceedingly sensitive, as in various forms of proctitis, and who would have difficulty retaining medicaments.[*]

It is important that both the pharmacist and the physician realize that conditions such as anal fissure or inflamed hemorrhoids may make rectal administration difficult or dangerous.

The problems related to the rectal dosage places certain limits on the administration of drugs by this route. The correct dose for the rectal suppository must be determined for each drug. In some cases the concentration of the drug or the total amount of the drug that must be given will be either too irritating or in greater amount than reasonably can be placed into a suppository. The dose of 400 to 500 mg. of a drug may be considered as a maximum, making allowance for increasing the weight of the suppository to 3 Gm. In any case, the availability of the drug from the medication base is dependent on physical characteristics of the finished dosage form. The suppository base and the drug cannot be considered separately because mixture of drug with vehicle usually changes the physical properties of the latter.

As Reigelman and Crowell have shown,[19] diffusion of the drug to the surface for absorption is one of the rate-limiting steps. They demonstrated the important effect of particle size of the suspended drug and the apparent effect of surface-active agents on the mucous fluid secreted over the absorbing surface. Another influence which can be projected is the lowered availability of the drug when it is bound to components of the base either through physical interaction with the surface-active agents present or through

* Smith, A.: Technic of Medication, p. 126, Philadelphia, Lippincott, 1948.

preferential solubility of the drug in the base. The effect of percentage of saturation on the release of the drug from the solutions has been thoroughly presented by Allawala and Reigelman.[1] The reasoning may be easily followed that a drug that is very soluble in theobroma oil and present in a low concentration will have a smaller tendency to escape to the aqueous solution than will one that is slightly soluble and present in the theobroma oil at saturation level.

The absorption of drugs from the colon as described by Schanker[23] and the kinetics of rectal absorption as determined by Reigelman and Crowell[19] agree in principle, so that it might be said that the absorption of drugs from the colon and that from the rectum are quite similar. However, one should keep in mind that the area to which rectal retention enema is applied is much greater than that of the suppository, since the latter makes contact only with the rectal ampulla. The real anatomic difference, with perhaps a physiologic advantage, is that the rectum is supplied with the lower and the middle hemorrhoidal veins which pass directly into the general circulation. The upper hemorrhoidal vein along with venous supply for the digestive tract pass into the hepatic portal system. Thus, medications and food products assimilated in the alimentary tract circulate through the liver before reaching the general system. Drugs which are modified in activity or concentration by the liver are thought to act more rapidly if they are spared immediate action by the liver. Bucher showed that more than one half (50 to 70%) of the rectally administered drug was absorbed directly into the general circulation.[3]

Among the many drugs which have been found to produce useful systemic effects in rectal dosage are aspirin, aminophylline, chloral hydrate and tribromoethanol, as well as many of the barbiturate and the alkaloidal salts.

The results of a most interesting recent study[33] which makes a distinct contribution to the understanding of rectal absorption are shown in Figure 7-2, which compares the blood serum levels of lincomycin in 10 subjects, after a single 500-mg. dose. The commercial capsule was given orally with about 6 fluid ounces of water and the fasting period

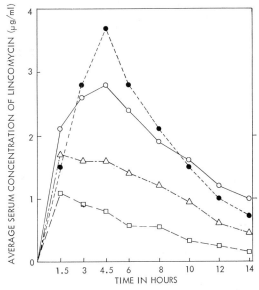

Fig. 7-2. Average serum concentrations of lincomycin in 10 subjects common to three studies in adult volunteers. *Key:* •----• capsule, oral, fasting, study A; o———o solution rectal, preceded by enemas, fasting, study B; △—•—△ solution, rectal, without enema, nonfasting, study C; □——□ suppository, rectal, without enema, fasting, study A. (Wagner, J. G., Carter, C. H., and Martens, I. J.: J. Clin. Pharmacol. *8:* 158, 1968)

continued for 4 hours post medication. The rectal solution was prepared by dilution with water of the 500-mg. aliquot of the lincomycin solution to make 10 ml. The cleansing enema was given before retiring for the night and the 10-ml. aqueous lincomycin solution was administered rectally by means of an infant rectal syringe in the morning. The fasting period was overnight and for the 4-hour period after medication. The suppository contained 500 mg. of lincomycin (as the hydrochloride) in a mixture of Carbowax 6000, 45 per cent, Carbowax 1500, 25 per cent and sufficient deionized water to make (with the drug) 100 per cent. The dramatic differences between the drug serum concentrations produced by the rectal suppository and the rectal solution are partially explained by the fact that the suppository was given without a cleansing enema. The cleansing of the rectum allowed greater spreading of the 10 ml. within the rectal area than was possible when either the suppository or the solution was administered without the cleansing enema.

Other factors that influence availability from the rectal-colon area include the degree of ionization and the lipid:water partition of the undissociated form. The pH of the colon was demonstrated by Schanker[23] as 6.8 to 7.0, and it was found to have little buffer capacity. Thus in the colon the dissolved drugs determine the existing pH according to their own properties of dissociation. Therefore, weak acids and bases are absorbed, whereas those that are highly ionized are absorbed slowly. Schanker further showed that acidic drugs were absorbed more readily when the rectal contents were made more acidic. Weak organic electrolytes that are highly lipid-soluble were found to be absorbed more readily.

Schanker's work is further confirmed by a study comparing the rectal and the oral administration of tetracycline and penicillin. Wagner and co-workers[34] dissolved the drug in 5 ml. of water for administration by infant rectal syringe. The tetracycline absorption by the rectal route was 9 per cent of the oral dosage. This acidic solution was not appreciably changed by the low buffer capacity of the rectal contents and thus only a small portion of the drug was available for absorption as the un-ionized form. The penicillin in this form was absorbed at 13.5 per cent of the oral dosage, and this is explained in the same manner. By comparison, the rectal lincomycin (Fig. 7-2) was absorbed at 58 per cent of the oral dosage, owing to its relatively neutral characteristics. The tetracycline hydrochloride was found to be very irritating because of the highly acidic solution, causing a short retention time (average of 74 minutes) as compared to the average of 473 minutes for the sodium penicillin solution administered to the same patients in a crossover experiment.

TESTING OF THE SUPPOSITORY

The *U.S.P. XVIII* in its definition of suppositories states that the preparation should melt, soften or dissolve at body temperature.[32] Also, on page 4 of the General Notices section of the *U.S.P.* under Ointments and Suppositories there is the statement . . . "the proportions of the substances constituting the base may be varied to maintain a suitable consistence under different climatic conditions, provided the proportion of active ingredients is not varied." The official procedure for determining the melting temperature of fatty substances (Class II) can be used to determine the melting range of the simple suppository, but it does not prove to be satisfactory for those suppositories containing a significant amount of suspended particles. Nor is the melting procedure satisfactory for the definition of "softening or dissolving at body temperature."

Setnikar and Fantelli[24,25] painstakingly reviewed the proposed methods for describing the physical properties of suppositories and have suggested an improved test procedure. This procedure for liquefaction time appears to answer many of the problems not previously solved by any one procedure. A comparison of the liquefaction times with the clinical experiences should be made, as was done by Hennig,[11] to make the results of this test significant.

Setnikar and Fantelli described the mechanical and the physicochemical conditions present in the human rectum which they thought important for a test procedure to reproduce. These were: (a) an average temperature of 36.9° C. (36.2° to 37.6° C.); (b) water not present in the liquid state but represented in the semisolid feces (which contain about 80% of water); (c) water content somewhat variable due to diffusion from the body fluids (osmotic force attracts the water, and high force may result in irritation and pain); (d) practically no peristaltic movement; (e) pressure on the contents varying from zero to 50 cm. of water, and (f) possible presence of feces.

The apparatus (Fig. 7-3) is prepared by placing a length of moistened inflated cellulose dialysis tubing through the cylinder and over the ends, securing the end of the tubing with elastic bands. Water is circulated through the cylinder and the height of the apparatus adjusted so that the lower half of the tubing is collapsed. When the temperature of the water has been adjusted to 37° C., the suppository is dropped into the open end of the tube. Then the apparatus is lowered about 30 cm. to obtain the desired pressure of water. The liquefaction time is determined

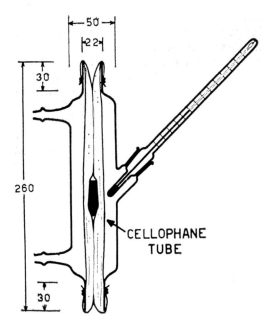

FIG. 7-3. Apparatus for measuring the liquefaction time of rectal suppositories; the dimensions are in millimeters. The thermometer scale is divided into tenths of a degree and a scale ranging from 32 to 45° is adequate. (Setnikar, I., and Fantelli, S.: J. Pharm. Sci. *51*:566-571)

when the suppository has completely melted.

A comparison of melting points and liquefaction times of some suppository bases is given in Table 7-1. More detailed compositions for the suppository bases are listed in Chapter 12 of *American Pharmacy,* 6th Edition.

SUPPOSITORY BASES

In suppositories, the function of materials other than medication is to present an acceptable and usable dosage form. For example, the difficulty of handling a rectal evacuant dose of glycerin is overcome by the addition of soap to make a firm gelled mass which can be inserted readily. The suppository base also may be required for dilution of the drug to a nonirritating concentration. Thus, the irritant local action and the volatility of chloral hydrate are reduced to acceptable levels by incorporation into a suppository. Other possible functions of the base are to stabilize or to control the rate of release of the drug. This may be demonstrated by the following example. The poor gastric dissolution of aminophylline from a compressed tablet form and its consequent slow rate of assimilation may

TABLE 7-1. SUPPOSITORY BASES: COMPARISON OF MELTING CHARACTERISTICS*

BASE	MELTING POINT (° C.)	LIQUEFACTION (° C.)	LIQUEFACTION TIME (min.)	SOFTENING POINT (° C.)	COLLAPSING WEIGHT AT 25°C. (Kg.)
Theobroma Oil	34	34	6	29	3.4
Witepsol H12†	36	36	9	32	4.7
Witepsol W35†	36.5	37	10	31	4.0
Witepsol E79†	38.5	38.5	#	33	4.7
Myrj 52‡	51	47	31	42	>5
Tween 61‡	39	39	#	25	0.5
Glycerinated Gelatin USP	50	50	32	25	0.5
Carbowax 4000§	59	59	30	55	>5
Carbowax 6000§	62	63	45	56	>5
Carbowax 6000§ with 20% water	54	61	27	51	2.0

* Data from Setnikar and Fantelli.[24,25]

† Reported by Setnikar and Fantelli as Imhausen products, Chemische Werke Witten, Ruhr, Germany. (Riches-Nelson Inc., Greenwich, Conn., Agents.)

‡ Atlas Chemical Co., Wilmington, Delaware.

§ Union Carbide Chemicals Co., New York, New York.

No liquefaction, softening after 10 to 20 minutes.

be obviated by use of a suppository preparation containing a dispersion of finely powdered drug in a suitable base.

A general classification of suppository bases is possible on the basis of their physical properties. The oleaginous class includes cocoa butter and fats with similar properties and contrasts with the "water-soluble" class which includes the polyethylene glycols and glycero-gelatin. An intermediate "hydrophilic" class is proposed to include all those not included in the other two as well as those surfactants and mixtures which disperse themselves or the medication in water.

Theobroma oil (cocoa butter) is the principal suppository base and is often thought of as the base to be used when none is specified. It is a firm solid of cream color which, on warming, begins to soften at 30° C. and melts to a thin oil at about 34° C. Unlike many fats and oils, cocoa butter is generally uniform, having a faint, agreeable odor. Its composition is also different in that there are only a small number of glyceride types present and two of these constitute more than three fourths of the total. Meara[16] reported the composition of one representative sample of cocoa butter to be as follows:

	MOLE PERCENTAGE
Fully saturated triglycerides	2.6
Oleodipalmitin	3.7
Oleopalmitostearin	57.0
Oleodistearin	22.2
Palmitodiolein	7.4
Sterodiolein	5.8
Triolein	1.1

A consequence of the presence of the high proportion of disaturated triglycerides is marked polymorphism (the property of existing in several crystalline forms). When cocoa butter is heated to above the melting temperature (about 36° C.) and then chilled in a suppository mold, solidification does not take place until the temperature is well below 15° C. and crystallization takes place as a metastable form. If such a suppository is taken from the mold after such treatment and allowed to come to room temperature, it will be found to melt at about 23° or 24° C. The explanation of this phenomenon is that the stable crystal nuclei have been lost by heating the cocoa butter beyond the melting point. Should the suppository made from the overheated cocoa butter be allowed to remain cool for a sufficient length of time, its original melting temperature will be restored. The exact length of time will vary from a few days to more than a week according to the response of the melted mass to the rate of cooling and the presence of other components. Should it be necessary to heat cocoa butter, the melting should be done carefully, keeping temperature of the mass as low as possible and mixing well to keep the temperature uniform. The finely shredded fat is heated carefully to a creamy, pourable state, leaving nuclei of the stable crystals which, on cooling, encourage solidification to the original form.

A further complication results with cocoa butter suppositories when substances dissolve significantly in the fat and lower the melting temperature. It is well known that the freezing point of a solution is lower than that of the pure solvent and the freezing point depression is proportional to the concentration of the solute. The proportionality constant is the molal freezing point depression which is estimated as 15° to 16° C. for cocoa butter.*

Increasing the concentration of a soluble substance in the fat lowers melting temperatures of the mixture until the eutectic point is obtained. Further addition of the substance increases the melting temperature from the eutectic point up to the melting point of the added compound. Thus, the addition of white wax to the cocoa butter in amounts up to 3 per cent will give mixtures which have lower melting temperatures than the original cocoa butter (even after appropriate aging). Addition of white wax beyond 6 per cent is required to raise the melting temperature of the cocoa butter–wax mixture. Even larger proportions of wax will be required to make an acceptable suppository should other soluble components be present in amounts having a significant effect on the melting temperature.

The addition of a greater number of com-

* This value was calculated from the melting point determinations reported by Oesch[14] for dilute concentrations (about 0.05 molal) of phenol and procaine.

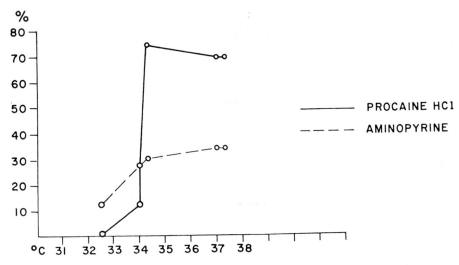

FIG. 7-4. The per cent of drug released from cocoa butter after 90 minutes as related to the temperature of the test. Abscissa: temperature in °C. (Sprowls, J. B.: American Pharmacy, ed. 6. Philadelphia, J. B. Lippincott, 1966.)

ponents may also have the effect of increasing the melting range. The suppository may have a liquid portion held by the crystalline matrix at ordinary room temperatures. On warming, additional components become melted until a significant portion has been melted and the solid form no longer exists. Thus, the melting point of the base is most significant when the medication is not appreciably dissolved in the base but is merely suspended in it. Figure 7-4 illustrates the availability of aminopyrine and procaine hydrochloride from cocoa butter in an in-vitro test as reported by Eckert and Muhleman.[8]

In determining these data, the procaine hydrochloride was suspended in the cocoa butter as a fine powder. It is evident that the procaine was able to transfer to the oil–water interface after the temperature had reached the melting temperature of the cocoa butter. The aminopyrine was released to the water and did not appear to be more than slightly temperature-dependent. It may be assumed that the aminopyrine was dissolved in the liquid portion of the suppository base and was transferred by diffusion to the oil–water interface.

Fatty Substitutes. A number of oleaginous substances have been suggested as substitutes for cocoa butter. Most recently the use of Illipe butter, or Borneo tallow, has been proposed.[20] This vegetable fat, because its melting temperature is slightly higher than that of cocoa butter, may be used more conveniently. The German Pharmacopoeia in 1959 recognized **Adeps Solidus** in its Third Supplement to the 6th Edition.[6] The monograph bearing this title describes neutral fatty compounds containing triglycerides of saturated vegetable fatty acids mixed with partial glycerides in various amounts to control viscosity and emulsifying ability of the base (see Table 7-1, p. 265). A number of items similar to Adeps Solidus are now available in the United States and include the Wecobee series* and the Witepsol series.† These bases are reviewed by Pennati and Steiger-Trippi.[18]

In general, oleaginous compounds of the types described are used in the same way as cocoa butter; however, they have an advantage in that the formation of unstable polymorphic forms with lower melting points does not take place easily. They have increased ability to emulsify water and glycerin and are stable to oxidation. However, Hennig[11] and others have shown that drugs are absorbed at different rates from these bases and from cocoa butter. Therefore, this is another indication of the need for clinical

* Drew Chemical Co., Boonton, N.J.
† Riches-Nelson, Inc., Greenwich, Conn.

TABLE 7-2. PHYSICAL PROPERTIES OF SELECTED POLYETHYLENE GLYCOLS
FOR SUPPOSITORY USE*

SERIES NO.	AVERAGE MOLECULAR WEIGHT	SPECIFIC GRAVITY	FREEZING RANGE ° C.	SOLUBILITY AT 20° C. (GM. PER 100 ML.)		
				WATER	METHANOL	ETHANOL
300 (N.F.)	300	1.125	−15 to −8	completely miscible		
400 (U.S.P.)	400	1.125	4– 8	completely miscible		
1,500	†	1.15	38–41	73	48	1
1,540 (N.F.)	1,450	1.15	42–46	70		
4,000 (U.S.P.)	3,350	1.204	53–56	62	35	1
6,000	6,750	1.207	60–63	50		
20,000	17,500	1.215	53‡	§		

* Abstracted from "Carbowax" Polyethylene Glycols, Union Carbide Chemicals Corporation, 1958.
† Mixture of equal parts polyethylene glycol 300 and polyethylene glycol 1,540.
‡ Softening point reported because of the high viscosity of the melt.
§ Data not available.

comparison of results, as opposed to reliance on in-vitro data.

WATER-SOLUBLE SUPPOSITORY BASES

Glycerinated Gelatin. The general formula and procedure for making Glycerinated Gelatin Suppositories are described in *U.S.P. XVIII,* and may be outlined as follows:

Water and the medicinal agents ..	10 Gm.
Glycerin	70 Gm.
Gelatin	20 Gm.

The ingredients are mixed in the order in which they have been given, taking particular care that the medication is dissolved and the gelatin added without formation of lumps or incorporation of air. Solvation of the gelatin requires heat and time. Tice[31] suggested that a salt-water bath be used to increase the temperature and reduce the time for the gelatin to dissolve. If an electric hot plate is used, care must be taken so that the high temperature does not cause the mixture to burn, especially since the glycero-gelatin mixture does not conduct heat readily from the bottom to the rest of the mixture. The mass should be well stirred, but with care that air bubbles are not entrapped. Either Gelatin A* or Gelatin B* may be used to make the suppositories, according to the compatibilities of the medication. Propylene glycol or Polyethylene glycol 400 may be used to replace the glycerin for drugs requiring such

* Kind and Knox Gelatin Co., Camden, N. J.

solvents. Sometimes the gelatin content is increased to as much as 30 per cent to make a firmer suppository, especially when it is to be used for rectal insertion.

Glycerinated gelatin base is most often used for local application of antibacterial agents to the vaginal tract where it is intended that the solution be retained for prolonged action of the drug. The hygroscopic tendency of the glycerin makes it necessary that the suppository be protected from external moisture and, at the same time, requires sufficient water to be present in the glycerinated gelatin suppository to prevent irritation of the mucous tissues. It is recommended that the glycerinated gelatin suppository be moistened with water before insertion to take away the initial "sting" caused by the hygroscopic agent.

The polyethylene glycols were developed in Germany during the 1930's as the result of the need for "ersatz" materials. They were patented in the United States and Germany in 1938 as water-soluble ointment and suppository materials.[2] The solid polyethylene glycols have molecular weights above 1,000 (as shown in Table 7-2). The viscous solutions formed when they are used are less likely to leak from the body cavity to which they have been applied. As is the case with glycerinated gelatin, water must be compounded in the suppository or the suppository dipped in water before insertion in order to overcome the possibility of irrita-

TABLE 7-3. POLYETHYLENE GLYCOL SUPPOSITORY BASES

BASE NO.	1*	2*	3†	4‡	5‡	6‡	7‡
Polyethylene glycol 400			30				
Polyethylene glycol 1,000				96	75		
Polyethylene glycol 1,540	33		30			70	30
Polyethylene glycol 4,000		33	40	4	25		
Polyethylene glycol 6,000	47	47				30	50
Water	20	20					20

* Sperandio, G. J., and Hassler, W. H.: J. Am. Pharm. Assoc. (Pract.) *14*:26, 1953.
† Hassler, W. H., and Cacchillo, A. F.: J. Am. Pharm. Assoc. (Sci.) *43*:683, 1954.
‡ Collins, A. P., Hohman, J. R., and Zopf, L. C.: Am. Prof. Pharm. *23*:231, 1957.

tion caused by water being drawn from the tissues to dissolve the base and release the medicament. Formulators have suggested the use of a coating containing a local anesthetic, and another suggestion which has been made is to include a waxy material such as cetyl alcohol. The former suggestion adds therapeutic complication and the latter suggestion makes a product that is dissolved slowly. The problem of irritation is emphasized in the arguments against the use of these bases, whereas the proponents of the use of the base find that irritation is a minor consequence. There is reason to believe that the level of irritation will vary with individuals, medications, formula modifications and conditions of use.

Cacchillo and Hassler[4] reported that the 2-hour blood salicylate level after administration of acetylsalicylic acid averaged as follows: water-soluble suppository, 93 per cent of the level after oral administration; cocoa butter suppository 66 per cent and glycero-gelatin suppository, 53 per cent. Sperandio and Hassler[27] compared the polyethylene glycol base with cocoa butter by making suppositories of water-soluble barbiturates and determining the onset of action and the duration of action in rats. The onset of barbiturate action was more rapid from cocoa butter suppositories and the duration of action was longer from polyethylene glycol suppositories.

Some examples of formulas proposed for polyethylene glycol bases will be found in Table 7-3.

As these formulas indicate, considerable variation is possible in the proportions of high molecular weight and low molecular weight polyethylene glycols to be used. With certain drugs it may be possible to use a single solid polyethylene glycol.

Difficulties in compounding are usually reduced by mixing several of these bases to yield the desired properties. An example of the difficulties encountered is the formation of a gelatinous mass which occurs when aminophylline is melted with polyethylene glycol 4,000 (Guida).[9] Addition of 10 per cent or more of the lower molecular weight polyethylene glycols 400 or 1,500 facilitates formulation by retarding the gel formation during the melting stage so that the mass may be poured into the suppository mold. Addition of the low molecular weight polyethylene glycol compounds and water aid in the formation of a more plastic mass; however, these compounds may lose water unless the more hygroscopic glycerin or propylene glycol is added. A firm plastic property is desired to prevent formation of a crumbly mass. A large proportion of insoluble medication or use of the higher molecular weight polyethylene glycols (particularly polyethylene glycols 4,000 and 6,000) may lead to the formation of a dry crystalline mass that is easily crumbled.

The "hydrophilic" suppository bases as defined in this chapter are those mixtures of the oleaginous and the water-soluble materials which make suitable mixtures, which emulsify water to make w/o emulsions or which disperse themselves in water. Examples of single substances that are included in this class are Polyoxyl 40 Stearate (Myrj 52*), Polyoxyethylene sorbitan monostearate (Tween 61*) and Polyoxyethylene oxypropylene stearate (G2162*).

Mixtures of cocoa butter with various

* Atlas Chemical Industries, Wilmington, Delaware.

emulsifying agents have been made. It is relatively easy to add 2 per cent of cholesterol or 10 per cent of wool fat to cocoa butter, which will allow the incorporation of a significant proportion of water (up to 25%) in the form of a w/o emulsion. It is difficult to see how a true o/w emulsion system may exist in a solid dosage form that would be suitable for suppository use. The external continuous phase should be of a solid or semisolid material that melts or dissolves.

Mixtures of oil emulsifying agents with fatty bases must of necessity produce a "quasi emulsion" to form a solid suppository. On contact with the mucous fluids, they are hydrated to form a creamy fluid which spreads over the cavity and in time releases the basic medication. There is insufficient in-vivo data available to confirm this, but in-vitro release data by Eckert and Muhleman[7] indicate that water-soluble drugs dispersed in w/o emulsions are not as readily available as the same drugs suspended in anhydrous vehicles.

A great deal of caution is advised in the use of surfactants with drugs intended for rectal absorption,[1, 7, 9, 16] since there are many reports of interactions of these compounds with active drugs. Each combination should be considered on its own merits and clinical testing is indicated for assurance of therapeutic efficacy.

Tardos et al.[28,29] have reported increased absorption of atropine sulfate, morphine sulfate, pilocarpine hydrochloride and pentamethazol as measured by a pharmacologic test when cocoa butter base was modified by the addition of Span 60* at 3 per cent or Tween 60* at 1 per cent. With atropine sulfate it was reported that the addition of nitroglycerin 0.01 per cent or 0.05 per cent further increased the pupillary response. Using suppositories without the surface-active agent, no increased response was observed on the addition of the local vasodilators.

A review of drug absorption from suppositories appears in the 6th edition of *American Pharmacy*. T. W. Schwarz, the author of the portion on Suppositories, draws the following conclusion:

* Atlas Chemical Industries, Wilmington, Delaware.

In comparing the various results of in-vivo tests, one is struck with the lack of agreement in them. It is evident that no one vehicle can be established unequivocally as superior to others and no principle in the choice of base holds up throughout the multitude of reports. The discrepancies may well be due to the different drugs used. They may also be due in part to the variances in experimental set-ups and the condition of the test subjects or animals.*

METHODS OF MANUFACTURE

The method of manufacture of suppositories depends on the number of units to be made, the materials to be used and the equipment at hand. In general there may be considered to be two methods—the hot or the fusion process and the cold process. All of the suppository bases and many of the added medicaments can be processed by melting the mixture and pouring it into molds. The cold process may be subdivided further into the *hand rolling method* and the *compression method,* which differ in the manner in which the suppositories are formed.

The hand rolling method is the molding of the suppository with the fingers after the formation of a plastic mass. This method has the advantage of requiring only the minimum of equipment—a mortar and a pestle, a spatula and a pill tile or an ointment slab. Usually no more than 10 or 12 doses are made at one time by this method and no excess of materials need be measured, since, with good technic, the loss of materials will be slight.

The finely powdered drugs are mixed in a mortar with an equal weight of finely grated cocoa butter, by the levigation technic. The remaining cocoa butter is added by portions in finely divided form, with thorough mixing after each addition. The pestle should be used to force the mass together and against the sides of the mortar. The cocoa butter under this pressure becomes plastic and mixing is possible. Should the mass fail to become plastic, it may be warmed very gently to a temperature not to exceed 30° C. by placing the mass protected with paper between the hands and kneading the mass with the fingers.

The uniformly mixed semiplastic mass must be further kneaded into a cohesive plastic mass that can be formed into suppositories.

* Sprowls, J. B.: American Pharmacy, Ed. 6, pp. 313-326, Philadelphia, Lippincott, 1966.

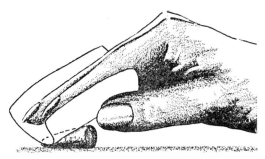

FIG. 7-5. Hand rolling the suppository.

formed, it is rolled into a cylinder. The entire mass should be weighed at this time to record the total amount and to calculate the size of the dose desired. The mass which is handled with the spatula or with a thickness of filter paper between the fingers and the suppository mass, is further rolled out on the pill tile into a cylinder of the approximate diameter of the suppository. Then the cylinder can be divided into the number of doses to be made. As the unit portions of the cylinder are cut off, they are shaped quickly into the desired form (Fig. 7-5). The mass will quickly solidify and lose its plasticity, but this is not a problem because the portion can be kneaded (using the paper in the palm of the hand) to restore the plasticity so that shaping may be completed. The use of small amounts of starch as a dusting powder is permissible to prevent "stickiness" of the suppository mass. Proper or "ideal" temperature control usually obviates the need for starch, but this may not always be possible when liquid components are present in the mass.

By keeping the mass within a lintless paper towel or filter paper the fingers and hands are prevented from coming into direct contact with the mass while kneading. The proper consistency is reached by working quickly and forcefully. With this mixing procedure, the plastic mass is easily mixed and formed. However, when it is worked slowly or intermittently, the plastic portion will revert back to its normal, solid form.

Once the cohesive plastic mass has been

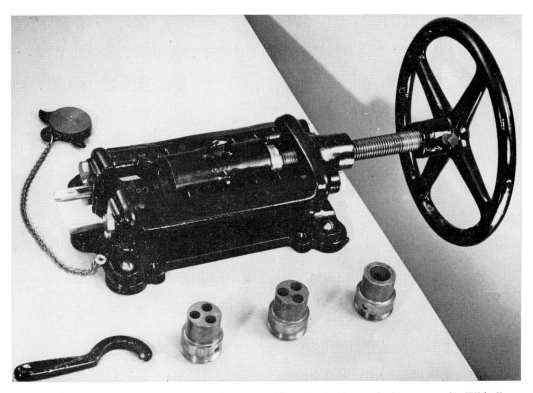

FIG. 7-6. The Armstrong Suppository Machine No. 3 (formerly known as the Whitall-Tatum Press), showing compression chamber, separate dies, end plate and locking wrench. (Formerly made by the Armstrong Company, Lancaster, Pa.)

The cone and the pointed cylinder are the shapes most easily formed by the hand rolling procedure. Uniformity of weight, shape and length are most important considerations. The appearance of the dosage form is of psychological importance to the patient, since he may prejudge the efficacy of the medication solely on his impression of the neatness and uniformity of the preparation.

The finished suppositories regain the usual firmness of the cocoa butter base when they are allowed to stand for a period of ½ hour in a cool room. They are packaged after the hardening period in order to prevent such deformations as would otherwise occur in wrapping and packaging operations.

The compression method requires the formation of a uniform mixture prior to placing the mass into the chamber for molding. One should follow the procedure described in the previous section for making the uniform mixture of medication with cocoa butter. In this method, three or four additional suppositories must be made for each lot so that excess material is available to expel the suppositories from the mold.

First, one must find the weight of the base for each suppository. This is done in the following manner (assuming cocoa butter as the base).

The cocoa butter is placed in a granulated form in the chamber of the machine to which the appropriate mold has been attached. Molds are available for 5-Gm. vaginal and for 1-Gm. or 2-Gm. rectal suppositories. The compression chamber is placed in the frame and the pressure wheel turned to close the chamber. Then crushed ice is placed on the chamber and the mold for a few minutes. After chilling the mass to approximately 10° C., the pressure wheel is turned to extrude the base from the chamber into the mold against the end plate. After the air is expelled from the base, there is a considerable increase in pressure on the wheel. At this point the pressure wheel is reversed slightly, the end plate removed and pressure re-applied carefully to eject the molded suppository. The trimmed suppository is weighed to determine the weight of the cocoa butter needed to fill the mold.

The temperature of the compressed mass is the critical factor for ease of manufacture. Under pressure the material will flow into the mold, solidify and contract sufficiently when not under pressure to be ejected in solid form. For plain cocoa butter this temperature range is about 5° to 10° C. The temperature range must be increased for those masses containing significant amounts of insoluble powders and reduced when materials lowering the melting range of the mass are present.*

Many of the suppository bases proposed in this chapter may be formulated with drugs and excipients permitting the use of the compression method. The mass should have sufficient plasticity to flow into the mold under pressure and to congeal when the pressure

*The novice is advised to read the operating instructions for the compression machine and to make a practice lot using plain cocoa butter.

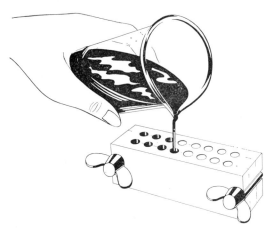

FIG. 7-7. Pouring of Suppositories (Witepsol, Chemische Werke Witten, 1961)

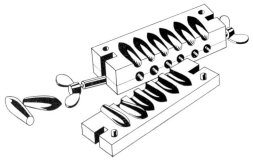

FIG. 7-8. Suppository mold having longitudinal partition. (Witepsol, Chemische Werke Witten, 1961)

is removed so that a solid form may be ejected. The use of plasticizing agents and control of the temperature for compression make the use of many other materials possible.

The fusion method is used with all of the suppository bases and may be used for all but the most heat-sensitive drugs. It is the method used for making gelatin-base suppositories and Glycerin Suppositories, *U.S.P.* because each of these materials requires a high temperature. Also, the suppository formulas using a polyethylene glycol base quite often are prepared by melting all constituents together and pouring the liquefied mass directly into the mold. The molds are usually at room temperature or higher if a slow rate of cooling is required to allow air bubbles to rise to the surface and, thus, aid in formation of a more stable form.

In the procedure for cocoa-butter-base suppositories, only enough heat to cause the mass to become pourable should be used. Insoluble powders may be mixed with grated cocoa butter in a mortar with a pestle, or a portion of the melted mass may be poured as a levigation agent on the powders while they are mixed with the spatula on an ointment slab. Once a smooth mixture has been made, the mixture of powder and base is placed in a beaker to be melted with the remainder of the base. The mixture is stirred to prevent settling of the powders as it is poured into the chilled molds. The molds should be overfilled by 3 to 4 mm. to allow for contraction on cooling. One should expect the formation of a dimple in the center of the molded suppository, as suppository materials contract on solidification and, thus, allow convenient removal from the molds.

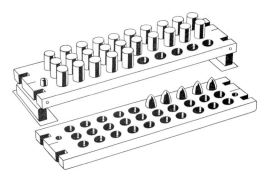

Fig. 7-10. Suppository mold of transverse partition design, open. (Witepsol, Chemische Werke Witten, 1961)

Comparison of Methods of Manufacture. Reports have been made from time to time of variations in absorption of drug caused by the use of different procedures. Tardos *et al.*[28,29] reported a difference between suppositories made by the compression method and those made by fusion, for two of the bases tested (Myrj 52 with Carbowax).[28] The differences may occur because the drug is not solubilized or dissolved in the excipient when the suppository is made by mixing and compression. Gunnar Hopp[12] compared melted and compressed suppositories; for those suppositories made by compression he reported increased oxidation, which he attributed to metal from the machine entering the suppository and acting as a catalyst to oxidative changes. Many of the suppository bases are subject to such oxidative changes, and, therefore, care should be taken particularly to avoid iron contamination.

SPECIAL DISPENSING AND COMPOUNDING PROCEDURES FOR SUPPOSITORIES

Incorporation of Insoluble Powders. Powdered material should be reduced until it will pass completely through a 120-mesh sieve. A microcrystalline powder is preferred where possible. In general, the partially melted suppository base should be used as the levigation agent; however, in formulas containing more than 10 per cent of powder a liquid levigation agent is added to about one half the weight of the powder. A vegetable oil is preferred for use with the fatty bases and one

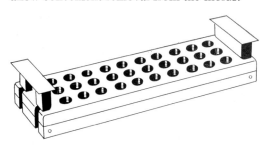

Fig. 7-9. Suppository mold of transverse partition design, closed. (Witepsol, Chemische Werke Witten, 1961)

of the liquid components (glycerin, polyethylene glycol 400 or water) is chosen for the water-soluble bases.

Castor oil is used to aid the incorporation of extracts, particularly when alcohol is used to soften the hardened pilular extract. Usually the alcohol will have evaporated almost completely before the softened material is finally incorporated, otherwise there will be: (a) the possibility of irritation; (b) migration to the surface of the alcohol-soluble constituents on storage; (c) change in medicament release because of solvent effect of alcohol or migration of drug.

For the incorporation of large amounts of powder into suppositories the same rules should be followed in the choice of a levigation agent as are followed in the preparation of ointments. An additional requirement is that the levigation agent be nonirritating to the mucous surface of the cavity.

Care should be taken in the fusion process that the suspended powders continue to be dispersed uniformly throughout the suppository mass until it has congealed. The mass is heated until it has just reached a creamy, pourable consistency and is stirred while being poured. When properly handled, congealing takes place relatively quickly, thus preventing separation. Lehman[15] reported that the addition of aluminum stearate to the fatty bases aided suspension of the powders during the critical phase by increasing the viscosity of the melted base.

Lubrication. The suppository mold generally does not require lubrication if the surface is clean and polished. The mass should have sufficient contraction to free the molded form on cooling, and time should be allowed for the complete contraction. Should difficulty indicating requirement of a lubricant occur, the choice should be made of a light mineral oil coating for the water-soluble bases. For fatty bases, water which will condense from the atmosphere as a very thin film on the chilled mold is usually the best lubricant. Aqueous soap solutions may be applied as a light film of a very dilute solution.

Dusting Powders. Suppositories properly formulated and properly made need no dusting powders. Should extemporaneously compounded suppositories require a powder, it is suggested that starch be used and then in a minimum amount. Excess powder, particularly of a type which is not easily wetted, may interfere with release of the medication.

Lowered Melting Temperature. A characteristic lowering of solidification and melting temperatures occurs when a significant concentration of soluble drug is mixed with the base. Theobroma oil is particularly sensitive, because of the low-melting polymorphic forms which are possible and its high molal freezing point depression. The problem may be solved without change in the formula by requiring that the finished suppository be stored in a "Cool Place"* to maintain the solid form until use. The use of beeswax or spermaceti in amounts sufficient to raise the melting temperature is not without difficulty, as the method of treatment of the drug-theobroma oil-wax mixture prior to and during congealing will determine the melting temperature of the finished suppository. Also, there is the possibility of a change in the melting temperature on storage, as theobroma oil reverts to a higher melting polymorph.

Use of Plastic Molds. A few years ago plastic molds were introduced as a replacement of the traditional metal molds. The plastic mold does not have the mechanical strength, loses polish more easily so that sticking is more of a problem, and does not conduct heat as readily as the metal mold. These disadvantages have been set aside partly by the use of thin shells of plastic in two pieces that allow molding of the suppository and dispensing it in the mold which serves as its package. The patient may easily remove the suppository and discard the shell at the time of use. Many commercial suppository formulas may be conveniently packaged in this way with economic efficiency. Its use on a small scale will depend on the availability of a smaller molding tray. Currently, the molding tray holds 288 of the plastic shells (Fig. 7-11).

PREPARATIONS BY THERAPEUTIC CLASS

Rectal Evacuants and Enemas. The normal process of defecation removes most of the fecal matter from the rectum. However,

* Defined in *NF XIII* and *USP XVIII* as 8° to 15° C.

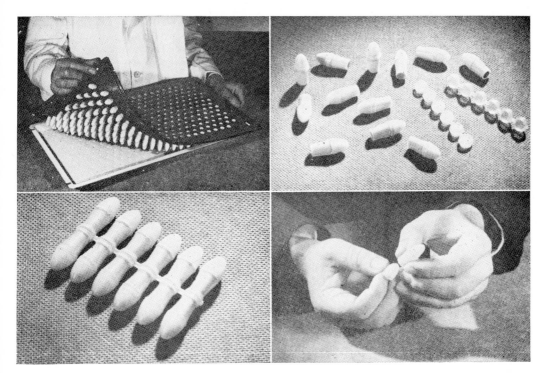

Fig. 7-11. Suppository molding using plastic shells. (*Top, left*) Placing the mat ready for molding. (*Top, right*) The filled shells ready for mounting on stems. (*Bottom, left*) The molded and capped suppositories. (*Bottom, right*) The user removing the suppository from its shell. (Chemical and Pharmaceutical Industry Co., Inc.)

when the fecal matter that remains interferes with examination of the tissues (as in sigmoidoscopy), the attending nurse uses an aqueous saline solution or a mild soap solution in an enema. The retention enema is a special form of enema injected into the lower colon when the medication indicates. An example is the use of hexylresorcinol in water for the treatment of whipworm (Trichuris) infestations.[13]

1. ℞
    Hexylresorcinol 0.2% in water   500 ml.
    Sig: Rectal retention enema. Retain one
    hour.

The large volume enema is very probably a most effective cleansing procedure but it requires considerable nursing skill as well as time and effort. The retention enema in particular becomes more difficult to manage as the volume of liquid is increased. For this reason, as well as the seriousness of the infection, it is suggested that the hexylresorcinol

retention enema as above be used only in the hospital.

Small volume retention and cleansing enema preparations have been used both in and out of the hospital because in many cases these allow the patient to self-administer the procedure. Pre-packed and disposable items make the procedure more convenient for the nurse.

2. ℞
    Fleet's Phospho-Soda ....145 ml.
    Sig: Use as directed before the next office
    visit.

This preparation is a hypertonic sodium phosphate solution with glycerin present. The osmotic effect of the solution causes irritation and a flow of fluid from the tissues; the defecation reflex occurs as a result of the large volume of fluid presented to the proctocolonic cavity. Within minutes after instillation of this preparation, the person is no longer able to prevent the expulsion of the contents of the lower colon and the rectum. The effectiveness of this cleansing procedure depends on whether or not sufficient softening and loosening of the contents was effected in the time allowed for the procedure. For the more sensitive rectum, or when stool softening is the main consideration, an oil preparation is available (90 ml. volume).

Suppository preparations also are widely used to stimulate the defecation reflex. The most widely used is the Glycerin Suppository, which causes the evacuant action by abstracting water from the adjacent tissues, thus producing the stimulant and lubricant actions desired. The sodium stearate content is varied somewhat by the manufacturer, in order to adjust the degree of firmness and the amount of water (and hence the hygroscopic power) as related to the stability of the preparation. Therefore the several brands of Glycerin Suppositories vary in firmness and in the degree of irritation elicited upon use.

A suppository developed a few years ago produces rectal stimulation and evacuant action by the formation of carbon dioxide gas when it comes in contact with the aqueous fluids in the rectum. This suppository is made somewhat larger (about 6 Gm.) so that the mechanical stimulant effect is increased because of its size. The formula below (℞ 3) serves as an example of this type of preparation. The polyethylene glycols of high molecular weight are the least hygroscopic of the water-soluble suppository base materials and, when mixed with the salts, may be formed into the desired shape by using compressed tablet technology.

3. ℞
    Sodium biphosphate . . . . 290 mg.
    Sodium bicarbonate . . . . 168 mg.
    Carbowax 4000
    Carbowax 6000   aa qs ad   6 Gm.
    Ft rectal suppository, d t d #15
    Sig: Moisten with cool water before insertion.

A number of rectal evacuant preparations are available that contain surface-active agents and other irritant substances. The several examples shown above demonstrate the wide variation possible in such preparations. As the proctologist is acutely aware, there are individuals for whom the glycerin suppository is as effective a cleansing agent as the larger volume enema is for the less sensitive patient.

Hemorrhoidal Treatment. In contrast to rectal evacuants, the preparations used in treatment of the irritated rectum are soothing materials. These ointments and suppositories are intended to provide temporary relief in cases of pain associated with some hemorrhoids.[10] A wide variety of medications are included in ointments and suppository preparations to provide not only emollient and anesthetic activity, but the not-so-well-documented effects of antiseptics, astringents, antispasmodics and vasoconstrictors as well. Several of the well advertised products contain materials that are not recognized in standard pharmacology texts and are under attack by the Federal Trade Commission for misleading claims. These claims include the "shrinking of piles" and the alleviation of the itching pain associated with minor hemorrhoid conditions. There are physicians who use medications of this type in treatment in spite of comments such as:

There is at present no satisfactory evidence that medicated anorectal suppositories have more than placebo effects in the treatment of anorectal disorders. Where there is pain, however, suppositories containing local anesthetics may possibly be useful; controlled trials are needed to determine their effectiveness and safety.*

In another report[31] these conservative attitudes are repeated, with specific comments concerning the choice of efficacious treatment. In the latter report it is suggested that the suppository has an advantage over the ointment in that the solid object is retained higher in the rectum and closer to the condition to be treated. Use of vasoconstrictor agents, astringents and antispasmodics and antiseptics is reported as being only "marginally effective." The action of vasoconstrictor drugs applies only to capillaries and arteries and does not affect the veins.

The most effective treatment for painful, irritated hemorrhoids includes the softening of stools to prevent mechanical damage while the "sitz" bath, cold compresses to the area, and rest allow the healing process to take over.

* The Medical Letter, *10*:107, 1968 (December 27).

Physicians have had success in the treatment of these minor conditions with ointments and suppositories. The following prescription serves as an example:

4. ℞
    Benzocaine 5%
    Oxyquinoline sulfate 0.8%
    Menthol 0.4%
    Bismuth subgallate 6.0%
    Zinc oxide 4.0%
    Peru balsam
    Castor oil   aa 2.0%
    Lanolin, anhyd. 8.0%
    Petrolatum   qs ad .... .100%

    Sig: apply to hemorrhoids as directed.

Various commercial products have many different combinations of the several active ingredients or of medications similar to those in the formula above: It is suggested that the student modify this formula in several ways using other oleaginous suppository and ointment bases to compare the physical properties. The "long fibre" type of petrolatum is usually specified for the ointment form, and this is supplied with a special applicator on the ointment tube, which allows the introduction of the ointment within the anal sphincter.

When either the ointment or the suppository is to be used, simple cleansing procedures should be included in the instructions to the patient, which should cover the nature of cleansing agents, the frequency of application and the use of protective pads to prevent staining of the clothing.

Systemic Effects by Rectal Route. The range of drugs that may be prescribed for rectal administration to obtain systemic effects is demonstrated in the following example.

5. ℞
    Chlorpromazine HCl............5 mg.
    Dispense suppositories no. 15.

    Sig: Use for nausea as required.

Chlorpromazine HCl is available as Compazine® in a number of dosage forms in addition to the rectal suppository. The drug is water soluble and is readily released for assimilation from the hydrogenated vegetable oil base. It is also light sensitive and subject to oxidative degradation and therefore is protected by a foil-plastic package. The pharmacist should use this opportunity to explain to patient the proper use of the medication.

6. ℞
    Aspirin   0.5
    Cocoa butter qs
    Ft rectal suppos. Dispense 30 of such.

    Sig: Insert one as directed at bedtime

Aspirin by the rectal route is indicated for the arthritic patient in order to spare gastric irritation or to allow the drug to be absorbed during the night and thus prevent "morning stiffness." The cocoa butter substitutes such as Wecobee have been used as well as the Carbowaxes (see Table 7-2). The solid polyethylene glycol bases have been shown to permit more rapid absorption,[4,5] but care is needed to prevent moisture damage to the aspirin. It has been suggested that suppositories with the poylethylene glycol base be dipped into water before use to reduce the irritation caused by the hygroscopic material.

In this formula, the use of cocoa butter substitute Wecobee SS* is suggested, first because its higher melting temperature allows the preparation to be stored at room temperature (up to 30° C.) without softening, and second, because the chilled preparations would collect moisture by condensation when brought to room temperature before use. Care should be taken that the specifications for the cocoa butter replacement include the hydroxyl value as well as the usual physical characteristics. The hydroxyl value indicates the presence of the mono- and diglycerides and contributes greatly to the solvent effect of the base on the drug and the ability of the base to mix with and spread over the mucous surfaces. Therefore variations in the hydroxyl value for a given base will result in differences in the absorption rate for the drug.[11,22]

7. ℞
    Nembutal Sodium® Abbott ....120 mg.
    Dispense 20 rectal supp.

    Sig: i at bedtime.

The manufacturer's literature states that cocoa-butter-modified spermaceti is used as the base for this drug. On melting, the water-soluble drug is released from the oleaginous base with very little difficulty. The previous comments on the incorporation of wax into cocoa butter apply specifically to this preparation. The wax should be melted and the

* Drew Chemical Co., Boonton, N.J.

cocoa butter added in several portions with only enough heat to effect a creamy consistency. The incorporation of powders has been discussed previously (p. 273).

8. ℞
   Cafergot® (Sandoz) supp. 15

   Sig: Use for the initial signs of migraine.

The active components, ergotamine tartrate and caffeine, are water soluble and readily released from the cocoa butter base. Tartaric acid is added and apparently is required to aid the dissolution and subsequent absorption of the drugs.

9. ℞
   Aminophylline . . . . 450 mg.
   Dispense Rectalad (Wampole) no. 15

   Sig: Use as directed.

This commercial preparation is an aqueous solution of the drug in a special package that allows self-administration as a rectal retention enema. Aminophylline by this route is rapidly absorbed;[21] a comparison should be made with the work reported by Wagner.[33,34] The rectal suppository forms also are available using either the cocoa butter base or a Carbowax base, and each formula has its particular advantages.

10. ℞
    Furacin® (Eaton) vaginal suppositories
    Dispense 24

    Sig: Use as directed.

This medication is also available as urethral inserts and several topical applications. The suppository base Tween 61* is a polyethylene sorbitan monostearate mixed with about 10 per cent of glyceryl monolaurate to stiffen the base. This self-emulsifying material softens in aqueous body fluids (as noted in Table 7-2). Other water-soluble antiseptics and spermatocidal agents may be formulated and compounded with this base, but contact with water must be avoided, since moisture allows dosage forms incorporating this material to stick to the molds. If the molds are dry and cool (8° to 15° C.), the melted mass may congeal without moisture condensation on the surface and the attendant difficulties this creates.

* Atlas Chemical Industries, Wilmington, Delaware.

REFERENCES

1. Allawala, N. A., and Reigelman, S.: J. Am. Pharm. Assoc. (Sci.) 42:267, 1954.
2. Bochmuhl, and Middendorf, U. S. Pat. 2,149,005, 1937.
3. Bucher, K.: Helv. physiol. pharmacol. acta 6:821, 1948.
4. Cacchillo, A. F., and Hassler, W. H.: J. Am. Pharm. Assoc. (Sci.) 43:683, 1954.
5. Collins, A. P., Hohman, J. R., and Zopf, L. C.: Am. Prof. Pharm. 23:231, 1957.
6. Deutsches Arnzeibuch VI, 3rd suppl., 1959.
7. The Drug and Therapeutic Bulletin 7:41-43, 1969 (May 23).
8. Eckert, V., and Muhleman, H.: Pharm. acta helv. 33:649, 1958.
9. Guida, A. F.: An "In Vitro" Method for the Study of Theophylline Release from Suppository Bases, Thesis Univ. Kansas, 1952.
10. Handbook of Non-Prescription Drugs, pp. 113-119, American Pharmaceutical Association, 1969.
11. Hennig, W.: Ueber die Rektale Resorption von Medicamenten, Zurich, Juris Verlag, 1959.
12. Hopp, G.: En Sammenliknende undersokelse over grunnmasser og fremstillings-metoder for suppositorrer, Oslo, 1961
13. Kallet, A. (ed.): The Medical Letter 9:99, 1967 (Dec. 15).
14. Kremers, E., and Urdang, G.: History of Pharmacy, ed. 2, Philadelphia, Lippincott, 1951.
15. Lehman, H.: Schweiz. Apoth. Zeit. 97:555, 1959.
16. Meara, M. L.: J. Chem. Soc. 1949, 2154.
17. Oesch, P.: Ueber die Herstellung und Prufung von Suppositorien, Zurich, Ernst Lang, 1944.
18. Pennati, L., and Steiger-Trippi, K.: Pharm. acta helv, 33:663, 1958.
19. Reigelman, S., and Crowell, W. J.: J. Am. Pharm. Assoc. (Sci.), 47:115, 123, 127, 1959.
19a. Robinson, G. D.: J. Obstet. Gyn. (Brit.) 32:496, 1928.
20. Robertson, J. S.: J. Pharm. Sci. 50:21, 1961.
21. Rudolfo, A. S., et al.: Am. J. Med. Sci. 237:585, 1959.
22. Samelius, Y., and Åström, A.: Acta pharmacol. tox. 14:240, 1958.
23. Schanker, L. S.: J. Pharmacol. Exper. Ther. 126:283, 1959.
24. Setnikar, I., and Fantelli, S.: J. Pharm. Sci. 51:566, 1962.

25. Setnikar, I., and Fantelli, S.: J. Pharm. Sci. 52:38, 1963.
26. Smith, A.: Technic of Medication, Philadelphia, J. B. Lippincott, 1948.
27. Sperandio, G. J., and Hassler, W. H.: J. Am. Pharm. Assoc. (Pract.) 14:26, 1953.
28. Tardos, L., Weisman, L. J., and Ello, Pharmazie 14:526, 1960.
29. Tardos, L., Ello, Magda, and Jobbagyi: Acta Pharm. Hung. 29:22, 1959.
30. Taylor, A. B.: Am. J. Pharm. 24:211, 1852.
31. Tice, L. F., and Abrams, R. E.: Am Prof. Pharm. 18:327, 1952.
32. United States Pharmacopeia XVIII, Mack, 1970.
33. Wagner, J. G., Carter, C. H., and Martens, I. J.: J. Clin. Pharmacol. 8:154-163, 1968.
34. Wagner, J. G., Leslie, L. G., and Gove, R. S.: Int. J. Clin. Pharmacol. 2:44-51, 1969.

Chapter 8

Aerosols

John J. Sciarra, Ph.D.*

INTRODUCTION

The application of the principles of aerosols or pressurized packaging to medicinal and pharmaceutical products is of relatively recent occurrence. While it is true that several spray-on antiseptics, burn preparations and local anesthetics were available during the early years of the aerosol industry, it is only during the past 5 or 10 years that serious interest has been given to the formulation of suitable pharmaceutical and medicinal aerosols. In 1967, over 41 million units of medicinal and pharmaceutical aerosol products were produced in the United States. This represented an increase of 9.7 per cent from the 1966 figure (over 37 million); an increase of 17 per cent from 1965 figure (over 35 million) and a 40 per cent increase from the 1964 figure (over 28 million). When it is noted that less than 1 million units of these products were produced in 1952, the newness of the development and the increased interest in this area is quickly ascertained. Figure 8-1 traces the growth of aerosols in the United States from 1958 to 1967.

Pressurized containers for pharmaceutical products actually were used for many years on a small scale and for special purposes. Many will recall the physicians' use of ethyl chloride for minor surgery.[27] This product consisted of ethyl chloride (acting as both propellant and active ingredient) packaged in a glass ampul fitted with a valve. When the ethyl chloride ampul was held in the warmth of the hands, the vapor pressure of the ethyl chloride increased. After the valve was opened, the liquid ethyl chloride escaped.

* Director of the Graduate Division and Professor of Pharmaceutical Chemistry, St. John's University, College of Pharmacy.

Since the boiling point of ethyl chloride is 12.3° C., it reverted quickly to the vapor state. This caused a freezing of the skin and tissues with resultant local anesthetic effect.

A host of aerosol products have evolved which are of interest to the pharmacist from both a commercial and a scientific viewpoint. Ever since the first aerosol products were developed, the community pharmacy has been a major outlet for their distribution. These products include insecticides, hair lacquers, room deodorants, shave creams, perfumes and colognes, as well as some of the more specific pharmaceutical and medicinal aerosols such as the burn preparations, the local anesthetics, the steroids, the first aid products, the antiasthmatic and migraine preparations, the dental creams, etc. which are part of the daily armamentarium of the professional pharmacist. The products have been formulated utilizing different aerosol systems—each system designed to serve a specific purpose. This newer method for the dispensing of medicinal and pharmaceutical products has many advantages over the more conventional methods and, in some instances, has made popular products that cannot be dispensed or applied efficiently by any other method—for example, hair lacquer.

From a scientific viewpoint, aerosols are important to the professional pharmacist since they have become another dosage form. Since aerosols have invaded the domain of the pharmaceutical field and are sold to such a large extent by the pharmacist both over-the-counter and on prescription, it is the responsibility of the professional pharmacist to equip himself with as much knowledge as possible in regard to aerosol products.[67] In this way he can render another professional

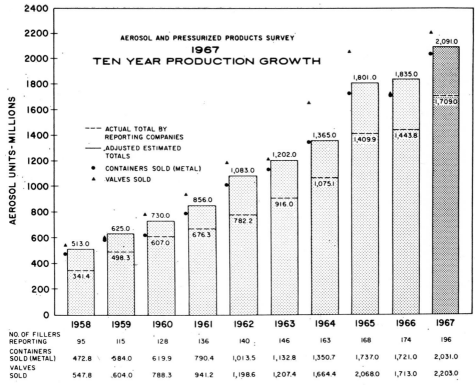

FIG. 8-1. Growth of the aerosol industry (C.S.M.A.).

service to both patient and physician. A knowledge of aerosol formulation and components is essential in order to discuss these products intelligently. As the technology increases in this field the pharmacist may well find himself compounding a number of aerosol prescriptions extemporaneously.[68]

DEFINITIONS

The term *aerosol* is defined as a system consisting of a suspension of fine solid or liquid particles in air or gas. As such, smoke, fog, dust or moisture suspended in the atmosphere, etc., can be classified as aerosols. While this is generally accepted as the classical definition of the term, a more recent definition includes as aerosols those products which depend on the power of a liquefied or a compressed gas to expel the contents from the container. This is slightly different from the definition advanced by the Chemical Specialties Manufacturers Association which includes only those products utilizing a liquefied gas propellant.[8] Terms such as "pressure pack," "pressurized packaging,"

"pressurized product" etc. are also used to describe this type of product. It is in the light of the newer definition that the term *aerosol* is used in this chapter.

Originally, the term *aerosol* referred to liquid or solid particles of a specific size range, but this concept is falling into disuse. However, one current system for the classification of aerosol products is based on particle size: for example, *space sprays* dispense the active ingredients as a finely divided spray with the particles no larger than 50 microns in diameter, while those sprays having particles considerably larger are classified as *surface coating sprays*.[50] The latter generally produce a wet or a coarse spray and are used to coat a surface with a residual film. Finally, the aerated foam system completes this classification of aerosol products. This system is used when a foam, such as is found in shaving creams, rather than a spray, is desired. The characteristics of the foam depend on the nature of the formulation and will be described in greater detail in a later portion of this chapter.

All of the existing aerosol products can be encompassed within the above classification. Medicinal and pharmaceutical aerosols are included in the general definitions. However, the principles and the considerations involved in the formulation of aerosol products used for a therapeutic response are quite different from those regarding other aerosols and, in addition, differences exist between those aerosols intended for internal administration and those for topical administration. Therefore, it is advantageous from the viewpoint of discussion as well as formulation to distinguish between these types of aerosol products.

Medicinal aerosols may be defined as those aerosol products containing therapeutically active ingredients dissolved or suspended in a propellant or a mixture of a solvent and a propellant and intended for administration as fine solid particles or liquid mists via the respiratory system or the nasal passages. They are intended for local action in the nasal areas, the throat and the lungs as well as for prompt systemic effect when absorbed from the lungs into the bloodstream (inhalation or aerosol therapy). The particle size must be considerably below 50 microns and, in most instances, should be between 3 and 6 microns for maximum therapeutic activity.

Pharmaceutical aerosols may be defined as aerosol products containing therapeutically active ingredients dissolved, suspended or emulsified in a propellant or a mixture of solvent and propellant and intended for topical administration or for administration into one of the body cavities such as the ear, the rectum and the vagina. Ophthalmic preparations may also be included in this definition.

In this chapter, pharmaceutical and medicinal aerosols will be discussed in the light of the preceding definitions, but several other definitions have been advanced. Kanig[37] defines both medicinal and pharmaceutical aerosols as "those which are administered internally or externally and which have a therapeutic effect in the cure or alleviation of any human or animal disease or condition."

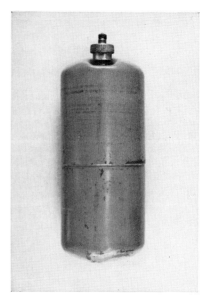

FIG. 8-2. Original aerosol "bug bomb."

HISTORY

Aerosol products were first introduced in the United States about 1942[49] when the well-known aerosol insecticide was developed as a result of the investigations of Goodhue[29] and Sullivan[30] of the United States Department of Agriculture. The insecticidal aerosols produced a fine spray, and particles of insecticide remained suspended in air for a relatively long period of time, making them extremely effective against insects and household pests. These preparations were used by members of the Armed Forces throughout the world, especially in malaria infested jungles and swamps, and their effectiveness has been well established. They were generally in high pressure cylinders, since the propellant available at the time was dichlorodifluoromethane which has a vapor pressure of 70 pounds per square inch gauge (psig) at 70° F.* Interstate Commerce Commission regulations necessitated a heavy, bulky steel container for the shipment of these products in interstate commerce. Figure 8-2 illustrates a typical product of this kind. Following World War II, newer propellants, valves and

* The term psig represents the uncorrected gauge pressure and is to be distinguished from psia which represents pounds per square inch absolute—that is, corrected to include atmospheric pressure (14.7 psig).

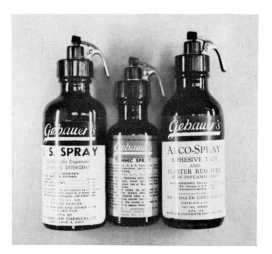

FIG. 8-4. Early pressurized products.

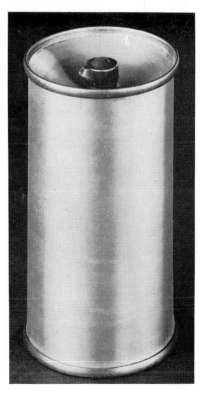

FIG. 8-3. "Beer can" type aerosol container. (Continental Can Company)

containers were developed so that a spray possessing the proper particle size could be produced using a pressure of 35 to 40 psig. In 1947, an amendment to the Interstate Commerce Commission regulations permitted pressures of 40 psig at 70° F. in thin-walled containers. The lower pressure made possible the use of a "beer-can" type of container (Fig. 8-3) which could be mass-produced at a considerably lower price than the heavy-walled containers.

Aluminum and stainless steel containers were developed for use with medicinal and pharmaceutical products as well as for several perfumes and colognes.[19] The development of the low-pressure and the ultra low-pressure (15-25 psig) aerosols made possible the use of glass and plastic-coated glass containers.[43] Plastic containers have been developed but have not been utilized to any great extent.

With the development of the standard 1-inch opening for tin plate containers, various

valves were designed to dispense the product in many different ways, such as a fine stream, a fine mist, a coarse spray, a foam etc. An important milestone—essential for medicinal aerosols—was the development of a metered-valve. Following this, many other metered valves were developed utilizing different principles so that today metered valves are commercially available for dispensing quantities of concentrate from as low as 50 mg. to as much as 1 ounce.

While the work of Goodhue and Sullivan formed the basis for the modern-day aerosol, the dispensing of products from a pressurized container antedates many of the current aerosol products. In fact, the first commercial aerosols were pharmaceutical proprietaries.[73] The various products covered by Gebauer in his basic patents were pressurized products.[25,26] Ethyl chloride, tannic acid and surgical soap were marketed in this manner. Several of these products are shown in Figure 8-4. Several antiseptic solutions were developed utilizing carbon dioxide as the propellant.[46] The atomizer has been on the medical scene for about one hundred years and represents an early development for the administration of substances in aerosol form.[65] In fact, the atomizer was used to a great extent to aerosolize hair lacquers prior to the use of liquefied gases for this purpose. While many of these atomizers and similar devices were cumbersome and bulky to use, they were the only devices available for this purpose. Chapter 13 indicates the use of atomizers, nebulizers, vaporizers etc.

While the method of inhalation or aerosol therapy is not new, formulation and development of a convenient, effective self-spraying unit is the result of recent endeavors. The ancients recorded the efficacy of the vapors from burning leaves and herbs; within the past 30 years, the smoke from burning stramonium leaves has been used in the treatment of asthma. The burning of sulfur candles to disinfect the air and the spraying of operating rooms with germicidal materials are well-known and effective means for fumigation and sterilization. A patient partaking of the beneficial effects of salt air at a beach may be utilizing aerosol therapy unknowingly when the minute salt particles in the air produced by the atomization forces of the breakers are inhaled.

The first medicinal aerosol product appeared in the United States in 1955. This product—Medi-Haler Epi (Riker Laboratories)—was intended for local action in the lungs and was effective in relieving the symptoms of asthmatic attacks. Following this, other products were developed for use as antiasthmatics, treatment of the symptoms of angina pectoris, nasal vasoconstrictors and treatment of migraine headaches.

Pharmaceutical aerosols were first developed in the early 1950's and included local anesthetics, antiseptics, spray-on bandages, topical creams and ointments, burn preparations and, toward the end of the 1950's, several vitamin preparations.

PHARMACEUTICAL AND MEDICINAL AEROSOLS

Before considering other aspects of pharmaceutical and medicinal aerosols, an examination of the advantages of aerosol products may be desirable.

General Advantages

1. The product is more convenient to use, since the package is a compact unit and the product can be applied or administered easily and quickly.

2. Since the medication is sealed in a pressurized container, there is no danger of contamination of the product with foreign materials, and, at the same time the contents can be protected from the deleterious effects of both air and moisture.

3. If the product is packaged under sterile conditions, sterility is maintained throughtout the life of the product.

4. Through use of metered valves, accurate dosage can be obtained.

Advantages of Pharmaceutical Aerosol Preparations

1. The irritation produced by the mechanical application of a medicinal over an abraded area of the skin is reduced and, sometimes, eliminated by a spray-on aerosol.

2. Finely powdered drugs such as antibiotics can be conveniently administered from this type of container.

3. There is no danger of contamination of the unused portion of the aerosol medicament from an infected wound, as is possible with conventional packages.

4. Since the medicinal is applied directly from the container to the affected area of the skin, there is no waste or messiness such as accompanies the use of an applicator or a cotton swab.

5. Liquefied gas aerosols dry rapidly, due to the cooling effect of the vaporization of the propellant, which may be desirable in certain cases.

6. The medication can be applied in an extremely thin layer directly over the affected area, resulting in faster absorption and more efficient utilization of a given amount of medication.

Advantages of Medicinal Aerosols (Inhalation Therapy)

1. Some medicinals formerly given as an injection can be administered by inhalation, thereby making possible self-medication at home by the patient in place of administration by medically trained personnel in the office or hospital.

2. The dangers of giving medicinals by injection (trauma, embolism, sterile abscesses etc.) are avoided, since inhalation therapy will often replace an injectable product.

3. The use of medicinals by inhalation does away with the necessity for elaborate sterile preparations required for parenteral administration.

4. Response to drugs administered by inhalation is prompt, faster in onset of activity

as compared with response to drugs given orally and, with most drugs, approaches intravenous therapy in rapidity of action.

5. Since the drugs are absorbed directly into the blood stream via the lungs, there is no decomposition or loss of drug in the gastrointestinal tract such as occurs when the drug is administered orally.

MODE OF OPERATION OF AEROSOLS

Aerosol systems may be classified as follows:
- A. Liquefied gas
  1. Two-phase systems
     a. Space spray
     b. Surface spray
     c. Dispersion or suspension system
  2. Three-phase systems
     a. Two layer system
     b. Foam system
        (stabilized foam)
        (quick-breaking foam)
- B. Compressed gas systems
  1. Solid stream dispensing
     a. Insoluble inert gas
  2. Foam dispensing
     a. Soluble inert gas
  3. Spray dispensing
     a. Soluble inert gas
     b. Insoluble inert gas
- C. Separation of propellant from concentrate systems
  1. Piston type
  2. Flexible bag type
  3. Atomizer type
- D. Co-dispensing systems

LIQUEFIED GAS SYSTEMS

When an aerosol preparation stands at room temperature in a closed container, some of the propellant will change from a liquid to a gas and fill the empty space in the container. An equilibrium is soon reached between the number of molecules going from liquid to vapor and from vapor to liquid. Equilibrium is established when the pressure within the container becomes equal to the vapor pressure of the propellant. This vapor pressure is exerted equally in all directions and is independent of the quantity present.

When the valve of the container is opened, the pressure forces some of the liquid up the dip tube and through the valve. When the liquid material comes into contact with the warm air at atmospheric pressure, the propellant portion of the formulation instantly changes to a gas and, in so doing, dispenses the active ingredients as a fine spray. The volume of head space within the container is increased as the product is discharged. This causes a temporary drop in pressure as a result of the expansion of the gas in the vapor phase. Some of the liquid propellant now changes to the vapor phase, thus, quickly restoring equilibrium and original pressure. (This is a significant difference from compressed gas aerosols.)

Two-Phase System. Space sprays and surface sprays function as indicated in the preceding paragraph. The two types of spray

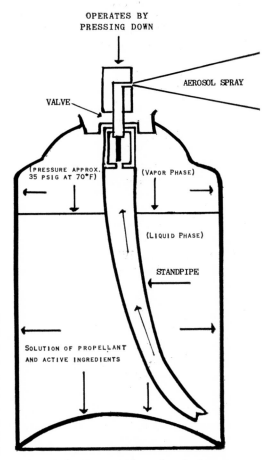

FIG. 8-5. Cross section of typical space or surface spray.

differ in regard to pressure within the container: the space spray has a pressure of 30 to 40 psig, producing a fine mist so that the particles remain suspended in air for at least 40 to 60 minutes; the surface spray is slightly lower in pressure and is used to coat a surface with active ingredients rather than suspending particles in air. Residual insecticides, mothproofers, paints and paint removers make up some of the surface sprays. Figure 8-5 shows a typical two-phase system applicable for use as either a space or a surface spray.

The active ingredients are dissolved in the propellant or a mixture of propellant and solvent. When the valve of the aerosol is depressed, active ingredients and propellant, or propellant and solvent are released. Propellant and solvent vaporize quickly, leaving behind the finely subdivided active ingredients. This system has been used to great advantage for both medicinal and pharmaceutical aerosols. However, several problems in formulation become immediately apparent. For the most part, the therapeutically active ingredients are not directly soluble in the propellants and must be dissolved through use of a suitable cosolvent. The solvents available for this purpose are limited to those showing very little, if any, irritation and toxicity when used topically or by inhalation. Lack of adequate data on toxicity for many solvents further complicates the formulation of such products. Ethyl alcohol, mineral oil, glycerin, propylene glycol, polyethylene and polypropylene glycol, acetone and ethyl acetate are a few of the solvents that have been used. When one considers solvents for inhalation, the list is considerably narrowed.

Several of the antiasthmatic aerosols such as Nebair,* Asthma Nephrin,† and Isuprel HCl Mistometer,‡ are examples of solution type aerosols in which about 30 per cent ethyl alcohol has been added as a cosolvent for the aqueous solution of the salt in water.

DISPERSION OR SUSPENSION SYSTEM. Insoluble materials can be suspended in a liquefied gas propellant through the use of suitable dispersing agents. Several aerosols containing insoluble materials have been developed and consist primarily of talcum, dispersing agents such as isopropyl myristate, and propellant. Paint aerosols are included in this category. Antibiotic and steroid aerosols are further examples of this type. In several medicinal aerosols containing epinephrine and ergotamine the therapeutically active ingredients are suspended in the propellant. In use, the propellant evaporates, leaving behind the finely dispersed active ingredients. This system is a useful method for the application of antibiotics and other medicinal agents. Decadron Respihaler§ and Medihaler-Epi‖ exemplify this system.

Three-Phase System. This system is characterized by the presence of a greater quantity of water than is found in a two-phase system. Since water is not miscible with the propellants that are generally used, separation will occur unless an emulsion is formed. Depending on the type of formulation desired, one of the two following systems may be employed.

TWO-LAYER SYSTEM. The active ingredients are dissolved in water or an aqueous base, and, when propellant is added, two immiscible layers are formed. Depending on the density of the propellant, the propellant either will float on top of the aqueous solution or will fall to the bottom of the container. The propellant is one phase; the second phase consists of the aqueous solution; finally, some of the propellant vaporizes and fills the head space to make up the third phase. The propellant vaporizes due to the decrease in pressure as the contents of this three-phase aerosol diminish, and the gas passes through the aqueous solution (if the propellant is the heavier layer) and restores the pressure in the head space. Only a small quantity of propellant is used in aerosols of this type, and only aqueous solution is dispensed. The absence of propellant from the dispensed solution necessitates the use of a specially designed nozzle to produce the proper spray. Figure 8-6 shows such an aerosol.

Several products utilize a hydrocarbon

---

* Isoproterenol HCl and Thonzonium bromide (Warner-Chilcott Laboratories).

† Racemic Epinephrine HCl (Thayer Laboratories, Inc.).

‡ Isoproterenol HCl (Winthrop Laboratories).

§ Dexamethazone (Merck, Sharp and Dohme).

‖ Epinephrine bitartrate (Riker Laboratories).

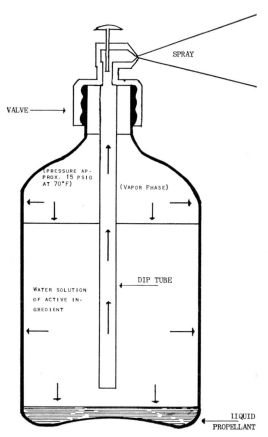

FIG. 8-6. Three-phase glass aerosol.

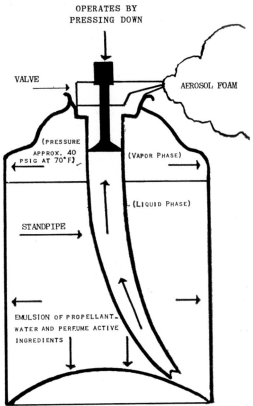

FIG. 8-7. Foam type aerosol.

such as isobutane or propane as the propellant. The hydrocarbons are used in the same way as are the fluorocarbons for this purpose, except that the hydrocarbon is lighter than water and floats on top of the aqueous layer. Several household cleaners and mothproofers are examples of three-phase aerosols.

This system has not been utilized to date for pharmaceutical and medicinal aerosols. It should be useful for the dispensing of various antiseptic solutions. Through use of a suitable actuator and baffle (similar to a nebulizer) the desired type of spray may be obtained.

FOAM SYSTEM. Foam aerosols operate on essentially the same principle as the two-phase system except that the propellant is partially emulsified with the active ingredients. When the valve is depressed, the emulsion is forced through the nozzle and, in the presence of warm air and at atmo-

spheric pressure, the entrapped propellant changes to a gas and whips the emulsion into a foam. Foam products operate at about 35 to 40 psig at 70° F. and contain about 6 to 10 per cent of propellant as compared with about 80 to 90 per cent of propellant for spray products. Figure 8-7 shows a foam type aerosol. When the container is supplied with a dip tube (as shown in Fig. 8-7), the container is held upright during use. Some products do not contain a dip tube, and, therefore, the directions specify that the container be inverted prior to use. It is important that the directions be followed; otherwise, the propellant may escape without dispensing the active ingredients. Another important consideration is that these products must be shaken before use. As these are emulsion type products, there is a certain amount of separation of active ingredients and propellant so that shaking is required to produce a homogeneous mixture. This is another significant difference from most of the compressed gas aerosols which specify that the container is not to be shaken and is to be held upright during use. Shave creams and shampoos are examples of foam type aerosols. While it is highly unlikely that this system will be useful for medicinal aerosols, it has been used for the formulation of pharmaceutical aerosols. The product is dispensed as a foam which can then be applied to the affected area. In this manner the medicinal agent can be applied either to a limited area or to a larger area with very little, if any, irritation due to application of the medicinal. A recent advance in this area is the development of the "quick-breaking" foam. The product is dispensed as a foam, but, in contact with skin areas, the foam quickly collapses, leaving only the solution of medicinal agent. This makes possible the application of medicinals to wounded or abraded areas without the necessity of rubbing to disperse the medicinal. This is highly desirable when applying medicinals to such areas.

COMPRESSED GAS AEROSOLS

Depending on the nature of the formulation and the type of valve used, a compressed gas can be used to dispense the product as a solid stream, a fine mist or a foam.

In aerosol products of this type an inert gas such as nitrogen, carbon dioxide, nitrous oxide etc. is used as the propellant. (Fig. 8-8) As the name indicates, the gas is compressed in the container, and it is the expansion of the compressed gas which provides the push or the force necessary to expel the contents from the container. This is essentially the same principle as the liquefied gas aerosol except that there is little or no reservoir of gas, so that as the contents of the container are expelled the volume of the gas will increase causing a drop in pressure according to Boyle's Law.

$$P = k \frac{1}{V} \text{ where } P = \text{pressure}, V = \text{volume of gas.}$$

Solid Stream Dispensing. Nitrogen is used as the propellant for this type of product. Nitrogen is essentially insoluble in the mixture of active ingredients so that only the concentrate is dispensed and none of the gas. This makes possible the dispensing of a product in its original form and is suited for

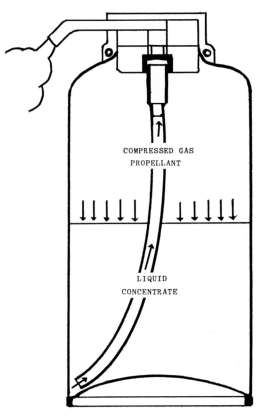

FIG. 8-8. Compressed gas aerosol.

the dispensing of hair dressings, ointments and creams, cosmetic creams, cough syrups, vitamins, foods, and other products. It is because of the lack of solubility and the fact that the product is to be dispensed as a stream and not as a spray that one is cautioned not to shake a compressed gas aerosol containing nitrogen prior to use. The concentrate is generally semisolid in nature and the dispensing characteristics are largely dependent on the viscosity of the product and the pressure within the container.[44] Since there is no liquefied gas present, compressed gas aerosols operate at a substantially higher initial pressure of 90 to 100 psig at 70° F. This higher initial pressure is necessary to ensure adequate pressure for the dispensing of most of the contents from the container. The amount of product retained in the unit after exhaustion of the pressure varies with the viscosity of the product and loss of pressure due to seepage of gas during storage.

In order to determine the dispensing char-

TABLE 8-1. PETROLATUM AS A COMPRESSED GAS AEROSOL*

COMPOSITION OF BASE		PHYSICAL APPEARANCE	DISPENSING CHARACTERISTICS
PETROLATUM % W/W	LIQUID PETROLATUM % W/W		
0	100	Limpid oily liquid	A
10	90	Limpid oily liquid	A
20	80	Limpid oily liquid	A
30	70	Viscous oily liquid	A
40	60	Viscous oily liquid	A
50	50	Jellylike semisolid	B
60	40	Jellylike semisolid	C
70	30	Jellylike semisolid	D
80	20	Viscous semisolid	E
90	10	Viscous semisolid	E
100	0	Viscous semisolid	F

* Nitrogen at 90 psig.
A — Too limpid, does not adhere to skin surface.
B — Flowed evenly, may be a little too limpid, does not adhere to skin surface.
C — Produced a product having most of the desired characteristics.
D — Could be dispensed, may be too viscous.
E — Could be dispensed, too viscous to be spread over skin surface.
F — Could not be dispensed.
From Sciarra, J. J., Tinney, F. J., and Feely, W. J.: The formulation of topical pharmaceuticals in aerosol packages, Drug Standards 28:20, 1960.

acteristics of several commonly used ointment bases when formulated as a compressed gas aerosol, Sciarra, Tinney and Feely[72] used a petrolatum base and a polyethylene glycol base. These were packed into aerosol containers utilizing nitrogen as the propellant. Tables 8-1 and 8-2 show the results of their investigation.

Several problems arise during the formulation of compressed gas aerosols because all of the product cannot be dispensed from the container, and, in the case of extremely viscous materials, the product does not flow readily, resulting in cavitation and subsequent loss of gaseous propellant.

Foam Dispensing. This system is similar to

TABLE 8-2. POLYETHYLENE GLYCOL AS A COMPRESSED GAS AEROSOL*

COMPOSITION OF BASE		PHYSICAL APPEARANCE	DISPENSING CHARACTERISTICS
PEG 4,000 % W/W	PEG 400 % W/W		
0	100	Limpid liquid	A
5	95	Viscous liquid	C
10	90	Very viscous liquid	C
20	80	Jellylike semisolid	D
30	70	Viscous semisolid	D
40	60	Very viscous semisolid	F
50	50	Very viscous semisolid	F

* Nitrogen at 90 psig.
A — Too limpid, does not adhere to skin surface.
C — Produced a product having most of the desired characteristics.
D — Could be dispensed, may be too viscous.
F — Could not be dispensed.
From Sciarra, J. J., Tinney, F. J., and Feely, W. J.: Drug Standards 28:20, 1960.

the liquefied-gas foam system except that nitrous oxide and carbon dioxide are used as the propellants. Recently, a mixture of a liquefied gas (octafluorocyclobutane) and nitrous oxide has been introduced for use in whipped creams and toppings. These gases are soluble in the product concentrate (which is generally an emulsified product) and, when the aerosol is dispensed, some of the soluble compressed gas is emitted with the concentrate. This will cause a whipping of the cream. In this type, shaking of the container prior to use is desired in order to mix some of the gas with the active ingredients.

Spray Dispensing. This system is similar to a two-phase system except for the propellant. A compressed gas such as nitrogen, carbon dioxide or nitrous oxide is used. Since the compressed gases do not possess the dispersing power of the liquefied gases, a mechanical breakup actuator is used and a wet spray can be produced. Nitrogen is used to dispense an aqueous solution of an iodine

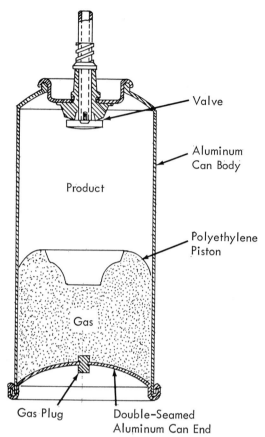

FIG. 8-10. Piston aerosol container. (American Can Company)

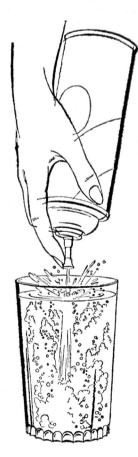

FIG. 8-9. Self-agitating aerosol product (Daylight Industries, Inc.)

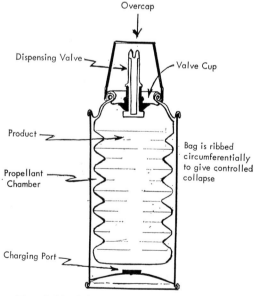

FIG. 8-11. Schematic view of Sepro container. (Continental Can Company)

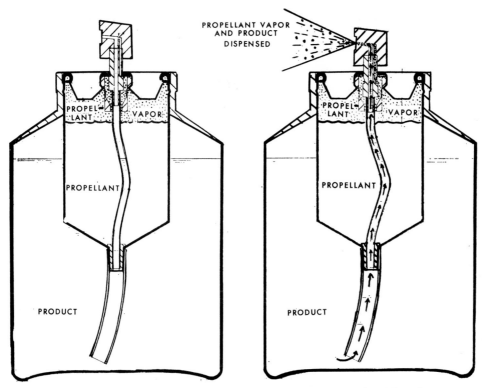

FIG. 8-12. Preval system in rest (*left*) and in operating position (*right*). Note the separate passageways for propellant vapor and product in actuator. (Precision Valve Corporation)

complex; nitrous oxide has been used to dispense a barbecue sauce, while carbon dioxide is used to dispense a de-icer spray. Webster[83] has investigated the use of some of the soluble compressed gases as propellants for products requiring a fine spray. The major advantage of this type of system is that the propellant has greater compatibility with aqueous liquids.

A recently developed compressed gas aerosol system is unique in that it makes use of three variables, namely the viscosity of the product, the orifice of the valve and the pressure within the container, to dispense the product as a fast moving "jet" stream which becomes self-agitating if it is directed into milk or water.[20] In this process, a soluble compressed gas is used to dispense the product as an aerated foam into a liquid diluent. As the foam comes into contact with the diluent, the gases trapped within the foam expand, resulting in a complete mixture of the concentrate with the diluent. While the soluble compressed gases have greater dis-

persing power, nitrogen also can be used advantageously. The principle has been applied to several flavored syrups (chocolate, strawberry etc.) with success. At the present time, the system is used principally in the dispensing of food and beverage concentrates,[65] but it may be used for dispensing many pharmaceutical syrups, elixirs and other liquid products. Figure 8-9 shows the dispensing of such a product.

Additional systems have been developed during the past several years that are capable of separating the propellant from the other ingredients used in the formulation. These systems are useful in that they overcome any incompatibilities between the propellant and the rest of the formulation, which makes possible the use of aerosols containing water as the solvent and also aerosols of a relatively high viscosity.

Piston System. This system, termed "Mira-Flo" by American Can Company, consists of a thin-walled aluminum container fitted with a polyethylene piston.[62] The system is

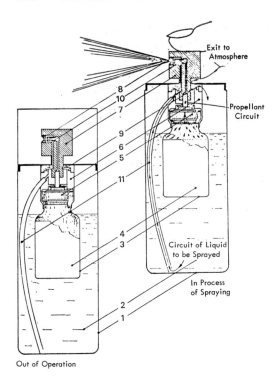

Exit to Atmosphere

Propellant Circuit

Circuit of Liquid to be Sprayed

In Process of Spraying

Out of Operation

FIG. 8-13. Innovair system in rest (*left*) and in operating position (*right*). Note that the dip tube is outside the propellant cartridge. (Geigy, Inc.)

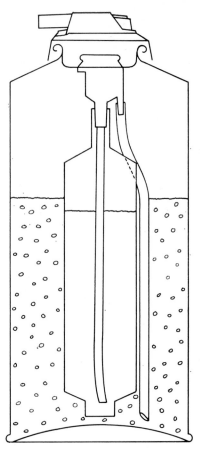

FIG. 8-14. System for codispensing of aerosol products.

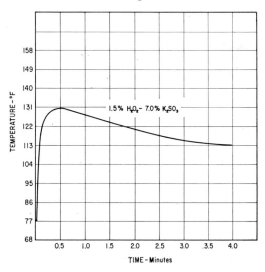

FIG. 8-15. Heat production H_2O_2—K_2SO_3 by oxidation reduction reaction. (E. I. Du Pont)

limited to viscous liquids, ointments and creams. The container is filled with the product through the 1-inch opening and the valve is fitted into place. The propellant, generally nitrogen or Propellant 12, is added through a small opening located in the bottom of the container. The opening is then sealed with a rubber plug. Figure 8-10 illustrates this system.

Flexible Bag System. A flexible polyethylene or multicomponent plastic bag is fitted inside of a standard three-piece tin-plated container.[80] The bag, which is filled with the product, is accordion-pleated and does not come into contact with the walls of the container. After the valve is sealed into place, the propellant is added in a manner similar to that in the piston type system. A "Sepro" container (Continental Can Company) is illustrated in Figure 8-11. This system can be used to spray limpid liquids or to dispense semisolids.

Atomizer Type Systems. Two systems,

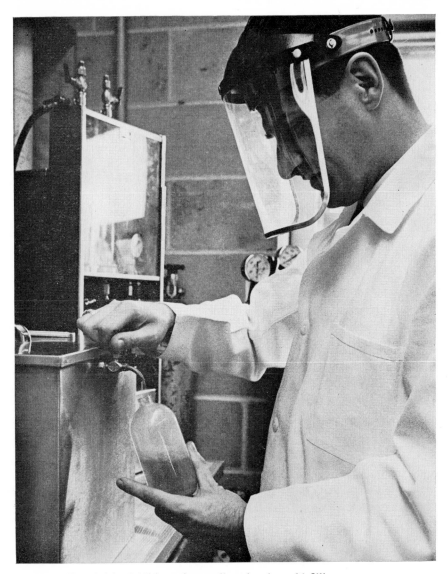

Fig. 8-16. Addition of propellant by the cold filling process.

based on the Venturi principle, recently have become available. These systems utilize a propellant cartridge that allows the propellant to be dispensed as a vapor. The vapor, passing over a capillary tube immersed in the product, draws the product into the actuator, where both propellant vapor and product are mixed and emitted as a fine mist. Figures 8-12 and 8-13 show the operation of these systems.

Co-dispensing Systems. A recent development in aerosol technology has made it possible to dispense thermal foams. Isolating two chemical reactants capable of liberating heat in a single container and allowing them to mix in the proper portions at the time of dispensing results in the liberation of a thermal foam. This system has been developed primarily for use with shave creams, but it can be applied to pharmaceutical ointments, lotions and body rubs. A typical system is shown in Figure 8-14. A solution of hydrogen peroxide is placed within the inner polyethylene bag. The outer container is filled with the foam formulation, propellant and a reducing agent such as potassium sulfite or a

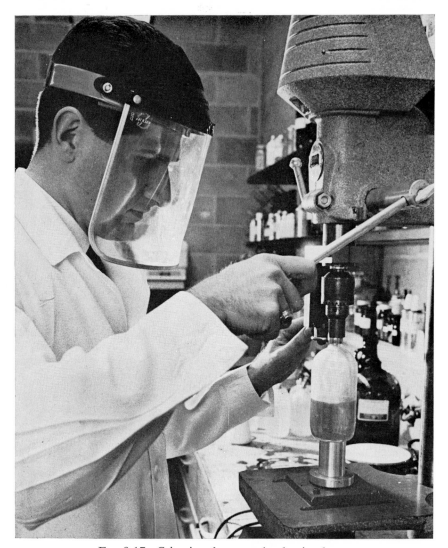

Fig. 8-17. Crimping the aerosol valve in place.

mixture of potassium sulfite and potassium thiosulfate. The valve is designed to dispense a given amount of foam formulation and hydrogen peroxide, which are then mixed together in the valve chamber. The following reaction then takes place:[5]

$$H_2O_2 + SO_3^= \rightarrow H_2O + SO_4^=$$

This reaction results in the liberation of 87.7 K cal./mole, which heats the foam as shown in Figure 8-15. Several different types of valves have been developed for this application and are based on upright or upside-down dispensing.

MANUFACTURE OF AEROSOL PRODUCTS

A propellant compound can be liquefied either by lowering the temperature below its boiling point or by an increase in pressure. When the propellant is kept below its boiling point or at a pressure above its vapor pressure, the propellant will be in the liquid state. This is essentially the basis for the two methods used to fill liquefied gas aerosol products.

LABORATORY PROCEDURES

Cold Process. In the cold process, the active ingredients are chilled and weighed

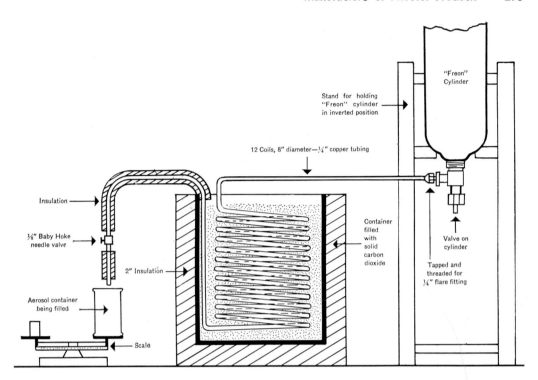

CAUTION: Outlet valve on cylinder and valve on filling line should <u>never</u> both be closed at the same time, thereby trapping liquid which may expand and rupture line. One or both valves should <u>always</u> be open.

NOTE: Aerosol container to be filled is cooled before filling by immersing in finely ground solid carbon dioxide.

FIG. 8-18. Laboratory cold filling of aerosols. (E. I. Du Pont.)

into an open container. Then the cold propellant is metered into the container and the container is sealed by crimping the valve in place. This unit is then heated in a water bath to 130° F. to test for leaks and to test the strength of the container. Figure 8-16 shows the addition of the propellant component to the concentrate and Figure 8-17 illustrates the crimping of the valve onto the aerosol container. A schematic diagram of the cold filling apparatus is shown in Figure 8-18.

This method is fast but is not generally suited for aqueous and emulsion type products, since the concentrate will freeze and solidify at these low temperatures (−40° F.).

Pressure Process. This process can be used for aerosol products of all types. The concentrate is prepared in the usual manner and placed into the aerosol container at room temperature (Fig. 8-19). After the valve is crimped into place, the trapped air is evacu- ated from the container via a vacuum pump or evacuated at the same time that the valve is inserted through use of a combination crimper and vacuumizing unit. The propellant is added through the valve, utilizing the vapor pressure of the propellant to force it through the valve. This is shown in Figure 8-20, a diagram of the apparatus is given in Figure 8-21. Since a relatively large amount of propellant must be forced through a small valve opening, newer techniques utilize the pressure of nitrogen or another compressed gas on the propellant to force the propellant through the valve openings.

The development of "under-the-cap" filling technics has made possible filling speeds in excess of what may be accomplished with cold filling equipment. The pressure filling process has become the method of choice for most aerosol products.

The differences between these two methods have been summarized by Herzka and Pickthall[36]:

Cold Process	Pressure Process
1. Not suitable for small to medium production runs at moderate speeds.	1. Suitable for small to medium production runs at moderate speed.
2. Propellant losses are likely to occur.	2. Propellant losses are insignificant.
3. Unsuitable for inflammable propellants.	3. Suitable for inflammable propellants.
4. The moisture content of the pack is likely to increase during filling.	4. Filling is completely anhydrous.
5. Heat has first of all to be removed from the product and the propellant and then replaced in order to bring the temperature of the pack to 130° F.	5. No heat has to be removed initially and less heat is therefore needed to bring the temperature of the pack to 130° F.
6. The product must have reasonable viscosities at low temperature and must be unaffected by refrigeration. Therefore, it is unsuitable for water-based products.	6. Suitable for water-based products.

Herzka, A., and Pickthall, J.: Pressurized Packaging (Aerosols), ed. 2, p. 115, New York, Acad. Press, 1961.

In the pressure process, provision must be made to evacuate or remove all of the air from the container, otherwise the air trapped within the container will increase the final pressure. According to Dalton's Law of Partial Pressures, the total pressure, P will be equal to the sum of the pressure due to air, p_1, and the vapor pressure of the propellant, p_2.

$$P = p_1 + p_2$$

Since the propellant is added prior to sealing the valve in the cold process, the air is expelled by the partial vaporization of the propellant. Both of these methods are used satisfactorily in the laboratory and in production for the filling of all types of aerosol products. The method of filling the compressed gas products is similar to the pressure process, and the gas is added through the valve through use of a specially designed nozzle and a reducing gauge set to the desired pressure as shown in Figure 8-22. For soluble compressed gases, the contents must be shaken during the gassing operation, either mechanically or by hand, to ensure adequate solution of the gas in the concentrate.

LARGE-SCALE PRODUCTION OF AEROSOL PRODUCTS

Since aerosol technics are quite different from the usual pharmaceutical procedures, it may be advantageous to discuss the procedures involved in the large-scale production of aerosol products briefly, with special emphasis on medicinal and pharmaceutical aerosols.

The filling of aerosol products is accomplished through the use of specialized equipment. An aerosol filling plant combines the standard manufacturing and filling equipment found in most pharmaceutical plants with the specialized equipment necessary to pressurize aerosol products, and facilities devoted exclusively to the filling of all types of aerosol products are available.

A manufacturer who wishes to market an aerosol product can do so in one of two ways. The entire operation may be set up and the manufacturing and the packaging operations done by the pharmaceutical company. On the other hand, the services of a custom or contract filler or loader may be secured and the complete operation be performed by the custom filler. If desired, the manufacturer may supply the concentrate, and the custom filler will package the product as an aerosol.

Production equipment is based on the two principles previously discussed—the cold method and the pressure method. The concentrate is manufactured according to generally accepted procedures and taken to the concentrate filler. From this point, specialized aerosol filling equipment is used. A discussion of the nature of the equipment is beyond the scope of this chapter. Pharmaceutical and medicinal aerosols can be produced on equipment of either the rotary type

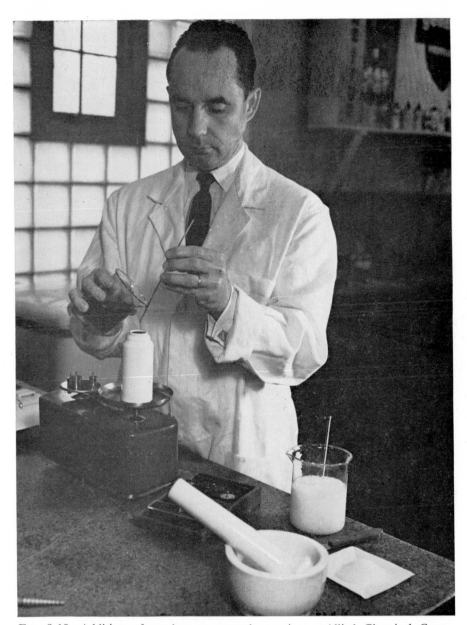

Fig. 8-19. Addition of product to aerosol container. (Allied Chemical Corp., Industrial Chemicals Div.)

(Fig. 8-23) or the straight-line type (Fig. 8-24).

Figure 8-23 illustrates the "under-the-cap" pressure filler. This pressurizes aerosols in three stages. The product concentrate is added to the container and the valve is dropped into place. The container is then fed to the "under-the-cap" filler. In the first stage or vacuum phase, a seal is made on the rim of the container, and as vacuum is applied the valve is raised allowing for removal of air trapped in the container. The propellant is added during the second stage and flows under the valve cup and into the container. In the final stage, the valve is released and crimped into place. Pharmaceutical and medicinal aerosols are generally filled in a completely enclosed, air-conditioned room

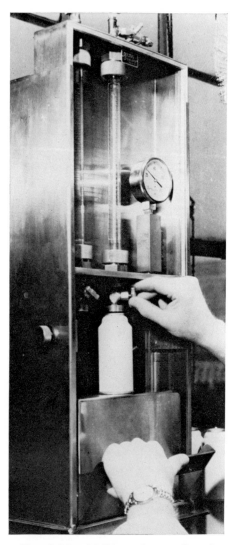

FIG. 8-20. Addition of propellant by pressure filling process. (Builders Sheet Metal)

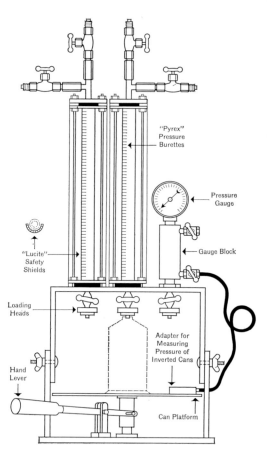

FIG. 8-21. Laboratory pressure filling apparatus. (E. I. Du Pont)

kept under positive pressure. Strict quality control procedures should be adhered to at all times.

PHYSICOCHEMICAL PROPERTIES OF PROPELLANTS

The propellant is one of the most important components of the aerosol package. It is said to be the heart of the aerosol. It provides the necessary force to expel the contents; it causes the product to be dispensed as either a foam or a spray, depending on the formulation.[1] Also—with the exception of the compressed gas propellant—it serves as a solvent for certain active ingredients.

According to the Chemical Specialties Manufacturers Association, a propellant is "A liquefied gas with a vapor pressure greater than atmospheric pressure (14.7 psia) at a temperature of 105° F." This includes substances which in themselves cannot be used as propellants but which will give a satisfactory vapor pressure when they are mixed with a liquid of high vapor pressure. This definition is not all-inclusive, since it does not cover the compressed gases. Since the vapor pressure of some of the compressed gases approaches 800 psig, for practical purposes, they cannot be used as liquefied gases. For purposes of this chapter the *propellant* includes:

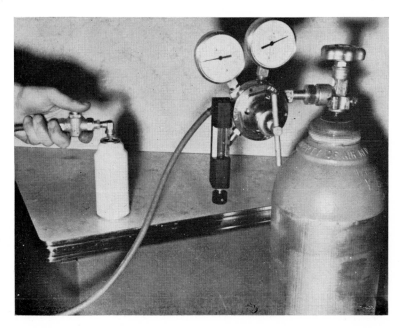

FIG. 8-22. Compressed gas filling in the laboratory. (Builders Sheet Metal)

1. Liquefied gases
   A. Fluorinated hydrocarbons (halo-
      carbons)
   B. Hydrocarbons
2. Compressed gases

LIQUEFIED GAS PROPELLANTS

Fluorinated Hydrocarbons. The liquefied gases used as propellants are essentially chlorinated fluorinated hydrocarbons of the methane and the ethane series and, more recently, the butane series. These compounds have been used for many years as refrigerants. Their low boiling points and vapor pressures make them ideal for this purpose. These properties are the basis for their use as aerosol propellants. Compounds such as trichloromonofluoromethane (Propellant 11), dichlorodifluoromethane (Propellant 12) and dichlorotetrafluoroethane (Propellant 114) are examples of some of the propellants utilized in aerosol products. Each propellant has a constant vapor pressure at any given temperature and by varying the propellant, vapor pressures from about 5 to 140 psig at 70° F. can be obtained. The wide range in vapor pressure of these compounds, their relatively nontoxic property, their nonin-

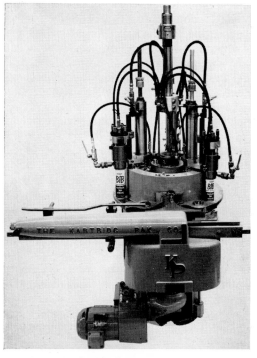

FIG. 8-23. Under-the-cap automatic pressure filler. (The Kartridg Pak Co.)

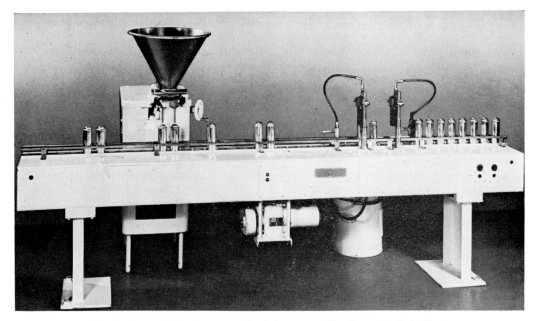

FIG. 8-24. Straight-line aerosol equipment. (The Kartridg Pak Co.)

flammability and their nonirritating characteristics make them safe and effective propellants. The U. S. Food and Drug Administration has already approved several products containing propellants of these types for spraying into the mouth or the nose. Each new product must be fully investigated before it is given approval. Propellant C-318 and Propellant 115, known as octafluorocyclobutane and chloropentafluoroethane, respectively, are reported to be nontoxic, stable and suitable for use in food aerosols. They have been granted approval by the Food and Drug Administration for use in whipped creams and toppings.

NOMENCLATURE. The fluorinated hydrocarbons (halocarbons) are derived from relatively simple chemical compounds (methane, ethane and butane), but it is awkward to refer to substituted compounds by their complete chemical names—for example, dichlorodifluoromethane, dichlorotetrafluoroethane, etc. For this reason, the refrigeration industry has adopted a numbering system which is used to designate the various fluorinated hydrocarbon propellant compounds.[1]

1. All propellants are designated by three digits.

2. The first digit on the right is the number of fluorine atoms in the compound.

3. The second digit from the right is one *more* than the number of hydrogen atoms in the compound.

4. The third digit from the right is one *less* than the number of carbon atoms in the compound. When this digit is zero, it is omitted from the number. Therefore, two digit numbers indicate methane derivatives.

5. The number of chlorine atoms in the compound is found by subtracting the sum of the fluorine and the hydrogen atoms from the total number of atoms which can be added to the carbon chain.

6. In the case of isomers, each has the same number, and the most symmetric one is indicated by the number alone. As the isomers become more and more asymmetric, the letter *a, b, c* etc. follows the number.

7. Where the compound is cyclic, a *C* is used before the number. The following is an example of the use of this system.

PROPELLANT 12—This contains two fluorine atoms (last digit) and no hydrogen atoms (second digit from right is one more than number of hydrogen atoms). Since it is a two-digit number (zero is understood before the first digit), this compound is a

TABLE 8-3. NUMERICAL DESIGNATIONS OF FLUORINATED HYDROCARBONS

CHEMICAL NAME	CHEMICAL FORMULA	NUMERICAL DESIGNATION
Trichloromonofluoromethane	CCl_3F	11
Dichlorodifluoromethane	CCl_2F_2	12
Monochlorodifluoromethane	$CHClF_2$	22
Dichlorotetrafluoroethane	$CClF_2CClF_2$	114
Monochlorodifluoroethane	CH_3CClF_2	142b
Difluoroethane	CH_3CHF_2	152a
Octafluorocyclobutane	$CF_2CF_2CF_2CF_2$	C-318
Chloropentafluoroethane	$CClF_2CF_3$	115

methane derivative. Since four atoms can be attached to this carbon and only two fluorine atoms are present, there must be two chlorine atoms. Therefore, the compound is dichlorodifluoromethane.

$$\begin{array}{c} Cl \\ | \\ F-C-F \\ | \\ Cl \end{array}$$

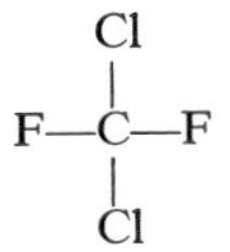

Table 8-3 indicates the relationship between the chemical name and the number of some of the commonly used propellants. In the following discussion these compounds will be referred to as Propellant 11, Propellant 12 etc. In the United States these compounds are available under the following trade names:

Freon—Freon Products Division, E. I. du Pont de Nemours and Company

Genetron—Industrial Chemicals Division, Allied Chemical Corp.

Isotron—Industrial Chemicals Division, Penwalt Corp.

Ucon—Union Carbide Chemicals Company, Union Carbide Corp.

PHYSICAL PROPERTIES OF PROPELLANTS. Several of the more important physical properties of the fluorinated hydrocarbons are in Table 8-4.

Vapor Pressure. The fluorinated hydrocarbons are gases at room temperature but their vapor pressure is low enough so that they may be liquefied easily. Vapor pressure is defined as the pressure exerted by a gas or a vapor when it is in contact with the liquid or the solid phase of the same material.[10] This is constant for any given material at a given temperature. The fluorinated hydrocarbons are unique in that they exhibit a range of vapor pressures when blended.

Figure 8-25 shows the extent of vapor pressures obtainable with the various available fluorinated hydrocarbons.

As the temperature of the fluorinated hydrocarbons is increased, the vapor pressure will increase, since a greater number of molecules will exist in the vapor state at elevated temperatures as compared with lower temperatures. Since an equilibrium exists between the number of molecules changing from the vapor state to the liquid state and from the liquid state to the vapor state, a temperature is soon attained where the propellant can exist only in the gaseous state. This is known as the critical temperature. However, aerosols of the liquefied gas type depend on the condition that the vapor phase be in equilibrium with its liquid state. For practical purposes, the vapor pressure considerations very seldom exceed temperatures of 130° F. Figure 8-26 shows the effect of temperature on the vapor pressures of a number of different propellant compounds, and Figure 8-27 shows this same relationship with commonly used propellant blends. The effect of varying the amount of each component of the propellant at various temperatures is shown in Figure 8-28.

While the vapor pressure of the propellants remains constant at any given temperature, the vapor pressure can be "custom-made" by blending various propellants having different vapor pressures. This has been shown graphically in Figures 8-27 and 8-28, however, it is possible to calculate this relationship. Roault's Law states that the vapor pressure of a solution is dependent on the vapor pressure of the individual components.[11] For ideal solutions, the vapor pressure is equal to the sum of the mole fractions

TABLE 8-4. PHYSICAL PROPERTIES OF FLUORINATED HYDROCARBONS

		PROPELLANT						
		11	12	114	152a	142b	C-318	115
Molecular weight		137.38	120.93	170.93	66.05	100.50	200.00	154.5
Boiling point (1 atm.)	°F.	74.7	−21.6	38.39	−11.2	15.1	21.1	− 37.7
	°C.	23.7	−29.8	3.55	−24.	− 9.4	− 6.1	− 38.7
Freezing point	°F.	−168	−252	−137	−179	−204	−42.5	−159.0
	°C.	−111	−158	− 94	−117	−131	−41.4	−106.0
Vapor pressure (psia)*	70° F.	13.4	84.9	27.6	76.4	43.8	40.1	117.7
	130° F.	39.0	196.0	73.5	191.0	112.0	106.7	−266.8
Liquid density (Gm./ml.)	70° F.	1.485	1.325	1.468	0.911	1.119	1.513**	1.291**
	130° F.	1.403	1.191	1.360	0.813	1.028		
Liquid viscosity (centipoise)	70° F.	0.439	0.262	0.386	0.243	0.330	0.42**	0.26**
	130° F.	0.336	0.227	0.296	0.186	0.250		
Surface tension (dynes/cm.)	77° F.	19	9	13	—	—	7**	5**
Solubility of propellant in water (weight %)	77° F.	0.11	0.028	0.013	0.32	0.14	0.066	0.066
Solubility of water in propellant (weight %)	77° F.	0.011	0.009	0.009	0.17	0.054	0.014	—
Limits of inflammability (volume per cent in air)		noninflam.	noninflam.	noninflam.	5.1-17.1	9.0-14.8	noninflam.	noninflam.
Toxicity (U.L. rating system)		5A	6	6	5A	5A†	6‡	6

* psig + 14.7 = psia   † Probable   ‡ Preliminary Value   ** at 77° F.

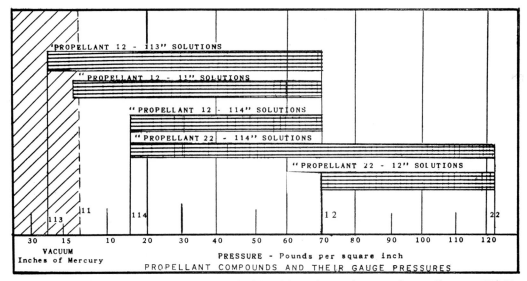

Fig. 8-25. Range of vapor pressures obtainable with various mixtures of propellants at 70° F.

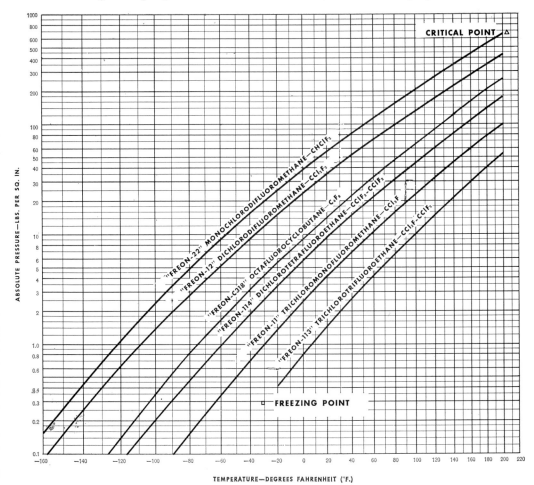

Fig. 8-26. Vapor pressure versus temperature. (E. I. Du Pont)

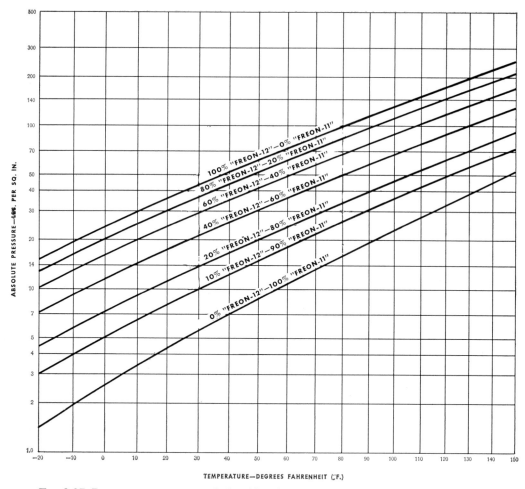

FIG. 8-27. Pressure-temperature relationship of Freon 12/11 solutions. (E. I. Du Pont)

of each component present, multiplied by the vapor pressure of the pure compound at the desired temperature. Expressed mathematically:

$$p_a = \frac{n_a}{n_A + n_B} p_A o = N_A p_A o$$

where

P_a = partial vapor pressure of Component A
$P_A o$ = vapor pressure of pure Component A
n_A = number of moles of Component A
n_B = number of moles of Component B
N_a = mole fraction of Component A.

Similarly:

$$p_b = \frac{n_b}{n_B + n_A} p_B o = N_B p_B o$$

The total vapor pressure of the system is then obtained by

$$V. P. = p_a + p_b$$

This is best shown by referring to the following example:

Calculate the vapor pressure at 70° F. of a solution consisting of 60 per cent by weight of Propellant 114 and 40 per cent by weight of Propellant 12.

To calculate the moles of each substance present:

$$moles = \frac{Weight}{M.W.} = \frac{60}{170.9}$$

$$= 0.3511 \text{ moles Propellant 114}$$

Similarly:

$$\frac{40}{120.9} = 0.3309 \text{ moles Propellant 12}$$

Total number of moles:

0.3511 + 0.3309 = 0.6820 moles of
Propellant 114/12

Mole fraction of Propellant 114:

$$\frac{\text{Moles of Propellant 114}}{\text{Total Moles}} = \frac{0.3511}{0.6820} = 0.5149$$

Mole fraction of Propellant 12:

$$\frac{\text{Moles of Propellant 12}}{\text{Total Moles}} = \frac{0.3309}{0.6820} = 0.4851$$

Partial pressure of Propellant 114:

Mole fraction × V.P. = 0.5149 × 27.6
= 14.21 psia Propellant 114

Partial pressure of Propellant 12:

Mole fraction × V.P. = 0.4851 × 84.9
= 41.18 psia Propellant 12

Total pressure of system:

14.21 + 41.18 = 55.39 psia (absolute)

To obtain gauge pressure:

55.39 − 14.7 = 40.69 psig (gauge)

The results of these calculations generally
differ slightly from the experimental results,

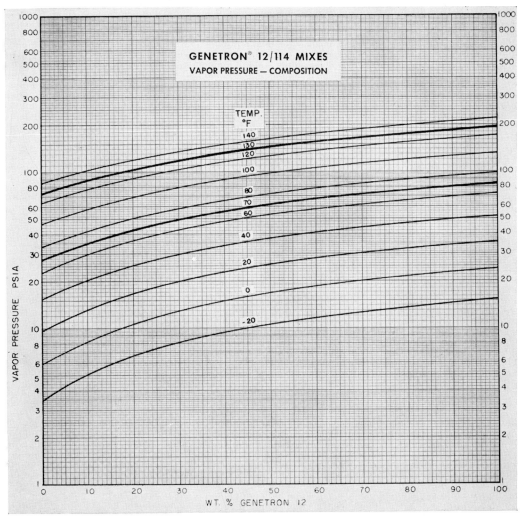

FIG. 8-28. Vapor pressure: composition of Genetron 12/114 mixes. (Allied Chemical
Corp. Industrial Chemicals Div.)

since it is assumed that the solutions are ideal in behavior. As the second component becomes smaller and smaller, the behavior approaches ideal conditions.

In any given series of fluorinated hydrocarbons, as the number of fluorine atoms increase, the boiling point will decrease and the vapor pressure will increase. This can be seen from Table 8-4.

Density. These materials vary in density from 0.911 to 1.513 Gm./ml. Generally, the density of the compound increases as the number of fluorine atoms increase. This holds true for any given series of compounds. In many instances, the amount of propellant to be used in a given formulation is expressed in terms of weight. However, it is sometimes more convenient to measure these quantities on the basis of volume, and the density would be used to calculate the volume from the weight. Figure 8-29 shows the densities of the

various aerosol propellants at different temperatures.

For the most part, the liquid density is important. In the case of liquefied gases, the density of the propellant in the vapor state is equally important. Depending on the size of the container, the weight of the propellant in the vapor state becomes significant. Figure 8-30 shows the vapor densities of Propellants 11 and 12.

Heat of Vaporization. When an aerosol product is dispensed from a container, the volume of the head space increases, causing a temporary drop in pressure. Immediately, some of the molecules in the liquid state change to the vapor state to restore the original pressure. In so doing, heat changes take place. If the discharge is rapid, then this heat change is noticeable in that the temperature of the package is lowered. The heat of vaporization for Propellant 11 and

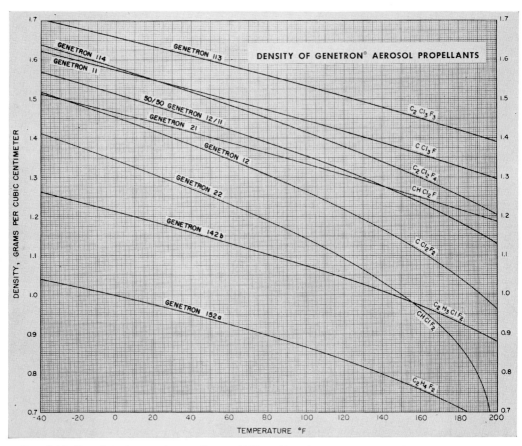

FIG. 8-29. Density of aerosol propellants. (Allied Chemical Corp., Industrial Chemicals Div.)

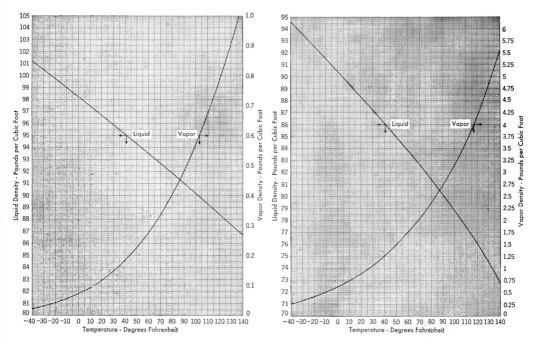

FIG. 8-30. Saturated liquid and vapor density. *Left,* Propellant 11. *Right,* Propellant 12.
(Allied Chemical Corp., Industrial Chemicals Div.)

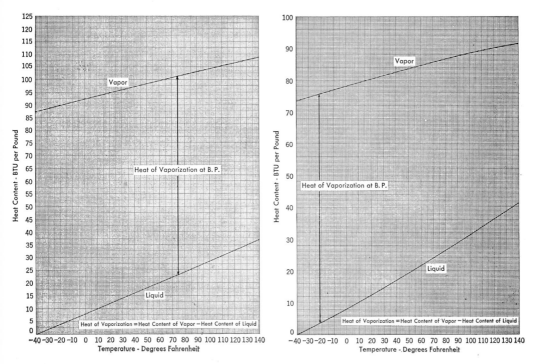

FIG. 8-31. Saturated liquid and vapor heat content. *Left,* Propellant 11. *Right,* Propellant 12.
(Allied Chemical Corp., Industrial Chemicals Div.)

Propellant 12 is shown in Figure 8-31. In the cold filling process a knowledge of the heat changes involved are important so that proper equipment may be utilized.

Solubility Characteristics. The fluorinated hydrocarbons are relatively nonpolar organic liquids and are good solvents for materials of similar types. They are not miscible with the highly polar compounds such as water. The fluorocarbons have solvent qualities similar to those of the chlorinated solvents such as carbon tetrachloride. However, there is enough difference so that direct comparison is not too helpful. The solvent power of the fluorinated hydrocarbons ranges from poor for the highly fluorinated compounds such as Propellants 12 and 114 to fairly good for those containing less fluorine—such as Propellant 11. Fluorinated compounds containing other halogens are usually better solvents than the completely fluorinated compounds. Generally, compounds with a low molecular weight are more soluble in the fluorinated hydrocarbons than those with high molecular weight.

CHEMICAL PROPERTIES. The fluorinated hydrocarbons are noted for their chemical inertness. They are, for the most part, nonreactive. The general reaction which may take place involves the carbon-to-halogen bond. It has been established that the fluorine

strated by measuring bond distances. Generally, the shorter the bond distance, the greater the energy required to rupture the bond. Table 8-5 gives some of the carbon-to-chlorine bond distances.

The reaction becomes important in the presence of water, for hydrolysis will take place, resulting in the formation of acids which are corrosive to the metal container and the metallic parts of the valve. Propellant 11 shows a greater rate of hydrolysis than the other compounds and, therefore, cannot be used for aqueous preparations.

$$CCl_3F + H_2O \rightarrow HCl + CHCl_2F$$

Table 8-6 contains selected information as to the hydrolysis of some of the commonly used propellants. From this table it can be seen that, in regard to hydrolysis, Propellant 11 is the least stable, and, while Propellants 12 and 114 are stable, the completely fluorinated Propellant C-318 has about 1/20 the hydrolysis rate of Propellant 12. The hydrolysis rate is increased in the presence of alkaline materials and, therefore, is a function of the hydroxyl ion concentration. An increase in temperature will also increase the rate of hydrolysis.

Another reaction which has been the cause of corrosion in metal containers is the reaction of Propellant 11 with ethyl alcohol:

$$CCl_3F + C_2H_5OH \longrightarrow \underset{\text{acetaldehyde}}{CH_3CHO} + HCl + CHCl_2F$$

$$CH_3CHO + 2C_2H_5OH \longrightarrow \underset{\text{acetal}}{CH_3CH(OC_2H_5)_2} + H_2O$$

$$C_2H_5OH + HCl \longrightarrow C_2H_5Cl + H_2O$$

linked with a carbon atom increases the stability of the other halogens attached to the same carbon atom. This may be demon-

It has been estimated that this reaction takes place to the extent of about 7 per cent. The acetaldehyde and acetal are corrosive in action. Sanders[60] has noted that this is a typical free radical reaction and requires the presence of a catalyst. It was concluded that this reaction could be prevented by the addition of a suitable stabilizer. This led to the formulation of a "stabilized" Propellant 11S which is Propellant 11 with the addition of a stabilizer such as nitromethane. This is sufficient to prevent the reaction.

Propellants 11, 12 and 114 are commonly used in all aerosol formulations. They are suitable for use in pharmaceutical and medicinal aerosols as well. Propellant 11 has

TABLE 8-5. STABILIZING EFFECT OF
FLUORINE ATOMS

COMPOUND	FORMULA	CARBON–CHLORINE BOND DISTANCE (Å)
Methylene chloride	CH_2Cl_2	1.77
Carbon tetrachloride	CCl_4	1.76
Propellant 22	$CHClF_2$	1.73
Propellant 12	CCl_2F_2	1.70

TABLE 8-6. RATE OF HYDROLYSIS OF SEVERAL COMPOUNDS
(Grams of Propellant Hydrolyezd/Liter of Water/Year)

	ONE ATMOSPHERE PRESSURE—86° F.			
COMPOUND	WATER ALONE	WATER + STEEL	WATER + COPPER	1 PER CENT SOD. CARB.
Propellant 11	< 0.005	19.0	0.18	0.12
Propellant 12	< 0.005	0.8	0.005	0.04
Propellant 21	< 0.01	5.2	0.38	330
Propellant 114	< 0.005	1.4	0.005	0.01
Propellant 22	< 0.01	0.14	0.02	220

Note. The hydrolysis rate of Propellant C-318 was found to be 2.2 mg./liter of 10 per cent Sodium Hydroxide solution/year.

a greater solvent range than the others; however, hydrolysis in aqueous media limits its use. Propellant 12 is used to a great extent for medicinal aerosols, since the desired particle size is produced when used with a specially designed applicator.

Recent investigations by Tinney and Sciarra[71] have shown that Propellants 142b and 152a are suitable for use in medicinal aerosols. Propellant 142b and Propellant 152a have been found to be good solvents for some of the commonly used medicinal agents such as ephedrine, atropine and tripelennamine. These propellants are less prone to hydrolysis than Propellant 11 and cause less irritation. While Propellant 152a tends to be slightly more inflammable than some of the other propellants, the quantity of propellant used in medicinal aerosols is extremely small so that inflammability is not considered to be a problem.

An additional feature of the fluorinated hydrocarbons is their noninflammability. In fact, they have been used as fire extinguishers. The vapors are heavier than air and will form a blanket around the flame with the exclusion of oxygen. This unique property is shown in Figure 8-32.

Hydrocarbon Propellants. The hydrocarbons (butane, propane and isobutane) have not been utilized to date for pharmaceutical and medicinal aerosols. While their low order toxicity makes them suitable for use, their odor, taste and high degree of inflammability discourage their use for this purpose. However, mixtures of hydrocarbons and fluorinated hydrocarbons have been investigated and found to be less inflammable than the pure hydrocarbon.[54]

COMPRESSED GAS PROPELLANTS[38]

Of the nonliquefied compressed gas propellants, nitrogen has found the greatest use. Its insolubility and inertness have made it the propellant of choice when dispensing certain pharmaceutical products in their original form such as vitamins, ointments and creams. It is possible that the future development of suitable actuators and baffles may allow the use of nitrogen and other compressed gases as propellants for medicinal aerosols. Since the size of the particles must be well below 10 microns for inhalation therapy, an efficient baffle is necessary. Present-day technology in this area precludes the use of the compressed gases for this purpose.

Other compressed gases finding use for pharmaceutical preparations are nitrous oxide and carbon dioxide. These are known as soluble compressed gases and are used for a variety of purposes. Being soluble in the product concentrate, they cause the product to expand when emitted from the container. If the product is emitted through a foam type valve, a foam is produced. A fine mist can be obtained through utilization of a mechanical break-up actuator and a nonfoaming product concentrate. The type of formulation will determine the dispensing characteristics of the product. Formerly, a compressed gas propellant was used to push the material through the valve and dispense it in its original form. Nitrogen was used for this purpose. Recently, it was found that by using a soluble compressed gas and a spray nozzle, the product could also be dispersed as a wet spray.

The pressure developed by a compressed gas is dependent largely on the temperature and the amount of gas present. The ideal gas

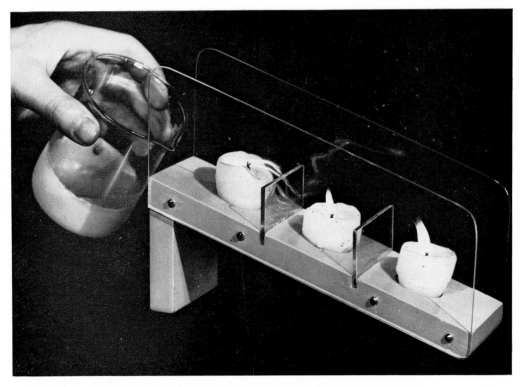

FIG. 8-32. Propellant vapor extinguishing a flame (Du Pont)

formula may be used to express the relationship:

$$PV = nRT$$

where P = pressure in atmospheres, V = volume in liters, n = moles of gas (Gm./M.W.), R = universal gas constant (0.08205 liter atmospheres/degree/mole) and T = absolute temperature (°C. + 273).

This can be used to calculate pressure changes taking place as a compressed gas aerosol is dispensed. Whereas a liquefied gas aerosol maintains a constant pressure throughout the life of the product, a compressed gas aerosol will show a drop in pressure. For example, 6 fluidounces of a tooth paste concentrate are placed in an 8-fluidounce container and pressurized with nitrogen to 90 psia; when 2 fluidounces of product have been dispensed, the pressure falls to approximately 45 psia (Boyle's Law). If the product contained a soluble compressed gas, the pressure change would not be as great.

Some physical constants for the commonly used compressed gases are shown in Table 8-7.

Nitrogen is chemically inert and has been used for many years to prevent the oxidation of pharmaceuticals. This property adds to its effectiveness as an aerosol propellant. Nitrogen is generally prepared by liquefaction of air followed by separation of the nitrogen from the oxygen and the other components of air.

It is used mainly for those aerosol products intended for dispensing as a solid stream in their original forms. As such, it is useful for many semisolid preparations and viscous liquids.

Nitrous oxide is stable in the presence of most oxidizing agents. It is generally used in combination with carbon dioxide as a propellant for whipped cream and toppings. It is used in the formulation of a veterinary product for mastitis, to dispense the product as a foam.

Carbon dioxide is considered to be a stable and relatively inert gas. However, it is

TABLE 8-7. PHYSICAL PROPERTIES OF COMPRESSED GAS PROPELLANTS

	PROPELLANT			
	CARBON DIOXIDE	NITROUS OXIDE	NITROGEN	AIR
Chemical formula	CO_2	N_2O	N_2	$N_2 + O_2$
Molecular weight	44	44	28	29
Boiling point, °F.	−109*	−127	−320	——
Vapor pressure, psia, 70° F.	852	735	492†	——
Solubility in water,‡ 77° F.	0.7	0.5	0.014	0.017
Limit of inflammability	nonflam.	nonflam.	nonflam.	nonflam.
Toxicity, U.L. rating system	5	——	6	6
Density (gas) Gm./ml.	1.53	1.53	0.96699	——

* Sublimes.

† At Critical Point (−233° F.).

‡ Volume of gas at atmospheric pressure soluble in one volume of water.

soluble in water to which it imparts an acid pH.

In many food products such as fruit-flavored syrups the acid pH is desired, since it imparts a tart taste to the product. In addition to its use as a food propellant, carbon dioxide has been used to formulate the de-icer type aerosol sprays.

TOXICITY OF PROPELLANTS

The Underwriters' Laboratories have investigated the toxicity of several of the fluorinated hydrocarbons and reported their find-

TABLE 8-8. UNDERWRITERS' LABORATORIES CLASSIFICATION OF TOXICITY

CLASSIFICATION	DEFINITION
1	0.5 to 1 vol. %, serious injury in 5 minutes
2	0.5 to 1 vol. %, serious injury in 30 minutes
3	2 to 2.5 vol. %, serious injury in 1 hour
4	2 to 2.5 vol. %, serious injury in 2 hours
4-5	Less toxic than 4 but more toxic than 5
5a	Much less toxic than 4 but more toxic than 6
5b	Data indicate classing as 5a or 6
6	20 vol. %, no injury in 2 hours

From Reed, F. T.: Toxicity of propellants, American Perfumer 75:42, 1960.

ings for groups. The Laboratories system of classification is given in Table 8-8. Table 8-9 gives the classifications for some commonly used chemicals, and Table 8-10 presents the results of the Underwriters' Laboratories studies.[55] Propellants 12, 114 and 152a have been placed in Group 6 and are rated as less toxic than carbon dioxide. Considering that air is a member of Group 6, it is apparent that materials classified in Group 6 may be used safely as propellants.

However, a danger to the manufacturer of the propellants and to the aerosol loader would exist should these materials displace the oxygen in the air. Since the propellants will not support life, precautions must be taken to ensure an adequate air supply.

Since many of these products are used topically, skin sensitization to the commonly used propellant compounds should be con-

TABLE 8-9. TOXICITY RATING OF SEVERAL COMMONLY USED SUBSTANCES

COMPOUND	U. L. CLASSIFICATION	MAXIMUM ALLOWABLE CONCENTRATION
SO_2	1	10 ppm
NH_3	2	100 ppm
CCl_4	3	25 ppm
CH_3Cl	4	100 ppm

From Reed, F. T.: American Perfumer 75:42, 1960.

TABLE 8-10. CLASSIFICATION OF
PROPELLANT COMPOUNDS

PROPELLANT	U. L. CLASSIFICATION	MAX. ALLOWABLE CONCENTRATION
11	5a	1,000 ppm
12	6	1,000 ppm
21	5	1,000 ppm
22	5a	1,000 ppm
114	6	1,000 ppm
142b	5a	——
152a	6	——
C-318	6	1,000 ppm
CO_2	5a	5,000 ppm
N_2O	—	——
N_2	6	——
Air	6	——
Propane	5b	1,000 ppm
n-Butane	5b	1,000 ppm
i-Butane	5b	1,000 ppm

Adapted from Reed, F. T.: American Perfumer
75:42, 1960.

sidered. Very little data are available on these compounds as to skin sensitization. However, to date, very few, if any, cases of skin sensitization have been reported. In rabbit-eye tests which were conducted, Propellants 11, 12 and 114 caused no reaction. While the concentration of propellant used in each test was low, lack of toxicity was indicated for this group of compounds.[55]

The liquefied gas propellants are refrigerants and may cause frost-bite if they are sprayed on a skin area for a prolonged period of time. This is unlikely to occur, since the initial chilling effect would serve as a warning. Very little is known as to the quantitative temperature changes taking place on the skin when an aerosol product is sprayed over an affected area. Studies by Dunne[15] led to the following conclusions:

1. The chilling effect of a system is generally less than that of the pure propellant. However, at propellant concentrations of 70 per cent and above, the chilling effect may be greater than that of the pure propellant.

2. The chilling effect increases as propellant concentration increases.

3. The chilling effects of propellant-solvent systems, for a given solvent, are in the same relative order as the pure propellants.

These effects were studied further by Broderick and Flanner.[6]

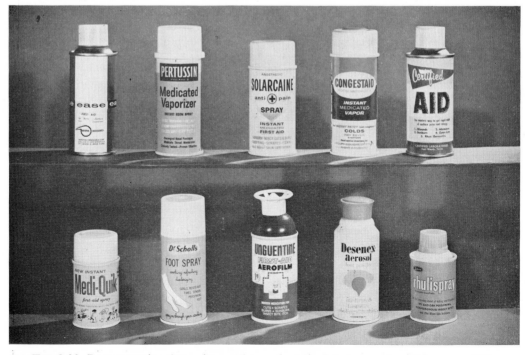

FIG. 8-33. Representative three-piece and two-piece tinplated aerosol containers used for pharmaceuticals.

AEROSOL CONTAINERS

The containers used for pharmaceutical and medicinal aerosols are similar to the usual type of aerosol containers. Aerosol or pressure containers generally fall into one of the following categories:

1. Metal
    A. Tin-plated steel
        a. Side-seam (three-piece)
        b. Two-piece or drawn
    B. Aluminum
        a. Two-piece
        b. Extruded
    C. Stainless steel
2. Glass
    A. Uncoated glass
    B. Plastic-coated glass
3. Synthetic resins and plastics

All of the materials listed above have been used in the construction of aerosol containers. Pharmaceutical and medicinal aerosols are packaged in many of these containers. Figures 8-33 to 8-35 illustrate the variety of different containers used for pharmaceutical aerosols.

AEROSOL VALVES

During the development of the aerosol industry many new and challenging problems were encountered. As the various aerosol products were developed the shortcomings of the technology in various areas became apparent. However, once a problem presented itself, ways and means to overcome the difficulties were immediately investigated. The development of various types of propellant compounds and the technology involved in the development of the various aerosol containers have been discussed in the preceding sections. The development of the aerosol valve was not different. Here, too, many problems were apparent, since the valve must perform various functions.[4]

1. The valve must be capable of releasing the product promptly and of stopping the flow quickly.

2. It must be capable of dispensing the product in the desired physical form, whether or not this requires a change in the original form. For example, insecticides are dispensed as fine sprays or mists, shaving creams as foams, and tooth pastes in their original form. While the nature of the formulation and the type of propellant used have an influence on the dispensing characteristics, it is the valve which ultimately determines the form of the dispensed product.

3. Certain applications require that the flow of product be accurately controlled—that is, only a given amount of product must be dispensed. This is especially needed for medicinal aerosols and several pharmaceutical aerosols.

Various aerosol valves have been developed and include the following:

1. Non-metered valves
    A. Liquefied gas
        a. Spray
        b. Foam
    B. Compressed gas
        a. Spray
        b. Foam
        c. Solid stream

2. Metered valves
    A. Liquefied gas
        a. Spray
        b. Foam
    B. Compressed gas
        a. Spray
        b. Foam
        c. Solid stream

Most of the valves listed above are available for use on both metal and glass containers. A few can be used only on metal containers, due, mainly, to certain restrictions placed on the size of the valve proper.

Spray Valves. Most spray valves are composed of certain basic parts, consisting essentially of an orifice which opens into a chamber. There are generally two or three of these orifices and chambers in each valve. The discharge rate of the product is controlled, for the most part, by the size of the smallest internal orifice while the dimensions of the external orifice generally determines or influences the degree of atomization. As the liquid passes from one orifice to another, it expands, causing a drop in pressure which results in a partial vaporization of the liquid. This process is repeated at the other orifices, the vaporization of propellant becoming more violent at

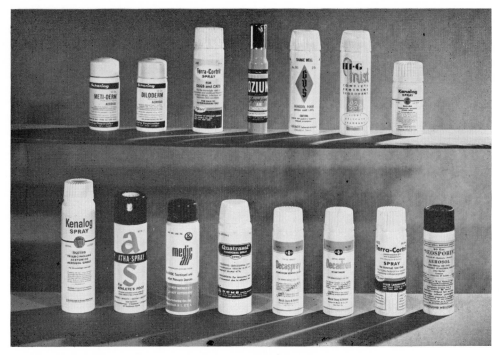

FIG. 8-34. Representative aluminum aerosol containers used for pharmaceuticals. (Peerless Tube Company)

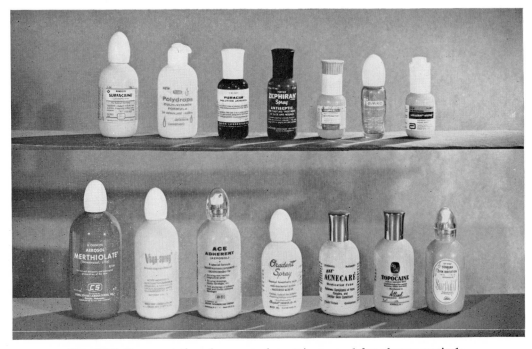

FIG. 8-35. Representative glass aerosol containers used for pharmaceuticals.

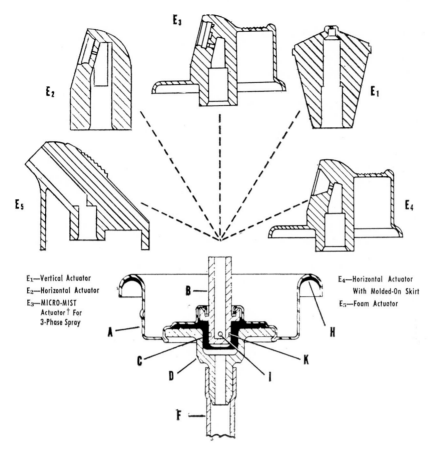

FIG. 8-36. Typical aerosol valve. *A,* Valve cup. *B,* Valve core. *C,* Valve seat. *D,* Valve cup. *E,* Actuators. *F,* Dip tube. *H,* Gasket. *I,* Dual orifice. *K,* Groove. (Risdon Manufacturing Co.)

each orifice and resulting in a complete atomization of the product at the final orifice. This spray type valve will dispense the contents of the container continuously as long as the valve is left in the open position.

In addition to the orifices, the valve is made up of an actuator button, a valve core, a natural or synthetic rubber gasket seal, a valve cup, a stainless steel or nylon spring, and a dip tube. Figure 8-36 shows such components and their relation to each other. The gasket prevents the liquid phase of the product from flowing through the valve stem by sealing it when the valve is in the closed position. Tension on the valve stem is maintained by the spring. When finger pressure is applied at any point on the side of the actuator, the valve core is deflected from the seat. This exposes the orifice to the product

concentrate, thus allowing access to the expansion chambers within the valve core. Other valves operate by depressing the actuator rather than by a tilting action.

The product and the propellant come into intimate contact with most parts of the valve and steps must be taken either to choose materials that are not affected by the propellant or the product concentrate or to protect those components which will be affected with suitable coatings. Through use of an appropriate actuator the product can be dispensed in a variety of ways using this type of valve.

Foam Valves. The valve described in the preceding paragraphs can also be used for foam products. However, a simpler type is useful and allows for a greater flow rate. These valves generally consist of a valve stem inserted through a rubber or rubberlike gasket. When the valve stem is tilted or depressed, the valve seat is no longer in contact with the rubber gasket and the product is allowed to flow through the openings.

Metered Valves. A valve that dispenses a predetermined quantity is highly desirable for medicinal aerosols the dosage of which must be controlled within narrow limits. These valves may be designed in one of the following ways:

1. Double chamber system
2. Stainless steel ball check
3. Flexible chamber type
4. Rigid chamber type[42]

The valves are capable of accurately dispensing from 50 to 150 mg. of propellant with active ingredients. This amount will vary somewhat, depending on the density of the concentrate. These valves can be used only with liquefied gas propellants. They have been used successfully for perfumes, colognes and medicinal aerosols. In addition, they are useful for both spray and foam products, depending on the formulation and the actuator. Other types of metered valves can be used for both liquefied and compressed gas aerosols.

PHARMACEUTICAL AEROSOLS

These products have been developed as fine sprays, foams, powders and semisolid preparations. Since they are used topically, local irritation is an important consideration. Other considerations, as outlined by Porush[75] are as follows:

1. Compatibility of component ingredients
2. Wetness or spray characteristics, including rate of propellant and cosolvent evaporation
3. Stability of the drug in contact with the container and valve parts
4. Effect of the aerosol solution and drug on the container and the valve (including corrosion of metals and deterioration of gaskets)
5. Appraisal of dermal toxicity
6. Clinical evaluation of the drug

The classification of various ointment bases and the absorption of medicinals from these bases have been discussed elsewhere.[19] How-

ever, in regard to the use of pharmaceutical aerosols, it is of interest that, according to Fuller, Hawkins and Partridge,[22] the fundamental consideration in the absorption of substances from ointments is "the ratio of the surface of the preparation to its volume." If the surface is relatively large—as in a thin film layer—the delay from oil preparations is small; this is found when ointments are smeared over a large surface. In this connection it seems that an aerosol ointment preparation is advantageous, since it will coat a large area of the body with a very thin film of medication.

Particle size is always important in ointment preparations. It is of even greater importance when the ointment is to be applied to irritated, or diseased skin or denuded areas. The smaller the particle size of the medicament, the less is the preparation likely to cause further irritation. Such a reduction in particle size can be accomplished by a liquefied gas aerosol formulation in which the dispersion of particles from the actuator is within the range of 30 to 50 microns or less. With the reduction both in particle size and in thickness of the material to be applied to a given area, penetration of medication into the ducts of the skin can be accomplished without vigorous rubbing.

Ethyl alcohol is a good cosolvent and is useful in many types of pharmaceutical aerosols. It is miscible with the usual propellants and is relatively free of dermal toxicity. However, alcohol is not suitable for application to large areas of broken, abraded skin or burned areas, since it causes a stinging sensation. Other cosolvents such as propylene glycol, polypropylene glycol, isopropyl myristate, polyethylene glycols, some fixed oils, glycerin, liquid petrolatum, hexylene glycol and several of the diethylene glycol monoalkyl ethers may be used. General formulas which can be used as a starting point for the formulation of two-phase pharmaceutical aerosols follow:

		by weight
1.	Active ingredients	10%
	Propellants 12/11 (50:50)	90%

This can be used to formulate medications for athlete's foot, burn remedies, wound medication etc. The amount of active ingredients may be varied to suit individual needs.

	by weight
2. Active ingredients	1-5%
Solvents	10%
Propellants 12/11 (50:50)	85-89%

This can be used for the products listed under Formula 1. The solvents tend to decrease the chilling effect as well as to leave behind a thin film or residue, depending on the nature of the solvent.

An emulsified or foam system has been used to great advantage for the dispensing of therapeutically active ingredients which may be irritating or otherwise harmful if inhaled. It is also useful for those applications in which the chilling caused by the rapid evaporation of the propellants presents a problem. For the most part, foam aerosols contain a considerably smaller quantity of propellant. Depending on the type of formulation, the foam may be quick-breaking or stabilized. The quick-breaking foam formulation is useful when products are used to cover a large area or when rubbing is not desirable—as in treatment of extensive areas that have been burned or denuded. The mechanical application of medication together with the abrasion caused by spreading the product over the affected area may cause further damage. The stabilized foam preparation is useful for many topical preparations when penetration of the active ingredients is enhanced by rubbing. Many sterol and steroid preparations are dispensed in this manner.

In an attempt to determine some of the principles involved in the formulation of emulsion type topical preparations, Sciarra, Tinney and Feely[72] investigated several typical ointment bases in combination with surfactants. One series consisted of an ointment base and a propellant while the other series consisted of an ointment base, a propellant and a surface-active agent. The dispensing characteristics are shown in Tables 8-11 and 8-12.

The addition of a surface-active agent to the propellant/ointment base mixture increased the stability of most of the products insofar as separation of ingredients is concerned. In those cases where a foam type spray was produced, the foam quickly collapsed, releasing the base in its original form. This is believed to be an ideal method for the administration of medicinal ingredients over a large area, since no spreading or rubbing is required in order to bring the base and the medicinal agents in contact with the affected areas of skin. No attempt was made during this study to alter the propellant concentration in order to produce different types of sprays and foams.

Further investigations were carried out in the laboratories of Allied Chemical Corporation, Industrial Chemicals Division, as to the formulation of quick-breaking foams.[82] A basic formulation for a quick-breaking foam is as follows:

Ethanol	46.0-66.0%
Surfactant	0.5- 5.0%
Water	28.0-42.0%
Propellant	3.0-15.0%

The proportion of surfactant in a quick-breaking foam is between one half and one twentieth of that employed in formulations for the stabilized foam products.

According to investigations carried out in the laboratories of the E. I. du Pont de Nemours and Company, nonaqueous aerosol foams may also be formulated.[59] Glycols and glycol derivatives have been substituted for water in conventional formulations. By proper selection of the glycol, the surfactant and the propellant, foam stability may be varied to obtain very stable foams or quick-breaking foams. The use of aerosol foams has been suggested for vaginal foams, ointment bases, burn preparations and other topical aerosols.

A suggested starting formulation for non-aqueous foams is as follows:

Glycol	86%
Emulsifying agent	4%
Propellant 12/114 (40:60)	10%

An ointment base formulation may consist of:

Polyethylene glycol 400	86%
Propylene glycol monostearate S.E.	4%
Propellant 12/114 (40:60)	10%

TABLE 8-11. LIQUEFIED GAS AEROSOLS WITHOUT SURFACTANT

COMPOSITION OF BASE	% W/W	COMPOSITION OF PROPELLANT	% W/W	PHYSICAL APPEARANCE	SPRAYING CHARACTERISTICS
Liquid petrolatum Petrolatum	90 10	Propellant 12 Propellant 114	20 80	Thin opaque liquid; no separation on standing	Produced a fine thin spray*
Liquid petrolatum Petrolatum	80 20	Propellant 12 Propellant 114	20 80	Thin opaque liquid; no separation on standing	Produced a fine thin spray*
Liquid petrolatum Petrolatum	70 30	Propellant 12 Propellant 114	20 80	Thin opaque liquid; no separation on standing	Produced a fine thin spray
Liquid petrolatum Petrolatum	60 40	Propellant 12 Propellant 114	20 80	Viscous opaque liquid; no separation on standing	Produced a fine thin spray
Liquid petrolatum Petrolatum	50 50	Propellant 12 Propellant 114	20 80	Viscous opaque liquid; separated on standing	Did not produce an acceptable spray
PEG 400	100	Propellant 12 Propellant 114	20 80	Thin opaque liquid; showed separation on standing	Did not produce an acceptable spray
PEG 400 PEG 4,000	90 10	Propellant 12 Propellant 114	20 80	Thin opaque liquid; showed separation on standing	Did not produce an acceptable spray

* Variation of propellant concentration may yield proper spray.
From Sciarra, J. J., *et al.*: Drug Standards *28*:20, 1960.

TABLE 8-12. LIQUEFIED GAS AEROSOLS WITH SURFACTANT

COMPOSITION OF BASE	% W/W	SURFACTANT	% OF TOTAL, W/W	PHYSICAL APPEARANCE	SPRAYING CHARACTERISTICS
Liquid petrolatum Petrolatum	70 30	Tween 20*	10	Opaque liquid; little separation on standing	Gave a fine spray
Liquid petrolatum Petrolatum	70 30	Tween 80†	10	Opaque liquid; little separation on standing	Gave a fine spray
Liquid petrolatum Petrolatum	65 35	Tween 20	5	Opaque liquid; no separation on standing	Gave a fine spray #
Liquid petrolatum Petrolatum	65 35	Tween 80	10	Opaque liquid; no separation on standing	Gave a foam type spray
Liquid petrolatum Petrolatum	60 40	Tween 20	10	Opaque liquid; no separation on standing	Gave a foam type spray
Liquid petrolatum Petrolatum	65 35	Span 80‡	5	Opaque liquid; no separation on standing	Gave a foam type spray
Liquid petrolatum Petrolatum	70 30	Miranol MSA§ modified	5	Opaque liquid; no separation on standing	Gave a foam type spray
Liquid petrolatum Petrolatum	80 20	Arlacel 165‖	10	White viscous liquid; no separation on standing	Gave a foam type spray
PEG 400 PEG 4,000	90 10	Tween 20	10	White viscous liquid; separated on standing	Gave a foam type spray
PEG 400 PEG 4,000	90 10	Arlacel 165	10	White viscous liquid; separated on standing	Gave a foam type spray

* Polyoxyethylene sorbitan monolaurate; Atlas Chemical Industries, Inc., Wilmington, Delaware.
† Polyoxyethylene sorbitan mono-oleate; Atlas Chemical Industries, Inc., Wilmington, Delaware.
‡ Sorbitan mono-oleate; Atlas Chemical Industries, Inc., Wilmington, Delaware.
§ Moranol Chemical Co., Irvington, N.J.
‖ Glycerol monostearate; Atlas Chemical Industries, Inc., Wilmington, Delaware.
Propellant consisted of 50% W/W Propellant 11 and 50% W/W Propellant 12.
From Sciarra, J. J., et al.: Drug Standards 28:20, 1960.

Antibiotic preparations have been formulated using a foam type aerosol. The following is a general formula which may be used for this purpose:

Foam base	90%
Active ingredients	2%
Propellant 12/114 (40:60)	8%

A typical stabilized foam base is composed of the following:[47]

Part A	Myristic acid	1.33%
	Stearic acid	5.33%
	(triple pressed)	
	Cetyl alcohol	0.50%
	Lanolin	0.20%
	Isopropyl myristate	1.33%
Part B	Triethanolamine	3.34%
	Glycerin	4.70%
	PVP	0.34%
	Water, purified	82.93%

It is prepared according to standard pharmaceutical technics and pressurized using the pressure method.

The suspension or the dispersion system has been used to great advantage in the dispensing of powders, including antibiotics and steroids. The propellant quickly evaporates and leaves behind the finely dispersed powder. Major difficulties which accompany the formulation of this type of aerosol product are valve clogging brought about by an agglomeration of the insoluble particles and the settling out of the therapeutically active ingredients. These problems have been overcome through the use of specially designed aerosol valves together with suitable lubricants and dispersing agents. In regard to the latter, isopropyl myristate has been used to the greatest extent in preventing the agglomeration of the insoluble particles. Other substances which have been used successfully or are currently under investigation are liquid petrolatum, propylene glycol, lanolin and its derivatives, stearic and myristic acids and stearic and myristic alcohols. Most of the usual pharmaceutical suspending and dispersing agents, such as acacia, tragacanth, methylcellulose etc., cannot be used, since they are incompatible with the propellants.

An example of this type of system is as follows:

Active ingredients (insoluble)	0.5%
Suspending and dispensing agents	0.5%

Inert powder such as Talc (350 mesh)	10.0%
Propellant 12/11 (50:50)	89.0%

This can be used for dispensing a variety of topical preparations including medications for athlete's foot, first aid preparations and antibiotics.

CLASSIFICATION OF AEROSOL PHARMACEUTICAL PREPARATIONS

A recent survey of aerosol pharmaceutical products found that aerosol pharmaceuticals were available for many different uses.[63,69] A listing of pharmaceutical aerosols which supplies the name of the manufacturer, as well as type of aerosol, composition and use, is also given.[69]

Local Anesthetics. A variety of chemical compounds having local anesthetic properties have been utilized as the active ingredients for this type of aerosol. Benzocaine, ethyl chloride, tetracaine, naepaine, cyclomethylcaine and pramoxine hydrochloride are only a few of the local anesthetic agents which have been used. In addition, Propellant 114 alone, ethyl chloride and Propellant 114 and Propellants 12/11 have been used for their local anesthetic properties.

Antiseptics, Germicides, Disinfectants and First Aid Preparations. The nature of the active ingredients used in aerosol preparations of this type varies from the simplest of antiseptic agents such as iodine to some of the more complex agents such as antibiotics, quaternary ammonium compounds and organic mercurials.

Adhesive Tape Removers and Bandage Adherents. The adhesive tape removers consist of a solvent such as ethyl alcohol, acetone or isopropyl myristate, oleate, stearate etc. dissolved in the propellant. Rosin, benzoin and other resinous materials are used for the bandage adherents. The tape removers are useful in that they allow for the easy removal of surgical tape with a minimum of irritation.

Body Rubs. There are basically two types of preparations used as body rubs. One type consists of a silicone incorporated into a suitable base, while the other consists of an alcohol, such as ethanol or isopropanol, and a propellant. These products are generally used for the prevention of bedsores in bed-ridden patients.

Burn remedies consist chiefly of a local anesthetic in combination with antiseptic agents such as sulfur, hexachlorophene, benzyl alcohol, tannic acid etc. In addition, cooling and soothing agents such as menthol and chlorobutanol are generally present. A typical burn formulation follows:[7]

Benzocaine	1.00%
Camphor	0.10%
Menthol	0.10%
Pyrilamine maleate	0.25%
Hexachlorophene	0.02%
Acetulan*	1.00%
Oleyl alcohol	4.00%
Dipropylene glycol	1.00%
Propellant 152a/11	92.53%

The effectiveness of an antibiotic spray powder in the local treatment of burns has been noted by Garnes *et al.*[24]

Dermatologic Products. This is a rather broad classification and includes those products used as antipruritics, anti-inflammatory agents, in the treatment of acne or poison ivy and related conditions etc. Many of these preparations utilize a steroid—generally cortisone or one of its derivatives—as the therapeutically active ingredient. Other products make use of antihistaminics. These products are extremely effective, since they allow for maximum penetration of the active ingredients with a minimum of waste. In most cases, a thin film of medication is applied over the affected areas, and, in the case of foam preparations, the medication is applied only to the affected area without waste. Several studies indicating the effectiveness of many different dermatologic aerosols have been reported.[23,57,81,84]

Foot Preparations. The aerosol method is an ideal method for the application of foot preparations. In the treatment of athlete's foot, shoes, stockings and affected areas can be sprayed easily with medication. The usual ingredients for athlete's foot remedies are undecylenic acid and one of its salts (such as zinc undecylenate) although many other ingredients are being used. Other foot preparations make use of a talcum powder with or without an antiseptic agent such as hexachlorophene.

* American Cholesterol Products.

Spray-on Protective Films. One of the first formulations for a spray-on protective film utilized polyvinyl pyrrolidone and vinyl acetate copolymers:[76]

PVP/VA E-335 resin	5.0%
Polyethylene glycol 600	0.2%
Ethanol, anhyd.	24.8%
Propellant 12/11 (30:70)	70.0%

Many medicinal agents such as antibiotics and antiseptics can be incorporated with this basic formulation. On application, the solvent and the propellants vaporize, leaving behind a thin transparent film, which, in addition to providing protection, allows for the visual inspection of the affected area. Since this is a "breathing film," the possibility of infection by anaerobic bacteria is minimized. Other protective preparations utilize a silicone which provides a water-resistant film over the affected area.

Pharmaceutical Inhalants. The vapor from an inhalant type product is designed to give prompt relief from the symptoms of nasal and bronchial congestion. Generally, the vapors of therapeutically active ingredients are produced through the utilization of a vaporizer (see Chap. 13). Recently, aerosol products have become available for this purpose. In use, an enclosed area is sprayed with the medicinal ingredients. The force of the liquefied gas propellant disperses the medicinal agents throughout the area in the manner of a vaporizer. In addition, these products can be used to spray a small amount of the medicinal on a handkerchief and the vapors are then inhaled.

A typical formulation may contain the following:[79]

Triethylene glycol	0.3%
Dipropylene glycol	0.5%
Deltyl Extra	0.2%
S.D.A. Ethanol No. 40	15.0%
Aromatic Oil	1.0%
Propellant 11/12 (50:50)	83.0%

Other Applications. Many reports have indicated the variety of pharmaceutical products which can be dispensed in aerosol foam.[16,31,53,61,64] These products include eye, ear, nose, throat and dental preparations. Many of these products are currently under investigation and in various stages of development. However, problems as to formulation, valve design, necessary applicators etc. must be solved before they can become commercially available.

MEDICINAL AEROSOLS

Inhalation therapy may be defined as the administration via the respiratory system of medicinal agents which are in the form of fine solid particles or liquid mists. In recent times, physicians have administered penicillin and other antibiotics by way of the respiratory tract. Many drugs have been administered by this method as indicated by Dautrebande,[12–14] Amsler,[2] Grant,[32] Sulsenti[78] and Sciarra.[65] Neuroth[48] discussed the use of several devices suitable for the production of aerosol particles.

In 1955, the first aerosol medicinal product was introduced in the United States. This preparation consisted of a self-contained pressurized unit which utilized epinephrine as the therapeutically active agent. In use, the product dispensed finely subdivided particles of epinephrine. The particles were in the range of 10 microns and below, with 90 to 99 per cent less than 5 microns.[52] According to Dautrebande, for true inhalation therapy the particles must be well below 0.5 microns and, in many instances, of submicronic size.[13]

In order to understand fully the therapeutic efficiency of inhalation therapy, a review of the respiratory system is desirable. However, a detailed discussion of this subject is not within the scope of this chapter. Those parts of the respiratory system to which inhalation therapy is applicable have been reviewed by Sciarra and Lynch[70] and are illustrated in Figure 8-37.

Since it is known that the particle size of therapeutic aerosols affects their clinical usefulness, many investigations have been carried out to determine the particle size that is most effective for a given therapy. Particle size determines the site of deposition in the lungs and, hence, clinical effectiveness. According to Abramson[28] and Findeisen,[18] particles larger than 30 microns were deposited in the trachea; those 10 to 30 microns in size reached the terminal bronchiole; those ranging from 3 to 10 microns reached the alveolar duct, while those particles in the range of 1 to 3 microns reached the alveolar sacs. It has been further reported that particles less than 0.5 microns in size reached the alveolar sacs and were expired. Other workers have reported different values. Also, the per cent retention of the particles must be considered.[45] Landahl[39] reported that particles of 60 microns or more were collected in the trachea with less than one per cent for particles less than 6 microns. Particles larger than 20 microns failed to reach

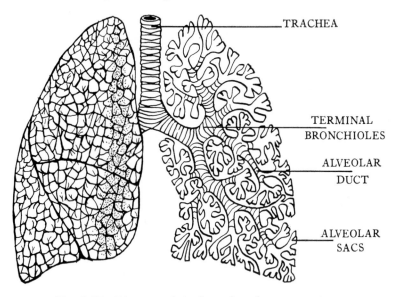

FIG. 8-37. Diagram of the bronchopulmonary system.

TABLE 8-13. PARTICLE SIZE OF ISOPROTERENOL AND EPINEPHRINE AEROSOL SUSPENSIONS

	MASS MEDIAN DIAMETER,* (microns)	MASS OF PARTICLES WITH DIAMETERS		
		< 5 microns, %	< 7 microns, %	< 10 microns, %
Lot No. 1. (Iso)	3.5	70	88	98
Lot No. 2. (Iso)	2.7	78	92	99
Lot No. 3. (Iso)	2.9	77	92	99
Lot No. 4. (Epi)	3.5	73	93	100

* As determined by the "light scatter decay method" (analysis of the change in light intensity of a Tyndall beam as an aerosol settles under turbulent conditions). From Porush, I., et al.: Pressurized pharmaceutical aerosols for inhalation therapy, J. Am. Pharm. A. (Sci.) 49:71, 1960.

TABLE 8-14. EFFECT OF INTERNAL PRESSURE OF ISOPROTERENOL SUSPENSION ON PARTICLE SIZE DISTRIBUTION EMITTED

	PRESSURE (psig)	MMD (microns)	MASS WITH DIAMETERS		
			< 5 microns, %	< 7 microns, %	< 10 microns, %
Sample A.	80	1.9	99.6	100.0	100.0
	45	3.7	69.0	89.0	98.6
Sample B.	80	2.5	83.1	95.4	99.6
	45	4.0	66.2	89.0	98.9

From Porush, I., et al.: J. Am. Pharm. A. (Sci) 49:71, 1960.

the terminal bronchiole, while those larger than 6 microns failed to reach the alveolar duct. Those particles less than 2 microns failed to reach the region of the alveolar sacs. However, it is more or less agreed in regard to material to be deposited in the alveoli for therapeutic value, that those particles less than 0.5 microns must be considered. The importance of particle size in aerosol therapy has been indicated by Lovejoy.[40]

Freedman,[21] Grater and Shuey,[33] Harris,[34] Seltzer[73] and Zohman and Williams[85] all reported significant therapeutic improvements when patients suffering from chronic asthma were treated with liquefied gas aerosols containing either epinephrine or isoproterenol. In a study of the effects of various nose drops and sprays on vasomotor rhinites of pregnancy, it was found by Barton[3] that a liquefied gas aerosol containing phenylephrine seemed to be the most effective agent. The author concluded that the beneficial results obtained from this product were due to the efficient method of propelling the medication into the nasal and the nasopharyngeal spaces. Administration of ergotamine in the form of a liquefied gas aerosol has been shown by various investigators such as Finch,[17] Ryan,[58]

and Speed[77] to be an effective and efficient way of introducing the drug into the circulation.

Many medicinal agents lend themselves to administration by inhalation. In fact, a drug given by intravenous injection can, in most cases, be reformulated into a suitable aerosol, provided that the drug is capable of being deposited in the respiratory tract and is non-irritating. Such drugs as epinephrine, isoproterenol, octyl nitrite, phenylephrine and ergotamine have been successfuly formulated into liquefied gas aerosols. The particle sizes of isoproterenol and epinephrine produced by liquefied gas aerosols have been investigated by Porush et al.[52] and some typical results are given in Table 8-13. Table 8-14 illustrates the relationship between internal pressure and particle size. These products have met with a great deal of success and have been readily accepted by both physician and patient.

Some typical formulations of medicinal aerosols follow:[75]

Angina Spray
Octyl nitrite	1.00%
Propellant 12/114	99.00%

Asthma Spray

Isoproterenol hydrochloride	0.25%
Ascorbic acid	0.10%
Ethanol	35.75%
Propellant 12/114	q.s.

Asthma Spray

Epinephrine	0.25%
Hydrochloric acid, 3N	0.50%
Ascorbic acid	0.15%
Water	1.00%
Ethanol, absolute	33.10%
Propellant 12	25.00%
Propellant 114	40.00%

Figure 8-38 illustrates several medicinal aerosols which are available.

VETERINARY AEROSOL PRODUCTS

Aerosol products offer many advantages to the veterinary field. In addition to the generally accepted advantages of aerosol products, veterinary aerosols (1) provide increased penetration of medicinal agent through the animal's fur; (2) facilitate administration of the medicinal agent and (3) minimizes loss of medication from the affected area through activity of the animal, since the ingredients are finely dispersed.

Veterinary products have been developed for use as deodorants, repellants, grooming agents, antiseptics and germicides, and for the treatment of several specific conditions such as pinkeye, mastitis, foot rot and ringworm. Many of the pharmaceutical aerosols previously covered are applicable to veterinary use; however, only those products developed specifically for veterinary use will be included in this section.

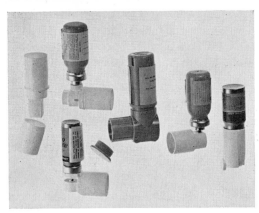

Fig. 8-38. Medicinal aerosols.

Antiseptic and Germicidal Veterinary Aerosol Products. These products are intended for the treatment of a variety of conditions from a simple wound or abrasion to foot rot and ringworm. The active ingredients generally consist of antibiotics and antiseptic and germicidal ingredients. A rather recent development—an aerosol product intended for the treatment of mastitis—consists of the following ingredients per dose:

Dihydrostreptomycin	250 mg.
Neomycin	100 mg.
Polymyxin B	71,000 Units
Methylparaben	5 mg.
Propylparaben	1.25 mg.
Milk-miscible vehicle to	2.5 ml.

The active ingredients are added to the milk-miscible vehicle and, after packaging, the product is charged with nitrous oxide. By means of a metered valve, a measured dose of 2.5 ml. is dispensed through a special teat tube. In use, the teat tube is inserted into the teat canal. The valve is actuated by pressing down and allowing the medication to flow through.

An aerosol preparation suitable for treatment of pinkeye in cattle and sheep contains:

Methyl violet	0.06%
Furfuryl alcohol	0.60%
Tetrahydrofurfuryl alcohol	0.03%
Urea	0.60%
Isopropanol	14.60%
Propylene glycol	9.11%
Propellant 12	37.50%
Propellant 11	37.50%

A typical flea, lice, and tick spray may contain the following:

Pyrethrins	0.06%
Piperonyl butoxide	0.48%
Malathion	0.50%
Methoxychlor	0.50%
2,2 Thiobis (4 chloro-6 methyl phenol)	0.10%
Petroleum distillate	23.36%
Methylene chloride	10.00%
Propellant 11	27.50%
Propellant 12	37.50%

SPECIAL TESTING OF AEROSOL PRODUCTS

Like other pharmaceutical and medicinal products, aerosol products of a medicinal

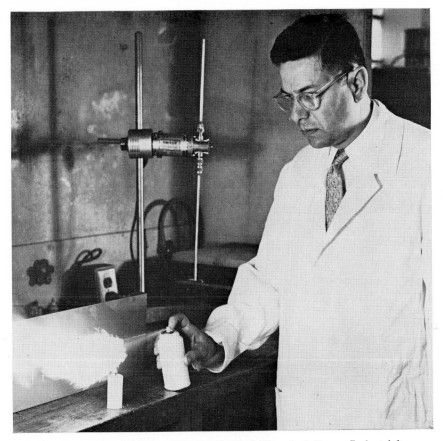

FIG. 8-39. Flame-extension test. (Allied Chemical Corp., Industrial Chemicals Div.)

nature require a "new drug" application. Hauser[35] has discussed some of the data which are necessary.

The various components used to package aerosol products must be thoroughly inspected by the quality control department. In addition to the general analytic control procedures used in the manufacture of non-aerosol products, several special tests are required for aerosol products.

All aerosol products must pass a "flame-extension test"—that is, when the aerosol product is sprayed toward an open flame, the flame will not extend more than a given length. In Figure 8-39 a typical aerosol preparation is subjected to this test. Additional tests are required to determine the explosiveness of the product using the "open" or the "closed" drum apparatus. The vapor pressure of the final product must also be determined.

It has previously been indicated that all aerosols are heated to 130° F. in order to test for leaks and strength of container. In the case of pharmaceuticals and medicinals, an exemption from this test is permitted for those products which will undergo decomposition at this temperature. Many of these tests are described in detail in a publication of the Chemical Specialties Manufacturers Association.[9]

For spray products, the spray pattern is extremely important. The application for which the product is intended will determine the requirements of the spray. The spraying characteristics are dependent on the nature of the formulation, the pressure and the amount of propellant present, as well as on the valve and the actuator. In many instances, faulty manufacturing procedures can be detected through an examination of the spray pattern. Some contract fillers routinely ob-

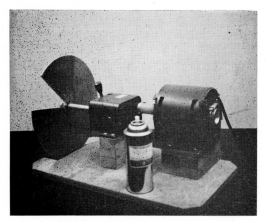

FIG. 8-40. Apparatus for the determination of spray pattern of aerosols.

serve the spray pattern of each aerosol container produced. A typical apparatus for the determination of the spray pattern can be seen in Figure 8-40.

These are only a few of the necessary tests. The entire filling operation for pharmaceutical and medicinal aerosols should be closely supervised. Mason and Hart[41] discuss some of the differences in filling and control procedures between pharmaceutical and non-pharmaceutical aerosol products.

Pharmaceutical and medicinal aerosols have established themselves as a dosage form which has many unique features and a technology of its own. Since this is a relatively new dosage form and requires the use of a liquefied or compressed gas, studies must be initiated to determine the behavior of many medicinal agents in contact with the propellants. In addition, the pharmacologic activity must be determined for both new and old drugs, since the mode of administration is different. As this information becomes available, it will be possible to utilize aerosols more extensively as a dosage form.

REFERENCES

1. Anon, Aerosol News 3:7, 1958.
2. Amsler, R., and Malaboeuf, J.: Present role of aerosols in the treatment of various pulmonary diseases, Sem. hop. Paris 37: 856, 1961.
3. Barton, R. T.: Western J. Surg. 66:347, 1958.
4. Beard, W. C.: Valves in Shepherd, H. R.: Aerosols: Science and Technology, p. 119, New York, Interscience, 1961.
5. Boden, H.: Hot shave lather technology, Bull. No. A-74, E. I. Du Pont, Wilmington, Del., 1968.
6. Broderick, G. F., and Flanner, L. T.: The chilling effect of propellant/alcohol mixtures, Proc. C.S.M.A. 51st Mid-Year Meeting, May, 1965.
7. Burn Remedy, GAPF-22; 23, Allied Chemical Corp. Industrial Chemical Div., 1968.
8. Chemical Specialties Manufacturers Association, Glossary of Terms Used in the Aerosol Industry, New York, 1966.
9. C.S.M.A. Aerosol Guide, New York, Chemical Specialties Manufacturers Association, 1966.
10. Daniels, F., and Alberty, R. A.: Physical Chemistry, ed. 2, p. 125, New York, Wiley, 1961.
11. Ibid., 148.
12. Dautrebande, L.: Characteristics of liquid aerosols, Physiol. Rev. 32:214, 1952.
13. ———: Studies on Aerosols, p. 104, Washington, D. C., Dept. of Commerce, 1958.
14. ———: Studies on aerosols, Arch. int. pharmacodyn. 129:455, 1960.
15. Dunne, T. F.: Determination of possible chilling effects of propellants, Aerosol Age 4:36, 1959. (May)
16. ———: Aerosols as a pharmaceutical dosage form, Aerosol Age 6:22, 1961. (April)
17. Finch, J. W.: Oral inhalation therapy, Med. Times 88:1029, 1960.
18. Findeisen, W.: Ueber des abetzen kleiner in der Luft suspendierter Trichen in der menschlichen Lunge bei der Atmung, Pfluger's Arch. ges Physiol., 236:367, 1933.
19. Foresman, R. A., Jr.: The Metal Container in Shepherd, H. R.: Aerosols: Science and Technology, p. 57, New York, Interscience, 1961.
20. Fox, I., and Palley, S.: U. S. Patent No. 2,977,231, 1961.
21. Freedman, T.: Medihaler therapy for bronchial asthma, Postgrad. Med. 20:667, 1956.
22. Fuller, A. T., Hawkins, F., and Partridge, M. W.: Rate of absorption of sulfonamides in vitro and in vivo after local application, Quart. J. Pharm. Pharmacol. 15:127, 1942.
23. Gant, J. Q., and Gould, A. H.: Steroid-antibiotic aerosols: a practical modality in otitis externa, Med. Ann. D. C. 30:528, 1961.

24. Garnes, A. L., Corbin, E. E., and Prigot, A.: Local therapy of burns with a neomycin-bacitracin spray powder, Antibiot. Med. 7:291, 1960.

25. Gebauer, C. L.: U. S. Patent No. 2,171,-501, 1939.

26. ———: U. S. Patent No. 711,045, 1902.

27. ———: U. S. Patent No. 668,815, 1901.

28. Glasser, O.: Medical Physics, Vol. 2, p. 823, Chicago, Year Book Pub., 1950.

29. Goodhue, L. D.: Insecticidal aerosol production: spraying solutions in liquefied gases, Industr. Eng. Chem. 34:1456, 1942.

30. Goodhue, L. D., and Sullivan, W. N.: U.S. Patent No. 2,321, 023, 1943.

31. Graham, J. J.: Packinging pharmaceutical aerosols, Drug Cosmetic Industry 87:36, 1960.

32. Grant, I. S.: Practitioner 181:698, 1958.

33. Grater, W. C., and Shuey, C. B.: Medihaler in asthma, Southern M. J. 51:1,600, 1958.

34. Harris, M. C.: The use and abuse of the pocket nebulizers in the treatment of asthma, Postgrad. Med. 23:170, 1958.

35. Hauser, J.: New drug applications for aerosol pharmaceuticals, Aerosol Age 5:30, (June), 30 (July) 1960.

36. Herzka, A., and Pickthall, J.: Pressurized Packaging (Aerosols) ed. 2, p. 115, New York, Acad. Press, 1961.

37. Kanig, J. L.: The present status and future of medicinal aerosols, Aerosol Age 6:35, 1961. (May)

38. Kleniewski, A.: Use of nitrogen in aerosols, Aerosol Age 13:40, 1968. (Sept.)

39. Landahl, H. D., Tracewell, T., and Lassen, W. H.: Retention of airborne particulates in the human lung, A.M.A. Arch. Industr. Hyg. 3:359, 1951.

40. Lovejoy, F. W., Jr., et al.: Importance of particle size in aerosol therapy, Proc. Soc. Exp. Biol. Med. 103:836, 1960.

41. Mason, A. P., and Hart, J. W.: The filler's role in pharmaceutical aerosols, Soap and Chemical Specialties 36:127, 159, 1960.

42. Meshberg, P.: Metered valves for dispensing products propelled by immiscible gases, Aerosol Age 6:36, 1961. (Dec.)

43. Mina, F. A.: Mode of action of ultra-low pressure aerosols, Drug and Cosmetic Ind. 75:625, 1954.

44. ———: Pressure-Viscosity-Time Factors in Dispensing Aerosol Liquids, Proc. C. S. M. A. 45th Annual Meeting, p. 72, 1958.

45. Mitchell, R. I.: Retention of aerosol particles in the respiratory tract, Am. Rev. Resp. Dis. 82:627, 1960.

46. Mobley, L. K.: U.S. Patent No. 1,378,481, 1921.

47. Neomycin Foam, A.T.P. Bull. No. 32, New York, Allied Chemical Corp., Industrial Chemical Div., 1958.

48. Neuroth, M. L.: Aerosols, newest of old therapy, Am. Prof. Pharm. 26:223, 309, 1960.

49. Package for Profit, p. 3 Wilmington, Del., Freon Products Division, E. I. duPont, 1967.

50. Ibid., p. 10

51. Phillips, T. W., and Holler, F. C.: The Propellant 12/Propellant 11/Vinyl Chloride System: Vapor Pressures and Liquid Densities, Tech. Bull., Allied Chemical Corp., Industrial Chemicals Div., Morristown, N. J.

52. Porush, I., Thiel, C. G., and Young, J. G.: Pressurized pharmaceutical aerosols for inhalation therapy, J. Am. Pharm. Ass. (Sci.) 49:70, 1960.

53. Prussin, S. B.: The potential of pharmaceutical aerosols, Drug Cosmetic Industry, 84:584, 734, 1959.

54. Reed, F. T.: Propellants in Shepherd, H. R.: Aerosols: Science and Technology, p. 224, New York, Interscience, 1961.

55. ———: Toxicity of propellants, Am. Perfumer 75:40, 1960.

56. Reingold, G.: Can making and can making materials (personal communication).

57. Robinson, H. M.: Prednisolone (Meti-Derm) as an aerosol for dermatoses, A.M.A. Arch. Derm. 79:103, 1959.

58. Ryan, R. E.: A new approach to the symptomatic treatment of migraine, A.M.A. Arch. Otolaryng. 72:325, 1960.

59. Sanders, P. A.: Non-aqueous aerosol foams, Aerosol Age 5:33, 1960. (Nov.)

60. ———: The Reaction of Trichloromonofluoromethane with Ethyl Alcohol, Proc. C.S.M.A. 46th Mid-Year Meeting, p. 66, 1960.

61. Schering's Diloderm foam aerosol, Aerosol Age 5:27, 1960. (June)

62. Schultz, R. S.: Free piston container, Soap and Chemical Specialties 38:127, 1962.

63. Sciarra, J. J.: Development of pharmaceutical and medicinal aerosols in the United States, Aerosol Age 6:65, 1961. (Dec.)

64. ———: Aerosols and the pharmacist, J. Am. Pharm. Ass. (Pract.) 19:672, 1958.

65. ———: Aerosol therapy, Aerosol Age 1:14, 1956. (Sept.)

66. ———: A new approach to the development of pressurized food products, Proc. C.S.M.A. 49th Mid-Year Meeting, p. 60, 1963.

67. ———: The importance of aerosol technology to the community pharmacist, Aerosol Age 4:66, 1959. (Dec.)

68. ———: Extemporaneous preparation of pressurized pharmaceutical products, Aerosol Age 12:85, 1964 (May); 12:55, 1967. (June)

69. Sciarra, J. J., and Eisen, H.: Dermatological pharmaceutical aerosols, Am. Perfumer 77:57, 1962.

70. Sciarra, J. J., and Lynch, V.: Aerosol inhalation therapy, Drug Cosmetic Industry 86:752, 1960.

71. ———: in Herzka, A.: International Encyclopaedia of Pressurized Packaging (Aerosols), New York, Pergamon Press, 1966, p. 610.

72. Sciarra, J. J., Tinney, F. J., and Feely, W. J.: The formulation of topical pharmaceuticals in aerosol packages, Drug Stand. 28:20, 1960.

73. Seltzer, A.: A useful device for treating acute allergic drug reactions, Med. Ann. D. C. 27:131, 1958.

74. Shepherd, H. R.: Aerosols: Science and Technology, p. 2, New York, Interscience, 1961.

75. ———: Aerosols: Science and Technology, p. 387, New York, Interscience, 1961.

76. Spray-on Protective Film, GAPF-18; 19, N. Y., Allied Chemical Corp., Industrial Chemical Div., 1968.

77. Speed, W. G.: Ergotamine tartrate inhalation, Am. J. Med. Sci. 240:327, 1960.

78. Sulsenti, G.: Cortisonic agents by aerosol in otorhinolaryngology, Arch. ital. otol. 71:559, 1960.

79. Technical Manual Aerosol Formulations, Givaudan-Delawanna, Inc., New York, 1968.

80. Irland, L. F., and Kinnavy, J. W.: The Sepro can, Drug and Cosmetic Ind. 101: No. 2, 42, 1967.

81. Walker, M. H.: A hydrocortisone-pantothenylol aerosol foam for skin therapy, J. Am. Podiat. Ass. 52:198, 1962.

82. Wallace, T. A., Jr.: Quick breaking aerosol foams, Am. Perfumer 75:85, 1960.

83. Webster, R. C.: Compressed gas propellants for non-food products, Aerosol Age 6:20, 1961. (June)

84. Yontef, R.: Prednisolone aerosol, Med. Times, Dec. 1958.

85. Zohman, L., and Williams, H. M., Jr.: Comparative effects of aerosol bronchodilators on ventilatory function in bronchial asthma, J. Allergy 29:72, 1958.

Chapter 9

Formulation and Prescription Problems: General Considerations and Inorganic Compounds

Joseph R. Robinson[*]

Dispensing pharmacy has undergone a number of significant changes in a relatively short period. It seems obvious that as today's pharmacist becomes less involved with compounding prescriptions, he must now fulfill the role to which he is best qualified—drug and dosage form consultant to the patient and physician. Pharmacists are still concerned with the theory, technology and stability of dosage forms, but they are becoming increasingly aware of the necessary involvement of the patient. This requires that each and every prescription must be evaluated and judged, not only in terms of the technology required to prepare it or its jurisprudence and physicochemical compatibility, but also as to how the prescription is related to the disease state, the medical history, total drug therapy and idiosyncrasies of the patient. In some areas, such as self-medication (O.T.C. items), the pharmacist is frequently the only person aware of what the patient is taking and must relate this self-medication to his medical background and total drug therapy in order to serve in an advisory capacity concerning this self-medication. Therefore, today's pharmacist, when dispensing a finished prescription, be it compounded or premade, must be sure the product is: (1) stable from a physico-chemical standpoint; (2) therapeutically active for the intended purpose; and (3) compatible with the patient's idiosyncrasies,

physiological condition and total drug background.

The purpose of this and the next chapter is to present some of the possible problems a pharmacist might encounter in compounding and filling prescriptions, as well as suggested ways to overcome these problems. The discussions are from a physicochemical standpoint and hence fall under points 1 and 2 in the preceding paragraph. Point 3 is discussed in Chapter 11. It should be obvious that this cannot be a complete review of all potential problems because there are an infinite number of these. What is attempted is to provide a sufficient background on incompatibilities, as well as some of the more common problems, so that the student can extrapolate from these discussions to his particular situation.

GENERAL CONSIDERATIONS

Receipt of the Prescription. Chapter 1 includes a description of the information that should be present on each prescription. Upon receipt of the prescription, it may be desirable to obtain additional facts that will help in its evaluation. It is essential that the pharmacist know what the prescription is intended for, as well as any other problems the patient might have. This does not mean the pharmacist is infringing on the duties of the physician, but it does suggest that the pharmacist use all the information he has available in tailoring the drug and dosage

[*] Assistant Professor of Pharmacy, School of Pharmacy, University of Wisconsin

form to the patient. Thus, a good up-to-date family medication record is essential in today's pharmacy, and although it takes a little more time to keep adequate records, it is well worth the effort. There are numerous instances in which a patient's medication record of prescriptions, including refills and O.T.C. items, has been the key in diagnosing untoward biologic problems and sometimes preventing serious complications. The important point is that the pharmacist obtain as much information as possible from whatever sources are available *before* filling the prescription.

The Prescription.   It has been mentioned that interpretation of a prescription includes jurisprudence, physicochemical compatibility and relation to the patient. Experience teaches that the reason why incompatibilities are frequently not discovered in time is that many pharmacists do not have a logical procedure in evaluating a prescription, or they begin compounding immediately without sufficient prior thought. This may seem like the obvious method in filling a prescription, but unless a specific procedure is established and followed at all times, serious prescription errors can arise.

1. Check patient's name, address and age, and note anything that might be useful—e.g., if the patient has an out-of-state address, is a child, animal, etc.

2. Check the date, mainly to prevent use of an illegal prescription and to be sure the patient hasn't saved the prescription from a previous illness.

3. Check the physician's name, address, signature and registry number. A quick glance through at this point should satisfy the pharmacist as to its legality.

4. Examine the prescription and decide for what purpose the prescription is to be used. In actual practice, one obtains much of this information from the patient. Evaluate each ingredient as to the size of dose and function in the prescription, and ultimately evaluate all ingredients together to determine: if they serve a purpose in the prescription, and if there any incompatibilities— physical, chemical or therapeutic.

5. At this point, evaluate the type of dosage form and again check on dosage regimen by determining: if it is a D.T.D.

or a divide, and what the dosing schedule is.

It might seem that the preceding steps involve a laborious procedure. This is, in fact, not true, and with experience this procedure requires a minimum of time. It is most important to realize that actual filling of the prescription comes *only* after these steps have been completed and represents only a small part of dispensing a completed prescription.

POTENTIAL PROBLEMS IN THE PRESCRIPTION

Overdosage.   Errors in placement of decimal point or very large overdoses occasionally occur in a prescription and are usually easy to spot. In most cases, however, a number of things must be taken into account to determine that an overdosage exists, such as age and weight of patient, dosage regimen and type of dosage form.

It is unfortunate that prescriptions frequently do *not* contain the age of a patient, and they almost never contain the weight of a patient. The age of the patient is useful in calculating the dose for an infant or child and is seldom used beyond this. Average doses are not determined by age but by weight, and most dose rules for children are based on an average weight or body surface area for a particular age. Weight, therefore, is an important factor to consider, and this can be appreciated more fully by considering a prescription for an adult midget.

Certain precautions must be taken with respect to drug therapy for infants. Young children, and especially infants, may not have fully developed enzyme systems to metabolize a particular drug, and hence the biologic effect can be entirely different and sometimes opposite to that of an adult. The important point is that children and infants should not always be considered as small adults (as is done when considering them on the basis of weight or body surface area) in evaluating dose and dose regimen. In some specialty areas, the children's rules for dose calculation cannot be used, and the pharmacist must rely heavily on the specialist's expertise. For example, in ophthalmology, weight or surface area average cannot be used.

The type of dosage form is usually not of great importance in evaluating correct dose, but it should be remembered that with rectal administration of drugs, one can usually tolerate a slightly higher dose owing to leakage from the rectum and loss by other routes. In addition, some drugs undergo significant decomposition or loss by the oral route, and hence only a fraction of the dose is absorbed. The dose for intravenous or intramuscular injection of drug must be evaluated with this in mind.

As a general rule of thumb, on a per dose basis, more than twice the recommended dose is considered an overdose. If available, the total daily dose should also be used and consideration given to whether the patient will be taking the medication on a long- or short-term basis in evaluating the dose and dose regimen.

Overdosage is not restricted to internal medication, and a number of drugs applied externally have an upper limit in which they can be applied to the body. Phenol, for example, should not be used above a concentration of 1 per cent on cutaneous membranes.

All cases of suspected overdosage should be referred to the prescriber.

Clarity and Intent of the Prescription. Occasionally, the desired drug is not clearly written and/or the physician has prescribed a drug that does not coincide with the patient's illness. In any situation involving an ambiguity, the physician should be contacted. Many trade-name drugs, unfortunately, have names that are similar in sound and spelling. The pharmacist must be absolutely positive of the drug intended before dispensing a prescription.

Nonspecific Problems. In this and the next two chapters, a number of potential problems in dispensing pharmacy are explored. These problems range from mildly irritating to disastrous, from both the patient's and pharmacist's point of view, if they are not caught in time.

TREATMENT OF SUSPECTED PROBLEMS

Incompatibilities, although relatively few in number in today's pharmacy, can present a very great problem. When an interaction occurs, there is the potential for a decrease or loss in therapeutic activity, as well as the possible production of a new species (in the case of chemical incompatibility) that could produce undesirable biologic effects.

To correct suspected incompatibilities, there are two possible approaches: (1) Assume responsibility, correct the incompatibility, and dispense without contacting the physician; or (2) formulate alternative methods to overcome the incompatibilities, present them to the prescriber, and let him make the decision.

The question that arises at this point is what are the circumstances when a pharmacist uses his own judgment and accepts the responsibility, and at what point should he consult the physician. We can make a broad generalization that whenever alterations are made in a prescription that do not change either the dosage form, therapeutic intent, or availability, it is usually not necessary to consult the physician. Most pharmacists, if for no other other reasons than professional courtesy and to demonstrate expertise, consult the physician in most instances. Also, in some states, substitution laws may be so written as to require consultation with the physician in each instance.

It is important to realize that at no time should the pharmacist jeopardize the patient-physician relationship. Therefore, should a problem arise in a prescription, it is usually unnecessary to inform the patient that the physician has erred.

Some specific examples will help to clarify the previous discussion:

Secundum Artem (According to the Art). Mixing order, packaging, and method of preparation are entirely in the hands of the pharmacist. If altering any of these reduces or eliminates the incompatibility, consultation with the physician is not necessary.

Additional Ingredients. It is frequently necessary to add ingredients in order to prepare an acceptable, stable preparation—e.g., the preparation of an emulsion requires an emulsifying agent and frequently a stabilizer; diluents such as magnesium oxide are used to prevent eutectic materials from interacting; stiffening agents are added to cocoa butter suppositories to maintain consistency, and so on. Although at first glance it seems that additives such as these fall under the secundum artem class, this need not be so because addition of these agents can alter the availability of the drug and must, therefore, be added with caution. Perhaps the most striking example is the choice of suspending agent for a topical preparation. Some suspending agents form protective films when applied to the skin, and this is undesirable in certain skin conditions (excessive sebum production) and desirable in others. However, in general, physician approval in this situation is not necessary.

Change in Vehicle or Dosage Form. This should always be done with prior approval of the physician because the availability may be different in the new vehicle or dosage form. Consider as an example a topically applied steroid prescribed in an emulsion vehicle; for a weeping skin condition substitution of an oleagenous base obviously affects the rate of absorption through the skin, and therefore, consultation with the prescriber is essential.

In all of these foregoing examples, there is the practical point that the physician may have described to the patient the type of dosage form to expect, and any obvious alteration can lead to patient-pharmacist-physician interaction if prior approval is not obtained.

It is sometimes necessary to either increase or decrease the volume of the prescription and make corresponding alteration in the dosing schedule. This type of problem, although not explicitly requiring approval, should be pointed out to both physician and patient.

It is sometimes necessary, if all else fails, to dispense the incompatible ingredients separately. This is a useful approach only if more convenient methods cannot be found.

Only a few situations that might arise with physicochemical incompatibility have been described here. The important point is that the pharmacist anticipate an incompatibility before mixing and then know how to treat it or prevent it in order to dispense the prescription.

With respect to therapeutic incompatibilities, it is much more difficult to give guidelines in treating potential problems. Therapeutic incompatibility as implied here means the relationship of the drug to a particular patient, including the patient's idiosyncrasies, total drug profile and adverse drug reaction.

In this situation, the pharmacist gives the prescriber all the information concerning the patient and drug he has at his disposal, and no real decision by the pharmacist is usually necessary.

It is important not to imagine incompatibilities that do not exist, but it is far worse either not to recognize a problem or to recognize one and not act. Pharmacists occupy one corner of a triangle with the patient and physician occupying the other two corners. The rapport a pharmacist enjoys with a physician and patient is based in large part on their mutual respect. If the patient and physician feel they can depend on the pharmacist for advice and counsel concerning drugs and dosage forms, then rapport is established and the pharmacist fulfills his role as drug consultant.

PHYSICOCHEMICAL INCOMPATIBILITIES

If roughly 97 per cent of prescriptions filled by the retail pharmacist are of the premade type, why should an extensive discussion of stability and physicochemical incompatibility be necessary? A number of reasons justify this treatment—for example, premade liquid dosage forms are frequently mixed with other premade liquid dosage forms, and there is the potential for interaction not only to lead to a decrease (or perhaps a complete loss) of biologic activity, but also the new species formed could possess pharmacologic properties much different from the original compound, and in some instances could be toxic. In addition, the pharmacist is responsible for storing drugs and dosage forms, and a knowledge of the effect of storage conditions on the stability of drugs is therefore essential. Finally, even though only 2 to 3 per cent of the total prescriptions filled are of the compounded type, this small percentage is enough to warrant a thorough discussion of stability and incompatibility.

STORAGE CONDITIONS

It seems worth while at this point to put the cart before the horse and discuss storage conditions and containers as they pertain to stability of pharmaceutical dosage forms. As mentioned earlier, pharmacists are responsible for storing drugs and dosage forms, and storage conditions can play an important role in the stability of the product. Changes such as color fading, altered rate of release from a dosage form, and drug degradation can be significantly inhibited or prevented completely by proper storage conditions. In general four atmospheric conditions can create problems: gases, light, heat and moisture.

Gases. The two gases most often responsible for stability problems are oxygen and carbon dioxide. Many drugs are prone to oxidation by atmospheric oxygen, and hence an inert atmosphere can be placed above a pharmaceutical product to protect it from oxidation. This works well for unit dose containers, but for multiple dose containers added protection is sometimes necessary. This is accomplished by the addition of a suitable antioxidant. Antioxidants usually act in the form of a free radical or an oxygen scavenger to retard oxidation, and they can be classified as water-soluble or oil-soluble (Table 9-1).

Carbon dioxide is another atmospheric contaminant that can cause stability problems. When dissolved in aqueous media, carbon dioxide establishes an equilibrium according to the following scheme:

$$CO_2 \text{ (solution)} \underset{}{\overset{H_2O}{\rightleftharpoons}} H_2CO_3 \overset{H_2O}{\rightleftharpoons} H_3O^+ + HCO_3^-$$

producing an acid pH. Freshly distilled water has a pH near neutrality, but on standing it is converted to an acid pH of around 5.5. For drugs that are sensitive to acid pH this can present a problem. Additionally, absorption of CO_2 into an alkaline solution produces carbonate, which can precipitate out with the proper cation:

$$CO_2 + OH^- \overset{OH^-}{\rightleftharpoons} HCO_3^- \rightleftharpoons CO_3^= + H_2O$$

Very little can be done by the retail pharmacist to guard against carbon dioxide and oxygen absorption except to use tight closures and minimum time during transference.

Light. Degradation of drugs by light can take place in a variety of ways—for example, production of free radicals due to energy in the form of light or acceleration of reaction rates by light-induced sensitization. The most common problem due to light is color fading of dosage forms, which generally is not a serious incompatibility but certainly can disturb the patient. Without resorting to chemical means to overcome this problem, the pharmacist can use proper lighting conditions in his storage area and amber containers to minimize the effect of light.

Temperature and Humidity. At one time or another, pharmacists have observed what happens when moisture comes in contact with powdered material. The most obvious example is the agglomeration of common table salt. One can extrapolate this physical instability to pharmaceutical dosage forms. Unfortunately, this and related physical instabilities are not the only problems that arise when moisture comes in contact with a dosage form.

Liquid Dosage Forms. There are numerous examples of physical instability of liquid preparations due to the incorporation of moisture. Such phenomena as viscosity changes (of particular importance in ophthalmic preparations) and perhaps precipitation from pseudoanhydrous vehicles are good examples. Additional examples that can be more serious bear mentioning. Consider the problem of a sustained release suspension composed of a coated active ingredient that is suspended in a pseudoanhydrous vehicle. The coating around the active ingredient must be water-permeable so that the drug is available to the body, and the pseudoanhy-

TABLE 9-1. EXAMPLES OF ANTIOXIDANTS USED IN PHARMACEUTICAL PRODUCTS

Water-soluble	Oil-soluble
Metabisulfite/bisulfite	α, β or γ Tocopherol
Hydroquinone	Propyl gallate
Ascorbic acid	Butylated hydroxy toluene (BHT)
Thiourea	Butylated hydroxy anisole (BHA)

drous vehicle is a palatable base containing a minimum amount of water. Naturally, a product such as this has an expiration date. However, any additional water will hasten the release from the coat and destroy the sustaining effect. This problem is also present with suspensions of slightly soluble drugs in which the dosage regimen depends on the drug being in an insoluble form rather than a solution. Any moisture in the system will dissolve more of the drug.

Although physical problems are numerous and have the potential to affect the therapeutic efficacy of a product, chemical reactions in homogeneous and heterogeneous liquid dosage forms present a greater range of complications. Chemical reactions can be of many types—for example, interactions with other components of the system or perhaps hydrolytic degradation. These interactions have been covered in Chapter 4.

Many commercially available liquid preparations contain humectants to prevent the product from drying out or to enhance flavor, and they can attract moisture, particularly in areas of high humidity.

Solid Dosage Forms. Solid dosage forms, such as tablets and capsules, represent the largest fraction of products in pharmacy. Although active ingredients are generally more stable in solid heterogeneous systems than in liquid homogeneous or heterogeneous systems, this by no means indicates that tablets and other solid dosage forms do not exhibit stability problems.

Problems due to the deliquescence or efflorescence of drugs are well known to the pharmacist. These properties alone suggest that we should keep drugs and dosage forms in well-closed containers impervious to water vapor. Unfortunately, this is not the only problem we must concern ourselves with. In particular, when drugs and dosage forms that are "dry" are kept under conditions of high humidity and high temperature, significant physical and chemical changes can occur that seriously hamper the efficacy of the drug.

Considerable attention has been paid to the effect of water on physical changes in a solid dosage form. It is well known that color fading, friability, and changes in disintegration time or dissolution rate are markedly influenced by moisture. This is of great importance from a therapeutic standpoint because a reduction or loss of effectiveness can occur.

All the interactions discussed under the section on liquids occur with solid dosage forms as well. The point that needs to be stressed is that only small changes in moisture content are necessary to cause changes. For example, it has been shown[4] in a study of vitamin A, thiamin and ascorbic acid in three polyvitamin formulations that a reduction in moisture content from 3 to 1 per cent led to a corresponding reduction in thermodegradation rate by 70 to 80 per cent.

It should be stressed that the water we have been speaking about need not come from the atmosphere. Numerous studies have shown that the water of hydration or crystallization associated with many common solid diluents yields sufficient water to cause degradation. In addition, many drugs and drug diluents are hygroscopic and attract water to the product.[5] For these reasons, pharmacists should store drugs in areas of controlled humidity and temperature.

Containers. Of great importance to the entire picture of drug stability is the container; this is particularly true with the unit dosage form. The container must protect the product from environmental conditions of temperature, humidity, light and atmospheric gases while at the same time it must be inert to the contents. The packaging trend away from the use of glass toward plastics of varying polymer composition requires that extensive studies be carried out to determine the degree of container protection. There are numerous reported studies indicating that many polymer films are permeable to water vapor—for example, penicillin tablets stored in polystyrene containers were found to degrade because of water vapor transmission through the containers.[2]

In addition to the container material, selection of the best possible container closure for a specific drug is also of importance. Some factors to be considered are type of product to be packaged, its hygroscopicity, and product reaction with the cap and/or cap liner. In general, metal caps are preferred to plastic caps as closures for dry products because high humidity can cause plastic caps to expand. In addition, studies have indicated that metal caps are better barriers to moisture vapor transmission than plastic caps.[1]

SOME PHYSICAL INCOMPATIBILITIES

Eutectic Formation. Eutectic formation occurs when two chemicals are mixed and the resulting mass softens or liquefies. In general, there is no decrease in therapeutic effectiveness when two agents are eutectic, and for this reason when eutectic-forming agents are present in small amounts they are allowed to react and then are adsorbed onto other solids or dissolved in a liquid preparation. When the eutectic ingredients are not present in small amounts and it is desirable to prevent or retard the reaction, inert protectants such as magnesium oxide and magnesium carbonate can be added to each ingredient separately and then combined.

Cementation. Insoluble drugs are frequently encountered, and it is necessary to prepare a suspension of the drug. Frequently, the suspended material settles to the bottom of the bottle and forms a cake or "cement" that is difficult or impossible to resuspend. The reasons for this caking are numerous, usually involving an interaction between suspending agent and some other agent in the prescription. For example, acacia in the presence of bismuth salts forms a cement. Interactions such as these between the suspending agent and any of the ingredients in the prescription should be avoided.

Color Changes. These changes are caused by chemical changes and can be observed not only in compounded prescriptions but also in commercial products. The most usual cause for this phenomenon is light absorption, although there can be chemical causes, for example, pH change.

Gas Generation. Although in-situ gas generation (CO_2) is desirable in effervescent dosage forms, it is undesirable in any other circumstance. Usually ammonia or carbon dioxide is the offending gas, and if the incompatibility is not corrected in time an explosion can result. For slow reactions this can be particularly dangerous because the explosion can occur after the patient has obtained the prescription. A classic example of this type of problem is the mixing of carbonate salts—e.g., bismuth subcarbonate—with an acid. The acid can come from the vehicle or from an ingredient.

Immiscible Liquids. This problem is discussed in Chapter 4.

REVIEW OF OXIDATION-REDUCTION ACID-BASE REACTIONS AND SOLUBILITY

Most physicochemical incompatibilities can be ascribed to one of three causes: oxidation-reduction reactions, acid-base reactions, or insolubility. Before discussing specific inorganic and organic compounds it seems advisable to discuss these three areas. The discussion here emphasizes inorganic compounds, since organic compounds are discussed in Chapter 10.

Oxidation-Reduction. The process of transferring electrons from a reducing agent to an oxidizing agent is known as oxidation-reduction reaction. Schematically this appears as:

$$R \rightleftharpoons R^+ + e^- \qquad \text{reducing agent is oxidized}$$
$$O + e^- \rightleftharpoons O^- \qquad \text{oxidizing agent is reduced}$$
$$R + O \rightleftharpoons R^+ + O^- \text{ overall redox reaction}$$

The tendency for electron transfer between an oxidizing agent and a reducing agent can be described quantitatively by considering the voltage that develops during the reaction. Spontaneous reactions develop positive potentials and nonspontaneous reactions develop negative potentials. The larger the numerical value of this potential the more spontaneous if positive and inert if negative. If we divide the oxidation-reduction reaction into two halves (half-cell reactions), one for oxidation and one for reduction, we can determine the potential for the entire reaction:

$$E° \text{ overall} = E°½, \text{oxidation} + E°½, \text{reduction}$$

From the overall standard potential we can get an indication of the feasibility of reaction. The standard potentials ($E°$) for reactions can be obtained from the lists shown in Table 9-2.

Problems arise from oxidation-reduction reactions not only because the biologic activity of these agents can be altered, but also because some of the reactions occur

TABLE 9-2. STANDARD POTENTIALS FOR SOME INORGANIC REACTIONS*

Half-Cell Reaction	$E°\frac{1}{2}$ (Volts)
$L_i \rightleftharpoons L_i^+ + e^-$	3.02
$Na \rightleftharpoons Na^+ + e^-$	2.71
$Al \rightleftharpoons Al^{3+} + 3e^-$	1.67
$3OH^- + H_2PO_2^- \rightarrow HPO_3^{2-} + 2H_2O + 2e^-$	1.60
$2OH^- + SO_3^{2-} \rightleftharpoons SO_4^{2-} + H_2O + 2e^-$	0.93
$3H_2O + H[H_2PO_2] \rightarrow H_3PO_3 + 2H_3O^+ + 2e^-$	0.59
$S^{2-} \rightleftharpoons S + 2e^-$	0.51
$Fe \rightleftharpoons Fe^{2+} + 2e^-$	0.44
$Fe \rightleftharpoons Fe^{3+} + 3e^-$	0.036
$H_2 + 2H_2O \rightleftharpoons 2H_3O^+ + 2e^-$	0.00
$H_2S + 2H_2O \rightarrow S^0 + 2H_3O^+ + 2e^-$	−0.14
$SN^{2+} \rightarrow SN^{4+} + 2e^-$	−0.15
$Bi + 3H_2O + Cl^- \rightarrow BiOCl + 2H_3O^+ + 3e^-$	−0.16
$H_2SO_3 + 5H_2O \rightarrow SO_4^{2-} + 4H^3O^+ + 2e^-$	−0.17
$2S_2O_3^{2-} \rightleftharpoons S_4O_6^{2-} + 2e^-$	−0.17
$Cl^- + Ag \rightarrow AgCl + e^-$	−0.22
$2Cl^- + 2Hg \rightarrow Hg_2Cl_2 + 2e^-$	−0.27
$Bi + 3H_2O \rightarrow BiO^+ + 2H_3O^+ + 3e^-$	−0.32
$4OH^- \rightarrow O_2 + 2H_2O + 4e^-$	−0.40
$2I^- \rightarrow I_2 + 2e^-$	−0.54
$3I^- \rightarrow I_3^- + 2e^-$	−0.54
$4H_2O + HAsO_2 \rightleftharpoons H_3AsO_4 + 2H_3O^+ + 2e^-$	−0.56
$ClO^- + 2OH \rightleftharpoons ClO_2^- + H_2O + 2e^-$	−0.66
$H_2O_2 + 2H_2O \rightleftharpoons O_2 + 2H_3O^+ + 2e^-$	−0.68
$Fe_2^+ \rightarrow Fe_3^+ + e^-$	−0.77
$2Hg \rightarrow Hg_2^{2+} + 2e^-$	−0.79
$Ag \rightarrow Ag^+ + e^-$	−0.80
$Hg \rightarrow Hg^{2+} + 2e^-$	−0.85
$Hg_2^{2+} \rightarrow 2Hg^{2+} + 2e^-$	−0.92
$HNO_2 + 4H_2O \rightarrow NO_3^- + 3H_3O^+ + 2e^-$	−0.94
$2OH^- + Cl^- \rightarrow ClO^- + H_2O + 2e^-$	−0.94
$2Br^- \rightarrow Br_2 \ (Ag) + 2e^-$	−1.09
$2H_2O + Cl^- \rightarrow HClO + H_3O + 2e^-$	−1.49

* From Discher, C. A.: Inorganic Pharmaceutical Chemistry, John Wiley and Sons, 1964.

with explosive violence. A classic example is the mixture of potassium permanganate and sugar. A partial list of some potentially dangerous pharmaceuticals is shown in Table 9-3.

TABLE 9-3. POTENTIALLY DANGEROUS PHARMACEUTICALS WHEN MIXED TOGETHER

Oxidizing Agents	Reducing Agents
Nitrates	Sugars
Hypochlorites	Acids
Peroxides	Sulfites
Permanganates	Bisulfites
Chromic acid	Glycerin
Perborates	Charcoal
Halides	Hydriodic acid

Acids and Bases. According to the Bronsted-Lowry definition of acids and bases, an acid is a substance that can give up a proton, i.e., a proton donor; a base is a substance that can accept a proton, i.e., a proton acceptor. When the base accepts a proton, it becomes an acid. In losing its proton, the acid becomes a base. A conjugate pair, therefore, is an acid and a base related to each other by the absence or presence of a proton.

Neutralization is the transfer of the proton from the acid of one conjugate pair to the base of a second conjugate pair:

$$HA_1 + A_2 \rightleftharpoons HA_2 + A_1$$

In aqueous systems water serves as the base of the second conjugate pair.

Of importance is an understanding of

the strengths of acids and bases. A useful measure of acid and base strength is the ionization constant for the acid and base. Consider the introduction of an acid into water with the resulting equilibrium being established:

$$HA + H_2O \rightleftharpoons H_3O^+ + A^-$$

for which we can write the equilibrium constant

$$K = \frac{[H_3O^+][A^-]}{[HA][H_2O]}$$

Because the water concentration is large and does not change appreciably with the change in concentration of the other constituents, it can be considered a constant and can be included in the equilibrium constant

$$K_a = K[H_2O] = \frac{[H_3O^+][A]}{[HA]}$$

where K_a is the acid ionization constant. A similar treatment for bases can be used to obtain the base ionization constants K_b.

Ionization constants for several inorganic acids are shown in Table 9-4.

There are much weaker acids than those listed in Table 9-4, such as aliphatic alcohols and phenols. Although they are weak acids, they can still participate in chemical reactions owing to their dissociation (see Chapter 4).

It is apparent from Table 9-4 that all acids can be considered strong or weak. Strong acids are highly ionized with the reaction proceeding to completion. Weak acids are feebly ionized, and the reaction does not go to completion.

Perusal of Table 9-4 indicates that acids can be placed in three categories: hydro-acids, hydrated cations as acids, and hydroxy acids.

Hydro Acids. Examples of these acids are

TABLE 9-4. IONIZATION CONSTANTS OF SOME INORGANIC ACIDS AT 25° C*

ACID	K_a	pK_a
Ammonium ion	5.6×10^{-10}	9.26
Arsenious	6.0×10^{-10}	9.22
Boric	5.8×10^{-10}	9.24
Carbonic (1)	4.5×10^{-7}	6.4
(2)	5.6×10^{-11}	10.2
Hexaquo aluminum (III) ion	1.3×10^{-5}	4.85
Hexaquo chromium (III) ion	1.5×10^{-4}	3.82
Hexaquo calcium (II) ion	$\sim 10^{-13}$	13.0
Hexaquo iron (II) ion	5.0×10^{-9}	8.3
Hexaquo iron (III) ion	6.3×10^{-3}	2.22
Hexaquo zinc (II) ion	2.0×10^{-10}	9.7
Hydrochloric	$\sim 10^{+7}$	-7.0
Hydrocyanic	7.2×10^{-10}	9.14
Hydrofluoric	7.2×10^{-4}	3.14
Hydrogen peroxide	2.4×10^{-12}	11.6
Hypochlorous	3.6×10^{-8}	7.44
Hypophosphorous	1.0×10^{-2}	2.0
Nitrous	4.5×10^{-4}	3.34
Phosphoric (1)	5.0×10^{-2}	1.3
(2)	5.9×10^{-8}	7.2
(3)	4.8×10^{-13}	12.3
Silicic	2.0×10^{-10}	9.7
Sulfuric (1)	~ 100	-2.0
(2)	1.0×10^{-2}	2.0
Sulfurous (1)	1.7×10^{-2}	1.76
(2)	6.2×10^{-8}	7.20

* From Discher, C. A.: Modern Inorganic Pharmaceutical Chemistry, John Wiley and Sons, 1964.

the simple hydrides, hydrochloric acid and water. Their acid strength is controlled mainly by two factors. Within a given family of elements, acid strength increases with increasing ionic radius because the proton is held less firmly and therefore dissociates more readily. Horizontally across the periodic table, as atomic weight increases so also does acid strength owing to increasing electronegativity.

Hydrated Cations as Acids. In aqueous solution these agents ionize in the following manner:

$$[M(H_2O)_x]^{n+} + H_2O \rightleftharpoons [M(H_2O)_{(x-1)}(OH)]^{(n-1)+} + H_3O^+$$

The acid strength is determined by charge, valence shell type and ionic radius. As an example, consider the aquo cations of aluminum, magnesium and sodium. Ionic radius increases from aluminum to sodium, whereas charge decreases in the same order. Only the aluminum ion, with its high charge and small radius, allows ionization of a proton.

Hydroxy Acids. This is the largest group of acids, and their acid strength depends very much on other groups attached on the molecule. If there are no nonprotonated oxygens on the molecule, the acid is weak, such as boric acid [$B(OH_3)$] and phenol [C_6H_5OH]. Acids with two or three nonprotonated oxygens are strong acids, such as sulfuric acid [$O_2S(OH)_2$] and perchloric [$O_3Cl(OH)$] acid.

Bases. Bases are usually anions such as OH^- or OAc^-, or neutral molecules such as water. In order for the hydroxide ion to act as a base, the cation associated with it must be moderately electropositive and possess a closed valence shell—for example, NaOH and $Ba(OH)_2$.

Salts as Acids and Bases. Both anions and cations must be considered in deter-mining acidity and basicity of a salt. Of interest in this discussion is the ultimate pH of salts in water. Water can function as both an acid and a base, depending on the salt involved—for example:

$$Na^+OAc^- + H_2O \rightleftharpoons HOAc + OH^- + Na^+$$

The extent of reaction of either or both of a salt's ions and water depends on the acid-base properties of the ions. Table 9-5 gives a classification of salts on the basis of acid-base strength of the cation and anion involved.

Class 1 and class 4 salts are usually neutral. Class 2 salts are alkaline when placed in water, with the degree of alkalinity proportional to the strength of the base. Class 3 salts are acid in nature. Naturally, the acid-base strength of these salts is determined by the extent of hydrolysis.

Solubility. Chapter 4 on solutions should be reread by the student at this point. Briefly reviewing, dissolution involves breaking of solvent-solvent and solute-solute bonds, and formation of solute-solvent bonds. Pharmaceutical solvents have as their principal attractive forces van der Waals and dipole-dipole interactions. Solute forces are the ion-ion, dipole-dipole and induced dipole-induced dipole types. The ion-ion type is exemplified by salts, metal oxides and metal hydroxides. These compounds are considered completely ionic. Dipole-dipole forces are not as strong as ionic forces, and hence these species have lower melting points; boric acid is an example. Induced dipole-induced dipole (sometimes referred to as van der Waals force) is the weakest of all and is considered to be the force present in gases such as neon, nitrogen and hydrogen,

TABLE 9-5. ACID-BASE STRENGTH OF SALTS IN WATER

CLASS	CATION		ANION	
	CLASSIFICATION	EXAMPLE	CLASSIFICATION	EXAMPLE
1	Weak acid	Na^+	Weak base	Cl^-
2	Weak acid	Na^+	Strong base	OAc^-
3	Strong acid	NH_4^+	Weak base	Cl^-
4	Strong acid	NH_4^+	Strong base	OAc^-

which accounts for their compressibility into liquids.

Dissolution is a solute-solvent interaction process. The types of interaction present can be classified as: induced dipole-induced dipole, dipole-induced dipole, dipole-dipole, ion-dipole and ion-induced dipole.

With respect to inorganic compounds, the most important category is the ion-dipole attraction. These ion-dipole interactions may be considered as a solvation process of the ions of solute by the solvent. When water is the solvent, the process is known as hydration. The hydration process can be pictured as dipolar molecular wedging between the oppositely charged ions and reducing the attractive forces of the solute. The important points to consider for these interactions are: (1) dielectric constant and dipole moment of the solvent, (2) size of the solvent molecule, (3) charge of the ion and (4) size of the ion.

Water with a high dielectric constant, high dipole moment and small size is an excellent solvent for ionic species. Methyl and ethyl alcohol are also small molecules and are capable of solvating the solute. Polyvalent ions are readily solvated and, in fact, form stable hydrates—for example, Al^{+++}, Mg^{++} and Fe^{++}—which indicates their strong attraction for the water dipole.

Some general solubility rules can be formulated. (1) When both anion and cation of an ionic compound are univalent, the attractive forces are relatively easy to overcome and therefore the compounds are quite soluble. (2) If one of the two ions is monovalent and the other bi- or trivalent, the resulting compound will still have appreciable water solubility if the cation is an ammonium ion or alkali metal or if the anion is an acetate, nitrate or oxyhalogen ion. (3) When both anion and cation are bivalent or trivalent, the compound is usually insoluble because the attractive forces are too difficult to overcome. There are exceptions to these generalities, but they hold true in a sufficient number of cases to make them useful.

From the preceding discussion of solute-solvent interactions, we can make the following observations: (1) Inorganic compounds (acids, bases and salts) in general tend to be soluble in polar solvents such as

TABLE 9-6. SOLUBILITY OF SALTS IN WATER

SPARINGLY SOLUBLE	SOLUBLE
Bromides, chlorides and iodides of lead, mercury and silver	Ammonium, potassium and sodium salts
Sulfides of all metals except the alkaline earth and alkali metals which are soluble [$(NH_4)_2S$, Na_2S, CaS, BaS]	Chlorides, except silver chloride, mercurous chloride and certain oxychlorides (zinc oxychloride)
Sulfates and chromates of barium, lead, mercury, silver and strontium	Acetates, nitrates and nitrites
Hydroxides, oxides, carbonates, phosphates, oxalates and carbonates of all metals, except the *alkali* metals and the ammonium ion (NH_4)	

water and insoluble in nonpolar solvents such as benzene, ether and chloroform. (2) Salts with weak crystal forces and a high tendency to hydrate are water-soluble, whereas salts with strong crystal forces and a slight tendency to hydrate are sparingly soluble in water.

The solubilities of some selected salts are shown in Table 9-6.

THE ELEMENTS

The organization and presentation of this section entails the discussion of the elements in a given group as to their physical and chemical properties. Because incompatibilities are due mainly to inorganic-organic reactions, it seems more valuable to be aware of the physicochemical properties of the inorganic compounds to determine if an incompatibility exists rather than attempt to memorize the infinite number of possible reactions.

Group 1 and 1A: the Alkali Metals. Ammonium is included in Group 1 because many of its properties are similar to those of the alkali metals. Not included in this discussion are rubidium, cesium and francium because they have virtually no pharmaceutical application.

Members of this series have in common one valence electron that is easily removed, overlying an inert gas structure. Ease of removal of this electron increases with increasing atomic radius as reflected by the decreasing ionization potential when progressing from lithium to cesium. The ions of the alkali metals are extremely stable and thus redox incompatibilities are nonexistent.

Owing to the inertness of the alkali cations, their chemical properties can be ascribed to the anion present. Thus, sodium hypochlorite is an oxidizing agent because of the hypochlorite ion, and sodium hydrogen sulfate is an acid owing to the hydrogen sulfate ion.

Almost all alkali metal salts are water-soluble, and in fact, the salts of this series are more water-soluble than the salts of any other periodic group. In general, these cations form water-soluble salts with all the univalent and divalent anions. Salts formed from trivalent anions—e.g., PO_4^{-3}—tending to be much less soluble. Table 9-7 illustrates this solubility difference.

From the information in Table 9-7 it appears that ammonium salts are more soluble than lithium salts, lithium salts are more soluble than sodium salts, and sodium salts are more soluble than potassium salts. With the exception of the ammonium ion, the

TABLE 9-7. SOLUBILITIY OF SALTS OF THE ALKALI METALS

SALT	SOLUBILITY GM./100 ML.
Potassium nitrate	31.6
Potassium chloride	34.0
Potassium sulfate	11.11
Potassium phosphate	Sl. sol.
Sodium nitrate	87.5
Sodium chloride	35.8
Sodium sulfate	18.89
Sodium phosphate	11.11
Lithium chloride	78.
Lithium nitrate	71.45
Lithium sulfate	35.0
Lithium phosphate	0.039
Ammonium nitrate	192.4
Ammonium chloride	37.0
Ammonium sulfate	76.0

TABLE 9-8. COMPARISON OF ENERGY OF HYDRATION OF ALKALI IONS WITH THE SOLUBILITY OF THEIR CHLORIDES AND SULFATES

	Li^+	Na^+	K^+
Hydration energy (Kcal./mole)	124.4	97.0	77.0
Solubility of chlorides (Gm./100 ml.)	78.0	35.8	34.0
Solubility of sulfates (Gm./100 ml.)	35.0	18.89	11.11

solubility differences can be explained on the basis of hydration energy* of these ions as shown in Table 9-8.

Lithium. Lithium salts are rarely used in pharmacy, a notable exception being lithium carbonate, which is coming into prominence in psychiatric work.

Sodium and Potassium. Sodium and potassium are normal constituents of body fluids, and thus they are employed medicinally as fluid and electrolyte replenishers and in physiologic salt solution. Sodium and potassium salts can frequently be interchanged, but there are differences between them. For example, potassium salts generally tend to have greater solubility in polar organic liquids such as ethanol, and are less deliquescent (hygroscopic) than sodium compounds.

Ammonium. Ammonium salts differ from potassium and sodium salts in a number of important ways. Because the ammonium ion is an acid ($pK_a = 4.86$), its salt solutions are acid to neutral (the degree of acidity being dependent on the anion present), whereas sodium and potassium salt solutions are neutral to alkaline. In addition, the stability of ammonium compounds is a function of the anion—ammonium salts of weak acids (boric acid) are unstable at room temperature, whereas salts of strong acids (hydrochloric acid) are stable at room temperature.

Some additional observations can be made concerning this group of cations: (1) Lithium salts (chlorides, bromides, and iodides) are often deliquescent and are freely soluble in alcohol and glycerin. (2) When these

* Hydration energy is an indication of the relative affinity of these ions for water. In ions having the same valence, the smaller ions (smaller ionic radius) have a more intense field than the larger ions and therefore greater hydration energy.

cations are combined with anions from weak acids, they form salts whose aqueous solutions are alkaline. This alkalinity is frequently the cause of precipitation of free alkaloid from alkaloidal salts, which generally require an acid pH for stability. (3) Ammonium salts decompose with the liberation of ammonia in strongly alkaline solutions, the rate of this decomposition increasing with an increase in temperature.

Group 1B: the Coinage Metals. The properties of elements in Group 1B are significantly different from those of the alkali metals, which are also in the first period. Some pertinent comparisons can be made. Whereas alkali metals are very reactive chemically the coinage metals are low in the e.m.f. series and thus are not very reactive. Alkali halides are water-soluble and are not hydrolyzed, whereas copper, silver and gold halides are nearly insoluble in water and are easily hydrolyzed. Oxides and hydroxides of alkali metals are strongly basic, whereas the coinage oxides and hydroxides are weakly basic. Finally, the alkali metals seldom form complexes with anions, whereas all the coinage metals form complexes—for example, $Ag(CN)_2^-$ and $Au(NH_3)_2^+$.

Group 1B elements have a tendency toward covalent bond formation with increasing atomic number, and most salts of this group are insoluble in water. This series of elements is quite prone to oxidation-reduction reactions.

Copper. Copper forms two series of salts, cuprous (Cu^+) and cupric (Cu^{++}), but only the cupric is pharmaceutically important. Cupric chloride, sulfate and acetate are soluble in water, whereas most other salts are insoluble. Many of the insoluble cupric salts —e.g., tannates, carbonates and phosphates —are soluble in acid solutions. Aqueous solutions of cupric salts are slightly acid owing to hydrolysis of the salt.

Silver. This metal forms only one series of salts, the monovalent silver ion (Ag^+). Most silver salts are water-insoluble with the exceptions of nitrate, sulfate (1 per cent), chlorate, lactate and acetate (1 per cent). Because silver salts are easily reduced, exposure of these salts to sunlight results in darkening because of their conversion to free silver. Silver nitrate is an excellent oxidizing agent and is easily reduced to metallic silver (the darkening that occurs when this compound is placed on the skin is due to reduction to free silver). Silver precipitates proteins, alkaloids and tannins. Silver salts in alkaline solution are converted to silver oxide.

Mild silver protein is a frequently used, hygroscopic salt that is freely soluble in water. Solutions of silver salts, especially silver protein, tend to decompose on exposure to light so that they should be freshly prepared and well protected.

Gold. This very inactive metal forms two series of salts, aurous (Au^+) and auric (Au^{+++}), all members of which are unstable and are easily converted to gold. In alkaline solutions, auric salts are converted to auric hydroxide, which precipitates.

Groups 2 and 2A. These metals, including beryllium, magnesium, calcium, strontium, barium and radium, constitute part of the alkaline earth metals, the remaining members being zinc, cadmium and mercury. All elements of this group are bivalent, and two electrons are available for removal. The ionization potentials of these elements indicate that as molecular weight increases, ease of removal of the electron increases. Thus, salts of these metals are usually ionic, although they tend to become covalent as the ion size becomes smaller. Redox incompatibilities are absent with these elements because their ions are extremely stable.

Salts of these metals are not as soluble as those of the alkali metals, and in general, the solubility of a single anion with the alkaline earth metals will follow $Ca > Sr > Ba > Ra$, with the sole exception of the hydroxides, in which the series is reversed. The most soluble salts of this group are with the monovalent anions (F^-, Cl^-, I^-, NO_3^-) and the least soluble with divalent and trivalent anion (SO_4^{2-}, CO_3^{2-}, PO_4^{2-}). Exceptions to the univalent solubility rule are the bicarbonate and hydroxide compounds, which are insoluble.

The solubilities of most of the alkaline earth salts (which are given in Table 9-9) appear to follow their energies of hydration. Note that solubility of the magnesium salts does not follow hydration energy, in that they are less soluble than the calcium salts,

TABLE 9-9. SOLUBILITIES OF SALTS OF THE ALKALINE EARTH METALS

	BARIUM	STRONTIUM	CALCIUM	MAGNESIUM
Atomic weight	137	87	40	24
Hydration energy Kcal./mole	325.2	346	385	459.1
Fluorides Gm./100 ml.	0.16	0.012	0.0016	0.00076
Chlorides Gm./100 ml.	35.7	52.9	74.5	54.5
Bromides Gm./100 ml.	101	102	96	96.5
Iodides Gm./100 ml.	203	177.8	200	148
Nitrates Gm./100 ml.	9.3	60.8	121.8	73.2
Sulfates Gm./100 ml.	0.00023	0.01	0.2	34.4
Hydroxides Gm./100 ml.	3.89	0.77	0.17	0.001

with the single exception of magnesium sulfate, which is quite soluble. Magnesium sulfate (Epsom salt) is hydrated even in the solid state, and when placed in solution, separation of the ions is relatively simple.

All the univalent salts of these cations are deliquescent and are highly hydrated. These compounds should therefore be well protected during storage.

The major incompatibilities of these elements are acid-base reactions that occur when the salts are placed in solution with salts of organic acids or with other inorganic salts—for example:

$$SrBr_2 + 2Na\ salicylate \longrightarrow 2NaBr + Sr(salicylate)_2\downarrow$$
$$Ca(OH)_2 + 2Na\ phenobarbital \longrightarrow Ca(phenobarbital)_2\downarrow + 2NaOH$$
$$CaCl_2 + Na_2SO_4 \longrightarrow CaSo_4\downarrow + 2NaCl$$

Beryllium. This element has no apparent pharmaceutical importance.

Magnesium. Salts of this element are used for many purposes. The trisilicate is used as an antacid, the sulfate (Epsom salt) as a cathartic. The trisilicate salt, when in contact with acid of the stomach, is converted to magnesium chloride and gelatinous trisilicic acid. This hydrated gel can adsorb alkaloids and other drugs and is therefore a potential danger in reducing the biologic activity of drugs. Magnesium oxide, because it is inert, is frequently used as a protectant to separate potential eutectics. It is highly hydroscopic and hydrates readily. Light magnesium oxide, having a smaller particle size, hydrates readily, whereas the heavy magnesium oxide (large particle size) is hydrated less easily and therefore is preferred.

Talc, another magnesium-containing compound, is chemically hydrated magnesium silicate. Owing to its inertness and ready adherence to skin, it is frequently employed in topical dusting powders.

Calcium. Salts of calcium are hygroscopic, and in fact, calcium chloride is used commercially as a drying agent to remove water. The chief incompatibility of the calcium ion is that of precipitation. It forms water-insoluble compounds with carbonate, hydroxide, sulfate, oxalate and phosphate. Soluble salts of calcium are gluconate, lactate and hypophosphite.

Calcium carbonate is a frequently used antacid preparation because of its ability to neutralize acid. A purified form of calcium carbonate is known as prepared chalk or drop chalk.

Strontium. The lactate of strontium has been used with calcium to promote remineralization of bones. Aside from this the element has little pharmacologic importance.

Barium. The barium ion is very toxic. Barium sulfate, which is used as a diagnostic aid, is insoluble in water, and the usual form of administration is therefore an aqueous suspension. The solubility of barium salts parallels that of calcium salts.

Group 2B. All Group 2B metals form normal divalent ions, and mercury also has a monovalent ion. They are less reactive than Group 2A elements, owing in part to their smaller size, and they exhibit covalency much more than the Group 2A elements. This is reflected in the solubility of their salts. All transition metal cations exhibit an attraction for water, and this attraction increases with the charge on the cations—monovalent least, and the tri- and tetravalent most. As the energy of hydration increases, the bonding between the cation and water changes. In the alkali and alkaline earth metals, water of hydration apparently occupies holes in the crystal lattice (weakly bound), whereas in the transition and heavy metals the water appears to be definitely bound to the specific cation in many of the salts. This type of binding is a factor in causing many of the divalent and trivalent cation hydroxides to be amphoteric.

The principal amphoteric hydroxides are $Zn(OH)_2$, $Sn(OH)_2$, $Pb(OH)_2$, $Al(OH)_3$ and $Cr(OH)_3$. These hydroxides dissolve in alkaline solution to produce their respective ions:

$Zn(OH)_4{}^{2-}$	Zincate ion
$Sn(OH)_3{}^-$	Stannite ion
$Pb(OH)_3{}^-$	Plumbite ion
$Al(OH)_3{}^-$	Aluminate ion
$Cr(OH)_4{}^-$	Chromite ion

They also dissolve in acid to form salts.

Zinc. This metal is bivalent in all its compounds. The zinc ion enters into a number of reactions—e.g., soluble carbonates, phosphates and borates produce white precipitates of basic zinc carbonate, phosphate or borate from solutions of zinc salts. In addition, zinc salts readily form insoluble hydroxides in neutral and slightly alkaline media:

$$ZnSO_4 + 2XOH \longrightarrow Zn\overset{\displaystyle OH}{\underset{\displaystyle OH\downarrow}{\big<}} + X_2SO_4$$

For this reason, zinc salts should be buffered when dispensed as solutions. Frequently, insoluble compounds of zinc are desired; thus, zinc sulfides are prepared in situ (white lotion):

Sulfurated potash + zinc sulfate → potassium sulfate + zinc mono- and disulfides.

Solutions of zinc salts undergo partial hydrolysis, for example:

$$ZnCl_2 + HOH \rightleftarrows ZnOHCl \text{ (solid)} + HCl$$

The formation of HCl in this reaction indicates that these salts are acidic in solution. The foregoing reaction occurs readily with zinc salts of the halides and acetates, whereas the nitrate and sulfate salts do not hydrolyze as readily and, therefore, form more stable solutions.

Zinc salts can also be precipitated when combined with salts of organic acids—for example:

$$ZNSO_4 + 2Na \text{ salicylate} \rightarrow Zn \text{ (salicylate)}_2\downarrow + Na_2SO_4$$

Because of this basicity, divalent ions such as zinc or calcium can crack or invert an O/W emulsion prepared from a fatty acid—for example:

$$2R\overset{\displaystyle O}{\overset{\displaystyle \|}{C}}-ONa + Ca^{++} \longrightarrow Ca\,(O-\overset{\displaystyle O}{\overset{\displaystyle \|}{C}}-R)_2\downarrow + 2Na^+$$

A classic example of an acid-base reaction due to zinc is the formation of insoluble zinc borate when solutions of zinc sulfate and sodium borate are mixed. Substitution of boric acid for sodium borate overcomes this incompatibility.

In addition to precipitating organic acids, zinc salts also precipitate the larger molecules containing a dissociating proton, such as acacia, proteins and tannins. They precipitate these species not only by virtue of salt formation, but also by dehydration of the large hydrated molecule.

Cadmium. The ion of cadmium resembles that of zinc in its biologic action but is more toxic. In general, it has little pharmaceutical use.

Mercury. This element forms two series of compounds, one of which has an oxidation state of $+1$ (mercurous) and one an oxidation state of $+2$ (mercuric). Mercurous salts in general tend to convert to the more stable mercuric series and are easily reduced to the free metal by most reducing agents, even by light and moisture. Soluble mercurous salts, for example the nitrate, are easily hydrolyzed in alkaline solution to form basic salts. Soluble iodides precipitate the yellow mercurous iodide from a solution of mercurous ion.

The mercurous ion consists of two mercuric ions plus two electrons that form a covalent bond between them:

$$[Hg:Hg]:$$

Mercurous chloride then may be pictured as having a linear covalent structure:

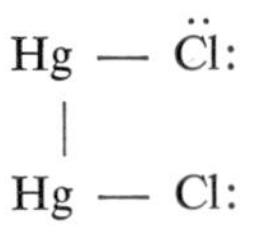

$$Hg — \ddot{C}l:$$
$$|$$
$$Hg — \ddot{C}l:$$

This covalent structure contributes greatly to the insolubility of these compounds, accounts for their decreased toxicity compared to the mercuric salts. In summary, concerning mercurous salts: (1) They are easily reduced to free mercury, and this is hastened by light and moisture; (2) they are readily converted to the more soluble and more toxic mercuric ion; and (3) soluble mercurous salts hydrolyze to form insoluble basic salts.

Mercuric salts are similar to mercurous salts in that they are readily hydrolyzed to form insoluble basic salts:

$$Hg(NO_3)_2 + HOH \longrightarrow Hg \underset{OH \downarrow}{\overset{NO_3}{<}} + HNO_3$$

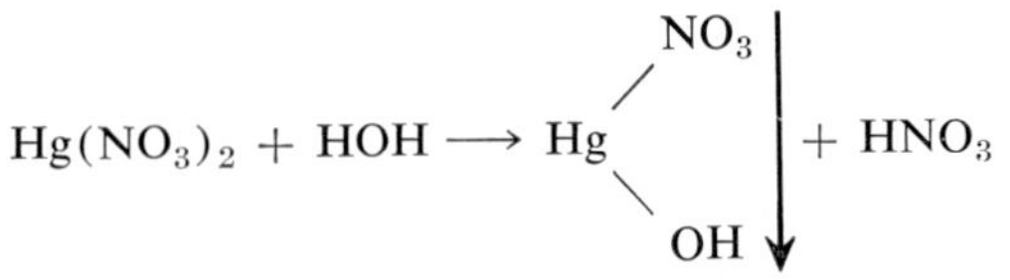

This reaction is increased in alkaline media. Of the soluble salts, mercuric chloride has the least tendency to hydrolyze in solution because of its low degree of ionization and, therefore, its small concentration of mercuric ion.

Mercuric iodide is $\frac{1}{10}$ as soluble as mercuric chloride, but it is solubilized in an excess of potassium iodide by forming a soluble complex salt, potassium mercuric iodide, according to the following equation:

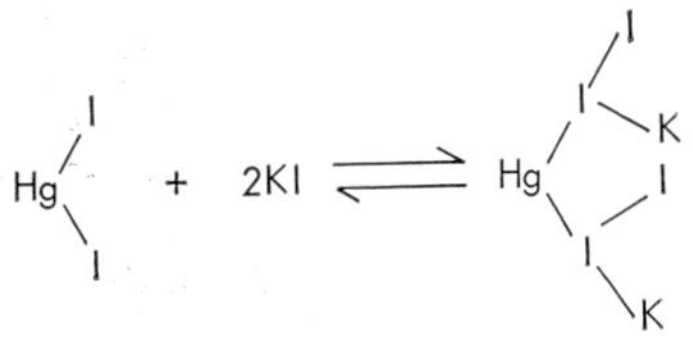

The addition of KI to these solutions in order to solubilize mercuric salts is justifiable. However, these solutions turn yellow on standing owing to liberation of iodine, and the addition of a small quantity of sodium thiosulfate prevents this. Potassium mercuric iodide is an alkaloidal precipitant.

A comparison of the solubility of the salts of these metals is shown in Table 9-10.

TABLE 9-10. SOLUBILITY OF SALTS OF ZINC AND MERCURY

ZINC SALT	SOLUBILITY GM./100 ML.	MERCURY SALT	SOLUBILITY GM./100 ML.	
			MERCUROUS	MERCURIC
Acetate	30	Acetate	0.75	25
Borate	Soluble			
Fluoride	S.S.	Fluoride	Decomposes	Decomposes
Chloride	432	Chloride	0.00021	6.9
Bromide	447	Bromide	0.000004	0.61
Iodide	437	Iodide	S.S.	S.S.
Nitrate $3H_2O$	327	Nitrate	Decomposes	S.S.
Nitrate $6H_2O$	184			
Sulfate	86.5			
Sulfate · $6H_2O$	Soluble	Sulfate	0.06	Decomposes
Sulfate · $7H_2O$	96.5			
Sulfides	Insoluble	Sulfide	Insoluble	0.000001
Hydroxide	Insoluble	Hydroxide	Insoluble	Insoluble

Groups 3 and 3A: the Rare Earth Metals. The first two elements of this series, boron and aluminum, are the only ones of interest to the pharmacist. In general, the tendency of this group to covalent bond formation is greater than that of the preceding groups owing to the small ion size and greater charge. As one descends in Group 3, the elements show increased metallic character with a decreasing tendency toward covalency. This can be seen by the increasing basicity and the decreasing hydrolysis of the hydroxides. Boron trihydroxide (boric acid) is a weak acid, and aluminum hydroxide is a weak base.

Boron. All boron compounds are toxic. Boron compounds of interest to us are boric acid, sodium tetraborate and sodium perborate. With few exceptions boron is trivalent, and its oxide and hydroxide are acidic. However, although boron hydroxide (boric acid) is a weak acid in water, when dissolved in glycerin it behaves as a strong monobasic acid. The chemical behavior of boron compounds is very similar to that of carbon.

Aluminum. This element has all three valence electrons in the third energy level and thus is always trivalent (Al^{+++}). The chemical properties of aluminum can be ascribed to its small size and high nuclear charge. It has a strong tendency to form complex ions with water:

$$Al^{+++} + 6H_2O \longrightarrow Al\,(6H_2O)^{+++}$$

This great attraction for water results in high heat of hydration and hydration energy.

One important property of aluminum ions is hydrolysis of the strong acid salts to produce an acidic aqueous solution. The process may be viewed as the formation of hydroxyl complexes by successive ionization of the water molecules:

$$Al(H_2O)_6{}^{+++} + H_2O \rightleftharpoons Al(H_2O)_5OH^{++} + H_3O^+$$
$$Al(H_2O)_5OH^{++} + H_2O \rightleftharpoons Al(H_2O)_4(OH)_2{}^+ + H_3O^+$$
$$Al(H_2O)_4(OH)_2{}^+ + H_2O \rightleftharpoons Al(H_2O)_3(OH)_3 + H_3O^+$$
$$Al(H_2O)_3(OH)_3 \rightleftharpoons Al(OH)_3\downarrow + 3H_2O$$

This also occurs with anions of weak acids as well, because alkali carbonates or soluble sulfides cause precipitation of the water-insoluble aluminum hydroxide.

Aluminum salts formed with highly electronegative ions such as F^-, NO_3^- and SO_4^{--} are ionic compounds. All the halide salts are water-soluble with the exception of fluorides, and almost all the univalent salts of aluminum are water-soluble, as well as many of the bivalent anion salts. With trivalent species such as PO_4^{---}, the salts are insoluble.

The most frequently used aluminum salts —the chloride and the sulfate—produce highly acid solutions, and for use on the skin these agents should be buffered. Because of the hydrolysis and acidity of $AlCl_3$, the aluminum chlorhydroxy complex is frequently substituted.

Aluminum hydroxide gel is a colloidal suspension of $Al(OH)_3$ that is used as an antacid. The colloidal system is destroyed by heat, freezing, electrolytes and dehydrating agents. In addition, on drying, the particle size of aluminum hydroxide increases rapidly, which greatly reduces the adsorbing and reacting power of the compound.

The double sulfates of aluminum with either potassium or ammonium (alums) are used as styptics.

The remaining members of this series and of the 3B series have little pharmaceutical application.

Groups 4 and 4A. Carbon, silicon, titanium, zirconium and hafnium are members of this grouping. Carbon and silicon are characteristically nonmetallic in chemical behavior and have a maximum valence of four. In addition, carbon can exhibit a valence of two. The bonding of both carbon and silicon is primarily covalent in the tetravalent ions and is considerably ionic in the divalent carbon ion.

Titanium, zirconium, and hafnium are transition elements that have valences from two to four, the tetravalent form being most prevalent. The halides of titanium and zirconium both behave as Lewis acids.

Carbon. This element is the basic building block of organic chemistry, and these compounds are discussed at length in Chapter 10. Of interest to us here are the inorganic carbon compounds—charcoal and carbon dioxide. Charcoal can be obtained from different sources, and hence one can obtain wood and bone charcoal. The most widely used charcoal for pharmaceutical purposes is activated charcoal, which is a fine, black, odorless and tasteless powder that is completely insoluble in water. The primary use of charcoal is to adsorb gases and toxins, and it is therefore a digestive aid. Activated charcoal can adsorb not only gases but also drugs, which could lead to a decrease or loss in activity of some drugs, particularly the alkaloids. Charcoal is rapidly oxidized by the most mild oxidizing agents.

Carbon dioxide is a gas at room temperature, and when dissolved in aqueous solution it imparts an acid taste to the solution. It is frequently generated in situ by mixing sodium bicarbonate and an organic acid such as citric or tartaric acid in water:

$$NaHCO_3 + \text{citric acid} \rightarrow H_2CO_3 + \text{Na citrate}$$
$$\uparrow\downarrow$$
$$H_2O + CO_2$$

The weak acid produced from CO_2 in water is carbonic acid (H_2CO_3). In the presence of a base, carbonic acid is converted to the monobasic bicarbonate ($NaHCO_3$), or to the dibasic carbonate (Na_2CO_3). The carbonate and bicarbonates of ammonium and alkali metals are soluble, whereas the carbonates of other metals are usually insoluble.

Silicon. This element is tetravalent in all its compounds. A widely used silicon compound is magnesium trisilicate, which is used as a protective agent for the stomach. Purified siliceous earth (SiO_2) has little chemical reactivity and is therefore sometimes used as a filtering aid where it acts as an adsorbent.

Titanium. The only pharmaceutically important compound of this metal is titanium dioxide. Because of its very high refractive index (2.70), it is used as an opacifying or refractory material in many cosmetics such as sunscreen agents.

Zirconium. Salts of zirconium have been used in antiperspirants and other topical preparations because of their astringent properties, but owing to increased incidences of skin granulomas they have been deleted from most products.

Hafnium. This element has no pharmaceutical importance.

Group 4B. Because germanium has little pharmaceutical importance, our discussion is limited to tin and lead, elements that have valences of either two or four. As the atomic weight increases, the elements become metallic in their properties. Lead is definitely metallic whereas germanium is nonmetallic; tin has one nonmetallic allotropic form and another metallic form. The chemical activity increases as we progress down the period, with lead being most active. The hydroxides in the tetravalent state of this group are all very weak acids.

Tin. Stannous and stannic ions in the form of solutions of their soluble salts react with alkaline solutions to precipitate the insoluble hydroxides; they are also precipitated by carbonates. Stannous fluoride is used in dentistry in an aqueous solution, which on standing hydrolyzes to yield an acidic solution that slowly precipitates the insoluble stannous hydroxide. For this reason, only freshly prepared solutions of stannous fluoride should be used.

Lead. This element exists in two oxidation states—the divalent plumbous ion (Pb^{++}) and the tetravalent plumbic ion (Pb^{++++}). Salts of divalent lead such as acetate, nitrate and chlorate are soluble, whereas halogen derivatives are only slightly soluble. Solutions of lead salt react with carbonates and hydroxide to produce insoluble products. Soluble chromates also react with lead to produce lead chromate. Table 9-11 gives the solubility of some lead salts in water.

Lead preparations are used primarily as astringents and act by virtue of the lead ion

TABLE 9-11. SOLUBILITIES OF SOME LEAD COMPOUNDS

	(in Gm./100 ml.)
Soluble	
Acetate	62.5
Nitrate	50.0
Subacetate	6.25
Slightly Soluble	
Chloride	1.075
Bromide	0.50
Iodide	0.074
Fluoride	0.0625
Sulfate	0.0443
Borate	Insoluble
Arsenate	Insoluble

reacting with the proteins of the skin forming an insoluble lead proteinate.

The most serious problem encountered with solutions of lead salts is stability. The chloride, nitrate, acetate and subacetate are all hydrolyzed in solution, and they react quickly with carbon dioxide in the water and precipitate out as the basic lead carbonate.

Groups 5 and 5A. This group includes nitrogen, phosphorus, vanadium, niobium and tantalum, but only nitrogen and phosphorus are of any importance to pharmacy. Both elements are nonmetallic. Nitrogen in combination with carbon, oxygen, and hydrogen is usually joined by covalent bonds. All these elements possess five valence electrons in the outer shell. Nitrogen usually has three covalent bonds and an unshared electron pair whereas phosphorus forms five covalent bonds.

The major compounds of nitrogen and phosphorus are organic and are discussed in Chapter 10.

Group 5B. Arsenic, antimony and bismuth are the metallic elements of Group 5, bismuth having the most metallic properties and arsenic being essentially nonmetallic. Of these elements the compounds of arsenic and bismuth are the most important pharmaceutically.

All these elements react with halogens to form covalent tri- and pentahalides, which are readily hydrolyzed by water to the hydrogen halides and oxyacids in arsenic, and to hydroxy and oxychlorides in antimony and bismuth.

All three elements form oxides with oxygen and sulfides with sulfur. As atomic number increases, the acidity of the oxide decreases until the last members of the group are basic.

Arsenic. The three forms of arsenic are elemental arsenic, trivalent arsenic and pentavalent arsenic. The elemental form of arsenic is seldom used today in medicine.

Trivalent arsenic is a common form of the element, and although mainly nonmetallic it can form compounds in which it acts as a cation. The halides such as arsenic trichloride are good examples of this. Arsenic trichloride is readily hydrolyzed in water to produce orthoarsenous acid:

$$AsCl_3 + 3H_2O \rightleftharpoons 3HCl + H_3AsO_3$$

Orthoarsenous acid is readily converted to the oxide (arsenic trioxide), which is slightly soluble in water. The solubility of arsenic trioxide is increased in the presence of acid or alkali. Solutions or arsenous acid (arsenic trioxide) are generally prepared by adding HCl or $KHCO_3$ to the medium. Arsenic trioxide is weakly acidic and therefore reacts with alkali to form the metallic arsenites. It can also act as a base and react with Lewis acids (halogens) to form halides.

Pentavalent arsenic also forms acids and oxides. Orthoarsenic acid is easily dehydrated to arsenic pentoxide just as orthoarsenous acid is converted to arsenic trioxide.

Arsenites and arsenates of alkali metals are soluble, but most other metal salts are insoluble.

Antimony. Antimony potassium tartrate (tartar emetic) is essentially the only antimony compound of pharmaceutical importance. Aqueous solutions of this compound are precipitated by most metals and form insoluble potassium tartrate with acids.

Bismuth. In contrast to the arsenicals, which are usually used in medicine as solutions, bismuth compounds are highly insoluble and are administered as powders or suspensions.

Bismuth oxides are weakly basic and therefore combine with acids to form salts that are easily hydrolyzed. Hydrolysis of bismuth salts leads to many of the incompatibilities associated with these compounds. For example, bismuth subnitrate readily hydrolyzes to liberate nitric acid:

$$2BiONO_3 + H_2O \rightleftharpoons (BiO)_2\,OHNO_3 + HNO_3$$

Bismuth chloride hydrolyzes as follows:

$$BiCl_3 + H_2O \rightleftharpoons BiOCl + 2HCl$$

Suspensions of bismuth salts are therefore acidic and have the incompatibilities of acids —the liberation of carbon dioxide from carbonates; acid-base reaction, such as the liberation of water-insoluble salicylic acid from salicylates; and the liberation of iodine from iodides, which in turn, is converted into dark brown bismuth iodide.

Bismuth compounds are also easily reduced to metallic bismuth in the presence of organic reducing agents such as hypophosphates and glycerin. This reaction is facilitated by an alkaline media. Bismuth compounds should therefore be protected from light, and reducing agents must be omitted.

Groups 6 and 6B. The main similarity between the elements in Group 6 is that they have six valence electrons, and only when all six are involved in bonding are similarities between the subgroups (A and B) found. In this case, the resemblance of the B subgroup is nearer to the typical elements than the A subgroup. This is true in Groups 4 to 7, whereas the reverse is true for Groups 1 to 4.

The main difference in the members of this group lies with oxygen and the remaining elements, which have oxidation states of -2, 0, $+2$, $+4$ and $+6$. Oxygen has only -2, -1 and 0 oxidation states. These elements are among the most electronegative in the periodic table, with electronegativity decreasing as one goes down the group. Oxygen and sulfur are generally nonmetallic, whereas selenium and tellurium are metalloid.

Members of this group form monoatomic anions—for example, oxides and sulfides—and can therefore exhibit both ionic and covalent bonding. In addition, the members of this group form hydrides (H_2O, H_2S), which decrease in stability and increase in acidity as molecular weight increases. The sulfides, selenides and tellurides of alkali and alkaline earth metals are water-soluble, but salts of other metals are water-insoluble.

The most common oxide forms of these elements are XO_2 and XO_3, which are the anhydrides of the corresponding acids H_2XO_3 and H_2XO_4. The acidity of oxyacids of a given element is greatest when the oxidation number is highest. Thus, sulfuric acid (6) is more acidic than sulfurous acid (4).

Sulfur. Natural sulfur is available in three forms, precipitated, sublimed and washed. Elemental sulfur in these forms is insoluble in most solvents. The difference between these forms lies in their particle size and purity. For example, precipitated sulfur is a fine, pale yellow microcrystalline powder that is odorless and tasteless, whereas sublimed sulfur (flowers of sulfur) is a yellow crystalline powder having a faint odor and taste.

Selenium. This element and its salts are quite toxic and have biologic actions similar to those of arsenic. Selenium compounds are used in shampoo preparations to treat seborrheic dermatitis of the scalp.

Tellurium and Polonium. These have no pharmaceutical importance.

Group 6A. The elements of this group, chromium, molybdenum and tungsten, are all metallic. The oxides of these elements are acidic and form chromates, molybdates and tungstates.

Chromium. The three forms of chromium are divalent, trivalent and hexavalent chromium. The divalent form (chromous) is relatively unstable and is easily converted to the trivalent form (chromic). When chromic salt solutions are treated with alkaline hydroxides, insoluble chromic hydroxide precipitates.

Molybdenum and Tungsten. These elements have no pharmaceutical importance.

Groups 7 and 7B. Included in this grouping are fluorine, chlorine, bromine, iodine and astatine. These elements are only one electron short of the noble gas configuration and thus can form the uninegative ion (X^-) or a single covalent bond ($-X$). These elements are completely nonmetallic in their chemical behavior. The solubility of the halides usually follows their atomic weights; thus, silver iodide is less soluble than silver bromide, which is less soluble than silver chloride.

Iodine. This element is a black solid with a slight metallic luster. It sublimes without melting and has slight solubility in water (0.33 Gm./liter at 25°C.). Iodine is an oxidizing agent that reacts with many organic and inorganic chemicals—e.g., hypophosphates and volatile oils. Iodine solution is prepared with the aid of potassium iodide. Care must be used in making iodine preparations because the element sublimes; thus if heat is necessary, it must be applied cautiously.

Group 7A. Group 7A elements include manganese, technetium and rhenium, of which only manganese is pharmaceutically important.

Manganese. This element can exhibit several valence forms.

Name	Valence
Manganous	2
Manganic	3
Manganite	4
Manganate	6
Permanganate	7

Only manganous and permanganate valence forms are important in pharmacy.

Manganese in its lower state of oxidation (manganese dioxide) is a powerful reducing agent. Typical reactions of manganous salts are: alkaline solutions producing the white precipitate of manganous hydroxide, alkaline carbonates precipitating white manganous carbonate, and sulfides precipitating manganous sulfide.

Manganous ions are solubilized by complex formation with agents such as the citrates.

Group 8. Iron, cobalt and nickel are classified as transition elements. The remaining transition elements— ruthenium, rhodium, palladium, osmium, iridium and platinum—have no pharmaceutical importance.

Iron, cobalt and nickel have two electrons in the outermost shell and a partially filled next inner shell. The outermost electrons are used to form divalent ions and one of the inner electrons is used to form the trivalent ion.

Iron. Iron has two forms of interest in pharmacy, the ferrous (Fe^{++}) and ferric (Fe^{+++}) states. Ferrous salts in the solid state are only slowly oxidized by atmospheric oxygen, but in solution they are rapidly converted to the corresponding ferric salts, which are usually less water-soluble. The ferrous ion is readily precipitated from solution by carbonates and phosphates. Ferric salts generally produce acidic solutions owing to hydrolysis. Hydroxides and carbonates precipitate the ferric ion, and in addition, ferric salts produce dark precipitates with tannins. In general, a pH below 4 is required to maintain ferric ions in solution.

Precipitation of iron salts or their hydroxides can be prevented in many cases by the addition of complexing agents. Such substances as lactate, citrate, pyrophosphates, amines, sugars and polyhydroxy alcohols form coordination complexes with ferrous and ferric ions that are soluble. Examples of these complex iron salts are: (1) soluble ferrous phosphate (contains sodium citrate to solubilize), (2) iron and ammonium citrate, (3) ferric pyrophosphate with ammonium citrate, (4) ferric citrochloride (ferric citrochloride tincture), (5) saturated ferrous carbonate, (6) iron glycerophosphate, (7) iron peptonate, (8) iron tartrate, and (9) saturated iron oxide.

This type of complex formation can be considered an incompatibility—e.g., Fe^{+++} ions form deeply colored complexes with phenolic compounds such as phenols, cresols, salicylic acid and salicylates.

The oxidizing action of ferric ion and the reducing action of the ferrous ion produces numerous incompatibilities. For example, hydroxy acids, mercurous salts, phenols and other easily oxidized substances are readily acted on by ferric ions, especially under the influence of light.

REFERENCES

1. Blaug, S. M., Hickman, E., and Lach, J. L.: J. Am. Pharm. Ass. (Sci.) 47:54, 1958.
2. Bull, A. W.: J. Pharm. Pharmacol. 7:806, 1955.
3. Discher, C. A.: Modern Inorganic Pharmaceutical Chemistry, New York, Wiley, 1964.
4. Tardif, R.: J. Pharm. Sci. 54:281, 1965.
5. Yamamoto, et al.: Arch. Pract. Pharm. 19: No. 1, 1959.

GENERAL REFERENCES FOR THE INORGANIC SECTION

Discher, C. A.: Modern Inorganic Pharmaceutical Chemistry, New York, Wiley, 1964.

Soine, T. O., and Wilson, C. O.: Rogers' Inorganic Pharmaceutical Chemistry, ed. 8, Philadelphia, Lea and Febiger, 1967.

Cotton, F. A., and Wilkinson, G.: Advanced Inorganic Chemistry, ed. 2, New York, Interscience, 1966.

Chapter 10

Pharmaceutical Formulation Problems of Organic Compounds

Dale E. Wurster, Ph.D.*

In this chapter a large number of the various types of chemical and physical problems encountered in the formulation of drug products and the compounding of prescriptions are discussed. The information given here will also be most useful as a theoretical background for solving the many chemical problems associated with I.V. solution additives. Unfortunately, it is not practical in a single chapter to discuss all the classes of chemical compounds employed in pharmaceutical preparations. However, a sufficient number of substances are treated to acquaint the student with the kind of information required to recognize and solve problems pertaining to drug stability in pharmaceutical systems. The student should also be aware of the fact that the information presented is fully as useful to explain compatibility as it is to explain incompatibility in these systems.

The problems mentioned are primarily chemical in nature, but some physical problems, particularly those related to solubility, are also discussed. The emphasis on solubility is justified, as many problems are the result of either the initial insolubility of a compound or the formation of a precipitate through chemical reaction or interaction.

To avoid unnecessary repetition, a comprehensive treatment of the kinetics of drug degradation is omitted from this chapter, since this information has already been treated in the text. Other calculations, such

* Professor of Pharmacy, University of Wisconsin

as those dealing with pH and solubility, are also omitted for the same reason. However, a few pertinent calculations are included to aid the student in relating the information given here with that given in other chapters.

Lastly, information pertaining to the stability of certain physical systems rather than chemical compounds per se can be found in the chapter dealing with the dosage form containing the particular physicochemical system. Thus, the correlation of the information given in this chapter with that in the other chapters serves to make evident to the student the solution of both chemical and physical problems of both the drug and the pharmaceutical system.

HYDROCARBONS
SATURATED HYDROCARBONS

This class of chemical compounds is represented in pharmaceutical dispensing by liquid petrolatum, petrolatum and paraffin. Although the actual number of substances of this class which are used is not great, the above-mentioned agents are employed extensively.

Solubility. The saturated hydrocarbons are nonpolar compounds and, therefore, are insoluble in water and other polar solvents. However, these substances are miscible with other nonpolar solvents such as ether, benzene, petroleum ether, chloroform, carbon disulfide and fixed oils as a result of induced dipole-induced dipole interactions.

Formulation Problems. Inasmuch as the alkanes are extremely unreactive substances, they give rise to no problems in prescriptions due to chemical reactions. However, they do cause many problems of a solubility nature. The members of the alkane series do not react with acids, alkalies or oxidizing or reducing agents. In order to bring about a change in their structure, either extremely high temperatures, strongly electrophilic (electron-seeking) reagents or both usually are required.

Problems in prescriptions involving the saturated hydrocarbons arise mainly from attempts to mix these nonpolar compounds with polar compounds. The same principles apply both in liquid preparations containing liquid petrolatum and in ointments containing petrolatum. In either case, if water is included, whether alone or with dissolved substances, compatibility can be attained only through emulsification.

ALCOHOLS

The alcohols may be considered as hydroxy derivatives of hydrocarbons. The substitution of a hydroxyl group for a hydrogen of a hydrocarbon causes profound changes in both the chemical and the physical properties with the change in solubility characteristics being particularly evident. Inasmuch as alcohols may contain one or more hydroxyl groups, they are classified as monohydroxy and polyhydroxy compounds.

MONOHYDROXY ALCOHOLS

Solubility. The alcohols are miscible with water by virtue of their ability to associate with water through hydrogen bonding. From a practical pharmaceutical standpoint, propyl and isopropyl alcohol represent the upper limits of solubility of alcohols in water, although normal butyl alcohol is soluble to the extent of 7.9 Gm. per 100 ml. and amyl alcohol to the extent of 2.7 Gm. per 100 ml. of water. As the alkyl chain of the monohydroxy alcohols is increased beyond certain limits (4 to 5 carbon atoms), these alcohols become increasingly less polar and lose their ability to compete with the more polar water molecules for a place in the association complex. They then are replaced by water molecules and become immiscible.

TABLE 10-1. SOLUBILITY OF SOME MONOHYDRIC ALCOHOLS

ALCOHOL	Water	Alcohol	Ether, etc.
Methyl alcohol ...	∞	∞	∞ eth.
Ethyl alcohol	∞	..	∞ eth., chl., me. al.
Isopropyl alcohol .	∞	∞	∞ eth.
n-Butyl alcohol ...	7.9[20]	∞	∞ eth.
Isobutyl alcohol ..	12.5[20]	∞	∞ eth.
n-Amyl alcohol ...	2.7[22]	∞	∞ eth.
n-Hexyl alcohol ..	0.59[20]	∞	∞ eth.

eth. = ether
chl. = chloroform
me. al. = methyl alcohol
∞ = soluble in all proportions

Alcohols are miscible with or solubilize other substances containing hydroxyl (—OH), amino (—NH_2) or imino (—NH) groups having hydrogen as the positive end of a dipole with which the alcohol can associate. Thus, the alcohols are capable of solubilizing substances such as alkaloids, carboxylic acids, phenols, resins, balsams, barbituric acid derivatives, etc. and may be added to aqueous preparations containing these substances to prevent precipitation.

Formulation Problems. Alcohol precipitates many substances such as tragacanth, acacia, agar, other plant gums that are carbohydrate in nature, albumin, gelatin and other proteins from aqueous solution. These substances are precipitated because the alcohol acts as a dehydrating agent. The alcohol possesses such an affinity for the water that the two readily associate and destroy the association existing between the gums and the water.

Many inorganic salts are precipitated from aqueous solutions by the addition of alcohol.

POLYHYDROXY ALCOHOLS

The polyhydroxy alcohols demonstrate the relationship that exists between the number of hydroxyl groups and the molecular weight of the compound. When the ratio of the hydroxyl groups to the carbon atom content is increased, the result is an increase in dielectric constant, polarity and solubility in water. The glycols, glycerin and carbohydrates are examples of compounds of this class which are used in pharmaceutical dispensing. Problems of a solubility nature are encountered when these substances are mixed with nonpolar substances that are incapable of association through hydrogen bond formation.

Carbohydrates. The carbohydrates include substances such as the sugars, the starches, the pectins, the celluloses and many other substances closely related to them.

SUGARS. The sugars which are used in pharmaceutical dispensing are classified according to their behavior toward hydrolytic agents (e.g., monosaccharides, disaccharides, etc.). These classes are also subdivided into groups, depending on whether they are reducing sugars (e.g., glucose, fructose, maltose, lactose) or nonreducing sugars (e.g., sucrose).

Solubility. The monosaccharides and the disaccharides are soluble in water in spite of their relatively large molecular weight, since they have a sufficient number of hydroxyl groups in the molecule to promote solubility. Water dissolves these substances by association through H-bond formation. They are slightly soluble in alcohol for the same reason, although to a much more limited extent.

Formulation Problems. Alcohol causes the precipitation of sugars from concentrated solutions. This may be explained on the following basis: the alcohol competes more efficiently for water, associates with it and forces the sugar out of solution.

The sugars are oxidized easily and, when triturated in the dry form with strong oxidizing agents such as permanganates, peroxides, picric acid, etc., they form explosive mixtures. The disaccharides are hydrolyzed by acids. In alkaline solution, the reducing sugars turn dark because of the formation of decomposition products.

GUMS. The plant gums acacia, agar, chondrus, sodium alginate and tragacanth are carbohydrate in nature and find use in pharmaceutical dispensing as dispersion stabilizers in polyphase systems such as emulsions and suspenions.

Solubility. These hydrophilic substances become hydrated to form gels due to the presence of the hydroxyl groups in the molecule. Their water solubility is thus attributed to their ability to associate through hydrogen bonding.

Most of the plant gums require a considerable amount of time to hydrate completely to form homogeneous preparations. Extemporaneous preparations can be made by triturating the gum with a small amount of water-soluble hydroxy compound such as alcohol or glycerin. They are insoluble in the alcohols, and, when triturated together, each small particle of the gum becomes surrounded with alcohol. On the subsequent addition of water, the alcohol and the water associate through hydrogen bonding, and the water is thus drawn through the mass so that each small particle of the gum is surrounded by water. Therefore, hydration of the gum takes place more readily and a homogeneous mucilage is obtained more rapidly than when water alone is used. This technic may be employed for acacia, tragacanth, methylcellulose, etc.

Formulation Problems. The gums are dehydrated and precipitated by alcohol with a resulting decrease in viscosity. Some are also precipitated by heavy metals.

AGAR. The chemical constitution of agar has been shown to be a magnesium or a calcium salt (or a mixture of these two) of a sulfuric acid ester of a linear polygalactose.[44]

Structure of Agar[1]

Agar is dehydrated and precipitated from aqueous preparations by the addition of alcohol. Tannin also has a dehydrating action on agar similar to that of alcohol, but is effective in a much lower concentration. Whereas the alcohol must be in excess of 30 per cent by weight, a 1 per cent concentration of tannic acid causes precipitation. There is also a difference between the two in the mechanism of dehydration. It is believed that the tannin is adsorbed on the surface of the colloidal particles in such a manner in this complex that the hydrophile portion of the tannin molecule is oriented toward the surface of the agar and the aromatic groups toward the dispersion medium, or water. The external nature of the agar is thus changed in a manner so as to curb or suppress hydration.[52] A small amount of alcohol will restore the hydrophilic property of the agar by removing the adsorbed tannin.[53]

Electrolytes in adequate concentration (0.1 N and above) compete with the colloid for the water which is present, thus causing dehydration and a decreased viscosity of sols. Due to the presence of the sulfuric acid ester in the molecule, agar ionizes to yield a negatively charged hydrophilic colloid which may form a coacervate with an oppositely charged colloid with a resulting decrease in viscosity.[54]

CHONDRUS (IRISH MOSS). This is chemically similar to agar and resembles agar in its physical and chemical incompatibilities. It forms a soft gel at 3 per cent and a firm one at 5 per cent concentration.

SODIUM ALGINATE. This is the sodium salt of alginic acid. Although the structure of alginic acid is incompletely known, it is believed to be a polyuronic acid. Alginic acid is insoluble in cold water and only slightly soluble in hot water. However, the magnesium, ammonium, potassium and sodium salts possess hydrophilic properties.[54] Sodium alginate is soluble 1:20 in water.

Structure of Alginic Acid[5]

Addition of soluble calcium salts to aqueous solutions of sodium alginate yields the insoluble calcium alginate which precipitates as a gel. A similar gel formation is obtained by all other metallic ions, with the exception of alkali, magnesium and ammonium ions. Sodium alginate solutions are compatible with sugars, soaps, glycols, glycerin, starch, proteins and a number of dispersion stabilizers.[65] At a pH of less than 4, precipitation occurs due to the formation of the insoluble alginic acid. Mineral and organic acids in small quantities are a source of this incompatibility. Above a pH of 10, sodium alginate is unstable, and there is a decrease in viscosity. Once again, alcohol in sufficient quantity (above 30 per cent w/w) causes precipitation from aqueous solution.

ACACIA. The acacia molecule contains d-galactopyranose, d-glycuronic acid, l-rhamnopyranose and l-arabofuranose, and exists in the form of the calcium, the magnesium and the potassium salts.[34, 70] It owes its acidity to the presence of d-glycuronic acid. Acacia is sufficiently acidic to cause effervescence with carbonates and bicarbonates. It is precipitated by heavy metal ions. Common precipitation incompatibilities occur with ferric chloride, lead subacetate, tannins and sodium borate. The precipitation occurring due to the alkalinity of the sodium borate may be retarded by the addition of glycerin. This yields a weak acid solution by forming a sodium glyceroborate and glyceroboric acid buffer system. Alcohol (above 35%) precipitates acacia by acting as a dehydrating agent.

Acacia is stated to contain an oxidizing enzyme[11] which is capable of causing incompatibilities with the easily oxidized phenolic compounds such as resorcinol, phenol, thymol, tannin, etc.* Other substances containing phenolic hydroxyl groups in their molecule (e.g., morphine) are affected similarly.[38]

TRAGACANTH. According to Norman,[63] tragacanth is composed of a water-soluble fraction (called tragacanthin) and bassorin, which swells in water. The water-soluble fraction consists of uronic acid and arabinose.[64] Rowson[79] showed that the bassorin contains methoxyl groups and is similar to pectin in composition.

Tragacanth is precipitated by alcohol (above 35%) and decomposed by alkalies.

CELLULOSE DERIVATIVES. Methylcellulose (Methocel) is used as a dispersion stabilizer in polyphase systems because of its ability to increase viscosity. Wide ranges in viscosity

---

* The mechanism of these oxidation reactions is probably similar to that brought about by tyrosinase. Tyrosinase is responsible for the black coloration observed in potatoes, bananas, etc., when they are exposed to air. The enzyme tyrosinase is capable of introducing a hydroxyl group in ortho position to the —OH group already present in phenols. o-Dihydroxylic phenols are readily autoxidizable in alkaline solution or in neutral solution.

are possible through the use of the various viscosity types.*

Solubility. METHYLCELLULOSE is water-soluble and forms viscous, transparent, neutral solutions. The water-solubility of methylcellulose is in marked contrast with the parent compound, cellulose. The difference in the water-solubility of these two substances may be explained on the following basis.

Cellulose is insoluble in water because of the intermolecular association existing between the cellulose molecules. This association between the cellulose molecules ties up the hydroxyl groups so that they are unavailable for association with water. When cellulose is methylated,† association between the cellulose molecules is hindered to such a degree that the ether and free hydroxyl groups are exposed and become available for association with water.

Representation of Random Distribution of Methoxyl Groups in a Dimethylcellulose

Formulation Problems. Methylcellulose is precipitated from aqueous solutions by heat. Thermal agitation causes the water molecules to move about more freely, and the weak association bonds are ruptured, thereby causing a decrease in the water-solubility of the methylcellulose. This effect of heat in decreasing the water-solubility also occurs in other alcohols.

and, therefore, are not affected appreciably by alkaline and acidic substances in prescriptions. However, dilute alkalies do cause a slight increase in viscosity.

Tannic acid interacts with methylcellulose and causes it to be precipitated from aqueous solution. Similar complexes which result in the precipitation of the methylcellulose are formed with other phenols such as resorcinol. Unlike the plant gums, methylcellulose in aqueous solution is not as readily precipitated by relatively high concentrations of alcohol.

Inasmuch as methylcellulose is nonionic, it is compatible with the commonly employed dispersion stabilizing agents, such as plant gums, soaps, bentonite, sodium lauryl sulfate and benzalkonium chloride.

ETHYLCELLULOSE (Ethocel) is the ethyl ether of cellulose. It does not hydrate in water but is solubilized in organic solvent systems such as one composed of equal parts of chloroform and isopropyl alcohol. It is used to form water-insoluble films to control both drug stability and drug release in granules and tablets. The water resistance of the films can be decreased by the inclusion of water-soluble substances such as methylcellulose, polyethylene glycols and polyvinyl alcohol.

CARBOXYMETHYLCELLULOSE (Cellulose Gum, CMC) can be represented as the product of the type of reaction such as that between alkali cellulose and sodium monochloroacetate in which a substitution of approximately 0.75 carboxymethyl group per anhydroglucose unit is obtained in the polymer.

Aqueous methylcellulose solutions are stable over wide pH ranges (pH 2 to 12)

* A 2 per cent solution of methylcellulose of the 100 cps viscosity type has a viscosity of 100 centipoises at 20° C. Methylcellulose is available in the following viscosity types: 15 cps, 25 cps, 100 cps, 400 cps, 1,500 cps and 4,000 cps. Two per cent solutions of these viscosity types yield solutions varying from low to very high viscosities.

† Within certain limits, an increase in the number of methoxyl groups per anhydroglucose unit increases the water solubility. Those cellulose derivatives containing an average of 1.3 methoxyl groups per anhydroglucose unit are water-insoluble. When the number of methoxyl groups per anhydroglucose unit varies between 1.3 to 2.6, the products are soluble in cold water; above 2.6 methoxyl groups per anhydroglucose unit, the compounds become less water soluble but they are more soluble in alcohol.

Like methylcellulose, carboxymethylcellulose is available in various viscosity grades (Hercules CMC-70-H, CMC-70-M and CMC-70-L). The sodium carboxymethylcellulose is easily hydrated with water as a result of both ion-dipole and dipole-dipole interactions. The pH of 1 per cent solutions of the viscosity-inducing agent is in the 6.5 to 8.0 range. Carboxymethylcellulose solutions are very stable to acid and do not precipitate until the pH is below 1.1. This pH would not be encountered normally in pharmaceutical preparations. Solutions of this agent also tolerate high concentrations of alcohol (up to 50%) without precipitating.

However, some problems are encountered when solutions of Cellulose Gum are mixed with solutions containing water-soluble salts such as aluminum sulfate, silver nitrate, ferric chloride and lead acetate. Several viscosity-inducing agents such as methylcellulose, pectin, sodium alginate and polyvinyl alcohol are compatible with aqueous solutions of carboxymethylcellulose, but delayed incompatibilities were observed with gelatin, acacia, chondrus and tragacanth.[17]

PHENOLS

Phenols are aromatic hydroxy compounds in which the hydroxyl group is attached directly to the aromatic ring. The presence of the aromatic ring greatly modifies the chemical and solubility properties from those observed in alcohols.

Solubility. Although the phenols are acidic, they are too weakly acidic to dissolve in water through an acid-base reaction, but they are solubilized in water through dipole-dipole interaction in the same manner as the alcohols. The introduction of more —OH groups into the aromatic ring increases the water-solubility, whereas nonpolar substituents decrease the water-solubility.

Cause of Acidity. The cause of acidity and the marked contrast in chemical properties between the phenols and the aliphatic alcohols are due to the presence of the acidic (electrophilic, electron acceptor) phenyl group. The unsaturated, electron-deficient phenyl group tends to withdraw the surplus electrons on the oxygen. In supplying a share of its *unshared* electron pair to the phenyl group, the oxygen becomes electron deficient. The electron pair of the oxygen-hydrogen bond, therefore, is held more closely to the oxygen. The oxygen-hydrogen bond is thus weakened and the proton held more loosely. This accounts for the acidic properties of phenols in which there is a tendency to ionize in aqueous solution by donating a proton to the more basic compound, water.

Phenols are only weakly acidic and do not ionize sufficiently to be highly soluble in

TABLE 10-2. SOLUBILITIES OF SOME PHENOLS

PHENOL	SOLUBILITY IN GM PER 100 ML.		
	Water	Alcohol	Ether, etc.
Betanaphthol	0.074[25]	12.5[25]	76.9 eth., s. chl., oils, alk., gly.
Catechol	45.1[20]	v. s.	s. eth., bz., chl., alk.
Chlorothymol	almost i.	200	50 chl.; 50 bz.; 66.5 eth.; s. alk.
Cresol	2.0[20]	∞	∞ eth.; s. chl., ord. org. solv.
Hexylresorcinol	0.05	v. s.	v. s. eth.
Phenol	6.7[16]	∞	v. s. eth.; s. chl., gly., alk.
Pyrogallol	62.5[25]	100[25]	83.3 eth.; sl. s. bz., chl.
Resorcinol	229[30]	243[25]	v. s. eth.; s. gly., bz.
Thymol	0.085[20]	357[20]	360 eth.; s. chl.; sl. s. gly.

alk. = alkali
bz. = benzene
chl. = chloroform

eth. = ether
gly. = glycerin
∞ = soluble in all proportions

water unless the aromatic ring has other acidic substituents which increase their acid properties, or other solubilizing groups (OH, NH_2) which increase their ability to associate. However, the phenols are sufficiently acidic to be readily soluble in dilute aqueous alkali hydroxides by virtue of the fact that they are capable of forming water-soluble ionized salts.

Unless they have other acidic substituents, they are weaker than carbonic acid and the water-insoluble phenols are precipitated from aqueous alkali solutions by carbon dioxide. Inasmuch as they are such weak acids, they do not decompose carbonates or bicarbonates.

The introduction of other acidic (electrophilic) groups into the aromatic ring increases the unequal sharing of the electron pair of the oxygen-hydrogen bond and makes the compound a stronger acid. This effect in increasing the acidity is illustrated clearly by trinitrophenol (picric acid), which is a much stronger acid than phenol itself. The pK_a values listed in Table 10-3 show the difference in acid strength between phenol, carbonic acid and trinitrophenol.

Chemistry. The result of the electron shifts is an increased electron density on the ortho carbon atom which, in turn, increases the electron density on the para and the other ortho carbon atoms. The ortho and the para positions thus react readily with electrophilic (electron-seeking) reagents; e.g., phenol is easily nitrated in the ortho and the para positions.

The electronic theory shows us that bases are capable of donating electrons and that acids are electron acceptors. When the phenomenon of oxidation-reduction reactions is taken into consideration, it is observed that

reducing agents donate electrons or a share in their electrons to the oxidizing agent. From the standpoint of the fundamental electronic concepts involved, an analogy can be drawn for bases and reducing agents and acids and oxidizing agents. Both bases and reducing agents, therefore, are electron donors, whereas acids and oxidizing agents are electron acceptors.[23, 76]

Consequently, phenols are reducing agents because the oxygen possesses unshared electrons and functions as an electron donor. It has long been known that oxidizing agents such as peroxides, permanganates, air, etc., are capable of oxidizing phenols to colored oxidative products, and these same reactions may give rise to problems in pharmaceutical preparations. Phenols give characteristic color reactions with ferric chloride. In this reaction, the iron functions as the oxidizing agent and is reduced to the ferrous state. Other important drugs classified under other chemical groups such as diethylstilbestrol, epinephrine, morphine, rutin, etc., which have phenolic groups in the molecule undergo similar reactions.

PHENOL is soluble in water to the extent of 6.7 Gm. per 100 ml. and is readily soluble in alcohol, glycerin and aqueous solutions of alkali hydroxides.

Phenol interacts with proteins to form water-insoluble complexes. This is the cause of the corrosive action of phenol on the skin.[27] Phenol should be removed from the skin with alcohol rather than water, due to its greater solubility in the former solvent. Phenol-in-oil solution does not cause the extensive tissue necrosis such as aqueous solutions cause, but its effectiveness against micro-organisms is also decreased. Phenol is precipitated from aqueous solution by soluble heavy metal salts. It forms liquid or soft masses with many organic compounds such as betanaphthol, camphor, chloral hydrate, menthol, lead acetate, pyrogallol, resorcinol, thymol, other organic compounds possessing low melting points and functional groups with which it can interact.

TABLE 10-3. pK_a VALUES

COMPOUND	pK_a	
Phenol	9.88	
Trinitrophenol	0.795	
Carbonic acid	6.45	(1st H)

The oxidation of phenol to colored decomposition products by peroxides, permanganates and other oxidizing agents takes place in the same manner as stated in the general discussion of phenols. Alkali hydroxides accelerate its oxidation and, thus, autoxidation by air in aqueous alkali solution occurs at a rapid rate.

CRESOL [$C_6H_4(CH_3)OH$]. Cresol is a mixture of the 3 isomeric cresols and is similar to phenol in its chemical properties. The effect of nonpolar substituents on the aromatic ring is shown clearly in the case of the cresols; thus we find that they are only about one third as soluble in water as phenol (approx. 2 Gm. per 100 ml.). Cresol is freely soluble in alcohol, glycerin, ether, fixed oils, solutions of alkali hydroxides and soap solutions.

CREOSOTE consists chiefly of cresol, oxycresol, methyl cresol and other phenols. It is only slightly soluble in water but is readily soluble in alcohol and fixed oils. It has reducing properties and is incompatible with oxidizing agents. Proteins and gums are precipitated by cresol. Color reactions are obtained with ferric salts.

BETANAPHTHOL is not very water-soluble (1:1,000) and it, too, illustrates the effect of decreasing the water solubility by increasing the molecular weight without an accompanying increase in the number of hydrophile groups. Betanaphthol is very soluble in alcohol, glycerin, fixed oils and dilute solutions of alkali hydroxides. In the presence of light

and air, betanaphthol is oxidized and turns pink to brown with the formation of colored oxidation products. Other oxidizing agents such as peroxides, permanganates, chlorates, etc., have a similar effect. In alkali hydroxide solutions, the oxidation reactions take place more readily. Soft masses or liquids are obtained when betanaphthol is triturated with phenol, menthol, camphor, etc.

RESORCINOL is much more soluble in water than is phenol and illustrates the ability of an increased number of hydroxyl groups to promote greater water-solubility. It is also soluble in alcohol and glycerin. In aqueous solution, resorcinol is oxidized and the solution assumes pink to red and brown colors because of the formation of colored oxidative products. Resorcinol is a reducing agent, especially in alkaline solution, and it is capable of reducing silver, mercury and copper

Resorcinol

salts. Even in ointments, for example, it is capable of reducing ammoniated mercury to free mercury. The free metal thus liberated causes the ointment to assume a blue to gray color. Blue to violet colors are obtained with ferric chloride. On trituration with substances such as camphor, menthol, phenol, betanaphthol, etc., soft masses or liquids result.

Hexylresorcinol (Caprokol) is almost insoluble in water (0.05 Gm. per 100 ml.) but is very soluble in alcohol and ether. It is also

soluble in glycerin and fixed oils. The introduction of the alky group produces decreased water-solubility as compared with resorcinol. Hexylresorcinol is similar to resorcinol in its chemical incompatibilities.

THYMOL (3-hydroxy-1-methyl-4-isopropyl benzene) is almost insoluble in water

(0.085 Gm. per 100 ml.). The decreased water-solubility as compared with phenol is due to the nonpolar substituents on the aromatic ring. Thymol is soluble in alcohol and dilute solutions of alkali hydroxides. It forms liquids or soft masses with camphor, menthol, chloral hydrate, phenol, etc.

CHLOROTHYMOL is similar to thymol in its properties.

TRINITROPHENOL (picric acid, 2,4,6-trinitrophenol) is a strong acid (p. 355). Explosions may result when picric acid in the dry form is triturated with substances which are oxidized easily, or when the acid is subjected to rapid heating or percussion. Picric acid precipitates proteins (gelatin, albumin, etc.) and most alkaloids. Because of this

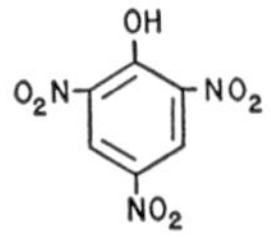

latter property, it is used as an alkaloidal reagent.

ALDEHYDES

Solubility. The lower members of the aldehyde series are soluble in water but those of C_5 and above are only slightly soluble or insoluble. Thus, these compounds have approximately the same limits of water-solubility as the monohydroxy alcohols.

Chemistry. The reactions of the aldehydes are a function of the carbonyl group. As illustrated in the following equation, there is a

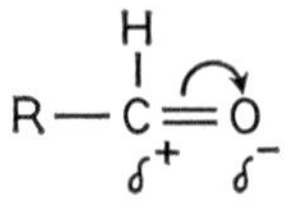

tendency for the electrons of the carbon-oxygen bond to break away from the carbon in favor of the oxygen.

This causes the carbon to become charged positively due to the electron deficiency, whereas the oxygen atom has gained a share of electrons and becomes charged negatively. As a result of the electron deficiency, the carbon becomes one of the reactive centers in the molecule and reacts with any reagent that has available electrons for attachment. In all the addition reactions of the aldehydes, it is observed that the more positive part of the reagent joins to the oxygen and the negative part joins to the carbon.

1. *Addition of sodium bisulfite:*

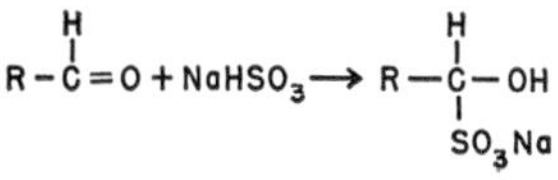

TABLE 10-4. COMPARISON OF WATER SOLUBILITY OF SOME ALDEHYDES AND ALCOHOLS

COMPOUND	SOLUBILITY IN GM. PER 100 ML. OF H_2O
Aldehyde	
Acetaldehyde	∞
Propionaldehyde	∞
Butyraldehyde	3.7
n-Valeraldehyde	sl. s.
n-Caproaldehyde	i.
n-Heptaldehyde	sl. s.
Alcohol	
Ethyl alcohol	∞
Propyl alcohol	∞
Butyl alcohol	7.9^{20}
Amyl alcohol	2.7^{22}
Hexyl alcohol	0.59^{20}
Heptyl alcohol	0.09^{18}

2. *Addition of HCN:*

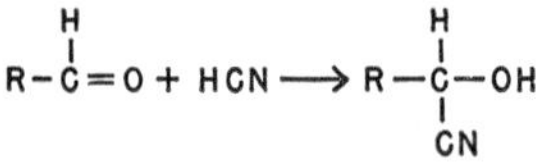

3. *Addition of hydroxylamine:*

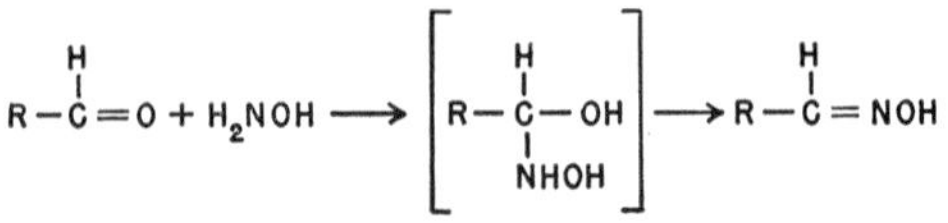

The carbonyl group also has an important effect on the hydrogen attached to the α-carbon atom. Since the carbon atom of the

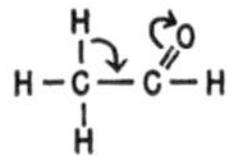

carbonyl group is deficient in electrons, it tends to withdraw the electrons bonding the hydrogen on the α-carbon atom. In this case, a tautomeric shift rather than resonance occurs because the hydrogen shifts from the carbon atom to the oxygen. However, this does account for the reactivity of the α-hydrogen. Thus, in the preparation of chloral, the hydrogen is substituted easily by chlorine.

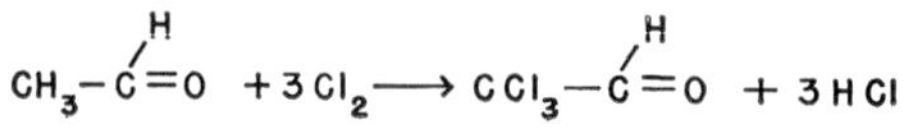

$$HC \overset{H}{\underset{H}{-}} C \overset{H}{=} O \rightleftharpoons H_2C = C \overset{H}{-} OH + Cl_2 \longrightarrow$$

Acetaldehyde

$$\left[HC \overset{H}{\underset{Cl}{-}} C \overset{H}{\underset{\boxed{Cl}}{-}} O\boxed{H} \right] \rightarrow HCl + H - C \overset{H}{\underset{Cl}{-}} C \overset{H}{=} O$$

$$HC \overset{H}{\underset{Cl}{-}} C \overset{H}{=} O \rightleftharpoons HC = C \overset{H}{\underset{Cl}{-}} OH + Cl_2 \longrightarrow$$

$$\left[Cl - C \overset{H}{\underset{Cl}{-}} C \overset{H}{\underset{\boxed{Cl}}{-}} O\boxed{H} \right] \rightarrow HCl + Cl - C \overset{H}{\underset{Cl}{-}} C \overset{H}{=} O$$

$$Cl - C \overset{H}{\underset{Cl}{-}} C \overset{H}{=} O \rightleftharpoons Cl - C = C \overset{H}{-} OH + Cl_2 \longrightarrow$$

$$\left[Cl - C \overset{Cl}{\underset{Cl}{-}} C \overset{H}{\underset{\boxed{Cl}}{-}} O\boxed{H} \right] \rightarrow CCl_3 - C \overset{H}{=} O + HCl$$
Trichloro-
acetaldehyde

Aldehydes are capable of addition reactions with water via the same mechanism as the other addition reactions. In aqueous solution, the following equilibrium is considered to exist, but the dihydroxy compound is usually too unstable to be isolated. However,

$$R - \overset{H}{\underset{}{C}} = O + HOH \rightleftharpoons R - \overset{H}{\underset{OH}{C}} - OH$$

the halogen-substituted aldehydes such as trichloroacetaldehyde (chloral) are capable of forming stable addition products with water.

$$CCl_3 - \overset{H}{\underset{}{C}} = O + HOH \longrightarrow CCl_3 - \overset{H}{\underset{OH}{C}} - OH$$

Chloral   Chloral Hydrate

Polymerization takes place with the aldehydes due to the polarization present in the carbonyl compounds, as previously explained.

Formulation Problems. In the presence of alkali, aldehydes undergo aldol condensation. The extent to which the reaction progresses is dependent on the concentration of the alkali. With strong alkali, aldehydes polymerize to form resins.

$$CH_3 - \overset{H}{\underset{}{C}} = O + CH_3 - \overset{H}{\underset{}{C}} = O \xrightarrow[\text{SOLUTION}]{\text{WEAK ALKALINE}} CH_3 - CH - CH_2 - \overset{H}{\underset{}{C}} = O$$
$$\qquad\qquad OH$$
Aldol

$$(CH_3 - \overset{H}{\underset{}{C}} = O)_n \xrightarrow[\text{ALKALI}]{\text{STRONG}} \text{ALDEHYDE RESIN}$$

PARALDEHYDE. Although it is an acetal rather than an aldehyde, paraldehyde is included at this point, since its incompatibilities are a result of the regeneration of acetaldehyde. Paraldehyde is a colorless transparent liquid possessing a pungent odor and a disagreeable taste. It is somewhat soluble in water (1 ml. in 8 ml.) and is soluble in all proportions in alcohol. Paraldehyde in the pure form is inert to oxidizing agents and

does not form addition products because the carbonyl group is no longer present. In dilute acid, however, acetaldehyde is regenerated. Thus, acid syrups and elixirs used as vehicles may promote the depolymerization of paraldehyde. The liberated acetaldehyde may then give rise to many incompatibilities, such as the formation of the usual addition products. Also, the acetaldehyde formed by this partial depolymerization reaction is now subject to oxidation, and both acetic and peracetic acids can be formed. The presence of the acid can then result in other problems such as the liberation of free iodine from iodides,[81,82] etc.

$$3CH_3 - \overset{O}{\underset{}{C}} - H \rightleftharpoons \quad \xrightarrow{H_2SO_4} \quad$$

Acetaldehyde   Paraldehyde

Because of its bad taste and odor, paraldehyde has not much popularity in present-day medicine, but it is actually one of the best and the least toxic of hypnotics.[28] Its use in the form of an emulsion has previously been recommended.[71]

CHLORAL HYDRATE. This is very soluble in both water and alcohol. The stability of this hydrated form of chloral may be ex-

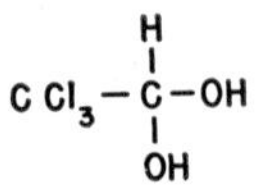

$$CCl_3-\overset{\overset{\displaystyle H}{|}}{\underset{\underset{\displaystyle OH}{|}}{C}}-OH$$

plained on the basis of the inductive effect of the halogen substitution on the α-carbon atom. Just as in the case of the chlorinated acetic acids, the electrophilic chlorine groups on the α-carbon atom tend to withdraw electrons. This inductive effect, together with the electromeric effect present in the carbonyl group, creates a center of low electron density on the carbonyl carbon atom so that addition reactions with nucleophilic reagents (electron donor) readily take place.

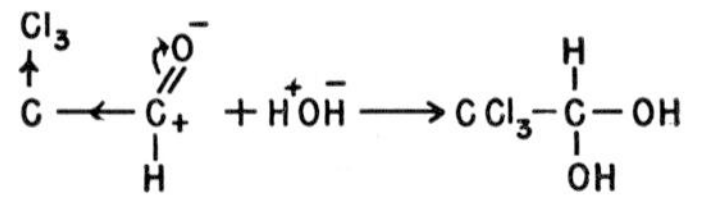

Chloral   Chloral Hydrate

In a similar manner, chloral forms chloral alcoholate by addition.[2,31] Chloral hydrate in aqueous solution is incompatible with alkaline substances and undergoes hydrolysis to form chloroform and the salt of formic acid. Due to this reaction, sodium phenobarbital, sodium diphenylhydantoinate and other salts which yield alkaline solutions may cause the hydrolysis of chloral hydrate and the subsequent precipitation of the free phenobarbital, etc.

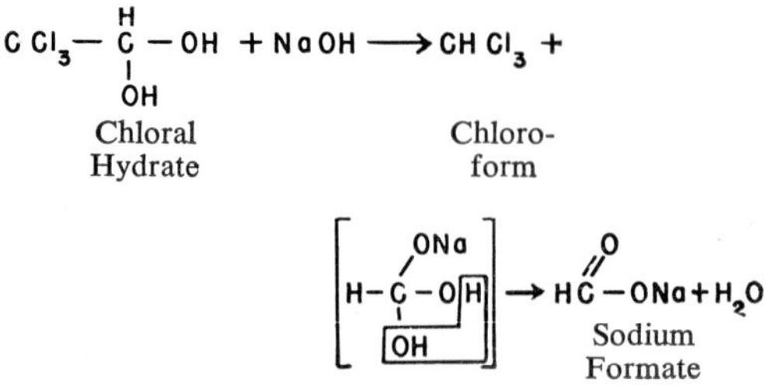

Chloral   Chloro-
Hydrate   form

Sodium
Formate

On oxidation, chloral hydrate yields trichloroacetic acid (CCl_3-COOH); on reduction, it yields trichloroethanol (CCl_3-CH_2OH).

Chloral hydrate forms soft masses or liquids when triturated with acetophenetidin, camphor, cocoa butter, menthol, phenol, thymol, salol and many other substances.

KETONES

Solubility. Like the aldehydes, the ketones have approximately the same limits of solubility in water as the monohydroxy alcohols. Those above C_5 are only slightly soluble or are insoluble in water.

Chemistry. Because the ketones contain a carbonyl group, many of them undergo the same addition reactions as the aldehydes; however, the substitution of an alkyl group for the hydrogen atom markedly decreases the additive reactivity of the carbonyl group. If one compares the activity of acetaldehyde and acetone in the formation of the bisulfite addition compound, it is observed that acetone reacts much less rapidly and to a lesser extent. This may be explained on the basis that the methyl group in acetone which has been substituted for the hydrogen atom in acetaldehyde is an electron-repellent group. This group then tends to decrease the electron deficiency of the carbonyl carbon atom, de-

TABLE 10-5. COMPARISON OF WATER
SOLUBILITY OF SOME KETONES
AND ALCOHOLS

Compound	Solubility in Gm. per 100 ml. of H_2O
Ketone	
Acetone	∞
Ethyl methyl	35.3[10]
Diethyl	4.7[20]
n-Propyl ethyl	v. sl. s.
Di-*n*-propyl	i.
Alcohol	
Ethyl	∞
Propyl	∞
Butyl	7.9[20]
Amyl	2.7[22]
Hexyl	0.59[20]
Heptyl	0.09[18]

creases the polarization of the molecule, and, consequently, the carbonyl carbon atom is less reactive with the electron donor reagents.

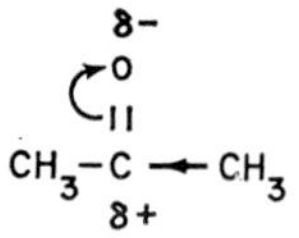

$$CH_3-\overset{\overset{\overset{\delta-}{O}}{\parallel}}{\underset{\delta+}{C}}\rightarrow CH_3$$

Because of their decreased polarization, the ketones are less susceptible to polymerization than the aldehydes.

In pharmaceutical dispensing, ketones give rise to few incompatibilities because they seldom appear as such in prescriptions, with the exception of camphor and, to a very limited extent, acetone. Since the polarizing effect of the carbonyl group does not lead to any important chemical incompatibilities, the problems encountered in the dispensing of those ketones which are used are due usually to insolubility or to the formation of eutectic mixtures.

ACETONE (dimethyl ketone) is soluble in water, alcohol, ether, chloroform and fixed

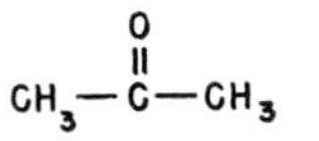

$$CH_3-\overset{\overset{O}{\parallel}}{C}-CH_3$$

oils. Although it has little application in the compounding of prescriptions, it is widely used in pharmacy as a solvent.

CAMPHOR is almost insoluble in water (approx. 0.1 Gm. per 100 ml.), but it is very soluble in alcohol, ether, chloroform, benzene and acetone. Problems of a solubility

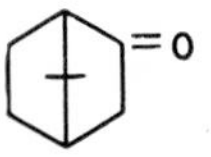

nature usually are due to the addition of water to alcoholic solutions of camphor, in which case the camphor is precipitated. Camphor may also be precipitated from camphor water by the salting-out effects of high concentrations of water-soluble salts. Camphor forms soft masses or liquids when triturated with chloral hydrate, phenol, menthol, thymol and many other substances. The liquefaction causes little difficulty in ointments but may be troublesome in external dusting powders.

CARBOXYLIC ACIDS

MONOCARBOXYLIC ACIDS (FATTY ACID SERIES)

Solubility. The monobasic carboxylic acids have approximately the same limits of solubility in water as the alcohols. The oxygen-hydrogen bonds of these acids are not polar enough to allow them to dissociate to a great enough degree to be solvated by water through an acid-base reaction. Therefore, the lower members of this series are soluble in water due to their ability to hydrogen-bond with water. As the alkyl chain is increased, the solubilizing influence of the carboxyl group is not sufficient to overcome the solvent-solvent interaction of water, and the molecule becomes insoluble.

TABLE 10-6. SOLUBILITIES OF SOME MONOCARBOXYLIC ACIDS
(FATTY ACID SERIES)

ACID	SOLUBILITY IN GM. PER 100 ML. OF		
	Water	Alcohol	Ether, etc.
Formic acid	∞	∞	∞ eth., gly.
Acetic acid	∞	∞	∞ eth.
Propionic acid	∞	∞	∞ eth., chl.
Butyric acid	5.62	∞	∞ eth.
Valeric acid	3.7[16]	∞	∞ eth.
Caproic acid	0.4	s.	s. eth.
Caprylic acid	0.25[100]	s.	∞ eth., chl.
Capric acid	sl. s.	s.	s. eth.
Lauric acid	i.	134[21]	v. s. eth.
Myristic acid	i.	44.9[21]	s. eth., chl.
Palmitic acid	i.	9.3[20]	s. eth.
Stearic acid	0.034[25]	2.5	v. s. eth.; s. chl.

eth. = ether   chl. = chloroform   gly. = glycerin

Although the monocarboxylic acids are weak acids, they form water-soluble ionized salts by reaction with alkali hydroxides, carbonates and bicarbonates. The alkali salts of the water-insoluble acids thus become soluble in water through an ion-dipole interaction. The alkali salts of the higher members of this series (C_{10} and up) are capable of lowering surface tension and are called soaps. When aqueous solutions of these water-soluble salts are acidified, the free acid separates out. All metals, other than the alkali metals, form water-insoluble salts with these higher acids.

The monocarboxylic acids are generally soluble in alcohol because of the ability of the two substances to hydrogen-bond. The acids of higher molecular weight are soluble in ether and other weakly polar solvents.

Chemistry. The substitution of acidic (electrophilic) groups for hydrogen in various

$$\underset{CH_2}{\overset{\overset{X}{\uparrow}}{}} \longleftarrow \overset{O}{\underset{}{\overset{\|}{C}}} \longleftarrow O \longleftarrow H$$

parts of the molecule profoundly affects the acidity of the compound. The acidic group is an electron acceptor and draws electrons toward it. This inductive effect causes a decreased electron density on the carbon atom of the carboxyl group. The electron pair of the oxygen-hydrogen bond, in turn, is held more closely to the oxygen and the proton is held less firmly. Therefore, the acidic strength is increased, as is observed by the decreased pK_a values in compounds with this type of substitution (Table 10-7). This effect is most pronounced when the substitution of an acidic group for a hydrogen takes place on the α-

TABLE 10-7. pK_a VALUES OF SOME MONOCARBOXYLIC ACIDS AND SOME CHLORINATED DERIVATIVES

ACID	pK_a
Formic	3.75
Acetic	4.76
Propionic	4.85
Chloroacetic	2.85
Dichloroacetic	1.3
Trichloroacetic	0.7
α-Chlorpropionic	2.83
β-Chlorpropionic	4.06

carbon atom and is diminished markedly the more remote the substitution becomes.[24] Because of the ability of electrophilic groups to withdraw electrons, the substitution of these groups on the α-carbon atom not only increases the acidity, but also has a "loosening effect"[86] on the carboxyl group, thereby causing an increased tendency to decarboxylate.

When a hydrogen is replaced with a substituent that releases electrons, the opposite effect is observed. Thus, when a methyl group replaces a hydrogen of acetic acid, the inductive effect is in the opposite direction and a slightly increased electron density in the carboxyl group results. The proton now is held more firmly, and the acid strength is decreased as in indicated by the increased pK_a values (Table 10-7).

$$CH_3 \longrightarrow CH_2 \longrightarrow \overset{O}{\overset{\|}{C}} \longrightarrow O \longrightarrow H$$

Formulation Problems. ACETIC ACID is soluble in water, alcohol and ether. It is a stronger acid than carbonic acid, thereby causing the liberation of CO_2 from carbonates and bicarbonates in aqueous solution [acetic acid $pK_a = 4.76$, carbonic acid $pK_a = 6.45$ (1st H)].

$$CH_3-\overset{O}{\overset{\|}{C}}-OH + NaHCO_3 \longrightarrow CH_3-\overset{O}{\overset{\|}{C}}-ONa + H_2O + CO_2\uparrow$$

$$2\,CH_3-\overset{O}{\overset{\|}{C}}-OH + Na_2CO_3 \longrightarrow 2\,CH_3-\overset{O}{\overset{\|}{C}}-ONa + H_2O + CO_2\uparrow$$

All of the common metal salts of acetic acid are soluble in water, with the exception of the silver and the mercurous salts, which are only sparingly soluble. Problems arise when alkali acetates are dispensed in aqueous solution with soluble inorganic salts other than those of the alkali metals. For example, a dark red color is observed in solutions containing the acetate ion when soluble ferric salts are added. This color is the result of the formation of ferric acetate, which then hydrolyzes and forms colloidal ferric hydroxide. The red ferric hydroxide is aggregated and precipitated on heating.

The other low members of this fatty acid series, such as propionic, butyric and valeric acids, are similar to acetic acid in their reactions.

OLEIC ACID ($C_{17}H_{33}COOH$) illustrates the effect of an increase in the alkyl portion of the molecule in decreasing the water solubility. This acid is insoluble in water, but it is soluble in alcohol and ether. The alkali metal salts of oleic acid are soluble in water due to the ion-dipole interaction between the solute and the solvent. On acidification of aqueous solutions containing soluble oleates, the original water-insoluble oleic acid separates out. Soluble heavy metal salts give rise to incompatibilities because of the formation of the insoluble oleate through double decomposition reactions. Since oleic acid is unsatu-

$$2\ C_{17}H_{33}\overset{\overset{O}{\parallel}}{C}-ONa + (CH_3-COO)_2Pb \longrightarrow$$

Sodium   Lead
Oleate   Acetate

$$2\,CH_3-\overset{\overset{O}{\parallel}}{C}-ONa + (C_{17}H_{33}COO)_2\,Pb$$

Sodium   Lead Oleate
Acetate   (insoluble)

rated, it is easily oxidized and absorbs iodine by addition across the double bond.

The higher members of this series such as stearic ($C_{17}H_{35}COOH$), palmitic ($C_{15}H_{31}$-COOH) and myristic acids ($C_{13}H_{27}COOH$) are similar to oleic acid in their reactions with the exception that they are all saturated, are not oxidized and do not absorb iodine. In aqueous solutions, the sodium salts of stearic and palmitic acids have a tendency to gel; the potassium salts exhibit a lesser tendency toward gel-formation.

TRICHLOROACETIC ACID (CCl_3—COOH) is a much stronger acid than acetic acid; in fact, it approaches the acidic strength of the mineral acids. This is due to the presence of

$$Cl \leftarrow \overset{\overset{Cl}{\uparrow}}{\underset{\underset{Cl}{\downarrow}}{C}} \leftarrow \overset{\overset{O}{\parallel}}{C} \leftarrow O\!\!:\!H$$

the 3 chlorine atoms which replace the 3 hydrogens on the α-carbon atom. Since the chlorine is an electron acceptor (electrophilic), it tends to withdraw electrons from the carboxyl group, thus causing the electron pair of the oxygen-hydrogen bond to be held more closely to the oxygen. This weakens the oxygen-hydrogen bond to such an extent that the hydrogen is held loosely and the compound readily dissociates. Trichloroacetic acid is very soluble in water in spite of its increased molecular weight (each chlorine being roughly equivalent to 3 carbon atoms). The molecular weight of trichloroacetic acid (163.40) lies between that of pelargonic (158.24) and capric (172.26) acids, both of which are water-insoluble. Therefore, it is obvious that the solubility of trichloroacetic acid in water is not a matter of association, as is the case with acetic acid, but arises from the fact that trichloroacetic acid readily dissociates by giving up its proton to the more basic compound, water. Water dissolves the acid through an acid-base reaction, whereby the water ruptures the covalent bond and produces ionization.

$$CCl_3-\overset{\overset{O}{\parallel}}{C}-O\!\!:\!H\ +\ H\!:\!\overset{\overset{\bullet\bullet}{}}{\underset{\bullet\bullet}{O}}\!\!:\!H\ \longrightarrow$$

$$CCl_3-\overset{\overset{O}{\parallel}}{C}-\bar{O}\ +\ H\!:\!\overset{\overset{\bullet\bullet}{}}{\underset{\bullet\bullet}{O}}\!\!:\!\overset{H}{}H$$

Trichloroacetic acid is incompatible with alkali salts of many weakly acidic substances which are water-insoluble in the free state—e.g., soaps, phenates, etc. Being a strong acid, it coagulates proteins (albumin, gelatin, etc.) and has a corrosive action on the skin. Because of this latter property, sometimes it is used to remove warts and corns.

DICARBOXYLIC ACIDS

As has already been pointed out in the chapter on solubilities, the intermolecular forces existing in organic compounds play an important role in the physical state and properties of the compound. These compounds, possessing strong dipoles, have high intermolecular cohesive forces due to the attraction of the positive end of a dipole in one molecule for the negative end of a dipole in another molecule.

Solubility. The dissolution of these acids in the inert solvent, water, necessitates the overcoming of the cohesive forces. Oxalic acid, possessing high intermolecular forces, exists as a solid and is less water-soluble than acetic acid, which is a liquid.

Chemistry. The pK_a values of the dicarboxylic acids show the effect of the additional

TABLE 10-8. SOLUBILITIES OF SOME POLYCARBOXYLIC ACIDS

ACID	SOLUBILITY IN GM. PER 100 ML. OF		
	WATER	ALCOHOL	ETHER, etc.
Oxalic acid	9.5	23.7	1.37 eth.; i. chl., pet. eth., bz.
Succinic acid	6.8^{20}	$7.5^{21.5}$	0.3 eth.; i. bz., chl.
Tartaric acid	139^{20}	19.85^{15}	0.4 eth.
Citric acid	133	116^{25}	2.26 eth.
Adipic acid	1.4^{15}	v.s.	0.6^{15} eth.

bz. = benzene   chl. = chloroform   eth. = ether   pet. eth. = petroleum ether

TABLE 10-9. pK_a VALUES OF SOME POLYCARBOXYLIC ACIDS

ACID	pKa_1	pKa_2
Oxalic acid	1.26	4.28
Succinic acid	4.19	5.63
Maleic acid	1.82	6.26
Fumaric acid	3.0	4.38
Tartaric acid	3.02	4.36
Citric acid	3.15	4.78 (pKa_3 6.4)

carboxyl group in the molecule. Oxalic and acetic acids are interesting in this respect, and it is observed that oxalic acid is the much stronger acid of the two. The additional carboxyl group attracts electrons so that the hydrogen on the other carboxyl group is held less firmly and dissociates more readily. The pK_a value for the second hydrogen is increased greatly by virtue of the fact that, after the dissociation of the first hydrogen, that carboxyl group then bears a negative charge

and repels electrons. The hydrogen of the second carboxyl group is thus held more firmly, as is shown by its pK_a value (see Table 10-9). The more remotely the carboxyl groups are spaced from each other in the molecule, the less prominent this inductive effect becomes (see succinic acid, Table 10-9).

Cis-trans isomerism also plays an important part in determining the acidity in the unsaturated dicarboxylic acids. When the carboxyl groups are close to each other in space (cis form), the inductive effect is greater than when they are farther apart (trans form) (see maleic and fumaric acids, Table 10-9).

HYDROXY-POLYCARBOXYLIC ACIDS

These acids are solids for the same reasons as listed for the dicarboxylic acids. In pharmacy, these acids are represented by tartaric and citric acids.

Solubility. These are weak acids and are soluble in water because they contain a large number of functional —OH groups relative to their molecular weight. They are soluble in water because of their ability to hydrogen-bond with the solvent. The salts of the alkali metals are water-soluble, but the normal salts of most other metals are insoluble.

Incompatibility. TARTARIC ACID (dihydroxysuccinic acid) is a weak acid but it is soluble in water, since it is capable of association with water. The normal alkali metal

salts of tartaric acid are soluble in water; most other metals form water-insoluble salts. However, the bitartrates of potassium and ammonium are only slightly soluble. A precipitate of potassium bitartrate is often obtained in solutions containing soluble potassium salts and tartaric acid. Acids also

oxidation products.[12, 29] Air oxidation can be prevented by the addition of 0.1 per cent sodium bisulfite, sodium sulfite, sodium thiosulfate or other antioxidants. The presence of oxidizing agents in the solution, of course, greatly accelerates the above reaction.

The salicylates yield color reactions with ferric chloride and copper salts.[85] The usual eutectic mixtures are encountered when salicylic acid is triturated with phenols, acids and alcohols.

ACETYLSALICYLIC ACID (aspirin) is practically insoluble in water (1 Gm. per 400 ml.) but is soluble in alcohol (1 Gm. per 5 ml.) and dilute aqueous alkali. In alkaline solution, it forms the water-soluble ionized salt.

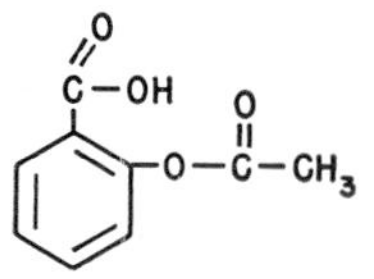

In general, acetylsalicylic acid should not be dispensed in aqueous solution since it undergoes hydrolysis to yield acetic and salicylic acids. However, if an aqueous preparation

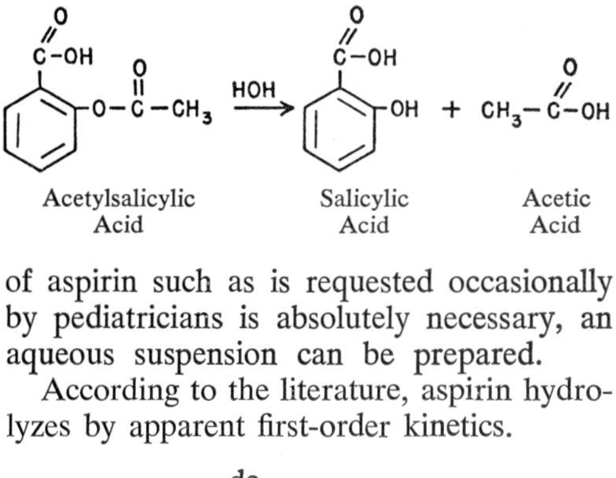

| Acetylsalicylic Acid | Salicylic Acid | Acetic Acid |

of aspirin such as is requested occasionally by pediatricians is absolutely necessary, an aqueous suspension can be prepared.

According to the literature, aspirin hydrolyzes by apparent first-order kinetics.

$$\frac{dc}{dt} = -kc$$

and upon integration

$$\log C = \log C_o - \frac{kt}{2.303}$$

where C is concentration, t is time and k is the rate constant (see Chapter 4).

The rate of hydrolysis is, of course, greatly influenced by both pH and temperature. The influence of pH is shown in Table 10-12.

TABLE 10-12. INFLUENCE OF pH ON THE HYDROLYSIS OF ASPIRIN

pH	k (DAYS^{-1})	$t_{\frac{1}{2}}$ (DAYS)
0.53	0.577	1.2
1.33	0.083	8.3
2.5	0.048	14.4
2.99	0.034	20.2
4.04	0.088	7.8
12.77	0.693	1.0

As shown in Table 10-12 the longest half-life (20 days) occurs at a pH of approxi-

$$t_{\frac{1}{2}} = \frac{0.693}{k}$$

mately 3.[22] Thus, the aspirin can be suspended in an acid vehicle such as citric acid syrup and remain sufficiently stable for a short period of use.

The influence of temperature on the hydrolysis rate is shown in Table 10-13.

From the information in Table 10-13, it is obvious that a liquid aspirin preparation has an increased half-life at a refrigerated temperature. If a plot of the logarithm of the rate constant (k) versus the reciprocal of the absolute temperature $(\frac{1}{T})$ shows a linear relationship, then the rate constants at other temperatures can be obtained by extrapolation (see Arrhenius equation, p. 176). Using the data in Table 10-13 in this manner, the rate constant at 15°C. and at pH 2.5 would be 0.018 days^{-1} and the half-life 38.5 days.

The hydrolysis rate is usually somewhat inhibited in nonaqueous or partially aqueous

TABLE 10-13. EFFECT OF TEMPERATURE ON THE HYDROLYSIS RATE

TEMPERATURE (°C.)	pH	k (DAYS^{-1})	$t_{\frac{1}{2}}$ (DAYS)
25	2.5	0.048	14.4
35	2.5	0.113	6.1
50.3	2.5	0.417	1.6
60.3	2.5	1.04	0.66

solutions containing other solvents such as alcohol, glycerin, and propylene glycol. After hydrolysis, the liberated salicylic acid or salicylate ions yield the typical color reactions with ferric salts.

The acetate and citrate salts of the alkali metals have previously been recommended

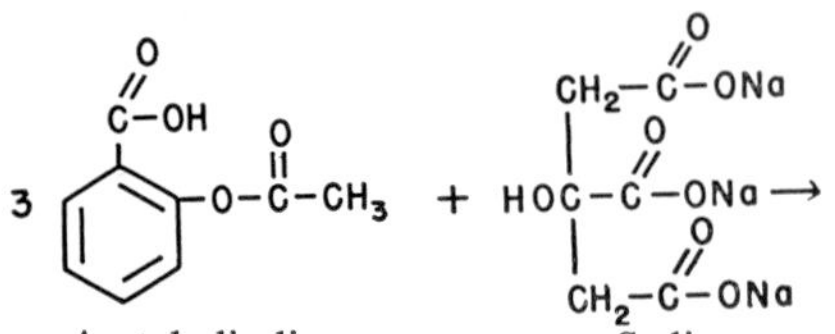

Acetylsalicylic Acid (water insoluble) + Sodium Citrate (water soluble) →

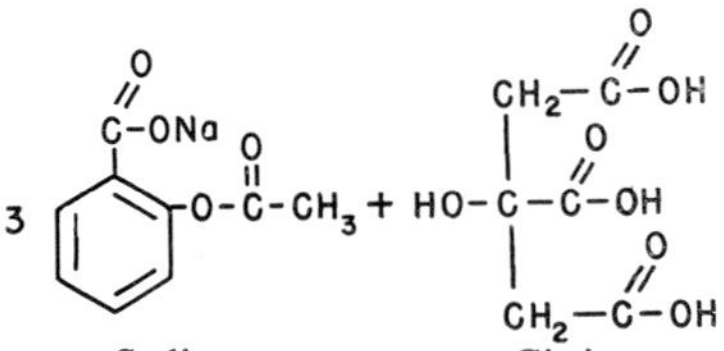

Sodium Acetylsalicylate (water soluble) + Citric Acid (water soluble)

as solubilizing agents for acetylsalicylic acid in aqueous solutions, but this is also a questionable practice, since hydrolysis still takes place. These salts yield alkaline solutions and form the water-soluble sodium acetylsalicylate. The acid citrate or free citric and acetic acids formed in the reaction are, of course, also water-soluble.

Acetylsalicylic acid is a stronger acid than carbonic acid and effervesces with carbonates and bicarbonates, liberating carbon dioxide.

Aspirin forms soft masses when triturated with acetanilid, acetophenetidin, aminopyrine, antipyrine, etc.

PROBENECID (Benemid; *p*-(dipropylsul-

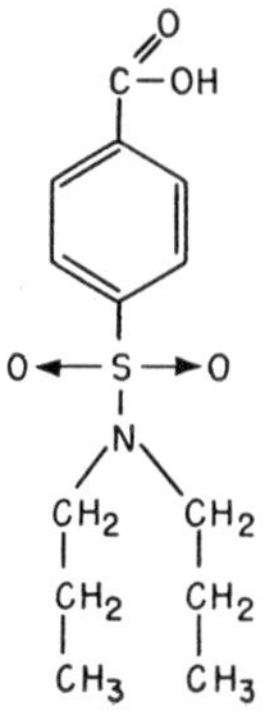

famyl)benzoic acid) can be classified both as an aromatic carboxylic acid and as a sulfonamide type compound. It is nearly insoluble in water and dilute acids but soluble in alcohol, acetone, chloroform and dilute alkalies. In medicine it is employed as a uricosuric agent in the treatment of gout and is used to prolong the activity of penicillin, *p*-aminosalicylic acid and phenolsulfonphthalein in the body.

TANNIC ACID (tannin, gallotannic acid) is a complex and heterogeneous group of astringent plant principles in which one or more of the hydroxyl groups of glucose are esterified with either gallic $[C_6H_2(OH)_3-COOH]$ or digallic $[HOOCC_6H_2(OH)_2-OCOC_6H_2(OH)_3]$ acid.[25] Tannic acid is very soluble in water, alcohol, glycerin and acetone. The presence of many —OH groups in its molecule, which enables this acid to hydrogen-bond with other —OH-containing compounds such as alcohol and water, explains its great solubility in these solvents. The alkali metal salts of tannic acid are water-soluble, but the salts of many other metals such as lead, tin, copper and iron are water-insoluble. The ferric salts yield the typical blue-black coloration and precipitate with tannic acid. This is due to the oxidation of the tannic acid by the iron. The presence of mineral acids and alkali citrates tends to prevent this reaction with ferric salts. The oxidation potential of iron is reduced by acid. With the alkali citrates, a Fe^{+++} citrate complex is formed which also reduces the oxidation potential of the iron (see p. 349).

Tannic acid precipitates practically all alkaloids from aqueous solution, but the precipitate redissolves on the addition of alcohol. Tannic acid reacts with proteins (gelatin, pepsin, albumin, etc.) and precipitates them from aqueous solutions.

In aqueous solution, tannic acid is oxidized and the solutions turn brown, presumably due to the formation of quinoid oxidation products of the phenolic compounds. The presence of oxidizing agents hastens the decomposition. Explosions may result from the trituration of tannic acid and strong oxidizing agents such as permanganates, iodine, chlorates, etc., in the dry form.

Tannic acid also precipitates antipyrine,

some neutral bitter principles, glycosides and the plant gums (p. 352).

ESTERS

An ester is an organic or inorganic acid in which the acid hydrogen has been replaced by an alkyl group.

ESTERS DERIVED FROM ORGANIC ACIDS

Solubility. The esters of the
$$R—\overset{\overset{O}{\|}}{C}—O—R$$
type derived from alcohols and organic acids exhibit approximately the same limits of solubility in water as the alcohols. Table 10-14 illustrates this similarity. The introduction of hydrophilic groups (—OH, —NH_2, etc.) into the ester molecule increases the polarity and the water-solubility in the same manner as it does in the case of the alcohols. Therefore, water-solubility is augmented due to the increased ability of these compounds to associate with water. A comparison of glycerol monoacetate (monacetin, CH_2OH—CHOH—CH_2OOC—CH_3) and propyl acetate, both of which contain the same number of carbon atoms, affords a good example of the effect of these groups in promoting water-solubility. Glycerol monoacetate is very soluble in water, whereas propyl acetate is much less soluble (Table 10-14). As the length of the alkyl group is increased, there is a decrease in the polarity and an accompanying decrease in the water-solubility. Many of the esters are soluble in alcohol, but the alkyl group may be increased to such an extent that they become

TABLE 10-14. A COMPARISON OF THE WATER SOLUBILITY OF SOME ESTERS AND ALCOHOLS

COMPOUND	SOLUBILITY IN GM. PER 100 ML. OF H_2O
Esters	
Methyl acetate	s.
Ethyl acetate	8.6^{20}
Propyl acetate	1.89^{20}
Alcohols	
Propyl	∞
Butyl	7.9^{20}
Amyl	2.7^{22}

practically insoluble in this solvent. The fixed oils (triglycerides), which contain the large alkyl group of the fatty acids, are a good example of this effect. Inasmuch as the esters are relatively nonpolar compounds, they are soluble in the other relatively nonpolar solvents such as ether, chloroform, carbon tetrachloride, etc.

Formulation Problems. The esters are neutral compounds which gradually hydrolyze in the presence of water into their corresponding alcohols and acids. The hydrolysis rate is increased by both acids and alkalies.

FATS AND FIXED OILS. The fats and fixed oils are glyceryl esters of fatty acids. Chemically, there is only a minor difference between fats and oils; the oils are liquid due to the increased unsaturation of the fatty acids. These glyceryl esters are relatively nonpolar compounds and are, therefore, insoluble in water and alcohol, but are soluble in other nonpolar solvents such as ether, chloroform, etc. Castor oil is soluble in alcohol due to the fact that the oil is composed mainly of the triglyceride of ricinoleic acid [$CH_3(CH_2)_5$-$CHOHCH_2CHCH(CH_2)_7COOH$] which is a hydroxy acid capable of associating with the alcohol.

Rancidity may develop in fats due to oxidative, hydrolytic or ketonic degradation, but usually it is attributed to the oxidative type which is induced and accelerated by the presence of air, light, heat, moisture and the presence of metal catalysts such as copper, zinc, etc. The products formed in the rancidification of fats include aldehydes, ketones, lactones, hydroxy acids, other acids of smaller molecular weight than the parent acid, carbon dioxide and water.[21] Because of the presence of free acids, rancid fats liberate iodine from iodides. Due to their unsaturation, some fats and all oils absorb iodine at their double bonds.

Other problems of a solubility nature arise when oils are used in preparations containing water. In such cases, one must resort to the process of emulsification in order to obtain a homogeneous preparation.

The fats and the oils are gradually saponified by alkalies on long standing and more rapidly with the aid of heat. All fixed oils contain a small amount of free fatty acids which readily form metallic salts, e.g., lime water is utilized in Calamine Liniment to form the calcium soaps of the free fatty acids of olive oil, which then form a water-in-oil emulsion.

RESORCINOL MONOACETATE (Euresol) is a water-insoluble liquid which is soluble in alcohol and most other organic solvents. It

illustrates the effect of esterification in decreasing the water-solubilizing properties of the hydrophilic hydroxyl group. Resorcinol is soluble in water since it contains 2 phenolic hydroxyl groups, and the ratio of the functional —OH groups to the molecular weight is well within the limits of water-solubility. However, after esterification of one of the —OH groups, the ability to associate with water is greatly decreased, so that the resulting ratio of —OH groups to the molecular weight falls beyond the limits of water solubility. Resorcinol monoacetate is soluble in dilute solutions of alkali hydroxides but it is rapidly hydrolyzed to resorcinol and acetic acid in this medium. In alkaline solution, resorcinol readily undergoes air oxidation to colored decomposition products. Oxidizing agents and heat accelerate this reaction.

BENZYL BENZOATE is insoluble in the more polar solvents such as water and glycerin, but is soluble in alcohol and the less polar sol-

vents ether and chloroform. Since it is insoluble in water, it is often used in the form of an emulsion for external application in the treatment of scabies. The official Benzyl Benzoate Lotion of the *N.F.* contains oleic acid and triethanolamine which form the triethanolamine soap as the emulsifying agent for the benzyl benzoate.

METHYLPARABEN AND PROPYLPARABEN. Methylparaben (methyl parahydroxybenzo-

ate) and propylparaben (propyl parahydroxybenzoate) are used for the preservation of pharmaceutical preparations which are subject to microbial deterioration. The methyl ester is soluble to the extent of 1 Gm. in 400 ml. of water, whereas the propyl ester is soluble only to the extent of 1 Gm. in 2,000 ml. This illustrates the subsequent decrease in water solubility which results when the alkyl group is increased in similar compounds. Inasmuch as both compounds contain the phenolic —OH group, they are readily soluble in dilute solutions of alkali hydroxides but are then hydrolzyed to the benzoate and the corresponding alcohol. These two compounds are also soluble in alcohol, ether and fixed oils.

ESTERS DERIVED FROM INORGANIC ACIDS

The esters derived from alcohols and inorganic acids show varying chemical and physical properties. The esters derived from nitric and nitrous acids are neutral, whereas those esters derived from sulfuric acid are strong acids.

Solubility. The nitric and the nitrous acid esters are soluble in alcohol, but they are insoluble in water. The sulfuric acid esters are strong acids due to the presence of the coordinate sulfur-oxygen bonds which create

strong dipoles in the molecule. The electron pair of the oxygen-hydrogen bond is held more closely to the oxygen, and the compound readily dissociates. These compounds are readily soluble in water, since they are solvated through an acid-base reaction. In alkaline solution, they form water-soluble ionized salts.

Esters derived from carbonic acid have only a limited use in pharmacy. They are usually water-insoluble and soluble in alcohol.

Formulation Problems. The esters derived from inorganic acids are readily hydrolyzed by alkalies to yield the parent alcohol and the alkali metal salt of the acid.

NITRITE ESTERS. *Ethyl* NITRITE. Ethyl Nitrite Spirit (spirit of nitrous ether, sweet spirit of niter). The spirit gradually hydrolyzes in the presence of water, light and air, and liber-

$$CH_3-CH_2ONO$$

ates nitrous acid. The nitrous acid present in the spirit is capable of liberating free iodine from iodides, nitrogen from ammonium salts and carbon dioxide from carbonates and bicarbonates. Color reactions are observed with

$$NH_4Br + HNO_2 \rightleftarrows NH_4NO_2 + HBr$$

$$NH_4NO_2 \longrightarrow 2H_2O + N_2\nearrow$$

many aromatic compounds such as acetanilid and acetophenetidin which yield yellow colors, antipyrine which exhibits a green color due to the formation of nitrosoantiyprine, and

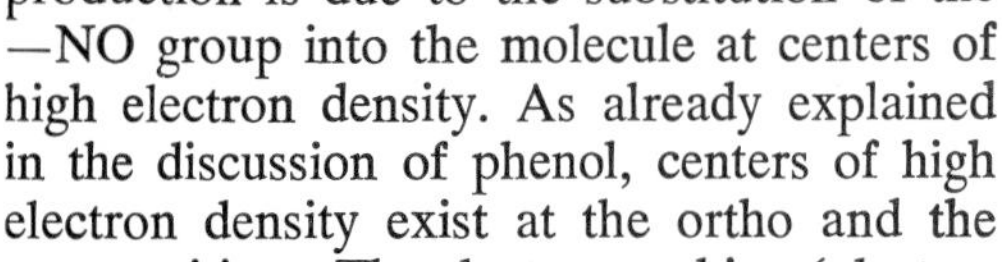

Antipyrine   Nitrosoantipyrine

phenolic substances with which reddish brown colors are produced. The cause of the color production is due to the substitution of the —NO group into the molecule at centers of high electron density. As already explained in the discussion of phenol, centers of high electron density exist at the ortho and the para positions. The electron-seeking (electrophilic) reagent thus reacts at these positions.

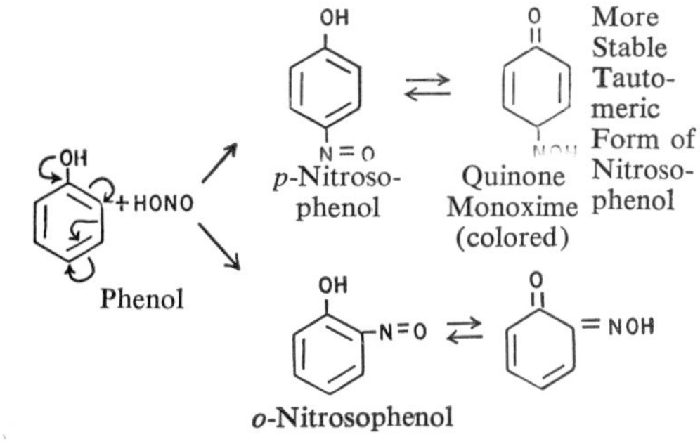

Phenol

p-Nitroso-phenol

Quinone Monoxime (colored)

More Stable Tautomeric Form of Nitroso-phenol

o-Nitrosophenol

In alkaline solution, the ethyl nitrite is rapidly hydrolyzed to ethyl alcohol and the nitrite salt.

$$CH_3-CH_2-O-N=O + NaOH \longrightarrow C_2H_5OH + NaNO_2$$

Amyl nitrite (CH_3—CH_2—CH_2—CH_2—CH_2—O—NO) has similar potential incompatibilities but it is always administered by the inhalation method so that the dispensing problems are eliminated.

NITRATE ESTERS. *Glyceryl Trinitrate* (Nitroglycerin, Glonoin)

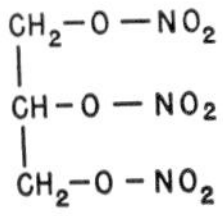

Erythrityl Tetranitrate (Erythrol Tetranitrate)

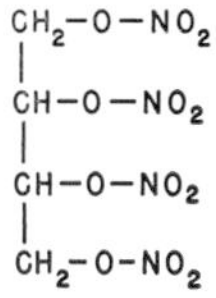

Mannitol Hexanitrate

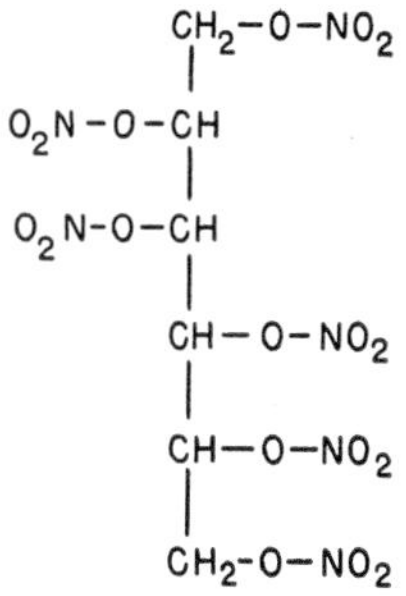

Pentaerythritol Tetranitrate (*Peritrate*)

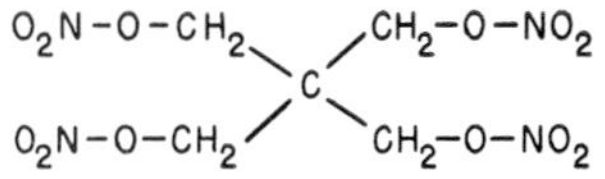

The nitrate esters cause little difficulty in prescription practice because usually they are dispensed in the dry tablet form. They are insoluble in water and soluble in alcohol. In the dry, undiluted form, they explode on percus-

TABLE 10-15. COMPARISON OF BOILING POINTS AND WATER SOLUBILITY OF SOME ALCOHOLS, ETHERS AND ALKANES

COMPOUND	B. P. (°C.)	SOLUBILITY IN GM. PER 100 ML. OF H_2O
Alcohols		
Propyl	97.19	∞
Butyl	117.7	7.9^{20}
Amyl	138	2.7^{22}
Hexyl	157.2	0.59^{20}
Heptyl	176	0.09^{18}
Ethers		
Dimethyl	−23.65	$3,700^{18}(cm.^3)$
Ethyl methyl ..	7.9	s.
Diethyl	34.6	7.5^{20}
Methyl-*n*-butyl .	70.3	v. sl. s.
Ethyl-*n*-butyl ..	91.4	i.
Alkanes		
Propane	−42.17	$6.5^{18}(cm.^3)$
Butane	−0.6 to −0.3	$15\frac{17}{772}(cm.^3)$
Pentane	36.2	0.036^{16}
Hexane	69.0	$0.0138^{15.5}$
Heptane	98.52	$0.0052^{15.5}$

sion and thus are marketed in the form of a 1:10 trituration with lactose. They are hydrolyzed readily by alkalies to the alcohol and the nitrate salt.

$$
\begin{matrix}
CH_2{-}O{-}NO_2 \\
| \\
CH{-}O{-}NO_2 \\
| \\
CH_2{-}O{-}NO_2
\end{matrix}
+\ 3\,NaOH \longrightarrow
\begin{matrix}
CH_2OH \\
| \\
CHOH \\
| \\
CH_2OH
\end{matrix}
+\ 3\,NaNO_3
$$

Glyceryl Trinitrate   Glycerol

CARBONATE ESTERS. *Creosote carbonate* (Creosotal) is a mixture of the carbonates of the constituents of wood-tar creosote. It is a colorless to yellowish, clear, viscid liquid. This compound is insoluble in water but is soluble in alcohol, chloroform and fixed oils. In the presence of alkalies, it is hydrolyzed to the carbonate and various phenolic constituents of creosote which are, chiefly, guaiacol and creosol (methyl guaiacol).

Guaiacol   Creosol

ETHERS

Solubility. The ethers are neutral, unreactive, organic compounds. When the boiling points and the water solubility of ethers are compared with those of alcohols of a comparable molecular weight, it is observed that the substitution of a nonpolar alkyl group for the hydrogen of the —OH group causes a great change in these physical constants. This type of substitution removes the hydrogen bond function of the —OH group causing the ethers to resemble in some respects the low-boiling nonpolar hydrocarbons. This also results in a decreased tendency to associate with water, which causes a decrease in their water-solubility. The boiling points of the ethers are also lower than those of alcohols of comparable molecular weight, since, as previously explained, the ethers, like the alkanes, are poorly associated, whereas the alcohols are highly associated through hydrogen bonding.

The ethers, being relatively nonpolar, are insoluble in the highly polar solvents but are readily soluble in the nonpolar solvents.

Formulation Problems. The ethers give rise to few incompatibilities since they are very unreactive and are used but sparingly per se in pharmaceutical preparations. Ethers may be cleaved by hydriodic acid to the corresponding alcohol and alkyl iodide, but this reaction requires drastic conditions (refluxing for 2 hours or more), not normally encountered in manufacturing procedures or pharmaceutical dispensing practice. This reaction may be considered to be an electrophilic attack by the hydrogen ion on the oxygen.[77]

$$R{-}CH_2{-}\overset{\circ\circ}{\underset{\circ\circ}{O}}{-}CH_2{-}R \longrightarrow R{-}CH_2OH + I^- + R{-}\overset{+}{CH_2}$$

$$HI$$

$$R{-}\overset{+}{CH_2} + I^- \longrightarrow R{-}CH_2I$$

ETHER (diethyl ether, $CH_3{-}CH_2{-}O{-}CH_2{-}CH_3$), although seldom used in the actual filling of prescriptions, is used extensively as a solvent in the pharmaceutical industry. Ether is an excellent extraction medium, as it is generally a good solvent for most organic compounds and dissolves only a very few inorganic substances. It is immiscible with water and separates out as a discrete upper layer. Because of the high volatility of ether, it is removed easily by distillation from extracts at a temperature (34.6° C.) which does not destroy the extracted principles.

When ether is exposed to air and light for long periods of time, it is oxidized to a nonvolatile peroxide which, on removal of the solvent, becomes explosive when heated. The following substances have been identified tentatively in the ether-peroxide mixture:

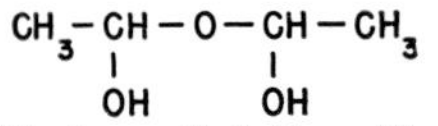

Dihydroxyethyl Peroxide 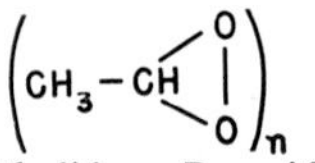   Ethylidene Peroxide Polymer

Ether is somewhat soluble in water (7.5 Gm. per 100 ml.) and is soluble in strong acids. The solubility in acids is due to the basic character of the oxygen. The oxygen possesses unshared electron pairs and is, therefore, nucleophilic. That is, it is capable of donating electrons. One pair of the unshared electrons thus coordinates with the proton of the acid to produce a salt, as shown in the following reaction.[50]

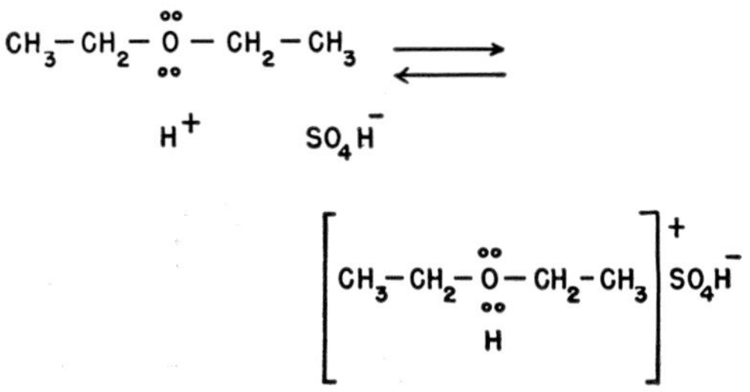

BASIC NITROGEN-CONTAINING COMPOUNDS

AMINES

The amines are derivatives of ammonia in which one, two or three of the hydrogens are replaced by an alkyl group. They are designated as primary, secondary or tertiary amines, depending on the number of hydrogens which are replaced.

Solubility. The amines have slightly higher

limits of solubility in water than the alcohols and other oxygen-containing compounds.

The lower amines are soluble in water due to the presence of the unshared electron pair on the nitrogen which makes it possible for them to associate with water through hydrogen bonding.[80]

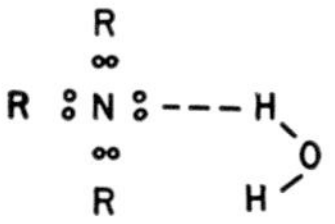

As the length of the alkyl chain is increased, they lose their ability to compete with water for a place in the association complex and become water-insoluble.

The water-insoluble amines are soluble in dilute acid solutions by virtue of the unshared electron pair contained on the nitrogen. This unshared electron pair coordinates with the proton of the acid to form a water-soluble ionized salt.

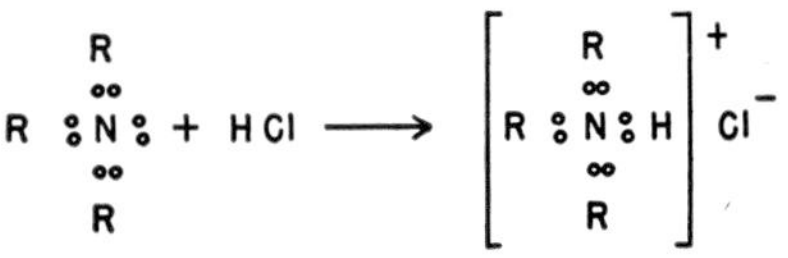

Thus, the acid salts

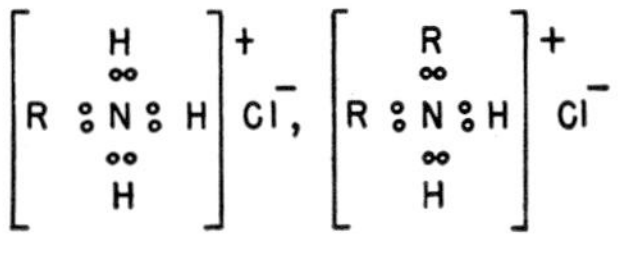

and

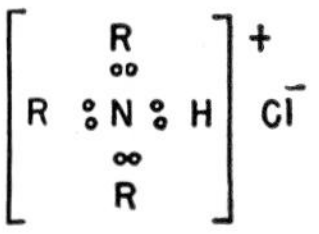

of these basic nitrogen compounds are water-soluble, since the highly polar compound, water, is able to rupture the ionic bonds and solubilize the compounds through an ion-dipole mechanism as it does in a similar manner with NaCl. Due to their ionic nature, these compounds are insoluble in the nonpolar solvents such as ether, chloroform, benzene, carbon tetrachloride, etc.

The basic nitrogen in a primary, secondary or tertiary amine is capable of carrying

TABLE 10-16. COMPARISON OF THE WATER
SOLUBILITY OF SOME AMINES AND
ALCOHOLS

COMPOUND	SOLUBILITY IN GM. PER 100 ML. OF H_2O
Amine	
Ethyl	∞
Propyl	∞
n-Butyl	∞
n-Amyl	s.
n-Hexyl	sl. s.
n-Heptyl	sl. s.
n-Octyl	sl. s.
n-Nonyl	sl. s.
Alcohol	
Ethyl	∞
n-Propyl	∞
n-Butyl	7.9^{20}
n-Amyl	2.7^{22}
n-Hexyl	0.59^{20}
n-Heptyl	0.09^{18}
n-Octyl	i.
n-Nonyl	i.

approximately 5 carbon atoms into aqueous solution.[56] The ratio of the number of basic nitrogen groups to the molecular weight of the compound is operative in the same manner as it applies in —OH-containing compounds, e.g., *n*-hexylamine [$CH_3(CH_2)_5$-NH_2] is only slightly soluble, whereas 1,6-hexanediamine [$NH_2(CH_2)_6NH_2$] is very soluble in water.

The aliphatic amines are more basic than ammonia, a fact which is borne out by their pK_a values. In fact, trimethylamine is capable of displacing the weaker base, ammonia.[15] However, when an acidic group (electrophilic, electron acceptor) replaces one or more of the hydrogens of ammonia, a decrease in the basicity is obtained. In this case, the electron pair bonding the nitrogen to the acidic group is held more closely to the acidic group, which, in turn, causes the unshared electron pair of the nitrogen to be held more closely to the nitrogen. This then decreases the ability of the nitrogen to hydrogen-bond with water and, also, decreases its ability to coordinate with the proton of an acid in salt formation. More specifically, in Table 10-17, it may be observed that aniline is much less

basic than the alkyl-substituted compounds. The basic —NH_2 (electron donor) group of aniline contains an unshared pair of electrons which it can share with the acidic (electrophilic) phenyl group.[51] In the light of the preceding discussion, it is obvious that in the following structure the unshared electron pair of the nitrogen is no longer as readily available either for hydrogen bonding with water or for coordinating with the proton of an acid

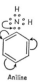

Aniline

to form a salt. The electronic shifts indicated in the above structure also account for the high reactivity of the ortho and the para positions with respect to electrophilic reagents. The ortho and the para positions are centers of high electron density and react with reagents which can accept electrons.

The effect of decreasing water-solubility by substituent groups which replace one or more hydrogens on the basic nitrogen is readily borne out when benzylamine and aniline are compared. Aniline is soluble in water to the extent of 3.4 Gm. per 100 ml.; whereas benzylamine, which contains one more carbon atom, is miscible in all proportions. The increased solubility of benzylamine over aniline in water is due to the fact that a methylene group is interposed between the phenyl group and the amino group so that the amino group in this case is not conjugated with unsaturation as in the case of

TABLE 10-17. pK_a VALUES OF SOME
ORGANIC BASES

BASE	pK_a
Ammonium hydroxide	9.26
Methylamine	10.7
Dimethylamine	10.72
Trimethylamine	9.87
Ethylamine	10.75
Diethylamine	11.1
Triethylamine	10.81
Pyridine	5.36
Aniline	4.66
Piperidine	11.2

aniline. This makes it impossible for the unshared electrons to shift and increase the covalency between the nitrogen and the aromatic nucleus.

Other acidic groups when substituted for a hydrogen of ammonia have a similar effect in decreasing the basicity of the nitrogen. The amides may be taken as an example. In this case, the shift of a pair of electrons from the double bond between the carbon and the oxygen tends to cause an electron deficiency on the carbon atom which, in turn, is satisfied

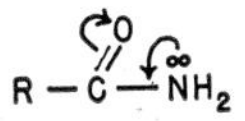

$$R-\overset{\overset{\displaystyle O}{\parallel}}{C}-NH_2$$

by the shift of the unshared electron pair of the nitrogen to cause an increase in the covalency between the nitrogen and the carbon. Since the oxygen has acquired a share of an electron pair, it has become negatively charged, and the nitrogen, having given up a share of an electron pair, has become positively charged. If the molecule were completely polarized, it could be represented by the following structure:

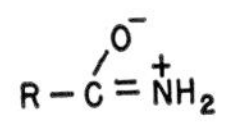

$$R-\overset{\overset{\displaystyle O^-}{\parallel}}{C}=\overset{+}{N}H_2$$

However, it exists in the more stable intermediate form or hybrid between the conventional structure and that shown above. Although water-solubility is not greatly affected in the case of the amides derived from ammonia, some decrease is observed: (n-nonylamine, $CH_3(CH_2)_7CH_2NH_2$ is slightly soluble in water; pelargonamide, $CH_3(CH_2)_7CONH_2$ is insoluble). The lower solubility, in this case, is caused by the decreased availability of the unshared electron pair of the nitrogen which is necessary for hydrogen bonding. A great decrease in the basicity of the nitrogen also is observed (see Table 10-17), and the amides have a neutral reaction to dilute acid solution. However, water-insoluble amides are sufficiently basic to dissolve in more concentrated acid solutions.

Actually, sufficient substitution of acidic groups for the hydrogens of ammonia may progress to the point where the nitrogen no longer retains its basic properties, and a re-

maining hydrogen on the nitrogen becomes acidic. Such is the case with succinimide

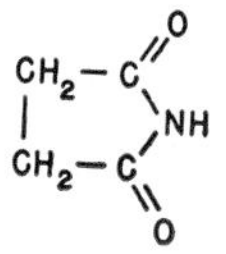

and phthalimide

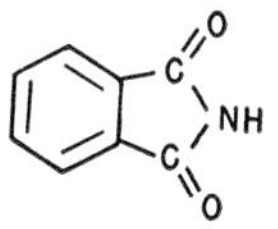

Phthalimide is practically insoluble in water but dissolves readily in alkali. The sulfonamides and the barbiturates, which will be discussed in detail later in the chapter, are also examples of nitrogen-containing compounds with sufficiently strong acidic substitution to cause a remaining hydrogen to become acidic.

ALKALOIDS AND CHEMICALLY RELATED COMPOUNDS

In this chapter, the reader will observe that alkaloids are not treated as a separate class of compounds possessing incompatibilities peculiar only to them but that the discussion includes many chemically related substances having similar incompatibilities.

Alkaloids. Because the substances of this group differ so greatly in chemical composition, and since no one definition is sufficient to include all the various compounds, pharmaceutical chemists have commonly resorted to an enumeration of some of the chemical and physical characteristics of alkaloids in lieu of a definition. (Synthetic substances may have similar properties to those alkaloids of vegetable or animal origin.) Therefore, they have been stated to be white crystalline substances—although a very few are colored (e.g., berberine), and some of the oxygen-free compounds are liquids (e.g., nicotine, coniine, etc.). Most of the compounds of this class react with alkyl halides to give crystalline addition products. They give characteristic reactions with the commonly termed "alkaloidal reagents." The free alkaloids are usually water-insoluble but soluble in dilute acid solutions and the organic solvents, whereas the alkaloidal salts are soluble in water and alcohol but insoluble in the less polar organic solvents such as ether, chloroform and the fixed oils (Table 10-18). However, in determining the water-solubility of the free base of alkaloids and other chemically related compounds, it must be borne in mind that the basic nitrogen is capable of carrying approximately 5 carbon atoms into solution.[56] Thus, such substances as antipyrine, aminopyrine, caffeine, etc., are water-soluble (p. 383).

The nitrogen which is contained in the molecule and which must be present in order for these substances to be labeled as alkaloids may occur in the form of primary, secondary and tertiary (either aliphatic or cyclic) amines. Other forms of nitrogen combinations such as acid amides, acid imides, cyanides, quaternary ammonium, amino-imine, diamino-imino, imine and triamine groups also may be present along with the *amines* in the alkaloid molecule.[26]

Although the presence of nitrogen is essential in alkaloids, they also contain many other functional groups which contribute to the activity of the compound from the chemical, the physical and the physiologic standpoint. These functional groups include primary, secondary and teritary alcohols, ketones, aldehydes, carboxylic acids, esters, methyl ethers, methylene ethers and phenols.[38]

Classification of Some Alkaloids and Chemically Related Compounds (Basic N-Containing Compounds)

I. Alkylamine Group

A. PRIMARY AMINE

1. *Tuamine* (2-aminoheptane)

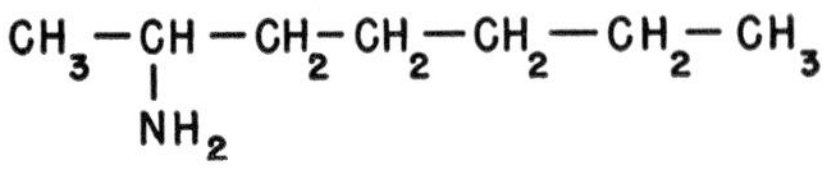

B. TERTIARY AMINES (Dimethylethylamino group)

1. *Diphenhydramine Hydrochloride* (Benadryl Hydrochloride; β-dimethylaminoethyl benzhydryl ether hydrochloride)

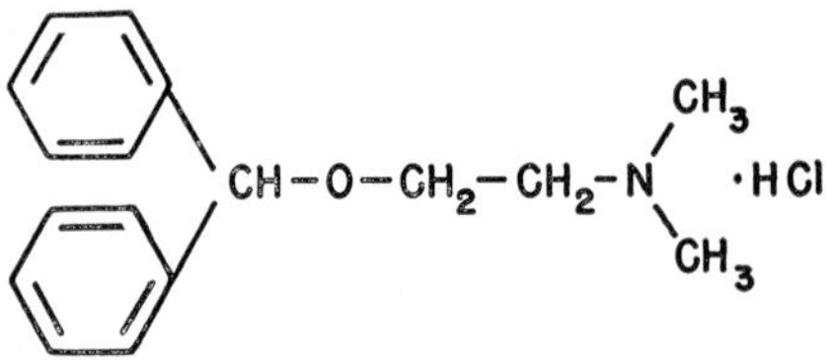

2. *Tripelennamine   Hydrochloride* (Pyribenzamine; pyridylbenzyl-dimethylethylenediamine hydrochloride)

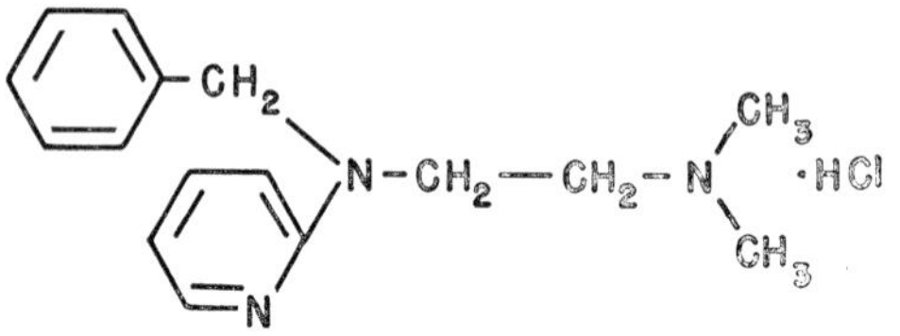

3. *Thenylpyramine   Hydrochloride* (Histadyl; Thenylene, N,N-dimethyl-N′ (2-thenyl)-N′ (2-pyridyl)-ethylenediamine hydrochloride)

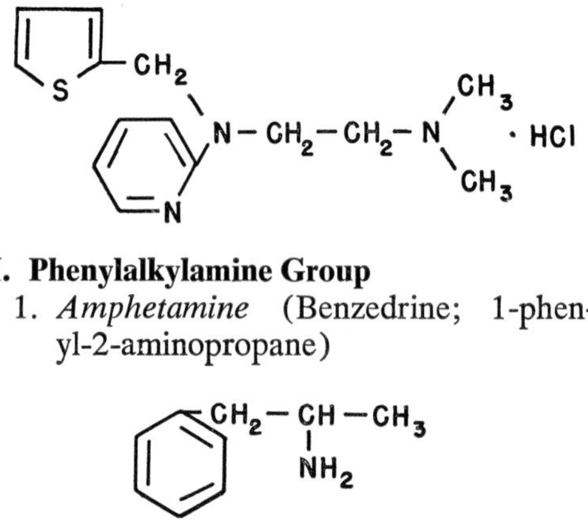

II. Phenylalkylamine Group

1. *Amphetamine* (Benzedrine; 1-phenyl-2-aminopropane)

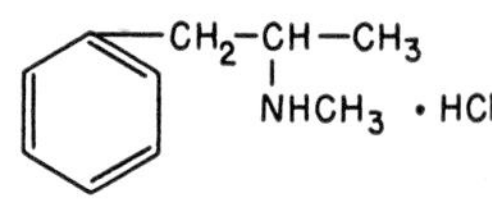

2. *Methamphetamine   Hydrochloride* (Desoxyephedrine Hydrochloride; 1-phenyl-2-methylaminopropane)

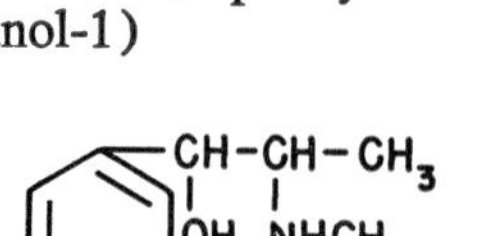

3. *Ephedrine* (1-phenyl-2-methylaminepropanol-1)

4. *Epinephrine* (Adrenalin; methylamino-ethanolcatechol)

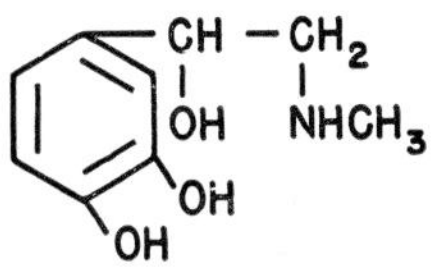

$$CH_3-CH_2-\overset{\overset{O}{\|}}{C}-C-CH_2-CH-N\overset{CH_3}{\underset{CH_3}{\diagup}}$$

(with two phenyl rings and a CH_3 branch on the central carbon)

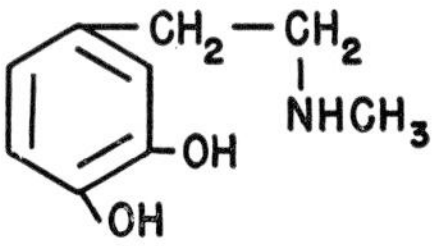

6. *Phenylephrine Hydrochloride* (Neosynephrine; α-hydroxy-β-methylamino-3-hydroxy ethylbenzene hydrochloride)

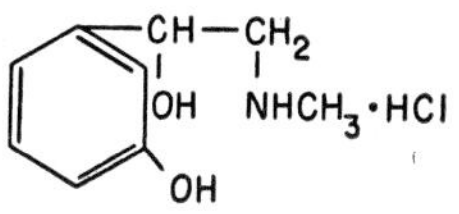

7. *Nethamine* (1-phenyl-2-methylethyl-amino-propanol-1)

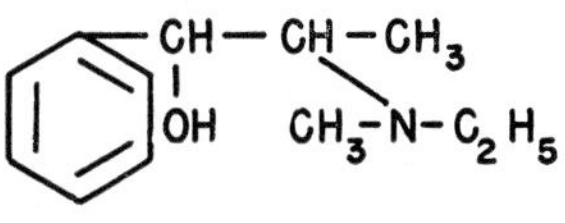

8. *Paredrine* (*p*-hydroxy-1-phenyl-2-amino-propane)

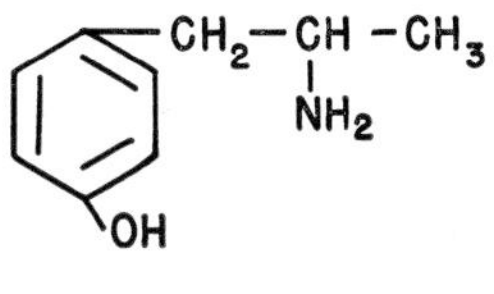

9. *Phenylpropanolamine* (Propadrine; 1-phenyl-2-amino-propanol-1)

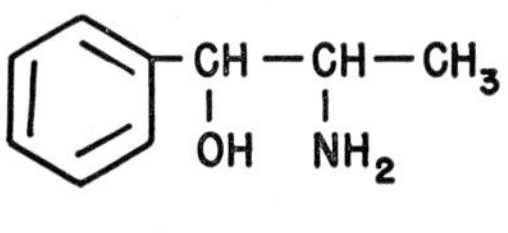

III. Diphenylalkylamine Group
1. *Methadon* (Dolophine; 4,4-diphenyl-6-dimethylaminoheptanone-3)

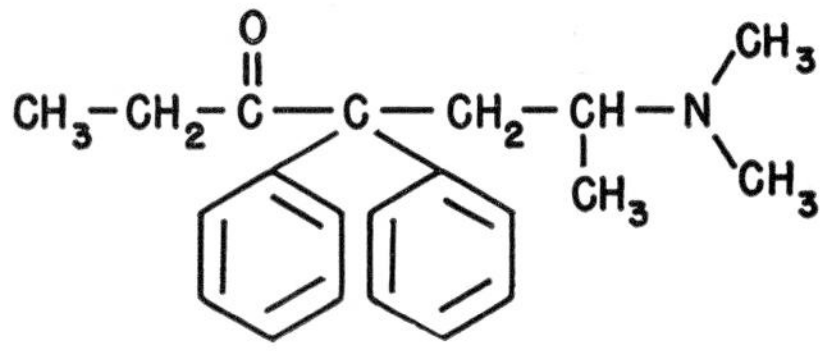

IV. Alkanolamine Group
1. *Triethanolamine*

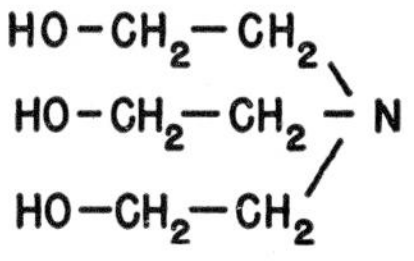

$$
\begin{aligned}
HO-CH_2-CH_2 \\
HO-CH_2-CH_2 \\
HO-CH_2-CH_2
\end{aligned}
\Big\rangle N
$$

A. *p*-Aminobenzoic Acid Derivatives
1. *Procaine Hydrochloride* (Novocain; *p*-amino-benzoyl diethylamino-ethanol hydrochloride)

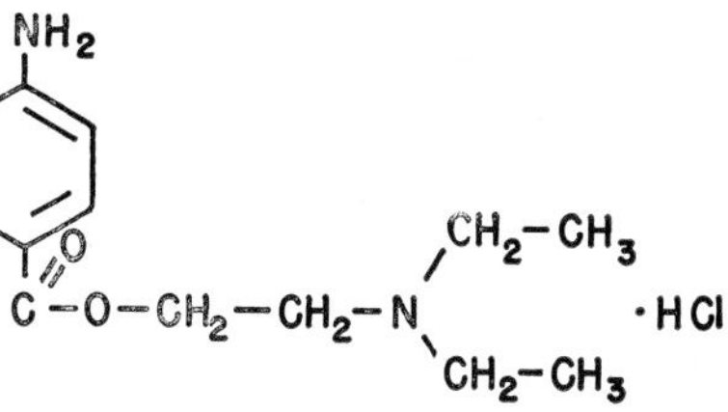

2. *Butacaine Sulfate* (Butyn Sulfate; *p*-amino-benzoyl-dibutylamino-propanol sulfate)

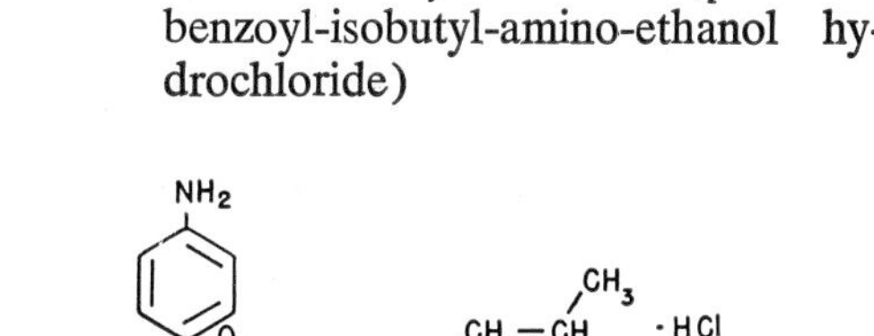

3. *Monocaine Hydrochloride* (*p*-amino-benzoyl-isobutyl-amino-ethanol hydrochloride)

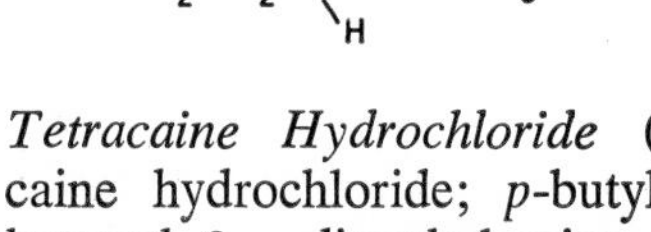

4. *Tetracaine Hydrochloride* (Pontocaine hydrochloride; *p*-butylamino-benzoyl-β dimethylamino-ethanol hydrochloride)

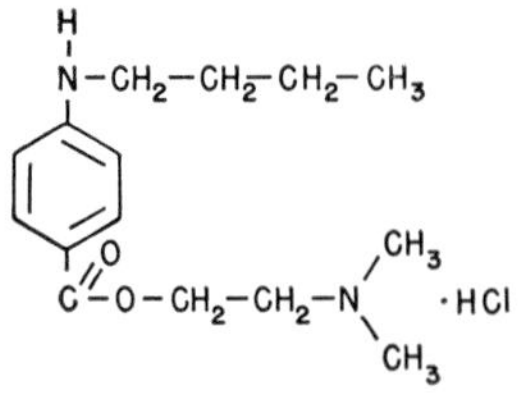

5. *Amylsine Hydrochloride* (Naepaine Hydrochloride; mono-*n*-amyl-amino-ethyl-*p*-amino-benzoate hydrochloride)

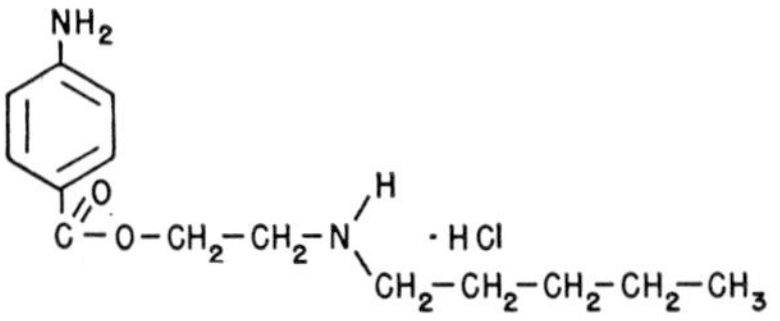

B. BENZOIC ACID DERIVATIVE
   1. *Intracaine Hydrochloride* (Diethoxin; β-diethylaminoethyl-*p*-ethoxybenzoate hydrochloride)

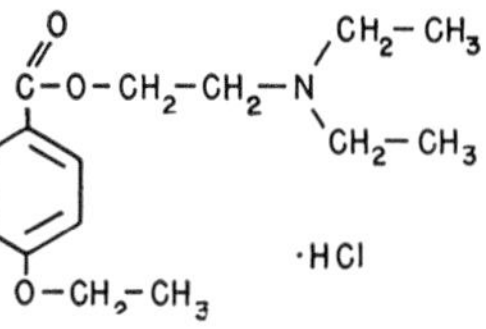

C. TROPIC ACID DERIVATIVE
   1. *Syntropan* (tropic acid ester of 3-diethylamino-2,2-dimethyl-1-propanol phosphate)

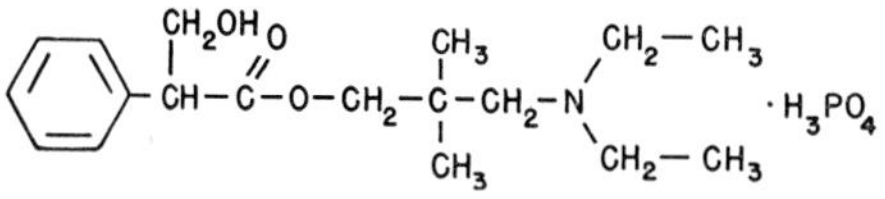

D. DIPHENYLACETIC ACID DERIVATIVE
   1. *Trasentine* (diphenylacetyldiethyl-amino-ethanol hydrochloride)

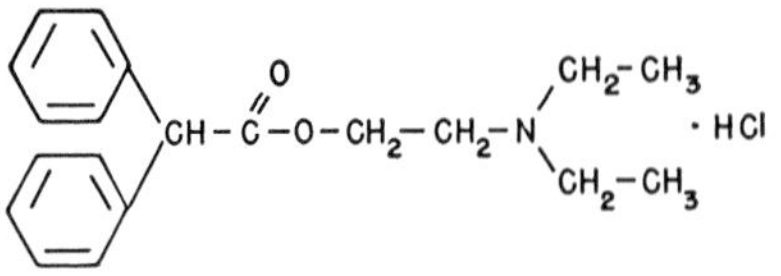

V. Pyridine Group
   1. *Pelletierine*

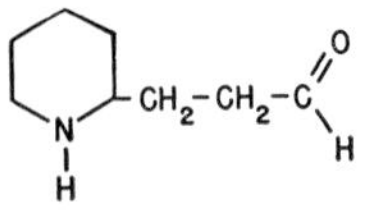

2. *Sparteine Sulfate*

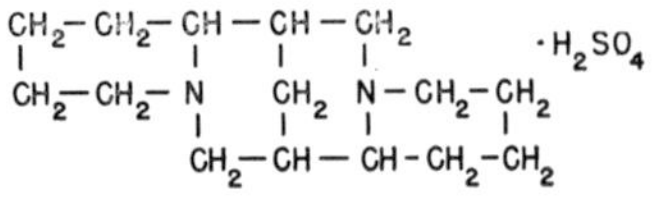

3. *Coniine*

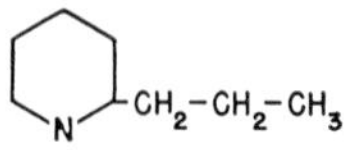

VI. Pyridine-Pyrrolidine Group
   1. *Nicotine*

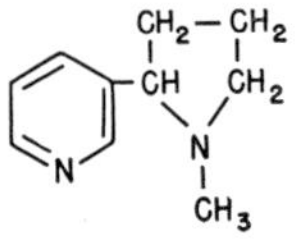

VII. Condensed Piperidine-Pyrrolidine Group (Tropine)
   1. *Atropine*

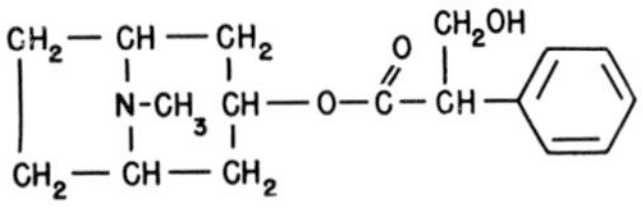

2. *Homatropine Hydrobromide*

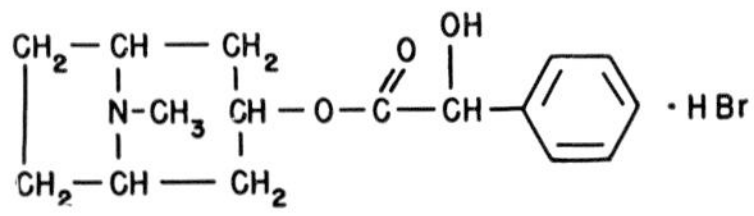

3. *Scopolamine Hydrobromide* (Hyoscine)

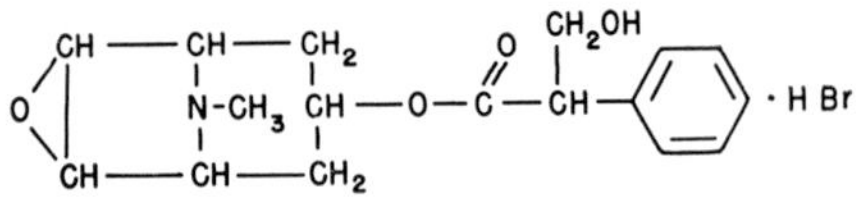

4. *Cocaine*

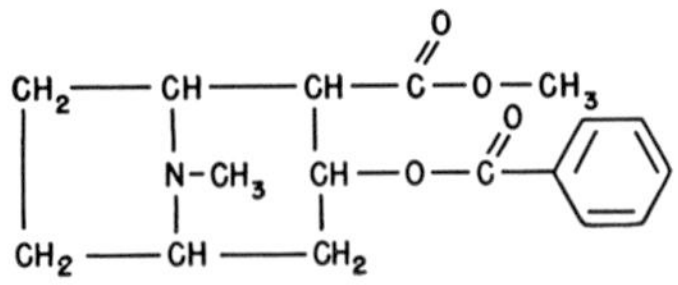

VIII. Quinoline Group

1. *Quinine*

2. *Quinidine Sulfate* (Dextro isomer of quinine)
3. *Totaquine* (Contains the total alkaloids of cinchona)
4. *Cinchonine Sulfate*

5. *Cinchonidine Sulfate* (Levo isomer of cinchonine)
6. *Pamaquine* [plasmochine; 6-methoxy-8-(1-methyl-4-diethylamino) butyl-aminoquinoline]

7. *Eucupin* (Isoamylhydrocupreine)

8. *Oxyquinoline*

IX. Isoquinoline Group

1. *Papaverine Hydrochloride*

2. *Morphine Sulfate*

3. *Codeine*

4. *Ethylmorphine Hydrochloride* (Dionin)

5. *Apomorphine Hydrochloride*

6. *Dihydromorphinone Hydrochloride* (Dilaudid)

7. *Dihydrocodeinone* (Mercodeinone, Hycodan, Dicodid)

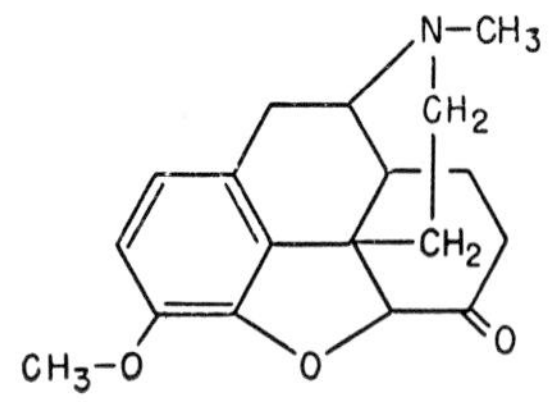

8. *Nalorphine Hydrochloride*
   (Nalline Hydrochloride)

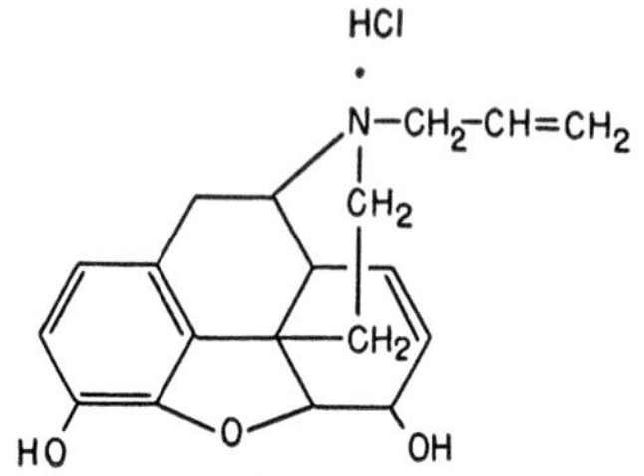

9. *Methyldihydromorphinone Hydrochloride* (Metopon Hydrochloride)

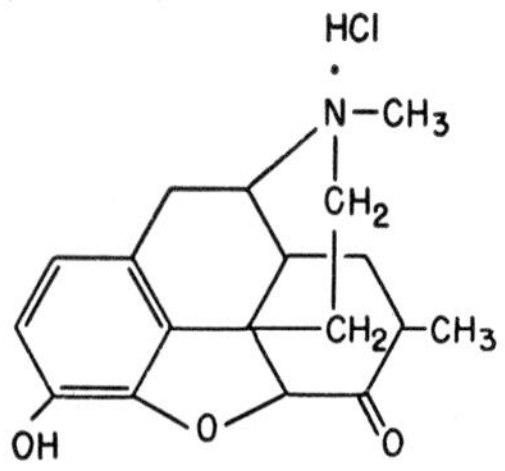

10. *Colchicine*

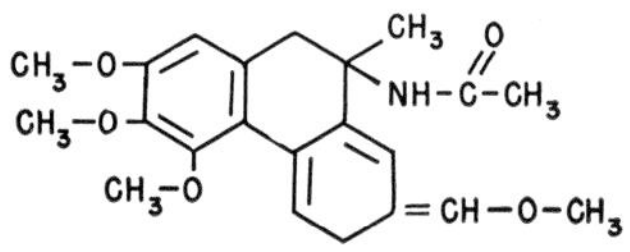

X. Indole Group

1. *Physostigmine Salicylate* (Eserine salicylate)

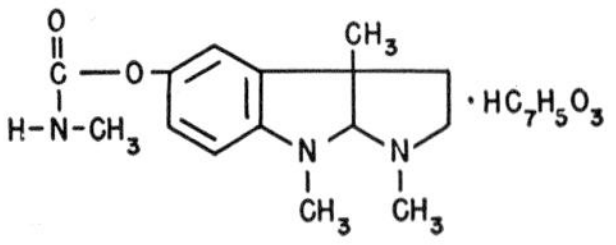

2. *Strychnine Sulfate*

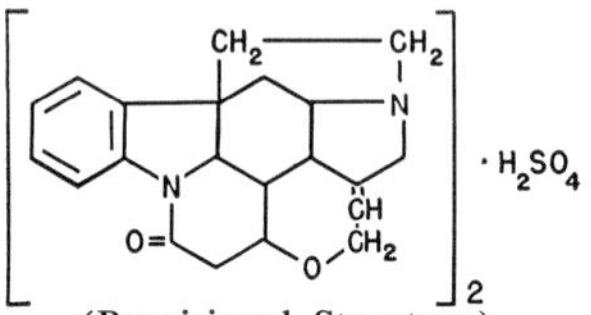

(Provisional Structure)

3. *Ergotoxine*[39]

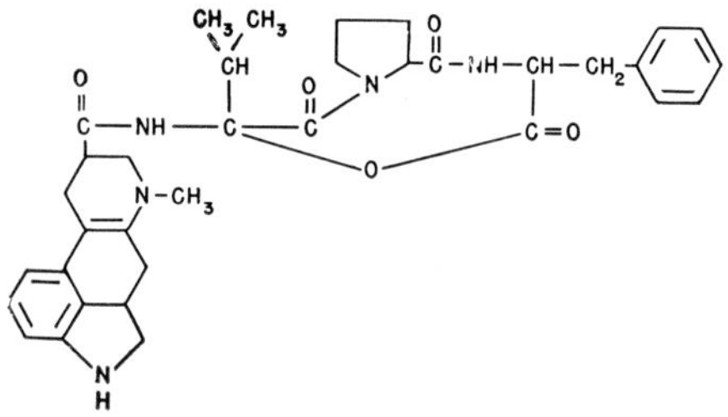

4. *Ergonovine Maleate*
5. *Ergotamine Tartrate*
6. *Reserpine*

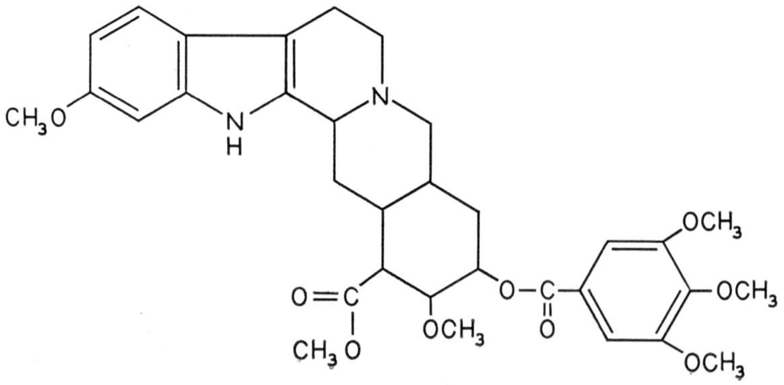

XI. Imidazole Group

1. *Pilocarpine Nitrate*

2. *Naphazoline Hydrochloride* (Privine Hydrochloride; 2(naphthyl-(1')-methyl)-imidazoline hydrochloride)

3. *Histamine Phosphate* (4-imidazolylethylamine phosphate)

XII. Pyrazole Group

1. *Antipyrine* (Phenazone; 1,5-dimethyl-2-phenyl-3-pyrazolone)

2. *Aminopyrine* (Amidopyrine, Pyramidon; 1,5-dimethyl-2-phenyl-4-dimethylamino-3-pyrazolone)

XIII. Piperidine Group

1. *Meperidine Hydrochloride* (Demerol Hydrochloride, Isonipecaine, Dolanthin, Pethidine; ethyl-1-methyl-4-phenyl piperidine-4-carboxylate hydrochloride)

2. *Piperocaine Hydrochloride* (Metycaine; benzoyl-γ-(2-methylpiperidino)-propanol hydrochloride)

3. *Surfacaine* (Cyclomethycaine; p-cyclohexyloxybenzoyl-γ-(2-methylpiperidino)-propanol hydrochloride)

4. *Diothane* (Piperidinopropanediol-diphenylurethane hydrochloride)

XIV. Aniline Group

1. *Phenacaine Hydrochloride* (Holocaine; ethenyl-p,-p'-diethoxydiphenylamidine hydrochloride)

XV. Purine Group

1. *Caffeine* (1,3,7-trimethylxanthine)

2. *Theophylline* (1,3-dimethylxanthine)

3. *Theobromine* (3,7-dimethylxanthine)

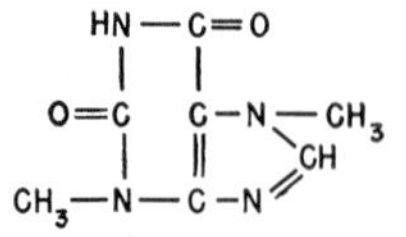

XVI. Guanidine Group

1. *Chloroguanide Hydrochloride*
   (Guanatol Hydrochloride; N_1-*p*-
   chloro-phenyl-N_5-isopropyl
   biguanide hydrochloride)

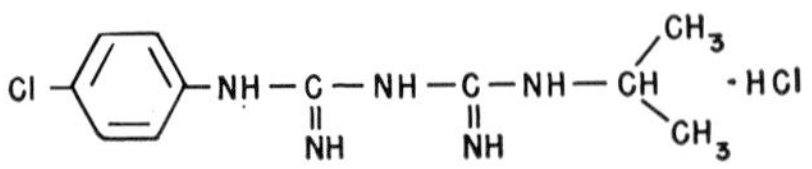

XVII. Phenothiazine Group

1. *Promethazine* (10-(2 dimethylamino-
   propyl)-phenothiazine)

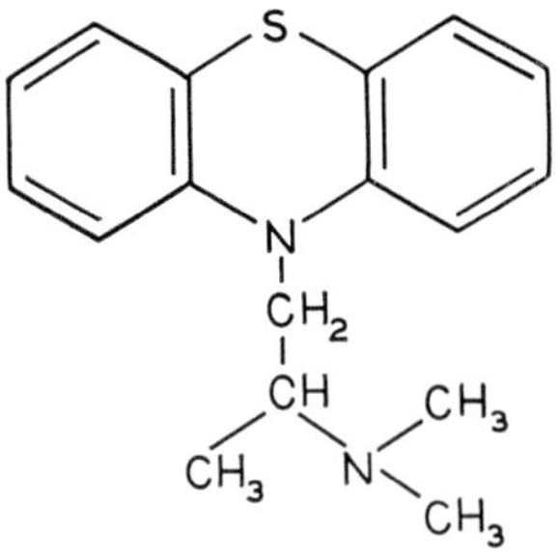

2. *Promazine* (10-(3 dimethylamino-
   propyl)-phenothiazine)

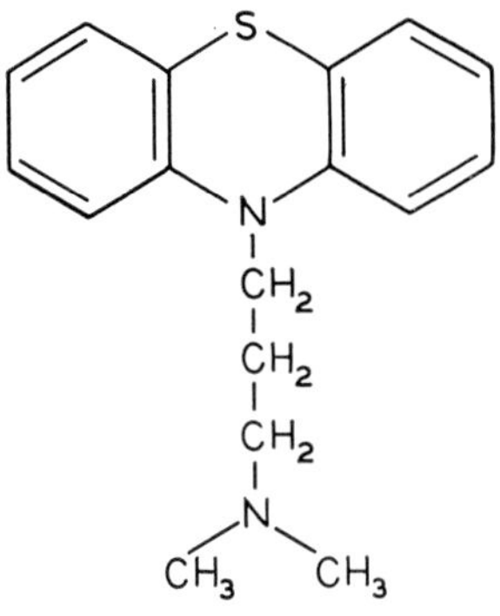

3. *Chlorpromazine* (Thorazine; 2-chloro-
   10-(3 dimethoyaminopropyl)-
   phenothiazine)

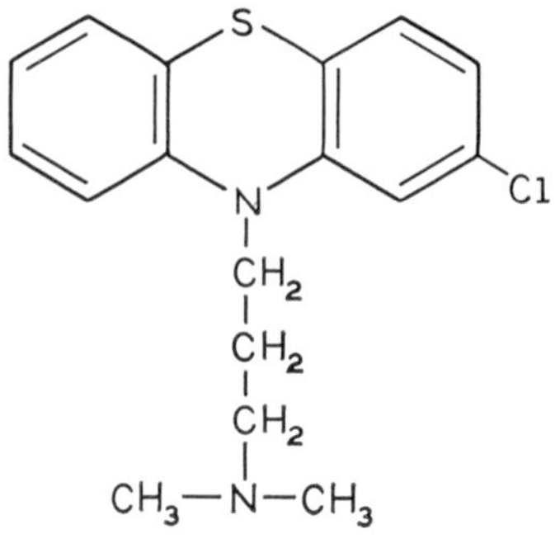

Formulation Problems. The alkaloids and chemically related compounds containing trivalent nitrogen are capable of forming water-soluble salts with acids. The unshared electron pair of the nitrogen coordinates with the proton of the acid to form the corresponding water-soluble ionized salt. Problems may thus result from attempts at dispensing these water-soluble mineral acid salts in an aqueous medium having an alkaline reaction, in which case the free base is precipitated, provided that it is not sufficiently water-soluble to remain in solution as such. This is perhaps the most frequently occurring type of incompatibility for this class of compounds. Included in the list of compounds which give an alkaline reaction in aqueous solution are the soluble hydroxides, carbonates, bicarbonates, the alkali citrates, tartrates, acetates, the sodium salts of barbiturates, the sodium salts of sulfonamides, etc. The following examples, while typical of the alkaloids, also are applicable to the chemically related synthetic compounds included in the previous classification:

1. Alkaloidal salt (HCl) + NaOH → free alkaloid + NaCl + H_2O
   (water-soluble)   (water-insoluble)
2. Alkaloidal salt (HCl) + sodium phenobarbital →free alkaloid + free phenobarbital + NaCl
   (water-soluble)   (water-insoluble)   (water-insoluble)
3. Alkaloid salt (HCl) + sodium citrate → free alkaloid + citric acid + NaCl
   (water-soluble)   (water-insoluble) (water-soluble)

TABLE 10-18. SOLUBILITIES OF SOME ALKALOIDS AND CHEMICALLY RELATED SYNTHETIC COMPOUNDS (BASIC N-CONTAINING COMPOUNDS)

	SOLUBILITY IN GM. PER 100 ML. OF		
	Water	Alcohol	Ether, etc.
1. Acetylcholine chloride	s.	s.	i. eth.
2. Aminopyrine, U.S.P.	5.5	66	7.6 eth.
3. Amphetamine (Benzedrine)	sl. s.	s.	s. eth.
4. Amphetamine sulfate (Benzedrine Sulfate)	s.	sl. s.	i. eth.
5. Amylsine hydrochloride (Amylcaine) ...	s.	sl. s.	i. eth.
6. Antipyrine	100	100	2.6 eth.
7. Apomorphine	sl. s.	s.	s. eth.
8. Apomorphine hydrochloride	2	2.47	0.053 eth.
9. Atropine	0.11^{25}	68.5	5.6 eth.; 64 chl.
10. Atropine sulfate	260	27	0.05 eth.; 0.16 chl.
11. Benzalkonium chloride (Zephiran Chloride)	s.	s.	i. eth.
12. Butacaine sulfate (Butyn)	100	s.	i. eth.; sl. s. chl.
13. Butyl aminobenzoate (Butesin)	0.00014	s.	s. eth., chl.
14. Caffeine	1.35^{16}	2.3^{16}	0.044 eth.; 14.2 chl.
15. Carbachol	100	2	i. eth., chl.
16. Chlorpromazine hydrochloride	100	66.6	s. chl., i. eth.
17. Cinchonidine	$0.019^{11.5}$	4.81	0.41 eth.; s. chl.
18. Cinchonidine sulfate	1.54	1.37	0.024 eth.; 0.16 chl.
19. Cinchonine	0.027^{20}	0.795^{20}	0.27 eth.; s. chl.
20. Cinchonine sulfate	1.55^{13}	17^{11}	0.043 eth.; 2.1 chl.
21. Cocaine	0.16^{25}	20^{25}	26.3 eth.; s. chl.
22. Cocaine hydrochloride	250^{25}	38.4^{25}	i. eth.
23. Codeine	0.83^{25}	62.5^{25}	8.0 eth.; s. chl.
24. Codeine phosphate	44.5^{25}	0.38^{25}	0.07 eth.
25. Codeine sulfate	3.3^{25}	0.1^{25}	i. eth., chl.
26. Coniine	1.1	∞	v. sl. s. eth.
27. Meperidine hydrochloride (Demerol Hydrochloride)	s.	sl. s.	i. eth.
28. Methamphetamine (Desoxyephedrine) ..	v. sl. s.	s.	s. eth.
29. Methamphetamine hydrochloride (Desoxyephedrine Hydrochloride) ...	s.	sl. s.	i. eth.
30. Dihydromorphinone hydrochloride (Dilaudid)	33	sp. s.	i. eth.
31. Diothane Hydrochloride	sl. s.	s.	i. eth.
32. Diphenhydramine hydrochloride (Benadryl)	s.	s.	i. eth.
33. Ephedrine	s.	s.	s. eth., chl.
34. Ephedrine hydrochloride	33	7.14	i. eth.
35. Ephedrine sulfate	s.	s. h.	i. eth.
36. Epinephrine	0.027^{17}	sl. s.	i. eth., chl.
37. Epinephrine hydrochloride	s.	s.	i. eth.
38. Epinine	sl. s.	sl. s.	....
39. Ergonovine (Ergometrine)	sl. s.	sl. s.	sp. s. chl.
40. Ergonovine maleate (Ergotrate)	2.77	.83	i. eth., chl.
41. Ergotamine	sl. s.	s.	s. eth., chl.
42. Ergotamine tartrate	0.2	0.2	....
43. Ergotoxine	v. sl. s.	s. h.	sl. s. eth.
44. Ethyl aminobenzoate (Benzocaine, Anesthesin)	0.04	20	50 chl.; 25 eth.
45. Ethyl morphine hydrochloride (Dionin) .	10	4	sl. s. eth., chl.
46. Eucupin (Isomylhydrocupreine)	i.	s.	s. eth.

TABLE 10-18. SOLUBILITIES OF SOME ALKALOIDS AND CHEMICALLY RELATED SYNTHETIC COMPOUNDS (BASIC N-CONTAINING COMPOUNDS) (*Continued*)

	SOLUBILITY IN GM. PER 100 ML. OF		
	Water	Alcohol	Ether, etc.
47. Chloroguanide hydrochloride (Guanatol Hydrochloride)	sp. s.	s.	i. eth.
48. Histamine	s.	sl. s.	
49. Histamine phosphate	25		
50. Homatropine hydrobromide	17.5^{25}	3.3	0.23 chl.; i. eth.
51. Intracaine hydrochloride (Diethoxin)	s.	s.	
52. Methacholine chloride (Mecholyl)	s.	s.	s. chl.
53. Methadone hydrochloride	s.	s.	i. eth.
54. Metycaine hydrochloride	s.	s.	s. chl.; i. eth.
55. Monocaine hydrochloride	sp. s.	sl. s.	sl. s. chl.; i. eth.
56. Morphine	0.03	0.39	0.02 eth.; s. chl.
57. Morphine sulfate	6.66	0.22	i. eth., chl.
58. Morphine hydrochloride	5.72	2.38	i. eth., chl.
59. Nalorphine hydrochloride (Nalline Hydrochloride)	s.	6.1	v. sl. s. chl.; i. eth.
60. Neostigmine bromide (Prostigmin Bromide)	100	s.	i. eth.
61. Neostigmine methylsulfate (Prostigmin Methylsulfate)	10	s.	i. eth.
62. Phenylephrine hydrochloride (Neosynephrine Hydrochloride)	s.	s.	i. eth.
63. Nethamine hydrochloride	70	14	
64. Nicotine	s.	s.	s. eth., chl.
65. Nicotine hydrochloride	s.	s.	
66. Oxyquinoline	i.	s.	
67. Oxyquinoline sulfate	s.		
68. Pamaquine naphthoate (Plasmochin)	i.	s.	s. acet.
69. Papaverine	v. sl. s.	v. s.	0.39 eth.
70. Papaverine hydrochloride	2.7^{18}	s.	i. eth.
71. Paredrine hydrobromide	s.		
72. Pelletierine	5	s.	s. eth., chl.
73. Pelletierine tannate	0.4	s.	sl. s. eth.; i. chl.
74. Phemerol Chloride	s.	s.	i. eth.
75. Phenacaine hydrochloride (Holocaine)	s.		i. eth.
76. Physostigmine (Eserine)	sl. s.	s.	s. eth., chl.
77. Physostigmine salicylate (Eserine)	1.33	7.71	0.57 eth.; s. chl.
78. Pilocarpine	s.	s.	sl. s. eth.; s. chl.
79. Pilocarpine hydrochloride	333	37^{25}	i. eth.; sl. s. chl.
80. Pilocarpine nitrate	10^{20}	6.2^{60}	i. eth., chl.
81. Naphazoline hydrochloride (Privine Hydrochloride)	s.	s.	v. sl. s. chl.; i. eth.
82. Procaine hydrochloride (Novocain)	100	3.33	sl. s. chl.; i. eth.
83. Phenylpropanolamine hydrochloride (Propadrine Hydrochloride)	s.	s.	i. eth., chl.
84. Quinine	0.064	154	73.8 eth.; s. chl.
85. Quinine hydrochloride	5.6^{25}	166^{25}	0.42 eth.
86. Quinine dihydrochloride	166.6	10.3	v. sl. s. eth.; sl. s. chl.
87. Quinine bisulfate	11.1	5.36	0.056 eth.; s. chl.
88. Quinine sulfate	0.14^{25}	1.16^{25}	sl. s. eth.
89. Quinidine	0.05^{15}	4^{20}	4.5 eth.; s. chl.
90. Quinidine sulfate	1.0^{15}	12	v. sl. s. eth.; s. chl.
91. Reserpine	1.	0.055	16.67 chl.; s. acids

TABLE 10-18. SOLUBILITIES OF SOME ALKALOIDS AND CHEMICALLY RELATED SYNTHETIC COMPOUNDS (BASIC N-CONTAINING COMPOUNDS) (*Continued*)

	Water	Alcohol	Ether, etc.
	\multicolumn{3}{c}{SOLUBILITY IN GM. PER 100 ML. OF}		
92. Scopolamine (Hyoscine)	10.5^{15}	v. s.	v. s. eth.; s. chl.
93. Scopolamine hydrobromide (Hyoscine Hydrobromide)	66.6^{25}	6.3^{25}	i. eth.; 0.13 chl.
94. Sparteine	0.304^{22}	v. s.	v. s. eth.; s. chl.
95. Sparteine sulfate	90.9^{25}	33.3^{25}	i. eth., chl.
96. Strychnine	0.016^{25}	0.9	0.018 eth.; s. chl.
97. Strychnine nitrate	2.4^{25}	0.83	i. eth.; 0.64 chl.
98. Strychnine phosphate	3.33	sl. s.	i. eth.
99. Strychnine sulfate	3.2^{25}	1.5^{25}	i. eth.; s. chl.
100. Surfacaine* (Cyclomethycaine)	1.0+	......	....
101. Syntropan†	s.	sl. s.	i. eth., chl.
102. Tetracaine hydrochloride (Pontocaine) ..	s.	s.	i. eth.
103. Tetraethylammonium chloride (Etamon Chloride)	s.	s.	i. eth.
104. Thenylpyramine hydrochloride (Histadyl, Thenylene)	s.	s.	i. eth.
105. Theobromine	0.03^{18}	0.023^{17}	sl. s. eth.
106. Theophylline	0.44^{15}	1.25	sl. s. eth.
107. Totaquine	i.	s.	s. chl.
108. Trasentine‡	s.	......	....
109. Triethanolamine	s.	s.	sl. s. eth.
110. Tripelennamine hydrochloride (Pyribenzamine)	s.	s.	i. eth.
111. Tuamine	sl. s.	s.	s. eth., chl.
112. Tuamine sulfate	s.	s.	sp. s. eth.

* As the hydrochloride.   † As the phosphate.   ‡ As the hydrochloride.

Other problems in the nature of precipitant reactions, of course, would be present when compounds of this class are dispensed in an aqueous medium containing any of the "alkaloidal reagents." However, this type is not too frequent, since these reagents are not employed commonly in present-day prescribing trends, although tannic acid and tannin-containing preparations are occasionally a source of difficulty.

Three methods of overcoming these precipitation reactions are aften listed as a possible means of correcting these incompatibilities:

1. Neutralization of the solution before the addition of the mineral acid salt of the basic N-containing compound.

2. Suspension of the insoluble precipitate with the aid of acacia, tragacanth, Methocel, etc.

3. The addition of alcohol or other water-miscible solvents such as glycerin or propy-lene glycol to solubilize the free base. Of these three methods, the last is most often used by the pharmacist. The addition of acid to neutralize the alkaline solution may lead possibly to other problems; the use of a suspending agent markedly changes the physical characteristics of the preparation and may not be desired, whereas the addition of a small amount of alcohol in preparations intended for internal administration solves the precipitation problem, does not change the pH and does not produce a visual change. Usually 10 to 35 per cent of alcohol is sufficient to dissolve the insoluble precipitate in all of the above incompatibilities.

The esters of this class, which include the local anesthetics such as Butacaine, Larocaine, Monocaine, Naphthocaine, procaine, Tetracaine, Tutocaine, Metycaine and Surfacaine, the alkaloids atrophine, homatropine, reserpine, scopolamine, cocaine and their synthetic substitutes, Syntropan and Trasentine, etc., undergo hydrolysis in aqueous medium to the corresponding alcohol and acid from which they are derived. The rate of hydrolysis (see page 367) is greatly accelerated at pH's near neutrality or on the alkaline side and by the application of heat, as in sterilizing. If these substances are buffered on the acid side (pH 3.0 to 5.0), the stability of their aqueous solutions is enhanced greatly.

As a general rule, it may be stated that alkaloids are incompatible with oxidizing agents. Some substances such as epinephrine, Epinine, Paredrine, Neosynephrine and physostigmine are even oxidized quite readily by the oxygen of the air. Therefore, an antioxidant such as sodium sulfite in a 0.1 per cent concentration is added to prevent this reaction and maintain their stability. These compounds are oxidized much more readily in an alkaline solution than in an acid solution. Thus, the use of buffers to maintain the solution at the proper pH aids materially in preventing their decomposition. The use of buffers to maintain the stability of these solutions by preventing precipitation, hydrolysis and oxidation reactions and to make them compatible with tissue fluids is of great importance in ophthalmic solutions and solutions intended for application to the mucous membranes of the respiratory tract.

Sorenson's modified buffer system at a pH of 6.8 (equal parts of an $M/15$ NaH_2PO_4 solution and $M/15$ Na_2HPO_4 solution = 6.81) has been recommended[39] as a buffer for atropine, ephedrine, eucatropine, homatropine and pilocarpine. The *United States Pharmacopeia*[54] recommends a 1.9 per cent boric acid solution for salts such as those of cocaine, piperocaine, procaine and tetracaine.

QUATERNARY AMMONIUM COMPOUNDS

The drugs of this chemical class include the parasympathomimetic agents acetylcholine chloride, methacholine chloride, carbachol, neostigmine bromide, neostigmine methylsulfate and benzpyrinium bromide, the parasympatholytic agents methantheline bromide, propantheline bromide, antrenyl, trycyclamol sulfate, and those possessing both parasympatholytic and sympatholytic activity such as tetraethylammonium chloride, hexamethonium bromide and hexamethonium

chloride. The surface-active and germicidal agents benzethonium chloride, benzalkonium chloride and cetylpyridinium chloride also belong to this chemical class.

Tetraethylammonium Chloride
(Etamon)

Hexamethonium Chloride* [Esomid Chloride; Hexameton Chloride; Methium Chloride; Hexamethylenebis (trimethylammonium chloride)]

  * Also available as Hexamethonium Bromide (Bistrium Bromide).

Acetylcholine Chloride

Methacholine Chloride (acetyl-β-methylcholine chloride)

Carbachol (carbaminoylcholine chloride)

Neostigmine Bromide (Prostigmine Bromide; dimethylcarbamic ester of 3-hydroxyphenyl-trimethylammonium bromide)

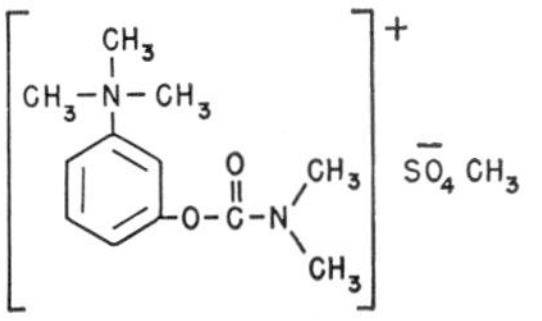

Neostigmine Methylsulfate (Prostigmine Methylsulfate; dimethylcarbamic ester of 3-hydroxyphenyltrimethylammonium methylsulfate)

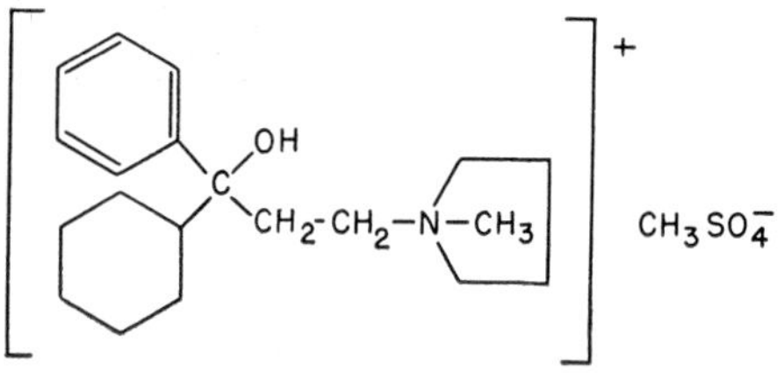

Tricyclamol Sulfate (Elorine Sulfate; 1-cyclohexyl-1-phenyl-3-pyrrolidino-1-propanol methylsulfate)

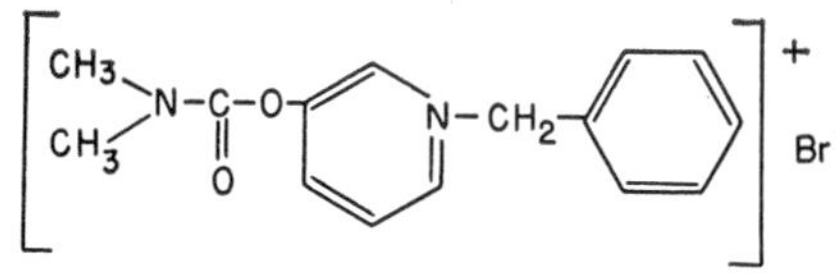

Benzpyrinium Bromide [Stigmonene Bromide; 1-Benzyl-3-(dimethylcarbamyloxy) pyridinium bromide]

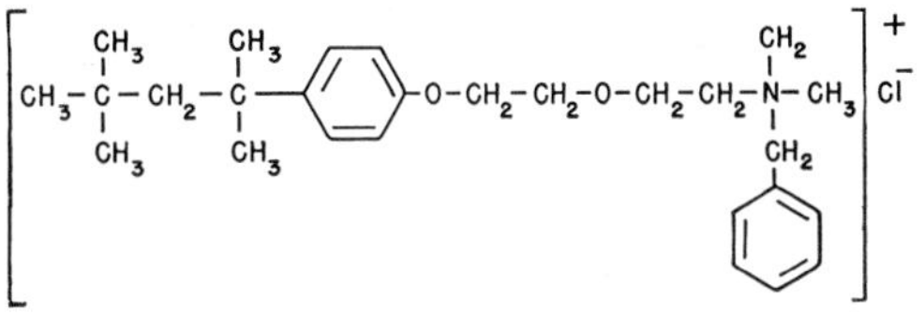

Benzethonium Chloride [Phemerol Chloride; p-(2-methyl-4-,4-dimethyl pentane-2) (phenoxy-ethoxy-ethyl) -dimethyl-benzylammonium chloride]

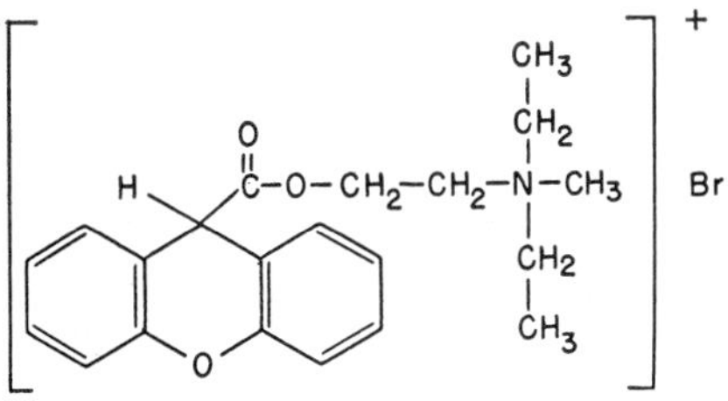

Methantheline Bromide (Banthine Bromide; β-diethylmethylaminoethyl-9-xanthenecarboxylate bromide)

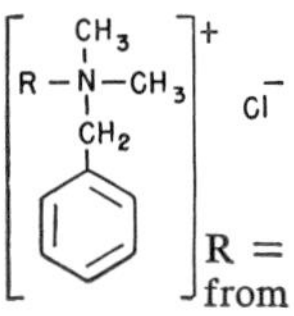

Benzalkonium Chloride (Zephiran Chloride; alkyldimethylbenzylammonium chloride)

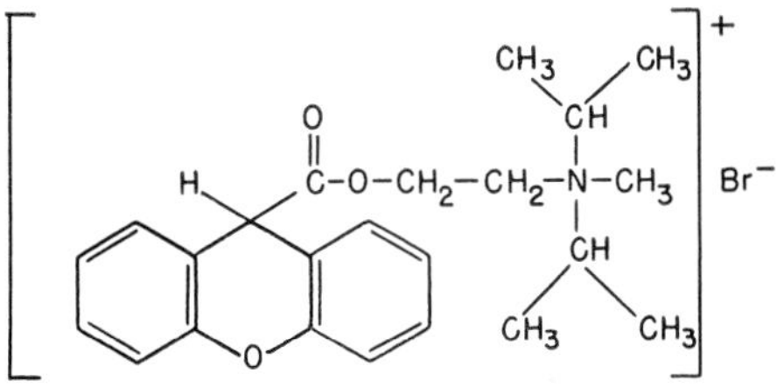

Propantheline Bromide (Pro-Banthine; β-diisopropylmethylaminoethyl-9-xanthenecarboxylate bromide)

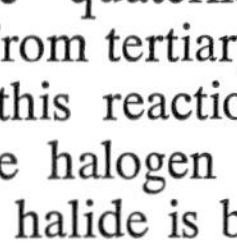

Cetylpyridinium Chloride (Ceepryn)

Solubility. The quaternary ammonium salts are derived from tertiary amines and an alkyl halide. In this reaction, the covalent bond between the halogen and the carbon atom of the alkyl halide is broken in such a manner that the halogen retains the electron which was contributed by the carbon atom to the covalent bond. The halogen thus retains its stable octet, and the carbon atom has lost an electron. The halogen gains an electron and becomes negatively charged. The alkyl radical, having lost an electron, is positively charged and accepts a share of the unshared electron pair of the nitrogen to complete its octet. The nitrogen, having given up a share in an electron pair, becomes posi-

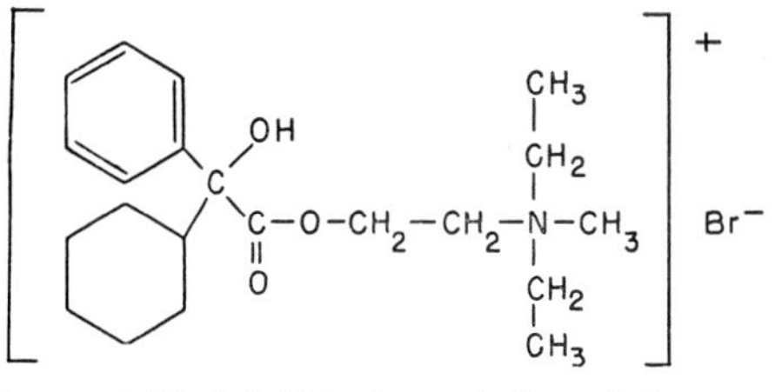

Antrenyl [diethyl (2-hydroxyethyl) methylammonium bromide α-phenyl-cyclohexaneglycolate]

tively charged and the solid, water-soluble, ionic salt is formed as indicated below.

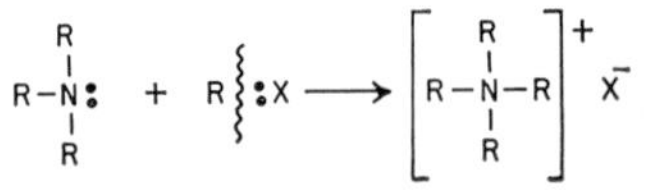

$$\underset{\underset{R}{|}}{\overset{\overset{R}{|}}{R-N:}} + R\left\{:X \longrightarrow \left[\underset{\underset{R}{|}}{\overset{\overset{R}{|}}{R-N-R}}\right]^+ \overset{-}{X}\right.$$

Tetraalkyl Ammonium Halide

BASE STRENGTH. The tetraalkylammonium hydroxides contrast sharply with ammonium hydroxide and the amine hydrates in that they are much stronger bases. These quaternary bases do not decompose with the loss of water, as do the amine hydrates and ammonium hydroxide, but dissociate to yield a high concentration of the hydroxyl ion and the tetraalkylammonium ion. As is indicated by the following structure, the quaternary ammonium bases are completely ionized and, therefore, are comparable in base strength with the hydroxides of the alkali metals.

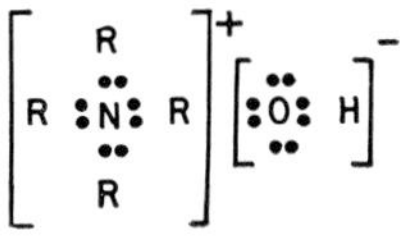

$$\left[\underset{\underset{R}{}}{\overset{\overset{R}{}}{R:N:R}}\right]^+ \left[:\overset{..}{\underset{..}{O}}:H\right]^-$$

Tetraalkylammonium
Hydroxide

Formulation Problems. These quaternary ammonium salts contrast with the hydrohalide salts of the amines in their behavior toward alkalies. They do not liberate the free amine on reaction with alkali. Although the following reaction may be considered as taking place, all of the substances present are completely ionized. Alkalies, therefore, are not a source of a solubility problems with the quaternary ammonium salts.

$$\left[\underset{\underset{R}{|}}{\overset{\overset{R}{|}}{R-N-R}}\right]^+ \overset{-}{X} + KOH \rightleftharpoons \left[\underset{\underset{R}{|}}{\overset{\overset{R}{|}}{R-N-R}}\right]^+ \overset{-}{OH} + KX$$

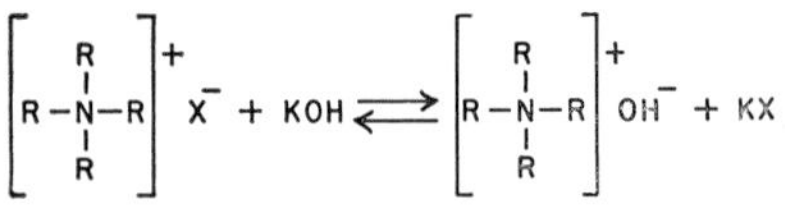

The surface-active agents and germicidals such as benzalkonium chloride, cetylpyridinium chloride and benzethonium chloride are cationic agents and their germicidal activity in aqueous solution is reduced greatly by such anionic agents as soaps, sodium lauryl sulfate and diocytl sodium sulfosuccinate. This decreased activity is due to the coacervation which takes place between oppositely charged anionic and cationic agents.

The parasympathomimetic agents of this group are chemically similar but give rise to few problems, because their therapeutic use does not often involve admixture with substances other than solutions to control the pH; e.g., neostigmine bromide and boric acid.

ACIDIC NITROGEN-CONTAINING COMPOUNDS

As explained in the discussion of the basic nitrogen-containing compounds, the nitrogen may be sufficiently substituted with acidic groups to weaken the nitrogen-hydrogen bond to such an extent that the remaining hydrogen becomes acidic. The proton may then be lost in basic solution with the formation of the water-soluble ionized salt (see p. 375).

SULFONAMIDES

The sulfonamide drugs afford a good example of the effect of this type of substitution. In this case, the sulfonyl group is sufficiently acidic to overcome the basicity of the nitrogen. An acidic group decreases the basicity of a basic nitrogen in the same way

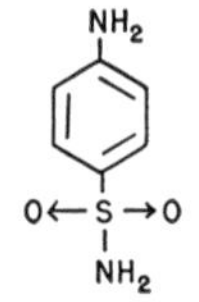

Sulfanilamide (p-aminobenzene
sulfonamide)

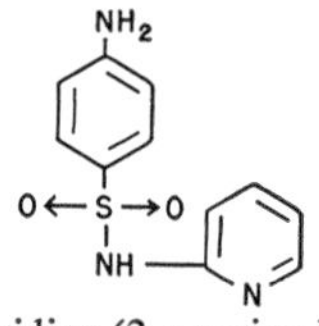

Sulfapyridine (2-p-amino-benzene
sulfonamidopyridine)

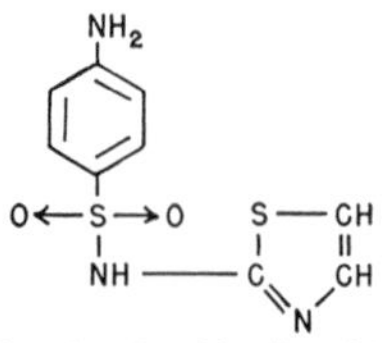

Sulfathiazole (2-sulfanilamidothiazole)

Sulfadiazine (2-sulfanilamidopyrimidine)

Sulfamerazine (2-sulfanilamido-4-
methyl-pyrimidine)

Sulfamethazine (2-sulfanilamido-4,6-
dimethyl pyrimidine)

Sulfaguanidine (*p*-amino-
benzenesulfonylguanidine)

Sulfisoxizole (Gantrisin; 3,4-dimethyl-
5-sulfanilamido-isoxazole)

Sulfaethylthiadiazole (5-ethyl-2-sulfanilamido-
1,3,4-thiadiazole)

Sulfamethoxypyridazine (3-sulfanilamido-
6-methoxypyridazine)

Succinylsulfathiazole
(Sulfasuxidine)

Phthalylsulfathiazole
(Sulfathalidine)

it increases the acidity of an acid—that is, by withdrawing electrons. In the case of the sulfonamides, the two coordinately bonded oxygen atoms cause the sulfur atom to become electron-deficient. In an attempt to satisfy this deficiency, the sulfur tends to withdraw electrons from the nitrogen. This, in turn, causes the pair of electrons bonding the hydrogen to the nitrogen to be held more closely to the nitrogen so that the hydrogen becomes bound loosely and is given up readily in basic solution to form the water-soluble ionized salt. This type of salt formation occurs only in those compounds which are derivatives of either ammonia or primary amines. Those compounds which are derivatives of secondary amines have no remaining hydrogen on the nitrogen, so salt formation is impossible.

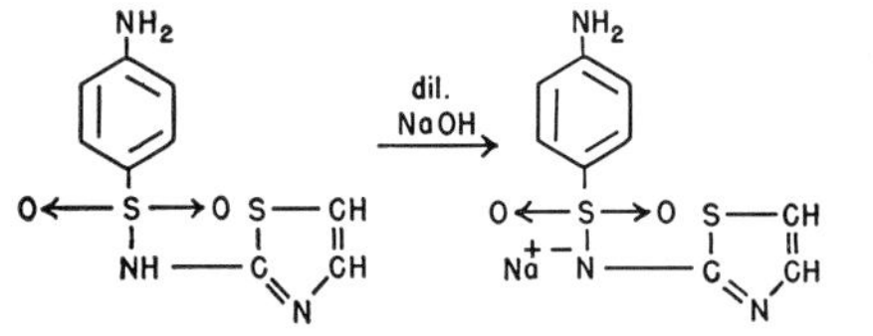

Sulfathiazole
(water-insoluble)

Sodium Sulfathiazole
(water-soluble)

Solubility. The sulfonamides which are weak acids are insoluble in water but soluble in dilute alkali. Due to the basic amino group, the sulfonamides are also soluble in solutions of mineral acids.

Formulation Problems. Most of the incompatibilities of the sulfonamides are of an acid-base nature resulting from attempts to dis-

Sodium Sulfathiazole
(water-soluble)

Ephedrine Hydrochloride
(water-soluble)

Sulfathiazole
(water-insoluble)

Ephedrine

pense the soluble sodium salts in a slightly acid medium. The sodium salts of the sulfonamides in aqueous medium have a pH of approximately 9 to 10.

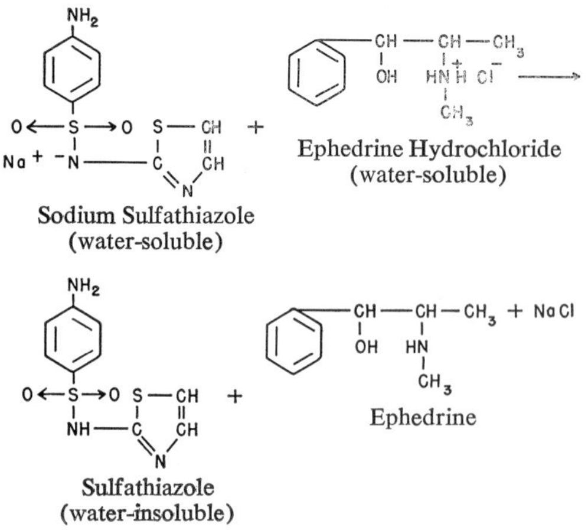

The following type calculation is most useful to determine the pH at which these weak acids (sulfonamides, barbiturates, hydantoinates, carboxylic acids, etc.) precipitate in solutions of given concentration:

$$pH = pK_a + \log \frac{S}{A}$$

To calculate the minimum pH required to prevent the precipitation of a 5 per cent aqueous solution of sodium sulfamethazine:

pK_a sulfamethazine = 7.37
Mol. wt. sulfamethazine = 278.33
Mol. wt. sodium sulfamethazine = 300.31
Solubility of sulfamethazine = 0.15 Gm./ 100 ml.

$$pH = 7.37 + \log \frac{\dfrac{50}{300.31} - \dfrac{1.5}{278.33}}{\dfrac{1.5}{278.33}}$$

$$= 7.37 + \log \frac{0.1664 - 0.0053}{0.0053}$$

$$= 7.37 + \log 30.3$$
$$= 7.37 + 1.48$$
$$pH = 8.85$$

A similar calculation for a 5 per cent solution of sodium sulfacetimide (pK_a 5.38, solubility 0.67 Gm./100 ml.) would show that precipitation does not occur until the pH goes below 6.14. From this it is evident that sodium sulfacetimide could be employed in solutions having the same pH as lacrimal fluid (7.4), whereas sulfamethazine could not. Obviously, the preceding equation is also useful in determining the concentration of a solution that can be employed at a given pH.

Aqueous solutions of the soluble sulfonamide salts are unstable in air, resulting in precipitates of the free sulfonamide due to the absorption of CO_2. Color reactions also are observed as the result of partial oxidation of the drug with the formation of complex, highly colored oxidative products. Oxidative changes in the solutions can be controlled by the addition of sodium sulfite (0.75 to 2.0%) and glycerin (1%).[42] The sodium salts are too alkaline for oral administration and may cause

TABLE 10-19. SOLUBILITIES OF SOME SULFONAMIDES AND THEIR SODIUM SALTS

SULFONAMIDE	SOLUBILITY IN GM. PER 100 ML. OF		
	Water	Alcohol	Ether, etc.
Sulfanilamide	0.4^{15}	3	s. dil. alk., dil. ac.
Sulfapyridine	0.03	0.2	s. dil. alk., dil. ac.
Sulfathiazole	0.06	0.5	s. dil. alk., dil. ac.
Sulfathiazole sodium	40	6.6	i. eth.
Sulfadiazine	0.012^{37}	sp. s.	s. dil. alk., dil. ac.
Sulfadiazine sodium	50	sl. s.	i. eth.
Sulfamerazine	0.016	sl. s.	s. dil. alk., dil. ac.; sp. s. eth., acet., chl.
Sulfamerazine sodium	33.3	sl. s.	i. eth., chl.
Sulfamethoxypyridazine	sl. s.	sp. s.	sp. s. acet., s. dil. alk., ac.
Sulfaguanidine	0.1	sp. s.	s. dil. ac.
Succinylsulfathiazole	0.0208	sp. s.	s. dil. alk.

dil. ac. = dilute acid   dil. alk. = dilute alkali   acet. = acetone

gastrointestinal disturbances. Some substances which cause the precipitation of the free sulfonamide are mineral acid salts of the sympathomimetic amines (ephedrine HCl, desoxyephedrine HCl, Paredrine HBr, etc.), mineral acid salts of the local anesthetics (procaine HCl, tetracaine HCl, etc.) and many other substances which yield acid solutions. If the substance (HCl salts, etc.) causing the precipitation of the free sulfonamide is in low concentration so that it remains soluble in water in the free form, the sulfonamide may be buffered at a stable pH and the precipitation prevented. However, some precipitation reactions of this nature occasionally are intended—e.g., nasal suspensions that contain 5 per cent sodium sulfathiazole and 2 per cent ephedrine hydrochloride, etc. can be prepared.

Many commercial preparations for intranasal therapy containing sodium sulfathiazole

(2.5%), d,l-desoxyephedrine hydrochloride (0.125%), anhydrous sodium sulfite (2.0%) and glycerin (1.0%) are clear, stable solutions. According to Hamilton et al., the water-soluble salts can be formed between the sympathomimetic amines and the sulfonamides. These salts were prepared by first heating the aqueous solution given above until all the ingredients dissolved and then adjusting to a pH of 8.7 with 0.6 N HCl.[30]

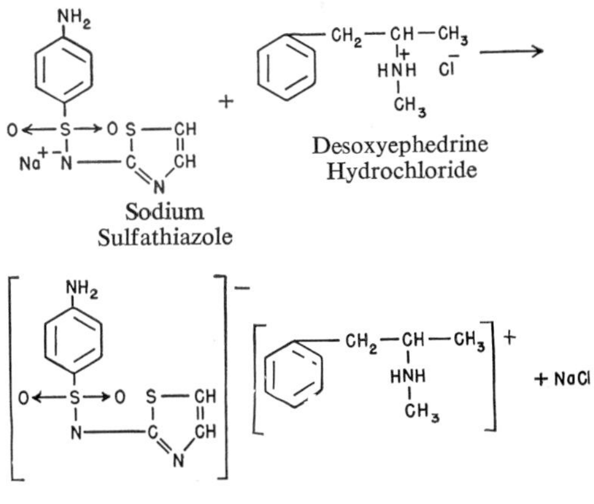

Sodium Sulfathiazole

Desoxyephedrine Hydrochloride

TABLE 10-20. pKₐ VALUES FOR CERTAIN SULFONAMIDES

SULFONAMIDE	pK_a
Sulfacetimide	5.38
Sulfadiazine	6.37
Sulfamerazine	7.06
Sulfamethazine	7.37
Sulfathiazole	7.12
Succinylsulfathiazole	4.5
Sulfisoxazole	4.96
Kynex	7.17

BARBITURATES

The barbiturates are another example of nitrogen-containing compounds with sufficient substitution of acidic groups for the hydrogens of the nitrogen to cause the remaining hydrogen to become acidic in nature.

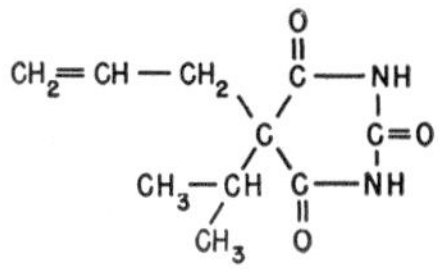

Alurate (5-allyl-5-isopropyl
barbituric acid)

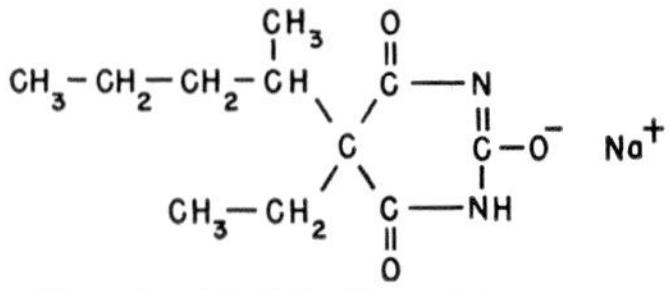

Pentobarbital Sodium [Nembutal;
Sodium-5-ethyl-5-(1-methyl-butyl)
barbiturate]

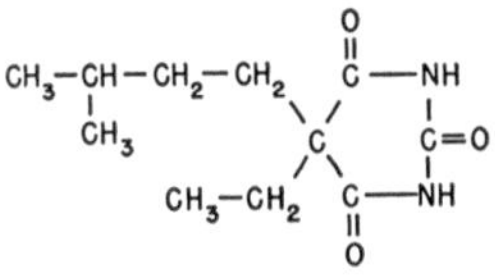

Amobarbital (Amytal, 5-isoamyl-
5-ethylbarbituric acid)

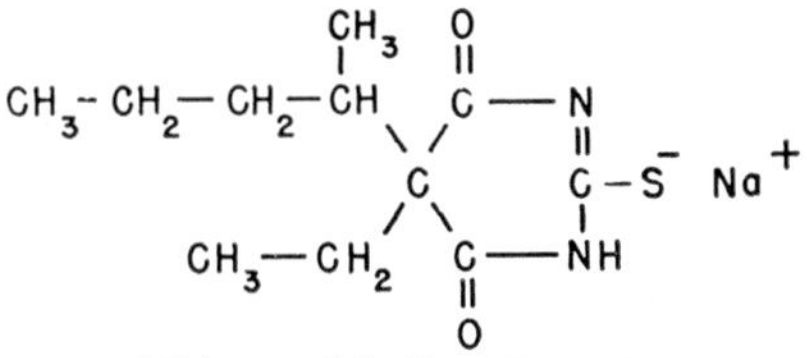

Thiopental Sodium [Pentothal
Sodium; Sodium 5-ethyl-5-
(1-methylbutyl) thiobarbiturate]

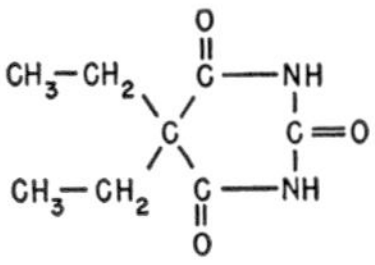

Barbital (5-diethylbarbituric
acid)

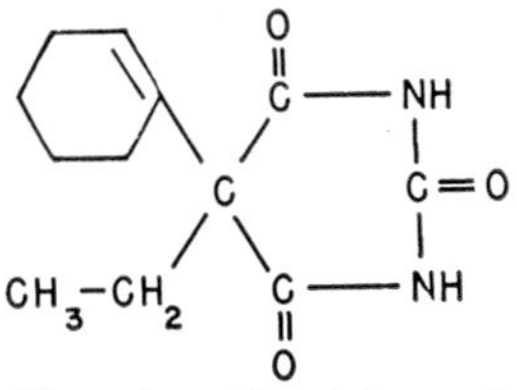

Phanodorn (5-cyclohexenyl-
5-ethyl barbituric acid)

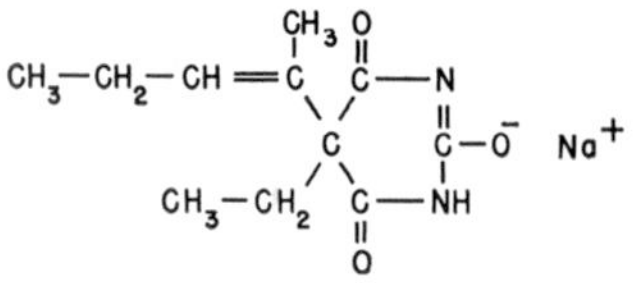

Delvinal [Sodium 5-ethyl-5-
(1-methyl-1-butenyl) barbi-
turate]

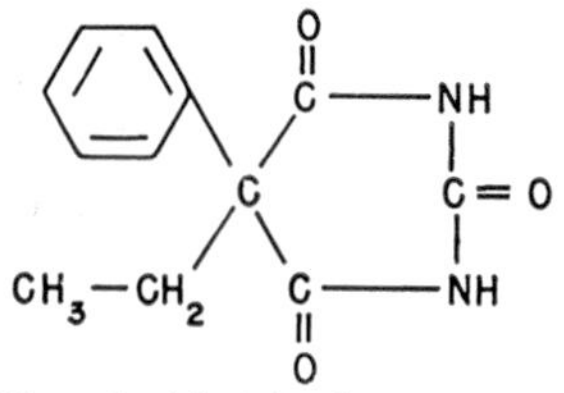

Phenobarbital (5-phenyl-5-ethyl
barbituric acid)

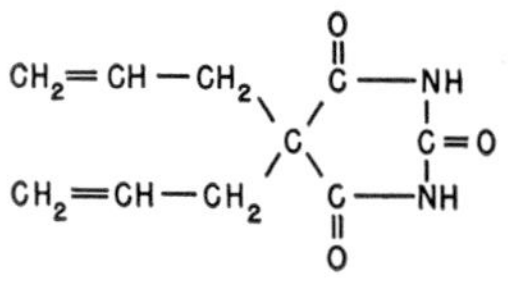

Dial (5,5-diallylbarbituric
acid)

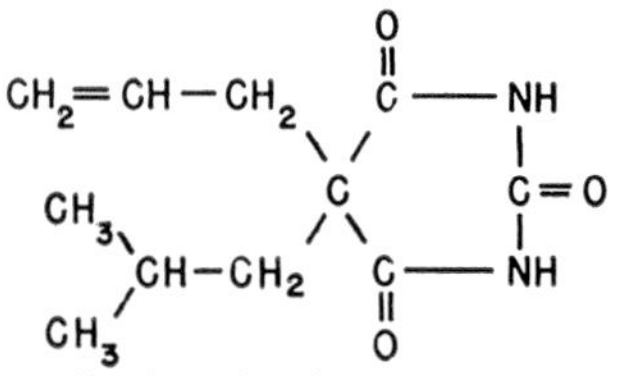

Sandoptal (5-isobutyl-5-allyl
barbituric acid)

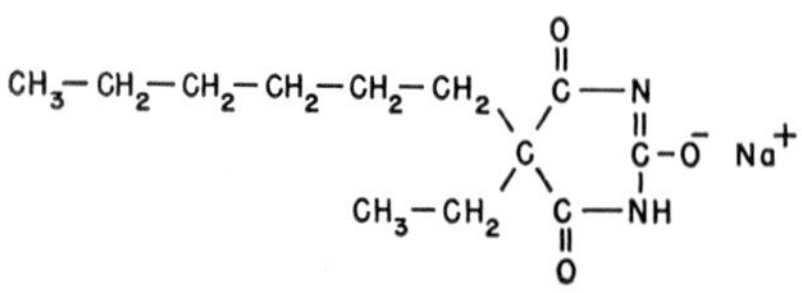

Ortal Sodium (Sodium 5-n-
hexyl-5-ethylbarbiturate)

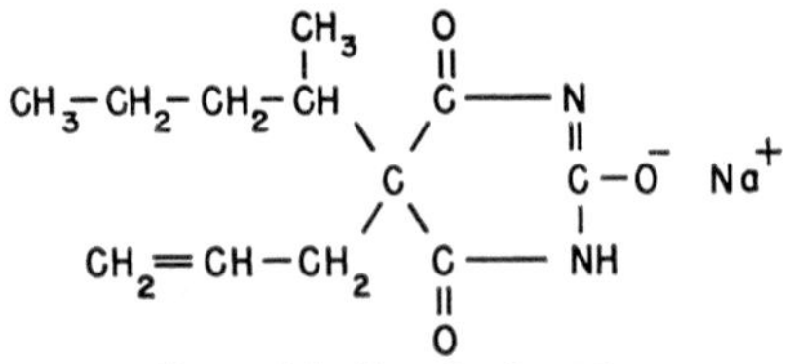

Seconal Sodium [sodium 5-
allyl-5-(1-methylbutyl) bar-
biturate]

As shown in the above structures, all of the important barbiturates are derivatives in which various groups are substituted for the hydrogens on the number five carbon atom. These barbiturates, which are derived from malonic acid and urea, are weak acids. As in the case of the imides, two acidic carbonyl groups must be substituted for the hydrogens of the nitrogen in order for the remaining hydrogen to become acidic. Here the effect of the individual carbonyl groups is the same

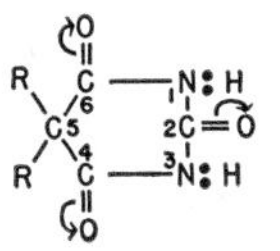

as in the acid amides (see p. 375). The tendency for a pair of electrons to shift from the double bond to form a stable octet on the oxygen creates an electron deficiency on the carbon atom. In an attempt to satisfy this deficiency, the carbon atom tends to withdraw electrons from the nitrogen. The unshared electron pair of the nitrogen thus shifts so as to increase the covalency between the nitrogen and the carbon. The electron pair bonding the hydrogen to the nitrogen, consequently, is held more firmly to the nitrogen, and the hydrogen in turn is held loosely. The combined effect of the two carbonyl groups makes the hydrogen so loosely held that the proton is removed easily in basic solution. This migrates to the oxygen of the carbon atom in number two position to yield the enol form which then reacts with the alkali to yield the water-soluble ionized sodium salt. The reaction may be illustrated as follows:

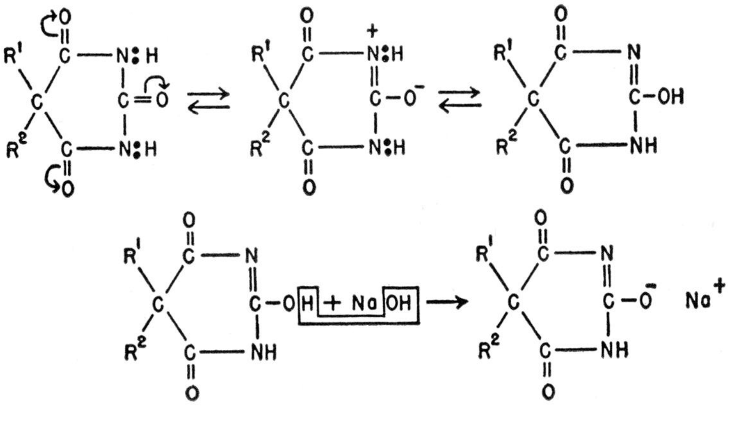

From the structure it can be observed that only the monosodium salt is formed with this class of compounds.

Solubility. The barbituric acid derivatives are soluble in alcohol and insoluble in water, but their sodium salts are readily soluble in both solvents.

Formulation Problems. The major problems of the barbiturate drugs are once again

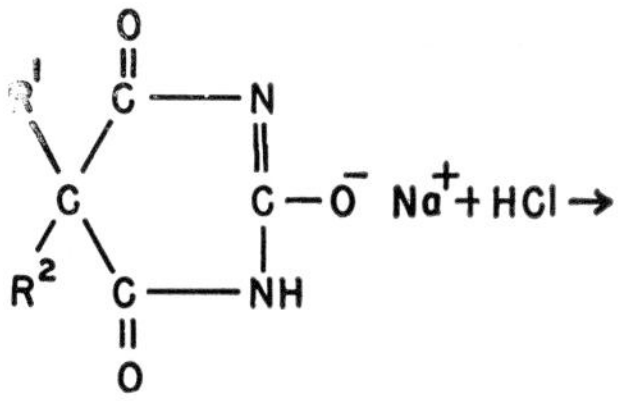

Sodium Salt of a Substituted Barbituric Acid
(water-soluble)

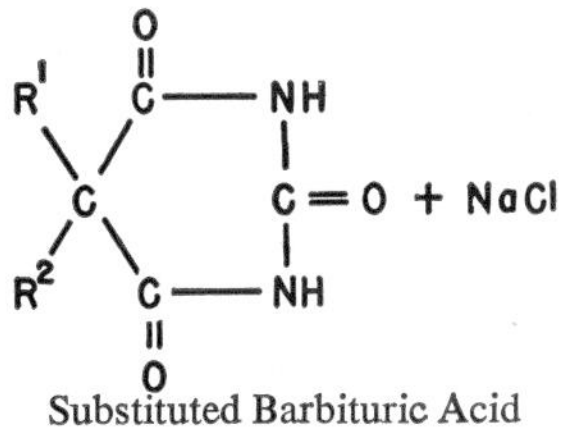

Substituted Barbituric Acid
(water-insoluble)

those of acid-base reactions. Aqueous solutions of the sodium salts of the barbiturates are alkaline in reaction, and, when acidified, the insoluble barbituric acid derivative is precipitated. This type reaction takes place whenever an attempt is made to dispense the soluble barbiturates in an aqueous medium containing alkaloidal salts, acid syrups, acid elixirs, salts of many of the vitamins of the

TABLE 10-21. SOLUBILITIES OF SOME BARBITURATES AND THEIR SODIUM SALTS

BARBITURATE	SOLUBILITY IN GM. PER 100 ML. OF		
	Water	Alcohol	Ether, etc.
Alurate	sl. s.	s.	s. dil. alk.
Amobarbital	v. sl. s.	s.	s. dil. alk.
Barbital, U.S.P.	0.69^{20}	6.6	2.85 eth.; s. dil. alk.
Barbital sodium	20	s.	i. eth.
Delvinal	s.	s.	i. eth.
Dial	v. sl. s.	s.	s. dil. alk.
Ortal sodium	v. s.	s.	i. eth.
Pentobarbital sodium	v. s.	s.	i. eth.
Phanodorn	v. sl. s.	s.	s. dil. alk.
Phenobarbital	0.1	10	6.6 eth.; s. dil. alk.; 2.5 chl.
Phenobarbital sodium	v. s.	s.	i. eth., chl.
Sandoptal	v. sl. s.	s.	s. dil. alk.
Seconal sodium	v. s.	s.	i. eth.
Thiopental sodium	v. s.	s.	i. eth.

B-complex and other substances having an acid reaction. Aqueous solutions of soluble barbiturates and thiamine hydrochloride, for example, result in the precipitation of the free barbiturate and a destruction of the thiamine activity due to the alkalinity of the soluble barbiturates. In all of the above precipitation reactions, alcohol may be added to solubilize the liberated barbiturate, or the free barbiturate may be substituted for the soluble barbiturate and again solubilized by the addition of alcohol. In the case of the soluble barbiturate-thiamine hydrochloride incompatibility, the free barbiturate and the alcohol always should be used to prevent the destruction of the thiamine by the alkalinity of the soluble barbiturate.

The soluble barbiturates are also incompatible with ammonium salts.[66] The following reaction takes place between these substances:

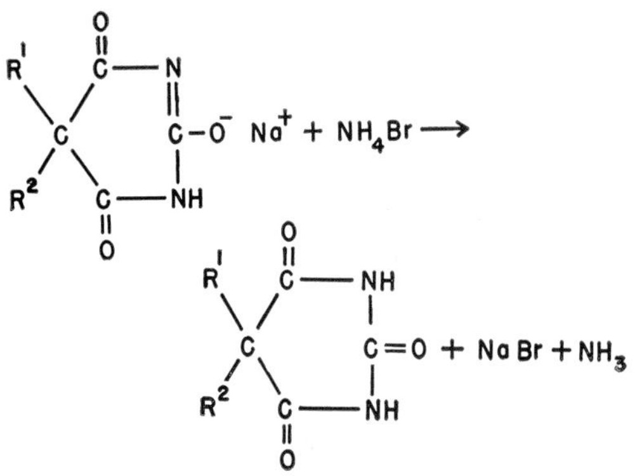

Aqueous solutions of the soluble barbiturates hydrolyze to form the R^1, R^2 acetyl urea and other therapeutically inactive substances. For example, aqueous solutions of phenobarbital sodium hydrolyze to form phenylethylacetylurea. The rate of decomposition is influenced markedly by the temperature and the pH of the solution. A 10 per cent solution of phenobarbital sodium at 39° C. showed 22 per cent decomposition in 1 month.[66] Soluble barbiturates are precipitated from aqueous solutions at pH's below 8.8[42] (see calculations p. 390).

HYDANTOIN COMPOUNDS

The hydantoin compounds are similar in structure and reactivity to the barbiturates, and the mechanism whereby they form soluble sodium salts is also the same as for the barbiturates.

Diphenylhydantoin sodium is soluble in water and alcohol. It has the same incompatibilities as the soluble barbiturates and is precipitated from aqueous solution as the free

TABLE 10-22. pK$_a$ VALUES FOR CERTAIN BARBITURATES

BARBITURATE	pK$_a$
Phenobarbital	7.41
Barbital	7.91
Amytal	7.94
Butethal	7.92

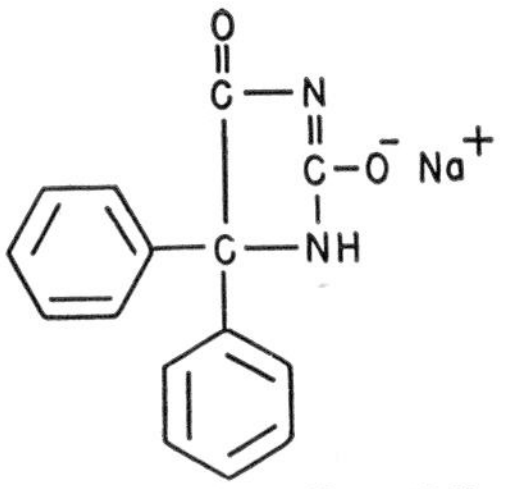

Diphenylhydantoin Sodium (Dilantin,
Soluble Phenytoin, sodium 5,5-
diphenylhydantoin)

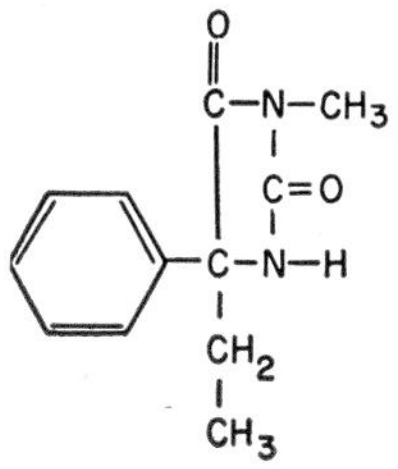

Phenantoin (Mesantoin; 3-methyl-5,5
phenylethylhydantoin)

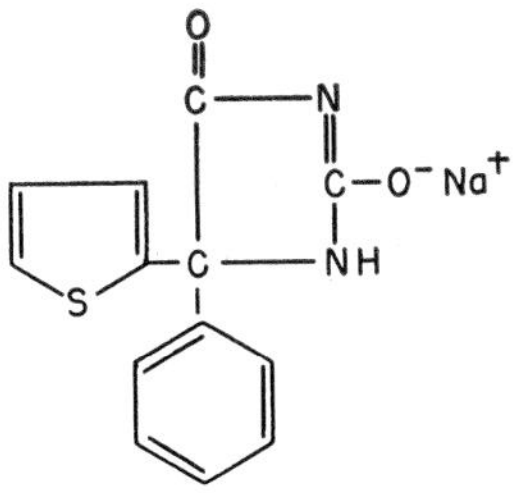

Phethenylate Sodium (Thiantoin
Sodium; Sodium 5-phenyl-5-
2-thienyl) hydantoinate)

diphenylhydantoin by acids and acid salts. Unless buffered to a pH of approximately 11.7, its aqueous solutions undergo hydrolysis, and precipitation of the free diphenylhydantoin occurs. Phenantoin and phethenylate are chemically similar to diphenylhydantoin.

DYES

The synthetic organic dyes or so-called "coal-tar dyes" are used in industry for the purpose of imparting colors to such substances as cloth, leather, paper, cellophane, wood, etc., and as coloring agents for pharmaceutical preparations. When used in pharmaceutical preparations, only certified colors which meet the specifications set forth in the Food, Drug and Cosmetic act may be used. Many dyes are also valuable therapeutic agents which are employed in medicine and surgery because of their antiseptic, germicidal and wound-healing properties.

Problems involving dyes are usually the result of chemical reactions leading to the loss of color or change in color. In order to understand the nature of these reactions, a certain amount of background in the theory of dyes is essential.

Theory of Color. The cause of color is attributed to the presence of certain chromophore groups within the color-producing molecule. These chromophores include the

$$-N=N-(azo), \quad =C=C(thio), \quad -N=O$$

(nitroso), $-\overset{+}{N}=\overset{}{N}-$ (azoxy), $\quad -\overset{+}{N}\overset{O^-}{\underset{O}{\diagup}}$

(nitro), $-CH=N-$ (azomethine), $=C=O$ (carbonyl) and $=C=C=$ (ethenyl) groups.

Other substituent groups called auxochromes, which cause a deepening of the color, may be present in the molecule. The auxochromes include the $-NR_2$, the $-NHR$ and the $-NH_2$ groups.

Although all organic molecules are capable of absorbing light to some degree, most of them absorb in the ultraviolet* region and appear colorless. In other words, they transmit or reflect those rays falling in the visual† region of the spectrum. According to modern concepts, the theory of light absorption is concerned with the vibrations of the electrons in the molecule in response to the stimulation by light waves of a certain specific oscillation frequency. Where the electrons are firmly bound in the molecule (e.g., as they are in a saturated hydrocarbon), their vibration rate is extremely high and they respond to and absorb light only of short wave length and high frequency, which falls in the far ultraviolet region. However, such is not always the case when the molecule contains unsaturated groups. The valence

* Below 4,000 Ångstrom units.
† Visual spectrum includes those wave lengths between 4,000 and 8,000 Ångstrom units (1 Å = 10^{-7} mm. or 10^{-10} m. or 0.000,000,0001 meter).

electrons of these unsaturated groups are held more loosely, or we may say that they are more mobile and are capable of being set in vibration by light of longer wave lengths. The absorption of light then may be in the visible region of the spectrum. In support of this theory, a simply constructed unsaturated compound usually absorbs light only in a single limited region of the spectrum and, therefore, has an absorption band of maximum intensity at a specific wave length. As the unsaturation and the complexity of the molecule increase, several absorbing centers may be created, giving rise to a complex absorption spectrum composed of several bands, a series of peaks or an extremely broad absorption band. The light of the visual spectrum which is not absorbed by the compound is transmitted or reflected, and the compound assumes the color of the unabsorbed light. Thus, if a compound absorbs all light of the visible spectrum except that viewed by the eye as red, it will appear to be that color. The various chromophore groups apparently differ in their activity; thus, it is observed that only one azo, thio, azoxy or nitro group as a substituent on a benzene ring is sufficient to yield a colored compound. Such is not the case with the remaining chromophoric groups listed on page 395. However, as a general rule, more than one chromophore group is required to yield a colored compound, and even in the above case the unsaturated benzene ring contributes to the color of the compound.

The auxochromes, while incapable in themselves of yielding colored compounds, possess the ability to augment the function of the chromophore group and cause an intensification of the color. According to Bury,[45] "the function of the auxochrome is to introduce the possibility of resonance" in the molecule. In the resonance structures, more mobility

is conferred on the valence electrons of the chromophore groups, which results in an increased light absorption in the longer wave lengths. In support of the resonance theory, Bury utilized the triphenylmethane dye, Dobner's violet, which shows resonance due to the possible existence of two equivalent structures. In order to show the importance of resonance in the production of color, fuchsonimine [$HN=C_6H_4=C(C_6H_5)_2$] is cited[16] as an example of a compound containing the same chromophore group (quinoid system) but lacking the p-amino group and is devoid of color, since it is incapable of resonance. Other structures capable of resonance include the diphenylmethane, amino and hydroxyazobenzene, indamine, indophenol, auramine, acridine, pyronine, azine, oxazine and thiazine dyes.[16] The chromophoric groups are unsaturated and are usually electron acceptors. The auxochromes are electron donors. The carboxyl, sulfonic acid groups and halogens have little effect either as auxochromes or chromophores.

In the dyeing industry, the term auxochrome has taken on another meaning from that originally intended. In this respect, auxochromes are referred to as groups in the molecule which confer on the compound the ability to dye a substance and yield a fast color; that is, they "facilitate the attachment of the dye to the fabric."[16] Many colored compounds not containing auxochromes are incapable of acting as dyes. When considered from this standpoint, the auxochromes fulfilling this function may be either acid or basic in nature. These auxochromes include the basic $-NR_2$, $-NHR$ and $-NH_2$ and the acidic $-SO_3H$, $-COOH$ and $-OH$ groups. The basic auxochromes are capable of causing an intensification or deepening of color; the acidic auxochromes do not possess this property. Dyes containing these groups may be classified as acidic and basic dyes, those forming salts with bases being acidic dyes and those forming salts with acids being basic dyes. The sulfonic acid derivatives are also prepared as a means of increasing the water-solubility of the dye. Certain groups when substituted in the auxochrome also cause a color change. When alkyl and aryl groups are substituted in the auxochrome, a deeper color is observed. These color-deep-

Dobner's Violet

ening groups are called bathochromes. If an acyl (e.g., acetyl) group is substituted in the auxochrome, the color becomes lighter and the substituent group is termed a hypsochrome.

Inasmuch as we are concerned at this point only with the chemical and the physical properties of these dyes, no attempt has been made to distinguish between those possessing therapeutic properties and those used purely as coloring agents.

Most of the dyes used in pharmacy, whether for their therapeutic or coloring properties, are salts of acid or basic dyes. The dye ion exhibits greater resonance than the parent molecule. The auxochromes are capable of forming ionizable salts. Any substance causing a decrease in the ionization will reduce the intensity of the color. This is the basis for many incompatibilities.

CLASSIFICATION OF DYES

I. Acridine Dyes

1. *Acriflavine* (Acriflavine base; a mixture of 3,6-diamino-10-methyl acridinium chloride and 3,6-diamino acridine)

2. *Acriflavine Hydrochloride* (a mixture of the hydrochlorides of 3,6-diamino-10-methyl acridinium chloride and 3,6-diamino acridine)
3. *Proflavine Dihydrochloride* (3,6-diamino acridine dihydrochloride)

4. *Proflavine Sulfate* (3,6-diamino acridine sulfate)

5. *Quinacrine Hydrochloride* (Mepacrine Hydrochloride, Atabrine; the dihydrochloride of 3-chloro-9-(4-diethylamino-1-methylbutylamino)-7-methoxy acridine)

II. Azo Dyes

1. *Scarlet Red* (Scarlet Red Medicinal, Biebrich Scarlet Red; o-tolyl azo-o-tolyl azo-β-naphthol)

2. *Scarlet Red Sulfonate* (Biebrich Scarlet, water-soluble; the disodium salt of azobenzenedisulfonic acid azo-β-naphthol)

3. *Pyridium* (Mallophene; phenylazo-2,6-diaminopyridine monohydrochloride)

4. *Serenium*   (2,4-diamino-4-ethoxy azo-benzene hydrochloride)

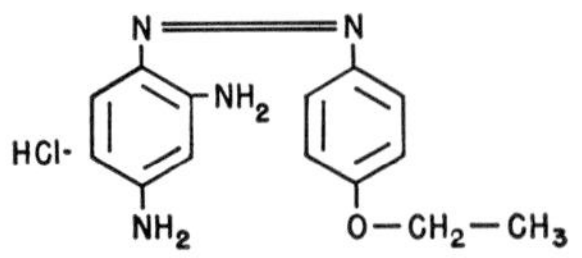

5. *Congo Red* (sodium diphenyl-diazo-bis-α-naphthylamine 4-sulfonate)

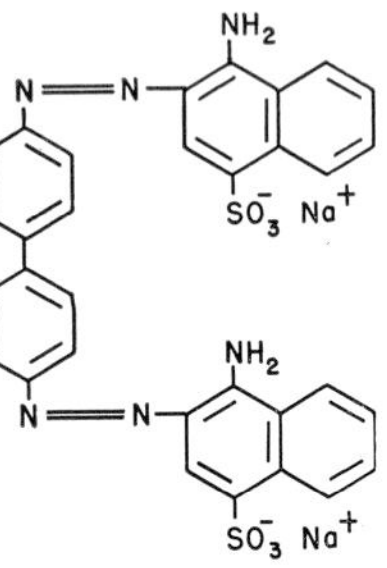

6. *F.D.&C. Red No. 1* (Ponceau 3R; the sodium salt of pseudocumylazo-β-naphthol-3,6-disulfonic acid)

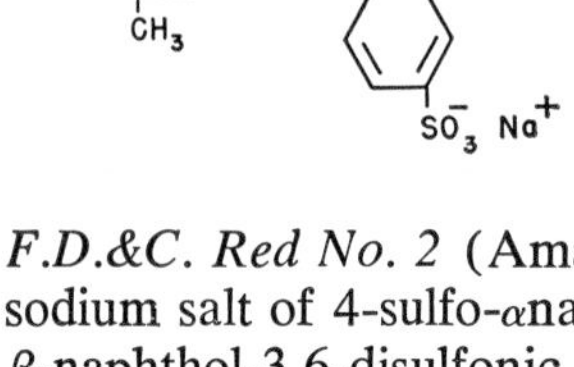

7. *F.D.&C. Red No. 2* (Amaranth; the sodium salt of 4-sulfo-αnaphthylazo-β-naphthol-3,6-disulfonic acid)

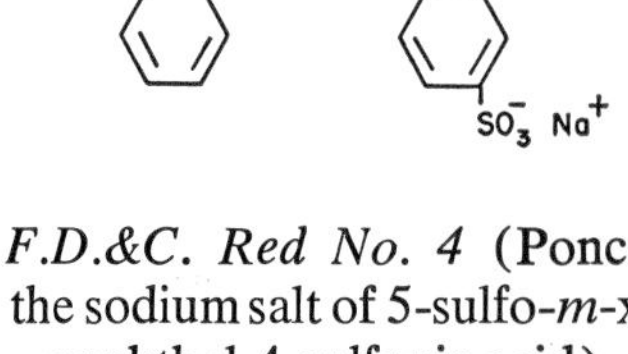

8. *F.D.&C. Red No. 4* (Ponceau SX; the sodium salt of 5-sulfo-*m*-xylylazo-α-naphthol-4-sulfonic acid)

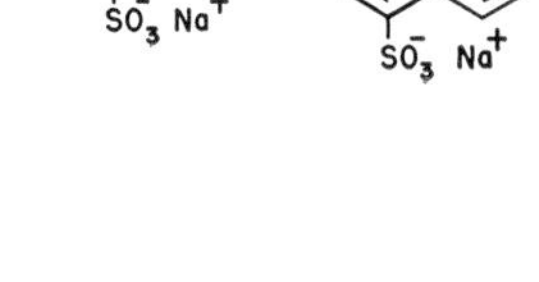

9. *F.D.&C. Red No. 32* (Oil red XO; *m*-xylylazo-β-naphthol)

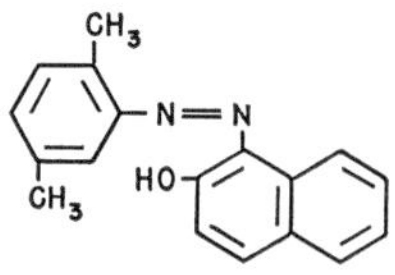

10. *F.D.&C. Orange No. 1* (Orange I, the sodium salt of *p*-sulfophenylazo-α-naphthol)

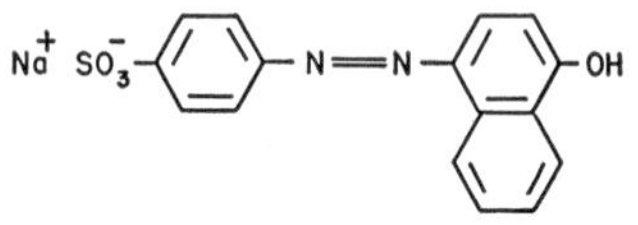

11. *F.D.&C. Orange No. 2* (Orange SS; *o*-tolylazo-β-naphthol)

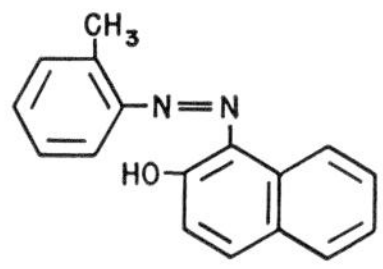

12. *F.D.&C. Yellow No. 3* (Yellow AB; phenylazo-β-naphthylamine)

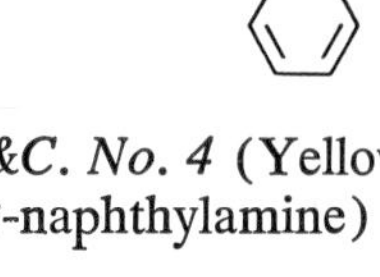

13. *F.D.&C. No. 4* (Yellow OB; *o*-tolyl-azo-β-naphthylamine)

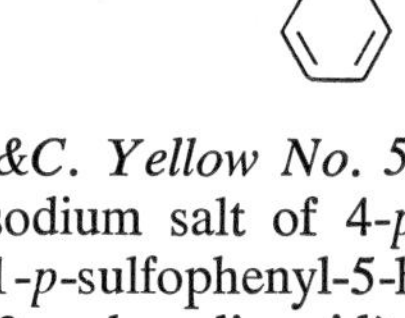

14. *F.D.&C. Yellow No. 5* (Tartrazine; the sodium salt of 4-*p*-sulfophenyl-azo-1-*p*-sulfophenyl-5-hydroxylpyra-zole-3-carboxylic acid)

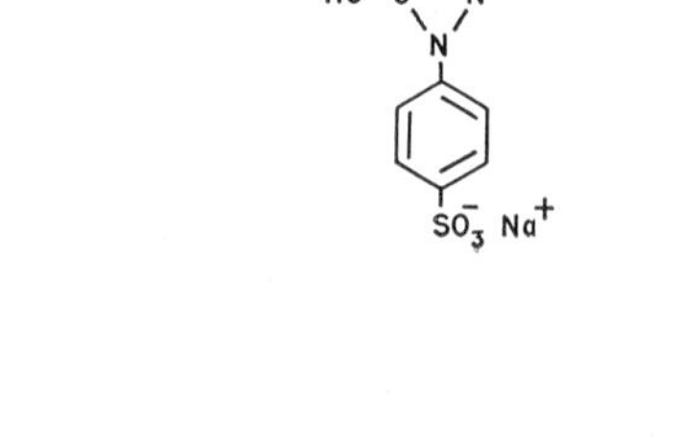

15. *F.D.&C. Yellow No. 6* (Sunset Yellow FCF; the sodium salt of *p*-sulfophenylazo-β-naphthol-6-monosulfonate)

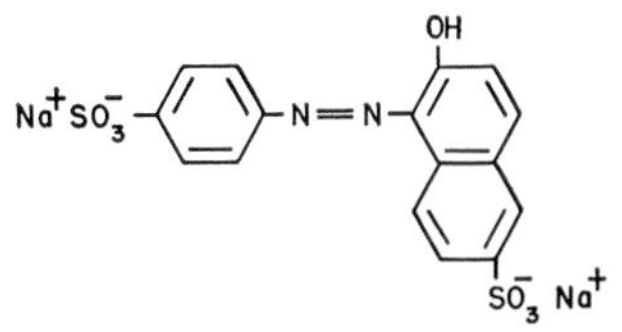

III. Phthalein Dyes

A. FLUORESCEIN (PYRONINE) DYES
   1. *Fluorescein Sodium* (Soluble Fluorescein, Resorcinolphthalein Sodium; the disodium salt of fluorescein)

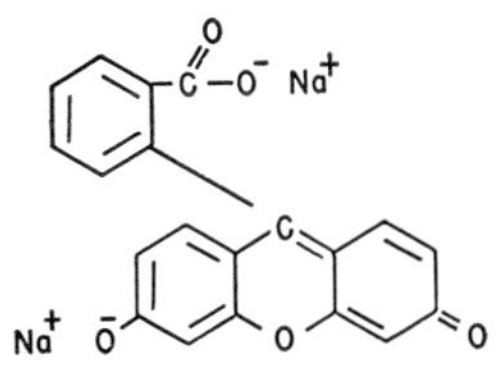

2. *Soluble Eosin* (the disodium salt of tetrabromofluorescein)

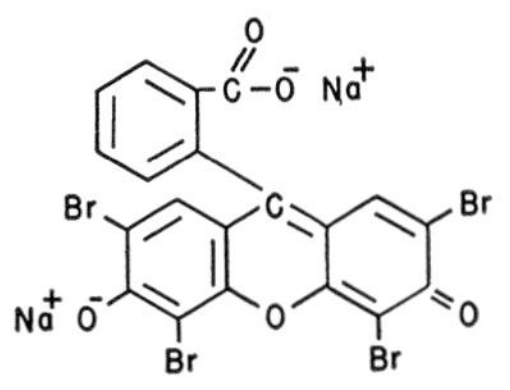

3. *Merbromin* (Mercurochrome; the disodium salt of 2,7-dibromo-4-hydroxymercurifluorescein)

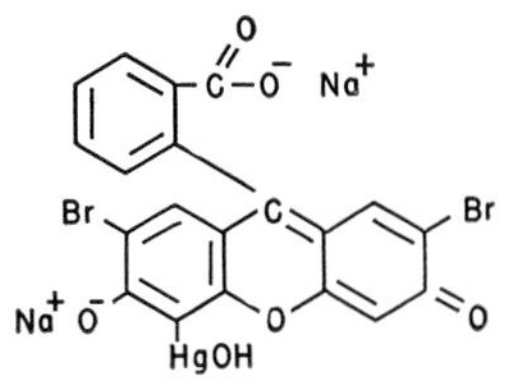

4. *F.D.&C. Red No. 3* (Erythrosin; the disodium salt of tetraiodofluorescein)

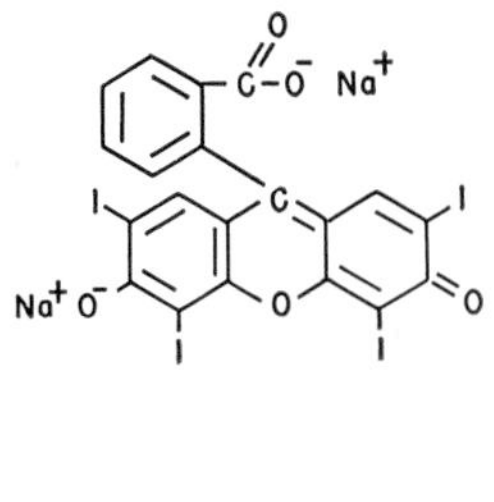

B. PHENOLPHTHALEIN DERIVATIVES
   1. *Phenolphthalein*

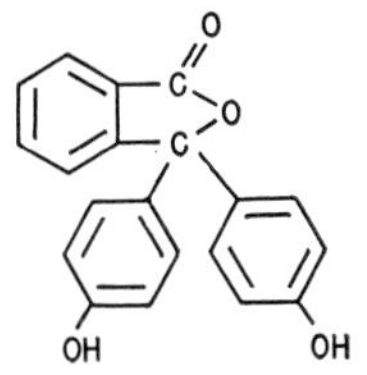

2. *Phenoltetrachlorophthalein*

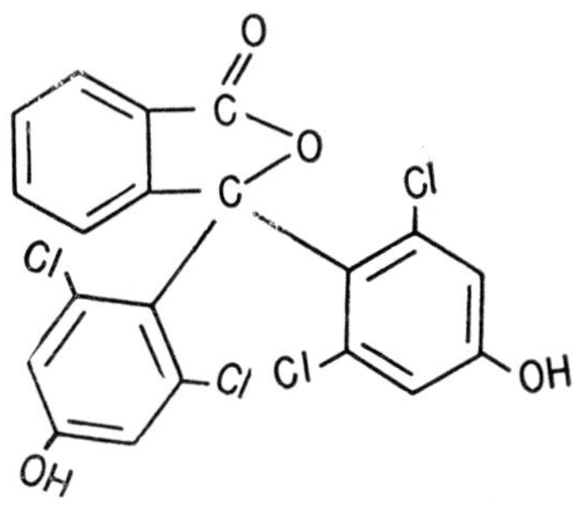

3. *Iodophthalein Sodium* (tetraiodophenolphthalein sodium; Iodeikon)

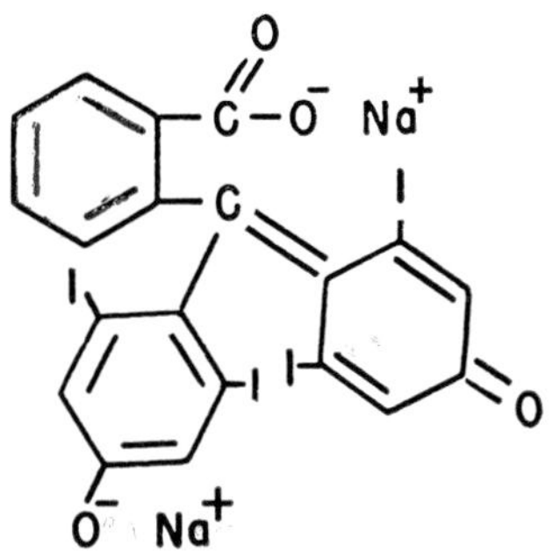

C. PHENOLSULFONPHTHALEIN DERIVATIVES
   1. *Phenolsulfonphthalein* (Phenol Red)

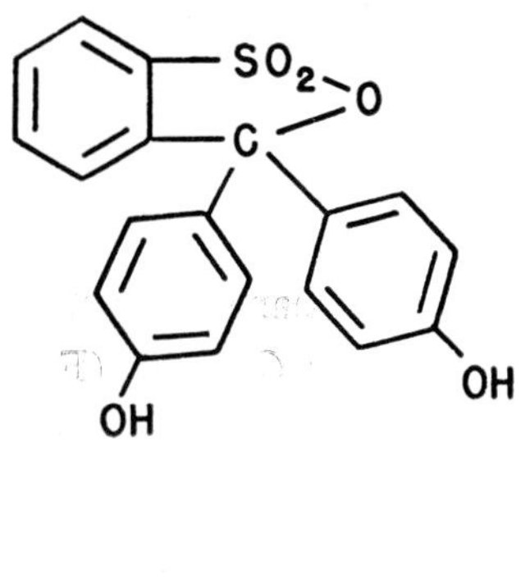

2. *Bromphenol Blue* (tetrabromophe-
nolsulfonphthalein)

IV. Thiazine Dyes

1. *Thionine* (Lauth's violet)

2. *Phenothiazine* (Thiodiphenylamine)

3. *Methylene Blue* (Methylthionine
Chloride; tetramethylthionine chloride)

V. Triphenylmethane (Rosaniline) Dyes

1. *Rosaniline Chloride* (Fuchsin, Magenta)

2. *Methylrosaniline Chloride* (Gentian
violet, crystal violet, methyl violet;
hexamethylparaosaniline chloride)

3. *Malachite Green* (tetramethyl-di-*p*-
aminotriphenyl carbinol chloride)

4. *F.D.&C. Green No. 1* (Guinea
Green; the monosodium salt of
dibenzyldiethyldiaminotriphenylcarbinol disulfonic acid anhydride)

5. *F.D.&C. Green No. 2* (Light Green
SF Yellowish; the disodium salt of
dibenzyldiethyldiaminotriphenylcarbinol trisulfonic acid anhydride)

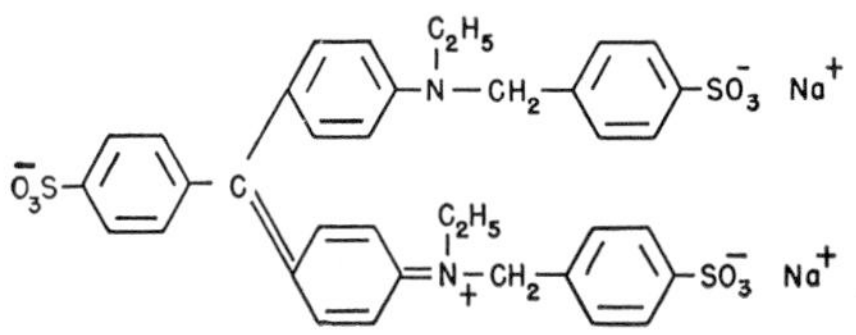

6. *F.D.&C. Green No. 3* (Fast Green FCF; the disodium salt of dibenzyldiethyldiaminohydroxytriphenylcarbinol trisulfonic acid anhydride)

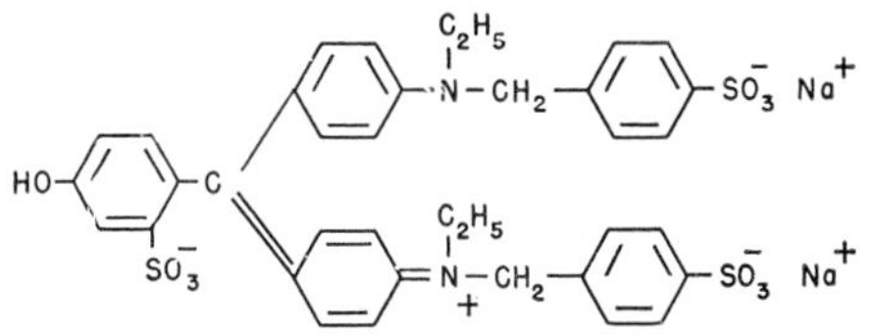

7. *F.D.&C. Blue No. 1* (Brilliant Blue FCF; the disodium salt of dibenzyldiethyldiaminotriphenylcarbinol trisulfonic acid anhydride)

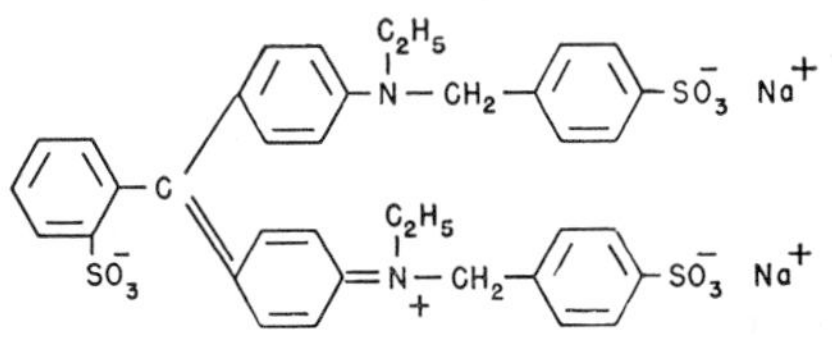

VI. Nitro Dyes

1. *F.D.&C. Yellow No. 1* (Naphthol Yellow S; the sodium salt of 2,4-dinitro-α-naphthol-7-sulfonic acid)

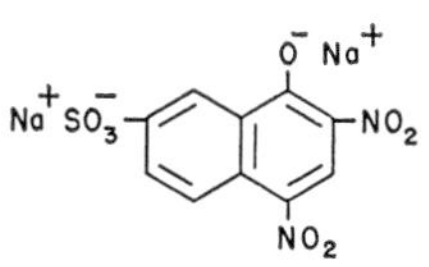

2. *F.D.&C. Yellow No. 2* (Yellow AB; the potassium salt of 2,4-dinitro-α-naphthol-7-sulfonic acid)

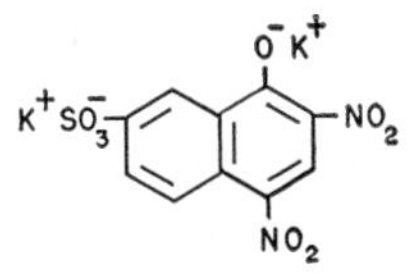

VII. Indigoid Dyes

1. *Sodium Indigotindisulfonate U.S.P.* (F.D.&C. Blue No. 2, Indigo Carmine; the sodium salt of the disulfonic acid of indigotin)

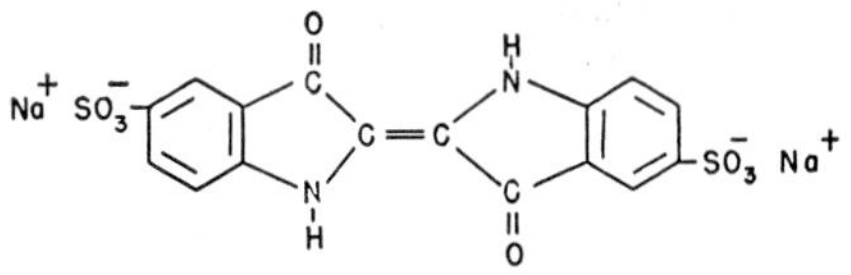

FORMULATION PROBLEMS

The incompatibilities of the various dyes may give rise to different problems, depending on their particular use. Relative to this point in the case of the medicinal dyes, we are concerned mainly with those reactions which result in a decreased therapeutic efficacy, whereas with the coloring agents we are concerned with those reactions in which a change or destruction of the intended color is noted. However, the causes of these incompatibilities may be similar in nature. For example, the precipitation of a medicinal dye from a solution decreases the therapeutic value of the solution (antiseptic, germicidal, cell proliferation activities, etc.) and, when a coloring agent is involved, causes a diminution of the intended color. Since the undesirable reactions are not entirely limited to the

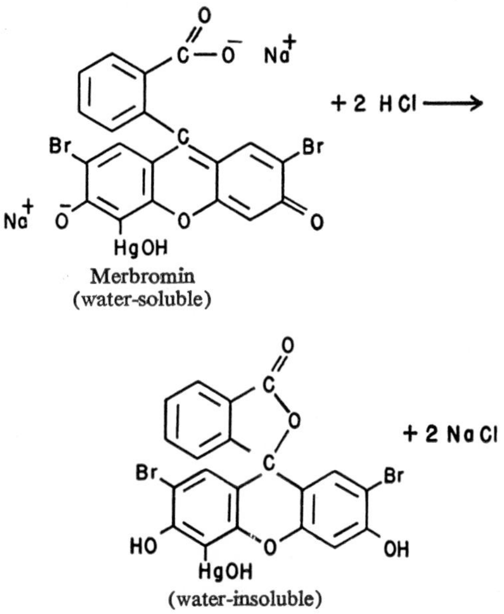

Merbromin
(water-soluble)

(water-insoluble)

TABLE 10-23. SOLUBILITIES OF SOME OF THE MORE IMPORTANT DYES USED IN PHARMACY

DYE	SOLUBILITY IN GM. FOR 100 ML. OF		
	Water	Alcohol	Ether, etc.
Acriflavine	33.3	sl. s.	n. i. eth., chl., f. oils
Acriflavine Hydrochloride	33.3	s.	n. i. eth., chl., f. oils
Amaranth, F.D.&C. Red No. 2	s.	sp. s.	s. gly.; i. eth.
Bismarck Brown	s.	s.	s. eth.
Bromphenol Blue	sl. s.	s.	sl. s. eth., dil. alk.
Congo Red	10	s.	i. eth.
F.D.&C. Blue No. 1, Brilliant Blue FCF	s.	s.	s. gly.; i. eth.
F.D.&C. Green No. 1, Guinea Green	s.	4.5	s. gly.; i. eth.
F.D.&C. Green No. 2, Light Green SF Yellowish	s.	s.	s. gly.; i. eth.
F.D.&C. Green No. 3, Fast Green FCF	s.	sl. s.	s. gly.; i. eth.
F.D.&C. Orange No. 1, Orange No. I	s.	0.3	s. gly.; i. eth.
F.D.&C. Orange No. 2, Orange SS	i.	s.	s. oils; sl. s. gly.
F.D.&C. Red No. 1, Ponceau 3R	s.	sl. s.	s. gly.; i. eth.
F.D.&C. Red No. 3, Erythrosin	s.	s.	s. gly.; i. eth.
F.D.&C. Red No. 4, Ponceau SX	s.	sl. s.	s. gly.; i. eth.
F.D.&C. Red No. 32, Oil Red XO	i.	sl. s.	sl. s. gly.; s. oils
F.D.&C. Yellow No. 1, Naphthol Yellow S	s.	sl. s.	s. gly.; i. eth.
F.D.&C. Yellow No. 2, Yellow AB	s.	sl. s.	s. gly.; i. eth.
F.D.&C. Yellow No. 3, Yellow AB	i.	sl. s.	sp. s. gly.; s. oils
F.D.&C. Yellow No. 4, Yellow OB	i.	s.	sl. s. gly.; s. oils
F.D.&C. Yellow No. 5, Tartrazine	s.	sl. s.	s. gly.
F.D.&C. Yellow No. 6, Sunset Yellow FCF	s.	sl. s.	s. gly.
Fluorescein Sodium	s.	sp. s.	i. eth.
Iodophthalein Sodium	14.3	sl. s.	i. eth.
Malachite Green	s.	s.	s. amyl al.
Merbromin	s.	i.	i. acet., chl., eth.
Methylene Blue	4.0	1.5	s. chl.
Methylrosaniline Chloride	3.0	10.0	6.6 gly.; s. chl.; i. eth.
Phenolphthalein	0.018^{20}	6.6	1.0 eth.; s. dil. alk.
Phenolsulfonphthalein	0.076	0.285	i. chl., eth.
Phenoltetrachlorophthalein	i.	s.	s. eth., acet., dil. alk.
Phenothiazine	i.	1.33	20.0 acet.; 5.0 chl.
Proflavine Dihydrochloride	10.0	s.	sl. s. eth., chl., liq. pet.
Proflavine Sulfate	0.334	sl. s.	n. i. eth., chl., liq. pet.
Pyridium	1.0	s.	i. acet., bz., chl., eth., oils
Quinacrine Hydrochloride	3.0	s.	n. i. eth.
Rosaniline	sl. s.	s.	i. eth.
Scarlet Red	i.	sl. s.	6.6 chl., s. f. oils, pet.
Scarlet Red Sulfonate	s.	sl. s.	sl. s. eth., i. bz., chl., f. oils
Serenium	s.	....	....
Sodium Indigotindisulfonate, U.S.P. F.D.&C. Blue No. 2	s.	sp. s.	s. gly.; i. eth.
Soluble Eosin	s.	s.	i. eth.
Thionine	i.	sl. s.	s. eth.

specific use of the compounds, no separation is made between the medicinal dyes and the coloring agents in the following discussion of their incompatibilities.

Although little has been written concerning the incompatibilities of the dyes, a study

of a few of their reactions will serve to acquaint the student with some of the problems which may arise in the dispensing of them. As a general rule, it may be stated that basic dyes are incompatible with those organic substances which yield a large negative

TABLE 10-24. RESISTANCE OF THE F.D.&C. CERTIFIED DYES TO VARIOUS CONDITIONS INFLUENCING THEIR COLOR STABILITY IN PHARMACEUTICAL PREPARATIONS

F.D.&C. CERTIFIED DYES	LIGHT	ACID	ALKALI	REDUCING AGENTS	OXIDIZING AGENTS
Water-Soluble Dyes					
F.D.&C. Blue No. 1, Brilliant Blue	good	moderate	moderate	good	poor
F.D.&C. Blue No. 2, Indigo Carmine	poor	good	moderate	moderate	poor
F.D.&C. Green No. 1, Guinea Green	poor	good	poor	good	poor
F.D.&C. Green No. 2, Light Green SF Yellowish	poor	good	poor	good	poor
F.D.&C. Green No. 3, Fast Green FCF	good	good	poor	good	poor
F.D.&C. Orange No. 1, Orange I .	moderate	moderate	moderate	poor	fair
F.D.&C. Red No. 1, Ponceau 3R .	good	good	good	poor	fair
F.D.&C. Red No. 2, Amaranth ..	moderate	good	good	poor	fair
F.D.&C. Red No. 3, Erythrosine ..	fair	poor	good	moderate	fair
F.D.&C. Red No. 4, Ponceau SX .	fair	poor	good	moderate	fair
F.D.&C. Yellow No. 1, Naphthol Yellow	moderate	good	good	fair	fair
F.D.&C. Yellow No. 2, Naphthol Yellow (K salt)	moderate	good	good	fair	fair
F.D.&C. Yellow No. 5, Tartrazine	good	good	good	poor	fair
F.D.&C. Yellow No. 6, Sunset Yellow FCF	good	good	good	poor	fair
Oil-Soluble Dyes					
F.D.&C. Orange No. 2, Orange SS	fair	....	....	poor	poor
F.D.&C. Red No. 32, Oil Red XO	fair	....	....	poor	fair
F.D.&C. Yellow No. 3, Yellow AB	poor	....	....	poor	poor
F.D.&C. Yellow No. 4, Yellow OB	poor	....	....	poor	poor

ion on ionization. Extending this point, we find that soaps, tannins, acidic dyes, etc., may yield precipitates with the basic dyes, although in many cases it is a very slow reaction. Conversely, the acidic dyes often yield precipitates with those substances which give rise to a large positive ion on ionization.

The sodium and the mineral acid salts of acid and basic dyes are prepared in order to facilitate the solution of the compound in water. When these salts are placed in an aqueous medium which destroys the salt, incompatibilities often result. For example, Merbromin is precipitated readily in an aqueous acid medium. Mineral acid salts of such substances as local anesthetics, sympathomimetic amines, etc., cause similar reactions. However, acidic dyes which are the sodium salts of sulfonic acid are not affected appreciably by acids or mineral acid salts of organic compounds (see Table 10-24). This behavior of the sodium salts of these acidic sulfonic acid dyes toward acid is explainable on the basis that sulfonic acids are strong acids so susceptible to ionization that they are capable of carrying large molecules into solution in water.

Acridine Dyes. The acridine dyes include acriflavine, acriflavine hydrochloride, pro-

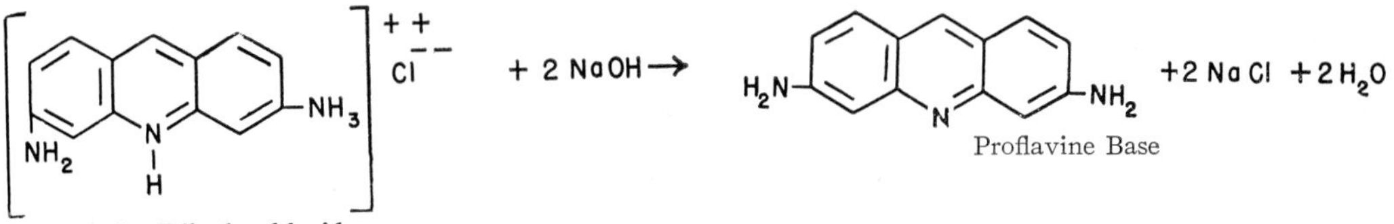

Proflavine Dihydrochloride

$$+ 2 NaOH \rightarrow$$

Proflavine Base

$$+ 2 NaCl + 2 H_2O$$

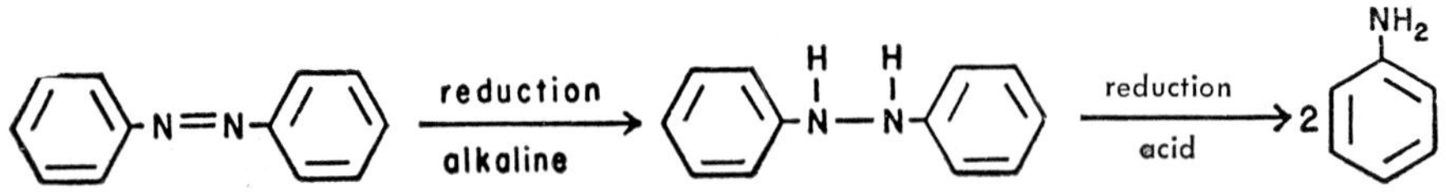

Azobenzene   Hydrazobenzene   Aniline

flavine dihydrochloride and proflavine sulfate. Acriflavine is incompatible with solutions containing chlorine, phenol, silver nitrate, mercuric chloride alkalies and sodium chloride.[67]

Aqueous solutions of proflavine dihydrochloride precipitate the yellow proflavine base on the addition of sodium hydroxide. Silver nitrate T.S. produces a precipitate of silver chloride with an aqueous solution of proflavine dihydrochloride.

Azo Dyes. On referring to the reactions of the azo compounds, it is observed that azobenzene is reduced readily in alkaline solution to hydrazobenzene and ultimately to aniline by acid reduction. Comparable reduction reactions also may take place with the azo dyes in the presence of reducing agents. On referring to Table 10-24, it will be ob-

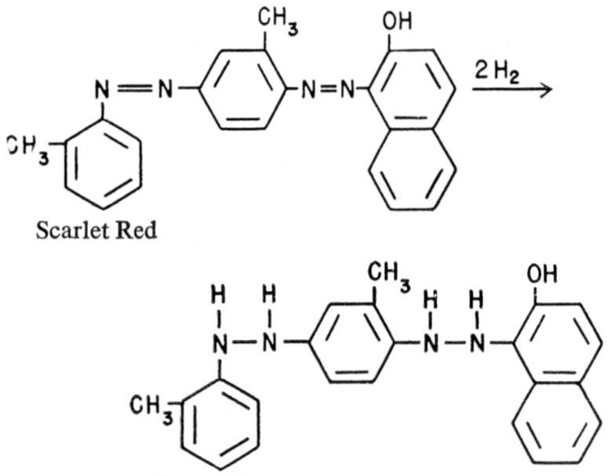

phthalein group and (3) the phenolsulfonphthalein group. They may also be classified as triphenylmethane dyes. The compounds of the first two groups are derivatives of phthalic anhydride and phenols; the members of the latter group are derivatives of sulfobenzoic anhydride. They are all used in pharmacy as dyes and indicators. In general, these compounds are water-insoluble but become water-soluble and highly colored on the formation of their sodium salts.

The reactions of the fluorescein compounds may be illustrated with fluorescein. The color of fluorescein is due to resonance which allows for the presence of the quinoid chromophore group in the molecule. Therefore, the indicated resonance structures (see p. 405) are possible in fluorescein. In alkaline solution, the following reaction takes place:

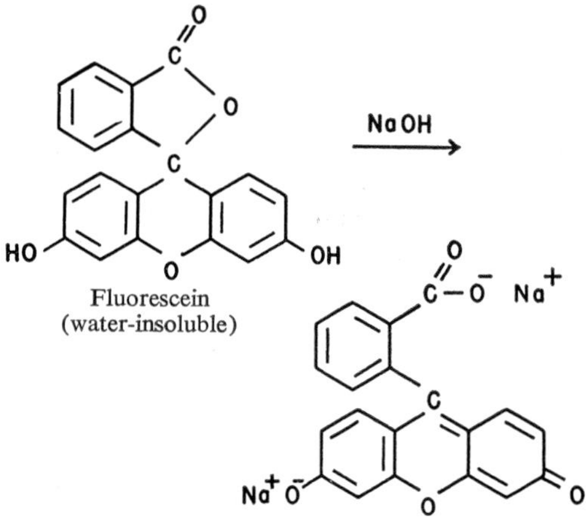

Scarlet Red

Leuco Form

Fluorescein
(water-insoluble)

Fluorescein Sodium
(water-soluble)

served that the F.D.&C. dyes (red 1, 2 and 4; orange 1 and 2; and yellow 3, 4 and 6) possess little resistance to color changes brought about by the presence of reducing agents. Scarlet red, for example, is converted by reduction to the leuco (colorless) compound.

Phthalein Dyes. The phthalein dyes may be divided into three groups: (1) the fluorescein (pyronine) group, (2) the phenol-

Phenolphthalein may be used to illustrate the formation of a salt and the production of color. An analogous reaction takes place with the phenolsulfonphthalein derivatives.

On the addition of alkali to a solution containing phenolphthalein (or similar compound), the water-soluble ionized disodium

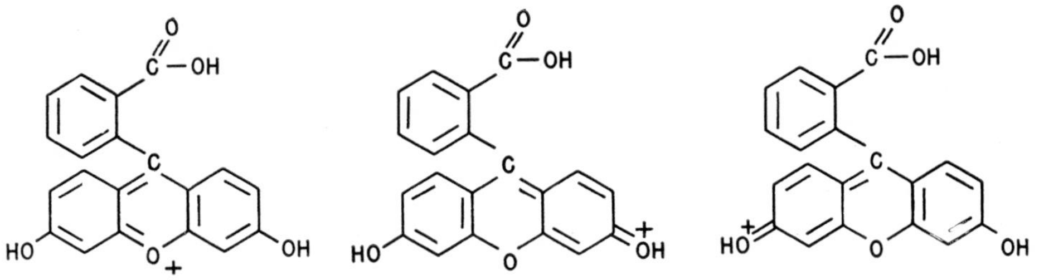

Fluorescein—Resonance Forms

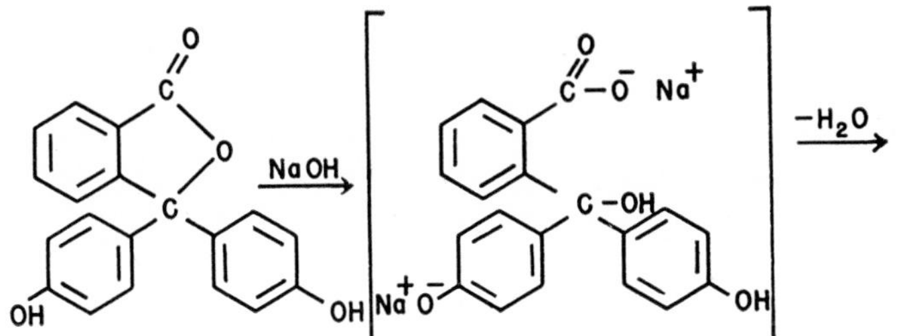

Phenolphthalein
(water-insoluble)

Colorless
Intermediate

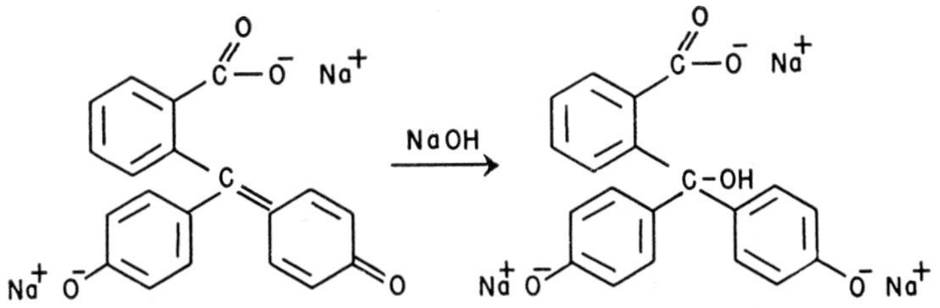

Disodium Salt
(water-soluble)
(red color)

Trisodium Salt
(colorless)

salt is formed and the solution turns red. The production of color is due to the splitting out of a molecule of water which results in the formation of the chromophore quinoid group. If more alkali is added, the trisodium salt is formed and the solution again becomes colorless. The loss of color is brought about by the destruction of the quinoid structure. The addition of acid reverses these reactions and the leuco form is again obtained.

Triphenylmethane Dyes. The triphenylmethane dyes owe their color to the presence of the chromophore quinoid group in the molecule. Because these dyes are reduced readily to the leuco form, problems may arise when they are mixed in solution with reduc-

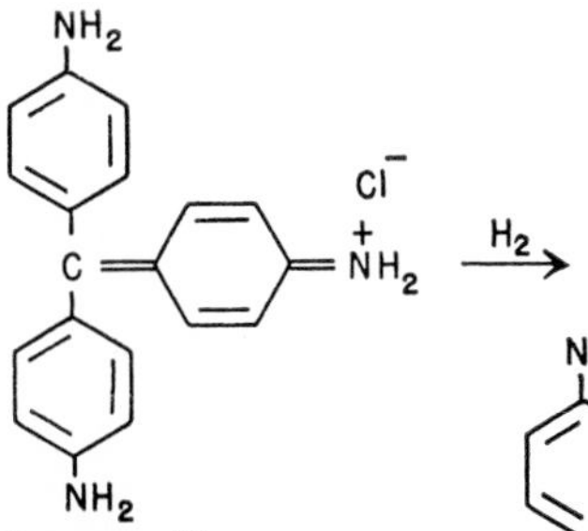

Pararosaniline
(color salt)

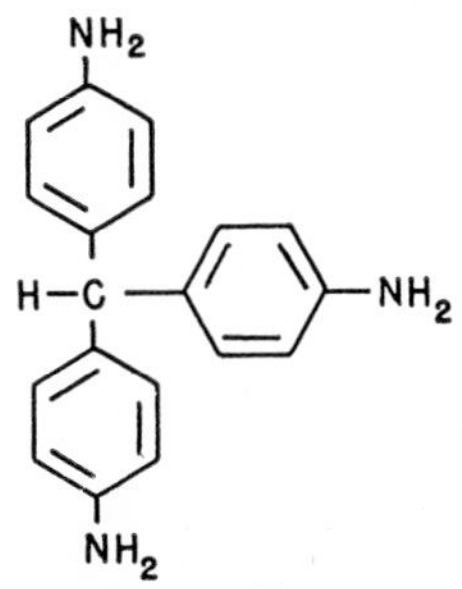

Leucopararosaniline
(colorless)

ing agents. The reaction with pararosaniline, shown on page 405, illustrates this phenomenon.

In the presence of alkali, the hydrochloride salts of the basic triphenylmethane dyes are converted to the colorless carbinol base. The colorless carbinol base may then be reduced to the leuco base.[73] This type of incompatibility is shown readily with malachite green and methylrosaniline chloride.

In addition to being incompatible with reducing agents and alkalies, methylrosaniline chloride (gentian violet, methyl violet, crystal violet) is incompatible with acids. The addition of acid causes the color to change from violet to green to yellow. The explanation of this color change lies in the fact that

the acid prevents the remaining basic groups from contributing to the resonance which is possible in the original structure.[74] Methylrosaniline chloride (gentian violet, crystal violet), a basic nitrogen-containing compound, yields a precipitate with tannic acid in a manner similar to that shown for alkaloids.

Thiazine Dyes. The thiazine dyes, which include thionine, phenothiazine and methylene blue, may resonate between several possible forms. Methylene blue is, perhaps, the most important of this group. Three of its possible resonance forms are shown below.

Methylene blue is reduced readily to the colorless compound. Other incompatibilities include color changes with acids and alkalies.

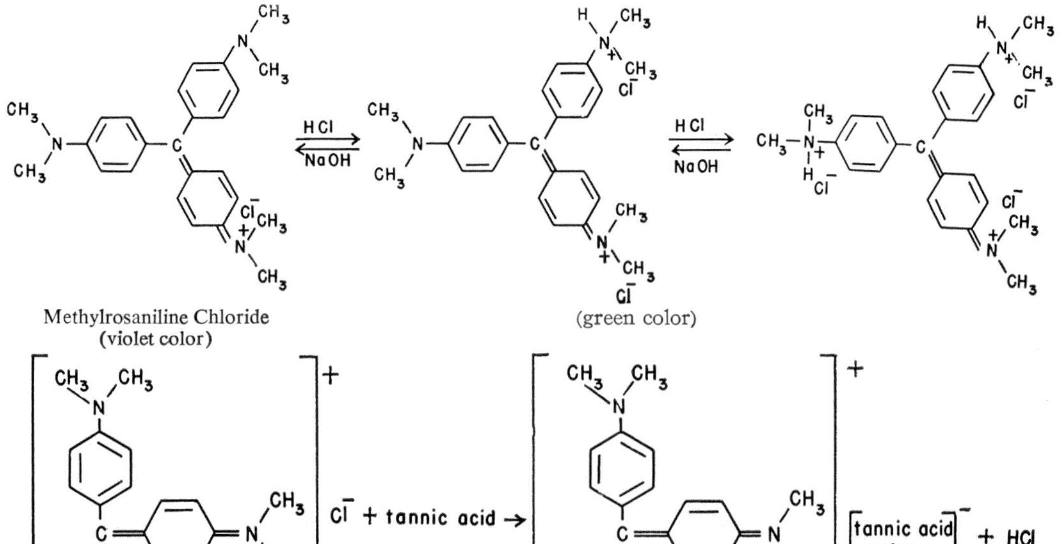

Methylrosaniline Chloride
(violet color)

(green color)

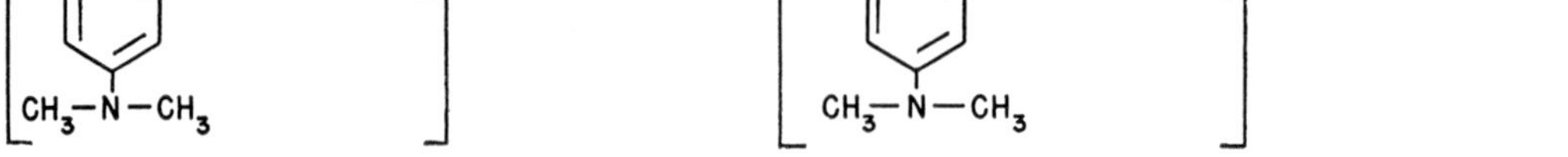

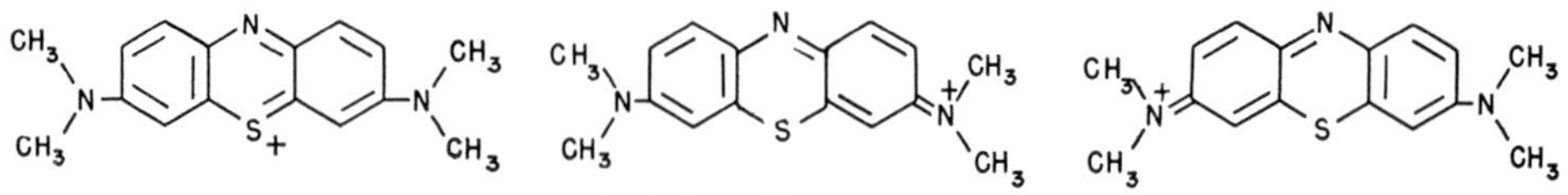

Methylene Blue

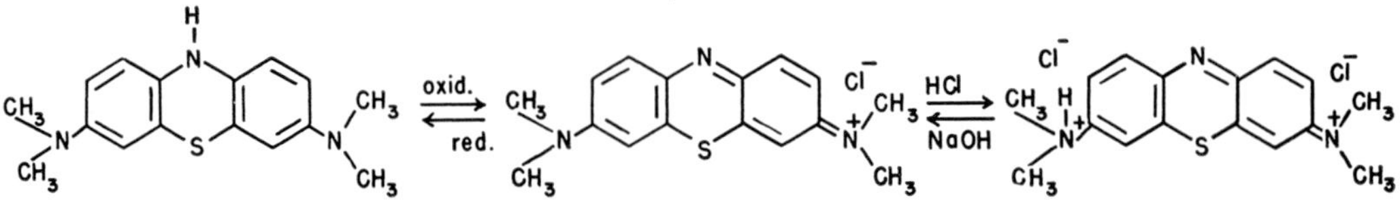

Methylene Blue

lighter blue color

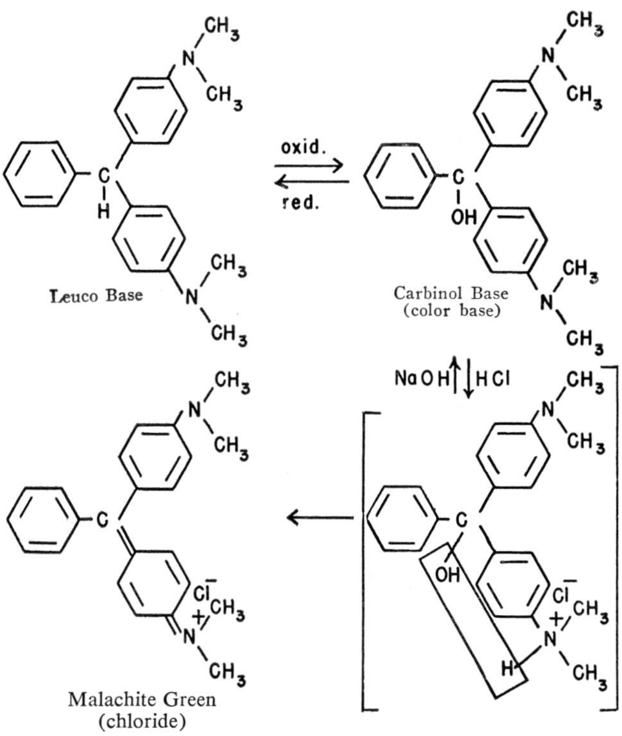
oxid.
red.
Leuco Base
Carbinol Base
(color base)
NaOH
HCl
Malachite Green
(chloride)

Acids cause the color to become a lighter shade of blue; a purple shade is obtained with alkalies. An excess of sodium hydroxide yields a violet precipitate on standing. These incompatibilities are shown in the following reactions. Other incompatibilities of a precipitation nature are caused by iodides, mercuric salts and tannic acid.

Nitro Dyes. The nitro dyes exhibit only a fair resistance to the influence of reducing agents. Aromatic nitro compounds are, of course, oxidizing agents and may be reduced to the corresponding amino compound. The nitro dyes are also susceptible to reduction and, thus, in Table 10-24 it is observed that the nitro dyes F.D.&C. No. 1 (Naphthol Yellow S) and F.D.&C. Yellow No. 2 (Yellow AB) manifest only a fair amount of resistance to the color changes brought about by reducing agents.

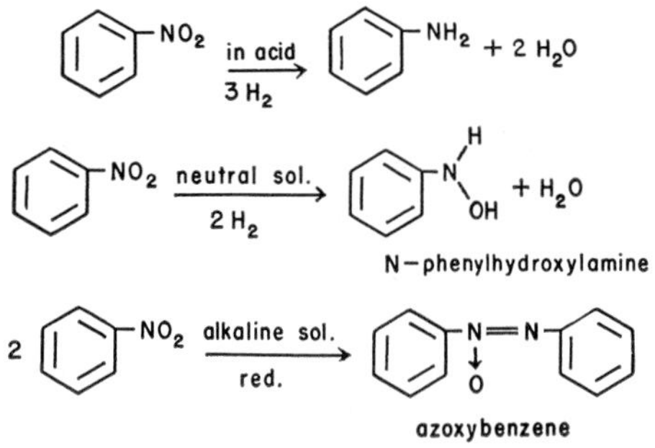
in acid
$3H_2$
+ $2H_2O$
neutral sol.
$2H_2$
+ H_2O
N-phenylhydroxylamine
alkaline sol.
red.
azoxybenzene

Indigoid Dyes. These dyes may be reduced to the leuco (colorless) form. The following reaction with indigo carmine (Sodium Indigotin Disulfonate, *U.S.P.*) illustrates the change brought about by reduction as shown on the following page.

On oxidation, the color of indigo carmine is changed from blue to green to light yellow.

From these reactions, it is observed that both oxidizing and reducing agents may be potential causative agents for incompatibilities for these dyes. However, in practical use it is found that indigo carmine has a moderate resistance to reducing agents but poor resistance to the activity of oxidizing agents (Table 10-24). Indigo carmine is precipitated by sodium chloride from aqueous solutions, and sodium hydroxide causes the color to change from blue to yellow.

ANTIBIOTICS

This group of therapeutic agents, which in the common pharmaceutical terminology has

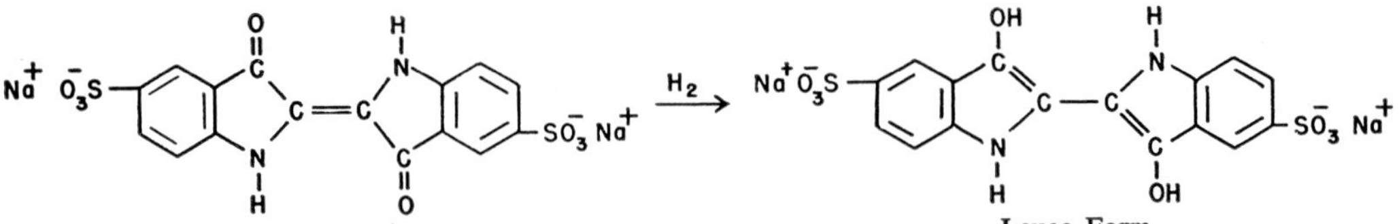

Indigo Carmine

Leuco Form

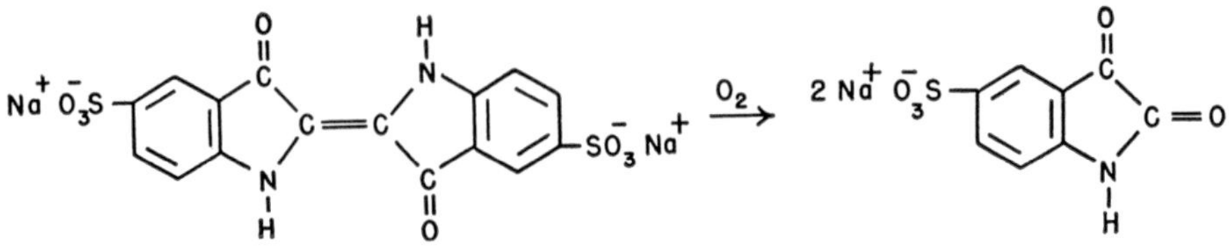

become known as the antibiotics, varies greatly in chemical composition. Because of the great differences in the chemical nature of the antibiotics, it is not logical to treat the subject of their incompatibilities as a class of compounds. The incompatibilities of each substance must be considered in an individual manner. Actually, the problems encountered by the practicing pharmacist in the compounding of these antibiotic substances tend to be reduced by the manner in which they are prescribed and used. However, it is essential for the pharmacist to know the reactions of these substances in order to understand not only the possible incompatibilities which may be encountered in compounding, such as the addition of antibiotics to parenteral solutions, but also the problems involved in product formulation, storage and the limitations of the various modes of administration. No attempt has been made in the following discussion to provide a complete list of the microorganisms against which the individual antibiotics are effective, since the therapeutic use of these agents is not within the scope of this chapter.

BACITRACIN

Bacitracin is a neutral polypeptide obtained from cultures of *Bacillus subtilis,* strain Tracy I. It is active against many gram-positive and certain gram-negative organisms and frequently is active against organisms which have become resistant to penicillin. It can be used by intramuscular injection against systemic infections, but its main use at the present time is by topical application against infections of skin, eye, nose and

throat. Bacitracin does not yield detectable blood levels when given by the oral route.

Solubility. Bacitracin is soluble in water and alcohol but insoluble in acetone, ether and chloroform.

Formulation Problems. Bacitracin can be precipitated from aqueous solution by high concentrations of soluble inorganic salts such as sodium chloride. It also is precipitated and inactivated by heavy metal ions[3] and tannic acid. Salicylic acid likewise causes bacitracin to be precipitated, but the precipitate maintains antibiotic activity. Aqueous solutions in general are unstable; however, in neutral or slightly acidic solution, activity is retained for long periods if the solution is refrigerated at 0° to 5° C. At 37° C., inactivation occurs in 2 weeks. In alkaline solution (pH 9 and above), the antibiotic is inactivated rapidly.

In the dry form, bacitracin is stable at temperatures up to 37° C. It is also stable in anhydrous hydrocarbon ointment bases but rapidly loses its activity in the water-miscible bases.[7] It is reported that bacitracin ointments containing polyethylene glycols and propylene glycol lose 50 per cent of their activity within a week at room temperature.[62]

CHLORAMPHENICOL

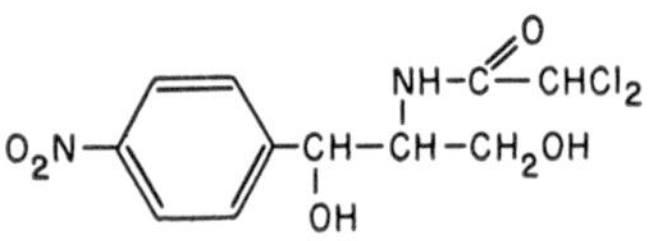

Chloramphenicol (Chloromycetin; D-*threo*-1-p-nitrophenyl-2-dichloroacetamido-1,3-propanediol) was obtained originally from cultures of *Streptomyces venezuelae* but is now prepared by chemical synthesis. It is a broad-spectrum antibiotic which is effective against certain gram-negative bacteria, spirochetes, rickettsia and larger viruses.

Solubility. Chloramphenicol is only slightly soluble in water (0.25%) but is soluble in alcohol, acetone, ethyl acetate and propylene glycol. The palmitate ester is very insoluble in water; thus the extremely bitter taste which characterizes the parent compound is decreased significantly so that the ester can be employed satisfactorily in aqueous suspensions for oral use. The sodium salt of the succinate ester is water-soluble.

Formulation Problems. Chloramphenicol is a much more stable compound than either penicillin or streptomycin; however, it is rapidly inactivated in dilute aqueous alkali. At pH 10.8, chloramphenicol is over 87 per cent inactivated in 24 hours at 25° C.[87] It is relatively stable in neutral and acidic solutions. In the dry form, the antibiotic is very stable at room temperature.

Cycloserine

Cycloserine (Seromycin, D-4-amino-3-isoxazolidone) is an antibiotic substance produced by *Streptomyces orchidaceus*[32] or *Streptomyces garyphalus*.[33] The compound is effective against the mycobacterium tuberculosis organism and is thus employed in the treatment of severe pulmonary tuberculosis.

Cycloserine is soluble in water (10 Gm. per 100 ml. at 25° C.). The compound is stable in alkaline but unstable in neutral and acidic solutions.

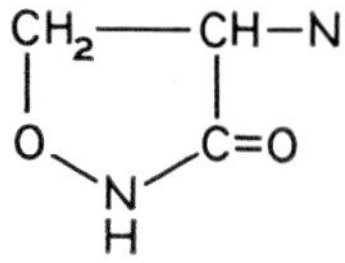

Erythromycin

Erythromycin (Ilotycin, Erythrocin) is a broad-spectrum antibiotic obtained from *Streptomyces erythreus*. It is somewhat similar to penicillin in antibacterial activity and allegedly does not produce the profound changes in the intestinal flora which is often observed with the use of other broad-spectrum antibiotics.[60]

The antibiotic has the following formula, and, since it contains basic nitrogen in the molecule, it is capable of forming salts with acids.

Solubility. The free base is poorly soluble in water (0.2%) but is soluble in alcohol, acetone, chloroform and ether. The hydrochloride salt is soluble in water (4.0%) but the stearate and the ethylcarbonate esters are water-insoluble. Because of their insolubility, these esters are not so bitter tasting as the free base or the soluble salts and, therefore, are particularly useful in pediatric preparations in the form of aqueous suspensions.

Formulation Problems. Erythromycin, both as the free base and in the soluble salt form, is destroyed rapidly in aqueous solution by both acids and alkalies. It is most stable in the range of pH 6 to 8 and is inactivated very rapidly at pH 4 and below. Therefore, the free base and the soluble salts are inactivated in the stomach unless given in the form of enteric-coated tablets. However, the insoluble stearate and the ethylcarbonate esters are not destroyed by the acid of the stomach and thus can be administered in the form of aqueous suspensions as previously stated.

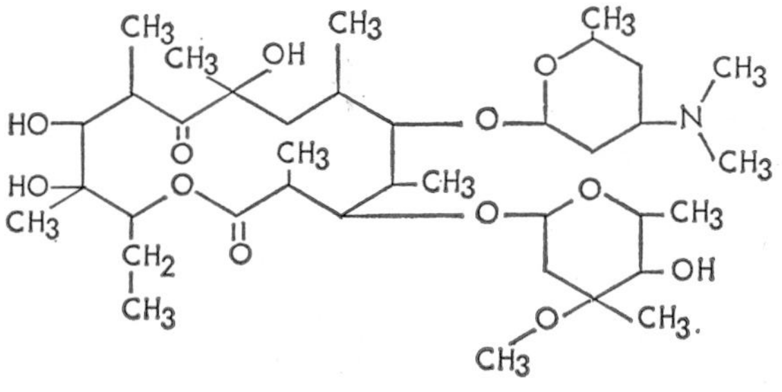

Erythromycin

KANAMYCIN

Kanamycin, like neomycin, is quite stable in aqueous solutions. Thus, it is relatively stable at room temperature and below over the wide pH range of 2 to 11. The influence of heat on the stability of aqueous solutions

Kanamycin

is readily shown, however, by the fact that at 100° C. and at pH's of 6 to 8, solutions are only stable for about 30 minutes. Kanamycin is water-soluble and is used in the form of the sulfate. The drug is administered orally in capsules and intramuscularly in solution.

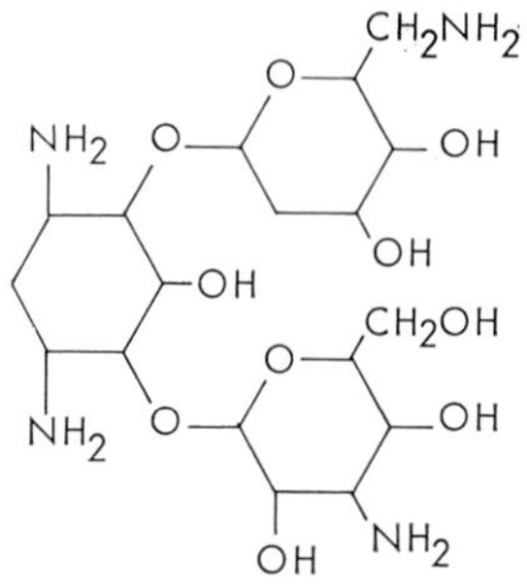

NEOMYCIN

Neomycin (Mycifradin) is a basic compound obtained from cultures of *Streptomyces fradiae*. It manifests antibiotic activity

Neomycin C

against both gram-positive and gram-negative bacteria and is particularly effective against staphylococci. Thus, it is widely used by topical administration, in both the solution and the ointment form, for the treatment of skin infections. It is also administered orally as an intestinal antiseptic.

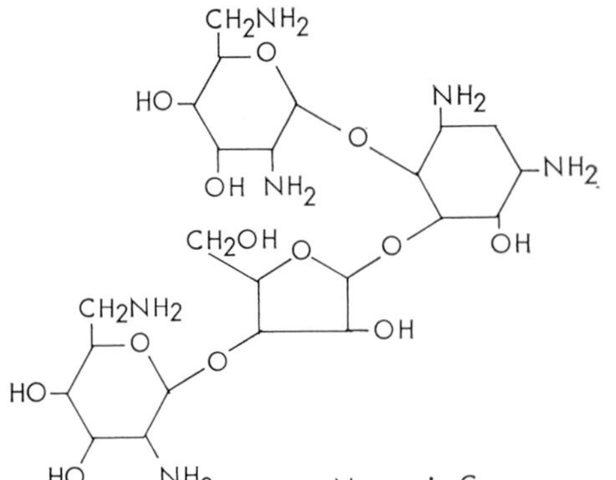

Solubility. Since Neomycin is a basic compound, it forms salts with acids. Neomycin Sulfate is soluble in water but insoluble in most organic solvents.

Formulation Problems. Neomycin is more stable in aqueous solution than many of the other antibiotic agents and is even active in alkaline solution.[4] Its stability range in solution is between pH 1.5 and 12.[1]

NOVOBIOCIN

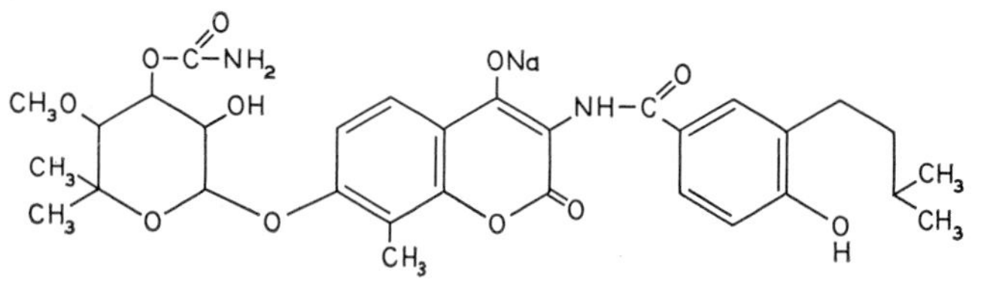

Novobiocin Sodium (Cathomycin So-

dium, Albamycin) is the salt of an acidic substance produced by the organism *Streptomyces niveus*.[36, 46] This antibiotic is effective against gram-positive organisms and is especially useful against resistant strains of staphylococci.

Novobiocin as the sodium salt is very soluble in water and is also soluble in alcohol, glycerin and propylene glycol. The antibiotic is relatively stable under both acidic and alkaline conditions and thus can be dispensed in liquid as well as dry solid dosage forms. Novobiocin (Cathomycin Calcium) is also available as the calcium salt. This salt is soluble in water (0.4 Gm. per 100 ml.), in alcohol (3.3 Gm. per 100 ml.) and in ether (0.22 Gm. per 100 ml.).

OLEANDOMYCIN

Oleandomycin phosphate is an antibiotic substance obtained from the growth media of *Streptomyces antibioticus*. This compound is effective against gram-positive organisms and is particularly useful against staphylococci, streptococci and pneumococci.

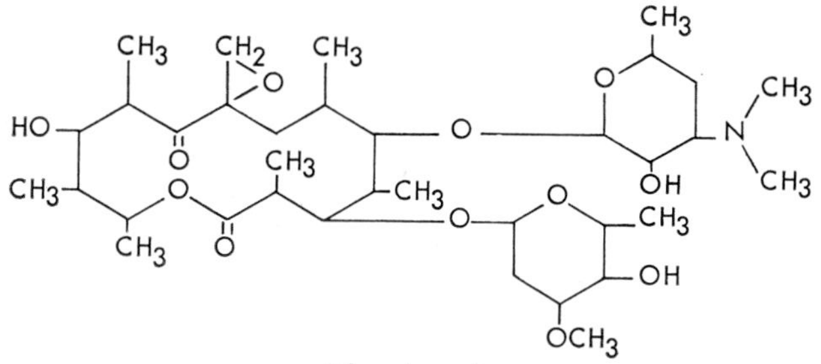

Oleandomycin

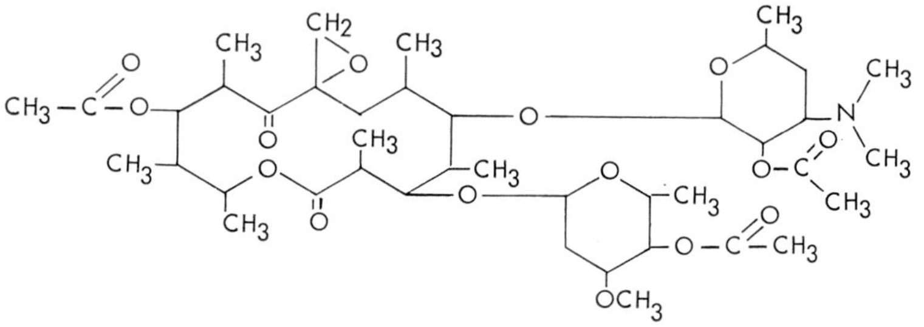

Triacetyloleandomycin

This antibiotic contains basic nitrogen[18] in its complex structure and thus is able to form water-soluble salts with acids. It is included in the macrolide group of antibiotics of which erythromycin is also a member.

Oleandomycin phosphate is soluble in water (45.4 Gm. per 100 ml.), in alcohol (33.3 Gm. per 100 ml.) and is slightly soluble in ether.

Triacetyloleandomycin (Cyclamycin, TAO), the triacetyl ester of oleandomycin, is only slightly soluble in water and ether but is soluble (10 Gm. per 100 ml.) in alcohol. Because of its decreased water solubility it is more stable in liquid preparations than salts of the parent compound and is often used in in the form of a suspension.

Penicillin

Penicillin is obtained as a growth product from the molds *Penicillium notatum* and *P. chrysogenum Thom* (Fam. Aspergillaceae). Penicillin G also has been prepared synthetically. The antibiotic substance obtained from these molds has been shown to be a mixture of chemically related substances. The fermentation liquors contain mainly penicillin G, smaller quantities of K and F, and variable amounts of the other penicillins. In various commercial procedures, the production of penicillin G has been increased by the process of adding certain precursors such as phenylacetamide and phenylacetic acid to the media, whereas the addition of S-allylmercaptoacetic acid to the fermentation broth yields penicillin O. All the known natural and synthetic penicillins are derivatives of the parent β-lactone structure shown below and differ only in the nature of the R radical.

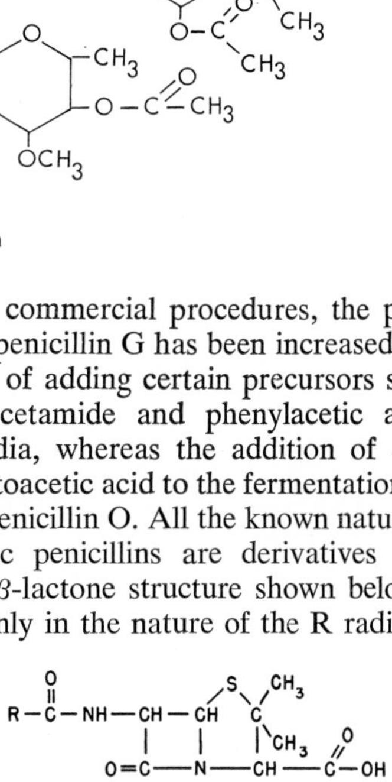

Parent Structure of Penicillin

The following are some of the more important penicillins.

Penicillin G R = 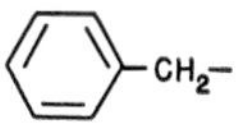 (Benzyl)

Penicillin F R = $CH_3-CH_2-CH=CH-CH_2-$ (Δ^2 Pentenyl)

Penicillin K R = $CH_3-(CH_2)_5-CH_2-$ (*n*-Heptyl)

Penicillin O R= $CH_2=CH-CH_2-S-CH_2-$

Penicillin V R= 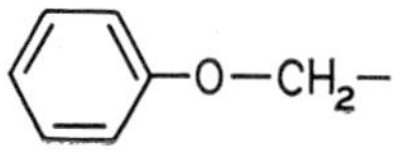

Penicillin X

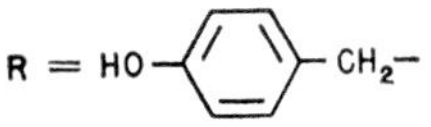

$R = $ HO—⟨benzene ring⟩—CH_2- (*p*-Hydroxybenzyl)

Methicillin (2, 6-dimethoxyphenyl)

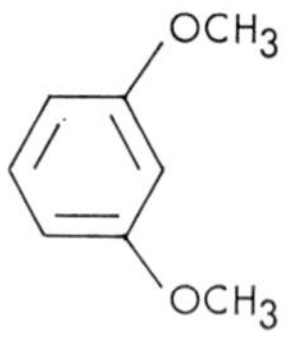

OCH₃ ... OCH₃

Oxacillin (Prostaphlin, Resistopen)
(5-methyl-3-phenyl-4-isoxazolyl)

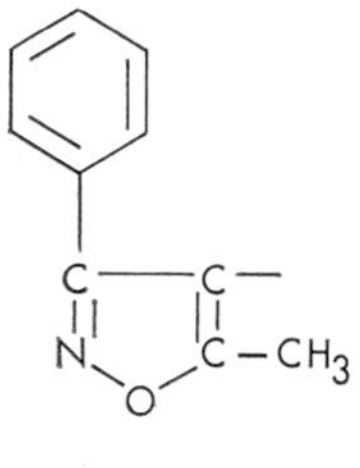

Phenethicillin (phenoxyethyl)

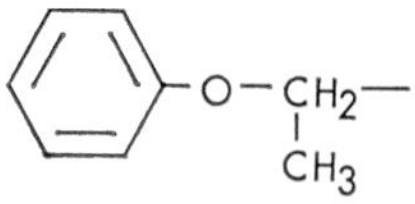

O—CH₂—
CH₃

Nafcillin Unipen (2-ethoxy-1-naphthyl)

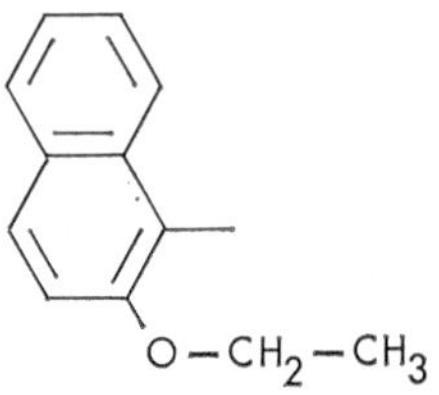

O—CH₂—CH₃

Ampicillin (α-aminobenzyl)

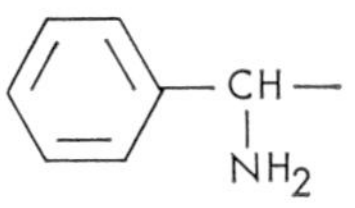

CH—
NH₂

Owing to the manner in which penicillin is prescribed and used, few incompatibilities are encountered in the actual dispensing of the drug. However, there are many important points concerning its stability which the pharmacist must know.

Solubility. The free acid of penicillin is insoluble in water and decomposes readily. The alkali and the alkaline earth metals all form water-soluble salts, but those salts derived from heavy metals are only slightly soluble in water. Penicillin is also soluble in glycerin and alcohol, but these solvents cause it to be inactivated. The salts derived from various amines such as procaine (Procaine Penicillin G) or N,N'-dibenzylethylenediamine (Benzathine Penicillin G; Bicillin) have poor water-solubility.

Formulation Problems. Aqueous solutions of penicillin readily decompose with a loss in potency even when refrigerated. In solutions having a pH of 5 or less, the free acid of penicillin is precipitated. Solutions having a pH 8.0 and above cause a rapid deterioration of the penicillin. The incompatibilities of penicillin in aqueous solution may thus be summarized as follows: (1) precipitated and inactivated by acids and heavy metals; (2) inactivated by alkalies (pH 8.0 and above), glycerin and alcohol; and (3) inactivated by oxidizing agents. Since penicillin is precipitated and inactivated by acids, it is incompatible in the acid medium of the stomach. In this case, the penicillin is inactivated before absorption can take place in the small intestine. This may be classed as a therapeutic or physiologic incompatibility. In order to facilitate the oral administration of penicillin, buffering agents such as aluminum hydroxide, calcium carbonate, anhydrous sodium citrate, etc., may be added to penicillin tablets or solutions to reduce the hydrogen ion concentration of the stomach. In this way, the destruction of the penicillin in the stomach is decreased. In the alkaline fluids of the

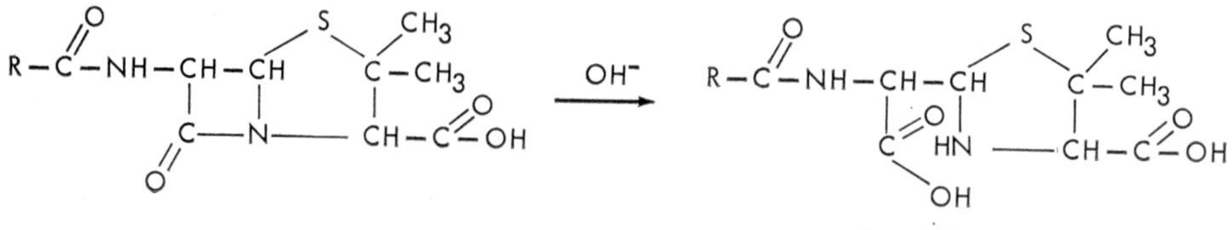

Penicilloic acid

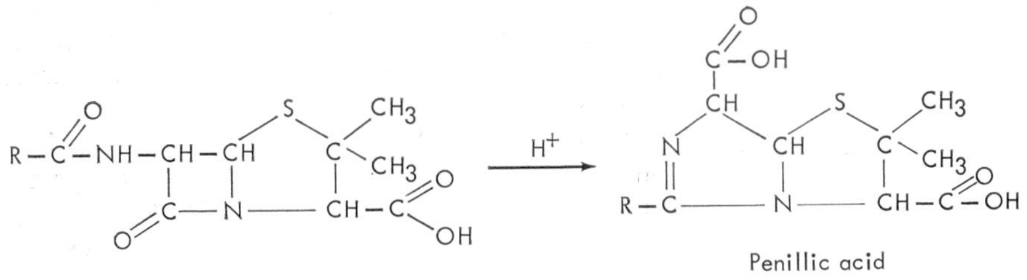

Decomposition of penicillin in acid solution

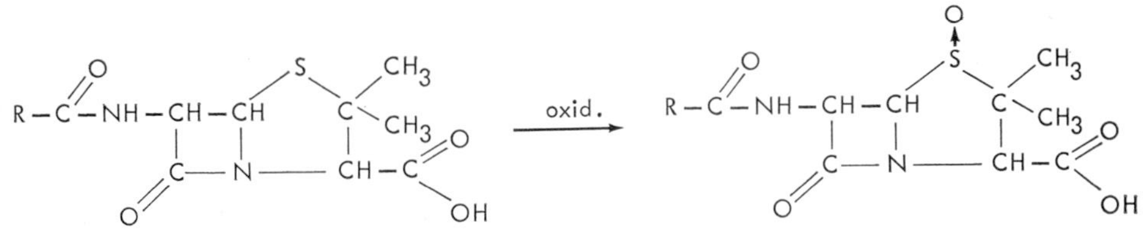

Mild oxidation of penicillin

body such as saliva, enteric juices and bile, the pH range usually falls between 5.0 and 8.0, and the drug is not destroyed so readily. The half-life at pH 6.67 is approximately 14 days. Even so, following oral administration with these precautions, roughly only about one fourth of the ingested penicillin is absorbed; thus, much larger doses are required with this route of administration.

The enzyme penicillinase also causes the type of decomposition reaction just shown. In the presence of solvents containing OH, esterification of penicilloic acid occurs.

Because of their water-insolubility, Procaine Penicillin G and Benzathine Penicillin G are more stable in an aqueous medium than the potassium salts. The aqueous suspensions are used both orally and parenterally and are stated to retain their activity for long periods of time. Therapeutically, these insoluble forms are of value because, after parenteral administration, they maintain higher and more constant penicillin blood levels than the more soluble forms.

Penicillin ointments remain active for a long period of time if they are compounded without first dissolving the drug in water but incorporated in anhydrous ointment bases. However, the area to which the ointment is to be applied governs to some extent the type of ointment bases used. When penicillin ointments are intended for application to mucous membranes, the drug, in the dry form, may be incorporated into a base which is capable of absorbing water. Solution of the penicillin then takes place in the aqueous fluids of the membranes to which the ointment is applied.

POLYMYXIN

The polymyxins are derived from various strains of the spore-forming soil bacterium *Bacillus polymyxa* (*B. aerosporus*). All the known members of the polymyxin group (A, B, C, D and E) are basic polypeptides and therefore are capable of forming water-soluble salts with inorganic acids. The polymyxins are effective against most gram-negative organisms. This antibiotic is used mainly by topical application but also can be given orally for infections of the gastrointestinal tract.

Solubility. Polymyxin B sulfate and the hydrochloride salts are soluble in water but insoluble in most organic solvents. As the free bases, the polymyxins are only slightly soluble in water and are insoluble in alcohol.

Incompatibility. The polymyxins are incompatible in aqueous solution with strong acids and alkalies. Such solutions rapidly lose their antibiotic activity even at room temperature. However, in less acidic and in neutral solutions (pH 2 to 7), the antibiotic is stated to be thermostable.[4, 75]

STREPTOMYCIN

Streptomycin is produced by the actinomycete, *Streptomyces griseus,* and is obtained as a growth product of this organism.

Chemically, streptomycin is an organic base composed of streptidine (1,3-diguanidino-2,4,5,6-tetrahydroxycyclohexane) and a disaccharidelike component streptobiosamine joined through a glycoside linkage.[13] The streptobiosamine portion of the molecule is composed of streptose and N-methyl-1-glucosamine. The structure of streptomycin is shown below ($C_{21}H_{39}N_7O_{12}$).

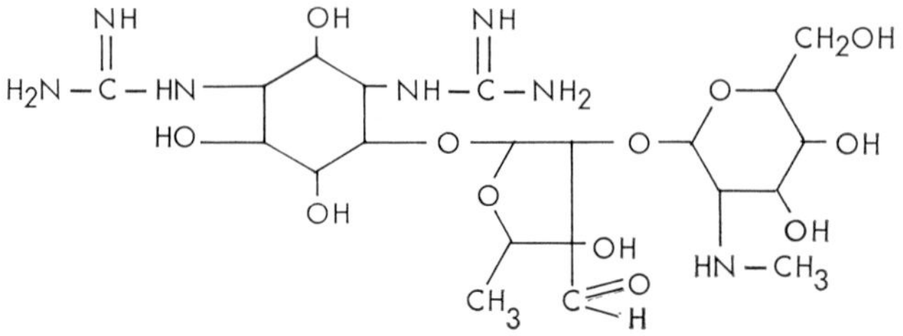

tetracycline (Declomycin) and rolitetracycline. Chlortetracycline is obtained from the organism *Streptomyces aureofaciens,* whereas oxytetracycline is obtained from *Streptomyces rimosus.* Tetracycline can be prepared by reductive dechlorination of chlortetracycline.[8,10] As is observed from their structures, these substances are amphoteric since they contain both acidic and basic groups in the molecule.

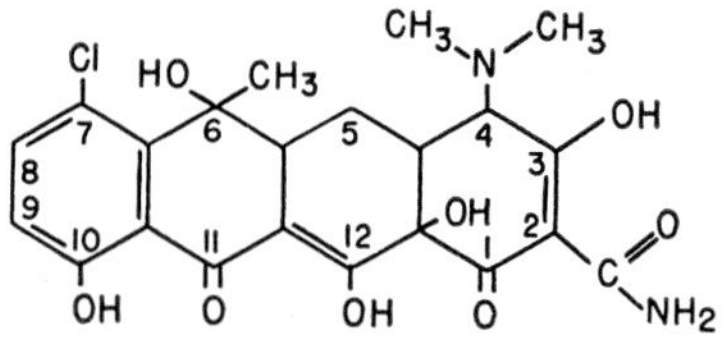

Streptomycin

Due to the presence of the basic nitrogen in the molecule, streptomycin forms salts with acids. It is available as the hydrochloride, the sulfate, the phosphate and the streptomycin calcium chloride complex known as streptomycin trihydrochloride calcium chloride [$(C_{21}H_{39}N_7O_{12}\cdot3HCl)_2CaCl_2$]. Reduction of the aldehyde group to a primary alcohol in the streptose portion of the molecule yields dihydrostreptomycin.

Solubility. Streptomycin and its salts are very soluble in water but insoluble in chloroform, ether and other nonpolar solvents.

Formulation Problems. In the dry crystalline form, it is quite stable at room temperature, but as a precautionary measure against decomposition is should be stored at temperatures not exceeding 15° C. The optimum pH for stability of streptomycin in water is 4.5 to 7.0. The approximate half-life for an aqueous solution at pH 6.6 at room temperature is 23.5 days. Dihydrostreptomycin is more stable to alkali than streptomycin.

TETRACYCLINES

The tetracyclines compose a group of chemically similar agents having similar broad-spectrum antibiotic activity. These agents are chlortetracycline (Aureomycin), oxytetracycline (Terramycin), tetracycline (Achromycin, Tetracyn) and demethylchlor-

Chlortetracycline

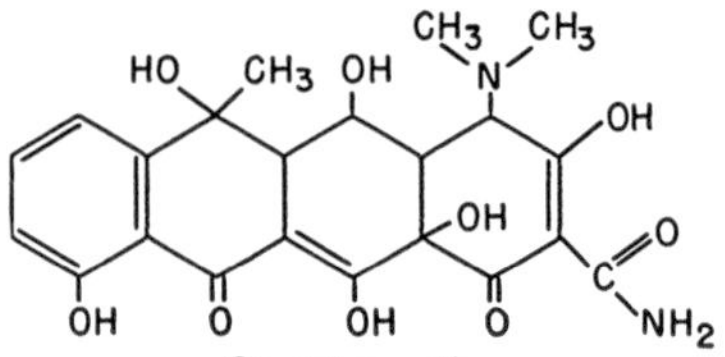

Oxytetracycline

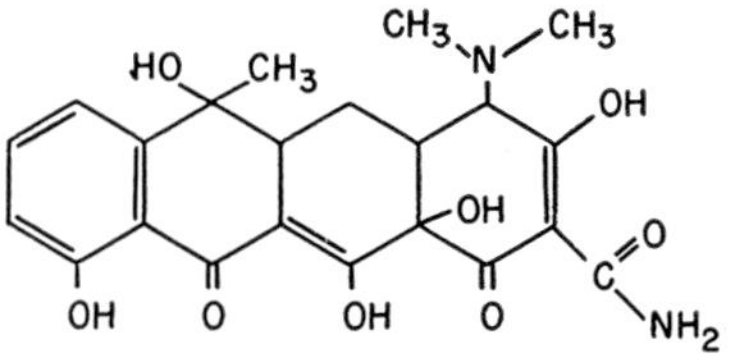

Tetracycline

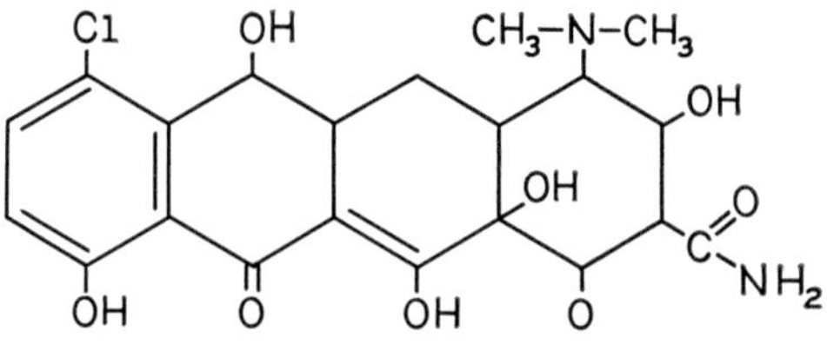

Demethylchlortetracycline

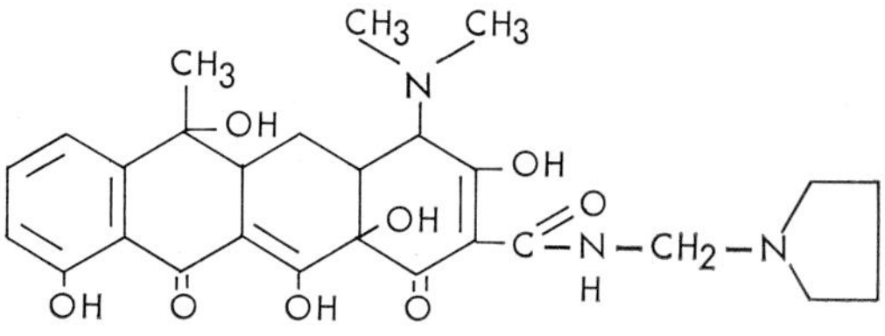

Rolitetracycline

They are thus able to form salts with either acids or alkalies. The acid salt is formed on the basic nitrogen of the dimethylamino group attached to the number four carbon atom. The monosodium salt is formed by reaction of the phenolic OH group in position 10 with alkali. The disodium salt of these compounds also can be prepared. In this case, salt formation occurs at positions 10 and 12.

Solubility. The free forms of the tetracyclines are only slightly soluble in water. However, the hydrochloride and the sodium salts are soluble in water but practically insoluble in acetone, chloroform and ether. Salts formed with other metals such as calcium and magnesium are water-insoluble.

Incompatibility. The tetracyclines are unstable in neutral and alkaline solutions. Therefore, it is not practical to use these agents in the form of their sodium salts in

TABLE 10-25. SOME STABILITY DATA FOR TETRACYCLINES IN AQUEOUS SOLUTIONS

COMPOUND	pH	TEMPERATURE (°C.)	HALF-LIFE ($t\frac{1}{2}$) (in hours)
Aureomycin	7.4	20	72
	8.0	20	29
	8.6	20	10
	9.2	20	2
	8.0	30	6
	8.0	40	2
Tetracycline	1.0	37	114
	2.5	37	134
	4.6	37	45
	7.0	37	26
	8.85	37	12
Terramycin	8.5	5	2424
	8.5	19.5	354
	8.3	37	33.2
	8.5	65	1.35
	4.5	37	47.8
	7	37	27.5
	8.3	37	34.4
	10	37	15

Epimerization (dimethylamino function at C4) of Terramycin solutions occurs in the pH range of 2.5 to 6.0 but is most rapid at pH 4.0. The epi form is only one-tenth as active as the natural form.

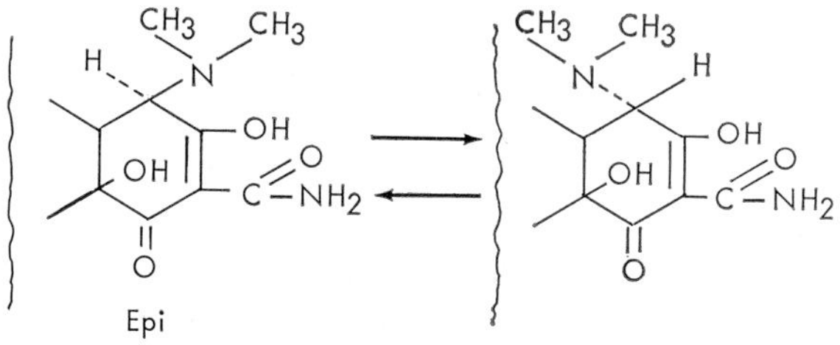

Epi

aqueous solutions. Tetracycline is somewhat more stable to alkaline conditions than is chlortetracycline; however, under more drastic conditions, a similar degradation of the molecule occurs.[9, 43, 83, 84] It has been shown that all of the tetracyclines are more stable in solution at pH 2.5 than at either pH 7 or 9 when heated to 100° C. for 15 minutes and that tetracycline was less inactivated at all three pHs than either chlortetracycline or oxytetracycline.[6] The hydrochloride salts of the tetracyclines are all stable in the dry state.

TYROTHRICIN

Tyrothricin is produced by the tyrothrix group of aerobic spore-forming soil bacteria *Bacillus brevis, B. mesentericus,* etc. It is composed of two crystallizable polypeptides known as gramicidin (20 to 25%) and tyrocidin (60%). These two substances can be separated by treatment with a mixture of acetone and ether. Gramicidin is soluble in this mixture and tyrocidin is insoluble.

Tyrocidin is believed to be a cyclic polypeptide having a molecular weight of approximately 2,500 and containing two molecules of aspartic acid, glutamic acid, or nithine, tryptophan, proline, tyrosine, leucine and valine, and three molecules of *d*-phenylalanine.

Solubility. Tyrocidin is strongly basic and forms water-soluble salts with hydrochloric acid. Gramicidin contains 6 tryptophan, 6 leucine, 4 valine, 4 alanine, 2 glycine and 2 unknown aminohydroxy compounds. Both of these polypeptides are nearly insoluble in water, but tyrothricin is soluble in alcohol.

Formulation Problems. Tyrothricin is used only topically, since it is apparently too toxic for systemic administration. The gramicidin allegedly causes hemolysis of the blood cells. To be effective, it is necessary that the tyrothricin come in direct contact with the offending organisms.

VITAMINS

The vitamins are a very important group of compounds in modern therapy and nutrition. Because most of the problems involving their stability and mode of administration have been solved, the practicing pharmacist does not encounter too many incompatibilities in the dispensing of them. Many of the previously existing difficulties have been overcome by the various types of preparations which are readily available from drug manufacturers. However, some incompati-

two groups: (1) the fat-soluble vitamins and (2) the water-soluble vitamins. The fat-soluble group includes vitamins A, D, E and K. The water-soluble group includes ascorbic acid and those of the B-complex.

A complete discussion of all the compounds possessing vitamin activity and their reactions is not appropriate in this chapter. Therefore, for the most part, only those reactions and properties which contribute to dispensing problems are discussed.

FAT-SOLUBLE VITAMINS

Vitamin A (antixerophthalmia vitamin) is a highly unsaturated alcohol found in the nonsaponifiable fraction of fish-liver oils and animal fats. The carotenoid pigments, known as provitamins, are found in the plant kingdom. The animal body is capable of converting many of these into vitamin A. Since both vitamin A and the carotenes are highly unsaturated, they are extremely sensitive to oxidation. In the absence of oxygen, they are quite stable to heat. Due to the relative ease with which they undergo oxidation and autoxidation, care should be taken that the emulsifying agents used in the preparation of emulsions of fish-liver oils do not contain oxidizing enzymes.[48] For example, the oxidase* present in acacia should be destroyed before the gum is used as an emulsifying agent.

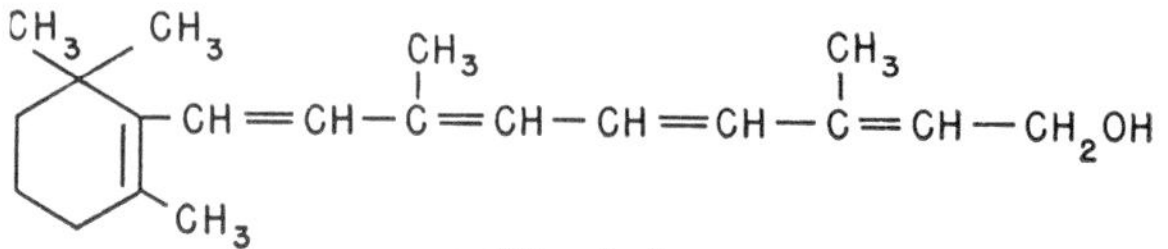

Vitamin A

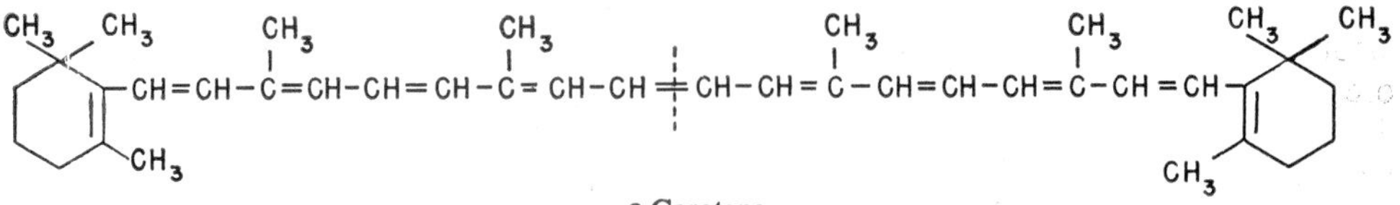

β-Carotene

bilities are created when physicians attempt to combine these preparations with other drugs.

The vitamins vary greatly in their chemical composition. On the basis of their solubilities and the manner in which they are dispensed, it is convenient to divide them into

Vitamin A and the carotenes are insoluble in water, but they are soluble in the nonpolar solvents of ether, chloroform, carbon disul-

---

* The oxidase is destroyed by drying the acacia at 103° to 105° C. (Kieft, J. P.: Pharm. Weekblad 76:1133, 1939) or by heating aqueous preparations to 100° C.

fide, benzene, petroleum ether and fats. The carotenes are practically insoluble in alcohol; however, vitamin A, due to the presence of the —OH group, is alcohol-soluble.

Vitamin D (antirachitic vitamin) is found in both plant and animal tissues. Ergosterol upon irradiation with ultraviolet light is converted to vitamin D_2 (calciferol). The compound originally designated as vitamin D was found to be a mixture of lumisterol and calciferol, of which only calciferol is antirachitic. The naturally occurring provitamin D, 7-dehydrocholesterol, yields vitamin D_3 on irradiation. This is identical with the

acetone and alcohol, but insoluble in water.

Vitamin E is found in vegetable oils such as wheat-germ oil, rice-germ oil and cottonseed oil. It is also present in leafy green and yellow vegetables and fruits such as lettuce and oranges. Animal tissues contain only very small amounts.

The tocopherols are water-insoluble but are soluble in the less polar solvents such as ether, chloroform and oils. Four closely related tocopherols of similar chemical composition, α, β, γ and δ, are known to possess vitamin E activity. In the absence of oxygen, the tocopherols are stable to heat up to

α-Tocopherol

natural vitamin D_3 of fish-liver oils. The animal body apparently is capable of synthesizing vitamin D from various sterols. At least 10 different provitamins D are now known to exist.

Vitamins D are relatively stable to heat and oxidation and, therefore, they are not inactivated by autoclaving at 120° C. in the absence of air. In the presence of air they are inactivated at this temperature. Vitamin D_2 (calciferol), on heating at 160° to 190° C. in the absence of air, yields pyrocalciferol

Vitamin D_2 (calciferol)

Vitamin D_3

and isopyrocalciferol, both of which are devoid of antirachitic activity.[78] Vitamin D is stable to alkali, as shown by the fact that it can be isolated from the nonsaponifiable fraction of fats. All of the known vitamins D in the pure state are white, odorless crystals which are soluble in fats, ether, chloroform,

200° C. and are not affected by hydrochloric or sulfuric acids at 100° C. The tocopherols are less resistant to alkalies and are destroyed gradually when allowed to remain in contact with alkalies for long periods of time. Sufficient stability to alkali is manifested by the tocopherols to make it possible to isolate them from fats by saponification. In an alkaline medium, the tocopherols are especially susceptible to oxidation. This oxidation results in a destruction of their vitamin E activity. Ultraviolet light also destroys their activity. Because of the ease with which they undergo oxidation, the tocopherols are effective antioxidants and are employed to prevent the oxidation of fats. The γ isomer is the most effective antioxidant, and the β isomer is more effective than the α isomer. The antioxidant activity is dependent on the free phenolic —OH group which is not necessary in the molecule for vitamin E activity.

Vitamin K (antihemorrhagic vitamin) occurs in plants and micro-organisms. Two naturally occurring vitamins K are definitely known. Vitamin K_1 is found in green plant materials such as alfalfa and spinach, and vitamin K_2 is found in most bacteria. The bacterial flora of the intestinal tract synthesize large amounts of vitamin K that provide an important source in humans.

Experimentation has shown that vitamin K activity is not lost when a hydrogen re-

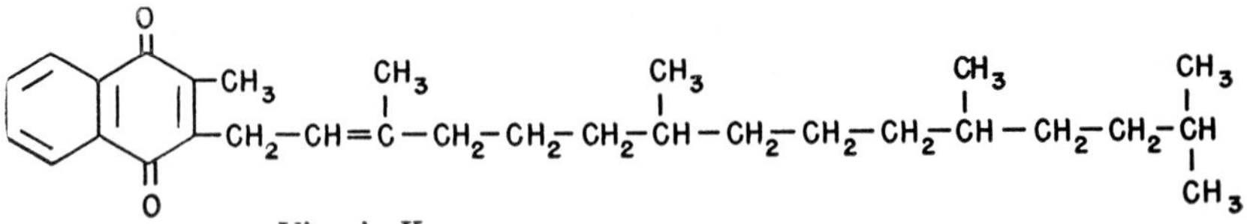

Vitamin K₁
(2-methyl-3-phytyl-1,4-naphthoquinone)

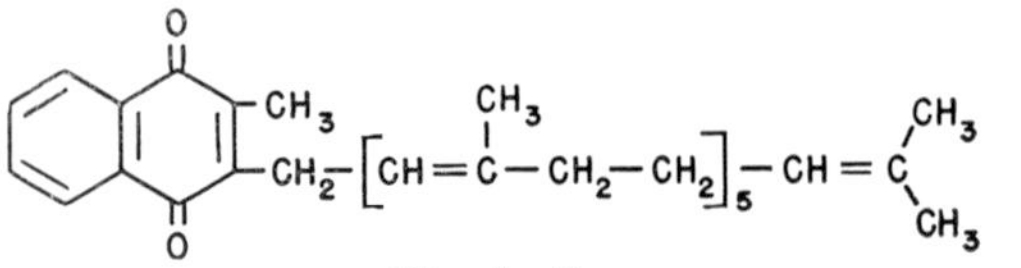

Vitamin K₂
(2-methyl-3-difarnesyl-1,4-naphthoquinone)

places the side chain in number 3 position. This compound, 2-methyl-1,4-naphthoquinone, also known as menadione, is official in the *U.S.P.* and is used extensively in medicine for its vitamin K activity. Other substituted naphthoquinones are known to possess vitamin K activity and have been used clinically. Menadione sodium bisulfite, which is a water-soluble derivative suitable for intravenous or intramuscular injection, is also included in the *U.S.P.*

The naturally occurring vitamins K and menadione are insoluble in water but soluble in fats, ether, chloroform, acetone and petroleum ether. The vitamins K are thermostable, but they are very sensitive to light (sunlight, artificial light and ultraviolet light) and alkalies. Reducing agents convert the natural vitamins K and menadione to hydroquinone derivatives.

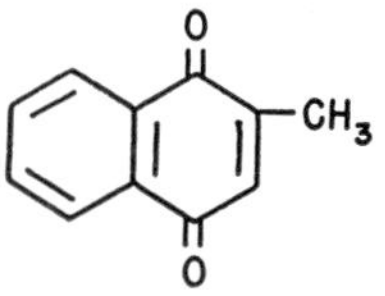

amounts, but increased quantities are present in the organs and the endocrine glands (liver, adrenal gland, thymus and pituitary). Humans are unable to synthesize the vitamin; thus it must be included in the diet. Excellent dietary sources include green vegetables, berries, apples and citrus fruits. The vitamin is also synthesized for commercial use.

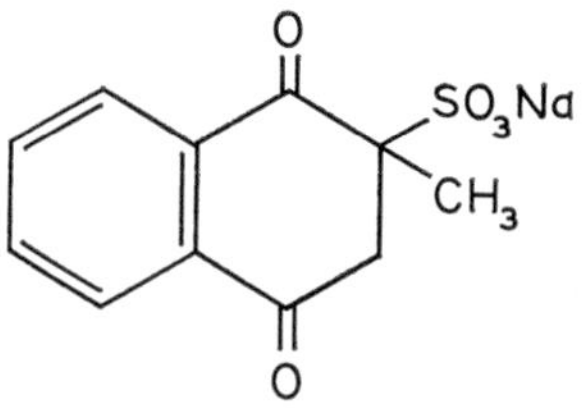

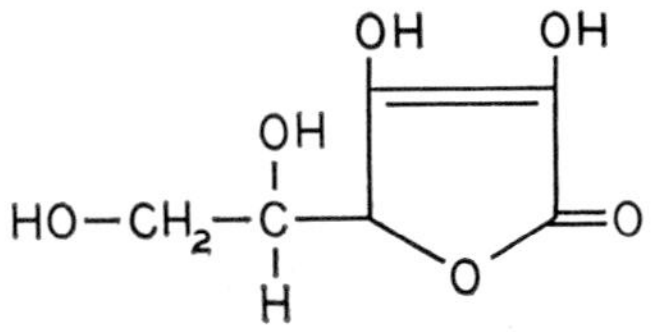

Ascorbic acid is an odorless, white, crystalline compound which is soluble in water (1 Gm. in 3 ml.) and alcohol (1 Gm. in 30 ml.) but insoluble in the nonpolar solvents ether, chloroform, fats, etc. Ascorbic acid is a monobasic acid, yields acid solutions and readily forms salts with metals. This acid is a strong reducing agent, and in aqueous solution it is readily oxidized and inactivated by the oxygen of the air. This oxidative destruction of ascorbic acid takes place rapidly in alkaline solution, but it is markedly decreased in acidic solution. Al-

Menadione
(2-methyl-1,4-naphthoquinone)

Menadione Sodium Bisulfite

WATER-SOLUBLE VITAMINS

Ascorbic acid (cevitamic acid, vitamin C), the antiscorbutic vitamin, is present in all living plant cells and is found in increased amounts in actively growing parts of the plant. Animal tissues contain only small

kalies, oxidizing agents, light, heat, riboflavin and traces of iron and copper are all capable of hastening the decomposition of ascorbic acid. In the dry crystalline form, ascorbic acid is relatively stable.

p-**Aminobenzoic acid** (PABA) occurs in the plant and the animal kingdoms in both free and combined form. Because of its wide distribution in nature, no deficiencies directly attributed to it have been observed in humans. Apparently, dietary sources and intestinal synthesis supply adequate amounts of this essential metabolite.

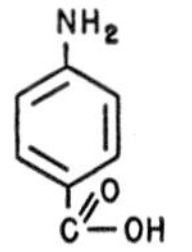

p-Aminobenzoic Acid

p-Aminobenzoic acid is a stable colorless substance which is soluble in water to the extent of 0.5 Gm. per 100 ml., freely soluble in boiling water and soluble (1:10) in alcohol. Its solubility in aqueous solution is increased by both alkali and mineral acids due to the presence of both the carboxyl and the amino groups which enable it to form the water-soluble ionized salts.

Biotin (vitamin H) is present in small amounts in all higher animals. Dietary sources include liver, kidney, eggs, milk, vegetables, grains and nuts. It occurs in the free state in plant sources and mainly as a chemically bound compound in animal tissues. The synthetic product is available commercially.

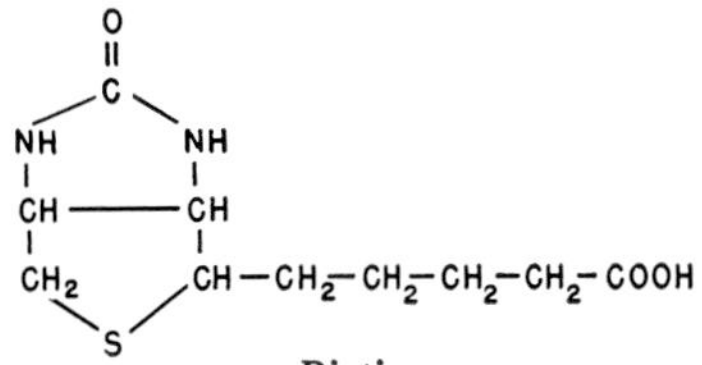

Biotin

Biotin is soluble in water and alcohol and insoluble in ether, chloroform and petroleum ether. The vitamin is relatively stable in acidic and basic solution and to heat. It is inactivated by oxidizing agents.

Choline (trimethyl-β-hydroxyethylammonium hydroxide) is a constituent of the phospholipids, sphingomyelin and lecithin. Dietary sources of the substance include egg yolk, liver, kidney and the germ of cereal grains. This substance, which is included in the B-complex, is a growth factor concerned biologically with transmethylation reactions in the animal body.

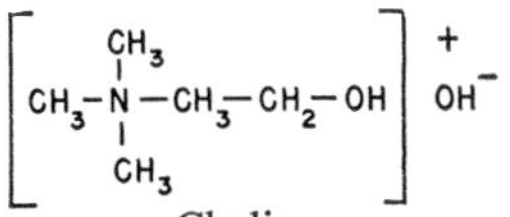

Choline

Choline is a colorless, viscid, hygroscopic, strongly alkaline liquid, very soluble in water and alcohol and insoluble in ether. It readily forms salts with acids (chloride, bromide, borate, picrate, etc.). The salts, which are hygroscopic, are also soluble in water and alcohol. Aqueous solutions of the salts are practically neutral.

Folic acid (pteroylglutamic acid, "*L. casei* factor," "vitamin M," pteridyl-*p*-aminobenzoyl-glutamic acid) is found in green leaves (spinach, etc.), mushrooms, yeast, liver and kidney. It is also prepared synthetically. Therapeutically, folic acid is used in the treatment of various macrocytic anemias.

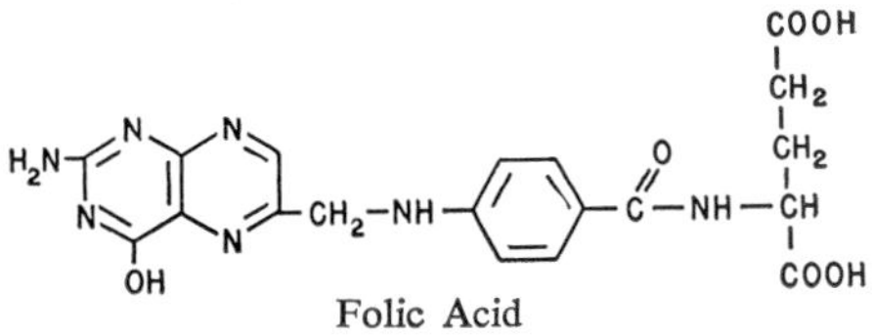

Folic Acid

The folic acid molecule is composed of a pteridyl group, *p*-aminobenzoic acid and *l*-glutamic acid. In foods it is found in the conjugated form containing additional molecules of glutamic acid. Folic acid is a stable, yellow, crystalline substance which, although only slightly soluble in water, is soluble in dilute alkali and acid due to the presence of carboxyl groups and basic nitrogen in the molecule. However, it is destroyed readily by boiling in acid solution.

Inositol (hexahydroxy-cyclohexane, meso-inositol) occurs naturally as a normal cell constituent in both plant and animal tissues and is prepared synthetically. In nature it occurs in many different forms. Some inositol occurs in the free state, but in plants it is present mainly in the form of the hexaphosphate; in the liver it is combined with a protein and is alkali-labile; in soybean it is found as a glycoside. Only the optically inactive form (meso-inositol) possesses biologic activity.

Inositol possesses a sweet taste and is soluble in water (approx. 16.5 Gm. per 100

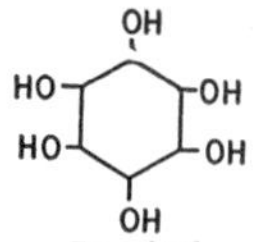

Inositol

ml.). It is insoluble in absolute alcohol and ether. Inositol is highly resistant to the action of both acid and alkali.

Nicotinic Acid and Nicotinamide. Nicotinic acid (niacin, P.P. factor, pellagra preventive factor, 3-pyridinecarboxylic acid) occurs in small amounts in all living cells.

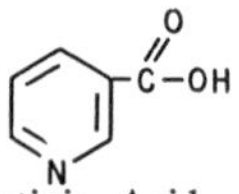

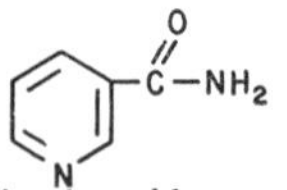

Nicotinic Acid   Nicotinamide

Dietary sources include liver, yeast, wheat germ and milk. Man is dependent on dietary sources for nicotinic acid, although considerable amounts probably are contributed through its synthesis by the bacterial flora of the intestines. In animal tissue it is found not as nicotinic acid but as the amide. A small amount of nicotinamide (niacinamide) is present in tissues in the free form, but the majority is present in the chemically bound forms of co-enzymes I and II. For commercial purposes, nicotinic acid and nicotinamide are prepared synthetically.

Chemically, nicotinic acid is the β-carboxylic acid of pyridine. It is very stable and may be heated without decomposition. Nicotinic acid is slightly soluble in water (approx. 1.65 Gm. per 100 ml.) and alcohol (approx. 1.25 Gm. per 100 ml.) and insoluble in chloroform and ether. The acid is readily soluble in dilute alkali and acid due to the carboxyl group and basic nitrogen which enable it to form the water-soluble ionized salt. Destruction of nicotinic acid does not occur even when the compound is heated in acid or alkaline solution.

Nicotinamide (niacinamide) is very soluble in both water and alcohol, but it is only slightly soluble in ether. In aqueous acid or alkaline solution it is converted to nicotinic acid by heating.

Pantothenic acid is present in all plant and animal tissues. Dietary sources include liver, kidney, heart, tongue, yeast, eggs, muscle tissue, rice bran and molasses. In both animal and plant tissue it is usually bound to protein; only a small amount of this acid occurs in the free form. It is also prepared synthetically.

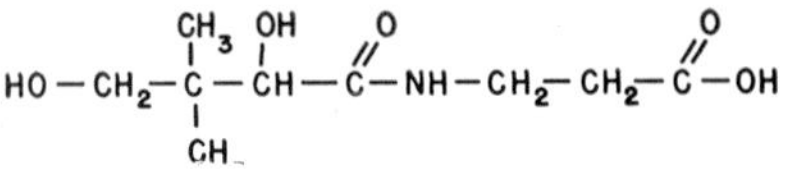

Pantothenic acid is a white, odorless, crystalline powder which is readily soluble in water but insoluble in alcohol. The vitamin is destroyed by heat, acids and bases. In aqueous acid or alkali solution it is hydrolyzed to β-alanine and α-hydroxy-β,β-dimethyl-γ-butyrolactone, as shown below:

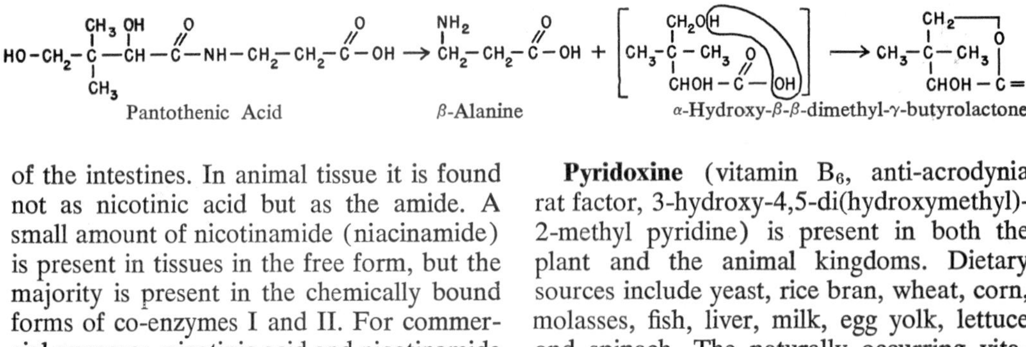

Pantothenic Acid   β-Alanine   α-Hydroxy-β-β-dimethyl-γ-butyrolactone

Pyridoxine (vitamin B_6, anti-acrodynia rat factor, 3-hydroxy-4,5-di(hydroxymethyl)-2-methyl pyridine) is present in both the plant and the animal kingdoms. Dietary sources include yeast, rice bran, wheat, corn, molasses, fish, liver, milk, egg yolk, lettuce and spinach. The naturally occurring vitamin is present in the form in which it is bound to protein. Only small amounts are found in the free state. It is prepared synthetically, as well.

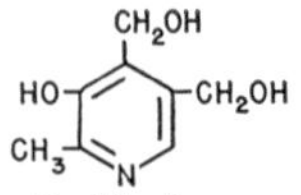

Pyridoxine 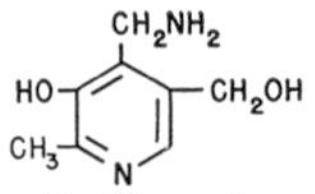   Pyridoxamine 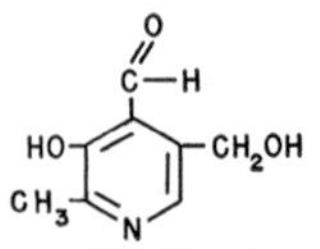   Pyridoxal

In higher animals, two other forms of the vitamin which possess activity equal to that of pyridoxine are the amine and the aldehyde analogs (pyridoxamine and pyridoxal). It is possible that other members of the B_6 complex also exist.[57]

Pyridoxine is a colorless, crystalline powder having a slightly bitter taste. It is soluble in water, alcohol and acetone but only slightly soluble in ether and chloroform. Due to the presence of the basic nitrogen in the molecule, it readily forms water-soluble ionizable salts with acids. The hydrochloride is the form which appears on the market and is most used. It is soluble in water (22.2 Gm. per 100 ml.) and alcohol (1.1 Gm. per 100 ml.). The aqueous solution of the hydrochloride has a pH of approximately 3.2. Pyridoxine is stable to heat and acid but is destroyed by light. Because of the phenolic —OH group in the structure, pyridoxine shows many reactions of the phenols; e.g., it yields an orange-red color with ferric chloride and undergoes air-oxidation in alkaline solution.

Riboflavin (vitamin B_2, vitamin G, lactoflavin; 6,7-dimethyl-9-(d-1'-ribityl-)isoalloxazine) occurs in all living cells of the plant and the animal kingdoms. It is found either as the free vitamin, the phosphate, or the adeninedinucleotide phosphate. Excellent dietary sources are heart, liver, kidney, muscle, eggs, milk, green leafy vegetable, whole grain and yeast. Commercial supplies of riboflavin are obtained by the synthesis of the vitamin.

Riboflavin is an orange-yellow crystalline compound which is only slightly soluble in water (12 mg. per 100 ml.) and ethyl alcohol (4.5 mg. per 100 ml.). It is insoluble in ether, acetone, chloroform and benzene. Because of the basic nitrogen in the molecule, it is capable of forming such salts as the monosuccinate, borate, phosphate and acetate which are more water-soluble than the parent compound. These more soluble salts have found use in pharmaceutical preparations.

Riboflavin is very soluble in aqueous alkaline solution by virtue of the acidic hydrogen of the imide group. The acidic hydrogen is replaceable by sodium and, therefore, in aqueous solution the water-soluble ionized salt is formed. However, the riboflavin is then quite unstable to light and heat. In aque-

Riboflavin

Irradiation in alkaline solution →

Lumiflavin (6,7,9-trimethyl-iso-alloxazine)

Irradiation in neutral or acid solution →

Lumichrome (6,7-dimethyl-alloxazine)

ous alkali, riboflavin is converted by irradiation to the biologically inactive, fluorescent, degradation product, lumiflavin. In acid solution (pH 1.0 to 6.0), riboflavin is quite stable to heat, but it yields the inactive lumichrome on irradiation.

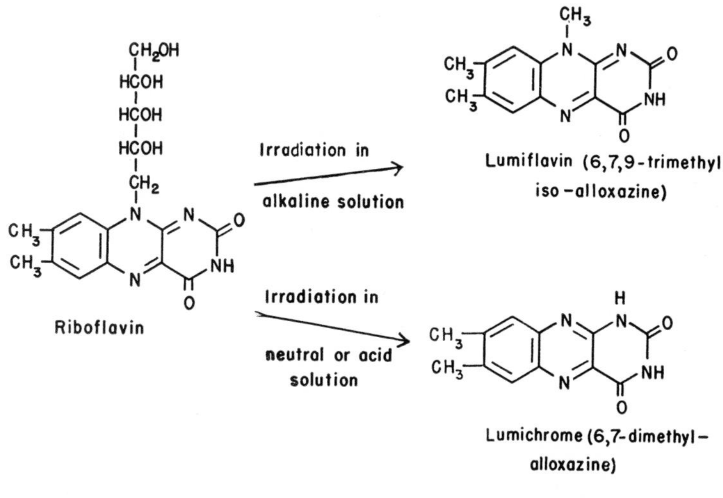

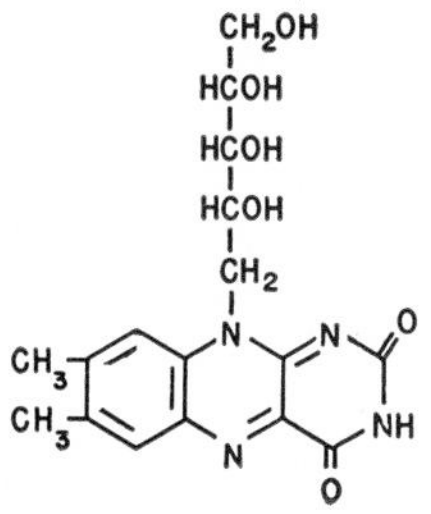

Reducing agents convert riboflavin to leucoriboflavin, but this reaction is easily reversible. The oxidation-reduction reaction on page 422 is of great importance in the

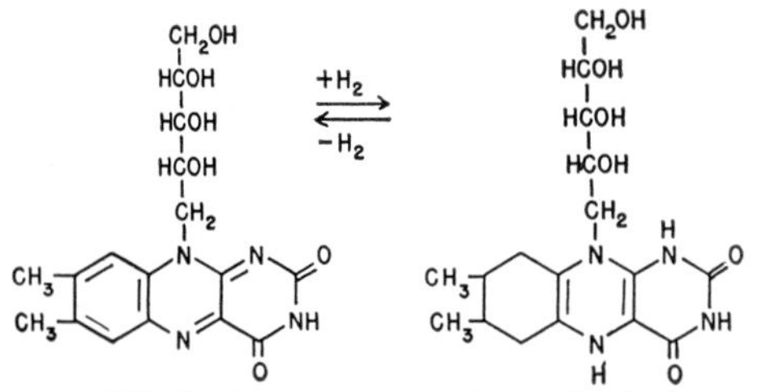

Riboflavin   Leucoriboflavin

function of riboflavin nucleotide in cellular respiration. Riboflavin is quite resistant to the action of oxidizing agents.

Thiamine hydrochloride (vitamin B_1, thiamine, thiamine chloride, aneurin, antineuritic vitamin, antiberiberi vitamin; 4-methyl-5-β-hydroxy-ethyl-N-{[2-methyl-4-amino-pyrimidyl-(5)]-methyl}thiazolium-chloride-hydrochloride). Thiamine occurs naturally in the free form, as a protein complex, as a phosphorus-protein complex, and as the pyrophosphoric acid ester (cocarboxylase). Dietary sources of the vitamin include pork, yeast, cereal grains, milk, peas, beans, fruits and nuts. It is prepared synthetically for commercial uses.

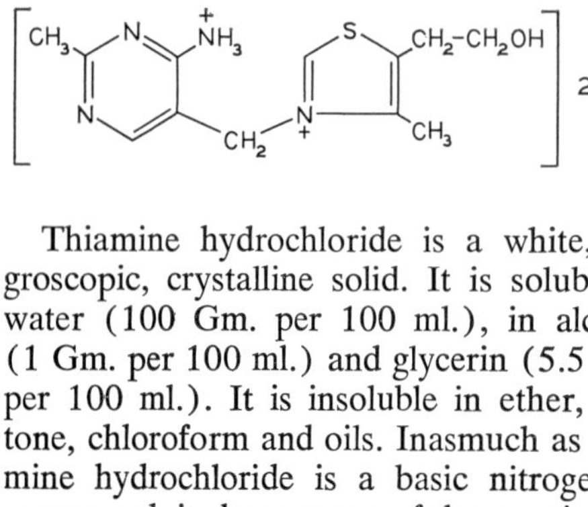

Thiamine hydrochloride is a white, hygroscopic, crystalline solid. It is soluble in water (100 Gm. per 100 ml.), in alcohol (1 Gm. per 100 ml.) and glycerin (5.5 Gm. per 100 ml.). It is insoluble in ether, acetone, chloroform and oils. Inasmuch as thiamine hydrochloride is a basic nitrogenous compound, it shows many of the reactions of the alkaloids and logically could be classified with them. It forms insoluble compounds with tannic, picric and phosphotungstic acids, potassium mercuric iodide, mercuric chloride and iodine.

In the dry crystalline form, the vitamin is stable, in strongly acid solutions it is quite stable; thus, aqueous solutions having a pH of 3.5 may be autoclaved at 120° C. without decomposition. However, weakly acid solutions (pH 5.0 to 6.0) are not stable to heat. In aqueous neutral or alkaline solu-

tions, thiamine hydrochloride is unstable—heat accelerates the decomposition. It is, thus, incompatible with alkalies and other basic substances. Many incompatibilities of this nature arise when the vitamin is dispensed in aqueous solution with substances such as sodium phenobarbital, alkali carbonates, bicarbonates, citrates, acetates, etc., all of which yield alkaline solutions.

Thiamine hydrochloride is very sensitive to both oxidation and reduction and it is, therefore, incompatible with oxidizing and reducing agents. On oxidation, the vitamin is converted to the biologically inactive, highly fluorescent thiochrome. This reaction

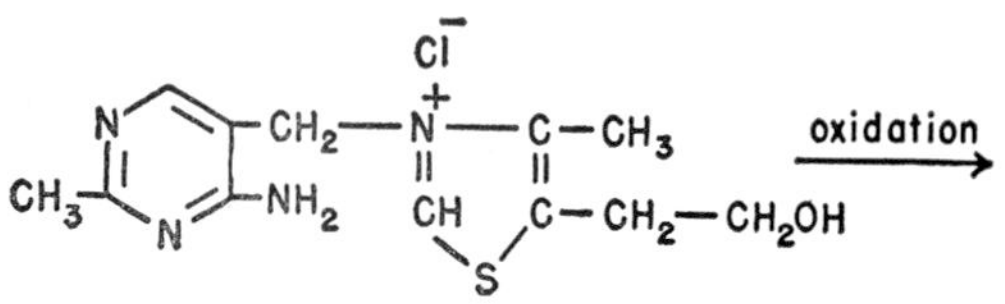

Thiamine

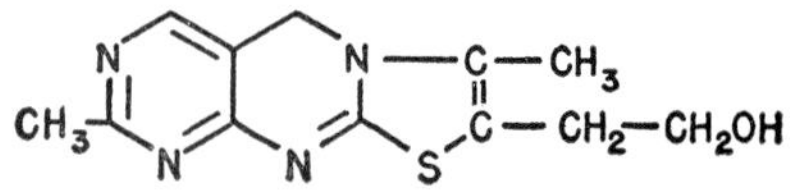

Thiochrome

is the basis for the photofluorometric method of assay for the vitamin. The reaction does not progress readily in strongly acid solution (pH 2.0), but the formation of the thiochrome is accelerated as the solution approaches neutrality (pH 7.0). After long periods of time, small quantities of thiochrome are formed even in alcoholic solutions of the vitamin.

Vitamin B_{12} (Bevidox, Cobione, Cyanocobalamin, Dodex) is obtained commercially from the fermentation products of such organisms as *Streptomyces griseus, S. olivaceus* and *S. aureofaciens*. In the normal daily diet, it is obtained from foods containing animal protein. It is considered to be an essential nutritional factor required for normal blood formation, neural function and growth. The main clinical uses for the vitamin at the present time are thus in the treatment of pernicious anemia both with and without neurologic complications, pain associated with neurologic disorders and growth retardation due to animal-protein deficiency.

The very complex chemical structure of vitamin B_{12} has been elucidated[19] and, as was accurately reported, in previous work, it has been shown to contain cobalt and a cyano group[46] and has an empirical formula corresponding to $C_{63}H_{90}N_{14}O_{14}PCo$. The cobalt is present in the form of a coordination complex in which the cobalt is trivalent and has a coordination number of six.[14] On acid hydrolysis (6 N HCl, 100° C.), 1-α-D-ribofuranosido-5,6-dimethylbenzimidazole is obtained from the vitamin, whereas more drastic conditions of acid hydrolysis yield one equivalent of 5,6-dimethylbenzimidazole. Other hydrolysis products which have been obtained from vitamin B_{12} are ammonia, phosphoric acid and D-1-amino-2-propanol.[58]

Vitamin B_{12} is soluble in water to the extent of 1.25 Gm. per 100 ml. at 25° C. and forms neutral, odorless and tasteless solutions. The vitamin is inactivated in aqueous solution by strong acids and strong alkalies. The maximum pH range for stability in solution is 4.5 to 5.0. In this range, solutions can be autoclaved without significant loss of activity. Vitamin B_{12} undergoes slow decomposition on exposure to both ultraviolet and visible light. It is stated to be unstable in aqueous solutions containing acacia, aldehydes (such as vanillin and those contained in synthetic fruit flavors), ascorbic acid, dextrose, ferrous gluconate, ferrous sulfate and sucrose.[59] It is stable in the dry form at room temperature provided that it is not exposed to strong light for extended periods of time.

REFERENCES

1. Abraham, E. P.: J. Pharm. & Pharmacol. *3*:264, 1951.
2. Adams, W. L.: J. Pharmacol. & Exper. Ther. *78*:340, 1943.
3. Anker, H. S., *et al.*: J. Bacteriol. *55*:249, 1949.
4. Antibiotics, p. 8, London, Pharmaceutical Press, 1952.
5. *Ibid.*, p. 67.
6. Bohonos, N., *et al.*: Antibiotics Annual, 1953-1954, p. 54, New York, Medical Encyclopedia, 1953.
7. Bond, G. C., Himelick, R. E., and MacDonald, L. H.: J. Am. Pharm. Ass. (Sci.) *38*:30, 1949.
8. Boothe, J. H., *et al.*: Antibiotics Annual, 1953-1954, p. 46, New York, Medical Encyclopedia, 1953.
9. ———: *Ibid.*, p. 47.
10. Booth, S. H., *et al.*: J. Am. Chem. Soc. *75*:4,621, 1953.
11. Bourquelot, E.: J. Pharm. Chim. *19*:473, 1904.
12. Brecht, E. A., and Rogers, C. H.: J. Am. Pharm. Ass. *29*:178, 1940.
13. Brink, N. G., Kuehl, F. A., and Folkers, K.: Science *102*:506, 1945.
14. ———: Science *112*:354, 1950.
15. Brown, H. C.: J. Am. Chem. Soc. *67*:378, 1945.
16. Bury, C. R.: J. Am. Chem. Soc. *57*:2,115, 1935.
17. Cellulose Gum, Hercules Powder Co., pp. 2-9, 1949.
18. Celmer, W. D., Els, H., and Murai, K.: Antibiotic Annual 1957-1958, p. 476, New York, Medical Encyclopedia, 1958.
19. Chem. & Eng. News *33*:3487, 1955.
20. Craig, L. C., Shedlovsky, T., Gould, R. G., and Jacobs, W. A.: J. Biol. Chem. *125*:289, 1938.
21. Daubert, B. F.: J. Am. Pharm. Ass. (Sci.) *33*:321, 1944.
22. Edwards, L. J.: Trans. Faraday Soc. *46*:723, 1950.
23. Gilman, H.: Organic Chemistry, vol. II, p. 1858, New York, Wiley, 1943.
24. ———: *Ibid.*, p. 1844.
25. ———: *Ibid.*, p. 1609.
26. Gisvold, O., and Rogers, C. H.: The Chemistry of Plant Constituents, p. 203, Minneapolis, Burgess, 1943.
27. Goodman, L., and Gilman, A.: The Pharmacological Basis of Therapeutics, p. 1079, New York, Macmillan, 1955.
28. ———: *Ibid.*, p. 169.
29. Grill, F.: J. Am. Pharm. Ass. *21*:765, 1932.
30. Hamilton, W. F., George, M. F., Simon, E., and Turnbull, F. M.: J. Am. Pharm. Ass. (Sci.) *33*:142, 1944.
31. Hargreaves, G. W.: J. Am. Pharm. Ass. *21*:571, 1932.
32. Harned, R. L., *et al.*: Antibiotics and Chemother. *5*:204, 1955.
33. Harris, D. A., *et al.*: Antibiotics and Chemother. *5*:185, 1955.
34. Hirst, E. L.: J. Chem. Soc. *1*:70, 1942.
35. Hirst, E. L., Jones, J. K. N., and Jones, W. O.: Nature *143*:857, 1939.
36. Hoeksema, H., *et al.*: J A. C. S. *77*:6,710, 1955.

37. Howard, M. E.: Modern Drug Encyclopedia and Therapeutic Index, ed. 6, p. 79, New York, Drug Publications, Inc., 1955.

38. Husa, W. J.: Pharmaceutical Dispensing, p. 544, Iowa City, Husa, 1951.

39. ———: Ibid., p. 650.

40. ———: Ibid., p. 551.

41. ———: Ibid., p. 458.

42. Husa, W. J., and Jatul, B.: J. Am. Pharm. Ass. (Sci.) 33:217, 1944.

43. Hutchings, B. L., et al.: J. Am. Chem. Soc. 74:3710, 1952.

44. Jones, W. G. M., and Peat, S.: J. Chem. Soc. 2:225, 1942.

45. Jordan, E. O., and Burrows, W.: Textbook of Bacteriology, ed. 14, p. 307, Philadelphia, Saunders, 1946.

46. Kaczka, E. A., Wolf, D. E., Kuehl, F. A., and Folkers, K.: J. Am. Chem. Soc. 73:3569, 1951.

47. Kaczka, E. A., et al.: J.A.C.S. 77:6404, 1955.

48. Kedvessy, G.: Chem. Zentr. II, 314, 1942.

49. Kuehl, F. A., Flynn, E. H., Holly, F. W., Mozingo, R., and Folkers, K.: J. Am. Chem. Soc. 68:536, 1946.

50. Luder, W. F., and Zuffanti, S.: The Electronic Theory of Acids and Bases, p. 120, New York, Wiley, 1946.

51. ———: Ibid., p. 83.

52. Lyman, R. A.: American Pharmacy, vol. 2, p. 196, Philadelphia, Lippincott, 1947.

53. ———: Ibid., p. 197.

54. ———: Ibid., p. 186.

55. McElvain, S. M.: The Characterization of Organic Compounds, p. 51, New York, Macmillan, 1953.

56. ———: Ibid., p. 51.

57. Melnick, D., Hochberg, M., Himes, H. W., and Oser, B. L.: J. Biol. Chem. 160:1, 1945.

58. Merck Service Bulletin, Vitamin B_{12}, Part I, Pharmaceutical Information, p. 2, 1953.

59. Ibid., p. 9.

60. New and Nonofficial Remedies, p. 134, Philadelphia, Lippincott, 1954.

61. Ibid., p. 112.

62. Nixon, W.: Pharm. J. 167:213, 1951.

63. Norman, A. G.: Biochem. J. 25:200, 1931.

64. ———: Ibid.

65. Osborne, G. E., and DeKay, H. G.: J. Am. Pharm. Ass. (Pract.) 2:240, 1941.

66. Osol, A., and Farrar, G. E.: U. S. Dispensatory, p. 868, Philadelphia, Lippincott, 1950.

67. ———: Ibid., p. 27.

68. ———: Ibid., p. 1043.

69. Peck, R. L., Graber, R. P., Walti, A., and Peel, E. W.: J. Am. Chem. Soc. 68:29, 1946.

70. Pfau, E.: Apoth. Ztg. 46:724, 1931.

71. Pfeiffer, C., and Williams, H.: J. Am. Pharm. Ass. (Pract.) 8:572, 1947.

72. Pharmacopeia of the United States, Sixteenth Rev., p. 826, 1960.

73. Pratt, L. S.: The Chemistry and Physics of Organic Pigments, p. 136, New York, Wiley, 1947.

74. ———: Ibid., p. 137.

75. Pratt, R., and DuFrenoy, J.: Antibiotics, p. 193, Philadelphia, Lippincott, 1953.

76. Remick, A. E.: Electronic Interpretations of Organic Chemistry, p. 37, New York, Wiley, 1949.

77. ———: Ibid., p. 235.

78. Rosenberg, H. R.: Chemistry and Physiology of the Vitamins, New York, Interscience, 1945.

79. Rowson, J. M.: Quart. J. & Yr. Bk. Pharm. 10:161, 1937.

80. Taylor, T. W. J., and Baker, W.: The Organic Chemistry of Nitrogen, p. 31, Oxford, Clarendon Press, 1937.

81. Toal, J. S.: Quart. J. & Yr. Bk. Pharm. 10:439, 1937.

82. ———: Ibid., 12:573, 1939.

83. Waller, C. W., et al.: J. Am. Chem. Soc. 74:4981, 1952.

84. ———: Ibid., 74:4978, 1952.

85. Wesp, E. F., and Brode, W. R.: J. Am. Chem. Soc. 56:1037, 1934.

86. Weygand, C.: Organic Preparations, p. 445, New York, Interscience, 1945.

87. Wilson, C. O., and Gisvold, O. T.: Textbook of Organic Medicinal and Pharmaceutical Chemistry, p. 642, Philadelphia, Lippincott, 1954.

Chapter 11

Therapeutic Incompatibilities

Peter P. Lamy, Ph.D.*†

More than 130,000 drug entities, drug combinations and drug dosage forms are listed in the *Physician's Desk Reference*.‡ Additionally, patients quite often use self-medication and a large number of over-the-counter (OTC) drugs are available to them. There is probably no complete list of OTC drugs; the *Pink Book*§ lists about 3,000 manufacturers, 600 classifications and approximately 21,000 brand-named products. These are not all OTC drug products, since this particular book also lists toiletries, baby items and others.

Cluff *et al.*[38] point out that no drug is completely harmless, even when used correctly, and all may produce an adverse reaction. Seidl *et al.*[172] observed that most physicians are ill-informed about adverse drug reactions. The Committee on Safety of Drugs for 1965 (England) concurs and stated:

"The public should be made increasingly aware that no effective drug is entirely without hazard to the patient, even a drug that can be bought without a prescription. Doctors, for their part, should bear in mind that drug-induced (iatrogenic) illness may be the result of self-medication by the patient."

The unexpected, unfavorable response to drug therapy is increasingly familiar to every physician. This might be ascribed to the constant addition of new and powerful drugs to the medical armamentarium, which in turn leads to the appearance of many new reactions of incredible diversity, or to an increase in the incidence of older, well recognized adverse reactions to drugs. Schimmel[168] reviewed the problem of adverse reactions to diagnostic and therapeutic agents or procedures and reported that approximately 20 per cent of hospitalized patients develop such untoward reactions.

Efforts are being made to shed more light on the possible undesirable effects of drug therapy. For example, the National Disease and Therapeutic Index (NDTI) is a continuous compilation of the incidence and treatment of diseases encountered in private medical practice in the United States. The Index correlates reports from about 1500 physicians on adverse drug reactions and possible drug interactions.

The use of many drugs for the treatment of a single disease has been prevalent throughout history.[96] Combinations of modern drugs, however, are totally different from the polypharmacy of the past. Every time a physician adds to the number of drugs in a particular therapeutic regimen, he may unintentionally devise a novel combination that has special risks. It is unfortunate that patients may be given several drugs at the same time without proper consideration of the possibility that one drug may interact with another. Often, there seems to be a psychological appeal in prescribing not just one but a combination of medically proven ingredients. "More" seems necessarily better than "less."[96]

How prevalent is combined drug therapy?

* Associate Professor and Director, Institutional Pharmacy Programs, University of Maryland, School of Pharmacy, Baltimore, Maryland.

† The author wishes to acknowledge the invaluable help in preparing this text by Mary Ellen Kitler, Ph.D., Postdoctoral Fellow, Department of Biostatistics, School of Hygiene and Public Health, Johns Hopkins University, Baltimore, Maryland, and David A. Blake, Ph.D., Associate Professor of Pharmacology, University of Maryland School of Pharmacy, Baltimore, Maryland.

‡ Medical Economics, Inc., Oradell, New Jersey, 1968.

§ Topics Publishing Co., New York, 1968.

A survey in a Baltimore hospital revealed that patients who were receiving a new type of penicillin also received, during the period of study, not less than six other medications. One patient received as many as 32 additional medications.[120] Seidl *et al.*[172] studied multiple drug therapy and reported that patients received an average of 14 different drugs during hospitalization. Bonnichsen *et al.*[26] found in a survey of fatal cases in Sweden that only in 58 per cent of all cases involving barbiturates was one single derivative detected. In 29 per cent of these cases, two derivatives were encountered, and in 13 per cent, more than two barbiturates were probably responsible for the particular fatality, and sometimes as many as five derivatives were identified.

To understand the importance of drug interactions in therapeutics, one must first recognize that single drugs occasionally produce severe illness and even death. Furthermore, it is usually not possible to predict an adverse effect or the seriousness of an interaction. When reactions do occur, they are most often unexpected.[38] It is necessary also to appreciate that there has been a marked increase in multidrug therapy, resulting in numerous potential dangers. For example, the combination of tolbutamide with sulfonamides may produce severe hypoglycemia. The efficacy of two or more antibiotics in the treatment of tuberculosis contrasts with the contraindication to the use of such combinations in most other infectious diseases because of the danger of superinfection by resistant organisms or because of actual antagonism between two antibiotics. In short, chemical agents can and do modify the effects of other substances, even though they appear to have no chemical similarity.

The use of multidrug therapy, however, has been the result of knowledge gathered on the usefulness and validity of combination therapy in tuberculosis, subacute bacterial endocarditis, hypertension, epilepsy and others. One of the most recent and successful examples of combined therapy is, of course, the use of multihormone therapy in birth control. Tranquilizers and analgesics are combined for relief of tension headaches and myalgia. Each of a particular group of diuretics has the ability to block sodium reabsorption in a different part of the renal tubule simultaneously, thus potentiating the net diuresis obtained. Essential to an understanding of drug interactions is also the fact that drug interactions are evident not only among drugs of different therapeutic actions but also among drugs used for the same therapeutic purpose. Perhaps the most important class of drugs illustrating this point is the antibiotics.

Jawetz,[94] in reviewing the use and misuse of antibiotics, found that physicians frequently use combinations of antibiotics, perhaps in the belief that this provides effective therapy that is also free of hazards. Most often, however, the therapeutic response is indifferent, and no advantage is gained by using multidrug therapy. At times, however, antibiotic combinations can be dangerous to the patient. Patients afflicted by pneumococcal meningitis, if treated only with penicillin, respond well to the treatment in 70 per cent of all cases, and fatalities occur in 30 per cent. When physicians employed combination therapy of penicillin plus chlortetracycline, a 79 per cent mortality rate was observed. Antibiotic combinations with synergistic actions are rare, unpredictable and quite specific, according to Jawetz.[94] Combinations can be used advantageously in (1) sepsis caused by gram-negative bacteria, in which treatment must begin before laboratory reports can be completed; (2) in mixed infections; (3) to delay emergence of resistant strains of organisms (this is the basis for use of isoniazid, aminosalicylic acid and streptomycin in tuberculosis); (4) to reduce the incidence or the intensity of adverse reactions; and (5) in cases where an effect can be produced that would not be obtainable by either drug alone —for example, in the treatment of methicillin-resistant staphylococcal infections.

The problem of drug reactions and interactions becomes more complex when one considers the many factors or independent variables other than the dose of the drug that can markedly influence the duration of action of a drug. A prolongation in the duration of action of a drug may, in turn, contribute to the toxicity of the drug itself or of a drug combination.

Such variables as (1) time interval between drug administration, (2) mode of administration, (3) sex difference, (4) age, (5) liver disease, (6) kidney disease, (7) vitamin deficiency, (8) nutritional status, (9) dehydration and (10) hypothermia singly or in combination can alter drug action. Most of these are probably self-evident, but it might be of interest to discuss at least one of these factors.

Hypothermia can lower the basal metabolism of man, thereby prolonging and intensifying drug action, even to the point of endangering life.[78] Many compounds possessing hypnotic-potentiating activity are able to lower body temperature to a significant degree.[202] Albert and Fazekas[4] found a lowered destruction of thiopental in humans in the presence of hypothermia. Brunton,[31] in 1874, pointed to the diminution of body temperature induced by chloral hydrate and the extraordinary effects of warmth in accelerating recovery from an overdose of this drug.

From this short discussion it becomes evident that, occasionally, a single drug but, more often, the use and presence of several drugs simultaneously in the body, produce adverse pharmacologic effects of obvious clinical importance. Each of the several drugs, moreover, may be used in a quantity that by itself would be sublethal, but the resulting combined action may well change the magnitude of response.

Most of our current knowledge of toxicities that may result from drug combinations has resulted from data obtained from animal studies and there is, unfortunately, no foolproof or generally acceptable method to ascertain their relevance to man. Blank[22] reports that the application to man of pharmacologic data obtained from animal studies presents numerous difficulties. The greatest difficulty arises from species differences in rates of biotransformation. Meperidine, for example, is metabolized in man at a rate of about 17 per cent per hour, so that an analgesic dose lasts for about 3 to 4 hours. In dogs, the rate of biotransformation of meperidine is about 70 to 90 per cent per hour. Phenylbutazone, which is slowly metabolized in man, about 15 per cent per day, disappears from mice, rabbits, dogs, guinea pigs and horses in a few hours.

The study of drug actions and interactions is also complicated by the fact that the haz-ards associated with the administration of drug combinations cannot be evaluated from the toxicity of the individual drugs or compounds. Routine clinical investigation of the pharmacology and toxicology of a drug in the laboratory provides, at best, only a limited basis for the prediction of a possible interaction with another drug.[121] This is especially true when the mode of action of a drug is uncertain and empirical interactions have not been performed. However, even though no firm bridge has been established between animal experiments and human reactions, such data can be used tentatively to evaluate multiple drug therapy in man.

Chloral hydrate, for example, has been found to interact in mice or rats with chlorpromazine,[2] imipramine,[15] benactyzine,[20] diphenhydramine,[79] atropine, physostigmine, tolazoline, naphazoline, methoxamine, epinephrine, norepinephrine, phenylephrine,[56] chlortetracycline,[142] quinine[145] and colchicine.[183] Although it cannot be predicted that similar reactions would occur in man, a knowledge of these reported interactions is important when similar drug combinations are prescribed.

It is apparent, then, that a drug is a tool that must be used with every degree of finesse. Its use can be beneficial or harmful, depending on the skill with which it is used. The physician is the only one who can determine whether the medical purpose for which he prescribes a specific drug is a desirable one. Sometimes, the physician may not be aware of a possible interaction, and, unfortunately, too often the physician may not know at all that his patient is using self-medication.

Friend[64] states that, once a physician has written a prescription, the pharmacist is generally the only professional practitioner to have contact with the patient before the medication is consumed. It is therefore of utmost importance that the pharmacist become more familiar with his patients, their allergies, their work and any other factors that might affect drug action. The ever-increasing problem of drug interactions or therapeutic incompatibilities demands that the pharmacist become familiar with these possible occurrences, enabling him to render complete professional service to physicians and patients alike.

SOME FACTORS INFLUENCING DRUG ACTION

Some reactions to certain drugs have been associated with heritable disorders, some of which are related to race. Seidl et al.[172] found that adverse reactions are more common in Caucasian than in Negro patients, and more common in women than in men. Howard and Tiedeman[87] seemed to discern a trend in the success rate of antihypertensive treatments in favor of Caucasians. Friend[63] found that approximately 11 per cent of all Negroes in this country have a deficiency in glucose-6-phosphate dehydrogenase in the red blood cells. This deficiency makes patients particularly susceptible to certain drugs, such as acetamide and phenacetin. If susceptible patients are treated with such drugs, hemolysis may occur, sometimes severe enough to cause anemia or jaundice. Pernicious anemia, on the other hand, is found much more in light-haired, blue-eyed individuals than in the darker races or Orientals. Furthermore, there is a highly significant association of pernicious anemia with blood group A.[62]

It is also known that enzyme levels in man vary with the age of the individual. Plasma cholinesterase, for example, is present at birth at a lower level than that seen in adults.[125] The level rises quickly for a few years and reaches its maximum at puberty. However, levels in females always stay lower than in males, and they decrease in both sexes with age.[100] The enzyme level, furthermore, can be positively correlated with body weight and with the thickness of the subcutaneous fat.[20]

The fatty tissue layers may sometimes play an important but unsuspected role in drug toxicity. Chlorophenothane (DDT), for example, is extensively stored in the fatty tissue[83,123] without causing undue effects. However, should a patient with relatively high levels of stored DDT start a crash diet, the insecticide may be mobilized and exert toxic effects.

Genetically different individuals (fraternal twins) have exhibited significant differences in the rate of antipyrine metabolism, whereas no differences were observed in identical twins.[193] Vesell and Page[192] have ascribed large variations in the duration of action of antipyrine to genetic factors in normal individuals not receiving other drugs. Large differences among individuals have also been reported in the half-lives of phenylbutazone[32] and dicumarol.[196]

Drug-induced hemolytic anemia such as that due to primaquine sensitivity, for example, is not a drug allergy mediated by an antigen-antibody reaction; the cause is an inherited defect of an enzyme (G-6-PD) in the red blood cell. When the defective cell is exposed to the action of certain drugs, mostly aniline derivatives, it may perish.[35,190] The occurrence of this effect requires a special sensitivity of the individual. There seems to be evidence that Negroes have a special susceptibility to the hemolytic effect of primaquine. Kalow[99] has listed other drugs that may act in a manner similar to that of primaquine, such as pamaquine, pentaquine, phenylhydrazine, acetanilid, antipyrine, acetophenetidin, sulfanilamide, sulfacetamide, nitrofurantoin, probenecid and tolbutamide. Wintrobe[200] pointed to quinine, phenothiazine, neoarsphenamine, mephenytoin and mephenesin, although he felt that it is not certain whether hemolysis caused by these agents is related to primaquine sensitivity.

The fava bean also contains an agent that is capable of causing hemolysis, the disease being called favism.[99] Favism seems to occur only in primaquine-sensitive persons. Peas and mushrooms may also cause this disease. Favism seems to be relatively frequent in some Mediterranean countries.

Geographic location has been shown to play an important part in drug action in other cases, too. Jaundice induced by oral contraceptives seems to have a particular geographic distribution, the majority of cases being reported from Finland, other Scandinavian countries and Chile.[146] This same peculiarity has been reported with reference to intrahepatic cholestasis of pregnancy.[119]

Modell[143] has referred to the extreme complexity of factors that must be considered in the evaluation of drug actions and interactions. Only recently this has been made even more complex by the recognition that environmental factors, such as pesticides and insecticides, may well influence drug action. It is often unrecognized that altitude may alter drug action.[149] For example, the digitalis dose should be reduced from one fourth to two fifths of the sea-level dose at altitudes above 10,000 feet.[124] As early as 1939, it was reported that aerospace conditions can affect therapeutic action.[53] A study of Cutting's[47] discussion of hazards in aviation medicine shows that airman duties are not contraindicated after oral use of iron preparations, but are contraindicated for 12 hours after their intravenous use.

This discussion should suffice to show that the pharmacist not only must be dosage-oriented but also must know his patient intimately in order to perform his duties to the fullest extent. Further, it should suffice to show the need for a much more clinically oriented pharmacist.

DRUG-INDUCED CHANGES AND DISEASES

The unexpected response of a patient to drug therapy is becoming increasingly common. Often, prior knowledge of this possibility may help alleviate patient anxiety or to properly assess adverse reactions. For ex-ample, many drugs can alter the appearance of urine or feces, which may lead to anxiety in the patient, or more importantly, it may lead to a false interpretation of the results of diagnostic tests. Drugs that may cause discoloration of the feces are listed in Table 11-1, and Table 11-2 lists those that discolor the urine.[23]

Other, more significant changes can be the by-product of drug action. It has been reported that thioridazine causes characteristic T-wave changes.[90,170] Changes in both T-wave configuration and the Q-T interval have also been reported following administration of ACTH and corticosteroids in the presence of bradycardia due to complete or partial A-V block.[1] Piperazine has been shown to cause E.E.G. changes in children.[17]

Although it can probably be assumed that the overwhelming literature on adverse reactions to oral contraceptives is well known, Table 11-3 lists some systemic diseases caused by drugs that may not be as well known.[131]

TABLE 11-1. DRUGS THAT MAY CAUSE DISCOLORATION OF THE FECES

THERAPEUTIC CATEGORY	COLOR IMPARTED TO FECES	DRUG(S) RESPONSIBLE
Analgesics (CNS)	Pink to red to black (resulting from internal bleeding)	Salicylates
Analgesics (urinary)	Orange-red	Phenazopyridine (Pyridium)*
Antacids	Whitish discoloration or speckling	E.g., Aluminum hydroxide preparations
Anthelmintics	Blue Red	Dithiazine (Delvex) Pyrvinium pamoate (Povan)
Antibacterial agents	Black	Bismuth sodium triglycollamate (Bistrimate)
Anticoagulants	Pink to red to black (resulting from internal bleeding)	All anticoagulants
Antiprotozoal agents	Black	Bismuth glycoloylarsanilate (Milibis)
Hematinic agents	Black	Iron preparations (e.g., ferrous sulfate)
Laxatives, cathartics	Can lead to a brownish staining of the rectal mucosa	1,8-Dihydroxyanthraquinone† (Dorbane; Doxan)

* Often used in combination with other antibacterials—e.g., Azotrex, AzoGantrisin.
† Often present in combination with dioctyl sodium sulfosuccinate—e.g., Dorbantyl, Doxidan. Also used in combination with calcium pantothenate (Modane)

TABLE 11-2. DRUGS THAT MAY CAUSE DISCOLORATION OF THE URINE

THERAPEUTIC CATEGORY	COLOR IMPARTED TO THE URINE	DRUG(S) RESPONSIBLE
Analgesics (urinary)	Orange to orange-red	Ethoxazene (Serenium) phenazopyridine* (Pyridium)
Antibacterial agents	Orange-yellow (in alkaline urine)	Salicylazosulfapyridine (Azulfidine)
	Discoloration (no specific effect)	p-Aminosalicylic acid and derivatives
	Rust yellow or brownish	Sulfonamides, Nitrofurantoin and derivatives, e.g., furazolidone (Furoxone)
Anticoagulants	Orange (in alkaline urine), pink or red to red-brown	Indanedione derivatives (e.g., anisindione (Miradon), phenindione (Hedulin)
Anticonvulsants	Pink or red to red-brown	Diphenylhydantoin (Dilantin), phensuximide (Milontin)
Antidepressants	Blue-green	Amitriptyline (Elavil)
Antidote to cyanide poisoning	Blue or green	Methylene blue
Antiprotozoal agents	Brown to black	Quinine and derivatives
	Rust yellow or brown	Pamaquine naphthoate (Plasmochin), primaquine, chloroquine (Aralen)
	Yellow	Quinacrine (Atabrine)
	Dark	Metronidazole (Flagyl)
Diuretics	Pale blue fluorescence	Triamterene (Dyrenium)
Hemostatic agents	Blue-green	Tolonium (Blutene)
Hematinic agents	Black	Iron-sorbitol-citric acid complex (Jectofer)
Laxatives, cathartics	Brown to black	Cascara, rhubarb
	Pink to red or red-brown	1,8-Dihydroxyanthraquinone† emodin (in alkaline urine) phenolphthalein‡
Skeletal muscle relaxants	Orange or purplish-red	Chlorzoxazone (Paraflex)
	Dark, brown to black or green on standing	Methocarbamol (Robaxin)
Tranquilizers	Pink to red or red-brown	Phenothiazines
Vitamins	Yellow	Riboflavin

* Often used in combination with other antibacterials—e.g., Azotrex, AzoGantrisin.
† Often present in combination with dioctyl sodium sulfosuccinate—e.g., Dorbantyl, Doxidan.
‡ May even produce a magenta coloration in alkaline urine.

TABLE 11-3. SYSTEMIC DISEASES CAUSED BY DRUGS*

CAUSATIVE AGENTS	DISEASE OR SYNDROME	SYSTEM
Anesthetics, mercurials, procaine amide penicillin, sulfonamides, sera, acetylsalicylic acid, insulin	Anaphylactic shock	Vascular
Antithyroid drugs, phenylbutazone, chloramphenicol, amphetamines, trimethadione, methylphenylethylhydantoin, diphenylhydantoin, tolbutamide, chlorpromazine HCl, aminopyrine	Hematoxic drug reactions	Hematologic
Chlorpromazine HCl, thiouracils, methimazole	Jaundice-intrahepatic obstruction	Hepatic
Hydralazine HCl (IV all cases)	Lupus erythematosus-like	Collagen
Oxygen in prematures	Retrolental fibroplasia	Metabolic
Penicillin, chlortetracycline HCl, meperidine HCl, mercurials, para-aminosalicylic acid, arsenic, acetylsalicylic acid, belladonna	Asthma	Pulmonary
Phenacemide, phenylbutazone, isonicotinic acid hydrazides	Hepatitis, hepatic coma	Hepatic
Sulfonamides, trimethadione, chelating agents	Nephroses	Renal
Autonomic blocking agents	Acute urinary retention	
Tranquilizers, particularly trifluoperazine, perphenazine, prochlorperazine, reserpine, rauwolfia; steroids, streptomycin sulfate, dihydrostreptomycin sulfate	Convulsive disorders and parkinsonism	Neurologic
	Psychoses, eighth nerve	

* Reprinted with permission of the author.[181]

TABLE 11-4. DERMATOLOGIC MANIFESTATIONS OF DRUG REACTIONS*

TYPE	MOST COMMON OFFENDERS
Allergic eczematous dermatitis	Sulfonamides, penicillin, mercurials, arsenicals, local anesthetics, quinacrine HCl, quinine, aniline dyes, arsphenamine
Bullous eruptions	Iodides, gold, salicylates, sulfonamides, phenolphthalein
Erythema multiforme and nodosum-like lesions	Bromides, iodides, salicylates, phenacetin, sulfonamides, penicillin, phenolphthalein
Exanthematic	Barbiturates, sulfonamides, heavy metals, arsenic, salicylates, foods adulterated with coloring, flavoring and preservative agents of coal tar origin, penicillin
Exfoliative dermatitis	Arsenicals, barbiturates, gold salts, mercurials, quinacrine HCl, belladonna
Fixed eruptions	Barbiturates, phenolphthalein, quinacrine HCl, sulfonamides, gold, phenacetin, antipyrine
Purpura	Barbiturates, gold salts, iodides, sulfonamides, arsphenamines
Urticaria	Organ extracts, penicillin, streptomycin, salicylates, sera, food adulterated with coloring, flavoring and preservative agents of coal tar origin

* Reprinted with permission of the author.[181]

Drug allergy is one of the most serious problems of therapeutics, and hypersensitivity represents a major problem in the use of some drugs. Although the incidence of hypersensitivity reactions is extremely low with most drugs, the list of known offenders, particularly those causing dermatologic manifestations, is growing steadily. Some of these are listed in Table 11-4.[131]

Certain diseases may also affect drug action. Usually, only large doses of isoniazid cause convulsion in man,[157] and only in rare cases do therapeutic doses of this drug induce an epileptiform state in a patient.[107] However, tuberculosis patients require an increased maintenance dose of an anticonvulsant during isoniazid therapy.

Pregnancy appears to influence drug metabolism. Kunelis et al.[108] suggested that the increased demand for protein anabolism during pregnancy may make the liver more sensitive to drugs, such as tetracycline, that depress this function. Schanker[167] described the epithelium of the mammary gland as a lipoid membrane separating blood of pH 7.4 from milk of a somewhat lower pH value. It seems that basic drugs, such as erythromycin, accumulate in the milk rather than in the plasma and therefore may be passed on to the baby. Completely un-ionized substances, such as ethanol and antipyrine, distribute evenly between milk and plasma.

Innumerable studies have been performed of the exchange of substances between mother and fetus. Cahen[34] believes that the placenta behaves as an inert barrier with lipoid properties toward most drugs and that any lipid-soluble drug, or any drug that crosses the blood-brain barrier, readily penetrates the placenta. Schanker,[167] although essentially in agreement with this view, cautions that there is only a "hint that the placental barrier is lipoid in character."

Although Hale[70] demonstrated in 1935 the teratogenic effect of vitamin A deficiency in pigs, and although sulfonamides,[13] insulin,[129] antibiotics[59] and hypocholesterolemic agents[163] were also shown to cause teratogenic effects in animals, it was only comparatively recently that clinicians began to investigate the etiology of fetal malformations induced by drugs.

Cahen[34] reports that some drugs cross the placental barrier and are embryotoxic, but regardless of the dose, do not produce malformations. He lists several drugs for which there is strong evidence that they cause congenital malformations in man, such as thalidomide, antimetabolites, steroids, hormones, and hypoglycemic agents. On the other hand, many drugs cause malformations in animals that have not been observed in man. Among these are sodium fluoride, salicylates, phenylbutazone, chlorcyclizine, acetazolamide and certain antibiotics. Many of these drugs, of course, have been used for years in therapeutics without any reports of abnormal development in the human fetus. Analgesics, meperidine, chloral hydrate, barbiturates and anticoagulants cross the placental barrier but do not seem to cause fetal deformation.

MacAulay and Charles[132] note that interest in transfer of drugs through the placenta is now oriented toward rate of transmission rather than mere presence. This may be important, they point out, in the prevention of intrauterine infection in the case of premature rupture of the membranes. Apgar[7] listed some relationships observed between maternal medication and fetal or neonatal changes. She cautions, however, that "only a few are proved beyond a shadow of a doubt, but until further data are collected, caution should be exercised in administering these substances to pregnant women" (Table 11-5).

INTERACTIONS OF DRUGS WITH ALCOHOL

In rabbits, rats, dogs and mice, ethanol has been found to interact with innumerable depressant drugs, usually producing a potentiation. Alcohol has been reported to enhance the effects of pentobarbital,[50,67] phenobarbital,[95] thiopental,[179] secobarbital,[155] hexobarbital,[55] amobarbital,[57] barbital[69] and cyclobarbital.[165] Bonnichsen et al.[26] reported that only about two-thirds of the "normal" lethal concentration of barbiturates were found in human fatalities due to overdoses of barbiturates when ethanol was present.

Chlorpromazine,[180] reserpine,[30] promazine,[54] promethazine,[130] hydroxyzine,[60] meprobamate,[8] chlordiazepoxide,[203] imipramine,[80] and benactyzine[85] have all been reported to interact with alcohol in animals.

TABLE 11-5. POSSIBLE RELATIONSHIPS BETWEEN MATERNAL MEDICATION AND FETAL
OR NEONATAL CHANGES*

MATERNAL MEDICATION	FETAL OR NEONATAL EFFECT
Oral progestogens	Masculinization and advanced bone age
Androgens	
Estrogens	
Cortisone acetate	Anomalies, cleft palate(?)
Potassium iodide	Goiter and mental retardation
Propylthiouracil	
Methimazole	
Iophenoxic acid	Elevation of P.B.I.
Sodium aminopterin	Anomalies and abortion
Methotrexate	
Chlorambucil	
Bishydroxycoumarin	Fetal death; hemorrhage
Sodium warfarin	
Salicylates (large amounts)	Neonatal bleeding
Streptomycin	Possible 8th nerve deafness
Sulfonamides	Kernicterus
Chloramphenicol	"Gray" syndrome, death
Sodium novobiocin	Hyperbilirubinemia
Erythromycin	Liver damage(?)
Nitrofurantoin	Hemolysis
Tetracyclines	Inhibition of bone growth, discoloration of teeth
Vitamin K analogues (in excess)	Hyperbilirubinemia
Ammonium chloride	Acidosis
Intravenous fluids (in excess)	Electrolyte abnormalities
Reserpine	
Hexamethonium bromide	Neonatal ileus
Morphine	Neonatal death
Phenobarbital (in excess)	Neonatal bleeding, death
Sulfonylurea derivatives	Anomalies(?)
Phenformin hydrochloride	Lactic acidosis(?)
Phenothiazines	Hyperbilirubinemia(?)
Meprobamate	Retarded development(?)
Chloroquine phosphate	Retinal damage or death(?)
Quinine	Thrombocytopenia
Thalidomide	Phocomelia, death, hearing loss
Vaccination, smallpox	Fetal vaccinia
Vaccination, influenza	Increased anti-A and -B titers in mothers
Antihistamines	Anomalies(?), infertility(?)
Thiazide diuretics	Thrombocytopenia

* Apgar, V.: Drugs in pregnancy, J.A.M.A. *190*:840, 1964.

The interaction of morphine with alcohol results in more than just an additive effect,[60,69] whereas only an additive effect is obtained when acetanilid and alcohol interact.[82] Other drugs known to interact with alcohol in animals are epinephrine,[141] scopolamine, atropine[55] and quinine.[145]

Lamy and Block[116] have suggested that antianginal agents, certain antibacterial agents, anticoagulants, antidiabetic agents, antihistamines, antihypertensive agents, monoamine oxidase inhibitors, phenothiazine derivatives, sedatives, hypnotics and tranquilizers all could interact with alcohol. Obviously, however, the severity of the possible interaction depends on the dose of alcohol ingested by the patient.

Graham[67] reported that the severity of symptoms of ethanol-barbiturate combinations was greater if the ethanol had been consumed in the form of hard liquor (such as whiskey or gin) rather than as beer, cider or in another dilute form, although the total quantity of alcohol consumed did not differ. Graham[67] also commented that drinkers of hard liquors suffered from a much more severe coma than drinkers of beers and wines, and he attributed this fact to the irritation of the gastric and duodenal mucosa by hard liquor. The irritated mucosa, in turn, would promote the absorption of any drugs subsequently administered.

Newman and Abramson[144] also observed that different alcoholic beverages are absorbed at differing rates and that wines, with their high buffer capacity, are absorbed less rapidly than are distilled liquors. Horwitz et al.[86] warn, however, that Chianti contains enough tyramine in 400 ml. to provoke a pressor response. Much smaller amounts of tyramine are apparently present in certain beers, and the authors suggested that beer drinkers would be intoxicated before a dangerous tyramine level would be reached.

Two other interactions of alcohol are of interest. Paraldehyde has frequently been used in the treatment of alcoholism, particularly in delirium tremens. However, evidence is accumulating suggesting that paraldehyde may be contraindicated for this purpose.[105,155,195] Weatherby and Clements[195] reported on a particularly interesting study, regarding the importance of the order of administration of drugs in relation to therapeutic interactions. When ethanol was administered to mice, followed by a paraldehyde injection, a very high mortality rate was observed. In contrast, when paraldehyde ad-

ministration preceded ethanol intake, no fatalities occurred, and the authors believed that fatalities were avoided because of the rapid elimination of paraldehyde.

Lawrence,[122] reviewing the possible effect of alcohol on patients receiving drugs, cautions that the diabetic patient should control his alcohol intake with great care. Alcohol may reduce the patient's need for insulin, and this seems particularly true if the patient suffers from hepatic damage or if large quantities of alcohol are consumed. Wood[201] ascribed this interaction to the carbohydrate-sparing action of alcohol, in which energy obtained from the metabolism of alcohol decreases the metabolic need for sugar.

INTERACTIONS OF DRUGS WITH FOODS

The importance of possible interactions of drugs with different foods has only recently been recognized. Block and Lamy[24] have reviewed some of the foods implicated in these interactions (Table 11-6).

The interaction between monoamine oxidase inhibitors and food substances containing tyramine is well recognized. Cheese is the food most commonly incriminated in these interactions. However, some patients consume cheese while on monoamine oxidase inhibitor therapy without ill effects, which can be explained by the fact that the tyramine content of cheese is related to maturation time, bacterial flora and details of manufacture. Cheddar cheese often contains suffi-

TABLE 11-6. INTERACTION OF SOME DRUGS WITH FOODS

Drugs	Foods
Antibacterial agents: tetracyclines	Milk, dairy products
Anticoagulants	Leafy green vegetables
Antihypertensive agents	Foods containing pressor amines (aged cheese, broad beans, pickled herring, chocolate, chicken liver, licorice)
Cardiac glycosides	Milk, dairy products, licorice
Diuretics, oral	Licorice
Monoamine oxidase inhibitors (antidepressants, pargyline)	Foods containing pressor amines (see under "Antihypertensive agents")
Thyroid	Soy bean preparations, vegetables of Brassica sp. (Brussels sprouts, cabbage, cauliflower, kale, turnips)

TABLE 11-7. INCOMPATIBILITIES OF COMMONLY USED DRUGS FOR
INTRAVENOUS ADMINISTRATION*

AGENT	INCOMPATIBLE AGENTS
Antibiotics	
Amphotericin B†	Potassium penicillin G, tetracyclines
Cephalothin	Calcium chloride or gluconate, erythromycin, polymyxin B, tetracyclines
Chloramphenicol	B-complex vitamin preparations, hydrocortisone, polymyxin B, tetracyclines, vancomycin
Methicillin‡	Tetracyclines
Nafcillin	B-complex vitamin preparations
Potassium penicillin G	Amphotericin B, metaraminol, phenylephrine, tetracyclines, vancomycin, ascorbic acid
Polymyxin B	Cephalothin, chloramphenicol, heparin, tetracyclines
Tetracyclines§	Amphotericin B, cephalothin, chloramphenicol, heparin, hydrocortisone, methicillin, potassium penicillin G, polymyxin B
Vancomycin	Chloramphenicol, heparin, hydrocortisone, potassium penicillin G
Pressors	
Ephedrine	Hydrocortisone
Epinephrine	Mephentermine
Mephentermine	Epinephrine
Metaraminol	Potassium penicillin G
Phenylephrine**	Potassium penicillin G
Miscellaneous	
Aminophylline	Acidic solutions, B-complex vitamin preparations, barbiturates, calcium or magnesium salts, vancomycin
B-complex vitamin preparations	Aminophylline, chloramphenicol, hydrocortisone, nafcillin
Barbiturates and tranquilizers	Many drugs
Calcium chloride or gluconate	Cephalothin, sodium bicarbonate, tetracyclines
Heparin	Tetracyclines, polymyxin B, vancomycin
Hydrocortisone	B-complex vitamin preparations, chloramphenicol, ephedrine, tetracyclines, vancomycin
Sodium bicarbonate	Calcium chloride or gluconate, lactated Ringer's solution

* The Medical Letter 9:17, 1967. (August 25)

† Specific instructions for reconstitution are provided by the manufacturer. The agent should always be administered alone.

‡ Physical stability or biologic potency may change after reconstitution. The agent should be administered alone soon after it is diluted.

§ The agent should not be mixed with solutions that contain calcium. Ringer's solution may be used as a diluent because the pH of the solution is acid.

** Bisulfite is used as an antioxidant in commercial preparations of this agent. Bisulfite slowly inactivates penicillin G.

Reprinted with permission of the duplicate letter.

cient tyramine to produce hypertension, but individual samples vary widely in tyramine content. The major hazard of monoamine oxidase inhibitors is the occurrence of a hypertensive crisis. Orally ingested amines such as tyramine are normally inactivated by hepatic monoamine oxidase. Inhibitors of monoamine oxidase impair this mechanism, thus allowing access of amine to the systemic circulation, possibly causing a hypertensive crisis.[152]

Saw-Lan Ip[166] and Sjoequest[177] found a high content of 5-hydroxytryptamine in bananas and warned against their addition to the diet of patients being treated with monoamine oxidase inhibitors. Sjoequest also included caffeine-containing drinks such as coffee and cola in a list of foods and drinks that have been implicated in interactions with monoamine oxidase inhibitors.

Another possible means by which food could affect drug action should not be overlooked, although it cannot be classified as an interaction. Levy and Jusko[127] have reported that the absorption of riboflavin is enhanced in the presence of food, probably because of a decrease in the intestinal transit rate, which causes the vitamin to be retained for a longer period at the absorption sites in the small intestine. As Kitler[103] pointed out, the transit rate of a drug through the gastrointestinal tract can be affected by foods and assumes importance when a drug either dissolves at an unusually slow rate or is absorbed only at a particular site along the tract.

PHYSICAL AND CHEMICAL INTERACTIONS OF DRUGS

Physical and chemical interactions of drugs have come to demand a much more increased and specialized knowledge on the part of the pharmacist with the increased use of I.V. admixtures. Although simple interactions such as the reaction of alkaloids with the tannins in wild cherry syrup are well known to every pharmacy student, interactions of commonly used drugs in I.V. admixtures still have defied categorization. The increased use of I.V. admixtures has, in part, been reviewed by Lamy *et al.*,[117] and possible interactions have been reported by Meisler and Skolaut[138] and Pelissier and Burgee.[148] A most extensive listing of intravenous additive incompatibilities has also been published by Skolaut.[92]

Although physical evidence of an incompatibility in an I.V. admixture does not necessarily mean therapeutic inactivation, the fact that a given combination of drugs is not designated incompatible in Table 11-7 does not imply that the combination is actually compatible, because different batches of drugs or fluids may vary widely as to pH and other factors.[137]

DRUG INTERACTIONS WITH DIAGNOSTIC TESTS

Many therapeutic regimens are based on clinical findings obtained with the aid of diagnostic tests. Those involved in the prescribing, preparing or administering of therapeutic agents must be aware of the influence that many drugs may have on clinical laboratory values. Hicks[81] has presented an excellent summary of possible interactions. Based on this discussion, Burgee[191] has prepared these data in the form of a quick reference table (Table 11-8).

TABLE 11-8. EFFECTS OF DRUGS ON LABORATORY VALUES

TEST	DRUG	EFFECT
Urine: acetone	Sulfobromophthalein, phenoisufonphthalein	Increase value
Kidney function	Sulfobromophthalein	Interferes with reading of phenolsulfonphthalein test (24 hours required between drugs)
Urine diacetic acid	Phenothiazines & salicylates	Increase value
albumin	Penicillin (massive doses), salicylates, tolbutamide, x-ray contrast media	Increase albumin excretion causing false positive
amino acids	Cortrophin (ACTH), cortisone, sulfonamides, epinephrine, insulin	Increase excretion of amino acids Decrease excretion of amino acids

TABLE 11-8. EFFECTS OF DRUGS ON LABORATORY VALUES *(Continued)*

TEST	DRUG	EFFECT
catecholamines	Erythromycin, methyldopa, quinidine, tetracyclines, hypertensive agents, B-complex vitamins, epinephrine-like agents used in asthma	Increase catecholamine content
Blood: enzymes		
acid phosphatase	Androgens, prostate massage	Increase blood level
Alkaline phosphatase	Methyldopa	Variable effect
Serum amylase	Morphine, codeine, meperidine	Increase level up to 24 hours
	Alcohol	Increase level
SGOT	Opiates, salicylates, methicillin, ampicillin	Increase level
	Methyldopa	Variable effect
Liver function	Anabolic steroids, barbiturates, estrogens, morphine, probenecid, phenozapyridine, iopanoic acid	Increase retention of sulfobromophthalein
Serum bilirubin	Caffeine	Decreases level
	Methyldopa	Variable effect
Blood ammonia	Sodium salts	May cause decrease
	Ion exchange resin (*e.g.,* Kayexalate)	May cause increase
Prothrombin time	Barbiturates	Increase prothrombin activity
	Antibiotics, globulin, salicylates, sulfonamides, hydroxyzine	Decrease prothrombin activity
	Methyldopa	Variable effect
Serum albumin	Penicillin (massive doses), salicylates, tolbutamide, x-ray contrast media	Increase values
Blood urea nitrogen	Chloral hydrate, triamterene, methyldopa	Increase BUN
	Glucose infusion	Decreases BUN
Serum proteins	Sulfobromophthalein	Elevated value
	Ammonium salts	Decreased value
Serum calcium	Heparin, insulin	May decrease levels
Serum sodium	Calcium salts, potassium salts, steroids	May increase levels
	Diuretics, paracentesis	May decrease levels
Serum potassium	Hyperventilation, corticotropin (ACTH) steroids, sulfates and phosphates	Decrease levels
Serum phosphorus	Epinephrine, insulin, general anesthetics	Decrease levels

TABLE 11-8. EFFECTS OF DRUGS ON LABORATORY VALUES *(Continued)*

TEST	DRUG	EFFECT
Serum chloride	Acetazolamide, bromides, ion exchange resins, steroids	Increase values
Serum copper	Iron and cobalt preparations	Increase values
Serum iron and iron binding capacity	Corticotropin (ACTH) and steroids	Decrease values
	Iron-dextran complex	Increase values
Blood cholesterol	Corticotropin (ACTH), cortisone, vitamin A, bromides	Usually raise level
	Androgens, thyroid, heparin, clofibrate	Decrease level
Blood glucose	Oral contraceptives	Decrease glucose tolerance curve
	Corticotropin (ACTH)	Increases level
Protein-bound iodine	X-ray contrast media	Increase values for as long as 10 years
	Barium sulfate, oral contraceptives, estrogens, amebicides (*e.g.,* Floraquin, Vioform), suntan oil, mouthwashes, vitamin preparations, iodized salt	Increase values
	Liothyronine, testosterone, corticotropin (ACTH), chlorates, cortisone, mercurial diuretics, salicylates, sulfonamides	Decrease values
	Sulfobromophthalein	Variable effect
Serum uric acid	Dicumarol, piperazine Corticotropin (ACTH), aspirin (large doses)	Decrease values
	Nitrogen mustard, aspirin (small doses), chlorothiazide, pyrazinamide	Increase values
	Methyldopa	Variable effects
Serum creatinine	Ascorbic acid, sulfobromophthalein, phenolsulfonphthalein	Increase level
Blood cross match: direct Coombs test	Methyldopa, cephalothin, penicillin	False positive (up to one year)
Cerebrospinal fluid protein	Local anesthetics	False elevated reading

The pharmacist should be constantly alert for newly reported interactions. It was recently reported, for example, that chlordiazepoxide may act as an antithyroid drug[11] and that, therefore, patients treated for anxiety and emotional disorders with this drug may show a depressed ^{131}I uptake when a thyroid function test is performed.[76]

Sometimes, radiologists mix antihistamines with contrast media, causing a reduction in the pH of the media, resulting in precipitation of the organic iodide.[134] At other times, an interaction may occur that is difficult to trace. If cork stoppers are used for containers of serum that is to be analyzed for calcium content, the calcium may be leached from the stoppers and cause elevated levels of calcium to be reported.[185]

ALTERATION OF ABSORPTION BY DRUGS

The rate and/or extent of drug absorption from the gastrointestinal tract may be markedly affected when other preparations are used concurrently by a patient. Most drugs are weak organic electrolytes. Antacids or acidifiers may bring about an alteration of the environmental pH and thus cause a shift in the proportion of the drug present as the un-ionized moiety. The pH-partition hypothesis of Shore et al.[175] considers the biologic barrier between the gastrointestinal lumen and the plasma to be permeable mainly to the un-ionized form of the weak electrolyte. Being dependent on the concentration of the un-ionized drug moiety present, absorption is therefore pH dependent and can be altered by concurrently administered preparations.

The amount of drug available for absorption from the gastrointestinal tract can also be affected by adsorption of the drug onto the surface of solids. Finely divided solids in suspension, such as aluminum hydroxide gel or milk of magnesia, could adsorb a portion of the drug and render it unavailable for absorption. Sorby and Liu[186] showed that the rate and extent of promazine absorption are decreased significantly in the presence of an attapulgite clay–citrus pectin mixture.

The formation of complexes with metal ions, present in milk or antacids or similar preparations, might also render a drug unavailable for absorption. This occurs when tetracyclines complex with divalent or trivalent metals.[113] Lamy and Shangraw,[118] in reviewing pharmaceutical aspects of some antibiotics, recounted the difficulties encountered in the development of tetracycline capsules, in which dicalcium phosphate was used as a filler. Metal-antibiotic chelation occurred, making some of the drug unavailable for absorption.

Surfactants, too, may affect the rate and/or extent of absorption of a drug. Kitler[103] remarked that the influence of surfactants on the rate and extent of drug transfer has been extensively investigated.[25,128,187] Both increased and decreased absorption of drugs has been shown, and in some instances the surfactants had no influence on the absorption of drugs whatsoever. Surfactants could increase the amount of drug absorbed by solubilizing the drug or by directly affecting the permeability of the gastrointestinal epithelium. In the case of solid dosage forms or suspensions, the surfactant might increase the rate of dissolution of the solid by increasing the contact between the particulate matter and the bulk fluid of the gut.

ALTERATION OF EXCRETION BY DRUGS

The elimination processes of some drugs are influenced by the administration of agents that affect the acidity or alkalinity of urine. A difference in pH between plasma and tubular fluid can result in a considerable difference in the fraction of undissociated weakly acidic or weakly basic drug, and it is usually the undissociated moiety of the drug that most readily diffuses between the two compartments.

Milne et al.[140] have shown that the pH of the tubular fluid, the pKa and the partition coefficient of a drug can influence renal tubular transfer of many drugs.

The importance of a knowledge of the pKa of a drug was shown by Block and Lamy[25] (Table 11-9).

Change in urinary pH can also alter the rate of urinary excretion. When a drug is in its un-ionized or undissociated form, it more readily diffuses from the urine into the blood. In an acid urine, there is a larger pro-

TABLE 11-9. SOME DRUGS WHOSE RENAL EXCRETION COULD VARY WITH CHANGES IN URINARY pH*

DRUG	APPROXIMATE pK$_a$	PER CENT OF DRUG IN IONIZED FORM† WHEN URINARY pH IS		
		4.0	6.0	8.0
Atropine	4.4	71.53	2.45	0.02
Imipramine	9.5	99.99	99.97	96.94
Mecamylamine	11.2	99.99	99.99	99.94
Meperidine	8.7	99.99	99.80	83.37
Perphenazine	7.8	99.98	98.44	63.09
Phenylbutazone	4.4	28.47	97.55	99.98
Quinine	8.4	99.99	99.60	71.53
Salicylic acid	3.0	90.91	99.90	99.99
Sulfadiazine	6.5	0.32	24.04	96.94
Sulfamethylthiadiazole	5.2	5.93	86.32	99.84
Sulfisoxazole	4.8	13.68	94.06	99.94
Tolazoline	10.3	99.99	99.99	99.50

* Drugs with a pKa > 9.0, such as imipramine, mecamylamine, and tolazoline, do not generally show a marked change in passive urinary excretion because urinary pH rarely exceeds a value of 8.0.
† Calculated from the following:
   For bases, % Ionized = 100/[1 + antilog (pH-pKa)]
   For acids, % Ionized = 100/[1 + antilog (pKa-pH)]

portion of an acidic drug in the undissociated form, and as a result more of the acidic drug diffuses back into the blood, resulting in prolonged activity of the drug. Milne et al.[139] report that such acidic drugs as nitrofurantoin are excreted faster when the urinary pH is alkaline. An acid urinary pH, on the other hand, results in faster excretion of such basic drugs as amphetamine, imipramine and triptyline.

Similarly, it has also been demonstrated that the renal clearance of salicylates is increased when sodium bicarbonate or other alkalinizing agents are administered concurrently.[84] Similar sensitivity to urinary pH has been shown with phenobarbital,[194] phenylbutazone analogs[68] and sulfadiazine.[151] It is generally accepted that elimination of sulfonamides can be accelerated by concurrent administration of sodium bicarbonate.[150] Phenylbutazone, moreover, can potentiate the hypoglycemic effects of acetohexamide by interfering with the renal excretion of the active metabolite, hydroxyhexamide.[58]

Beckett and Wilkinson[16] report that chlorpheniramine and its isomers show a dependence not only on urinary pH but also on the rate of urinary flow. Beckett et al.[15] also showed that the renal excretion of amphetamine and methylamphetamine depends on urinary pH.

Portnoff et al.[154] and Kostenbauder et al.[106] administered 3 to 4 Gm. of ammonium chloride for 2 to 3 hours until a urinary pH of 4.5 to 5.0 was achieved, followed by smaller doses to maintain pH at this level. To achieve a urinary pH of 8.0, they administered sodium bicarbonate hourly at a dose of 4 Gm., followed by smaller maintenance doses. This indicates that large doses of alkalinizers or acidifiers must be used in order to change urinary pH.

INTERACTIONS OF OTC DRUGS

The problem of drug interaction becomes more complex when OTC drugs are considered.[24,116] Whereas one can be reasonably

TABLE 11-10. NEW OTC PRODUCTS, 1959–1965

CATEGORY	NUMBER OF NEW DRUGS
Analgesics	113
Antacids and gastrointestinal products	137
Cough and cold products	343
Laxatives and evacuants	70
Sleeping aids and tranquilizers	29
Tonics	106
Vitamins and hematinics	529

TABLE 11-11. SELECTED OTC PRODUCTS THAT COULD CAUSE INTERACTIONS
WITH LEGEND DRUGS*

INGREDIENT(S)	PRODUCT	INGREDIENT(S)	PRODUCT
ANALGESICS		*Nasal Sprays and Nose Drops*	
3	A.S.A. Compound	4	Alconefrin
3	Alka-Seltzer	2,4	Bena-Fedrin
3	Anacin	2,4	Contac
3	Ascriptin	2,4	Drilitol
3	Aspirin	2,4	NTZ
3	BC	4	Neo-Synephrine
3	Bufferin	4	Paredrine sulfathiazole susp.
2,3	Cope	2	Privine
3	Doan's Pills	2,4	Sinex
3	Ecotrin	4	St. Joseph's Nose Drops for children
3	Empirin Compound		
3	Excedrin	2,4	Super Anahist
3	Fizrin	4	Vasoxyl
3	Measurin		
3	Midol	*Tablets and Capsules*	
3	Pabirin	3,4	4-Way Cold Tablets
3	P-A-C Compound	2,4	Allerest
2	Pamprin	2,4	Bronitin
3	Phensal	4	Bromo-Quinine
5	Pre-Mens	2,4	Bronkaid
3	Resolve	2,3,4	Cheracol Cold Capsules
3	Stanback	2,4	Chexit
3	Vanquish	2,4	Citrisun
3	Zarumin	2,4	Colchek
		2,4,5	Contac
REMEDIES FOR BRONCHIAL ASTHMA, COUGH AND COLD, HAY FEVER AND RHINITIS		2,3	Coricidin
		2,3,4	Coricidin-D
		2,4	Coryban-D
		2,4	Dondril
Inhalation Products		2,3,4	Dristan
4	Adrenalin chloride	2,4	Fedrazil
4	AsthmaNefrin	2	Thephorin
4	Breatheasy	2,3	Thephorin-AC
4	Bronkaid Mist	2,4	Theracin
4	Epinephrine solution	2,3,4	Triaminicin
4	Medihaler-Epi	2,4	Tri-Span
4	Primatene Mist	2,4	Tussagesic
		2,3,4	Ursinus Inlay-Tabs
Liquids		4	Zantrate
2,3,4	Coldene		
1	Creo-terpin (25% alcohol)	*SLEEP AIDS*	
2,4	Noscomel	2	Dormin
2,4	Novahistine, Novahistine DH	2	Nytol
4	Orthoxycol	2	Relax-U-Caps
2	Robitussin-AC	2,5	San-Man
2,4	Romilar CF	2,5	Sleep-Eze
4	Sudafed	2,5	Sominex
2	Super Anahist Cough Syrup		
1	Terpin Hydrate, Terpin Hydrate with Codeine, Terpin Hydrate with Dextromethorphan (42% alcohol)	*ANTIMOTION SICKNESS*	
		2	Bonine
		2	Dramamine
		2	Marezine
2,4	Triaminic	5	Mothersill's Remedy
2,4	Triaminicol		
4	Trind		

*Key: 1=alcohol; 2=antihistamine; 3=aspirin, salicylates; 4=sympathomimetic amines; 5=belladonna alkaloids and related compounds.

certain of at least the active constituents of a legend drug, the composition and strength of an OTC drug are often vague or cannot be ascertained at all. The proliferation of OTC products will make this problem even greater in the future. Table 11-10 shows the number of new OTC drugs that have been introduced in the recent past.

The pharmacist must not only be aware of any interactions, but he must also be willing and able to communicate this knowledge to physicians and, more importantly, to the patient.

Many drugs are available as OTC preparations in low dosages, but the same drugs, in a somewhat higher dose, are available only on prescription. One might mention Coricidin, Chlor-trimeton, Sudafed, Contac and others. Table 11-11 lists some OTC preparations and the active ingredient in the particular dosage form that could be the cause of an interaction with a prescription drug.

Classification of OTC products by use might be helpful in anticipating interactions, and Table 11-12 shows selected categories of OTC drugs.

Over-the-counter preparations serve a useful purpose by the alleviation of symptoms resulting from minor ailments. It has been stated that a drug may be sold without prescription if it is safe, if adequate indications for use are available to the patient, and if adequate directions for use are included on the label. However, many therapeutically undesirable interactions of OTC drugs with legend drugs (Table 11-13) have been published in the literature. Many of these are reported here, although in some instances the

original report may be based on only one or two individual notes.

Table 11-13 shows that thyroid preparations may interact with soy bean preparations. It should be noted that several baby foods and some of the present-day diet liquids contain partially hydrogenated soy bean.

Contrary to the widely held belief, aspirin is not innocuous. Interactions of aspirin could occur with antianginal agents, antibacterial agents, anticoagulants, antifungal agents, antihypertensive agents, hypoglycemic agents and monoamine oxidase inhibitors. In addition to the well known "aspirin intolerance," this drug has been implicated in abnormal renal function in rheumatoid arthritis, analgesic nephropathy, massive gastric hemorrhage, abnormal hemostasis due to hypoprothrombinemia, pancytopenia and encephalopathy.[77] Untoward reactions to aspirin are found in one fifth as many instances as penicillin reactions.[156] Aspirin intolerance is characterized by asthma, rhinitis and nasal polyps, and it is induced by aspirin but not by sodium salicylate.[164]

Glaucoma is a disease of the eye marked by heightened intraocular pressure, which may ultimately lead to blindness. Increased intraocular pressure may result from administration of belladonna alkaloids, and an attack of acute glaucoma may be precipitated by any of these alkaloids. Yet Table 11-11 lists a number of widely used OTC preparations that contain belladonna alkaloids, and the pharmacist must be ready to caution any patient suffering from glaucoma against the use of these preparations.

TABLE 11-12. SELECTED CATEGORIES OF OTC DRUGS THAT MAY CAUSE INTERACTIONS

CATEGORY	INTERACTING INGREDIENTS
Analgesics	Aspirin, salicylates
Antacids	Calcium, magnesium
Antihistamines, cold tablets & capsules	Antihistamines, aspirin, belladonna alkaloids
Cough syrups, elixirs, expectorants	Alcohol, antihistamines
Diarrhea remedies	Clays and other adsorbents
Laxatives	Surfactants
Motion sickness products	Antihistamines, belladonna alkaloids
Nasal sprays and drops	Sympathomimetic amines
Sleeping aids	Antihistamines
Tonics	Alcohol

TABLE 11-13. INTERACTION OF LEGEND DRUGS WITH OTC DRUGS

LEGEND DRUG	OTC DRUGS THAT MAY INTERACT
Antibacterial, antifungal agents	
Furazolidone	Phenobarbital
Griseofulvin	Ammonium chloride, aspirin and other salicylates, methenamine
Sulfonamides	
Tetracyclines	Colloidal antacids
Anticoagulants	Antihistamines, aspirin and other salicylates, mineral oil, phenobarbital
Anticonvulsants (hydantoin derivatives)	Phenobarbital
Antidepressants (see also monoamine oxidase inhibitors)	Adsorptive agents (attapulgite, bentonite, charcoal, colloidal antacids, kaolin)
Antidiabetic agents	Aspirin and other salicylates
Antihistamines	Sympathomimetic amines, sedatives (bromides, scopolamine and scopolamine aminoxide preparations)
Antihypertensive agents	Antihistamines, sympathomimetic amines
Bronchodilators	Antihistamines, sympathomimetic amines
Cardiac glycosides	Absorbable antacids, drugs containing large amounts of calcium
Monoamine oxidase inhibitors	Adsorptive agents (attapulgite, bentonite, charcoal, colloidal antacids, kaolin)
Oxytocics	Sympathomimetic amines
Phenothiazine derivatives (antihistamines, antiemetics, tranquilizers)	Adsorptive agents (attapulgite, bentonite, charcoal, colloidal antacids, kaolin), antihistamines, sedatives (bromides, scopolamine and scopolamine aminoxide preparations)
Sedatives, hypnotics and tranquilizers	Antihistamines, bromides, phenobarbital, scopolamine and scopolamine aminoxide preparations
Sympathomimetic amines	Antihistamines
Thyroid	Iodides, iodine-containing drugs used orally (iodochlorhydroxyquin) Soy bean preparations
Uricosuric agents	Aspirin and other salicylates
Vitamins, fat-soluble (A, D, E, K)	Mineral oil (chronic usage)

Table 11-11 also lists many remedies for bronchial asthma, cough, cold, hay fever and rhinitis that contain a sympathomimetic amine as a decongestant. The catecholamines challenge the pancreas and facilitate glycogen breakdown, causing an increase in blood sugar levels. The sympathomimetic amines, therefore, directly oppose the action of insulin, which facilitates glucose uptake and utilization, thereby decreasing the blood sugar level. For this reason, products containing sympathomimetic amines are required to carry a prominent warning against their use in the presence of diabetes.

Knapp and Knapp[104] participated in a limited study designed to test the knowledge of randomly selected pharmacists of this possible interaction. Sixty-five pharmacists were approached by a patient who claimed to be a diabetic on insulin therapy. Fifty-eight pharmacists sold this patient a nasal decongestant containing a sympathomimetic amine. The re-

TABLE 11-14. SOME THERAPEUTIC INCOMPATIBILITIES OF SELECTED CARDIOVASCULAR DRUGS

CARDIOVASCULAR DRUG	PHARMACOLOGIC CLASSIFICATION	INCOMPATIBLE AGENTS	REASON FOR INCOMPATIBILITY	POTENTIAL HAZARD
Warfarin	Anticoagulant (vit. K antagonist)	Highly bound anionic drugs (clofibrate, ethacrynic acid, indomethacin, oxyphenbutazone, phenylbutazone, salicylates, sulfamethoxypyridazine, tolbutamide)	Displacement of anticoagulant from plasma albumin	Depressed prothrombin levels, hemorrhagic crisis
		Anabolic steroids (methandrostenolone)	Unknown	Exaggerated anticoagulant effect
		Chloral hydrate, glutethimide, griseofulvin, phenobarbital	Acceleration of inactivation rate of anticoagulant	Lessened anticoagulant effect
		Tolbutamide	Biotransformation of tolbutamide is inhibited	Hypoglycemic shock
Propranolol	Antiarrhythmic (beta blocker)	Adrenergic bronchodilators (epinephrine, isoproterenol)	Blockade of beta adrenergic receptors renders bronchodilators ineffective	Refractoriness to bronchodilator
		Cigarette smoking	Unknown	Hypertension and diminished cardiac output
		Hypoglycemic agents (insulin, tolbutamide)	Propranolol blocks the glycogenolytic action of endogenous catecholamines	Hypoglycemic shock
Reserpine	Antihypertensive (sympathetic depressant)	MAO inhibitors (pargyline, tranylcypromine, phenylzine)	Reserpine blocks storage mechanism for serotonin and NE thereby releasing transmitters in their active form since MAO is inactivated	Hypertensive crisis, cerebral vascular accident

Drug	Class	Interacting agent	Mechanism	Effect
Methyldopa	Antihypertensive (sympathetic depressant)	Antidepressants (amitriptyline, amphetamines, desipramine, imipramine, MAO inhibitors)	Methyldopa causes release of NE, which remains physiologically active in the presence of these agents	Severe CNS stimulation and hypertension
Guanethidine	Antihypertensive (sympathetic depressant)	Sympathomimetics (amphetamines, methylphenidate)	Guanethidine sensitizes the myocardium to effects of sympathomimetics	Cardiac arrhythmias
		Antidepressants (amphetamines, desipramine, imipramine)	Antidepressants inhibit NE-depleting action of guanethidine	Lessened hypotensive effect
Digitalis glycosides	Cardiotonics	Diuretics: thiazide type (hydrochlorothiazide), misc. (ethacrynic acid)	Hypokalemia produced by kaluretic agents results in potentiation of cardiotonic glycosides	Cardiac arrhythmias, ventricular fibrillation
		Reserpine	Reserpine potentiates negative inotropic action of digitalis glycosides	Severe bradycardia
		Quinidine	Quinidine inhibits the ability of digitalis to release intracellular potassium	Reduced digitalis effectiveness
		Calcium salts (intravenous)	Hypercalcemia potentiates cardiotonic action of digitalis glycosides	Cardiac arrhythmias, ventricular fibrillation
Quinidine	Antiarrhythmic (cardiac depressant)	Muscle relaxants peripheral tubocurarine succinylcholine	Potentiation of neuromuscular blockade by quinidine	Prolonged apnea

sults, as Knapp and Knapp remark, "speak directly to the question of safety and efficacy" (in respect to the pharmacist's role).

DRUG INTERACTIONS

General. Many excellent discussions and reviews of drug interactions have recently appeared in the literature.[24,73–75,89,135,136,147,155,188,189] Individual reports on specific interactions continue to appear at a rapidly increasing rate. It has been reported that digitalis is potentiated by hypokalemia, which may result from thiazide administration. Hypotensive drugs such as methyldopa may be antagonized by very small doses of sympathomimetic amines, which are often found in barbiturate-amphetamine mixtures.[121] The antagonism of respiratory effects of morphine by nalorphine has been discussed, as well as the interaction of morphine and D-tubocurarine.[18,19]

Blake[21] reported extensively on possible interactions of cardiovascular drugs (Table 11-14). Other authors have reinvestigated well known interactions and in an attempt to explain them in view of new scientific developments, Bellville and Fleischli[19] found that the interaction of morphine and nalorphine is related primarily to a difference in the intrinsic activity of the drugs, and not solely in their receptor affinity. Gibaldi and Schwartz[65] reemphasized that probenecid causes increased penicillin serum levels, probably not because it primarily diminishes tubular secretion of penicillin, but because there is a significant decrease in the apparent volume of distribution of penicillin in the presence of probenecid.

Much of the current literature is concerned with anticoagulant interactions. The combination of anabolic steroids and anticoagulants may in some cases result in an exaggerated anticoagulant response.[52] Williams and Moravec[199] have warned against the concurrent use of penicillin and heparin, because penicillin apparently antagonizes the effect of heparin. Phenylbutazone has been reported to potentiate the action of warfarin,[3,182] whereas phenobarbital decreases the biologic half-life of bishydroxycoumarin[171] by increasing the rate of metabolism of the anticoagulant.[162] Hansen et al.[72] suggest that phenindione should be the anticoagulant of choice in patients being treated with diphenylhydantoin, because it does not interfere with its metabolism. Cullen and Catalano[46] have reported that the anticoagulant activity of war-

TABLE 11-15. EFFECTS OF DRUGS ON THE ACTION OF ANTICOAGULANTS

ANTICOAGULANT ACTION INCREASED BY:	ANTICOAGULANT ACTION DECREASED BY:
Alcohol (chronic intake)	Alcohol (acute episode)
Anabolic steroids	Antacids (excessive amounts)
Antibiotics (broad spectrum)	Antihistamines
Bromelains	Barbiturates
Choloxin	Chloral hydrate
Clofibrate	Contraceptives, oral
Dextrans	Corticosteroids
Diphenylhydantoin	Diuretics
Methylthiouracil	Chlorthalidone
Oxyphenbutazone	Mercurials
Papain	Thiazides
Phenylbutazone	Ethchlorvynol
Pheniramine	Glutethimide
Propylthiouracil	Griseofulvin
Quinidine	Haloperidol
Quinine	Meprobamate
Radioactive compounds & x-ray media	Mineral oil (chronic intake)
Salicylates	Vitamin K
Sulfonamides	
Vitamin B complex	

farin is depressed by the administration of griseofulvin and ethchlorvynol, and D-thyroxine potentiates the pharmacologic effect of warfarin.[184] Many of these interactions have been reviewed by Hunninghake and Azarnoff,[88] and are summarized in Table 11-15.

When any of the drugs that increase anticoagulant action are added to a stabilized anticoagulant regimen, hemorrhage may occur. Conversely, when drugs that tend to decrease anticoagulant action are added to such a regimen, the anticoagulant dose must be increased to retain the desired therapeutic effect. More importantly, the anticoagulant dose must be decreased when these drugs are deleted from multiple drug therapy.

The anticoagulant interactions with other drugs may well be used to illustrate the incredible spectrum of possible interactions. However, interactions with anticoagulants most often occur because of displacement of the drug from binding sites, because of enzyme inhibition or because of enzyme induction. These three modes of interactions are probably those most frequently discussed recently, and they are therefore discussed in some detail here.

Drug-Protein Interaction. When two or more drugs capable of binding with the same protein are administered concurrently, competition for binding sites on the protein molecule may occur. Because the number of binding sites is limited, the drug that is bound more strongly displaces the drug bound more weakly.[6,7]

Plasma proteins differ widely in their ability to react chemically, depending on the composition of the amino acids and their physical properties.[66] A great number of substances interact with plasma proteins and, with few exceptions, most combine with albumin. The isoelectric point of albumin is 4.9, so that at physiologic pH (7.4) the molecule is negatively charged. Drug molecules, interacting with proteins, obey the same laws as do other substances, and interactions of the negatively charged protein molecule with cations can be expected. However, ionic combinations between oppositely charged groups occur regardless of the net charge on the protein, and a number of anions also interact with albumin at physiologic pH.

Drug-protein interactions represent a most important facet of drug metabolism.[48] They may be responsible for the pharmacodynamic action of a drug, as well as for the distribution and transport of drugs. Drug-protein interactions are significant because only the unbound drug is freely diffusible and, therefore, active. A drug-protein complex is generally confined to the circulating plasma, and its access to the sites of drug action, metabolism and excretion is hindered. Hence, changes in the proportion of drug bound to plasma protein can directly influence drug therapy. For example, aspirin can reduce the extent of plasma protein binding of penicillin analogues, resulting in higher levels of the unbound drug.[110] Aspirin has also been implicated in the alteration of protein binding of chlorpropamide.[176] Hemorrhagic crises can result in patients who are maintained on anticoagulants being treated with other agents that displace the anticoagulant from its protein binding sites. Thus, displacement of a drug from its binding sites may cause an unexpected level of therapeutic action. It may also cause a change in the duration of action, because the drug molecules, in the unbound state, will be exposed to drug metabolism and thus to possible inactivation.

The penicillins may be regarded as modified fatty acids containing a cyclic dipeptide as part of the long chain. Penicillin K, having an n-heptyl chain, shows a greater affinity for binding than does penicillin G, which has a benzyl chain. The barbiturates are substituted carboxylic acids. The anionic and substituent groups are separated by an intervening ring. Binding of the barbiturates increases with chain length and the thio analogs are bound more firmly than are the oxy analogs.[66]

Phenylbutazone and sulfinpyrazone can displace protein-bound sulfonamides,[6] and sulfamethoxypyridazine, sulfaethylthiadiazole and aspirin can reduce the binding of many penicillin derivatives.[111] Binding of sulfonamides to albumin, in turn, increases in the order of sulfanilamide > sulfapyridine > sulfadiazine > sulfathiazole > sulfamerazine.[66]

The salicylate ion is bound up to 80 per cent in normal plasma,[181] and this extensive binding probably is responsible for the ion's slow penetration into the brain.[29] Salicylic acid exhibits a strong tendency for binding, whereas salicylamide and acetylsalicylic acid show little tendency for binding. The carboxylic acid groups probably confer primary binding capacity on compounds, and the presence of *ortho* hydrogen donors or of alkyl substitution may enhance this capacity. On the other hand, hydrogen donors in the *meta* or *para* position decrease binding capacity.

Other drugs that are bound to serum proteins include sulfonylureas[97] and methotrexate.[12] Methotrexate is used in the treatment of psoriasis at doses lower than those used in leukemia. Caution must be used when this drug is administered because it is displaced from its binding sites by salicylates and sulfonamides. Anton[5] showed that albumin-bound sulfonamide is devoid of antibacterial activity.

A proposed mechanism for the action of clofibrate involves protein binding.[9] The free acid is bound to plasma proteins, and the clofibrate anion probably competes with other anions, including androsterone and thyroxine, for the same binding sites. These anions are probably displaced from their binding sites and are concentrated in the liver. Their combined effect, then, decreases lipid synthesis and indirectly, serum lipid levels.

Kunin[109,110] showed the potentially deleterious effect of extensive binding to serum proteins on the antimicrobial activity of some of the new semisynthetic penicillins. Inhibitors of serum binding may well have potential usefulness in clinical medicine. As was previously shown, the binding of some penicillins can be reduced by several drugs,[111] which in turn can lead to higher levels of the antibiotics. Renal clearance of highly bound sulfonamides might be increased by inhibition of their binding, augmenting the removal of slowly excreted sulfonamides should toxicity be encountered.

Drug distribution in the tissues of the body is also affected by binding of the drug to tissue components (proteins, phospholipids, etc.). The cardiovascular action of norepinephrine can be potentiated by certain antihistaminic agents.[91,93,98,174] Isaac and Goth[93] attributed this to an inhibition of the uptake of norepinephrine by various tissues, resulting in an increase in the concentration of unbound norepinephrine. Thus, there is a potential hazard in the administration of antihistaminic agents to patients already receiving monoamine oxidase inhibitors in that a hypertensive crisis might ensue.

Table 11-16 lists some of the drugs bound to plasma or tissue components whose binding is affected by the administration of other agents.

Enzyme Induction. The duration and intensity of drug actions are, to a great extent, determined by the speed of drug metabolism.[27] Most drugs are metabolized in the liver; others are metabolized in the plasma,

TABLE 11-16. DRUGS WHOSE BINDING TO PLASMA OR TISSUE COMPONENTS MAY BE AFFECTED BY OTHER AGENTS

BOUND DRUG	DISPLACING AGENT
Analgesics (e.g., salicylates)	Indomethacin, phenylbutazone, oxyphenbutazone
Antibiotics, antibacterials (e.g., penicillin, long-acting sulfonamides)	Coumarin anticoagulants, indomethacin, phenylbutazone, oxyphenbutazone, salicylates, sulfinpyrazone
Anticoagulants (e.g., coumarin derivatives, indanedione derivatives)	Chlorophenoxyisobutyric acid, clofibrate, indomethacin, phenylbutazone, oxyphenbutazone, salicylates, sulfonamides, D-thyroxine
Antidiabetic agents (e.g., sulfonylureas)	Coumarin anticoagulants, indomethacin, phenylbutazone, oxyphenbutazone, salicylates, sulfonamides
Cardiovascular agents (e.g., norepinephrine, guanethidine)	Antihistamines, sympathomimetic amines
Mepacrine	Pamaquine and other 8-aminoquinolines

kidneys and other tissues. Metabolism results in inactivation of drugs and, more important, in the conversion of lipid-soluble drugs into water-soluble forms for excretion by the kidney.[159] To accomplish this, enzymes act on drugs to remove methyl, alkyl or amino groups, to introduce oxygen or hydroxyl groups into aromatic rings, etc.[173] Conjugation is another pathway of metabolism. In the liver the transferase enzymes produce combinations of agents, such as bilirubin, with substances, such as glucuronic acid. This pathway results in a further increase in water solubility and faster elimination by the kidney.

Brodie *et al.*[28] suggested that lipid-soluble substances would remain in the body almost indefinitely unless they could be converted into water-soluble forms. Enzymes responsible for this metabolism, they thought, seem to have developed in order to convert lipid-soluble impurities in the food such as alkaloids, terpenes and steroids into water-soluble substances.

Drug-metabolizing enzymes are localized almost exclusively in smooth-surfaced microsomes. Microsomes are artifacts produced by the breakdown of the endoplasmic reticulum of liver cells, which can be brought about by the action of chemicals.[61] An increase in the activity of these enzymes is called "enzyme induction."[160] Thus, enzyme induction may be brought about by certain drugs that could stimulate their own metabolism or the metabolism of other drugs. More than 200 drugs, insecticides, carcinogens and other chemicals are known to stimulate the activity of drug-metabolizing enzymes in animals. Some of the drugs whose metabolism is stimulated by other drugs in man are listed in Table 11-17.

There seems to be no apparent relationship between the ability of drugs to induce enzymes and their action or structure. Most inducers are lipid-soluble at physiologic pH, but the quantity of inducer necessary to have an appreciable effect on the enzyme varies considerably.[39] Most inducers can be exemplified either by phenobarbital or by 3-methylcholanthrene. The two types differ in the course and intensity of induction.

When a drug-metabolizing enzyme is induced, the drug is metabolized more rapidly. If as a result of metabolism, a relatively inert metabolite is formed, enzyme induction will accelerate termination of drug action. Conney[39] lists zoxazolamine, meprobamate, carisoprodol, diphenylhydantoin and several barbiturates as exemplifying this condition in animals. On the other hand, when the metabolite is of comparable or of even greater potency than the original drug is, the pharmacologic effect may be magnified by the accelerated rate of the formation of the metabolite.

After Conney and Burns[40] reported that certain hypnotics, tranquilizers, antihistamines, analgesics and muscle relaxants could markedly increase the amount of drug-metabolizing enzymes in liver microsomes, Cucinell *et al.*[44] reported that diphenylhydantoin and bishydroxycoumarin plasma levels are lowered by phenobarbital, Chen *et al.*[37] noted that phenylbutazone accelerates the metabolism of aminopyrine, Remmer[158] observed that barbiturates and glutethimide accelerate dipyrone metabolism, Dayton *et al.*[49] reported that heptabarbital lowers plas-

TABLE 11-17. DRUGS WHOSE METABOLISM IN MAN IS STIMULATED BY OTHER AGENTS

DRUGS AFFECTED	AGENT
Griseofulvin	Phenobarbital
Anticoagulants, coumarin	Phenobarbital
	Chloral hydrate
	Griseofulvin
	Heptabarbital
Anticoagulants, indanedione	Haloperidol
Anticonvulsants, hydantoin	Phenobarbital
Aminopyrine, dipyrone	Glutethimide, phenylbutazone
Meprobamate	Meprobamate
Digitoxin	Phenobarbital

ma levels of coumarins and Busfield *et al.*[33] reported on the well known interaction of phenobarbital and griseofulvin.

Conney *et al.*[41] also listed as activating drugs—i.e., drugs that induce increased enzyme synthesis—aminopyrine and diphenhydramine, among others; Kato[101] added thiopental, glutethimide, chlorpromazine and meprobamate to this list. Consolo *et al.*[43] just recently found that desipramine increases urinary excretion of amphetamine when given intraperitoneally but not when given intracerebrally. Desipramine probably impairs the hydroxylation of amphetamine in the liver, thereby increasing the level of circulating amphetamine and eventually of brain amphetamine.

Repeated administration of a drug often results in the induction of enzymes that metabolize this particular drug. Chronic treatment with the drug, in other words, accelerates its own metabolism, lowers its blood level and decreases its effect. Alteration of liver microsomal activity may thus be responsible for the development of tolerance to certain drugs. It has been suggested that tolerance may develop to meprobamate,[51] tolbutamide[14] and glutethimide[169] as a result

TABLE 11-18. DRUGS THAT STIMULATE THEIR OWN METABOLISM DURING CHRONIC ADMINISTRATION*

DRUG	SPECIES
Phenylbutazone	Dog, rat
Chlorcyclizine	Dog
Probenecid	Dog
Tolbutamide	Dog
Hexobarbital	Dog, rat
Pentobarbital	Rat, rabbit
Phenobarbital	Dog, rat
Aminopyrine	Rat
Meprobamate	*Man,* rat
Glutethimide	*Man*
Chlorpromazine	Rat
Chlordiazepoxide	Rat
DDT	Rat
Citrus red No. 2	Rat
Methoxyflurane	Rat
2,3-Benzpyrene	Rat
9,10-Dimethyl-1,2-benzanthracene	Rat
Benzene	Rabbit

* Conney, A. H.: Pharmacol. Rev. 19:317, 1967.

of the ability of these agents to stimulate liver enzymes that metabolize these drugs. During long-term therapy with these drugs, the rate of metabolism will increase and there will be a loss in pharmacologic activity.

Conney[39] reported that the drugs listed in Table 11-18 stimulate their own metabolism during chronic administration.

The study of enzyme induction has assumed an important place in clinical medicine. By knowing which drugs induce enzyme formation, it should be possible to anticipate causes of clinical relapse and warn against potential activators, such as household and agricultural insecticides. Other benefits from an understanding of enzyme induction have already become apparent. In man, the major metabolic change of griseofulvin is a loss of a methyl group at position six. Comparison with erythromycin shows that this drug, too, is inactivated by demethylation.[133] Cephalothin is inactivated through loss of an acetyl group. A new analogue, with a pyridine in place of the acetyl group (cephaloridine), is less labile enzymatically, and a clinically more effective drug has resulted.[112]

Enzyme Inhibition. Just as a drug can accelerate the metabolism of another drug by stimulating liver microsomal enzymes, examples are known in which one drug can inhibit the metabolism of another drug by inhibiting these enzymes. Disulfiram, for example, is an inhibitor of liver aldehyde oxidase. If a drug that is largely biotransformed in the liver is administered concurrently with disulfiram, there may be danger that the serum level of this drug can be increased manyfold, even to the extent of toxic levels. Examples of drugs whose metabolism in man has been decreased by other drugs are listed in Table 11-19.

MAO inhibitors depress the metabolism of meperidine and sympathomimetic amines.[184] Plasma levels of bishydroxycoumarin are elevated in patients treated concurrently with oxyphenbutazone;[197] the anabolic steroid, methandrostenolone, has been reported to decrease the rate of metabolism of oxyphenbutazone;[197] and Solomon and Schrogie[185] showed that phenyramidol potentiates the anticoagulant action of bishydroxycoumarin by inhibiting its metabolism. Metyrapone is a specific inhibitor of adrenal steroid 11-

TABLE 11-19. DRUGS WHOSE METABOLISM IN MAN HAS BEEN DECREASED BY THE ADMINISTRATION OF OTHER AGENTS

DRUG AFFECTED	AGENT
Tricylic antidepressants (e.g., imipramine, desipramine, amitriptyline)	Monoamine oxidase inhibitors (e.g., tranylcypromine, phenelzine, isocarboxazid, nialamide, pargyline)
CNS depressants	
Hypotensive agents	
Sympathomimetics	
Antihistamines	
Anticonvulsants, hydantoin	Disulfiram
Anticoagulants, coumarin	Oxyphenbutazone, phenyramidol
Oxyphenbutazone	Methandrostenolone

beta-hydroxylase.[126] The fat-soluble vitamin K, menadione, potentiates the pharmacologic effect of corticosteroids, apparently by inhibiting the metabolism of cortisol by liver microsomes,[114] and SKF 525A decreases the metabolism of testosterone, estradiol, barbiturates and other compounds.[42]

Diphenylhydantoin is hydroxylated in the liver, only trace amounts of it being excreted in the urine. This drug is extensively metabolized by microsomal enzymes.[45] Bishydroxycoumarin increases the biologic half-life of diphenylhydantoin in man, presumably by inhibition of p-hydroxylation.[72] Phenyramidol also inhibits its metabolism,[183] and simultaneous administration of isonicotinic acid hydrazide and para-aminosalicylic acid also impairs its metabolism in man.[115]

Any drug that can have an adverse effect on the liver must be suspected of being able to change the metabolism of other drugs through a possible effect on the liver microsomal enzymes. Unexpected results of a specific therapeutic regimen may well be connected to hepatotoxic effects of another drug. Knowledge of drugs that may cause liver damage has therefore assumed increased importance. Popper et al.[153] studied 155 cases of hepatic damage induced by nonmedical chemicals and drugs and published the list displayed in Table 11-20, which could probably be substantially enlarged by careful study of the literature.

DESIRED INTERACTIONS

As has been shown, not all drug interactions are undesirable. The interaction of BAL with heavy metals has been clinically valuable for some time, as has been the use of protamine sulfate in reversing the action of heparin. More specific clinical benefits

TABLE 11-20. HEPATOTOXIC AGENTS

Aminosalicylic acid	Metahexamide
Arsenical (unidentified)	Methimazole
β-phenyl-isopropylhydrazine	Methyltestosterone
Chlorpromazine	Norethandrolone
Chlorpropamide	Oxyphenbutazone
Chlortetracycline	Penicillin
Diphenylhydantoin	Perphenazine
Erythromycin estolate	Phenylbutazone
Ethionamide	Polythiazide
Halothane	Pyrazinamide
Iproniazid	Tetracycline
Isocarboxazid	Tolbutamide
Isoniazid	Tranylcypromine
Mepazine	Urethan
Mercaptopurine	Zoxazolamine

might well result from a study of drug interactions.

Barbiturates, in animals, stimulate the enzymatic glucuronidation of bilirubin by liver microsomes. Catz and Yaffe[36] believed that, based on this observation, barbiturates might have some therapeutic value in hyperbilirubinemia. They treated infants having congenital nonhemolytic jaundice with phenobarbital. Jaundice disappeared in the infants under phenobarbital treatment, but when treatment was discontinued the jaundice reappeared. Recent observations suggest that induction of liver microsomal enzymes may also be of value in diseases marked by overproduction of steroid hormones. Werk *et al.*[198] administered diphenylhydantoin chronically to two patients with nontumorous Cushing's syndrome. Biochemical and clinical amelioration of the manifestations was observed by the authors.

Of great potential interest could be the concurrent use of triamterene or other pteridines, and methotrexate. It has been shown experimentally in mice that this might result in increased uptake of methotrexate to make a tumor more drug sensitive.[71,161] Such effects might be of relevance to the human situation in which the cells of chronic lymphocytic leukemia do not take up methotrexate and thus remain clinically insensitive to the drug.

CONCLUSION

The clinically oriented pharmacist will have to be well versed in drug actions, interactions and reactions. The problems arising from multidrug therapy will become more complex. Oral contraceptives will probably be taken for a substantial part of the life of a patient, and the effects of prolonged steroid therapy cannot yet be gauged with confidence. Probenecid might be prescribed for prolonged use, as may diphenylhydantoin. Aspirin, used by self-medication, is probably used by a major proportion of the population, and its interactions with other drugs are just beginning to be appreciated. The recognition of the effects that chemical contaminants of the environment may have on drug action is in its early stages. Continuous study of this field is therefore a must for pharmacy students and pharmacists.

REFERENCES

1. Aber, C. P., and Jones, E. W.: Brit. Heart J. *27*:56, 1965.
2. Absil, J., Buchel, L., and Simone, V.: Arch. Sci. Physiol. *20*:233, 1966.
3. Aggeler, P. M., O'Reilly, R. A., Leong, L., and Kowitz, P. E.: New Engl. J. Med. *276*:496, 1967.
4. Albert, S. N., and Fazekas, J. F.: Anesthesia analgesia. Current Res. Anesth. Analg. *35*:381, 1956.
5. Anton, A. H.: J. Pharmacol. Exp. Ther. *129*:282, 1960.
6. Anton, A. H.: J. Pharmacol. Exp. Ther. *134*:291, 1961.
7. Apgar, V.: J. Am. Med. Ass. *190*:840, 1964.
8. Aston, R., and Cullumbine, H.: Arch. Intern. Pharmacodyn. *126*:219, 1960.
9. Ayerst product literature for Atromid-S.
10. Balek, R. W., Kocsis, J. J., and Geiling, E. M. K.: Arch. Intern. Pharmacodyn. *3*:182, 1957.
11. Baron, J. M.: British Med. J., *1*:699, 1967.
12. Barrie, P., and Clark, P. A.: Brit. Med. J. *1*:1339, 1966.
13. Bass, A. D., Yntema, C. L., and Hammond, W. S.: Science *110*:527, 1949.
14. Beaser, S. B.: J. Am. Med. Ass. *187*:887, 1964.
15. Beckett, A. H., Rowland, M., and Turner, P.: Lancet *1*:303, 1965.
16. Beckett, A. H., and Wilkinson, G. R.: J. Pharm. Pharmacol. *17*:256, 1965.
17. Belloni, C., and Rizzoni, G.: Lancet *2*: 369, 1967.
18. Bellville, J. W., Cohen, E. N., and Hamilton, J.: Clin. Pharmacol. Ther. *5*:35, 1964.
19. Bellville, J. W., and Fleischli, G.: Clin. Pharmacol. Ther. *9*:152, 1968.
20. Berry, W. T., Cowin, P. J., and Davis, D. R.: Brit. J. Nutr. *8*:79, 1954.
21. Blake, D. A.: Cardiovascular drugs: dosage forms and therapeutic incompatibilities. Presented to the Eighth Annual Robert L. Swain Seminar, Baltimore, Md., 1968.
22. Blank, H.: Transact. St. John's Hosp., Dermatol. Soc. (London), *53*:2, 1967.
23. Block, L. H., and Lamy, P. P.: Am. Prof. Pharm. *34*:27, 1968.
24. Block, L. H. and Lamy, P. P.: J. Am. Pharm. Ass. *8*:66, 1968.
25. Block, L. H., and Lamy, P. P.: J. Am. Pharm. Ass. (submitted for publication).

26. Bonnichsen, R., Maehly, A. C., and Frank, A. J.: J. Forensic Sci. *6*:411, 1961.
27. Bousquet, W. E.: J. Pharm. Sci. *51*:297, 1962.
28. Brodie, B. B., Gillette, J. R., and La Du, B. N.: Ann. Rev. Biochem. *27*:427, 1958.
29. Brodie, B. B., and Hogben, C. A. M.: J. Pharm. (London) *9*:345, 1957.
30. Brodie, B. B., Shore, P. A., and Silver, S. L.: Science *175*:1133, 1955.
31. Brunton, T. L.: Anat. Physiol. *8*:332, 1874.
32. Burns, J. J., Rose, R. K., Chenken, T., Goldman, A., Schubert, A., and Brodie, B. B.: J. Pharmacol. Exp. Therap. *109*: 346, 1933.
33. Busfield, D., Child, K. J., Atkinson, R. M., and Tomich, E. G.: Lancet *2*:1042, 1963.
34. Cahen, R. L.: Clin. Pharmacol. Ther. *5*:480, 1964.
35. Carson, P. E.: Fed. Proc. *19*:995, 1960.
36. Catz, C., and Yaffe, S. J.: Am. J. Dis. Child. *104*:516, 1962.
37. Chen, W., Vrindten, P. A., Dayton, P. G., and Burns, J. J.: Life Sci. *2*:35, 1962.
38. Cluff, L. E., Thornton, G. F., and Seidl, L. G.: J. Am. Med. Ass. *188*:144, 1964.
39. Conney, A. H.: Pharmacol Rev. *19*:317, 1967.
40. Conney, A. H., and Burns, J. J.: Adv. Pharmacol. *1*:31, 1962.
41. Conney, A. H., Davison, C., Gastel, R., and Burns, J. J.: J. Pharmacol. Exp. Ther. *130*:1, 1960.
42. Conney, A. H., Schneidman, K., Jacobson, M., and Kuntzman, R.: Ann. N. Y. Acad. Sci. *123*:98, 1965.
43. Consolo, S., Dolfini, E., Garattini, S., and Valzelli, L.: J. Pharm. Pharmacol. *19*: 253, 1967.
44. Cucinell, S. A., Conney, A. H., Sansur, M., and Burns, J. J.: Clin. Pharmacol. Ther. *6*:420, 1965.
45. Cucinell, S. A., Koster, R., Conney, A. H., and Burns, J. J.: J. Pharmacol. Exp. Ther. *141*:157, 1963.
46. Cullen, S. I., and Catalano, P. M.: J. Am. Med. Ass. *199*:582, 1967.
47. Cutting, W. C.: Guide to Hazards in Aviation Medicine, pp. 28, 67. Washington, D. C., Federal Aviation Agency, 1962.
48. Davison, C., and Smith, P. K.: J. Pharmacol. Exp. Ther. *133*:161, 1961.
49. Dayton, P. G., Tracan, Y., Chenkin, T., and Weiner, M.: J. Clin. Invest. *40*: 1797, 1961.
50. Dille, J. M., and Ahlquist, R. P.: J. Pharmacol. Exp. Ther. *61*:385, 1937.
51. Douglas, J. F., Ludwig, B. J., and Smith, N.: Proc. Soc. Exp. Biol. Med., *112*: 436, 1963.
52. Dresdale, F. C., and Hayes, J. C.: J. Med. Soc. N. J. *64*:609, 1967.
53. Editorial: J.A.M.A. *113*:1237, 1939.
54. Eerola, R.: Acta Anaesthesiol. Scand. *7*:87, 1963.
55. Eerola, R.: Ann. Med. Exp. Biol. Fenniae (Helsinki) *39*:Suppl. 3, 1961.
56. Fastier, F. N., Speden, R. N., and Waal, H.: Brit. J. Pharmacol. *12*:251, 1967.
57. Fearn, H. J., and Hodges, J. R.: J. Pharm. Pharmacol. *5*:1041, 1953.
58. Field, J. B., Ohta, M., Boyle, C., and Remer, T. A.: New Eng. J. Med. *277*: 889, 1967.
59. Filippi, B., and Mela, V.: Minerva Chir. *12*:1047, 1957.
60. Forney, R. B., Hulpieu, H. R., and Hughes, F. W.: Experientia *18*:468, 1962.
61. Fouts, J. R.: Fed. Proc. *21*:1107, 1962.
62. Fraser, R. J. A.: Brit. Med. Bull. *15*:129, 1959.
63. Friend, D. G.: Clin. Pharmacol. Ther. *5*:533, 1964.
64. Friend, D. G.: J. Am. Pharm. Ass. *4*: 528, 1964.
65. Gibaldi, M., and Schwartz, M. A.: Clin. Pharmacol. Ther. *9*:345, 1968.
66. Goldstein, A.: Pharmacol. Rev. *1*:102, 1949.
67. Graham, J. D. P.: Toxicol. Appl. Pharmacol. *2*:14, 1960.
68. Gutman, A. B., Dayton, P. G., Yu, T. F., Berger, L., Chen, W., Sicam, L. E., and Burns, J. J.: Am. J. Med., *29*:1017, 1960.
69. Haggard, H. W., Greenberg, L. A., Rakieten, N., and Cohen, L. H.: J. Pharmacol. Exp. Ther. *69*:266, 1940.
70. Hale, F.: Am. J. Ophth. *18*:1087, 1935.
71. Hall, T. C., Godsil, A., and Wodinsky, I.: J. Clin. Pharmacol. Ther. *8*:219, 1968.
72. Hansen, J. M., Kristensen, M., Skovsted, L., and Christensen, L. K.: Lancet *2*: 265, 1966.
73. Hartshorn, E. A.: Drug Intelligence *2*: 58, 1968.
74. Hartshorn, E. A.: Drug Intelligence *2*: 174, 1968.
75. Hartshorn, E. A.: Drug Intelligence *3*: 4, 1968.
76. Harvey, R. F.: Brit. Med. J. *2*:52, 1967.
77. Hawkins, D., Pinckard, R. N., and Farr R. S.: Science *160*:780, 196?

78. Hegnauer, A. H., Shriber, W. J., and Haterius, H. O.: Am. J. Physiol. *161*: 455, 1950.

79. Heirich, M. A.: Arch. Intern Pharmacodyn. *92*:444, 1953.

80. Herr, F., Stewart, J., and Charest, M. P.: Arch. Intern Pharmacodyn. *134*:328, 1961.

81. Hicks, J. T.: Hosp. Form. Management *2*:19, 1967.

82. Higgins, J. A., and McGuigan, R. A.: J. Pharmacol. Exp. Ther. *49*:466, 1933.

83. Hoffman, W. S., Adler, H., Fishein, W. I., and Bauer, F. C.: Arch. Environ. Health *15*:758, 1967.

84. Hoffman, W. S., and Nober, C.: J. Lab. Clin. Med. *35*:237, 1950.

85. Holten, C. P., and Larsen, V.: Acta Pharmacol. Toxicol. *12*:346, 1956.

86. Horwitz, D., Lovenberg, W., Engelman, K., and Sjoerdsma, A.: J. Am. Med. Ass. *188*:1108, 1964.

87. Howard, J. H., and Tiedeman, G.: Clin. Pharmacol. Ther. *8*:502, 1967.

88. Hunninghake, D. B., and Azarnoff, D. L.: Arch. Intern. Med. *121*:349, 1968.

89. Hussar, D. A.: Hosp. Pharm. *3*:14, 1968.

90. Huston, J. R., and Bell, G. E.: J.A.M.A. *198*:16, 1966.

91. Innes, I. R.: Brit. J. Pharmacol. *13*:6, 1958.

92. Intravenous Additive Incompatibilities, Washington, D. C., Pharmacy Department, Clinical Center, National Institutes of Health, U. S. Department of Health, Education and Welfare, Public Health Service, March 1967.

93. Isaac, L., and Goth, A.: Life Sci. *4*:1899, 1965.

94. Jawetz, E.: Ann. Rev. Pharmacol. *8*: 151, 1968.

95. Jetter, W. W., and McLean, R.: A.M.A. Arch. Pathol. *36*:112, 1943.

96. Jick, H., and Chalmers, T. C.: Clin. Pharmacol. Ther. *5*:673, 1964.

97. Johnson, P. C., West, K. M., and Masters, F.: Metabolism *9*:1111, 1960.

98. Jori, A.: J. Pharm. Pharmacol. *18*:824, 1966.

99. Kalow, W.: Pharmacogenetics, Heredity and the Response to Drugs, W. B. Saunders Co., Philadelphia, 1962, p. 108.

100. Kalow, W., and Gunn, D. R.: J. Pharmacol. Exp. Ther. *120*:203, 1957.

101. Kato, R.: Ann. Soc. Lomb. Med.-Biol. *14*:777, 1959.

102. Kato, R., Chiesara, E., and Vassanelli, P.: Biochem. Pharmacol. *12*:251, 1957.

103. Kitler, M. E.: An investigation of various factors influencing drug transfer in an *in vitro* model, Ph.D. Thesis, Baltimore, Md., School of Pharmacy, University of Maryland, 1967.

104. Knapp, D. A., and Knapp, D. E.: The safety and efficacy of practicing pharmacists. Presented to the Conference of Teachers, Am. Ass. Coll. Pharm., Las Vegas, April 1967.

105. Kopf, R.: Arch. Intern. Pharmacodyn. *110*:56, 1957.

106. Kostenbauder, H. B., Portnoff, J. B., and Swintosky, J. V.: J. Pharm. Sci. *51*:1084, 1962.

107. Kramer, W.: Acta Tuberc. Scandinav. *38*: 51, 1960.

108. Kunelis, C. T., Peters, J. L., and Edmondson, H. A.: Am. J. Med. *38*:359, 1965.

109. Kunin, C. M.: Clin. Pharmacol. Therap. *7*:166, 1966.

110. Kunin, C. M.: Clin. Pharmacol. Ther. *7*:180, 1966.

111. Kunin, C. M.: Proc. Soc. Exp. Biol. Med. *117*:69, 1964.

112. Kunin, C. M., and Atuk, N.: New Eng. J. Med. *274*:654, 1966.

113. Kunin, C. M., and Finland, M.: Clin. Pharmacol. Ther. *2*:51, 1961.

114. Kupfer, D., and Peets, L.: Fed. Proc. *25*:658, 1966.

115. Kutt, H., Winters, W., and McDowell, F. H.: Neurology *16*:594, 1966.

116. Lamy, P. P., and Block, L. H.: Maryland Pharm. *43*:440, 1968.

117. Lamy, P. P., Davies, W. L., and Kitler, M. E.: Hosp. Pharm. *3*:12, 1968.

118. Lamy, P. P., and Shangraw, R. F.: Hosp. Pharm. *1*:13, 1966.

119. Larsson-Cohn, U.: Lancet *1*:679, 1967.

120. Lasagna, L.: Ann. N. Y. Acad. Sci. *123*: 312, 1965.

121. Laurence, D. R.: Prescrib. J. (London), *3*:46, 1963.

122. Lawrence, W. H.: Tenn. Pharm. p. 10, March 1968.

123. Laws, E. R., Curler, A., and Biros, F. J.: Arch. Environ. Health *15*:766, 1967.

124. Lehman, A. J., and Hanzlick, P. J.: Proc. Soc. Exp. Biol. Med. *30*:140, 1932-1933.

125. Lehmann, H., Cook, J., and Ryann, E.: Proc. Roy. Soc. Med. *50*:147, 1957.

126. Leibman, K. C.: Fed. Proc. *25*:417, 1966.

127. Levy, G., and Jusko, W. J.: J. Pharm. Sci. *55*:285, 1966.

128. Levy, G., and Reuning, R. H.: J. Pharm. Sci. *53*:1471, 1964.

129. Lichtenstein, H., Guest, G. M., and Warkany, J.: Proc. Soc. Exp. Biol. Med. 78:398, 1951.

130. Lish, P. M., Albert, J. R., Peters, E. L., and Allen, L. E.: Arch. Intern. Pharmacodyn. 129:77, 1960.

131. Lockey, S. D.: Adverse reactions to drugs, Scientific Exhibit at the Annual Convention of the American Medical Association, Chicago, Illinois, June 26-30, 1966.

132. MacAulay, M. A., and Charles, D.: Clin. Pharmacol. Ther. 8:578, 1967.

133. Mao, J. C. H., and Tardrew, P. L.: Biochem. Pharmacol. 14:1049, 1965.

134. Marshall, T. R., Ling, J. T., Follis, G., and Russell, M.: Radiol. 84:536, 1965.

135. Marvel, J. R., Schlichting, D. A., Dencton, C., Levy, E. J., and Cahn, M. M.: J. Invest. Dermatol. 42:197, 1964.

136. McIver, A. K.: Pharm. J. 199:205, 1967.

137. Medical Letter 9:17, August 25, 1967.

138. Meisler, J. M., and Skolaut, M. W.: Am. J. Hosp. Pharm. 23:57, 1966.

139. Milne, M. D., Rowe, G. G., Somers, K., Muehrcke, R. C., and Crawford, M. A.: Clin. Sci. 16:599, 1957.

140. Milne, M. D., Scribner, B. H., and Crawford, M. A.: Am. J. Med. 24:709, 1958.

141. Milosevic, M. P.: Arch. Intern Pharmacodyn. 106:437, 1956.

142. Milosevic, M. P., and Terzic, M.: Therapie 15:1009, 1960.

143. Modell, W. J.: Pharm. Pharmacol. 11:594, 1959.

144. Newman, H., and Abramson, M.: Science 96:43, 1942.

145. Orahovats, P. D., Lehman, E. G., and Chapin, E. W.: Arch. Intern. Pharmacodyn. 110, 245 1957.

146. Orellana-Alcalde, J. M., and Dominguez, J. P.: Lancet 2:1278, 1966.

147. Patient Care, Nov. 1967.

148. Pelissier, N. A., and Burgee, S. L.: Hosp. Pharm. 3:15, 1968.

149. Perry, C. J. G.: Clin. Pharmacol. Ther. 6:771, 1965.

150. Peters, L.: Pharmacol. Rev. 12:1, 1960.

151. Peterson, O. L., Finland, M., and Ballou, A. M.: Am. J. Med. Sci. 204:581, 1942.

152. Pettinger, W. A., and Oates, J. A.: Clin. Pharmacol. Ther. 9:341, 1968.

153. Popper, H., Rubin, E., Gardiol, D., Schaffner, F., and Paronetto, F.: Arch. Intern. Med. 115:128, 1965.

154. Portnoff, J. B., Swintosky, J. F., and Kostenbauder, H. B.: J. Pharm. Sci. 50:890, 1961.

155. Ramsey, H., and Haag, H. B.: J. Pharmacol. Exp. Ther. 88:313, 1946.

156. Registry of Adverse Drug Reactions. Report of the Drug Reaction Registry Subcommittee of the Greater Philadelphia Committee for Medical-Pharmaceutical Sciences J.A.M.A. 203: 85, 1968.

157. Reilly, R. H., Killam, K. F., Jenney, E. H., Marshall, W. H., Taussig, T., Apter, N. S., and Pfeiffer, C. C.: J. A.M.A. 152: 1317, 1953.

158. Remmer, H.: Proc. First Internat. Pharmacol. Meet., Stockholm, p. 235, New York, Macmillan, 1962.

159. Remmer, H.: Enzymes and Drug Action (Ed. by J. L. Mongar and A. V. S. de Reuck), Ciba Foundation Symposium Boston, Mass., Little Brown & Co., 1962.

160. Remmer, H., and Merker, H. J.: Ann. N. Y. Acad. Sci. 123:79, 1965.

161. Robert, D., and Hall, T. C.: J. Clin. Pharmacol. Ther. 8:217, 1968.

162. Robinson, D. S., and Macdonald, M. G.: Hosp. Form. Manage. 2:43, 1967.

163. Roux, C.: Compt. Rend. Soc. Biol. 155: 2255, 1961.

164. Samter, M., and Beers, R. F., Jr.: J. Allergy 40:281, 1967.

165. Sandberg, F.: Acta Physiol. Scand. 22: 34, 1950.

166. Saw-Lan Ip, F.: Lancet 1:91, 1966.

167. Schanker, L. S.: Adv. Drug Res. 1:72, 1964.

168. Schimmel, E. M.: Ann. Intern. Med. 60:100, 1964.

169. Schmid, K., Cornu, F., Imhof, P., and Keberle, H.: Schweiz. Med. Wchnschr. 94:235, 1964.

170. Schoonmaker, F. W., Osteen, R. T., and Greenfield, J. C., Jr.: Ann. Intern. Med. 65:1076, 1966.

171. Schrogie, J. J., and Solomon, H. M.: Clin. Pharmacol. Therap. 8:70, 1967.

172. Seidl, L. G., Thornton, G. F., Smith, J. W., and Cluff, L. E.: Bull. Johns Hopkins Hosp. 119:299, 1966.

173. Sherlock, S.: Ann. Rev. Pharmacol. 5: 429, 1965.

174. Sherrod, T. R., Loew, E. R., and Schloemer, H. F.: J. Pharmacol. Exp. Ther. 89:247, 1947.

175. Shore, P. A., Brodie, B. B., and Hogben, C. A. M.: J. Pharmacol. Exp. Ther. 119: 361, 1957.

176. Silver, A. A.: Personal communication, May 12, 1967.

177. Sjoequest, F.: Proc. Royal Soc. Med. 58: 967, 1965.

178. Smith, F. E., Reinstein, H., and Brave-man, L. E.: New Eng. J. Med. *272*:787, 1965.

179. Smith, J. W., and Loomis, T. A.: Proc. Soc. Exp. Biol. Med. *78*:827, 1951.

180. Smith, M. E., Evans, R. L., Newman, E. J., and Newman, H. W.: Quart. J. Alc. Stud. *22*:241, 1961.

181. Smith, P. K., Gleason, H. L., Stoll, C. G., and Ogorzalek, S.: J. Pharmacol. Exp. Ther. *87*:237, 1946.

182. Solomon, H. M., and Schrogie, J. J.: Biochem. Pharmacol. *16*:1219, 1967.

183. Solomon, H. M., and Schrogie, J. J.: Clin. Pharmacol. Ther. *8*:554, 1967.

184. Solomon, H. M., and Schrogie, J. J.: Clin. Pharmacol. Ther. *8*:797, 1967.

185. Solomon, H. M., and Schrogie, J. J.: J. Pharmacol. Exp. Ther. *154*:660, 1966.

186. Sorby, D. L., and Liu, G.: J. Pharm. Sci. *55*:504, 1966.

187. Swarbrick, J.: J. Pharm. Sci. *54*:1229, 1965.

188. Symposium on Clinical Effects of Interaction of Drugs, Proc. Roy. Soc. Med. *58*:943, 1965.

189. Symposium on Evaluation and Mechanisms of Drug Toxicity, Ann. N. Y. Acad. Sci. *123*:1, 1965.

190. Tarlov, A. R., Brewer, G. J., Carson, P. E., and Alving, A. S.: Arch. Intern Med. *109*:209, 1962.

191. The Union Memorial Hospital Pharmacy Formulary, Baltimore, Md. (S. Burgee, Director of Pharmacy Service).

192. Vesell, E. S., and Page, J. G.: Science *159*:149, 1968.

193. Vesell, E. S., and Page, J. G.: Science *161*:72, 1968.

194. Waddell, W. J., and Butler, T. C.: J. Clin. Invest. *36*:1217, 1957.

195. Weatherby, J. H., and Clements, E. L.: Quart. J. Stud. Alc. *21*:394, 1960.

196. Weiner, M., Shapiro, S., Axelrod, J., and Brodie, B. B.: J. Pharmacol. Exp. Ther. *99*:409, 1950.

197. Weiner, M. Siddigui, A. A., Bostanci, N., and Dayton, P. G.: Fed. Proc., *24*:153, 1965.

198. Werk, E. E., Jr., Sholiton, L. J., and Olinger, C. P.: Second Int. Congr. Hormonal Steroids, Milan. Abstracts, Int. Congr. Ser. No. III, p. 301, New York, Excerpta Medica Foundation, 1966.

199. Williams, J. T., and Moravec, D. F.: Hosp. Form. Manage. *1*:28, 1966.

200. Wintrobe, M. M.: Clinical Hematology, ed. 4, p. 611, Philadelphia, Lea & Febiger, 1956.

201. Wood, F. C.: J.A.M.A. *181*:358, 1962.

202. Wylie, D. W.: Proc. Soc. Exp. Biol. Med. *98*:716, 1958.

203. Zbinden, G., Bagdon, R. E., Keith, E. F., Phillips, R. D., and Randall, L. O.: Toxicol. Appl. Pharmacol. *3*:619, 1961.

Chapter 12

The Coordination of Health Care Services

Roy C. Darlington, Ph.D.*

A major function of the practicing pharmacist is his service as consultant to members of allied health professions. Students, teachers and practitioners of pharmacy are constantly reminded that this is an important objective of pharmaceutical education, and many believe that it is being accomplished. However, the results of reliable studies and surveys indicate that the consultative service rendered by pharmacists to physicians is minimal, and in regard to practitioners of the other health professions, it is practically nonexistent. Thus, the present status of this area of interprofessional relations seems to be at variance with the objectives of pharmaceutical education and the various organizations of pharmacy, unless certain basic facts are taken into account.

A perusal of the Codes of Ethics adopted by the American Pharmaceutical Association in 1852, 1922 and 1952 reveals that not until 1952 was there specific reference to the relations of pharmacists to members of any of the allied professions other than physicians.[9] Furthermore, the statement, "The pharmacist willingly makes available his expert knowledge of drugs to the other health professions," appeared first in the 1952 Code. These facts are especially significant because the A.Ph.A. Code is generally accepted as the professional Code of Ethics of the pharmacists of the United States.[10]

The curriculum of the representative college or school of pharmacy, medicine, dentistry, osteopathy, podiatry or veterinary medicine does not provide for adequate in-

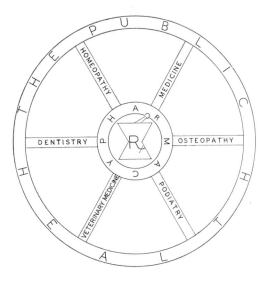

struction in the proper interrelationship of the allied health professions. As a result, the graduate pharmacist enters his profession with inadequate knowledge of the need that practitioners of the allied professions have for the consultative services he has to offer. Similarly, graduates of the allied health professions (including medicine) enter their respective professions unaware that it is the responsibility of pharmacists to provide these services. These conditions do not contribute to the attainment of the primary objective of all of the health professions—that is, the rendering of maximum service to public health.

If the health professions are to make a significant move toward ethical and professional responsibility, they must maximally coordinate their services. A prerequisite for

* Professor of Pharmacy and Chairman, Department of Pharmacy, Howard University.

interprofessional cooperation and functional coordination is interprofessional understanding. It is necessary that the practitioners of one health profession know the objectives, the qualifications, the responsibilities, the prerogatives and the limitations of each of these. The purpose of this chapter is to impart such knowledge to pharmacists.

MEDICINE

MEDICAL EDUCATION

Medical education began in the United States, as it did in Europe, with the apprenticeship system. By the year 1800, several medical schools associated with universities had been established. Within the next century, hundreds of medical schools were established in the United States. However, in 1908, when Abraham Flexner began his study of the schools of medicine in the United States and Canada, only about 10 per cent of the practicing physicians were graduates of medical schools.[11]

In the academic year 1966-1967, there were 84 approved medical schools and three approved schools of basic medical sciences in the United States. In addition there were 16 medical schools in development. There were 18,250 first-year applicants to these schools and 8,964 in the entering class. The total enrollment in all medical schools was 33,423, representing an increase of 588 over that of the previous year.[27]

When the Flexner report was published in 1910, only one of the 155 schools then operating required a baccalaureate degree for admission and only 16 required as much as 2 years of college work. Presently, 76 of the approved schools in which students can begin the study of medicine require at least 3 years of college preparation. Fourteen schools require the completion of a degree program for admission. In 1966 more than 86 per cent of the students admitted to medical schools in this country had completed four years of college.

GRADUATE MEDICAL EDUCATION

Internship and residency programs in hospitals provide graduate training for graduates of medical schools. These programs must be approved by the Council on Medical Education of the American Medical Association. There are two types of approved internship programs—straight and rotating.

The straight program provides 12 months of training on a single medical, surgical, pediatric, obstetric-gynecology, or pathology service in a hospital with an approved residency program in that specialty. The rotating program includes training for 12 or 24 months on two or more clinical services. One of the services must consist of not less than 4 months on the internal medicine service. In the internship of 12 months, the remaining time may be spent with or without emphasis on a specialty. The 2-year

TABLE 12-1. TYPES OF INTERNSHIP PROGRAMS OFFERED, 1957-1966

	ROTATING— NO MAJOR EMPHASIS		ROTATING WITH EMPHASIS ON A SPECIALTY*		STRAIGHT		FAMILY AND GENERAL PRACTICE		
	No.	%	No.	%	No.	%	No.	%	TOTALS
1957-58	842	77	34	3	217	20			1,093
1958-59	822	75	38	3	239	22			1,099
1959-60	816	75	33	3	246	22			1,097
1960-61	817	70	69	6	276	24	5		1,167
1961-62	737	61	107	9	359	30	9		1,212
1962-63	697	56	133	11	391	32	14	1	1,235
1963-64	661	52	153	12	432	34	17	1	1,263
1964-65	658	50	189	14	467	35	14	1	1,328
1965-66	641	45	251	17	531	37	17	1	1,440
1966-67	568	24	1,211	51	582	24	17	.5	2,378

*Listed in tables previous to this edition as mixed internships.

programs have been approved in 23 hospitals and were established for the purpose of preparing students for general practice. A third type of internship—family and general practice—is currently conducted on a pilot basis in 17 hospitals. These programs are designed to provide 2 years of training, equivalent to a 1-year internship and a subsequent 1-year residency (Table 12-1).

After completion of an approved internship program, graduate medical education may be continued in approved residency programs. There are 29 specialty fields in which training is offered, including the 23 conducted primarily in hospitals. Residency programs vary in length from 2 to 6 years, depending on the specialty and the demands of each of the 19 Specialty Boards that examine and certify the candidates within their jurisdictions.

MEDICAL LICENSURE

All the States and the District of Columbia require a license for the practice of medicine. Qualifications for the licensure of physicians educated in the United States, Canada, or Puerto Rico include graduation from an approved medical school and the passing of a licensing examination. Thirty-two states and the District of Columbia require a 1-year hospital internship. In addition, 4 years of preprofessional college education are required in 10 states, 3 years in two states, and 2 years in 38 states and the District of Columbia. Twenty-three states and the District of Columbia also require a basic science certificate.

All the states, except Arkansas, Louisiana and Nevada, have provisions for licensing graduates of foreign medical schools. All except six jurisdictions require full citizenship or legal declaration of intention to become a citizen. All jurisdictions give a written examination, 25 require also an oral examination, 27 require a basic science certificate, and 41 specify certification by the Educational Council for Foreign Medical Graduates. All except six states require one to three years of internship and residency training.

Annual renewal of licenses is required in 34 jurisdictions, biennial in 11, triennial in one. Licenses are not renewed in Kentucky, Massachusetts, Mississippi, New Jersey and Ohio. All licenses to practice medicine are issued by the states. The National Board of Medical Examiners also gives an examination that is accepted by most jurisdictions as a substitute for state examination. All jurisdictions, except Florida and Hawaii, provide some means of recognizing the licenses of other states, either through endorsement or reciprocity.[37]

MEDICAL PRACTICE

In 1966, 43 per cent of all physicians were located in the five states with the largest populations: New York, California, Pennsylvania, Illinois, and Ohio. As a rule general practitioners were distributed much more widely than specialists, whose members were concentrated in large cities.

The trend in medical practice is toward specialization. In 1923, the full-time specialists represented only 11 per cent of the practicing physicians in this country. At the end of 1966, 77 per cent were specialists. Thirteen per cent of all physicians were practicing as specialists in internal medicine and 10 per cent in surgery. An indication of the continuing preference for these specialties is the fact that 32 per cent of the 44,937 hospital trainees were majoring in these two specialties.

In December, 1966, the category of general practice represented 23 per cent of all physicians. This was 1 per cent less than the previous year. The unpopularity of general practice is indicated by the paucity of interns and residents in this area. Only 48 per cent of the available residencies were accepted and only 1.5 per cent of all trainees were in general practice (Table 12-2).[28]

An increasing number of physicians are entering research and teaching. A 1965 survey of a selected group of medical graduates (Class of 1955) disclosed that 12 per cent were in research and teaching, 65 per cent were in specialty practice, and 23 per cent were in general practice. About 31 per cent of those who chose to specialize were practicing internal medicine or surgery. Twenty-eight per cent were specializing in obstetrics-gynecology, pediatrics or psychiatry, and 41 per cent were engaged in one of the other specialties.[26]

TABLE 12-2. DISTRIBUTION OF PHYSICIANS IN THE US AND POSSESSIONS, DEC. 31, 1966

FIELD OF PRACTICE	ALL PHYSICIANS		ALL INTERNS, RESIDENTS AND FELLOWS			
	No.	% OF TOTAL PHYSICIANS	No. ON DUTY	% OF TOTAL MD'S IN THIS FIELD	% OF TOTAL ON DUTY	% OF RESIDENCIES FILLED IN THIS FIELD
General Practice	70,223	23	672	1	2	48
Internal Medicine	40,314	13	7,536*	19	17	85
Surgery	28,756	10	6,747*	23	15	90
Psychiatry	18,875	6	3,572	19	8	79
Obstetrics-Gynecology	17,444	6	2,629*	15	6	89
Pediatrics	16,417	5	2,924*	18	7	85
Radiology	10,189	3	1,773	17	4	80
Anesthesiology	9,110	3	1,199	13	3	70
Pathology	8,914	3	2,168*	24	5	60
Ophthalmology	8,735	3	1,184	14	3	96
Orthopedic Surgery	7,982	3	1,441	18	3	93
Totals	236,959	79	31,845	13	71	
Others	63,416	21	13,092	21	29	
Grand Totals	300,375	100	44,937	15	100	

*Includes Straight Internships.

The inability of the United States to produce enough physicians to meet its own needs has caused foreign medical graduates (FMG's) to occupy an important place in medical and hospital practice in this country. This group also includes American citizens who are graduates of foreign medical schools. Approximately 7,000 FMG's enter the United States each year. About 4,500 of these become interns or residents in approved hospital programs. In these programs they receive training and also assume major responsibilities for patient care. The remaining 2,500 enter other types of programs or receive training and provide patient care in hospitals whose programs are not approved by the American Medical Association. At present, there are more than 40,000 FMG's in the United States, comprising 14 per cent of the active physicians. Seventeen per cent of the new licentiates and 28 per cent of the interns and residents in approved training programs are FMG's (Table 12-3).[40]

The impact of specialization, the continuing shortage of physicians and the increasing numbers of FMG's on the availability and quality of health care are all cause for concern. If adequate medical services are to be provided under such conditions, the technical, the paramedical, the pharmaceutical, and other professional groups must work with medicine as a health team.

Practicing pharmacists render an important professional service through the dispensing of prescriptions in greater numbers each year (more than a billion prescriptions were dispensed in 1966).[34] They can provide an additional service of great importance by acting as consultants to physicians, who after all, are the principal prescribers.

TABLE 12-3. FOREIGN MEDICAL GRADUATES IN TRAINING PROGRAMS

	1959-60	1960-61	1961-62	1962-63	1963-64	1964-65	1965-66	1966-67
Interns	2,545	1,753	1,273	1,669	2,566	2,821	2,361	2,793
Residents	6,912	8,182	7,723	7,062	7,052	8,153	9,113	9,483
Others				1,024	1,791	1,925	2,355	2,566
Totals	9,457	9,935	8,996	9,755	11,409	12,899	13,829	14,842

DENTISTRY

DENTAL EDUCATION

Education for the profession of dentistry has evolved similarly to that of pharmacy and the other health professions—from the apprentice method with no formal academic requirements to the requirement of a professional degree preceded by a prescribed liberal arts education. Since the establishment of the first school (the Baltimore College of Dental Surgery) in 1840, the profession has developed from the level of apprenticeship training to the level of a comprehensively organized health profession.[20]

Dentistry has many national and local organizations, which publish an abundance of literature in the form of journals, scientific papers and survey reports. Some of the important national organizations vitally associated with dental education are the American Association of Dental Schools, the American Association of Dental Examiners, the National Board of Dental Examiners and the Council on Dental Education of the American Dental Association.[22]

The Council on Dental Education is responsible for the evaluation and accreditation of programs designed for the education and training of dentists and auxiliary dental personnel. During the 1967-1968 academic year, there were 50 operating dental schools, and five were in the process of development. Total enrollment was 14,955, and in 1967 there were 3,360 graduates. Graduates from 10 of the schools received the degree of Doctor of Dental Medicine, and the rest received the degree of Doctor of Dental Surgery or Doctor of Dental Science (D.D.S.).

Of the 4,200 freshmen students admitted to the dental schools in 1967, only 11 per cent possessed the minimum 2-year college educational requirement. Fifty-six per cent had earned a baccalaureate degree prior to enrollment. There were 1,374 dentists enrolled in advanced education programs during 1967-1968. There were also 937 dentists training as interns or residents.[4]

DENTAL PRACTICE

In 1967, there were more than 114,308 dentists in the United States, and more than 97,500 were active in the profession. More than 104,000 were members of the American Dental Association and its affiliated 54 societies in the states and dependencies and in its 462 societies in the nation's cities and counties.

More than 90 per cent of active dentists are engaged in private practice. About 8,500 are practicing in one of the eight recognized dental specialties, each of which has a national certifying board. More than one-half practice orthodontia (straightening of teeth), which was the first recognized dental specialty (1930). About one-fourth limit their practice to oral surgery, established in 1948. The remainder are engaged in periodontia (treatment of gums and underlying bone), pedodontia (children's dentistry), prosthodontia (preparation of artificial dentures), endodontia (root canal therapy), oral pathology and dental public health. There are presently fewer than 100 dentists in this country who are practicing in each of the latter two specialties.[3]

In its development, dental research has influenced dental practice considerably in the areas of diagnosis, prevention, restoration and treatment. As recently as the 1930's, dental practice was limited to relieving pain and treating lesions of teeth and tissues of the mouth. Today, with a health-conscious public that is much better informed concerning disease and is rightfully demanding better health service, the dentist must be concerned with the comprehensive management of oral, facial and speech defects and with oral structures and tissues as they relate to the total health of the individual. The dentist must not only prevent the occurrence and the progression of dental diseases, but also search for oral pathologic changes that provide early indications of systemic disease.[21] In other words, dentists have the responsibility of providing a complete health service to increasingly more persons by preventive and restorative practices in all conditions that can be diagnosed orally.

The demand for dental care will continue to increase because of population growth, improving economy, expanded dental insurance programs and rising educational levels. In 1968, when more than 3.5 billion dollars was spent by the public for dental care, more than half the population received no dental care.[8] If these persons are to receive professional service, dentistry must become more efficiently productive. Dentists can accomplish this only by utilizing to a much greater extent the auxiliary services of dental hygienists, dental assistants and dental technicians. They also must use effectively the services of the allied professions—medical and pharmaceutical, principally.

DENTAL LICENSURE

Dentists are licensed in all states and the District of Columbia by boards or committees. In all states except California and Pennsylvania, board membership is limited to dentists. Written and practical examinations are required for initial licensure in all states, and an oral examination is required in 24 states. All states except Arkansas, Hawaii, Indiana, Ohio and Utah license the graduates of accredited Canadian schools. No state board issues licenses to graduates of other foreign dental schools without additional training in U.S. dental schools.[38]

Approximately 99 per cent of eligible dental students take the theoretical examination administered by the National Board of Dental Examiners. At present, 45 licensing boards accept this examination in lieu of their written examinations.[31] Annual renewal of license is required in all but seven states, where the renewal period is biennial. At present, 11 states have no statutory provisions for recognition, by endorsement or reciprocity, of dental licenses issued by other states. The other 39 states and the District of Columbia have statutory provisions that are applicable at the discretion of the boards of dental examiners. It has been reported that in actual practice only nine states in any way recognize other dental licenses, and eight of these recognize only the licenses of states with which they have reciprocal agreements.[41]

PHARMACEUTICAL SERVICES

In 1966, more than 11 million new prescriptions were written by dentists, and it was predicted that they would write 18 million annually by 1970.[18] A recent survey indicated that almost 17 million prescriptions were written by dentists in 1964. The average number of prescriptions written during the 6-month period was nearly three times as high for specialists as for general practitioners. Oral surgeons, 99 per cent of whom prescribed, wrote the most prescriptions. Only 39.4 per cent of orthodontists prescribed, and they wrote the fewest prescriptions. General practitioners prescribed antibiotics most, and 93.7 per cent were prescribers. The percentage of dentists prescribing decreased as the age of the dentist increased. About 97 per cent of dentists under 40 years of age were prescribers and wrote the most prescriptions.[45]

It is relevant and significant that in 1969 35 of the 43 states that have approved Title XIX (Medicaid) programs have dental care programs. By 1975, the law requires that a state must be providing a comprehensive range of health services for all recipients in order to qualify for federal support under Title XIX. Thus, it can be expected that most, if not all, states will have comprehensive dental care programs by 1975.

It has been estimated that about 150 million dollars was spent for dental services under the existing Medicaid programs in fiscal 1968.[5] This fact and the trend of the prescribing practices of dentists make evident the increasing need and potential for pharmaceutical services. It is important that practicing pharmacists recognize this need and potential for service to a profession whose practitioners may legally prescribe for most conditions that can be diagnosed orally. Pharmacists must demonstrate their concern and competence as consultants.

Competence in this area requires that pharmacists understand the terminology, the therapeutic purposes and the dosage regimens of general practitioners and dentists who practice in a specialty. The necessities of dental therapy differ in many respects from those of medical practice. Because of these differences, dental prescriptions cannot be expected to contribute a large part of the dollar volume of prescription income. Moreover, because the therapeutic needs of many dental patients are short-term in nature, as few as two or three doses may be prescribed. For example, the dosage regimen for preoperative or postoperative treatment with drugs is usually of short duration. Furthermore, few such prescriptions are refilled. Pharmacists sometimes regard a dental prescription for six tablets or capsules or for 1 ounce of an oral liquid as a "nuisance prescription," but they should realize that such medication is a necessary adjunct to the rendering of an adequate service to the public health. They should utilize available house organs concerning dental therapeutic agents. They should encourage their local associations to sponsor joint meetings with local dental associations. They should initiate and sustain well planned consultative programs designed to make known the services they are prepared to offer. These programs should be directed especially to general practitioners, who represent more than 90 per cent of the practicing dentists. It is these dentists and the specialists in oral surgery and periodontology who most frequently use drug therapy in their practices. Information most useful to the dentist follows:

1. The procedure for procuring a narcotic registry number.

2. The procedure for writing conventional and special prescriptions (narcotic, etc.).

3. The legal requirements concerning oral (telephone) prescribing.

4. The legal requirements concerning the procurement of amphetamine, barbiturate and narcotic drugs for office use.

5. The formulation of special drug combinations for use in dentistry.

6. The availability of pharmaceutical specialties applicable to dental therapy.

7. The indications and the contraindications for the use of specific drugs in dental therapy.

8. The assistance that is available in the evaluation of currently available pharmaceutical specialties used by dentists.

In addition to serving as consultants concerning prescriptions, pharmacists should be familiar with the materials and the formulas used by the dentists in their offices.

PHARMACEUTICAL PREPARATIONS USED BY DENTISTS

Dentists purchase most of their office supplies from dental supply houses. Many of these products are promoted only to dentists, and pharmacists cannot buy them at a price less than that paid by the dentist. Therefore, it is impractical for pharmacists to serve as a source of supply for such products. It is possible for pharmacists to ascertain the needs of dentists in their neighborhood and to prepare some of their office supplies. However, pharmacists can serve dentists best by consultation concerning drugs that are available for dental therapy. In addition to the previously mentioned sources of information, booklets published by drug companies describe the drugs currently promoted to dentists. The number of such publications can be expected to increase, because young dentists are writing more prescriptions.

Practically all prescription drugs promoted to dentists are the same drugs used by physicians. For this reason, dentists, in taking a case history, attempt to learn what medicine, if any, the patient is receiving. By so doing, they avoid the risks of prescribing contraindicated drugs and of duplicating medicines. The following are some of the drugs now promoted to dentists.

Analgesics. The choice of an analgesic is determined by the severity of the pain. The following are prescribed most frequently.

Salicylates. A.P.C. capsules are used alone or in combination with codeine or an antihistamine.

Non-Narcotic Analgesics. Dextropropoxyphene—alone and in combination with compound aspirin or a tranquilizer and aspirin—is probably prescribed most often.[49]

Narcotic Analgesics. Meperidine hydrochloride (*U.S.P.*) is preferred to morphine for severe pain.

Anti-Infectives. Anti-infective drugs are used therapeutically to treat infections of the mouth. Indications for the use of these preparations are preoperative and postoperative prophylaxis in patients with a history of rheumatic fever, infectious hepatitis, kidney disease or diabetes. Although sulfonamides and the broad spectrum antibiotics are prescribed, penicillin tablets and lozenges are used most often. The following are examples of anti-infectives prescribed by dentists:

Phenoxymethyl penicillin tablets
  (*U.S.P.*) ....250 mg.
Potassium phenethicillin tablets ......250 mg.
Phenoxymethyl penicillin (125 mg.)
  with triple sulfa tablets (0.5 Gm.)
Buffered penicillin G tablets
  (*U.S.P.*) ....250 mg.
Penicillin lozenges ....5,000 units
Tetracycline hydrochloride capsules
  (*U.S.P.*) ....250 mg.

Antihistamines. Dentists use antihistamines prophylactically and therapeutically in cases of drug allergy. They prescribe them also for use before and after oral surgery to reduce postoperative edema and pain, and to improve the healing process. The rationale for the latter use is based on demonstrations that traumatic oral surgery increases the histamine content of the gingiva and the saliva.[50] Antihistamines prevent most of the reaction of the tissues to the increased amount of histamine. Liquid or solid oral dosage forms usually are prescribed. Because the preparations promoted to dentists are the same as those used by physicians and are so numerous and well known, examples of these are not given.

Anti-Inflammatory Agents. Tissue damage due to extractions and oral surgery is often followed by excessive inflammation. Such inflammatory responses can be harmful and delay healing. To prevent this type of reaction, some dentists use preoperative and postoperative treatment with corticosteroids. This is a low-dosage and short-term type of therapy. Pharmacists who recommend these drugs to dentists for use should also give them literature that explains the possible side effects and the contraindications for use. The following prescriptions are used by dentists.[46]

1. $\mathbb{R}$
    Prednisolone Tablets (*U.S.P.*)
    #24 ....2.5 mg.
    Sig.: 2 tabs. p.c. et h.s. for 2 days, then 1 tab. q 4 h

2. $\mathbb{R}$
    Prednisone (*U.S.P.*) ....2.5 mg.
    Chlorpheniramine maleate .....2.0 mg.
    Vitamin C .... 75.0 mg.[47]
    M. ft. Tab. #1
    D.T.D. #12
    Sig.: Take 1 tab. t.i.d. p.c. et h.s.

Hypnotics and Sedatives. Dentists use barbiturates and nonbarbiturate C.N.S. depressants to calm patients after operations and to make them less apprehensive before surgery. Usually, quick-acting sedatives are used.

3. $\mathbb{R}$
    Secobarbital sodium capsules (U.S.P.)
    #X ....gr. iss
    Sig.: i h.s. p.r.n.

4. $\mathbb{R}$
    Ethinamate tablets* ....0.5[51]
    Tab. No. VI
    Sig.: 2 tab. ½ h. before appointment

5. $\mathbb{R}$
    Pentobarbital sodium (*U.S.P.*) ...gr. iss
    Aspirin (*U.S.P.*) ....gr. v
    M. ft. Cap. #1
    Mitte #XII
    Sig.: i p.r.n. for pain and nervousness

Tranquilizers. Mild-acting tranquilizers of the neurosedative type are used with success by dentists. Unlike the barbiturates and many other sedatives, drugs of this type alleviate anxiety without lessening mental acuity.

Mild tranquilizers are especially useful in the treatment of the apprehensive and nervous patient who is having difficulty in adjusting to newly acquired dentures. They are also beneficial to many patients who are starting a long-range restoration or reconstruction program that will require dental appointments over a period of weeks or months. The anxieties of such patients are usually allayed by therapy with drugs such as the following:

6. $\mathbb{R}$
    Phenaglycodol ....200 mg.[52]
    No. 36 tablets
    Sig.: 1 tab. t.i.d.

7. $\mathbb{R}$
    Perphenazine tablets ....2 mg.[48]
    Sig.: 1 tab. q 4-6 h.

Vitamins. Because larger numbers of the populace are seeking dental care and because dental caries, gingivitis, glossitis and stomatitis may be early clinical signs of nutritional deficiencies, dentists are in a position to recognize the need for vitamin therapy.

Multivitamins, multivitamins with minerals, and B complex with C vitamins are used in cases that involve metabolic stress or significant dietary restrictions. These cases include patients with oral infections, those who are undergoing oral surgery and those who either are being fitted for dentures or have acquired them recently. Patients with a prolonged clotting time due to hypoprothrom-

*May be used in the presence of impaired liver or kidney function.

binemia often require vitamin K therapy when undergoing extraction or dental surgery. Among the vitamins presently prescribed by dentists are the following:

8. R̥
    Multiple vitamin caps. (therapeutic) No. 30
    Sig.: 1 cap. daily

9. R̥
    B complex with vit. C caps. No. 36
    Sig.: 1 cap. t.i.d.

10. R̥
    Multiple vitamin-minerals caps. (therapeutic) #24
    Sig.: 1 cap. A.M. and P.M.

11. R̥
    Menadione tablets
    (*U.S.P.*) No. 10 ....5 mg.
    Sig.: 1 tab. t.i.d.

HOMEOPATHY

DEVELOPMENT OF THE PROFESSION

The homeopathic concept of medical practice was introduced in 1796 by the German physician Samuel Hahnemann (1755-1843). He lived to see the profession practiced in many countries of Europe, Asia, South America and North America. The practice of homeopathy in the United States began in 1825 with the arrival of Dr. Constantine Hering, one of Hahnemann's disciples.[14] Dr. Hering is considered to be the father of Homeopathy in America. He established the first college at Allentown, Pennsylvania. When this college closed, he founded the Hahnemann Medical College in Philadelphia. This was the last college in this country to discontinue the teaching of courses in homeopathy to medical students.[25]

THE HOMEOPATHIC CONCEPT

This concept has its origin in a "Law of Cure" found in the writings attributed to Hippocrates (ca. 400 B.C.): "Through the like, disease is produced, and through the application of the like, it is cured."[15] It was this philosophy plus the results of his medical experiments that led Dr. Hahnemann to announce the Law of Similars (similia similibus curantur) as the Law of Cure, and thus launch the profession of homeopathy.

THE PRESENT STATUS OF HOMEOPATHY IN THE UNITED STATES

Education. Homeopathy is not taught in any institution that grants degrees. Professional education in homeopathy consists of a postgraduate course given each year for 2 weeks at Millersville State Teachers College in Pennsylvania. Physicians with the degree of M.D., M.B. (British), or D.O. (with unlimited practicing privileges) receive certificates on completion of the course. Other practitioners may take the course but they do not receive certificates. Homeopaths teach the course.

The most significant efforts in education have been made by the 11 Laymen's Leagues in as many cities. These Leagues conduct classes for laymen who are interested in learning about homeopathy. Instruction is by a layman or tape recordings and is given in 10 weekly meetings.[25]

Organizations of Homeopathy. There are five national organizations, two international organizations and 19 state and sectional societies with homeopaths as members. There are also about nine lay organizations working in the interest of homeopathy. The American Institute of Homeopathy, with business offices in Washington, D.C., is the national organization that represents the practitioners of homeopathy. The Institute publishes a bimonthly journal and is responsible for revision and publication of the *Homeopathic Pharmacopeia U. S.* The American Foundation for Homeopathy is the national organization that directs the professional and the laymen's educational programs. It also publishes much of the literature of the profession.

Practitioners of Homeopathy. Statistics concerning practitioners have not been published recently and were not published in 1967 by the profession or by the Government. However, it can be reported that in a metropolitan area with a population of 2 million there are about 21 practitioners of homeopathy and one homeopathic pharmacy. Only one of these homeopaths practices true homeopathy; the others use both allopathic and homeopathic methods of diagnosis and treatment. The one genuine homeopath does not prescribe, and the others together write an average of about 15 homeopathic prescriptions per day.[12] These facts indicate that homeopaths dispense rather than prescribe.

PHARMACEUTICAL SERVICES TO HOMEOPATHS

Based on membership in state societies, it appears that most practitioners of homeopathy are located in the states of California, New York and Pennsylvania. Homeopathic pharmacists provide prescription services, but the predominant service is that of manufacturing dosage forms to be dispensed by the homeopath. Those who practice only homeopathy need no other services. However, most homeopaths also practice allopathic medicine, and they therefore need additional pharmaceutical services. The regular pharmacist can provide consultative and prescription services in regard to the modern chemotherapeutic agents that most homeopathic pharmacies cannot afford to stock.

No profession can survive unless there is a demand for its services. The fact that homeopathy has survived indicates that there is still such a demand. As a consequence, it is necessary that information concerning these services be available to interested persons. A principal source of such information is the *Homeopathic Pharmacopeia of the United States*. The revised 7th edition was published in 1964. The *Homeopathic Pharmacopeia U. S.* has the same governmental status as the *U.S.P.* and serves homeopathy in the same manner that the *U.S.P.* serves medicine and pharmacy. All drugs or drug combinations that are official have been "proved" by testing on healthy human beings. There are no antibiotics, modern chemotherapeutic agents or injectables listed in the homeopathic pharmacopeia.

PREPARATION OF HOMEOPATHIC DOSAGE FORMS

The principal vehicles used in the preparation of liquid vehicles used in the preparation of liquid and solid dosage forms are:

1. Alcohol (*U.S.P.*)—used to prepare tinctures.

2. Dispensing alcohol (88% v/v)—used to prepare dilutions from tinctures.

3. Distilled water—used to prepare solutions of substances that have low solubility in alcohol.

4. Lactose—used to prepare solid dosage forms.

Great emphasis is placed on the use of fresh drugs in the preparation of tinctures and solutions. The moisture content of the drug is calculated as a part of the menstruum. The unit of medicinal strength is the dried drug. The pharmacopeia recognizes the following dosage forms.

Tinctures. These are designated by the sign "ø" (zero reduced) to denote the strongest liquid preparation. Unless otherwise indicated, they are 10 per cent preparations.

Aqueous Solutions. These are usually prepared in 10.0, 1.0 or 0.1 per cent concentrations, depending on the degree of solubility.

Dilutions. These are prepared by diluting tinctures with dispensing alcohol or by diluting solid forms with lactose. The official method of dilution is by the use of the decimal scale whereby the original quantity of medicine is divided progressively by ten. The first decimal (1$\times$) contains 1/10, the second decimal (2$\times$) 1/100, the third decimal (3$\times$) 1/1,000, and the fourth decimal (4$\times$) 1/10,000 of the original drug. Some practitioners designate this system of dilution by using D1 for 1/10, D2 for 1/100, D3 for 1/1,000, and D4 for 1/10,000 concentrations. A few homeopaths still use the centesimal system of dilution, which was recommended and adopted by Hahnemann. In this system each dilution contains 1/100 part of the preceding dilution. These dilutions are designated as follows: 1C (1/100), 2C (1/10,000), 3C (1/1,000,000) etc.

Triturations. These are tablets or powders prepared by dilution with lactose.

Tincture Triturations. These are prepared by adding the tincture to lactose, triturating and allowing it to dry. Because these triturations contain only the alcohol-soluble constituents of drugs, they are different from triturations prepared from the drug. To differentiate from drug triturations a minus sign is used above the figure denoting potency; for example, $\overline{\times}$ (1/10), $\overline{2\times}$ (1/100) etc.

Medicated Powders. These are prepared

by adding one part of a liquid preparation to 10 parts of lactose, triturating and allowing to dry. The strength of the medicated powder is one decimal more than the dilution used in its preparation.

Medicated Globules. These are made from sucrose or lactose, and they are medicated by saturation with liquid preparations. The excess of liquid is removed and the vial is inverted on a clean, white blotting paper until the globules no longer cling together.

Medicated Cones or Disks. These are made of cane sugar and egg albumen. They are formed into hemispherical masses, which are designated according to the diameter of the base in millimeters. The No. 6 size, which is most often used, will absorb about 2 drops of dispensing alcohol. They are used and dispensed in the same way as are medicated globules.[23]

Homeopathic Prescriptions. The following prescriptions were copied from the 1962 prescription file of a homeopathic pharmacy and are reproduced exactly as written. It is interesting to note that tablet triturates are prescribed by volume, as well as by number.[13]

℞
Mercurius dulcis . . . . 6×
Phytolacca dec. . . . . .6× equal parts
Disp. T.T. 125
Sig.: 2 Q2H Today then . . .
   2 Q3H

℞
Thuja . . . . 12×
Disp. T.T. oz. ii
Sig.: Four Tablets T.I.D.

℞
Valeriana ∅
Disp. 30 cc.
Sig.: gtt 20 HS

℞
Phosphorus . . . . 30× T.T.
Disp. oz. i
Sig.: Four tablets T.I.D.

℞
Glonoinum . . . . 6× T.T.
Disp. 500
Sig.: i PRN

℞
Carduus mar D2
Nux vomica D4
Valeriana . . . . ∅

Chelidon D2
   aa ad 50.0 cc
Sig.: gtt 20 T.I.D. ac

OSTEOPATHY

THE OSTEOPATHIC CONCEPT

The osteopathic concept as a system of medical practice was introduced by Andrew Taylor Still (1828-1917), who practiced as a physician and surgeon in the state of Missouri. From the time that he advocated a different approach to health and disease, and for 18 years thereafter, osteopathy was a one-man profession. In 1892 Dr. Still founded the first college of osteopathy at Kirksville, Missouri. The charter granted the corporation (American School of Osteopathy) and its board of trustees the right to confer the degree of Doctor of Medicine (M.D.). However, the degree Doctor of Osteopathy (D.O.) was chosen.

The osteopathic concept, as interpreted by the faculty of the Kirksville College of Osteopathy, emphasizes four general principles. From these are derived an etiologic concept, a philosophy and a therapeutic technic that is distinctive to osteopathy. However, it is emphasized that these are not the only features of osteopathic diagnosis and treatment. The four principles are as follows:

1. *The body is a unit.* Though heterogeneous in structure, the human body functions as a unit in both health and disease. Therefore, in the management of the patient, it is necessary to consider the patient as a whole.

2. *The body possesses self-regulatory mechanisms.* These mechanisms are operative in the: (A) production of natural and acquired immunity; (B) hemostatic regulation of vital functions: (C) repair of damaged tissues and (D) compensation for irreparable damage.

3. *Structure and function are reciprocally inter-related.* This relationship provides a basis for the structural etiology of disease and for the technics of manipulative therapy.

4. *Rational therapy is based on an understanding of body unity, self-regulatory mechanisms and the inter-relationship of structure and function.* All therapy is based

on an evaluation of the patient as a whole, and although special consideration is given to impairments arising in the musculoskeletal system, rational and appropriate therapy may include surgery, the use of drugs or any other properly recognized modality.[29]

OSTEOPATHIC EDUCATION AND TRAINING

A minimum of 3 years of prescribed liberal arts education followed by 4 years of professional study in an approved college of osteopathy is required for the degree of Doctor of Osteopathy (D.O.). Eighty-seven per cent of the 1969 entering class had one or more degrees. Almost all graduates (more than 99 per cent in 1967) serve an internship in an osteopathic hospital that has been approved by the American Osteopathic Association for training interns. Those who wish to become certified as specialists must have at least 5 years of training after service as interns. The successful completion of oral, written and practical examinations, which are administered by Certifying Boards, qualifies them as specialists. Presently there are 12 such boards.[35]

There are now six accredited colleges of osteopathy in this country. In 1969, there were approximately 1,997 students in these colleges, which had 427 graduates in 1969.[30]

OSTEOPATHY IN THE UNITED STATES

The first national organization (American Association for the Advancement of Osteopathy) was formed in 1897; in 1901 it changed its name to the American Osteopathic Association. The Association is a federation of divisional societies organized within the states and the territories of the United States. It publishes a scientific journal, an annual directory, a code of ethics and other publications for professional and lay use.[7]

Osteopaths are licensed to practice in all states and territories in accordance with the provisions of the licensing laws. The various laws provide for one of three types of licenses: Mississippi and Montana issue limited licenses that do not permit the use of drugs or surgery. Arkansas, Idaho, Louisiana, North Carolina, North Dakota and South Carolina issue limited licenses that permit the use of either drugs or minor surgery.

The other 42 states and the District of Columbia issue unlimited licenses that allow osteopaths the same privileges of practice granted medical doctors (M.D.'s).

There are approximately 13,000 D.O.'s in the United States. This does not include about 1,500 osteopathic physicians in California who, since 1962, have been classified as M.D.'s. About 97 per cent of those in active practice are located in the 42 unlimited states and the District of Columbia. General practitioners comprise 60.5 per cent; 16.7 per cent are general practitioners giving particular attention to a specialty; 12.6 per cent limit their practices to a specialty; and 10.2 per cent limit their practices to manipulative therapy.[24] More than half of all D.O.'s are located in five states—California, Michigan, Missouri, Ohio and Pennsylvania. Most are in private practice and are relatively young; 7 per cent are women. General practitioners tend to locate in small towns or cities. The specialists usually practice in large cities.

PRESCRIBING PRACTICES

A 12-month study in 1966 concerning the use of drugs in therapy by D.O.'s and M.D.'s revealed that osteopaths compare in many respects with medical doctors. The D.O.'s saw 17.3 patients per day and used 23 drugs to treat them. The M.D.'s saw 17 patients per day and used 20.7 drugs for treatment.[36] About 90 per cent of the more than 13,000 practicing osteopaths need the same pharmaceutical services required by medical doctors. No drugs or prescriptions are unique to osteopathy. Practicing pharmacists have the responsibility of establishing communication with the osteopaths in their communities. These practitioners need the consultative services of pharmacists even more than do physicians, because many are not detailed by representatives of drug companies to the extent that physicians are.

PODIATRY

Chiropody, which literally means the art of treating diseases of the hands and the feet, is now used synonymously with podiatry. Podiatry was formerly known as chiropody, and the graduates of such colleges received the degree, Doctor of Surgical Chiropody (D.S.C.). The approximately 8,100 practitioners licensed to practice in the 50 states and the District of Columbia deal solely with prevention, diagnosis and treatment of diseases of the feet. Hospitals, city health departments and clinics of the Veterans Administration use the services of podiatrists. As commissioned officers in the Medical Service Corps, podiatrists establish and supervise clinics of podiatry in the several branches of the Armed Forces. In 1959, a study conducted at an armed force training center revealed that 6 per cent of all recruits were referred to podiatrists for consultation and treatment.[19]

PODIATRIC EDUCATION AND PRACTICE

In 1968, almost 1,000 students were enrolled in the five accredited colleges of podiatry.[42] These colleges award either the degree of Doctor of Podiatry (Pod.D.) or Doctor of Podiatric Medicine (D.P.M.) after the completion of 2 years of prescribed liberal arts education and 4 years of professional education and training.[6] All states and the District of Columbia license podiatrists who pass qualifying examinations. Michigan, New Jersey and Rhode Island require the completion of a 1-year internship after graduation. Seven states and the District of Columbia have provisions for licensing foreign-educated podiatrists. Reciprocity is available to practitioners in all but nine of the states. Annual renewal of licensure is required in 42 jurisdictions and biennial in seven. No renewal is required in Mississippi.[1]

State laws vary, but as a rule, podiatrists are licensed to diagnose and treat most foot ailments by medical, surgical, physical and mechanical means. They use roentgenography, biopsy, urinalysis, and biologic and blood tests in diagnoses. They perform various types of surgery on the feet (no amputations). They do not treat systemic diseases. However, they are qualified by academic background to know when foot or lower-leg pathology indicates the possible existence of certain systemic diseases and the necessity for referral to a physician. They do not administer general anesthetics, but they inject local anesthetics. Thirty-seven states and the District of Columbia permit podia-

trists to prescribe all forms of medication. The other states place varying limitations on prescribing privileges.[2]

FORMS AND SOURCES OF DRUGS USED BY PODIATRISTS

The National Formulary (*N.F. XII*) contains the formulas for 15 specialty preparations used in podiatric practice. These include solutions, suspensions, ointments and a powder. They are representative of some of the topical medicines used by podiatrists.[33] In addition to the formulas for specialty preparations, *N.F. X* also included a list of more than 100 drugs and preparations used by podiatrists.[32] All the drugs necessary to compound these formulas are stocked by pharmacies, yet practically all podiatrists obtain their office supplies from supply houses, primarily because pharmacists make no effort to ascertain the needs of podiatrists.

PHARMACEUTICAL SERVICES REQUIRED BY PODIATRISTS

Educators and practitioners of podiatry have stated that the use of prescriptions is indispensable to a satisfactory and successful practice of podiatry. Therefore, the relation between podiatrists and pharmacists should be the same as that between physicians and pharmacists. Pharmacists should not prescribe and sell medicinals for the treatment of foot ailments that require diagnosis. They have a responsibility to assist in educating the public concerning foot health care. This responsibility dictates that pharmacists should inform their customers of the availability of podiatrists' services, and they should make referrals when necessary.

Podiatrists also want and need the consultative services of pharmacists concerning drugs and the writing of prescriptions. The need for these services is so great that at least one company sells booklets of prescriptions to podiatrists. These booklets contain 15 prescriptions, each of which is printed on a tear-off label. The advertisement states that this is a "dispensing service."[43] This service is obviously a responsibility of practicing pharmacists.

The following are examples of prescriptions used in the practice of podiatry.

Analgesics. In most cases, podiatrists can

administer effective local treatment to eliminate foot pain. However, oral medication occasionally is needed to relieve foot pain, which may vary from mild to severe.

For Relief of Mild Pain.

12. ℞
Acetophenetidin (*U.S.P.*) .... gr. iiss
Acetylsalicylic acid (*U.S.P.*) .... gr. iiiss
Caffeine (*U.S.P.*) .... gr. ss
M.ft. Cap. No. 1, D.T.D. No. 24
Sig.: ii q 4 h p.r.n. for pain

13. ℞
Pentobarbital sodium (*U.S.P.*) .... gr. ss
Acetylsalicylic acid (*U.S.P.*) ...... gr. v
M.ft. Cap. No. 1
Mitte No. 21
Sig.: i q 4-6 h. for pain

For Relief of Moderate Pain.

14. ℞
Acetophenetidin (*U.S.P.*) ...... gr. iiss
Acetylsalicylic acid (*U.S.P.*) .... gr. iiiss
Caffeine (*U.S.P.*)
Codeine phosphate (*U.S.P.*) aa. gr. ss
M.ft. Cap. No. 1, D.T.D. No. 16
Sig.: i not oftener than q 4 h p.r.n. for pain

15. ℞
Ethoheptazine citrate .... 75 mg.
Acetylsalicylic acid (*U.S.P.*) ... 325 mg.
M.ft. tab. No. 1, D.T.D. No. 24
Sig.: 1 or 2 tabs. 3-4 times daily for pain

For Relief of Severe Pain.

16. ℞
Meperidine HC1 Tablets (*U.S.P.*)...... ....
No. 9 .... 100 mg.
Sig.: Tab. i q 6 h. p.r.n. for pain

17. ℞
Methadone HC1 Tablets (*U.S.P.*)
.... 7.5 mg.
T.D. No. 10
Sig.: Tab. i not oftener q 6 h p.r.n. for pain

18. ℞
Dextropropoxyphene .... 32 mg.
Acetophenetidin (*U.S.P.*) .... 162 mg.
Acetylsalicylic acid (*U.S.P.*) .... 227 mg.
Caffeine (*U.S.P.*) .... 32.4 mg.
M.ft. Cap. No. 1, Mitte No. 20
Sig.: Cap. 1 or 2 q 6 h for pain

19. ℞
Levorphanol tartrate tablets (*N.F.*) 2 mg.
No. 12
Sig.: 1 q 8 h

Sedatives and Hypnotics. Patients who are apprehensive and restless before, during or after treatment or surgery may need the relief afforded by these drugs.

20. ℞
Pentobarbital sod. Cap. (*U.S.P.*) gr. iss
No. 6
Sig.: 1 cap. ½ h. before appointment

21. ℞
Secobarbital sod. Cap. (*U.S.P.*) ... gr. iss
No. 12
Sig.: 1 h.s. for sleep

22. ℞
Glutethimide Tab. (*N.F.*) 0.5
No. 10
Sig.: 1 tab. ut dict. p.r.n.

Anti-Infectives. Antibiotics and sulfonamides are used to treat infections of the feet and the lower part of the legs. They are also used prophylactically in foot fractures or foot surgery, with diabetic patients and those who have a history of rheumatic fever, infectious hepatitis or recent pulmonary disease. Although sulfonamides and broad spectrum antibiotics are prescribed, oral preparations of penicillin are used most frequently. The following are examples of preparations prescribed by podiatrists.

23. ℞
Buffered penicillin G Tabs. (*U.S.P.*) ....
No. 12 ....125 mg.
Sig.: 1 q 4 h. between meals

24. ℞
Potassium phenethicillin Tabs. .. 250 mg.
No. 12
Sig.: 2 stat., then 1 q 4 h. q.i.d.

25. ℞
Erythromycin Tab. (*U.S.P.*) ... 250 mg.
No. 12
Sig.: 1 q 6 h.

26. ℞
Phenoxymethyl penicillin for oral suspension (*U.S.P.*) .... 60 cc.
Sig.: 10 cc. t.i.d. 1 h. a.c.

27. ℞
Tetracycline HC1 Caps. (*U.S.P.*)
#16 .... 250 mg.
Sig.: 2 caps. q.i.d.

28. ℞
Triple sulfa Tabs. .... 0.5 Gm.
No. 36
Sig.: 4 tabs. stat., then 2 q.i.d. with full glass of water

VETERINARY MEDICINE

DEVELOPMENT OF THE PROFESSION

Veterinary medicine is a separate, self-governing profession with its own system of education, licensure and organization. As an organized medical profession it is relatively young, the first veterinary college in the United States having been established in Philadelphia in 1854. By 1900 about 30 veterinary schools had been organized, and with the exceptions of the state-supported institutions of Iowa, Ohio, Washington State and Cornell, New York, they were privately supported. More than 10,000 veterinarians were graduated from the privately supported colleges before the last one, located in Washington, D.C., closed in 1927. At present there are 18 veterinary schools in the United States and three in Canada; all are associated with a college or a university and are accredited by the American Veterinary Medical Association (A.V.M.A.).

The national demand for veterinarians has increased as the population has grown and as the veterinarian's role in our society has broadened. Veterinarians are in demand in many health-related areas, such as public health, laboratory animal medicine, military forces, animal disease control agencies, meat inspection service, and biomedical research, in government, universities and industrial laboratories. In 1964, more than 45 per cent of the graduates entered health activities other than private practice. It has been estimated that there will be a shortage of 20,000 veterinarians by 1985.[16]

VETERINARY MEDICAL EDUCATION

The 18 schools and colleges of veterinary medicine in the United States have their roots in the schools of agriculture. Most were outgrowths of departments of veterinary science. With the exception of Tuskegee Institute and the University of Pennsylvania, all the veterinary colleges and schools are located in land-grant or state-operated institutions. Seven of the state-supported veterinary schools have been established since the end of World War II.

Presently, most veterinary colleges require a minimum of 2 years of college education for entrance to the 4-year professional program. The University of Pennsylvania requires 3 years and the Universities of Oklahoma and Oregon require 4 years of preprofessional college education. Although individual courses vary, all professional curriculums include 2 years of basic sciences and 2 years of clinical veterinary medicine and surgery. Because of the limitations of physical facilities and personnel, most colleges admit fewer than 100 students in the freshman class. In 1969, there were approximately 3.5 applicants for each available opening.[53]

In most colleges, students are required to gain practical experience by working at least one summer session with a practitioner. Several colleges have internship programs that students must complete before they receive degrees. Each year about 1,100 graduates receive the degree of Doctor of Veterinary Medicine (D.V.M. or V.M.D.) from the 21 colleges. About 10 per cent of veterinary students, many faculty members and others engaged in research are doing graduate work in the fields of anatomy, microbiology, pharmacology, physiology, public health and veterinary pathology. On completion of these studies, they receive the degree of Master of Science or Doctor of Philosophy.

VETERINARY MEDICAL LICENSURE

Each state has an examining board, which administers written, oral and practical examinations to candidates for licensure. Approximately 30 states use objective tests prepared by the National Board of Veterinary Medical Examiners (established in 1950) and the Professional Examination Service of the American Public Health Association. It is expected that increasingly more states will use these examinations. Other statistical data concerning the profession of veterinary medicine are shown in Table 12-4.

THE AMERICAN VETERINARY MEDICAL ASSOCIATION (A.V.M.A.)

The A.V.M.A., which is the professional organization of American and Canadian veterinarians, was founded as the United States Veterinary Medical Association on June 9, 1863, in New York City. It assumed its present name in 1898. The Association is composed of 63 constituent associations representing veterinarians in the 50 states,

TABLE 12-4. DATA CONCERNING
VETERINARY MEDICINE IN 1969

Veterinarians in the United States	26,472
Membership in A.V.M.A.	18,960
Canadian membership in A.V.M.A.	560
Graduates from 18 U.S. colleges (1968)	1,061

VETERINARY DISTRIBUTION

Department of Health, Education and Welfare	492
U.S. Armed Forces	1,068
U.S. Department of Agriculture	3,329
State regulatory agencies (disease control and meat inspection)	1,430
Industry	313
Teaching and research	2,158
Laboratory animal medicine	850
Large animal practice	1,529
Small animal practice	5,947
Mixed animal practice	7,795
Poultry practice	87
Miscellaneous activities	more than 1,000

the Canadian provinces, the U.S. territories and possessions, the Federal Government and the Armed Forces. The Association has its headquarters in Chicago and maintains a bureau in Washington, D.C.

The Association publishes the *Journal of the American Veterinary Medical Association* (semimonthly), *The American Journal of Veterinary Research* (monthly) and a Directory (biennially). Specialty Boards in veterinary medicine recognized by the A.V.M.A. are the American College of Veterinary Pathologists, the American College of Laboratory Animal Medicine, the American Board of Veterinary Public Health, American Board of Veterinary Radiology, American College of Veterinary Microbiologists, American College of Veterinary Surgeons and American Board of Veterinary Toxicologists.

VETERINARY MEDICAL PRACTITIONERS

Most veterinarians are currently engaged in the following fields of work:
1. Animal health protection
   a. Farm animals
   b. Pets and recreational animals
2. Government service
   a. U.S. Department of Agriculture
   b. Department of Health, Education and Welfare
   c. Food and Drug Administration
   d. Food hygiene
   e. Department of Defense
3. Institutional work
   a. Teaching
   b. Research
4. Comparative medicine
5. Laboratory animal medicine
6. Radiological health[17]

SERVICES REQUIRED FROM PRACTICING PHARMACISTS

Pet veterinarians have the greatest need for the services of practicing pharmacists. These practitioners serve persons who are emotionally motivated to seek care for their pets, and who therefore readily accept prescriptions, whereas farmers are primarily interested in the dollar value of the animals that must be treated. Because most farm calls are for the treatment of emergency illnesses or to give injections for immunization, the medicines are usually administered by veterinarians. Despite these facts, pharmacists can provide some services if satisfactory communication is established. Pharmacists should especially know that the *U.S.P.,* the *N.F.* and other pharmaceutical textbooks are including increasingly more information concerning drugs used by veterinarians.

PHARMACEUTICAL PREPARATIONS USED BY FARM VETERINARIANS

Biologicals are the most important of the injections used by farm veterinarians. The quality of these preparations is controlled by the U.S. Department of Agriculture through its Animal Inspection and Quarantine Division of Agricultural Research Service, U.S.D.A. Approximately 125 kinds of veterinary biologicals were produced in 1959 by 65 companies.[39] Veterinarians use antisera, vaccines, bacterins, antitoxins, toxoids and other injectables in the prevention, diagnosis and treatment of diseases of animals. Examples of the preparations used follow.
1. *Antisera*
   Anti-anthrax serum
   Antibacterial serum bovine (bovine origin)
   Antibacterial serum equine (equine origin)
   Anti-blackleg serum bovine (bovine origin)

Hog cholera antiserum (porcine origin)
Swine erysipelas antiserum (equine origin)

2. *Antitoxins*
Botulinus antitoxin (Types A, B and C)
Tetanus antitoxin

3. *Bacterins*
Mixed bacterin, avian (chicken formula)
Leptospira pomona bacterin

4. *Toxoids*
Tetanus toxoid (alum precipitated)

5. *Vaccines*
Anthrax spore vaccine
Rabies vaccine

6. *Diagnostic Antigens*
Leptospira antigen
Pullorum disease antigen, stained, polyvalent
Tuberculin (intradermal)

PHARMACEUTICAL PREPARATIONS USED BY PET VETERINARIANS

The oral and the topical medications used to treat pets are similar to or identical with those used in the treatment of human beings. However, the doses and the nomenclature of many of these drugs differ. In addition, pharmacists should be aware of the unusual reactions of cats to certain drugs.

The dosage regimen of animals is determined by body weight. As a rule, the dose for cats is half that of the human adult, and the dose for the average dog (about 45 lbs.) is the same as that for the human adult. Cats are very sensitive to the opium alkaloids and their derivatives, and phenolic compounds are usually not applied topically. Prescriptions representative of the compositions of pharmaceutical specialties promoted to pet veterinarians are shown in Table 12-5.[44]

TABLE 12-5.

MEDICAL CATEGORY	PRESCRIPTION		REMARKS
Antihistaminic	Prophenpyridamine maleate	10 mg.	Used for eczema, pruritus, mange and other dermatoses
	Sulfur	20 mg.	
	Dl-methionine (*N.F.*)	30 mg.	
	M.ft. Cap. No. 1		
	Mitte No. 24		
	Sig.: Give one t.i.d.		
Sedative-Expectorant	Codeine phosphate (*U.S.P.*)	gr. iv	Used to treat coughs and colds
	Sodium citrate (*U.S.P.*)	℥ iss	
	Ammonium chloride (*U.S.P.*)	gr. xx	
	Ipecac syrup (*U.S.P.*)	℥ ii	
	Tolu balsam syrup (*U.S.P.*) q.s. ad	℥ iv	
	Sig.: ℥ i q 4 h		
Sedative-Expectorant	Ethylmorphine hydrochloride (*N.F.*)	gr. v	Used to treat bronchitis and tracheitis (should not be administered to cats)
	Potassium guaiacolsulfonate (*N.F.*)	℥ ss	
	Potassium citrate (*N.F.*)	℥ iss	
	Citric acid (*U.S.P.*)	℥ ss	
	Alcohol (*U.S.P.*)	5%	
	Orange syrup (*U.S.P.*) q.s.ad	℥ iv	
	Sig.: ℥ i t.i.d.		
Dermatologic	Iodoform (*N.F.*)	1%	Used to control capillary bleeding
	Tannic acid (*N.F.*)	3%	
	Potassium alum		
	Boric acid (*U.S.P.*) aa	5%	
	Exsiccated ferrous sulfate (*U.S.P.*)	6%	
	Talc (*U.S.P.*) q.s.ad	℥ i	
	Sig.: Use topically as directed		

TABLE 12-5 *(Continued)*

MEDICAL CATEGORY	PRESCRIPTION		REMARKS
Dermatologic	Neomycin sulfate (*U.S.P.*)	0.5%	Used for superficial skin infections or abrasions
	Pantothenylol	2%	
	Hydrophilic ointment (*U.S.P.*) q.s.ad	30.0	
	Sig.: Apply to affected area b.i.d.		
Dermatologic	Bismuth subgallate (*N.F.*)		For minor skin conditions or first-degree burns
	Oil of cade (*U.S.P.*) aa	1%	
	Resorcinol (*U.S.P.*)	5%	
	Bismuth subnitrate (*N.F.*)	9%	
	Calamine (*U.S.P.*)	10%	
	Zinc oxide (*U.S.P.*)	17%	
	White ointment (*U.S.P.*) q.s.ad	30.0	
	Sig.: Apply as directed		
Antihistaminic Bronchodilator	Phenylephrine HCl (*U.S.P.*)	04	For respiratory conditions complicated by congested mucosa, bronchospasm and cough (use with caution for cats)
	Chlorprophenpyridamine maleate		
	Dihydrocodeinone bitartrate (*N.F.*) aa	008	
	Chloroform (*U.S.P.*)	04	
	Menthol (*U.S.P.*)	004	
	Alcohol (*U.S.P.*)	10%	
	Aromatic elixir (*U.S.P.*) q.s.ad	120	
	Sig.: 10 cc. t.i.d.		
Antispasmodic Bronchodilator	Dextromorphan HBr (*N.F.*)	2	For cough associated with bronchial constriction
	Methoxyphenamine HCl	3	
	Sodium citrate (*U.S.P.*)	6	
	Cherry syrup (*U.S.P.*) q.s.ad	90	
	Sig.: 2 cc. q 4 h		
Geriatric Formula	Diethylstilbestrol (*U.S.P.*)	1.8 mg	Used in geriatrics; recommended for preoperative and postoperative use; also for weakened and deficient states due to any cause
	Methyltestosterone (*U.S.P.*)	36.0 mg.	
	Vitamin B$_{12}$		
	Thiamin HCl (*U.S.P.*) aa	18.0 mg.	
	Nicotinamide (*U.S.P.*)	90.0 mg.	
	Riboflavin (*U.S.P.*)		
	Pyridoxine HCl (*U.S.P.*)		
	Calcium pantothenate (*U.S.P.*) aa	9.0 mg.	
	Cherry syrup (*U.S.P.*) q.s.ad	90.0 cc.	
	Sig.: Give 5 cc. t.i.d.		
Hematinic vitamin	Desiccated liver (*N.F.*)	0 250	Used for anemias, malnutrition and anorexia; also as a tonic following removal of intestinal parasites
	Ferrous gluconate (*U.S.P.*)	0 120	
	Thiamin HCl (*U.S.P.*)	0 003	
	Riboflavin (*U.S.P.*)	0 001	
	Nicotinamide (*U.S.P.*)	0 005	
	M.ft. Cap. No. 1		
	T.D. No. 36		
	Sig.:Give 2 b.i.d.		
Anti-arthritic	Methylprednisolone Tab. No. 24	2 mg.	Recommended for use in certain skin, otic and ocular diseases; also used in allergic and stress conditions
	Sig.: Give one t.i.d. for 4 days; then one b.i.d.		

TABLE 12-5 *(Continued)*

MEDICAL CATEGORY	PRESCRIPTION		REMARKS
Anti-infective	Potassium penicillin G (*U.S.P.*) 200 M units Sulfadiazine (*U.S.P.*) Sulfamethazine (*U.S.P.*) Sulfamerazine (*U.S.P.*) M.ft. Cap. No. 2 D.T.D. No. 12 Sig.: One Capsule ½ h. a.c. I b.i.d.	0|167 0|167 0|167	Used for treatment of abscesses, pneumonia and other susceptible infections
Anti-infective	Tetracycline HCl Capsules (*U.S.P.*) #16 Sig.: Give two capsules q 6 h	125 mg.	Used to treat peritonitis, hemorrhagic septicemia, parotitis, otitis media and other infectious processes
Gastrointestinal agent	Neomycin sulfate (*U.S.P.*) Sulfaguanidine (*N.F.*) Sulfadiazine (*U.S.P.*) Sulfamerazine (*U.S.P.*) aa Kaolin (*N.F.*) Pectin (*N.F.*) Peppermint water (*U.S.P.*) q.s.ad Sig.: ℥ i b.i.d.	gr. v ℥ ii gr. viii ℥ vi gr. viii ℥ iv	Used for diarrheal conditions associated with infectious enteritis, distemper, leptospirosis and parasitic infestation
Gastrointestinal agent	Bismuth subcarbonate (*U.S.P.*) Phenyl salicylate (*N.F.*) aa Zinc phenolsulfonate (*N.F.*) Pepsin (*N.F.*) Methylcellulose (*U.S.P.*) ¼ % Lactated pepsin elixir (*N.F.*) q.s.ad Sig.: Give 2 to 4 cc. t.i.d.	0|5 0|3 1|0 120|0	An antacid, astringent and protectant for use in conditions where gastrointestinal irritation exists
Gastrointestinal agent	Aluminum hydroxide gel (*U.S.P.*) Sig.: 5 to 10 cc. q 2-4 h.	240.0	Used in treatment of peptic ulcers; also for relief of symptomatic hyperacidity
Gastrointestinal agent	Pentobarbital sodium (*U.S.P.*) Belladonna extract (*N.F.*) M.ft. Capsules No. 20 Sig.: Cap. 1 t.i.d.	0|3 0|2	Used in treatment of spastic states of gastrointestinal, biliary and urinary tracts
Bronchial anti-asthmatic	Aminophylline (*U.S.P.*) Dried aluminum hydroxide gel (*U.S.P.*) Phenobarbital (*U.S.P.*) D.T.D. No. 15 Sig.: Give 1 tab. daily	0|1 0|15 0|015	Used to treat asthma, ascites, edema and cardiac dyspnea
Tranquilizer	Chlorpromazine HCl Tablets (*U.S.P.*) Mitte No. XII Sig.: Tab. 1 q 12 h.	25 mg.	For use in treatment of hysteria, car sickness and vomiting

TABLE 12-5 *(Continued)*

MEDICAL CATEGORY	PRESCRIPTION		REMARKS
Tranquilizer-corticosteroid	Prednisolone *(U.S.P.)* Hydroxyzine HCl *(N.F.)* M.ft. Cap. No. 1 Mitte No. 12 Sig.: Cap. 1 b.i.d. for 3 days; then 1 daily	5 mg. 10 mg.	Used in treating a variety of allergic conditions complicated by anxiety and tension; e.g., chronic urticaria, keratitis, pruritus, kennel cough, eczemas and keratoconjunctivitis
Ophthalmic preparation	Hydrocortisone acetate *(U.S.P.)* Neomycin sulfate *(U.S.P.)* Benzalkonium chloride Phenacaine HCl *(N.F.)* Hydrophilic petrolatum *(U.S.P.)* q.s.ad (Dispense in ophthalmic tube) Sig.: Apply o.u. b.i.d.	1% 0.5% 1:5000 1% 15.0	For treatment of ocular inflammation and infection
Muscle relaxant	Mephenesin Tablets *(N.F.)* #21 Sig.: Give one t.i.d.	500 mg.	For treatment of spastic conditions associated with disease or injury to a joint; also used in chorea, arthritis and strychnine poisoning

REFERENCES

1. An Abstract of Laws, Opinions and Decisions Relating to Podiatry, Am. Podiat. Ass., p. 84a, 1968.
2. *Ibid.,* p. 91.
3. American Dental Directory, p. 3, Chicago, American Dental Association, 1967.
4. Annual Report on Dental Education 1967-68, Part I, p. 3, Chicago, American Dental Association and American Association of Dental Schools, 1968.
5. Council of Dent. Ed., J.A.D.A., 78: 970, 1969.
6. Blauch, L. E.: J. Amer. Pod. Assn., 55: 204, 1965.
7. Brewster, R. E.: Careers in Osteopathy, Guidance Leaflet No. 23, p. 8, Washington, D.C., U.S. Government Printing Office, 1961.
8. Bureau Report: Summary of survey of dental practice, J.A.D.A. 79:1447, 1969.
9. Burlage, H. M., Lee, C. O., and Rising, L. W.: Orientation to Pharmacy, p. 271, New York, McGraw-Hill, 1959.
10. Deno, R. A., Rowe, T. D., and Brodie, D. C.: The Profession of Pharmacy, p. 9, Philadelphia, J. B. Lippincott, 1959.
11. Flexner, A.: Medical Education in the United States and Canada, p. 3, New York, The Carnegie Foundation for the Advancement of Teaching, 1910.
12. Furr, W. B.: Private communication, August, 1968.
13. Furr, W. B., and Furr, E. B.: Private communication, June, 1962.
14. Green, J. M.: The Heart of Homeopathy, p. 24, Washington, D.C., American Foundation for Homeopathy, 1961.
15. *Ibid,* p. 4.
16. Health Manpower Act of 1968, p. 152, Washington, D.C., U.S. Government Printing Office, 1968.
17. *Ibid.,* p. 180.
18. Hillenbrand, H.: Dentists will write 18 million ℞'s by 1970, A.P.P. 28:23, 1962.
19. Hockstein, E. S.: The role of the podiatrist in the Naval Service, J.A.P.A. 51: 488, 1961.
20. Hollinshead, B. S.: The Survey of Dentistry, p. 95, Washington, D.C., American Council on Education, 1961.
21. *Ibid.,* p. 239.
22. *Ibid.,* p. 241.
23. The Homeopathic Pharmacopeia, ed. 6, p. 33, Boston, American Institute of Homeopathy, 1941.
24. Information and Statistics Relating to Doctors of Osteopathy and Osteopathic Institutions, American Osteopathic Association, 1967.
25. Lavelle, M. B.: private communications, June and August, 1962.

26. Mason, H. R.: Private communication, May, 1968.
27. Medical Education in the United States, JAMA *202*:753, 1967.
28. *Ibid., 202*:778.
29. Mills, L. W.: Educational Supplement, J.A.O.A. *61*:393, 1962.
30. Mills, L. W.: Educational Supplement, J.A.O.A. *69*:485, 1970.
31. National Board Dental Examinations, p. 4, Chicago, American Dental Association, 1967.
32. National Formulary, ed. 10, p. 801, Washington, D.C., American Pharmaceutical Association, 1955.
33. National Formulary, ed. 12, p. 551, Washington, D.C., American Pharmaceutical Association, 1965.
34. National Prescription Audit, R. A. Gosselin and Company, 1966, p. 2.
35. 1970 Yearbook and Directory of Osteopathic Physicians, ed. 62, p. 25. Chicago, 1970. American Osteopathic Association.
36. Prescribing, Administering and Dispensing. Habits of the Osteopathic Physician, American Osteopathic Association, 1967.
37. Public Health Service Publication No. 1758, p. 41, Washington, D.C., U.S. Government Printing Office, October 1967.
38. *Ibid.,* p. 110.
39. Report of Committee on Government Operations, Veterinary Medical Science and Human Health, p. 159, Washington,

D.C., U.S. Government Printing Office, 1961.
40. Report of the National Advisory Commission on Health Manpower, Vol. I, p. 17. Washington, D.C., U.S. Government Printing Office, November, 1967.
41. Report of the National Advisory Commission on Health Manpower, Vol. II, p. 502, Washington, D.C., U.S. Government Printing Office, November, 1967.
42. Rubin, A.: Desk Reference, p. 14, Washington, D.C., A.P.A., 1968.
43. Rubin, A.: Desk Reference and Directory, p. 87, Washington, D.C., A.P.A., 1962.
44. Stephenson, H. C., and Mittelstaedt, S. G.: Veterinary Drug Encyclopedia and Therapeutic Index, ed. 9, p. 7, New York City, R. H. Donnelley Corp., 1961.
45. The 1965 Survey of Dental Practice, p. 26, Chicago, American Dental Association, 1966.
46. Therapeutic Agents for Dental Medicine/ Surgery, p. 18, Bloomfield, New Jersey, Schering Corporation, 1961.
47. *Ibid.,* p. 18.
48. *Ibid.,* p. 29.
49. Therapeutic Agents Useful in Dentistry, p. 4, Indianapolis, Eli Lilly and Co., 1961.
50. *Ibid.,* p. 11.
51. *Ibid.,* p. 21.
52. *Ibid.,* p. 26.
53. Todd, F. A.: Private communication, April, 1970.

Chapter 13

Prescription Accessories and Related Items

Walter Singer, Ph.D.[*]

The term *prescription accessories* was coined in 1949 to categorize a wide variety of nondrug items that are needed for the home care of the ill or convalescent patient.[6] Other designations that have been used for these and related items include medicinal adjuncts, sick-room supplies, convalescent aids, home health care supplies, home comfort aids and surgical supplies. Although prescription orders usually are not essential for legal dispensing, physicians do, on occasion, write specifications for wheelchairs, surgical supports and other devices in a form related to that used to prescribe drugs.

Recent reports[26,27,79,92,147,148] have pointed out economic and professional advantages for the pharmacist who establishes a prescription accessory department. Several[117,141,147,149] provide useful detail about inventory, sources of supply, rental forms and charges, promotion, proper delivery service and effective display within the pharmacy. A recent survey[24] shows that at the end of 1966, there were 22,911 pharmacies with convalescent aid departments; 5,659 of these were installed during 1966 and 12,876 of those already operating were enlarged during the same year. The considerable increase in sales over a 6-year period is shown in Table 13-1. Spectacular increases[32] are projected on the basis of future greater numbers in the 65 and older group and in the crippled/handicapped population. The shortening of the average stay in the hospital to less than 7 days means longer convalescence at home. Medicare is expected to cause a critical shortage of hospital and nursing home beds, resulting in more home care. That Medicare will pay, wholly or in part, for prescription accessories will certainly be a factor.

The dominant position of the pharmacist as a supplier is shown by the high percentage of total sales that continues to be made in pharmacies (Table 13-1). Clearly, society has delegated to the pharmacist the prime responsibility for informing the lay person or the prescriber when there is need for appliances or supplies to ensure correct use of medicaments, to provide desirable correlative care of the sick individual or to enhance his comfort. The pharmacist is expected to advise intelligently in the choice of a suitable accessory from among a variety of competitive products that are not necessarily equivalent. He must warn against dangers of misuse, as well as inform about correct use, maintenance and storage. The role of the pharmacist in this respect is underscored by the continued refusal of Congress to pass the FDA-supported Medical Device Safety Act. This act[31] would give the FDA authority to apply safety, reliability and effectiveness provisions to medical devices, surgical instruments, artificial organs and limbs, therapeutic instruments and devices, and other medical and hospital equipment before they are marketed, just as it does with drugs through its new drug regulations. Currently the FDA can remove from the market only devices that it can prove in court to be unsafe or mislabeled. Such belated action gives the unscrupulous a great opportunity to take advantage of the uninformed.

* Professor of Pharmacy and Dean, Albany College of Pharmacy, Albany, N.Y.

TABLE 13-1. SALES OF PRESCRIPTION ACCESSORIES IN PHARMACIES

ACCESSORY	SALES IN PHARMACIES (ADD 000)		PHARMACY % OF TOTAL SALES	
	1968*	1962†	1968*	1962†
Suspensories	$ 1,220	$ 1,190	90	92
Medicated plasters	3,440	4,100	90	91
Medical atomizers	1,100	1,500	89	90
Vaporizers	9,700	10,680	84	86
Eyecups, enamelware, etc.	1,550	1,830	81	82
Flat goods, water bottles, etc.	11,410	10,000	77	77
Ice bags, icecaps	1,060	880	73	73
Feminine bulb syringes	2,230	1,750	77	75
Infant bulb syringes	4,870	4,310	72	74
Folding syringes	7,000	4,330	73	71
Heating pads	16,350	13,000	66	67
Men's supporter belts	2,890	2,440	67	66
First-aid supplies	122,070	98,560	55	57
Other elastic goods	9,600	7,730	50	52
Trusses	4,810	3,670	49	49
Heat lamps	2,680	2,060	37	40
Fever thermometers	10,680	9,760	34	40
Athletic supporters	4,590	3,530	35	36
Invalid rings	790	820	35	34
Abdominal belts	2,810	2,320	28	29
Elastic stockings	8,430	6,380	23	22
Crutch tips, pads	960	800	18	19
Colostomy appliances, urinals	510	590	18	18

*Data from Leibson, R. A.: How drugstores scored on 340 product lines. Drug Topics *113*:29, Sept. 1969.

†Data from Olsen, P. C.: What customers spent for all products sold in drug stores, Drug Topics *107*:6, July 15, 1963; Olsen, P. C.: Pharmacies up five million dollars in first aid sales, Drug Topics *107*:40, July 1, 1963.

This chapter is oriented toward supplying basic and specialized information about properties and uses of prescription accessories to assist the pharmacist in meeting these multiple responsibilities now and in the future. Obviously, a suitable internship under a preceptor possessing knowledge in this area is a desirable complement to the discussions presented here. The choice of accessories to be discussed has been governed by several factors. Some devices deserve mention because of their widespread use. Most attention is given to devices whose complexity in design or use leads to opportunity for a professional service. Others, such as surgical appliances and hearing aids, require training in fitting or adjusting to the degree that quite extensive course work at specialized schools is almost mandatory to obtain sufficient useful information. These are discussed only briefly.

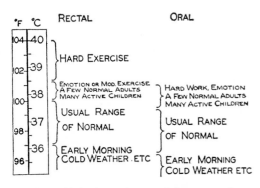

FIG. 13-1. An estimate of the ranges in body temperature found in normal persons. (From DuBois, E. F.: Fever and the Regulation of Body Temperature. Springfield, Ill., Charles C Thomas, 1948)

CLINICAL THERMOMETERS

Body temperature is commonly assumed to remain at so constant a level in health that a deviation from the limits of the accepted normal range is regarded by the physician and the layman as diagnostic of body malfunction. Fallacies in this concept have been pointed out.[120] A satisfactory approximation of the temperature of the internal organs can be made by insertion of a suitable thermometer into either the mouth or the rectum, these being closed cavities with fairly large blood vessels. Studies[11] of large samples of normal individuals have shown oral temperatures to range from 97.0 to 100.4° F. with 98.6° F. popularly accepted as average (Fig. 13-1). A diurnal variation of nearly 2° F. may occur with lowest temperatures during minimal activity between 2 and 6 A.M. and highest at active periods in the afternoon.[87] Rectal temperatures are said to be 1° F. higher than oral temperatures, although differences of only 0.7 to 0.9° F. are frequently encountered.[172] Values above 99.4° F. orally and 100.3° F. rectally are considered febrile, with perhaps 5 per cent chance of error in this respect.[11] Fever may have an emotional component, but, more frequently, elevation

of body temperature above normal is caused by an infectious process, inflammation of an area, brain injury, dehydration or certain drugs.[18]

Temperatures below 96.6° are considered subnormal. Malnutrition, shock, excessive perspiration or prolonged exposure to cold may lead to low body temperatures. Although the exact mechanisms by which changed levels of body temperature are produced and maintained are not known, such shifts are said to be due to "resetting the hypothalamic thermostat."[168] Physiologic aspects of body temperature, temperature regulation and fever have recently been well reviewed.[57,109] Body temperatures under different conditions are illustrated in Figure 13-2.

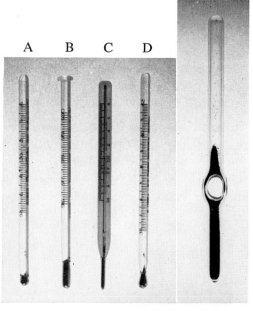

FIG. 13-3. (Left) Types of clinical thermometers. A. Security bulb. B. Basal thermometer with nailhead stem. C. Oral bulb, flat-type stem. D. Rectal bulb, centigrade scale. (Right) A model of the constriction chamber of a clinical thermometer. Powdered iron (appearing black) is used to represent the mercury. The central depression or "air bubble" is made by collapsing the heated wall of the stem so as to obliterate the center of the lumen. The openings around the depression are about 0.0006" in diameter in the clinical thermometer.

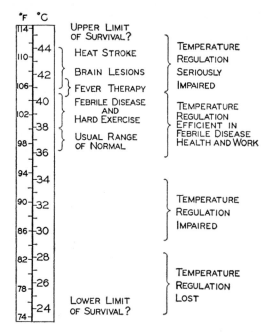

FIG. 13-2. Extremes of human body temperature with an attempt to define the zones of temperature regulation. (From DuBois, E. F.: Fever and the Regulation of Body Temperature. Springfield, Ill., Charles C Thomas, 1948)

Characteristics and Manufacture of Thermometers. The expert design of the clinical or fever thermometer (Fig. 13-3, *left*), which permits measurement of temperature with ease and accuracy, often is not appreciated by either the user or the pharmacist. The length is short enough to be supported in the mouth or the rectum without difficulty and to be easily carried about or stored, yet its scale may span as much as 18° F. In order to obtain maximum linear movement of the mercury with small changes in temperature, the thermometer bulb is made quite large, whereas the diameter of the stem capillary is only about 0.001 to 0.004 inches, approximately one tenth that of the human hair.[67] The stem tubing is triangular in cross-section, forming a prism so that the column of mercury is magnified as the user looks at it through the apex. Visibility is enhanced by the background furnished by an opaque strip of glass fused along the base of the triangle. Since the scale is not easily seen while the thermometer is still inserted orally or rectally, it is necessary to arrange to make the mercury column remain at its highest point even after the thermometer is returned to room temperature. This self-registering feature is provided by a small constriction chamber (Fig. 13-3, *right*) formed in the capillary about ½ inch above the juncture of the stem and the bulb. The heated expanding mercury must force its way through the two tiny openings that penetrate the chamber, but, as contraction of the mercury into the bulb starts on cooling, these thin columns of mercury break at the constriction, leaving the column level unchanged in the stem above. After the reading is taken, the mercury may be forced back down the stem by shaking the thermometer vigorously.

Oral, rectal and security (stubby) bulbs are available (Fig. 13-3). The oral bulb is cylindrical, elongated, and thin-walled for quick registration. The rectal bulb has a strong, blunt, pear shape, which aids in insertion into the rectum and retention by sphincter muscles. The short sturdy security bulb represents a compromise intermediate shape suited to either oral or rectal use. Acceptance of this bulb has increased markedly in recent years as the pharmacist has made known to the public its advantages of dual use and resistance to breakage.

Clinical thermometers are not machine-made. Glass blowers form each bulb individually and then join bulbs and stems in one of the first of many operations involved in producing a finished thermometer.[9,67,182] Exact reproducibility in size and shape of bulb is not possible in such handwork. Consequently each thermometer is unpredictably unique in the amount of mercury it contains. Each must have its scale determined individually by calibration. Thus, two thermometers, even though identified by the same catalog number and sold as equivalent, may have scale lengths and upper and lower limits that differ. Immersion in water baths thermostated to maintain known temperatures establishes the mercury levels for the scale limits of a given thermometer. "Pointing" machines automatically space and draw in intermediate scale markings on the waxcoated stem, which can then be etched by immersion in hydrofluoric acid. Suitable pigments are painted into the scale marks to increase visibility. The Fahrenheit scale is commonly used in this country, but many manufacturers make at least some of their styles available optionally with the Centigrade scale.

"Hard shakers" with too narrow constrictions and "retreaters" with too wide apertures are detected by appropriate tests and are discarded by reliable manufacturers. Thermometers are then stored in "seasoning vaults" for 4 to 6 months to allow the glass to achieve molecular stability. After this aging, the accuracy of calibration is rechecked in thermostated tanks before release for distribution. Some manufacturers season their thermometers before etching in the scale. Accelerated aging by heat treatment also is now practiced.[67] Minimum requirements for clinical thermometers have been developed by cooperative efforts of manufacturers, distributors and users along with the U. S. Department of Commerce. These are set forth in Commercial Standard 1-52 (CS1-52).* A revised standard should be available in 1970. Proposals include a new requirement that each thermometer be marked with a

* Available from the Superintendent of Documents, Government Printing Office, Washington, D.C.

serial number or code designation to indicate the date of calibration within 30 days. A certification that CS1-52 standards have been met or surpassed is packaged with each thermometer. Some may also certify to compliance with additional mandatory qualitative standards imposed by Massachusetts, Connecticut or Michigan. These thermometers bear an authorized seal-mark (MASS., CONN. or MICH.).

Accuracy of Thermometers. Because decisions as to therapeutic regimens to follow may be based on the presence or the absence of a few tenths of a degree of temperature, accuracy in a clinical thermometer is an obvious requirement. Rough checks of one thermometer against another may enable the pharmacist or user to detect gross variations, but precise determinations of accuracy are possible only in laboratories with special control equipment.

In a large study, 540 thermometers made by different manufacturers were selected at random from pharmacies at various widespread points in this country and compared by accepted technics with the accuracy limits prescribed by CS1-52, which all were certified to meet.[108] Almost 18 per cent exceeded the allowable error. For two brands, characterized as "of foreign manufacture" and as "promotional items," standards were not met, in one case, by 28 per cent (of 144 samples), and in the other, by 35 per cent (of 62 samples). In another study[17] nearly 20 per cent of 625 samples from 11 major companies failed to meet CS1-52 requirements. The

company with the best record had 95 per cent of its thermometers within accepted limits; one had only 36 per cent. Because companies are rated by name in the report, this study could serve as a purchasing guide for the pharmacist.

Clinical thermometers are relatively fragile. Many are shattered when dropped while they are being handled or shaken. Bulbs are broken by rinsing them with hot water. Less obvious and more dangerous are subtle changes in the constriction chamber; "retreaters," in which the level of the column drops before the reading is taken, can result from slight jarring. Decreases in accuracy may develop in improperly aged instruments. Separations may occur in the mercury column.* Figure 13-4 presents the results of a test of accuracy of 465 thermometers of a variety of brands and styles which were in actual use in a large general hospital.[82] If one assumes accuracy at end of manufacture, rigors of usage had evidently seriously damaged many of these thermometers. Retreaters, hard shakers, defective pigmentation and mercury separation also were found. It is probable that a large proportion of thermometers that are currently depended on for home use have been rendered similarly defective.

Use and Maintenance of Thermometers. Many manufacturers supply more or less detailed directions for use and maintenance with each thermometer packaged for individual sale. Additional instructive leaflets are available and helpful.[94] The pharmacist must be prepared to illustrate and supplement this information. He might proceed along the following lines, tailoring his approach according to the situation.

The pharmacist should advise as to the choice of bulb. Many laymen do not know there are different bulbs, let alone that one may have advantages of strength or sensitivity over another. This is also an opportunity to warn against rectal use of oral bulbs. The thermometer should be removed from its case and inspected in the presence of the purchaser to be sure that it is intact and that the bulb is of the type marked on the outside of

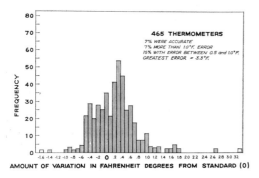

FIG. 13-4. Accuracy of thermometers in use in a hospital. (From Dimond, E. G., and Andrews, M. H.: Clinical thermometers and urinometers. J.A.M.A., *156*: 125, 1954)

* Take hold of the bulb end and shake toward the top, then reverse and shake toward the bulb. This should mend the break unless other damage has been done to the thermometer.

the package. Identification and explanation of the constriction chamber (the "air bubble") may prevent return of an irate client with the mistaken claim that he was given a faulty instrument. Holding the bulb for a few moments will make the mercury rise enough to permit a demonstration of how to read a thermometer. This will also illustrate why the bulb should not be held when a reading is being made. The pharmacist should instruct the client to: stand with back to light; hold the end opposite the bulb between the thumb and index finger of one hand and support the thermometer with the other hand, being careful not to touch the bulb; look down at the apex of the triangle toward the engraved scale and rotate the thermometer slightly back and forth until the mercury column appears at maximum width; locate the top of the column with respect to the scale reading. The pharmacist must explain the scale markings. While the major degree lines are easily interpreted, the fact that each of the four intermediate graduations represents 0.2° F. is not always clear to the user. If the individual finds it difficult to see the mercury column, the pharmacist should suggest a style especially modified for easier reading. Thermometers with flat stems, colored backgrounds in the stem, or glass balls that appear blue only when the column is in position to be read fall into this category.

The shaking down of the column should be demonstrated: hold the nonbulb end between thumb and index finger and swing arm down ending with a snap of the wrist as though shaking water off the fingers. The layman should be warned against trying to shake down a thermometer by jarring the hand against a solid object; this may damage the constriction. Suggest that shaking down the thermometer be done over a bed as protection in case it slips from the fingers. If a client seems apprehensive about this, demonstrate a style with a whirling device in which centrifugal force is utilized to carry down the mercury (Fig. 13-5).

Other information the pharmacist may wish to volunteer is found in recommended procedures for the use and maintenance of thermometers. Temperatures should not be taken for 20 to 30 minutes after drinking, eating, smoking or exercise, because such ac-

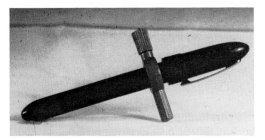

FIG. 13-5. Thermometer case with whirling attachment

tivities may raise body temperature (or lower it, in the case of cold drinks). Always be sure the column of mercury is at 97° F. or less before inserting the thermometer. For oral temperatures, the bulb (oral or security) should be moistened with cool tap water and placed under the rear edge of the tongue and rotated two or three times. The tongue should be held down and the lips should be closed gently over the stem Breathing should be nasal to avoid entry of air into the mouth. The individual should remain at rest. The reading should be taken after 3 minutes. The thermometer should be replaced in the mouth for another minute, and reread. This is repeated until two consecutive readings agree. Nichols et al.[172] have shown that it may take as long as 10 to 12 minutes to register maximum oral temperature in afebrile adults; 7 minutes is the minimum time suggested. A similar study[170] with afebrile children suggests 10 minutes is generally needed to allow the orally placed thermometer to reflect body temperature for youngsters 7 to 12 years of age. After 4 minutes, only 10 per cent of the 40 children tested had reached their maximum temperature. Kravitz,[135] however, claimed equilibration for oral temperatures (i.e., no change in three consecutive readings) occurred in 3 to 4 minutes. After the final reading, the thermometer is shaken down, and then cleaned and disinfected as described on page 485.

For rectal temperatures, the bulb (rectal or security) and the lower portion of the stem should first be lubricated for ease of insertion. In order of preference (for reasons of adverse influence on disinfection),[216] the lubricants to use are a water-soluble jelly,*

* K-Y Jelly, Johnson and Johnson, New Brunswick, N.J.

mineral oil or petrolatum. The thermometer is inserted gently and pushed with a minimum of force until the 98.6° F. mark passes the anal opening. About half the stem will now protrude. Studies by Nichols *et al.*[172] and Kravitz[135] indicate that 2 to 4 minutes should be ample time for registering maximum rectal temperature in adults or children. Longer insertion times may be required if the thermometer is cold or if the patient has poor circulation. An adult is probably most comfortable lying on his side. Babies should be held face down, perhaps across the knees, and the thermometer supported between the fingers throught the entire period. The thermometer is removed, wiped with cleansing tissue with the direction of motion being from the stem down over the bulb end and then read. Rectal thermometers are marked—by custom, apparently—to indicate 98.6° F. as "normal," although, as previously pointed out, normal rectal temperature may be 99.6° F. For the sake of clarity, both the actual temperature as read and the manner of taking the temperature should be reported to the physician.

It is thought that rectal injury by thermometer is common though rarely serious.[137,198] Wolfson[246] reported the death of a 10-day-old child following the jamming of a thermometer through the rectal wall, a subsequent barium enema examination and a laparotomy. Symptoms of traumatic intraperitoneal perforation of the rectum are immediate onset of severe abdominal pain, meteorism, restlessness, perhaps vomiting and hemorrhage, and not infrequently shock and peritonitis. Prophylaxis appears to be the only course. The rectal thermometer must be inserted carefully and correctly, and a small child or debilitated person should not be left unattended while his temperature is being taken.

Because of recognized inexactitudes, axillary or groin temperatures are taken only when neither the mouth nor the rectum can be used.[231] An oral or a security bulb is used. The axilla is wiped dry, the thermometer is placed in the axilla, and the arm is held close to the body to make as closed a cavity as possible. An enclosed space for the thermometer can be made in the groin by flexing the thigh on the abdomen. At least 10 minutes should elapse before the reading is made.[171]

An axillary or groin temperature is usually 1° F. lower than the oral, so 97.6° F. would be normal.

The temperature of the umbilicus has been measured[135] in an attempt to find another useful way to ascertain a normal body temperature. The dry bulb of an ordinary clinical thermometer (bulb type not identified) was inserted into the deepest recess of the umbilicus and the skin of the adjacent abdominal wall was compressed to cover and to seal off the bulb as much as possible. Readings stabilized in 3 to 5 minutes. Umbilical temperatures were lower than rectal and oral temperatures measured simultaneously. The differences were: in babies under 3 months, rectal temperatures averaged 0.54° F. higher, oral temperatures 0.20° F. higher; in older infants and children rectal temperatures averaged 0.85 to 0.97° F. higher and oral temperatures 0.62° F. higher. The method appears to have merit because it is safer than the rectal and more accurate than the axillary or groin procedure.

The Basal Thermometer. The basal thermometer is a specialized instrument helpful in estimating time of ovulation. Because it is probable that fertilization can occur only within the first 24 hours after release of the ovum from the graafian follicle, accurate knowledge of the occurrence of this event would permit timing of intercourse so as either to increase or to decrease the possibility of conception. Ovulation occurs once during each normal menstrual cycle, approximately 14 days before the next menstrual period. Basal temperature—the lowest temperature reached by the body of a normal healthy person while awake—typically passes through a biphasic cycle over the course of the menstrual cycle.[211] The temperature is initially low; a mid-cycle thermal shift occurs to a high level, where the temperature remains until it once again becomes low premenstrually (Fig. 13-6). The temperature rise indicates that ovulation has occurred 1 or 2 days before, will occur 1 or 2 days after, or is occurring at the moment of the temperature rise.[62] The temperature rise is said to be related to the presence of progesterone or some combination of progesterone and estrogen in the systemic circulation.[38,62] In spite of the lack of definitude, which has led some physi-

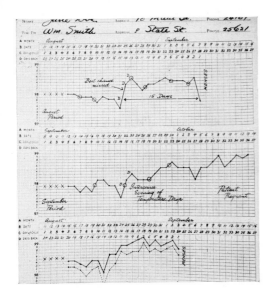

FIG. 13-6. Records of basal temperature.

cians to consider the method quite limited,[85, 211] others consider it reliable.[38,129,237]

An ordinary fever thermometer is not very satisfactory for measuring the small temperature rise of about 0.5° F. that is related to ovulation. The basal thermometer (Fig. 13-3) is easier to read, because its scale, ranging only from 96° F. to 100° F., is graduated to 0.1° F. rather than to 0.2° F. The bulb resembles an elongated security type. The proposed revision of CS1-52 adds specifications for basal thermometers. Temperature is taken either orally or rectally, once daily, immediately on awakening in the morning and before getting out of bed. Explicit directions and charts for recording these daily measurements are provided with the thermometer. Because each woman varies to some extent in her physical characteristics, each must determine her own menstrual rhythm by keeping this record for 3 or 4 months. Consultation with a physician is essential for proper interpretation of the chart.

Cleaning and Disinfecting Thermometers. The clinical thermometer should always be cleaned and disinfected after use to minimize the transfer of pathogens. The proper procedure for doing this has been the subject of numerous investigations.[102,173,215,216,248] Consideration of these reports leads to the fol-

lowing suggestions. After oral use, the thermometer should be wiped thoroughly with clean cotton wet with a solution of equal parts of tincture of green soap and water.* Wiping should start on the stem and proceed toward the bulb. After rinsing with cold running water, the thermometer should be immersed at least halfway up the stem for 10 to 15 minutes in a solution of 0.5 to 1.0 per cent iodine in 70 per cent alcohol, either ethyl or isopropyl. The 70 per cent alcohols without added iodine seem nearly as effective; so are aqueous solutions of 0.05 and 0.25 per cent iodine and 1.0 per cent potassium iodide.[215] A 0.1 per cent tincture of benzalkonium chloride has been found effective against the usual oral pathogens, whereas an aqueous 0.1 per cent solution was not.[248] Neither was reliable against the tubercle bacillus.[215,248] Certain synthetic phenolic disinfectants are useful in 2 or 3 per cent concentration.[248] Other strengths of alcohols—50, 95 or 100 per cent ethyl alcohol and 99 per cent isopropyl—are reported ineffective, as are certain iodophors containing 200 ppm available iodine solubilized with nonionic detergents. After suitable disinfection, the thermometer should be rinsed with cold water and wiped dry with clean cotton or tissue. Some suggest that a similar procedure should be followed immediately before use as well as after. Continued immersion in antiseptic solution is not recommended, because this may damage scale pigments. After rectal use, the thermometer should be wiped with dry, clean tissue to remove most of the fecal matter and the lubricant before reading it. The the same disinfection procedure can be followed because rectal pathogens are susceptible to it.[216] Greasy lubricants such as petrolatum and mineral oil interfere with disinfection.[216]

House and Henderson[121] have pointed out the impracticality of suggested disinfection methods for physicians on house calls. Over a 4½ year period (157 cases), they showed that it was adequate to thoroughly wipe a pathogen-carrying thermometer with cotton-

* In place of water, 95 per cent ethyl alcohol has been recommended for admixture here,[215] but the slight increase in effectiveness does not justify the added expense.

wool soaked in a suitable disinfectant. Among the satisfactory agents were 70 per cent ethyl alcohol, 1 per cent aqueous benzalkonium chloride and 0.5 per cent chlorhexidine in alcohol. Soap and water were ineffective.

Thermometer Cases and Accessories. A hard rubber or a plastic case resembling a fountain pen is usually furnished so that the thermometer may be stored safely. The case may or may not have an external clip for pocket use. Typically, there is an inner spring that grips the thermometer to keep it from striking the sides or falling out. Some cases are leakproof so that the thermometer can be stored in antiseptic solution. This may be justified in spite of damage to scale pigments when there is an extreme possibility of the transfer of infectious organisms, as in a series of house calls by physicians. Whirling devices are attached to some cases to help in shaking down the thermometers (see Fig. 13-5). An automatic battery-operated thermometer shaker that utilizes centrifugal forces developed by rotation is also marketed.* Elaboration in design of cases may add to the cost of the thermometer without real gain to the patient. The pharmacist and the user should avoid storing the thermometer near heat or in sunlight.

It is quite possible that the home into which the clinical thermometer is being taken may lack any or all of the following adjuncts to its effective use and maintenance: properly labeled disinfectant solution, cotton balls, tissues, tincture of green soap and a water-soluble lubricant. The pharmacist who is alert to his responsibilities for service will keep a supply of these items near his thermometers and will advise the need for them when it seems appropriate to do so.

Thermometers Broken in Situ. Clinical thermometers are frequently broken in situ, especially in the mouths of children. This immediately arouses concern, and advice is often sought from the pharmacist. Mehnert[155] surveyed the medical literature and commented on his failure to find a single report other than his own of serious injury related to the breakage of a thermometer in the mouth. In the case cited, the broken bulb

(rectal) had not been recovered after the accident. More than 2 years later, it was discovered that the tip had penetrated the hilum of the submaxillary gland. The released mercury had gravitated into the gland and also under the skin of the neck. Investigation of the cause of the pain and the tumor-like appearance of the region led to its discovery. Johnson and Koumides[128] reviewed the literature on metallic mercury poisoning for the past 70 years and reported a fatal case of suicidal self-injection of mercury. Metallic mercury is not dissolved appreciably if at all in the gastrointestinal tract. Little absorption occurs, even though the mercury may become dispersed in very fine droplets throughout the intestine.[10,65] Lack of toxicity is suggested by the once common oral administration of as much as 1 pound of mercury in the treatment of obstipation.[10,64] When a thermometer is broken in the mouth, primary concern should be directed toward the recovery of as much of the glass (and the mercury) as possible and stopping bleeding from cuts. It is advisable to give the white of egg as an antidote for mercury, perhaps thus erring on the side of caution. Soft bread to coat swallowed particles of glass to prevent damage to the intestines has been suggested. A physician should always be called. It may take as long as 14 days for all the mercury to leave the body in fecal matter.[10] Breakage of thermometers in the rectum seems less likely to occur and to involve snapping of stems rather than crushing of bulbs. Here the main problem is one of need for dexterity and care in removing the remnants of the thermometer. The inhalation hazard from mercury spilled from a broken thermometer is negligible.[60]

Electronic Thermometers. Temperature-sensing devices that react more quickly than do the usual mercury thermometers have been designed to permit measuring body temperature. Though expensive, the time saved may be enough to warrant suggesting their use in hospitals or physicians' offices. A thermocouple probe is inserted rectally, orally or into the axilla, and the body temperature is read on the machine dial in 7 to 30 seconds. The probe may be sterile and dispos-

* Ideal Easy-Shake, The Empire State Thermometer Co., Carlstadt, N.J.

able,* or it may be inserted into a disposable plastic shield for each use.† Accuracy to 0.2° F.* or to better than 0.25° F.† is claimed for these devices. Kravitz[135] has reported body temperature measurements using a thermocouple. It has been reported that temperatures taken at the eardrum with a thermocouple are more reliable indicators of a subject's condition than are rectal temperatures.[16]

RUBBER AND PLASTIC ACCESSORIES

A number of the devices designed to assist in making the sick more comfortable, in the irrigating of body cavities and the collecting of body secretions are made largely of rubber because this material is soft, tough, impermeable, easily formed and elastic—a unique combination of properties that only recently has been achieved in the synthesized elastomers, which can match rubber in most of these properties. The fascinating story of the introduction of rubber into European civilization and its subsequent growth to a position of top economic importance is recounted in detail in readily available encyclopedias.

PROPERTIES OF RUBBER

Natural rubber, an isoprene polymer $(C_5H_8)_n$, is obtained as an elastic solid from the latex (sap) of the rubber tree (*Hevea braziliensis*) or from similar sources. Latex‡ is a milky, sticky fluid containing about 35 per cent raw rubber (caoutchouc) as a colloidal aqueous suspension of globules. Latex concentrated to 60 per cent rubber and preserved with ammonia against spontaneous coagulation is itself commercially available. Alternatively, at the rubber plantation, a weak organic acid (formic or acetic) is added to latex to cause the rubber globules to come together to form a coagulum. The coagulum may be washed and rolled into thin sheets, which are dried in air to form a yellow-white crepe rubber. Sodium bisulfite is added during the processing to prevent browning due

* BTI Model 5000, Measurement Science Corporation, Brigham City, Utah.
† Office Electro-Temp, Electro-Medic, Inc., Neptune, N.J.
‡ An aqueous emulsion of synthetic rubber or of plastic is also called latex.

to oxidation. Sometimes the washed coagulum is rolled into heavy sheets, which are dried in hot smoke arising from burning wood. The smoke acts as a preservative and also turns the rubber brown. Latex, crepe rubber and smoked sheet seem to be ranked in this order of excellence as starting materials for rubber health goods.

The traditional production process for natural rubber has undergone modernization[22] in an effort to meet competition from synthetic elastomers. The current approach is to convert the rubber into a finely divided crumb form rather than into sheets. In the Hevacrumb process, castor oil (0.5 per cent) is used along with the acid to make the coagulum, which is then passed through three or four sets of creping rolls of decreasing gap widths to reduce the rubber to a fine crumb. The oil prevents the rubber crumbs from rejoining during milling. The crumbs are easily and quickly washed and dried, then automatically compressed into convenient sized bales and wrapped. The comminuted rubber processes make more effective purification possible, produce a rubber with more uniform properties and allow more scientific grading for quality.

Raw rubber has limited usefulness, since it softens and becomes sticky at summer temperatures while it is brittle at low temperatures. Also, it is dissolved by common organic liquids including gasoline. Cements, surgical adhesive tape, insulating tape and crepe soling are made from natural rubber. The principal treatment of rubber to improve its properties is vulcanization, i.e., heating with sulfur. Changes in properties with temperature are lessened and resistance to solvents is increased. Soft rubber contains 2 to 10 parts of sulfur, hard rubber 20 to 50 per cent. Accelerators such as thiuram sulfides, diphenylguanidine or other agents are added to speed up vulcanization. Materials such as zinc oxide, carbon black and clays are fillers added to modify stiffness, strength and resistance to abrasion and chemicals. Antioxidants—for example, phenyl-alpha or phenyl-beta naphthylamine—are needed to prevent deterioration. Solid pigments including lithopone and titanium dioxide, or soluble dyes of the phthalocyanine and the azo families are used to impart color. Proper choice of additives and suitable tailoring of the rubber for intended use are hidden aspects of quality which are difficult to evaluate in rubber health goods.

Plastics and synthetic rubbers have already replaced natural rubber in many uses[22,93] and are beginning to do so in the rubber health goods industry. The newly developed stereo-regulated elastomers such as polybutadiene and cis-polyisoprene may well be used when they become available in sufficient quantity. Excellent brief reviews of the nature and the properties of these materials have been published.[93,96,119] Neoprene, which is polymerized 2-chlorobutadiene-1,3, is used because it resists oil, sunlight and ozone deterioration. Plastics which make up part or all of a number of appliances are polyvinyl chloride, polystyrene, polyamide (Nylon) and polyethylene. Manufacturers use coined names for these plastics, often without otherwise identifying them in the descriptions of their products.

The Manufacture of Rubber Goods

The major steps in the manufacture of rubber goods are (1) the kneading of the warmed raw materials in specialized mixers until homogeneous; (2) the forming of the desired shape and (3) the curing, usually by heating. For purpose of description it is convenient to organize these items into groups according to the method of forming the shape, i.e., by molding, flattening into sheets or immersion of forms (mandrels) into fluid dispersions. This plan is deviated from (as in the case of elastic support items) where grouping according to a common therapeutic usage seems more fruitful. Also where apropos, nonrubber appliances are described.

Sheeting Goods

Sheeting may be made by forcing rubber mixtures to pass between heated rollers (calenders). Hospital film, a thin (.004 to .008 inches) transparent sheeting made by calendering, can be used to make pillow covers and the like, since it is readily cut to size and the cut ends can be sealed together with a hot iron. Dam is a similarly formed but thicker (approximately .015 inch) sheeting. Since it is used as an occlusive covering over wound dressings, dam is available in standardized widths and lengths with attached tie tapes.

Sheeting may also have a fabric base. The fabric, usually cotton, may be coated by the Macintosh process in which a naphtha solution of rubber is applied to the surface. A thinner sheeting known as rubberized voile is made by polymerizing neoprene within the meshes of the cloth. These supported and, therefore, stronger sheetings are used to make protective garments and protective coverings for mattresses.

Plastics, especially polyvinyl chlorides (Koroseal, Zonas), are used as sheeting materials because they have less odor and greater resistance to tearing than rubber. They also seem cooler to lie on. Unsupported sheeting of both film and dam thicknesses as well as the fabric type are available in rolls 36 to 54 inches wide and 25 or 50 yards long.

Rubber sheeting can be laundered with warm water and mild soap. It can be disinfected and odors removed with saponated cresol solution or formaldehyde solution. Autoclaving for not more than 20 minutes or immersion in boiling water for not more than 15 are also safe, especially if followed by a 12-hour period of nonuse to allow loss of absorbed water. Sheeting should not be folded sharply or wadded. It "fatigues" or loses its strength along creases formed from repeated folding, so it is recommended that sheeting be rolled rather than folded for storage.

Molded Goods

Water Bottles and Syringes. Water bottles, fountain syringes and combination syringe-water bottles are flat bags, essentially rectangular in shape (Fig. 13-7), all of which are molded in about the same way. Two pieces are cut from a sheet of heavy compounded rubber and placed against the inner faces of a two-piece mold. The mold is closed tightly and compressed air is admitted to keep the inner surfaces of the bag from sticking together while the mold is being heated to fuse the edges and to cure the rubber. The seam is usually covered and reinforced by cementing or fusing a thin strip of sheeting over it. The neck of a water bottle or a combination syringe has a threaded metal (usually brass) collar. The collar may be molded in as a part of the original operation or it

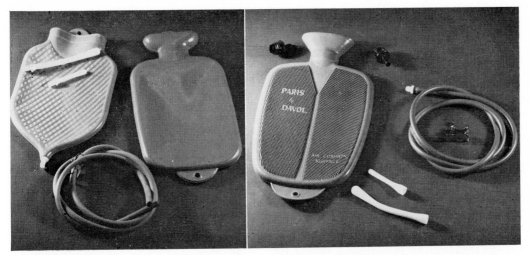

FIG. 13-7. (*Left*) Fountain syringe and water bottle. Slip-type pipes are shown; the larger is a vaginal tip, the smaller is an adult rectal tip. The shut-off on the tubing is the spring type. (*Right*) Combination syringe-water bottle. Screw-type pipes and a lever shut-off are shown. The water bottle stopple is lying at the left and the hollow syringe stopper at the right of the neck.

may be incorporated separately into a hard rubber ring which is cemented into the neck later. A hard rubber or a plastic stopple of standardized shape and thread is provided to close the bag. The combination syringe has in addition a specialized hollow stopper terminating in a short pipe to which tubing can be attached. The neck of the fountain syringe cannot be closed off and instead may be widened or funnel-shaped to make it easier to pour water into it. The base of the fountain syringe has a hard rubber or plastic outlet to which tubing may be attached. Accessories to the fountain and the combination syringe include tubing, a shut-off and tips or pipes (Fig. 13-7).

Most companies make three or four grades of quality in these articles. Cheaper bottles may be thinner walled and contain lower grade rubber with large amounts of mineral filler or of reclaimed rubber, making them less elastic and shorter-lived. Weight is not necessarily an indication of quality. Tubing is usually about 9/32 of an inch in internal diameter and 5 feet or slightly less in length but varies significantly in quality. Less expensive syringes have a simple spring or snap shutoff to stop flow through the tubing, while better ones have a more efficient and more easily operated lever type. Either two or three tips are furnished; there is usually a vaginal irrigator and an adult rectal and sometimes an infant rectal. These may be hard rubber, vinyl or nylon. Slip types which slide into the tubing are cheaper and more likely to allow leakage than the screw-on type. The packaging may become progressively more elaborate as the cost of the item increases. A guarantee against defective workmanship or material is given for periods of time which progress from 1 or 2 years up to 5 years for the more expensive bottles and syringes. While the pharmacist can readily point out quality differences to a prospective user when he is comparing items made by one company, it is more difficult to make a logical choice between equally priced items made by competitive suppliers. It is probable that significant differences do not exist.

Water bottles ordinarily are used as a means of applying dry heat to a limited body area in order to induce vasodilation and leukocytosis, relax muscles and connective tissue or hasten suppuration.[112] Reflex relief of congestion in internal organs may result. Hot moist applications are more effective for promoting drainage from wounds and skin lesions. Heat is contraindicated[112] when vasodilation will increase pain as in a swollen sprained ankle or an infected tooth. Heat should not be applied when it would be dangerous to hasten a suppurative process (as in appendicitis).

Because the water bottle seems to be such a simple device, the user may be unaware that there is a correct way to use it for maximum benefit with minimum danger. The water should be heated to 120° to 130° F. for an adult or to 110° to 120° F. for a child or an unconscious or an elderly person. The heated water should be placed in a pitcher and adjusted to temperature with a suitable thermometer before pouring it into the water bottle. The pharmacist may find it difficult to justify purchase of a thermometer along with a water bottle for short-term use. As an expedient he may suggest testing the water by hand; it should be uncomfortably hot but not unbearably so. Hot water from the tap may be over 140° F. and should not be run directly into the bag. The bottle should first be filled with hot water, stoppered and tested for leaks by applying pressure. The warmed bag should be emptied and then filled only to one half or three quarters of its capacity. A completely filled bag is uncomfortably heavy against the patient and, also, is unable to conform to body contours. Repeatedly filling the bottle to bulging with hot water will stretch it out of shape and hasten deterioration of the rubber. Next, the bottle should be placed on its side with the neck held up to prevent spilling while pressure of the hand along the flat surface squeezes the water up into the neck of the bottle, thus expelling the air and making the bottle more flexible. The stopple should be screwed in tightly and the bag turned upside down to be sure there is no leak at the neck. The outside of the bag should be dried and it should be wrapped in a towel or enclosed in a fitted cloth cover before placing it against the patient. This will decrease possibility of burning the skin and will also serve to absorb perspiration. Hot water bottles require refilling every 2 to 4 hours. After use the bottle should be drained completely and hung upside down by its tab until dry. Air should be blown in to keep the inside surfaces apart, the stopple inserted and the bag stored in its box in a cool place to protect it from heat, ozone and sunlight, which deteriorate rubber.

The *fountain syringe* is used to supply water or special solutions for enemas or for vaginal irrigations (douches). An enema is the injection of fluid into the rectum and the colon so as to cause contraction of the colon and the impulse to defecate[162] as a response either to the pressure sensations created or to irritants contained in the fluid. Enemas are given to relieve constipation (either real or fancied), to cleanse the bowel before surgery or before barium visualization, to help escape of gas from the colon or to inject fluids to be retained for local or systemic effects. Liquids used include tap water, normal saline, 1 to 2 per cent sodium bicarbonate or weak soap solutions. These may be warmed to about 100° F., but they should not be hot. About 1 quart of liquid is put into the bag for a cleansing enema. The hard rubber rectal tip is well lubricated, preferably with a water-soluble jelly, since petrolatum has an adverse effect on rubber. The newer plastic tips are said to have smooth surfaces slick enough to be inserted easily without prior lubrication. Air is eliminated from the tubing by allowing a small amount of solution to run out into a container. The inflexible hard tip must be inserted into the rectum very carefully and with due allowance for the inevitable involuntary protective spasm of the rectal sphincter muscles which will occur as the insertion starts. The adult rectum is about 5 or 6 inches long, so the tip should not be inserted more than 4 inches; 1 or 2 inches is usual for insertion for infants. The syringe is hung or held up so that the top level of the fluid is 18 to 24 inches above the patient's buttocks. The tube shut-off is released to allow fluid to flow slowly. The fluid should travel the entire length of the colon (about 5 feet), reaching the ileocecal valve in 5 to 8 minutes.[162] Because the capacity of the average adult colon is about 750 cc., between 500 and 1,000 cc. of enema fluid is needed to produce the pressure necessary to stimulate peristalsis. The patient should try to retain the fluid 5 to 10 minutes so that the feces may be softened. If the bag is held too high, the outflow will be too rapid and a small amount of fluid will initiate the defecation reflex without getting high enough to cleanse the colon or to soften the feces.

After use, the rectal tip should be wiped

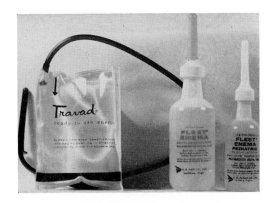

FIG. 13-8. Disposable enema units.

with clean tissue, washed and disinfected by immersion in saponated cresol solution or one of the synthetic phenol solutions* for not more than 15 minutes, followed by a 1-minute immersion in rubbing alcohol (70 per cent), and then dried. The bag and the tube should be rinsed out and hung up to dry before being returned to the box for storage. The shut-off should be removed from the tube, because kinked rubber deteriorates rapidly.

The pharmacist should know the purpose for which a syringe is to be used so he can give advice about its use and prevent misuse. For example, enemas, like cathartics, are contraindicated in the presence of undiagnosed abdominal pain and should not be employed regularly as a substitute for normal physiologic control of defecation.

Disposable enema kits are popular for home and hospital use because of convenience, safety and effectiveness.[180] They are plastic containers that may be compressed or otherwise manipulated so as to force their liquid contents into the lower bowels. Irritants (oxyphenisatin, soaps) or hypertonic agents (sodium phosphate, biphosphate and citrate) are the active components. There is no evidence[19] for a stool-softening action on the part of the surfactant ingredients or of mineral oil. There are two main types by volume: those containing 120 to 180 ml. and the miniature units (microenemas), which contain 5 or 6 ml. Examples of the former

* Two per cent Amphyl or O-syl (Lehn and Fink) is effective.

are the Fleet Enema,* Clyserol,† Lavema,‡ and Travad.§ Index‖ and Rectalad# are microenemas. Fleet Pediatric (75 ml.) and Rectalad Pediatric (2 ml.) are for use in children. The oil retention units made by Fleet and Clyserol contain mineral oil. Fig. 13-8 illustrates some units. Lack of information about the comparative merits of the kits[19] or of their general effectiveness relative to other evacuants[189] has been pointed out.

Vaginal irrigation is commonly done for cleansing purposes. The vaginal mucous membrane is folded and covered with protective secretions so it is not easy to clean the canal with washes. Kaminetsky[130] described vaginal biology to show that douches for healthy women are unnecessary because the normal vagina is self-lubricating and self-cleansing. He pointed out that persistent douching may upset the microbiological balance and cause irritation. The douche has clinical value[130] as an ancillary measure in the treatment of specific vaginitis and also to provide heat in treatment of postabortal and puerperal pelvic cellulitis. Because of the psychologic underpinnings of the cult of douching, the pharmacist would probably be unwise to counsel routinely against the practice.

Solutions containing boric acid, borax, alum, vinegar, lactic acid, surfactants, phenols and similar mildly antiseptic or acidic materials[78,136] are used, generally in volumes of 2,000 cc. or more.

The vaginal tip has a ribbed, somewhat bulbous end with a number of small openings around the bulb so as to give a spray effect. The user should lie on her back in the bathtub with the douche bag suspended not more than 3 feet above the body level. The syringe tip is inserted gently downward and backward until a resistance is felt. The lips of the vagina are pressed about the nozzle to prevent the fluid from escaping and the fluid allowed to run until a feeling of fullness indicates the

* C. B. Fleet Co., Inc., Lynchburg, Va.
† Clyserol Laboratories, Inc., Oklahoma City, Oklahoma.
‡ Winthrop Laboratories, N.Y., N.Y.
§ Flint Laboratories, Morton Grove, Ill.
‖ Johnson and Johnson, New Brunswick, N.J.
Wampole Laboratories, Stamford, Conn.

vagina is filled to capacity. After a moment, the lips of the vagina are released to allow the solution to run out. This process is repeated until the solution is used up. After use the equipment should be rinsed, dried and stored as described for the water bottle (p. 490).

The folding or travel style of fountain syringe (Fig. 13-9) is increasingly in demand because it can be fitted compactly into a small space for easy storage and carrying. The syringe is narrow but constructed with an inverted pleat along each edge so that addition of fluid to the bag everts the side panels to give an overall capacity of 2 quarts or more. The best grade of rubber (latex) is used for maximum extensibility and strength. To appeal to the feminine patron, these are made in a variety of colors and have attractive carrying cases.

Ice bags or caps may be made in molds in much the same fashion as water bottles, but a variety of shapes are made to permit application of dry cold to specific parts of the body (Fig. 13-10). The throat and spinal ice bag is long and narrow and may have tie tabs at each end so that it can be fastened in place around the throat or the abdomen. Some throat or tonsillectomy collars are permanently formed into a ring by metal springs incorporated along the perimeter. Molded icecaps are flat, somewhat circular in outline and have a large central opening for the ice. The English-type icecap is not molded, but is made of cloth rubberized by the Macintosh process. A thin layer of rubber is deposited

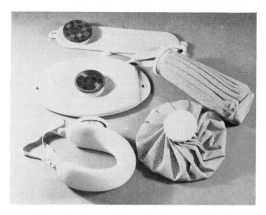

FIG. 13-10. Ice bags. (*Left, top*) Throat and spinal bag. (*Left, center*) Ice cap. (*Left, bottom*) Curved tonsillectomy collar. (*Right*) One of the two English-type caps has been flattened as it would be when used.

from a solution placed between two thicknesses of cotton cloth. Then an ornamental (usually checkered) cloth material is cemented to one surface to make a nonsweating exterior while the other surface is made moistureproof by painting on a rubber solution. A cylinder of this layered cloth is cemented to a circular bottom and fastened into a metal collar to form a multipleated bag which will stand erect or which can be flattened by telescoping the top into the bag (Fig. 13-10). Bags are made to be 6, 9 or 11 inches in diameter when flattened.

Ice should be broken up into small pieces, roughly walnut-size, and rinsed with water to melt off sharp edges before being put in the bag. The bag is filled one half to two thirds full, the air pressed out and the stopper screwed in. The outside should be dried and the bag tested for leaks. English icecaps do not require covering, but other styles do. The ice needs replenishing every 2 to 4 hours. After use the bag should be washed, dried and stored in a cool place.

The primary effects[162] of the moderate dry cold of the ice bag application include contraction of superficial blood vessels, pale cool skin, decrease in local perspiration, gooseflesh and, perhaps, shivering. Secondarily the superficial vessels dilate, the skin becomes warm and red, perspiration increases. Reflex effects, such as the stopping of nosebleeds by

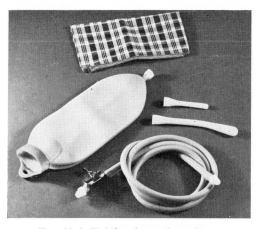

FIG. 13-9. Folding fountain syringe.

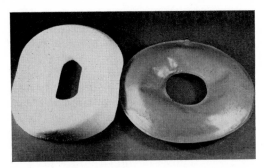

Fig. 13-11. Invalid cushions. (*Left*) A polyethylene foam type. (*Right*) An inflated ring.

cold application to the back of the neck, may be elicited. Therapeutic uses of dry cold seem quite limited.[52] Contraction of blood vessels may reduce circulating fluids in an area and relieve pain caused by pressure. Control of hemorrhage, checking of inflammation and prevention of suppuration may be achieved.[112] Reflex vasoconstriction of blood vessels in internal organs may occur. Moist cold is more effective than dry in most of these respects. Circulatory stasis and injured tissue are contraindications to application of cold.

Invalid Cushions. Persons who spend much of their time in a sitting or a recumbent position are more comfortable when their weight is distributed broadly and supported on air entrapped in rubber cushions. One type of invalid cushion (Fig. 13-11) is molded into an inflatable ring. Air is blown in through a simple type of air valve. Clients should be cautioned that the cushion is hard and uncomfortable if too full of air. The correct dimensions must be chosen so as to afford proper support of the paired tuberosities of the ischium upon which the weight of the sitting person rests.[153] Weight should be borne along the edge of the central hole. If the diameter of the opening is too small, the pelvic bones are forced apart; if it is too large, they are squeezed together. Since, in an adult, these bones are normally 4 to 6 inches apart, the 14-inch or 16-inch ring is usually satisfactory. The cushion should be inflated and sat on to test for leaks and for size. Circular cushions may become warm and uncomfortable as radiation from the body raises the temperature of the air in the

center opening. A horseshoe-shaped cushion which permits air circulation and, also, some adjustment of diameters is available but is quite expensive. Vinyl rings are now being marketed. Small oval inflatable rubber cushions, 8 by 10 inches, are designed for placement under ears, elbows or heels of bedridden patients with the intent of preventing development of ulcers which frequently result at these points where bony prominences may be pressed against the flesh.[25]

Cushions in which air is held as a foam within multiple rubber cells are now competitive in price with inflatable rings and offer the advantage of increased softness and greater flexibility in design. Foams may be made in several ways. Latex can be whipped in frothing units until a foam is produced. This is poured into molds, congealed and wet-vulcanized under conditions which prevent evaporation of the water contained in the gelled foam. Alternatively, latex may be frothed by gas that is rapidly liberated from hydrogen peroxide under catalysis by catalase; the foam is frozen, coagulated with CO_2 and then wet-vulcanized. The cushions generally available are the medium size (14½ by 12½ inches) and the large (16¼ by 13 inches). Polyethylene foam cushions are the plastic entry in this field.

In use, cushions may need to be covered to prevent excoriation of bare flesh on continued contact and rubbing. Those made of rubber should not come into contact with oily materials and should be stored under conditions conducive to preservation of rubber.

Some authorities[25,231] believe that doughnuts, air cushions and inflatable rings should be used at best only for temporary aid, because these supports cause a circle of pressure and may thus restrict circulation. Large soft pads placed next to the pressure points are recommended for long use. Pads are made from a number of materials, each claiming some specific advantages. Foam rubber cushions are widely available. A reticulated polyurethane foam pad,* 24 × 30 inches, allows good air circulation and free passage of fluids, does not support bacterial growth, is easily cleaned by ordinary washing, and

*Dermatec Comfort Pad, Parke, Davis and Co., Detroit, Mich.

can be autoclaved or cold-sterilized. However, it tends to compress markedly at pressure points,[25] and it may thus lose some of its supportive properties. Sheepskin has proven effective in the prevention of bedsores[90] and is now available in this country.* The natural fleece side is shorn to about 1 inch thickness, and the underside is tanned to a suede-like finish. The skins are about 36 inches wide and 42 inches long. The patient lies directly on the woolly side of the skin without intervening coverings or clothing. The pad is resilient and moisture-absorbent. It can be washed with mild soap and water and air-dried. A small amount of mineral oil rubbed into the leather side while it is still damp helps to keep the skin soft and pliable.[25] A synthetic fiber padding† made of Kodel polyester fiber is used in the same fashion as the sheepskin and may tolerate laundering better. An alternating pressure pad is sometimes used on top of a regular mattress. It has longitudinal air cells that are filled and emptied in alternate cycles of about 3 minutes with the intent of preventing prolonged pressure on any one area.[25] Probably the most effective system for preventing or curing pressure necrosis is a self-contained silicone gel block that has been recently marketed.‡ The 16-inch square pad consists of this viscoelastic material enclosed in a protective elastic membrane. The physical consistency of the gel warrants its being described as an "artificial fat." Paraplegic dogs that developed decubitus ulcers in 1 to 6 days while lying on steel, masonite, innerspring or polyfoam mattresses, or alternating pressure pad systems had no pressure problems after 38 days on the gel.[219,220] Clinical tests indicate usefulness as a wheelchair pad, as well as for a protectant for pressure points in bed patients. The pad may be washed with soap and water and is autoclavable. Torn covers are easily replaced. The high cost (nearly $300) will probably prevent wide use, in spite of the recognized expense and suffering that follow development of decubitus ulcers. The

supplier's brochure should be consulted for specifics of use, as well as for descriptions of other smaller and specially designed support cushions.

Urinary Appliances. Loss of urethral sphincter control results in urinary incontinence—the inability to prevent involuntary excretion of urine. There are numerous causes of incontinence,[125,244] including birth defects; disorders of central nervous system pathways; severe infection of the urinary tract; pressure from distended abdominal organs, tumor masses or the gravid uterus on the bladder; tension; traumatic or surgical injury; physiologic relaxation of urethral sphincters with age; loss of muscle control under heavy drug sedation; and cancer of the bladder or urethra. Sometimes, specialized treatments enable the individual to regain at least a measure of control. Urinary incontinence is much more prevalent in the male than in the female because incontinence frequently results from urethral sphincter damage during surgery to remove the hypertrophied or cancerous prostate of the aged male. The incontinent individual has emotional problems that arise from real or fancied social embarrassment.

A variety of rubber and plastic appliances are available for use of the incontinent ambulatory or bed-ridden male. The sheath style* looks like a prophylactic condom with a short open tube at the distal end. The appropriate size (small, medium or large) is rolled onto the penis and fastened down with a small rubber strap, with tape or with surgical cement. The sheath is then connected through a drainage tube to a collection bag. This system is used in nursing homes and hospitals to replace the Foley catheter. Another design has the sheath attached to an elastic athletic supporter. Snug fit over the penis is obtained by cutting down a cone-shaped thin rubber penile sheath that is inside the top of the main sheath. This prevents backflow and leakage when the individual sits down or reclines. A drain closure cap allows this appliance to be used without accessory tubing or bags as a limited capacity lightweight method of compensating for dripping or seepage rather than

*Nasco-Calstok, Modesto, Calif.; Bed-Ease Products, Yonkers, N.Y.

†Derma-Care, Pad, American Hospital Supply, Evanston, Ill.

‡Stryker Flotation Pad, Stryker Corp., Kalamazoo, Mich.

* Xterna-Cath, Faultless Rubber Co., Ashland, Ohio; Bardic URO sheath, Davol Rubber Co., Providence, R.I.

constant flow. A quite similar style uses a suspensory type of pouch and thus also provides support to the scrotum (Fig. 13-12, *top*). Most urinals consist of two parts—a top with an adjustable waistbelt and a lower portion or bag (Fig. 13-12, *bottom*). The top and bag may be directly joined by a screw-type connector, or they may be connected by a length of tubing to make it possible to suspend the bag from the side of a bed or to lay it on a low adjacent table. In ambulation, the bag is strapped along the mesial side of either thigh. Bags are elongated or oval and have capacities ranging from 5 ounces in the child's size up to 32 ounces, with 20 ounces being the size most used. A flutter-valve at the top of the bag prevents backflow of urine. Day-type urinals that lack the inner

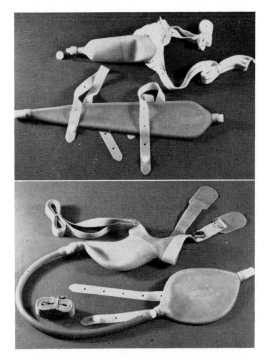

Fig. 13-12. Rubber urinal for male. (*Top*) The top has a cloth suspensory. The cap shown near the tip can be screwed on the drain closure to convert the top into a "drip" urinal. The elongated bag is screwed on the drain closure in usual usage. (*Bottom*) Urinal with tubing connecting top and bag. The use of the tubing is optional as the top and the bag may be screwed together directly. The top of this urinal is made of rubber.

penile sheath are lighter and more comfortable but are effective only when the individual is in an erect position.

A urinal must be cleansed and disinfected often. Both parts should be turned inside out, washed with soap and water, rinsed and kept inside out until thoroughly dry, after which the urinal should be dusted lightly with talcum powder. It should not be folded or hung up by its straps. Because of the need to allow time for drying the user should have at least two appliances. Immersion in weak hydrogen peroxide solution or a mild chlorine bleach for not more than 3 minutes helps to deodorize the rubber. Prolonged contact with these solutions causes oxidative deterioration of the rubber.

Urinals are labeled to indicate that health laws prohibit the acceptance of any used appliances for repair or exchange, and the pharmacist should be certain that each part of the equipment is in good order before releasing it to his client. He should also maintain a suitable stock of replacement parts.

Continued wearing of the penile bag tends to excoriate the constantly moist prepuce and glans penis. Strict personal hygiene and careful attention to technic[244] for using the appliance are necessary. The penis should be clean and dry. To lessen irritation, benzoin tincture should be applied over the penis and allowed to dry. The penile sheath is pulled on and compressed firmly with the hand to help to secure it. The urinal should be removed at least once a day and the penis washed thoroughly with mild soap and water. An antibacterial solution such as benzalkonium chloride (1:750) should then be applied and allowed to dry.

Female incontinence is especially difficult and uncomfortable to manage because the urinal has to be placed between the legs. Apparently it has not been possible to design an appliance that can be used when lying down. Consequently incontinent women usually use an indwelling catheter, generally the Foley, attached by flexible tubing to a collecting bag. The shorter and straighter urethra of women makes this a simpler and less potentially infectious method than in males in whom indwelling catheters are sometimes used.

Other methods for compensating for uri-

TABLE 13-2. BASIC DIFFERENCES BETWEEN A COLOSTOMY AND AN ILEOSTOMY*

	COLOSTOMY	ILEOSTOMY
Reason for doing:	Low-bowel obstruction: malignancy of colon or rectum; an inflammatory mass, as in diverticulitis	Severe ulcerative colitis
Location of stoma:	The colon	The ileum
Type of discharge:	Solid or semisolid feces	Liquid, irritating, small bowel content
Regulation and management:	Diet and irrigation	Low residue diet and an ileostomy bag
Restrictions on the patient:	May return to work and other normal activities (if radical surgery for cancer has been performed, sexual potency and/or fertility may be impaired in the male)	Same (sexual potency and/or fertility are unaffected except in a small percentage of males who have had the rectum removed)

* From Seide, D.: RN 23:37, 1960.

nary incontinence are worth noting. A male may use a penile clamp (Cunningham clamp) to mechanically compress the urethral wall. This is a small lightweight rubber-covered malleable metal frame that can be bent by hand for size adjustment and then clamped over the penile shaft by forcing the two wings together with a snap-button or spring-ratchet closing device. The pads that come in contact with the organ are made of soft sponge rubber. An inverted V in the lower half of the clamp exerts pressure directly on the urethra along the underside of the penis, while the heavy padding prevents excessive pressure, which would also quickly cut off blood flow.[125] The clamp is only for brief temporary use and should be repositioned at least every 2 hours to prevent damage to the urethra or circulatory obstruction.[244] Four sizes, infant to large, are available. The Kossler incontinence clamp,* made of nylon and padded, has similar uses though it differs in construction details.

Protective garments may be preferred to appliances. These are basically adult versions of disposable diaper panties used for babies. Skin care is a problem because urine is irritating. Frequent washing is necessary. Use of a neutral detergent followed by the application of oils, deodorizing powders or skin

* B. F. Goodrich, Akron, Ohio.

preparations containing waterproofing agents has been suggested.[112]

Enterostomy Outfits. The unique requirements of the patron who has undergone an enterostomy* offer the pharmacist a real opportunity for service. The two most common forms of this operation are the colostomy and the ileostomy. In the former a short portion of the lower end of the colon is pulled through the abdominal wall to form a stoma (opening) for intestinal drainage. In the latter, it is an end of the cut ileum which protrudes. See Figure 13-13 and Table 13-2. In either instance the individual will need specialized equipment to take care of the stoma and the discharges from it. Since normal control of defecation is often impossible, accessory kits for irrigation of the remaining portions of the intestine may be required. A wide variety of devices are now available, many of which have been designed in accord with suggestions from enterostomy patients themselves. The choice of appliance is generally made by consultation between the patient and physician before leaving the hospital. Instructions for use are given then also. The pharmacist may be expected to provide the equipment originally, to supplement instruc-

* An enterostomy is the artificial formation of a permanent opening into the intestine through the abdominal wall.

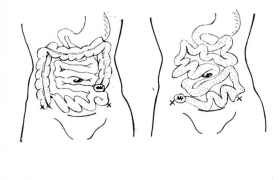

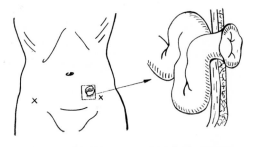

Fig. 13-13. Diagrams of typical enterostomies. (*Top, left*) The sigmoid and the rectum are removed in a typical colostomy. (*Top, right*) In a typical ileostomy the colon and a segment of the distal ileum are removed. (*Bottom, left and right*) The colostomy opening is made by pulling the colon through the abdominal wall, usually in the lower left abdominal quadrant as shown. The ileostomy stoma is generally formed in the lower right quadrant using the end of the cut ileum. (From Seide, D.: RN, 23:37, 1960)

tions for use and maintenance and to provide replacement parts as needed.

Colostomy care is the simpler of the two. Causes of common problems and ways to handle them have been described well.[132] By control of diet many patients can learn to have a regular well-formed stool once a day. Physiologic mechanisms by which fecal continence is maintained in the absence of lower sphincters are not well understood.[61] Leakage will be minor and the opening can be covered with a small gauze dressing or several folded tissues held in place by an elastic belt or girdle. Some feel more secure if the opening is covered by an impervious shield made of rubber plastic. Figure 13-14 illustrates one form of colostomy dome which is used in this way. The shield (a 75-mm.

vaginal diaphragm) is stretched over the flange lip of the flexible rubber colostomy ring (C ring). Two tissues are folded into the dome to absorb seepage. Surgical cement (natural rubber, zinc oxide and n-hexane) is applied to the skin and to the flat surface of the C ring. The skin and the C ring should be cleansed with benzine and thoroughly dried before applying the cement, and contact with excretion leakage should be avoided. After 1 or 2 minutes to allow the cement to set, the C ring is held in place against the body with gentle pressure until the cement dries. The elastic belt is snapped on the tabs of the C ring with appropriate adjustment to the desired tightness. Swimming and bathing are possible with the C ring in position, since the cement is waterproof. The C ring can be left in place for 4 or 5 days. It is removed by lifting one edge and peeling gently from the skin.

During the recovery period after surgery or during times of intestinal disorders with attendant diarrhea the patient will need to wear a bag to catch the excretions. A disposable plastic bag, 6 x 8 inches, can be attached with a rubber band over the flange of the C ring in place of the rubber cover. The bag is discarded as necessary. Units utilizing a soft rubber sponge against the body and no cement, and all-rubber models, some with inflatable cushions, are also available.

A number of patients are unable to master natural control of defecation after colostomy. A survey of some 92 colostomy patients[204] showed that 80 per cent had to cleanse the colon regularly by irrigations (enemas), commonly once daily, usually in the morning. An irrigating appliance is shown in Figure 13-14. The patient sits on or near the commode in the bathroom. Two or three pints of warm tap water (105° F.) are put into the assembled fountain syringe. The catheter (26F)* is attached to the tube by the tubing connector and threaded through the hole in the antisplash cup. The distal 3 or 4 inches of the catheter are lubricated with a water-soluble jelly or with petrolatum. The bag should be hung so that the water level is about 18 inches above the colostomy opening when the user is seated. The plastic drain sleeve is attached at its side opening to the large rub-

* See Table 13-3, p. 502, for catheter sizes.

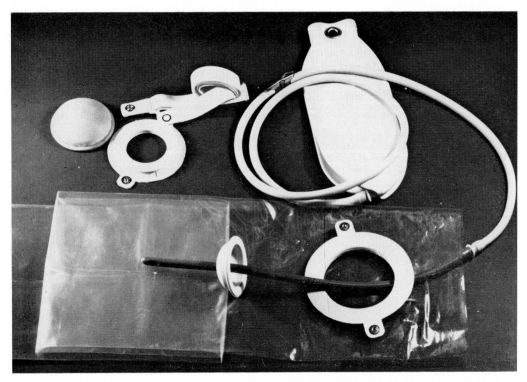

FIG. 13-14. A colostomy apparatus and irrigation set. (*Top, left to right*) The dome, the C ring and a folding-type fountain syringe. The tubing has a lever-type shut-off and is attached to a one-eyed catheter which is inserted into the top of the plastic drain sleeve and through the opening in the rubber ring by which the sleeve is fastened over the stoma. About 4 inches of the catheter has been pushed through the antisplash cup. See text for further description.

ber ring, then the flat surface of the ring is held against the body by a belt. The open end of the sleeve is suspended in the commode bowl. The water is allowed to run to expel air from the tube and to continue to flow slowly while the catheter is gently inserted to a depth of 2 to 4 inches. The antisplash cup is held against the body to prevent escape of fluid while the rate of flow is controlled as necessary by pinching the catheter. Fluid containing fecal matter is allowed to pass out of the opening off and on during the irrigation. Inasmuch as drainage may continue for 40 to 60 minutes after irrigation, the sleeve may be folded double and clamped to make a bag so that the user can move about. After use the components of the irrigation appliance should be washed with detergent, rinsed and allowed to dry. A somewhat different irrigation procedure that is

claimed to prevent spillage for 48 hours has been described.[205]

The ileostomy patient has additional difficulties because he has a constant and uncontrollable drainage of fluid. A detailed protocol for ileostomy management[163] points out that complete care of the patient requires knowledge of the placement and management of the stoma, the indicated appliance, and the treatment of problems that must follow the change in the physiologic function. A recent booklet provides useful explicit information.*

A permanent appliance must be worn. The available two-piece units (faceplate and pouch) are easier to center over the stoma,

* Larson, D.: Living Comfortably with Your Ileostomy (1968), The American Rehabilitation Foundation, 1800 Chicago Ave., Minneapolis, Minn.

and they offer the convenience of rapid change of pouch while the faceplate remains cemented to the body. However, they are bulkier than the more commonly used one-piece unit. The ileostomy appliance typically is a flat rubber or vinyl pouch with a disk-rimmed opening (faceplate) at one side near the top end and an open sleevelike continuation at the bottom end. Faceplates may be flat, concave, or convex as required for proper contact with the abdomen. The size of the hole is selected to allow a 2 mm. clearance around the stoma. The stoma must not be closely encircled by the relatively inflexible rim because there must be allowance for stomal stretching in order for solid objects in the stool to pass. The faceplate is cemented to the skin as described on page 497 for the C ring. Double-sided adhesive disks are sometimes used in place of cement. The bottom sleeve is folded back on itself and clamped to make a closed container; it is unfolded as needed to empty accumulated fluids. A waist-belt may be attached for additional support. Frequently, a clean bag is attached daily, and the soiled one is washed in warm soapy water, rinsed, allowed to dry and powdered on both internal and external surfaces with talcum or cornstarch. In 2 or 3 months, unpleasant odors permeate the appliance and force discarding the bag. Some patients prefer to use disposable plastic bags.

A questionnaire survey of over 400 patients with ileostomies[151] found that 85 per cent of the respondents had experienced skin problems near the stoma. Many of them reported irritation in the small circular area of unprotected skin between the inner rim of the appliance faceplate and the ileac stump. The duration of contact with the ileostomy drainage and the amount of proteolytic enzyme activity in the fluid determine the degree of irritation. Irritation may also result from fluid seepage beneath a loosened disk. The skin may be unable to tolerate the commonly used cements and solvents; reactions appear to be due to primary irritants rather than to allergens. Blisters may develop when the appliance rubs on the skin beneath it. Suggestions[151] included cementing to the body a soft sponge rubber pad that fits closely round the stump and serves as a base to which the rim of the pouch could adhere. Poorly fitted appliances had to be replaced. Karaya gum was reported to give the most relief of all ointments, pastes and powders that were tried.* A mixture of karaya gum and glycerin sets up into a solid that has both adhesive and protective properties.[218] This has been formed into flat washer-like rings† (2.5 mm. thick, varying internal and external diameters) that are applied to the faceplate of a permanent appliance and then pressed into place around the stoma without need of cement. The ring softens with body heat and adheres more closely with time. It is discarded when the appliance is changed. Advantages claimed[218] include: greater comfort, less skin irritation, better fit on uneven skin surfaces, and avoidance of irritants in cements and solvents. Zinc oxide ointment (*U.S.P.*) or aluminum paste (*U.S.P.*) are sometimes recommended for applications as protectants around the stoma,[208] but cements do not adhere well to these greasy preparations. Benzoin tincture may be applied to the skin around the stoma to alleviate irritation and to help in cementing the appliance in place, but compound benzoin tincture (*U.S.P.*) is said to be too irritating for this usage.[200]

Successful odor prevention and control are important to patients who have either a colostomy or ileostomy. Excessive passage of gas is a related problem. Recommendations[178] include a low-residue diet and avoidance both of gas-producing foods such as beans, cabbage, peas and fish, and of foods that produce frequent bowel movements, such as fruit, tomatoes and spinach. Because of individual variations, patients must determine by trial and error which foods to eliminate from the diet. Colostomy patients should completely empty the colon at regular intervals to avoid the excessive gas formation that is sometimes

---

* Sprinkle karaya gum lightly over the affected site. Allow it to form a sticky paste with the serum present, or add a small amount of water if necessary. Form a similar sticky paste on the appliance disk. Place the disk over the treated skin area. This will adhere and protect for about 24 hours. Somewhat longer adherence can be obtained by allowing the karaya gum to become firm on the skin and then using rubber cement to glue the appliance on this protective layer.

† Karaya Seal, Hollister Inc., Chicago, Ill.; Karaya Gum Discs, United Surgical Corp., Largo, Fla.; Sure-Seal, The Faultless Rubber Co., Ashland, Ohio.

associated with constipation. Oral use of chlorophyll tablets (100 to 200 mg. two or three times daily) and of activated charcoal (two tablets three times daily) has been both advocated[178] and deprecated.[200] Bismuth subcarbonate (600 mg. three times daily with meals) is claimed to have a striking effect in reducing bad odor both from feces and from the bag.[200] Soaking the appliance in a chlorophyll solution and putting two chlorophyll tablets or two crushed aspirin tablets into the empty pouch each time it is attached are said to reduce pouch odors.[178,200] Numerous products are marketed for this purpose. Strict appliance hygiene is probably the most important factor in reducing bag odors.

Some less common enterostomies such as the ileal-bladder, the wet colostomy and the ureterostomy present their own unique problems and require care and appliances that differ in some details from those for colostomies and ileostomies. Jeter[127] and others[179, 187,230] should be consulted for this information.

In the patient with an enterostomy, the pharmacist has a client who faces severe psychologic problems in adjusting to drastic changes in his way of life. During a study[86] of 41 patients with ileostomies, 46 per cent described various subjective problems such as sexual problems, fears of accidents, odor, straining themselves, and embarrassment. Successful adaptation by the patients depended on acceptance of the ileostomy by key figures in their lives such as family and employer. To help themselves to adjust to their disability, people with enterostomies have formed clubs in a number of localities. In addition to being able to provide practical guidance from first-hand experience, club members serve as successful figures with whom the new stoma patient can identify.[86] A national organization that has over 50 local chapters is the United Ostomy Association, Inc., with headquarters in Los Angeles. Another is QT, Inc. (Boston), which is named after surgical wards Q and T at Mt. Sinai Hospital, New York, where it was organized.[208] Each organization publishes helpful manuals and periodicals. Pharmacists frequently serve as guest speakers at local meetings and should seek out opportunities to become involved with these groups in order to contribute their specialized understanding and knowledge.

Bulb syringes are used to force fluids into body cavities such as the ear, the rectum or the vagina and to remove fluids from others —the nose for example. Syringes of this type consist of a hollow ball-like part, the bulb, and a hollow tip which may be either a prolongation of the bulb itself or a tube of different composition inserted into or otherwise joined to the bulb. Compressing the bulb expels the air so that fluid can be sucked up when pressure on the bulb is released and then forced out again on recompression. Bulbs are made by vulcanizing rubber or plastic in molds while inflating the warmed mixture either with air or with nitrogen generated by the action of heat on a pelleted mixture of sodium nitrite and ammonium chloride.

Bulb syringes are named according to the part of the body on which they are used.

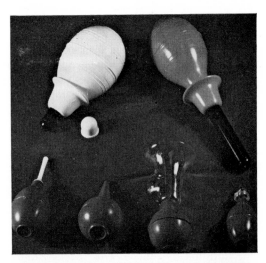

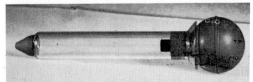

FIG. 13-15. Bulb syringes. (*Top, left*) Feminine bulb syringe with retracted pipe. (*Top, right*) Feminine bulb syringe, nonretractable pipe. (*Center, left to right*) Infant rectal syringe; ear syringe; breast pump; nasal aspirator. (*Bottom*) Asepto syringe with soft rubber tip.

However, the so-called ear syringe is quite adaptable to procedures other than irrigation of the ear. It is a one-piece unit with a relatively long, soft, flexible nozzle tapered to a small opening (Fig. 13-15). Capacities range from 1 to 3 ounces. Irrigation of the external canal of the ear is usually done for simple cleansing or to wash out impacted ear wax (cerumen) which has first been softened by a few drops of hydrogen peroxide solution, glycerin or olive oil.[145] A mixture of sodium bicarbonate (1.6 Gm.), glycerin (4 cc.) and water (q.s. to 30 ml.) is said to soften wax effectively.[112] Solutions of surfactants are marketed for this purpose,[100] but there have been reports of irritation from their use. Isotonic saline, 1 to 2 per cent sodium bicarbonate and tap water warmed to about 105° F. are among the fluids used for irrigation.

In an adult the ear canal runs upward and forward, then downward and forward to the eardrum.[112] The pinna should be lifted upward and backward to straighten the canal while the stream of fluid is directed with low pressure against the back wall of the canal. In an infant the eardrum is in an oblique position and covers part of the floor of the canal; in order to make the whole canal accessible to the fluid it is necessary to draw the auricle downward and backward.[112] Pressure on the bulb should be gentle and steady, since too much force can be damaging. The tip should be held so as not to block the canal in order to allow return flow into a catch basin. The amount of fluid to be used is judged by the clarity of the return flow and the appearance of the surface of the canal. Finally, the canal should be dried with pledgets of cotton. Unless ordered by a physician, irrigation of the ear is contraindicated when infection is present or when the eardrum is perforated.

Since air bubbles forced into the ear may produce loud sounds and discomfort, the bulb should be filled completely with fluid at the start. In general, this may be done readily, in the following way:[115] Compress the bulb and suck up liquid. Point the nozzle upward and squeeze until liquid starts to come out, then without releasing pressure put the tip back into liquid again. Now release pressure and the bulb will fill completely.

Rectal syringes are characterized by the long and narrow hard rubber or vinyl pipes which are slipped into the tip of the bulb (Fig. 13-15). The infant size has a bulb capacity ranging from 1 to 4 ounces and a pipe about 2 inches long; the bulb in the adult size holds from 5 to 8 ounces and the pipe is about 2½ inches long. These are used to introduce fluids to stimulate defecation, especially in infants; adults seem to prefer to use the fountain syringe for themselves. Constipation is seldom a real problem in children. Most often it is a diagnosis made by overworried parents who have been conditioned to believe that a daily bowel movement is a necessity. Pediatricians consider it wrong physically and psychologically for a parent to get into the habit of giving a child regular enemas.[221] They should be used only on special occasions with the advice of a physician. Authorities[115,192,221] differ in procedures to follow as well as in the types and amounts of fluid to use. Change of diet is advocated as a more fundamental approach to overcoming constipation.[212]

After use, the syringe should be wiped clean of lubricant and fecal matter and thoroughly washed with soap and water. It may be disinfected by contact with a 2 per cent solution of a synthetic phenol for not more than 15 minutes followed by thorough rinsing with water.[5] It should be stored with the usual precautions for preservation of rubber.

Feminine bulb syringes are used for vaginal douches. Bulb capacities range from 8 ounces to 10 ounces or more. The attached pipe is relatively large—about ½ inch in outside diameter and 5 to 6 inches long. It may be made of inflexible hard rubber or vinyl; it may be either straight or slightly curved. Less commonly, the pipe is flexible. The tip has multiple openings or a removable perforated screw cap to give a spraying action. A heavy soft rubber shield is fitted around and movable along the pipe. There may be a closure cap for the pipe.

In use, the syringe is filled completely with one of the usual douche solutions, and the tube is inserted so that its tip approaches the inner end of the vaginal canal (4 to 5 inches). Shallower insertion is advised if vaginal surfaces are inflamed. The shield should be adjusted to fit firmly against the vaginal entrance. The bulb should be squeezed very gently to force out its contents. Fluid will be retained in the vagina as long as the bulb is kept compressed. After the desired period of application the pipe is drawn partly out through the shield without allowing leakage, the compression slowly released and the fluid withdrawn into the bulb. The fluid can then be discarded and the irrigation repeated as desired. The syringe should be washed thoroughly with soap and water and may be disinfected by general procedures already described. It should be hung nozzle end down to drain and then properly stored when dry.

The feminine bulb syringe has some advantage over the fountain syringe in convenience of use and compactness. In fact, some are made so that the pipe may be retracted into the bulb for storage in a smaller space (Fig. 13-15). However, because of the possibility that a too forceful outflow will be generated by excessive pressure on the bulb, gynecologists generally do not recommend its use.

The same warning may be advanced to discourage the use of the family bulb (valve syringe). This is a rubber bulb with two valved openings, each attached to a flexible rubber tube. One tube is dipped into the irrigation fluid and the other, fitted with a rectal or a vaginal tip, is inserted into the cavity to be irrigated. The valves allow fluid flow in one direction only, so alternate constriction and release pumps fluid out of the reservoir through the bulb and into the body cavity. There is obviously danger of excessive force being used with this apparatus.

The *infant nasal aspirator* (Fig. 13-15) is a 1-ounce to 3-ounce bulb with a short acorn-shaped tip made of glass or clear plastic. It is used to suck mucus out of the nasal cavity if it has become so congested that the infant has difficulty breathing. This procedure is sometimes recommended as preferable to administration of nose drops or as desirable immediately prior to instillation of such drops.[212] The bulb is compressed, then the tip is inserted in the nostril while gradual release of pressure gently sucks out the mucus. This may be repeated 2 or 3 times with each nostril. An ear syringe is also useful for the same purpose. The Birmingham style nasal douche is not advocated for washing out the mucus, since the downward tilt of the nasal passages necessary for its action may cause flow of fluid into the Eustachian tubes and the ears. After use the aspirator should be washed, disinfected and stored as usual for rubber goods.

Breast pumps (Fig. 13-15) have a 1-ounce to 2½-ounce bulb into which is inserted a thick-walled, horn-shaped glass or plastic shield about 3 inches long, the open end of which flares out to a circle with a 2-inch diameter. One side of the neck is evaginated to form a shallow reservoir. In use the bulb is compressed and the shield is placed against the breast so as to enclose the nipple. On release of the bulb, milk is sucked out through the nipple. Recompression of the bulb allows the milk sacs to refill so that the procedure can be repeated until no further flow of milk is obtained. The milk may be desired for a baby who cannot nurse, in which case the pump should first be sterilized by immersion in boiling water for 10 minutes or should be otherwise suitably disinfected. Breast pumps may be used when a baby is weaned temporarily because of illness of the mother or because the baby is unable to suckle sufficiently to drain the breasts of milk at each feeding. It is necessary to empty the breasts completely, since failure to do so regularly will result in a drying up of the milk secretion. Manual expression of breast milk by the mother is a less traumatic and, therefore, a preferred procedure; a breast pump should not be supplied without advice from the physician in attendance.

TABLE 13-3. CATHETER, RECTAL AND COLON TUBE SIZES

French*	10	12	14	16	18	20	22	24	26	28	30	32	34
American	7	8	10	11	12	14	15	16	17	19	20	21	22
English	4	5	6	7	9	11	12	14	15	17	18	20	21
O. D. (inches)	.13	.15	.18	.20	.23	.26	.29	.31	.33	.35	.37	.40	.43

* One French unit equals 1 mm. in circumference.

The *urethral syringes* used currently are largely of the bulb type, the plunger type having been superseded by this more easily handled form. The syringe barrels are generally of glass for ready sterilization. The Asepto* urethral syringe is available in sizes ranging from ⅛ ounce to 1 ounce and with blunt or tapered glass tips as well as soft rubber tips. The neck of the bulb fits inside a flared end of the glass barrel (Fig. 13-15) and has thick walls the better to maintain its shape. The capacities of the bulb and the barrel are adjusted so that one full compression fills or empties the barrel without drawing fluid into the bulb. Two small side openings in the removable Bakelite plug in the neck of the bulb allow movement of air but hinder flow of fluid into the bulb. Other Asepto syringes are available with capacities up to 4 ounces, with special tips for attachment to catheters or hypodermic needles, or for irrigating the eye and other body cavities, so that they are of general utility.

The medicine dropper is a bulb syringe which the pharmacist handles so frequently that the usual forms require no description. The official medicine dropper is defined by the *United States Pharmacopeia*[240] as having a delivery end 3 mm. in external diameter and delivering water in drops weighing between 45 and 50 mg. at 15° C. Droppers vary in size and form of bulb and in length, curvature and style of tip; those to be used for instilling drops into the nose or the eye have blunt, flared or ball tips. Droppers attached to dropper bottles often are not standard. This may give the pharmacist cause to wonder if the amount of medication delivered in the number of drops stated on the prescription label is actually that intended by the prescriber. One manufacturer† advertises that his bottles have polyethylene tubes designed to deliver according to *U.S.P.* standards. It should be noted that these polyethylene droppers soften and collapse at autoclave temperatures and, thus, are not suitable for preparation of sterile ophthalmics. An interesting development is a flexible one-piece vinyl chloride medicine dropper* developed for one-time use in hospitals. These are actually reusable, since they are easily rinsed and can be boiled for 5 minutes or autoclaved for 10. The dropper meets *U.S.P.* specifications for size and for delivery of water.

MANDREL GOODS

Items such as catheters, tubing, rubber gloves and other rubber goods are often made by applying thin coats of rubber to the outside of forms (mandrels) immersed in fluid dispersions of rubber. A mandrel may be made of porcelain, glass, varnished wood or metal. In one method, the mandrel is dipped into a latex dispersion, then removed to allow drying of a thin layer of rubber on its surface. Successive dippings by hand or machine follow until the desired thickness is built up. In the electro-deposition or anode process, a metal mandrel is made a positively charged anode so that it collects on itself a coating of the electronegative rubber particles. Mandrel-made items are generally vulcanized by heat while still on the mandrel.

Tubing. High grade rubber tubing is made from latex by the anode process. Much of the tubing on the market is molded, often by an extrusion process, from rubber of varying quality and with formulations modified for specific purposes. It is often colored and may have exterior ribbing. That designated as "floating stock" is the purest form in the sense that it contains a low amount of sulfur and mineral fillers. While internal diameters of tubing usually range from 1/16 to ½ inch with wall thicknesses of 1/16 to ⅛ inch, tubings with dimensions different from these are made for specialized uses. Tubing is marketed in 25-foot or 50-foot rolls, in boxes or on reels. It is also available in shorter lengths—as 5-foot replacement tubing for fountain syringes, for example. Tubing has many uses, from general laboratory work to conducting intravenous solutions. Much tubing is now made of plastic rather than rubber.

Urethral catheters are tubes that are introduced into the urethra in order to drain the bladder or to inject fluids into it. The usual reasons for catheterization include: anatomic

* Becton, Dickinson and Company, Rutherford, N. J.
† Armstrong Cork Company, Lancaster, Pa.

* TFL Clinic Dropper, Thomas Fazio Laboratories, Auburndale 66, Mass.

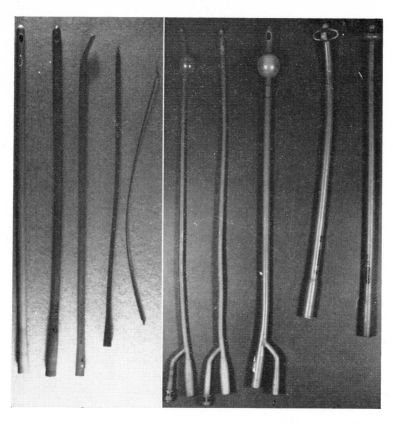

FIG. 13-16. (*Left*) Urethral catheters. From left to right: 30F Robinson 2-eye hollow tip x-ray opaque rubber catheter (eye on opposite side dotted in with white paint); 30F 1-eye solid tip rubber catheter: 24F 1-eye coude olive tip rubber catheter; 14F 1-eye Nylon woven catheter with male thread at tip; S-tip Nylon woven filiform with female thread to fit tip on Nylon woven catheter. (*Right*) Indwelling catheters. From left to right: Foley catheter, 18F, 5 cc. balloon inflated; Foley catheter, 18F, 5 cc. balloon, not inflated; Foley catheter, 30F, 30 cc. balloon inflated; Malecot tip catheter, 30F; Mushroom tip catheter, 30F.

obstructions of the urinary tract, temporary inability to void voluntarily (after surgery, for example), and incontinence. Pharmacists should be familiar with technics for inserting catheters[244] while recognizing that the procedure requires the skills and experience of a physician or a nurse. Catheters must be sterile and are inserted aseptically. Although opinions on the danger of catheterization vary greatly,[35,70] the catheter has been called the agent most commonly responsible for resistant urinary infections.[142] Lubrication is always necessary, a sterile, water-soluble jelly* being preferred to petrolatum or mineral oil for therapeutic reasons, as well as because less damage is done to rubber catheters.

Catheters are made of woven fabrics (silk, linen, nylon), metal, glass, synthetic rubbers (neoprene) and plastics (polyethylene, vinyl), as well as of hard or soft rubber. There is a growing trend toward the use of disposable plastic catheters that are supplied

*Lubafax, Burroughs Wellcome and Co., Tuckahoe, N. J.

presterilized and in individual envelopes. In order to provide the extremely smooth inner and outer surfaces necessary to limit damage on insertion and for unhindered flow of fluid, rubber catheters are made either by the anode process or by molding over glass tubing. Catheter sizes are designated according to scales named after the country of origin (Table 13-3). A catheter with an outside circumference of 20 mm. is identified as 20F or 20 Fr. on the French scale, which is the one most commonly employed. Sizes 8F to 12F are normally used for children, 14F to 22F for adults. Catheters are 10 to 12 inches long and are uniform in caliber throughout their length except for a funnel-shaped opening in some styles. The tip has varied shapes[244] such as round, coudé, filiform, spiral, bulb, olive and acorn, and it may be solid or hollow with one to several apertures (eyes) (Fig. 13-16).

Careful study of manufacturers' catalogs and of detailed texts[244] is necessary to become familiar with the many styles available and the reasons for selecting a particular one.

The kind and size selected depends on the size, shape and condition of the urethra through which the tube is to be passed, and whether the tube is to be left in place. Creevy[75] has identified five catheter styles that he says are satisfactory to fulfill all the needs of an active urologic practice. Short metal catheters or flexible, soft rubber catheters are generally used in women because the short straight urethra presents few problems. A fairly stiff nonelastic catheter, sometimes especially curved and tipped (coudé with olive tip, for example) is often easier to insert into male patients because of bends and strictures in the relatively long urethral passage. The filiform catheter has a long flexible tip that can be guided past strictures and that coils up in the bladder while the main body of the tube follows its lead. Sometimes, a wire stylet (mandrin) is used inside a rubber catheter to impart rigidity during insertion; the stylet is finally withdrawn, leaving the catheter in place. X-ray urethral catheters are impregnated with lead or bismuth salts so as to cast a shadow on the roentgenogram. Some catheters have calibrations on the outside so that the distance of insertion is readily determined. Double-channel catheters have two lumens and at least two eyes arranged to permit inflow and outflow for irrigation, which maintains patency of the tube and prevents obstruction to urinary drainage. Self-retaining, or indwelling, catheters have been designed to decrease the need for recurrent catheterization. Indwelling catheters have special tips that expand or can be expanded after reaching the bladder, thus providing resistance to involuntary withdrawal. The Foley catheter (Fig. 13-16) is the most used. It has a double lumen, the smaller additional one leading to an inflatable rubber bag (the balloon) near the tip. Balloons are generally of 5- or 30-ml. capacity. After insertion of the catheter, the proper volume of sterile water is injected with a hypodermic syringe into the lumen leading to the balloon. The catheter is thus kept in place until the bag is deflated by removing the water with a syringe. The 30-ml. bag is used for senile or aged patients who often try to pull out the catheter, after bladder muscle tone has degenerated, or sometimes to apply pressure for hemostasis

after operative procedures. Special hazards of indwelling catheters have been pointed out.[157,158]

Because of the specialized knowledge required for their use, and also perhaps because of their misuse in attempted self-abortions, catheters may be dispensed on prescription only.

Stomach tubes are 60-inch long, soft rubber or plastic tubes intended for passage into the stomach for purposes of removing its contents, for gastric lavage or for introducing liquid food or medication. These tubes have one eye near the open tip and a widely flared funnel opening at the other end. There is a depth mark 18 inches from the tip. In addition to this style, there is a design in which the tube is cut into two approximately equal lengths that are then joined through a valved aspirator bulb. Stomach tube sizes are designated according to the French scale. The small 22F size is used for children, and sizes 28F to 32F are used in adults. Although insertion of the stomach tube is usually performed by the physician, gastric lavage is a term familiar to pharmacists as a part of the emergency treatment of poisonings. It was once customary to first place the tube in ice to make it firmer and supposedly easier to insert. This is rarely done now with a rubber tube, and it is not at all necessary with one made of plastic.[72] Some recommend lubricating the tube with vegetable oil, though oils may increase the tendency to become nauseated. The tube is placed far back in the mouth of the sitting or recumbent patient. As he swallows, the tube is advanced until the marker is reached, indicating that the end is in the stomach. There is danger of damaging the larynx or perforating the esophagus or the stomach. If the patient is uncooperative, a smaller tube may be passed through the nose. Lowering the funnel end below the level of the tip will siphon out the stomach contents. The funnel is then held upright, and about 500 ml. of irrigating fluid (water at 105° F., usually) is added, keeping the funnel full. To siphon again, the funnel is inverted and lowered while there is still some fluid in it. This avoids the introduction of air, which may cause distention and pain. This alternate dilution and drainage is repeated until the wash fluid is clear or until a prescribed amount has been given. As much as 3 gallons may be used. Finally, the tube is pinched off at the patient's lips and quickly withdrawn. After use, the tube is cleaned and disinfected by the usual procedures satisfactory for rubber.

Duodenal tubes are used by insertion through the nose, usually into the upper part of the small intestine, to sample its contents or to remove gas and fluids to prevent or treat distention that follows abdominal surgery. Suction by an aspirating device is used in this procedure. The Levin tube is a flexible, soft-walled 4-foot tube, sizes 10 to 18F, with four side eyes near the tip and with concentric marking rings, usually 19, 23, 27 and 31 inches from the tip. The Cantor tube is an 18F, 10-foot tube with a small mercury-filled bag at its multiple-eyed tip. The "mushy" heavy balloon is intended to stimulate opening of the pyloric valve and to permit advancing the tube by gravity. The aspirator is started when the letter "S" on the tube is at the patient's nose. The Miller-Abbott[195] tube is a metal-tipped, 16F, 10-foot, double-lumen tube, one lumen opening into a small balloon near the tip. Markings on the tube indicate the distance the tube has been advanced. An eye at stomach level, as well as one at duodenal level, allows drainage of both. The tube is passed through the pyloric valve with the balloon deflated, then peristaltic action carries the inflated balloon and the tube along the intestine. Dam rubber reservoirs to accept aspirated fluids are located at the upper end. Many modifications of these basic designs, including some with magnet tips, are available.

Rectal tubes superficially look like large simple urethral catheters. They are made of flexible rubber or plastic with a funnel-shaped opening and with an eye near the end of the open tip. They are 20 inches long and are available in sizes 16F to 32F. In one enema method, a rectal tube is attached through supplemental tubing to an irrigating can or to a fountain syringe, and the tip end, lubricated with a water-soluble lubricant, is passed gently for a distance of 2 to 4 inches into the rectum. Higher insertion serves no purpose and may be dangerous. The larger the tube circumference, the more it stimulates the anal sphincter muscles to expel rectal contents. Also the enema fluid flows faster with more force in a larger tube. Recommended sizes[231] for adults are 26F to 32F for cleansing enemas, and 14F to 20F for retention enemas. The relatively long length of the rectal tube is intended to provide flexibility and also to allow some degree of control of rate of fluid flow by finger pressure. Danger of rectal perforation[137,164,198] exists with all enemas, but rectal tubes seem likely to be less traumatic than the hard inflexible tips usually supplied with fountain syringes. The pharmacist can do his patrons a service by advising them of the availability and use of rectal tubes. A rectal tube is sometimes inserted to provide an open passageway for the escape of gas when pre- or postoperative decompression of the lower bowel is necessary.[72] The tube is connected by other tubing to a water trap so that passage of gas may be confirmed by observing the bubbling in the water.

Colon tubes are larger and heavier-walled rectal tubes. They are 30 inches long and range in size from 22F to 32F. These tubes are used to remove feces from the lower colon by irrigation in much the same manner as are rectal tubes. They are also used to introduce fluid food into the lower bowel.

Rubber Gloves. Sterile rubber gloves are used by physicians and nurses to guard against contamination of wounds and to protect their hands from pathogens or unpleasant discharges while examining body areas. Surgical gloves are made from natural latex by the anode process to secure the thin walls necessary for freedom of motion and sensitivity of touch. Sizes from $6\frac{1}{2}$ to 10 allow for the desirable snug fit. The gloves may be sterilized by autoclaving for 15 minutes at 250° F. Procedures for obtaining maximum glove life have been worked out.[66] Washing with mild soap or detergent and rinsing are followed by drying inside and out. Holes are detected by visual inspection, air testing and electrical methods.[46] Before autoclaving, the gloves are powdered inside and out to prevent sticking on exposure to steam. Talcum or an absorbable powder prepared by processing cornstarch* is often used. Even ab-

*Biosorb, Ethicon, Inc., Somerville, N.J.

sorbable powder can cause granulomatous lesions and adhesions in the abdominal tract, and contamination of catheters, syringes and contrast media by glove powder has caused kidney damage during renal angiography.[249] The gloves are wrapped as individual pairs in muslin or in autoclave paper along with a packet of glove powder, which will be used when the gloves are donned. All air should be exhausted from the autoclave during sterilization. As little as 0.1 per cent of air remaining in the steam chamber doubles the rate of deterioration of the gloves.[66] Since the glove rubber temporarily loses its strength because of being heated, gloves should not be used for 24 to 48 hours after autoclaving. Ethylene oxide sterilization at 130° F. for 4 hours[74] followed by a post-sterilization rest period of 8 to 16 hours is also used. Gloves should be stored in a cool, dark place. Care must be taken to avoid puncturing gloves with the fingernails during handling. Surgical gloves are removed from the hands by rolling them inside out, rather than by pulling them off. Disposable polyethylene and polyvinyl gloves in presterilized unit packages are now relatively inexpensive and are becoming more widely used, especially as examining gloves.

Rubber gloves for household, garden or work use are also mandrel-made, but they usually are made by dipping procedures. The walls are thicker than those in surgical gloves, the fingers may be reinforced and roughened on the outside, and the inside may have a special lining for ease of donning. Small, medium, large and extra-large sizes are marketed. Synthetic rubbers such as neoprene, which resists oils and greases, as well as various plastics are widely used. Such gloves are appropriately stocked in a pharmacy, because they protect hands against detergents and common irritants.

Finger cots are rubber, finger-shaped shields used in lieu of gloves to protect fingers against corrosives or to provide a nonslip grip for work such as sorting or filing. Thin-walled cots are made from natural latex rubber by a mandrel process, and thicker ones for heavy work are made from neoprene. Usual sizes are small, medium, large and thumb. A cot that is too small can seriously interfere with blood cir-

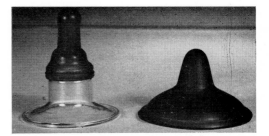

FIG. 13-17. (*Left*) Nipple shield. (*Right*) Breast shield.

culation. The pharmacist should discourage the use of finger cots as a waterproof covering over bandages, because they prevent ventilation.

Nipple and Breast Shields. A nipple shield (Fig. 13-17) is a round, slightly convex glass or plastic plate with a short central upwardly projecting tube to which a rubber nipple is securely attached. The nipple is mandrel-made. The shield is intended to be placed over sore nipples so that the pressure of the nursing baby's mouth is attenuated by the resistance of the rubber nipple. This device is not very satisfactory for either the mother or the baby, so it is used only when gross irritation or fissures are present. The breast shield (Fig. 13-17), made entirely of rubber and shaped much like the nipple shield, does not provide for nursing. It is worn to protect inflamed or irritated nipples from contact with clothing.

Condoms. The condom, or prophylactic, is a thin, nonporous sheath that is worn over the penis during coitus. A legal definition of the term prophylactic reads in part "any device, appliance or medicinal agent used in prevention of venereal disease."[186] Because of the public health aspect inherent in the use of condoms, many states have established standards of quality for these articles and test them regularly. About 16 states restrict their distribution to regular drug channels. Because condoms prevent the deposition of semen into the vaginal canal, physicians may prescribe their use when voluntary control of conception is necessary for obstetric or gynecologic reasons.

Sheaths made of rubber and of animal membranes are most widely available in this country.[232] A film[236] depicting the production of rubber prophylactics by a latex process is distributed without charge for showing to select groups. Glass mandrels are dipped into a dispersion of latex, heat-dried and re-dipped to make a sheath with a diameter ranging from 1½ to 2 inches and with a wall thickness of about 0.002 inches. A narrow bead is formed by rolling the open end on itself, leaving the tube slightly more than 7 inches long. Sheaths are heat-cured while on the mandrel. Dusting with talcum powder prevents sticking together of rubber surfaces. The sheaths are placed on metal mandrels and passed through an electrified bath to detect and eliminate those with holes. The individual condom is rolled into a flat ring which may then be sealed in aluminum foil or otherwise encased. Usual packages are paper envelopes, cardboard boxes or metal containers with 3, 12 or 36 condoms. In a cement process which is used by one company in this country, glass mandrels are dipped into a solution of crepe rubber in benzol or gasoline;[232] then the rubber is vulcanized at high temperatures. There is controversy as to the relative merits of the two processes. A special shape of prophylactic, the receptacle end condom, terminates in a short narrow pouch—about 1 x ¾ inches—which, in use, extends beyond the tip of the penis. This is claimed to reduce the possibility of breaking the sheath, since the semen is ejaculated into the open chamber rather than against an end which may be stretched tautly if the user of the regular condom does not allow a terminal margin. Receptacle end condoms may be dry or may be lubricated before packaging. The exact composition of the lubricant is a manufacturing secret, but the fluid is aqueous and generally contains glycerin and a preservative. Lubrication is intended to compensate for a possible dryness of the vaginal canal and is therefore stated to increase sensitivity.

Condoms made of animal membranes are about the same in general dimensions as those of rubber except that they may be slightly thinner walled. Details of manufacture are not available. These "skins" are made from a natural pouch, the "cul" or cecum of the lamb. The pouches must be cleaned and defatted to prevent deterioration and the development of noxious odors. Since they are not elastic, rubberized thread is sewn

along the rim of the open end. Skins are generally lubricated and rolled before packaging. Animal membranes are claimed to conduct heat better than rubber and, therefore, to interfere less with normal responses. They are more costly than those made from rubber.

Misbranding and adulteration provisions of the Federal Food Drug and Cosmetic Act apply to condoms which pass in interstate commerce. State regulations, where they exist, are often more specific. In California, for example, minimum dimensions of sheaths are specified and sample prophylactics must pass a water test.[186] Prophylactics are required to be labeled with the name and the address of the manufacturer and also with the date of manufacture. No prophylactic may be offered for sale when the dating indicates it was manufactured more than three years prior. Storage of prophylactics should be in a cool place removed from sources of heat or ozone.[186] Contact with petroleum jelly or oils can be expected to bring about deterioration of rubber prophylactics.

Diaphragms. The vaginal diaphragm is an occlusive device which the woman applies over the cervical opening prior to coitus. It is used only for contraceptive purposes. Diaphragms are generally made of thin latex rubber molded into a domed circular shape and rimmed with a steel spring enclosed in heavier rubber. Available models differ in shape, depth, kind of rubber and in type, thickness and tension of spring. When properly positioned, the lower part of the diaphragm rim rests in the posterior fornix and the upper part lodges behind the symphysis pubis so as to hold the diaphragm securely in place. The diaphragm does not allow sperm to be deposited directly at the cervical opening but it cannot be expected to prevent them from passing around its rim. A contraceptive jelly or cream must always be applied to its surfaces and rim so that sperm must travel in the spermicidal preparation for at least the diameter of the diaphragm before reaching the os. It is the increased duration of exposure to the spermicide which contributes to the effectiveness of this method.

To afford adequate protection the size and the type of diaphragm must be selected for the patient by the physician after a gynecologic examination to determine the depth of the vagina, the tone of the perineum and the condition of the pelvic organs.[225] The diaphragm which is either too small or too large is not properly supported and the penis may pass between it and the symphysis to release sperm at the cervical os. Because of the need for individual fitting and for instruction in proper insertion, Federal law stipulates that these devices may be dispensed only on prescription. Diaphragm sizes, designated in terms of the diameter in millimeters, range from 50 to 105 in increments of 5. Sizes 70 to 90 are those most commonly prescribed, with 75 the size most frequently called for.[225]

The wearer is taught to introduce the diaphragm with her fingers, or she may prefer to use an inserter specially designed for this purpose.[161] Most diaphragms may be used either dome up or dome down. Before insertion, about a teaspoonful of spermicidal jelly or cream is spread on the rim and over the side of the diaphragm which will contact the cervix or over both sides. The diaphragm may be inserted several hours prior to coitus and should be left in place for 6 to 8 hours after. It should be removed not longer than 24 hours after insertion. Removal is simply accomplished by hooking the tip of the index finger over the anterior rim of the diaphragm and pulling down and out. A cleansing douche may be taken at this time, although it is not necessary and, perhaps, undesirable. The diaphragm should be washed with mild soap and water, rinsed, dried thoroughly, dusted with talcum powder and stored in its container. It should be examined for holes or tears before use. Boiling the diaphragm or cleansing with antiseptic solutions is neither necessary nor recommended.[161]

Before dispensing a diaphragm the pharmacist should always examine it carefully for defects or deterioration. If the prescription does not carry complete information, he should ascertain if the patient desires an introducer and a vaginal cream or jelly. Kits containing these along with the diaphragm are available. A supply of talcum powder may be suggested as an adjunct to proper care of the diaphragm. Since a diaphragm may last about 2 years, the pharmacist may be well advised at the time of the original dispensing to tell the patient that permission of the prescriber will be needed when replacement is necessary.

Cervical caps are soft rubber, plastic or metal cups made to fit over the cervical opening. Suction may play a part in holding certain types in position. They are frequently left in place for days or even longer without injury.[233] Cervical caps may be used in some cases where anatomic abnormalities prevent the use of a diaphragm. Although they are in common use in Great Britain and Central Europe, they do not appear to be well-known to the lay public in the United States. They may be dispensed only on prescription.

Intrauterine Contraceptive Devices (IUDs, IUCDs). The placing of nonocclusive foreign bodies within the uterus to prevent pregnancy has been practiced for over 2,000 years.[183] The modern intrauterine contraceptive devices (Table 13-4) which are made of polyethylene or of stainless steel have been developed only since 1959, but statistics obtained from numerous clinical tests attest to their contraceptive competence.[4] There is abundant evidence that IUDs run a close second to the nearly 100 per cent effectiveness of oral contraceptives. The exact mechanism by which IUDs prevent pregnancy is not known. The most popular hypothesis is that the presence of a foreign body in the uterine cavity promotes hyperperistalsis of the oviducts so that the ovum reaches the unprepared uterus prematurely and cannot become implanted even if fertilized, because the zygote has not yet developed to the blastocyst stage.[152,199] Problems[4] with IUDs include spontaneous expulsion (often unnoticed by the user), bleeding and pain after insertion, pelvic inflammatory disease, and perforation of the uterus.[110] The devices are generally recommended only for parous women. It is postulated that their greatest value will be in impoverished and underdeveloped countries and that the use of IUDs in the United States will be primarily by women who lack the motivation or intellect for regimens requiring regular attention or for whom the oral contraceptives are psychologically or physiologically contraindicated.

TABLE 13-4. INTRAUTERINE CONTRACEPTIVE DEVICES*

DEVICE	COMPOSITION	CERVICAL APPENDAGE	NUMBER OF SIZES AVAILABLE	MANUFACTURER
Loop (Lippes)	Plastic	Nylon thread	4	Ortho Pharmaceutical Corp., Raritan, NJ
Margulies spiral (Gynecoil)	Plastic	Beaded plastic	2	Ortho Pharmaceutical Corp.
Hall-Stone ring	Stainless steel	None	1	Goshen Instrument Corp., Goshen, NY
Birnberg bow	Plastic	Nylon thread†	2	Marco & Son, Oakhurst, NJ
Double spiral (Saf. T. Coil 33)	Plastic	Beaded plastic or nylon thread	2	Julius Schmid, Inc., New York

*From AMA Committee on Human Reproduction: Evaluation of intrauterine contraceptive devices, J.A.M.A. *199*:647, 1967.
†Prior to 1966, the bow had no cervical appendage.

There are several types of intrauterine contraceptive devices (Table 13-4). The Hall-Stone ring is made of tight coils of stainless steel wire and is about 2 mm. in diameter. The Lippes loop has the form of two S's joined together. Two short nylon threads (the tail or cervical appendage) are fastened to one end. The Margulies spiral is shaped like a loosely wound watch spring with a long tail terminating in seven spherical beads set 6 mm. apart. The Birnberg bow looks like a bow knot with its loops spread open; a nylon thread cervical appendage is attached to recent models. The loop, spiral and bow are the most frequently used types. These flexible plastic IUDs are straightened out into a linear form by being placed into a small diameter plastic tube (the inserter) from which they are ejected by a plunger after insertion. When in situ in the uterus the device reassumes its original form. The tail extends into the vagina; this enables the patient to determine if the device has remained in place and also facilitates removal when necessary. Those without tails must be removed with a special hook. The spiral, loop and bow are made from a polyethylene plastic impregnated with a barium salt to make them radiopaque so that their in situ location can be verified by x-ray.[144] The time of insertion is important, it now being generally agreed that the optimal time is at or just before the end of the menstrual period to ensure insertion in a nonpregnant woman. The size of the IUD selected depends on the size of the uterine cavity. No device appears to be clearly superior or uniformly inferior, but the larger loops (size D) appear most promising[4] at this juncture. Currently, all IUDs are available only to physicians because the sterilized IUD must be inserted with due aseptic precautions by a specialist[152] to minimize potential pelvic inflammation or uterine perforation.

Surgical Appliances. The term surgical appliance encompasses trusses, surgical belts, orthopedic supports, braces, elastic hosiery and suspensories. There is ample evidence[77, 92,202] that the pharmacist can find spiritual and financial reward in servicing the public with these appliances if he is willing to allocate sufficient time, space and capital to the undertaking. It is not practical to attempt here an adequate explanation of the conditions for which anatomical supports are required or for descriptions of the myriad of appliances available or the techniques of fitting. Attendance at a specialized intensive training course that provides actual demonstrations and opportunity to practice applying supports is necessary.[79] Several surgical appliance companies offer such courses periodically. Generally they run about a week, and graduates are awarded a certificate. In addition to maintaining and extending his expertise through practice, the pharmacist will need to refer often to current books[56,59,97] and periodicals[118,228] dealing with this specialty area.

Some elastic support items are quite generally stocked by pharmacies owing to frequent requests for them for alleviation of relatively minor mishaps. Anklets, kneecaps, wrist and elbow supports, athletic supporters, suspensories, elastic hosiery and elastic bandages fall into this category.

Elastic bandages* may be made with rubber or elastomer threads woven into the fabric, or the elasticity may be due to a special knit of cotton fibers. These bandages are used chiefly to apply compression to sprains, varicose veins, burns or wounds, and rib fractures. The elasticity allows the bandage to give if swelling occurs under it, and interference with circulation is consequently minimized. All-cotton bandages do not readily deteriorate with exposure to light or heat, and washing restores the elasticity. Greater pressure may be applied with the rubber-containing bandages, but because they are somewhat occlusive the covered area gets warm. Replacing the rubber with a polyurethane elastomer fiber (spandex) is claimed to result in a lighter, cooler, softer, stronger and autoclavable bandage. This fiber (in brassieres) has been reported[229] to cause an allergic contact dermatitis. Elastic bandages are available in widths of 2 to 6 inches or more. The 2- or 2½-inch width is used for the wrist or foot, the 2½- or 3-inch width for the ankle or elbow, the 3- or 4-inch width for the knee or lower leg, and the 4- or 6-inch width for the shoulder. The usual length (stretched) is 5½ yards. Ends are fastened in place by flat metal clips furnished with each roll of bandage. Because clips are easily lost or broken, replacements should be stocked. Some brands are now marketed with clips that are permanently attached to one end.

A new form of elastic bandage† is made of nonwoven rayon with synthetic rubber strands running lengthwise through the backing. Because of a special adhesive substance in the backing, it sticks to itself, but not to skin. It does not slip about when being applied, and also the need for special clips is eliminated. The bandage is lighter, thinner and cooler than the woven ones. It may be steam-sterilized.

The pharmacist should study the instructions packaged with individual rolls of elastic bandages so that he can advise his clients on the proper method for applying the type of bandage selected. Too much or uneven compression can be harmful,[73] whereas a wrap that is too loose is useless.

Adhesive elastic bandages* are adhesive-coated cotton bandages with somewhat the same uses as those just described, as well as those more usual for regular adhesive tape. Widths vary from 1 to 4 inches and lengths (stretched) are up to 5 yards.

Elastic Hose. Elastic hosiery is worn to prevent or alleviate varicose veins.[59] These develop usually in individuals such as dentists or pharmacists who may be required to stand in one place for long periods of time. Alternate contraction and relaxation of leg muscles during walking help the return flow of blood to the heart against the force of gravity by massaging vein walls so as to squeeze the blood along through a series of valves which tend to direct it upward only. With continued standing, blood accumulates in the leg, venous pressure increases, the valves fail, the walls of the affected veins bulge and knot as they become distended by the blood and severe pain is felt. The compression and the massaging action of elastic bandages or hosiery are used to help the leg muscles in returning blood to the heart and thus give symptomatic relief and prevent further unsightly venous distention.

Elastic hosiery is knit from latex rubber thread covered with nylon, rayon or cotton. Brands and styles differ in details of design, in gauge of rubber thread used and in weight and type of knitting yarn.[59] An elastic stocking may have either two-way or one-way stretch, the latter lacking lengthwise stretch. One-way stretch stockings are generally of heavier weight and deliver maximum circular com-

---

* Ace Spandex Elastic Bandage, B-D Cotton Elastic Bandage, Becton, Dickinson and Company, Rutherford, N.J.; Comprol and Dyna-Flex Rubber Elastic Bandages, Johnson and Johnson, New Brunswick, N. J.; Readiflex Elastic Bandage, Parke, Davis and Co., Detroit, Mich.; Tensor Elastic Bandage, Bauer and Black, Chicago, Ill.

† Coban Elastic Bandage, 3M Company, St. Paul, Minn.

* Ace-hesive, Becton, Dickinson and Company.

pression which makes them better suited to treat severe or difficult cases. Men do not object to their bulkiness, but women find them unattractive and often refuse to wear them in public. Since there is no vertical give, the one-way stretch stocking must be fitted very carefully so as to provide uniform pressure. Failure to do so may cause edema or other complications in spots where too little pressure is being applied. Individual manufacturers supply diagrams to show the key parts of the leg to measure and corresponding tables to enable choice of the correct stock size. Snug measurements accurate to ⅛ inch should be taken without compressing the leg. If swelling occurs during the day, circumference measurements should be taken by the patient in the morning before arising.

Two-way stretch stockings are available in surgical (heavy) weight, service weight and in sheer light-weight styles. Fitting to the leg is easier, since the more the hose is stretched lengthwise the smaller its circumference becomes. A few measurements are taken to choose from among the 4 or 5 available sizes ranging from small to extra-large. As the thickness of the cloth decreases, therapeutic support does likewise. It is doubtful that the ultra-sheer style which vanity persuades women to choose actually provides adequate compression. They should be encouraged at least to wear a heavier stocking while at home.

Elastic stockings (Fig. 13-18, *top*) are available in lengths ranging from below-knee or garter styles to thigh hose, which allows for a choice according to need for support and to client preference. Some stockings have a full foot, but more often the toe and the heel, are cut out so that a pair of dress hose may be worn over them. Seamless elastic hose are popular because they are less noticeable when covered.

In order to prevent swelling of the legs, some wearers must put the elastic hose on in the morning even before standing up. The elastic stocking or hose is put on by rolling or folding it down until the foot may be inserted easily into the toe end and then rolling it back up the leg with a minimum of tugging and pulling. Dykes[88] has suggested that wearers should first put on lady's nylon hose, then pull the elastic stocking over it.

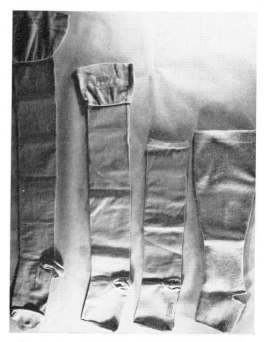

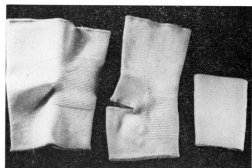

FIG. 13-18. (*Top*) Elastic hose. Left to right, overknee, lightweight, two-way stretch, full-foot seamless nylon elastic hose; similar with partial foot only; similar, underknee (garter) length; surgical weight, one-way stretch, garter length, rayon and cotton hose. (*Bottom*) Extremity supports. Left to right, knee support, ankle support and wrist support.

This reduces friction so the elastic stocking is easier to put on and also reduces discomfort and trauma to legs with recent skin grafts, stasis dermatitis, venous ulcers, scar epithelium or sensitive skin. Also, the stocking may last longer because direct contact with sweat is avoided. Men may need to cut a small hole in the toe of the nylon stocking to enlarge it for comfortable fitting.

Proper care of elastic stockings is important because the rubber is subject to deterioration from heat and other environmental factors. Contact with ointments, oils or lanolin should be avoided. Daily washing with soap and water, adequate rinsing and drying, and a period of nonuse between wearings add to the maximum life of the stocking. The wearer should purchase at least two stockings for each affected leg so as to enable him to alternate the use of the two sets.

Extremity Supports. Anklets, knee caps and elbow braces are made of rubber thread covered with cotton and woven into seamless surgical-weight tubes shaped to fit the areas that each is intended to support (Fig. 13-18, *bottom*). They are used most often to compress, support and immobilize sprains or wrenched joints. Sizes run from small to extra large, with fitting done by having the client try on the support. Hinged knee caps with jointed steel sidebars are available to supply lateral support when needed for severe sprains. Wristlets (Fig. 13-18, *bottom*) also are used to support a weak wrist and are available in leather, as well as in elastic cloth. Leather wristbands have one to three straps, depending on their width, and may be lined or unlined. Elastic and leather wristlets often are made in a single size that is adjusted to fit the wrist by use of snap buttons, buckles or Velcro fasteners.

Suspensories are used for a wide variety of conditions involving the scrotum and its contents.[59] Conservative treatment of varicocele, epididymitis and orchitis calls for wearing a suspensory. They are also used to support the scrotum after hydrocele treatment, hernia repair, prostatectomy and scrotal surgery. In each instance, the function of the suspensory is to hold up or to support the scrotum so as to relieve the pain and discomfort accompanying the afflictions just mentioned.

Suspensories consist of a pouch attached to a body belt (Fig. 13-19, *left*). Some also have leg straps which provide additional support though they may cause some discomfort to the wearer. Pouches are made of soft cotton knitted into a porous mesh to permit ventilation. The pouch should be the correct size to contain the entire scrotum comfortably. A pouch that is too small tends to bind and cut at the edges and to compress rather than to support. A pouch that is too large cuts into tissues around the scrotum and does not give good support. Since correct fit is determined only by observation from both front and side with the patient in a standing position, the original designation of size may be made by the attending physician. Pouch sizes range from small to extra large. Some styles have drawstrings which allow for minor adjustments. Belts may or may not be elastic but are always adaptable to a wide range of waist dimensions. Size designations do not refer to belt length but only to pouch capacity. Variations between suspensories

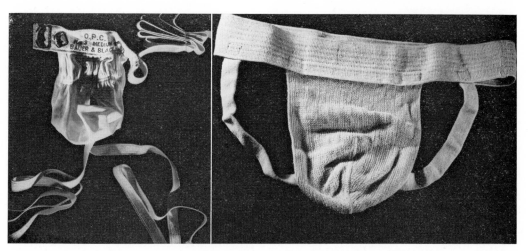

FIG. 13-19. (*Left*) Suspensory. This style with leg straps is especially suited for active or heavy-set men. (*Right*) Athletic supporter.

are found in weight of pouches, form of body belt and presence or absence of leg straps. Catalogs suggest that some styles are better for stout men and others are better for slender men.

Athletic supporters are worn usually as scrotal supports to combat fatigue and strain during sports or other tiring physical activities. They differ from suspensories in being made of elastic cloth (cotton or nylon) and in being designed to enclose all the genital organs within the pouch rather than only the scrotum (Fig. 13-19, *right*). Some are made with a nonelastic knitted mesh pouch. Both pouches and leg straps are generally an integral part of the appliance, but they are detachable in some styles. Belt widths vary from 1 inch up to 10 inches with the wider belts being used as abdominal supports, sometimes for a "slimming" effect. Sizes are in terms of waist measure, not pouch size, and run from small to extra large. Supporters are easily fitted, since the elasticity of the waistband allows for a range of 2 to 3 inches within each size. As with all appliances containing rubber, proper care to avoid contact with deteriorating agents will extend the period of useful service.

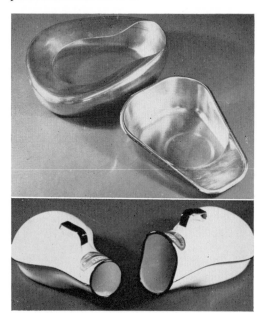

Fig. 13-20. (*Top*) Bedpan (*left*) and fracture pan. These are stainless steel. (*Bottom*) Male (left) and female enamel urinals.

SICKROOM UTENSILS

Proper care of a person confined to bed may require the use of several forms of pans or basins for collecting body excretions and discharges. This ware is made commonly of stainless steel or porcelain enamel and, sometimes, of glass, rubber or plastics.

Bedpans (Fig. 13-20, *top*) are fairly shallow pans which are slipped under the hips of a person lying in bed so as to collect his feces and urine. They are generally oval in shape and have a wide flat rim for supporting the weight of the individual. Both adult-size and child-size pans are made. A specially angled style* said to be less uncomfortable, is available. The fracture bedpan (Fig. 13-20,*top*) is smaller, flatter and easier to use with immobilized or overweight patients or children. Those of stainless steel are most suited to continued and rough use, as found in hospitals. Enamelware is acceptable for home use; though heavy, cold and easily chipped, it is easy to clean. Inflated rubber bedpans are warm and comfortable, but they are expensive and difficult to clean. Plastic bedpans† are light, warm, sturdy and easily cleaned, and so seem ideal for home use. Autoclavable pans are molded from polypropylene, nonautoclavable from polystyrene.

The purchaser may need instruction in the use and care of a bedpan. Steel or enamelware should be warmed before use by washing with warm water and then drying. It is advisable to spread several layers of newspaper under the patient's hips as a precaution against accidental spillage. Immediately after use, the pan should be cleaned, dried and made ready for reuse.

Commodes are straight-back chairs or wheelchairs with an open seat and a place beneath to hold a bedpan or other receptacle for feces or urine. Benton *et al.*[47] confirmed that many persons have difficulty defecating while on a bedpan. Straining to do so results in an increase in cardiac effort greater than that produced when the patient uses a commode, in spite of the energy expended by the patient in getting to and from the

* Relax Bedpan, The Jones Metal Products Company, West Lafayette, Ohio.

†Plasta-medic Manufacturing Inc., Pasadena, California; Jones-Zylon, Inc., West Lafayette, Ohio.

commode. Many styles of commodes are marketed. Some are made of aluminum tubing with legs that are adjustable to several heights.

Douche pans have the general appearance of fracture pans, but are flatter, shallower and more oblong. They are used to collect medicated solutions or washes following irrigations of body cavities.

Urinals are employed to collect urine. The two types—male and female—differ in shape (Fig. 13-20, *bottom*). The female type is little used because women seem to prefer a bedpan. Urinals are made from stainless steel, porcelain enamel, glass or plastic. Some are calibrated to facilitate measuring the volume of urine output when requested by the physician. They hold about 1,000 ml. in the horizontal position. Before use, urinals should be warmed in the same manner as bedpans and similarly cleaned after use. Autoclavable plastic urinals* are now available.

Hip or sitz baths[145] are taken to relieve urinary retention, tenesmus, pelvic pain, congestion and muscle spasm. Specially designed basin-like seats which may be placed on the standard toilet bowl and attached to the tub or sink water supply can be suggested for convenience and comfort greater than that resulting from the usual procedure of sitting in 6 inches of water in a bathtub.

Kidney basins, so named because of their shape, are also called emesis, pus and sputum basins, after the fluids commonly collected in them. The usual capacity is 500 to 1,000 ml. Inexpensive kidney basins of plastic or treated paper are available; these are disposed of after each use.

Other utensils and equipment that pharmacists should supply—because they are needed for taking care of bedridden patients —include wash basins, foot tubs, serving trays, feeding cups, water pitchers, drinking tubes or flexible straws, and graduated measures. Disposable kits containing some of these utensils packaged as units for sickroom use are now available. A number of miscellaneous items that can help to make home or hospital patients more comfortable have

been succinctly described in a small booklet.[15]

ELECTRIC HEATING PADS

For reasons of convenience and easy adjustment of temperature, electric heating pads are now popular for home use. Significant differences in design exist among the available models within any one brand of heating pad. For example, a pad may be constructed to be either moisture-resistant or wetproof; it may be a three-speed, a three-positive heat or a variable-heat pad. These terms are clarified in the descriptions that follow.

The pad usually consists of a heating element, at least two thermostats, a switch, a cordset, a plastic or rubberized cover and a cloth cover. The heating element is a resistance wire that is wound over an insulating core and then covered with an insulating layer of material to make a strand about 3 mm. in diameter. The strand is sewn to a flat piece of material (usually burlap) in either a spiral rectangular or a back-and-forth pattern that is designed to ensure a uniform distribution of heat over the whole pad. The thermostatic controls and the cordset are attached. The unit is then covered on both sides with a layer of soft cotton wadding backed with an open-mesh gauze layer, and the whole unit is sewn together along the edges. The flat pad is enveloped in a totally enclosed cover (usually a rubberized fabric, or sometimes vinyl) and sealed in a vulcanizing press or a high-frequency sealing machine to make it wetproof. These pads are immersed in water to meet quality-control standards for moisture leakage.*

In 1960 it was reported that 22 of 42 models selected for testing were not fully sealed against moisture, the fault usually being at the power-cord entrance.[13] A similar test[20] in 1966 found only 3 of 33 to be unacceptable. The construction of moisture-resistant pads differs from the wetproof in that the cover is not completely sealed; the pads are therefore not subjected to an immersion test.

---

* Plasta-medic Manufacturing Inc., Pasadena, California; Jones-Zylon, Inc., West Lafayette, Ohio.

* Standard for Electrically Heated Pads and Bedding, UL 130, Dec., 1954, Underwriters' Laboratories, Inc., Chicago, Ill.

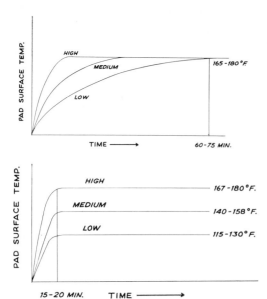

FIG. 13-21. (*Top*) Typical temperature-time characteristics of a three-speed electric heating pad. (From Little, L. D., and Wise, R. A., General Electric Co., Asheboro, N. Carolina) (*Bottom*) Typical temperature-time characteristics of a three-positive heat electric heating pad.

The switch selector on the three-speed pad may be marked low, medium and high; these refer not to the final temperature of the pad but rather to the rate of temperature rise. No matter which setting is used, the pad will eventually attain the same temperature (approximately 165 to 180° F.). Only the speed at which the pad heats up is controlled. The pad has two heater circuits that differ in resistance and by switching from one to another or by switching both circuits in parallel, the time required to obtain the desired temperature is varied (Fig. 13-21, *top*). One of the two thermostats operates the pad at the desired temperature, and the second one is in the circuit as a safety back-up in case the operating thermostat becomes defective and fails to open the circuit.[143] On the other hand, through different circuitry,[166] the three-positive (or fixed) heat pad does attain a separate and distinct surface temperature for each different switch selector position. Figure 13-21, *bottom,* shows temperature-time characteristics of such a pad. When a large series was tested,[20]

the following were reported: an average of 110° at the low setting, 145° at the high, about halfway between these for medium; 7 to 9 minutes for most models to reach 135° (90 per cent of high setting), about 11 minutes for a few.

Pads differ in design of control switch, there being push-button, slide, continuous rotary and click-stop rotary types. Push-button switches have been rated as the most convenient.[20] Switches may have a glow-light or raised "braille" markings to help in heat selection in the dark. Covers may be made of cotton, acetate, acrylic or nylon; they are generally washable and are often attractively patterned. Although 12 × 15 inches appears to be the standard size, both larger and smaller pads are available. Guarantees against defective workmanship and material range from 1 to 5 years. These factors, along with differences in basic construction features, are measures of quality or affect price. The wetproof pad is preferable because there is less danger of shock to the user who perspires heavily. Furthermore, the wetproof pad may be placed over a wet compress to supply steady warmth and moist heat which may be therapeutically desirable for inflamed areas of the skin, for example. On the other hand, the moisture-resistant pad must be kept dry; it must not be used with wet dressings. The three-positive heat pad is preferable to the three-speed pad, because the selectability of the correct heat is desirable for use over an extended length of time. The three-speed pad seems to be disappearing from the market.

The pharmacist should be sure that his client is warned about possible misuse of the electric heating pad. Precautionary statements are usually printed on the box; these should be emphasized when the pad is dispensed. Use of pins or other metallic means of fastening the pad in place is very dangerous because of the possibility of electric shock. For similar reasons, the pad should not be crushed or folded while being used nor should it be used if the vinyl cover shows signs of blistering, cracking or other damage. It is important to warn the user to examine frequently the skin area being heated for unusual redness or signs of burning. Cautions against going to sleep while using the pad should be voiced, since serious burns can result. Diabetics require special warning because they may be less sensitive to pain from intense heat and yet burn easily and badly because of poor circulation, particularly in the lower limbs[231] of the older diabetic.[84]

INHALATION THERAPY DEVICES

Inhalation therapy is defined[69] as therapy designed to restore toward normal, pathophysiologic alterations of gas exchange in the cardiopulmonary system. Adequate oxygenation and elimination of carbon dioxide are the usual aims. This is accomplished[69] "by means of the proper application of therapeutic gases including oxygen, helium-oxygen, and carbon dioxide mixtures; the use of pressure breathing devices, resuscitators, and respirators to promote artificial ventilation and respiration; the administration of aerosols to improve the airway of the pulmonary system by relieving bronchospasm, liquefying secretions, and combating infections; and the use of artificial airways to relieve obstruction." Archambault[36] has suggested a mission for the pharmacist in this relatively new medical service. Some selected aspects of inhalation therapy and associated equipment are discussed here. The pharmacist intending to remain up-to-date in this field should regularly read the official journal* of the American Association for Inhalation Therapy.

VAPORIZER-HUMIDIFIERS

Vaporizer-humidifiers are devices used to produce high humidity by putting a relatively large concentration of water in vapor or fine droplet form into an enclosed space such as a sickroom or a mist tent. Inhalation of moist warm air ("steam") is used to alleviate inflammation of the mucous membranes in acute colds and sinusitis, to liquefy thick tenacious mucus and to relieve coughing, croup, acute laryngitis and hoarseness.[145] Prolonged exposure to the low relative humidity of artificially heated rooms adversely affects the protective mechanisms of the respiratory tract and contributes to the in-

* *Inhalation Therapy,* J. B. Lippincott Co.

creased incidence of upper respiratory infection during cold weather.[107,160] Simple humidification may give relief to certain individuals with acute or chronic respiratory disease.[107] Volatile medications, such as compound benzoin tincture, that are sometimes used in these devices have not been shown to add anything beyond aroma to the vapor.[58]

Vaporizer-humidifiers may be classified into four types with respect to the method used to vaporize, aerosolize or nebulize water. These types are the electrolytic, the boiler, the cold steam and the ultrasonic nebulizer.

The basic components of the electrolytic and the boiler types are essentially similar—a jar to hold the water, an electrical unit to convert the water to vapor, a lid with an escape hole for the steam and a service cord to connect the electrical unit to regular house current. The jars are made of glass or a heat-resistant plastic such as polypropylene. The lids are usually made of hard plastic. A cup for medication generally is hollowed out of the portion of the lid immediately beneath the steam escape hole. A separate nozzle or steam spout is sometimes provided with the vaporizer. Most electrolytic models have an electrode assembly composed of the lid and of the two electrodes suspended in a cylindrical plastic chamber. When this is put into the main jar, water flows into the plastic chamber through a small hole in the chamber bottom. Only the relatively small amount of water in the chamber must be heated to boiling in order to produce steam. This makes for quicker starting and also greatly reduces the risk of burns or scalds, because the rest of the water in the jar does not get boiling hot. As the steam is generated, it rises through a series of holes at the top of the plastic chamber and escapes through the single large hole in the lid. For safety, automatic shut-off of the heating is assured by making the chamber too short to reach the bottom of the jar. When the chamber is empty, current flow between the electrodes is not possible even though there is still water in the jar. Because the water carries an electric current as long as the electrodes are in contact with it, the user must be cautioned always to disconnect the

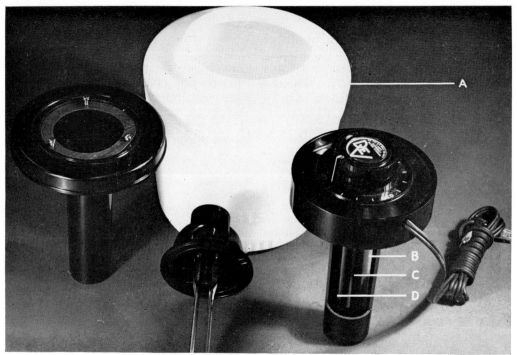

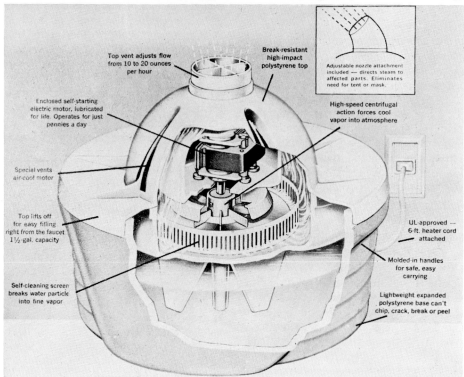

Fig. 13-22. (*Top*) Electrolytic vaporizer. The cap and the electrode assembly (lower center) have been removed from the chamber (*left*). Note that the chamber is shorter than the plastic jar with which it is used. Part of the cylinder of an adjustable-rate electrolytic model (*lower right*) was removed to show the electrodes. At the low setting the insulating plate is between the two electrodes. A, medicament cup; B, stationary electrode; C, insulating plate; D, movable electrode. (*Bottom*) Cold steam vaporizer-humidifier.

unit before lifting off the cover. Some models are designed to break the circuit automatically when the cover is raised.

The rate of steam production is proportional to the rate of current flow between the electrodes in the electrolytic models. This, in turn, depends on the quantity (and conductance) of the ions in the water. Failure to understand this relationship is frequently responsible for dissatisfaction on the part of the user. Tap water is rarely suitable. The high mineral content of hard water causes frothing, spilling over and a shortened duration of steaming. On the other hand, soft or distilled water conducts too poorly to produce enough steam. The preferred procedure is to use distilled water (or soft tap water) to which is added an amount of salt, borax or sodium bicarbonate adequate to impart the correct conductivity. Some companies provide small salt tablets with the vaporizer. It is usually necessary to start out with a very small amount of electrolyte and increase it with successive uses until the performance is satisfactory. A more selective control of rate of steaming is afforded by models in which the space separating the two electrodes can be widened or narrowed within set limits by turning a dial on the lid (Fig. 13-22, *top*). Increasing the distance between electrodes (turning dial toward *low*) results in a slower rate of steam production, because current flow is decreased. In electrolytic models, it is important to rinse the jar and the electrode chamber with tap water after each use so as to keep deposition of minerals to a minimum. Even if this is done, it is usually necessary after some 50 hours of operation to disassemble the electrode chamber in order to scrape accumulated mineral deposits from the electrodes.

In the boiler type, a sealed-rod heating element suspended from the lid dips into tap water in a small chamber within the jar and heats it to boiling. A thermostatic device cuts off the current flow before all the water is vaporized. This type has largely disappeared from the market.

In the cold steam (cool-mist) machine (Fig. 13-22, *bottom*) an electric pump sucks water from the reservoir tank up into a smaller chamber, where rapidly rotating metal vanes dash the water particles forcibly against a fine screen. The small droplets thus formed escape from the adjustable end or top vents.

The ultrasonic nebulizer, first released in 1964, utilizes high-frequency sound waves to produce large-volume, fine-particle aerosols. The frequency of vibration of the transducer crystal and the flow-rate of the air used to sweep the aerosol through the conducting tube to the patient control the droplet size and the volume of mist produced. The units are used with tents, face masks, incubators, IPPB respirators and special breathing systems in hospitals and occasionally in homes under special circumstances. Because of cost, they are not likely to be routinely stocked by pharmacists. Manufacturers'* brochures and selected references[83, 224] should be obtained for further information about ultrasonic nebulizers.

For optimum performance for home use, a vaporizer-humidifier should begin to produce vapor or mist within 2 or 3 minutes after being turned on. The vaporizer should produce moisture at a relatively high rate for about 2 hours in order to overcome the original dry condition of the room and furnishings and then slow down to a rate adequate to maintain the high moisture level. It should operate for at least 8 to 12 hours between refills; this requires a jar capacity of 1 to 1½ gallons. The vaporizer should shut off automatically before it becomes empty, and it should be safe and convenient to use —easy to fill, not readily tipped over and without burn or electrical shock hazards. Not all models satisfy these criteria to the same degree.[30]

Electrolytic, boiler and cool-mist vaporizer-humidifiers have been objectively compared.[30,107,222] The presence of heat in steam does not seem to offer therapeutic advantage over a cold fine aerosol. Cool-mist models are inherently safer because no heat is involved, but they do not humidify as fast as the electrolytic types, are noisier, and in hard-water areas, cause a white coating of minerals to be deposited on furniture. Most cool-mist models cost more than most electrolytics, but on the other hand, they use

* The DeVilbiss Co., Somerset, Pa.; Mistogen Equipment Co., Oakland, Calif.

about $\frac{1}{6}$ as much electricity. Boiler types do not require special additives and have less of a shock hazard than electrolytics, but they steam rather slowly.

Atomizers, Nebulizers, Insufflators

Atomizers and nebulizers are instruments used to apply liquids as sprays. However, they are not interchangeable in use. Atomizers are designed to form relatively coarse sprays for application to the nasal passages, throat and pharynx, whereas nebulizers emit fine sprays that reach the larynx and even the alveoli of the lungs. Construction characteristics and principles underlying their operation and use have been reviewed.[153,169,222] Chapter 8 contains a more detailed discussion of this subject.

Atomizers. All atomizers function according to the same basic plan. Liquid placed in a bottle is forced up and out through a dip tube because the pressure on the surface of the liquid is greater than that in the tube. As liquid emerges from the dip tube, it is dispersed into a spray by forcible impact with a rapidly flowing stream of air. The two basic atomizers—the vacuum and the pressure types—differ in the way in which the pressure on the surface is generated. In the vacuum type (Fig. 13-23), the air stream is conducted at high velocity over the exit end of the dip tube. Pressure in the tube is thereby reduced in accord with Bernoulli's principle,[169] and as a result, liquid is pushed up into the tube by the force of atmospheric pressure. Outside air enters the bottle through a small vent hole in the cap. In the pressure type (Fig. 13-23, *bottom*), part of the air stream is detoured through the container so as to reinforce the vacuum action by an additional pressure on the liquid surface. The container is not vented as this would negate the pressure effect. In atomizers for home use, the air stream is generated by squeezing a valved rubber bulb; those used in physicians' offices or in hospitals are often operated from a motorized air compressor. Vacuum-type atomizers have narrow air tubes and wide fluid tubes which result in the formation of large volumes of coarse spray. On the other hand, pressure atomizers, which are designed with wide air tubes and narrow fluid tubes, emit small volumes of a fine spray. Sprays from vacuum atomizers are intermittent, the flow stopping immediately on release of the bulb. Pressure atomizers tend to produce a more continuous spray.

The usual nose and throat formulations containing sympathomimetic amines, antiseptics, antihistamines and local anesthetics may be applied more effectively from atomizers, since sprays can reach throat and nasal surfaces which gargles and instillations from medicine droppers cannot.[153] The pharmacist probably should suggest the use of atomizers more frequently than he does. His clients will need advice in selecting from among the several styles the one suitable for the intended use. For example, certain atomizers are made with metal caps and outlet tubes because these are not easily broken and may be sterilized by flame or boiling. Unfortunately, many commonly used solutions either attack metal or deteriorate more rapidly in its presence. Commercial preparations compatible with metal atomizers are listed in Table 13-5. Atomizers designed so that the solutions contact only glass, plastic or hard rubber are more fragile and can be sterilized only by the relatively inefficient method of immersion in alcohol or other germicidal solutions. Some vacuum atomizers have twin outlet tubes and an adjustable spray tip which is convenient for directing the spray back of the soft palate.[169] These are particularly suitable for oleaginous* and viscous liquids.[169] Others with single tubes (Fig. 13-23 top) are easier to clean out if clogged and are recommended for solutions which tend to crystallize. Pressure atomizers generally produce a finer spray which carries the medication into deeper cavities of

---

* Oily vehicles are in disfavor because oil interferes with ciliary activity of mucous membranes and there is a risk of lipoid pneumonia if the droplets are inhaled.

Table 13-5. Atomizer Solutions Compatible with Metals

Furacin Nasal (Eaton)
Ephedrine Inhalant
Cepacol (Merrell)
Gluco-Fedrin (Parke, Davis)
Chloretone Inhalant (Parke, Davis)
S. T. 37 solution (Merck Sharp & Dohme)

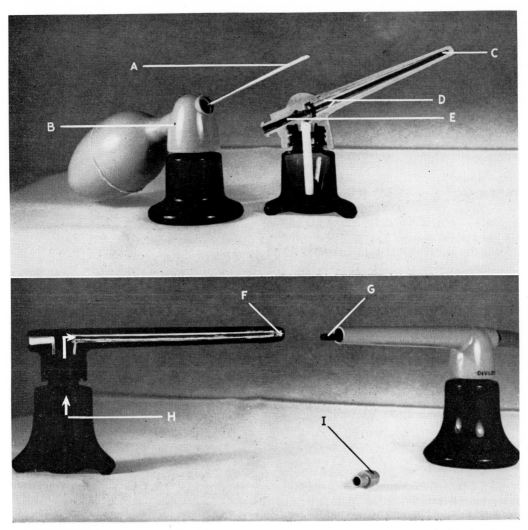

FIG. 13-23. (*Top*) Vacuum-type atomizer. The air stream is pumped through the air tube and does not enter the container. In order to show the air tube, the larger concentric tube through which the liquid flows has been unscrewed from the atomizer on the left, the one on the right has been sectioned. Atomization takes place at the tip where the air stream and the liquid meet. A, air tube (metal); B, vent; C, distal end of air tube; D, canal for liquid; E, proximal end of air tube. (*Bottom*) Pressure-type atomizer. (*Left*) In the sectioned atomizer the path followed by the air stream has been outlined with a light color. The course of the liquid is indicated by arrows. (*Right*) The tip has been unscrewed from the atomizer in order to show the end of the small plastic or hard rubber tube through which the liquid is forced. The air stream passes through the larger tube. F, atomizing chamber; G, tube for liquid; H, dip tube; I, removable tip.

the nose and the throat more readily than does the coarser spray from the vacuum types. A pocket-type atomizer operating on the vacuum principle produces a very fine mist almost equivalent to that from the nebulizer which it resembles in design. This compact and capped atomizer is convenient to carry, and, also, it operates with small volumes of solution—an advantage when the medication is potent and expensive.

Before spraying medication into the nose the patient should clear the nasal passages by blowing. The head is tilted back and the atomizer tip is placed in one nostril, leaving the other open. Some atomizers have a nasal guard which fits over the spray tip. The guard minimizes the danger of scratching the lining of the nares and limits back flow by partially plugging the nasal opening. Grooves on the surface prevent buildup of air pressure within the nasal cavities. For throat applications the nasal guard is removed and the tube of the atomizer is placed in the mouth with the tip directed toward the area to be sprayed. Atomizers tend to clog and are most easily opened up with the help of a fine wire such as a hypodermic needle wire.

Plastic spray bottles are commonly used for commercially available nasal and throat medications. When the flexible container is squeezed, the air inside is compressed and the increased pressure forces the fluid up a narrow-bore tube into a small hole in the tip at the same time that a stream of air is forced into the tip through two tiny holes. The shearing forces and the vacuum effect are similar to those already described for atomizers. Users sometimes complain that the bottle is not full, because they fail to realize that the air space is essential to the formation of the spray. Empty plastic containers are marketed for use with extemporaneous nasal preparations.

Nebulizers (Fig. 13-24) consist of a small vacuum-type atomizing unit enclosed in a larger container or flask. The spray is formed by forcing a fine jet of air over the tip of a capillary dip tube.[181] It is carried forward by the air current, which spreads out and slows up because the flask chamber is large and the outlet tube is wide. Consequently, only the smallest drops are carried through the outlet tube, larger ones striking the sides of the flask and falling back to the base of the dip tube. In some styles, this baffling action is enhanced by curving (Fig. 13-24, *left*) or offsetting the outlet tube. In some nebulizers (Fig. 13-24, *right*), the spray is made to strike against a baffle-plate placed about 2 mm. from its point of origin. This more efficient design[181] facilitates subdivision into finer particles and elimination of the large drops. Nebulizers are generally used with the vent hole open; closing it decreases the

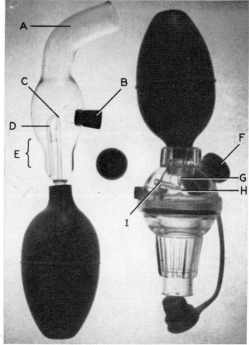

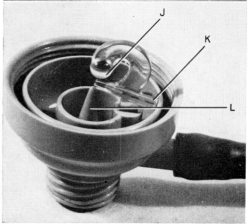

FIG. 13-24. Nebulizers. (*Top, left*) The nebulizer is used in the vertical position shown. A, outlet tube; B, vent stopper; C, air jet; D, capillary dip tube; E, approximate limits of liquid chamber. (*Top, right*) Nebulizer to be held in a horizontal position; thus, the base of the dip tube will extend into the liquid in the chamber. F, vent stopper; G, air jet; H, baffle; I, dip tube. (*Bottom*) Nebulizing unit with baffle-plate. J, baffle plate; K, capillary dip tube; L, air jet tube.

amount of spray formed. Nebulizers are made only of glass or of plastics, because metals accelerate the deterioration of agents commonly used in aerosols. Pocket-size models are available. Rubber bulbs are used to operate hand models. Small compressors or tanks of compressed oxygen, helium or other gases may be used in physicians' offices or in hospitals. Inexpensive adaptations of tire pumps to power hand nebulizers have been described.[111,185] A complete aerosol unit* (compressor, nebulizer and accessories) for home use is marketed. Ultrasonic nebulizers are described with the vaporizer-humidifiers (p. 519). With respect to size of particle produced and to some of their applications, they could as logically have been included in this section. Because of ventilatory impairment, some patients need also to use intermittent positive-pressure breathing (IPPB) machines during nebulization therapy.[184]

The mist or fog that flows out of the nebulizer is a suspension of a liquid in air and is classified as an aerosol. Nebulizers were first developed to apply bronchodilators directly to the lungs to palliate chronic bronchial asthma, chronic pulmonary emphysema and related conditions. Along with the local topical effect, there may be a pronounced systemic action, because these drugs may pass rapidly into the circulatory system.[190] Recent reviews[28,113] have stressed the limitations of and adverse effects from medications administered as aerosols, as well as the advantages and potentials of this dosage form.[54] Some authorities[42] believe the hand-bulb nebulizer is superior to Freon-propelled units for supplying medication to relieve bronchial constriction because a larger dose of drug may be provided with fewer adverse effects and more lasting benefit.

Particle size distribution, which depends on the design of the nebulizer and the way in which it is used, largely governs where the medication will impinge, how much will be retained or will be exhaled, and also the degree of absorption into the bloodstream.[54, 83,131,203,207] Particles 3 micra in radius and larger are taken out completely by the trachea, the bronchi, the bronchioles and the alveolar ducts.[95] Particles of 1 micron or more reach the alveoli and 97 per cent are retained, only 3 per cent being exhaled. Smaller particles, 0.3 to 0.4 micra in radius penetrate to the alveoli also, but 65 to 70 per cent of them are exhaled. Nebulizers should be constructed with suitable baffles to remove the large particles and to ensure delivery of small particles, most of which are the size optimum for deposition only in the bronchioles, the alveolar ducts and the alveoli. Particle radii ranging from 0.5 to 2.0 or 3.0 micra are suitable.[190,207] Disagreement concerning the precise relationship between particle size and retention in the lungs exists among workers in the field.[131]

Published performance data for commercially available nebulizers are scanty and are not in good agreement, perhaps owing to differences in experimental technics and to variations in the individual nebulizers used.[194,203] Most investigators have used the Vaponefrin* and the DeVilbiss† No. 40 nebulizers and have considered them to be satisfactory and about equivalent with respect to the average particle size produced. Of the particles produced by these nebulizers, 80 to 90 per cent were found to have a radius of 1.5 micra or less.[1,48] Reif and Holcomb[193] have listed relevant operating characteristics of nebulizers and have studied the effects of varying several cf these. Modell et al.[159] have reported that 97 per cent of the particles in the aerosol produced by the ultrasonic nebulizer have a mean particle radius of 0.4 to 1.55 micra. In view of the numerous claims for superiority of one design over another, it is unfortunate that a systematic comparison of all the available models and styles has not been made. Kanig[131] has reviewed methods of measuring particle size of aerosols and the difficulties therein.

Directions for using nebulizers are given on nebulizer boxes and inserts supplied with the medications used. The solution is added by dropper through the throat tube, 10 to 20 drops being used. The fluid level must be kept below the tip of the dip tube or

---

* Maxi-Myst Aerosol Unit, Mead Johnson and Co., Evansville, Ind.

* USV Pharmaceutical Corp., New York, N.Y.
† The DeVilbiss Company, Somerset, Pa.

atomization does not occur. Generally, the patient is directed to place the nozzle just inside his partially opened mouth, then to squeeze the bulb vigorously once or twice, inhaling deeply through the mouth with each compression. The vent is opened for maximum aerosol delivery. The inhalation of medication may be repeated several times at intervals of 1 or 2 minutes until relief is obtained. Swallowing the solution should be avoided so as to limit systemic effects. Gargling with warm water relieves the dryness that sometimes occurs. Patients should be told not to be concerned about the pink color that appears in the sputum as the drug is decomposed. Excess solution should be left in the nebulizer (capped) and not returned to the bottle, where it could hasten deterioration of the whole amount. A case[213] in which a nebulizer cork was accidentally aspirated with resultant bronchial blockage was attributed to features of the specific nebulizer, which is designed to facilitate storage of liquid within its chamber. The nebulizer should be cleaned at least once a week. Rinsing with cool water is generally adequate for plastic nebulizers; hot water damages them. Vinegar or rubbing alcohol may be used for glass nebulizers. It is sometimes necessary to unclog the jets with a fine wire.

Prigal[190] has pointed out the mixed blessings of the ease of aerosol administration and the almost instantaneous relaxation of bronchospasm obtained. Some asthmatics become psychologically addicted to the nebulizer and panic if they are without it or the medication, even temporarily. Others take the medication too frequently and in excess, thereby producing anxiety states and tolerance to the drug. The pharmacist should understand why these clients may sometimes become quite querulous. Some investigators[81,165] have reported that systemic effects from inhalation of nebulae of sympathomimetic amines are quite limited and have considered this to be evidence that only minor quantities are absorbed. Others[190,197] do not agree. A number of deaths have been attributed to "locked lung syndrome"[23] and to ventricular fibrillation[89] arising from excessive use of nebulized sympathomimetic compounds. Although asth-

matic patients with cardiovascular involvements or diabetes showed no ill effects from inhalation of epinephrine solutions,[81] Federal regulations require that sympathomimetics be labeled to indicate that they should not be used if high blood pressure, heart disease, diabetes or thyroid disease is present unless directed by a physician.

Powder insufflators or blowers are used to mix finely divided solid particles with air to form a spray for topical application. One form is shown in Figure 13-25 (*top*). Air from the compressed bulb whirls up fine powder in the reservoir, forming a cloud that is carried out through the outlet tube. This can be deposited as a uniform thin layer on nose, throat, ear, tooth socket or body surfaces. Powder blowers should be dispensed as accessories much more frequently than is customary in current practice.

Finely divided or micronized powders are sometimes inhaled orally or nasally to produce topical and systemic effects akin to those produced by liquid aerosols. Inhaled dusts are irritating,[44] and the vogue for this therapy has passed, taking with it most of the specialized devices that were designed for it. The Aerohaler used for applying isopropylarterenol sulfate* is illustrated in Figure 13-25, *bottom right.* A sifter cartridge of powdered drug is inserted in the assembled Aerohaler. When the user inhales through the mouthpiece or the nosepiece, a loosely rolling ball is pulled upward and forward, rapping against the cartridge so as to shake out some of the powder through two small holes in the cartridge plug. The dust is then inhaled. A pocket-type powder blower for applying micronized powders to both upper and lower respiratory tracts is available (Fig. 13-25, *bottom left*). For proper action, powder insufflators and the powders themselves must be kept dry to prevent clumping and clogging.

Oxygen therapy is generally an emergency procedure undertaken to compensate for inadequate oxygenation of the lungs (high altitude, bronchoconstriction, pneumonia, pulmonary edema, emphysema) or for inadequate circulatory transport of oxygen (cardiac decompensation, coronary occlu-

* Norisodrine Sulfate, 10 per cent and 25 per cent, Abbott Laboratories, North Chicago, Ill.

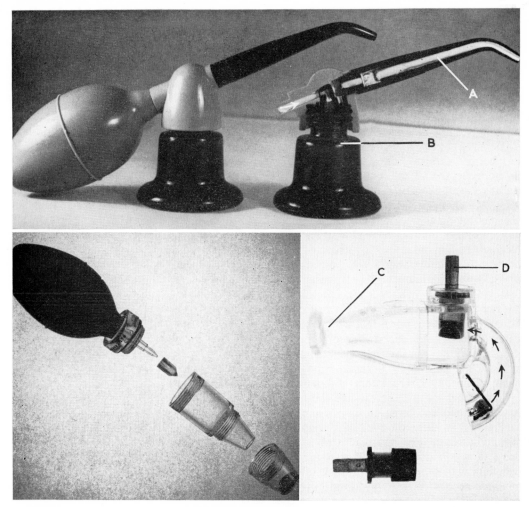

Fig. 13-25. (*Top*) Powder insufflator. Air (arrow) is forced into the bottle through a tube (B) ending well above the surface of the powder. The spray is forced up through the exit hole in the cap and passes out through the exit canal (A). The lumens of the air tube and the spray tube are painted a light color in the sectioned insufflator on the right. (*Bottom, left*) Pocket-type powder blower. In this disassembled blower the parts are (upper left to lower right): bulb and air jet tube; baffle, chamber; cap. The baffle slips down over the jet tip; air directed into it is deflected back against a micronized powder contained in the chamber so as to whip it up into a cloud of fine particles which floats out of the exit tube. (*Bottom, right*) Abbott Aerohaler. The arrows show the path followed by the ball when the user inhales through the mouthpiece (C). Sifter cartridge (D). A spare cartridge is also pictured.

sion, shock, carbon monoxide poisoning). A good review of the anatomy, physiology and pathophysiology of the respiratory apparatus is available.[42] The pharmacology and uses of oxygen and other therapeutic gases have been described in detail.[203,247]

A programed text[206] has proved useful for self-teaching of the precautions necessary as well as the purposes and methods of oxygen therapy.

In hospitals, oxygen may be supplied from a centralized pipe system or else from cylinders. Inventory costs are high[147] for a community pharmacy because cylinders must be purchased or a demurrage charge paid. Also a large assortment of accessory equipment must be stocked, including appropriate valves (flow regulators), pressure gauges and flowmeters to attach to the cylinders, adaptors, masks, tubing, humidifiers, mouthpieces, catheters, tents, floor stands and dollys.[147] Descriptive catalogs supplied by commercial distributors are informative.*

Details of technics of administering oxygen are best acquired by demonstration and by reference to specialized texts.[42,72,203] A comparative evaluation of oxygen therapy technics,[134] with respect to the relative oxygen concentrations achieved, the carbon dioxide concentrations developed and patient comfort, resulted in the following order of preference: (1) nasal cannula, (2) plastic face mask, (3) nasal catheter, (4) plastic face tent, (5) rubber oronasal mask, and (6) oxygen tent. More recently, Cherniak and Hakimpour[68] have shown that adequate oxygenation can safely be achieved with low flow rates of oxygen through nasal cannulae.

Barach[43] described portable apparatus using compensated regulators and refillable cylinders that make more feasible the use of oxygen therapy at home or for the ambulatory patient with chronic coronary and pulmonary disease. The pharmacist should be wary of recommending small, low-pressure cylinders with fixed orifices or with uncompensated needle valves or push-button valves, because oxygen flow rate falls progressively and sometimes very sharply as pressure within the cylinder falls. The literature accompanying a portable device should describe the actual oxygen flow delivered per minute and the tank capacity. Depending on the circumstances of use, the required flow rate ranges from 2 to 8 liters per minute.[72]

Although not without danger, oxygen therapy is seldom contraindicated through fear of toxicity. Untoward effects[113,247] include pulmonary atelectasis, oxygen apnea, retrolental fibroplasia (in premature infants exposed to high concentrations of oxygen at birth) and oxygen poisoning with both respiratory tract and central nervous system

effects. Water humidification should always be supplied because oxygen has a marked ability to dry and desiccate the respiratory mucosa.[113] It is absolutely necessary to keep open flames, sparks or heated elements away from oxygen equipment at all times.

Intermittent positive-pressure breathing (IPPB) devices are used to provide slight positive-pressure assistance during inhalation. The pressure may be needed to:[72,203] produce mechanical bronchodilation, improve distribution and deposition of aerosols, promote clearing of bronchial secretions, decrease work of breathing, and to regulate patterns of inspiratory and expiratory gas flows. The use of IPPB has greatly increased over the past few years because of the increasing incidence of chronic lung disease concomitant with increasing numbers of elderly individuals, heavy smoking and air pollution.[203]

Characteristics of available machines have been delineated in tabular form and in diagrams.[72,203] In the typical device, an automatic cycling machine forces either air or a therapeutic gas through appropriate connections to a tightly fitted mask or to a mouthpiece held between the teeth and sealed airtight with the lips. Machines may be powered by a compressed gas source or electrically. Machines[203] may be time-cycled (inflation ends at a preset time), volume-cycled (inflation ends when a preset volume has been delivered), or pressure-cycled (inflation ends when line pressure reaches a preset value). The IPPB device should have a variable sensitivity adjustment to permit the patient to initiate cycling with his own breathing motions.* The negative airway pressure produced by the patient's spontaneous inspiratory efforts starts the positive-pressure cycle, and gas flows into the lungs until the preset volume, pressure or time is reached. A valve is then actuated to shut off the inspiratory phase and passive expiration occurs. The design of the machine should allow for nebulizer attachments for aerosol

---

* Catalog 39-33-R, Oxequip, 8335 South Halsted St., Chicago, Ill. See reference 147 for other suppliers.

* Respirators that cycle automatically and do not follow the patient's spontaneous respirations are classified as ventilators (IPPV or PNPV machines).[208] Tracheal tubes or tracheostomy tubes rather than masks or mouthpieces are generally used for prolonged controlled ventilation procedures.

therapy and should provide for control of oxygen concentration when that gas is used.

A simple, relatively inexpensive IPPB device that is easy to operate and readily cleaned has been described.[184] A pressure source (compressor pump or compressed gas source) powers a nebulization assembly and a venturi device in a small hand-held unit. The patient closes his lips around the mouthpiece of the unit and with his thumb closes a small port in the handle, thereby directing compressed gas to both the nebulizer and the venturimeter. The venturi feature draws in extra air thereby increasing air flow and reducing oxygen concentration if compressed oxygen is used as the source of the power. When the patient feels his lungs are comfortably inflated, he releases his thumb and exhales passively through the handle. Design features provide safety by limiting or controlling the maximum pressures obtainable.

HYPODERMIC SYRINGES AND NEEDLES

A syringe is an instrument used to inject liquids into the body or to instill them into body cavities. Bulb syringes and gravity-flow (fountain) types are described with prescription accessories made of rubber. The forms and the uses of the plunger or hypodermic syringe are also of significant import to the pharmacist. The story of the development of the hypodermic syringe has been interestingly told.[241]

Because of the capacity for misuse inherent in instruments which are capable of injecting potent materials into the body, pharmacists clearly bear a great responsibility in their control of the distribution of hypodermic syringes and needles to lay and professional people. Federal regulation is lacking, but a number of states have laws which designate by whom and to whom they may be sold. For example, in California they may be dispensed only by registrants.[186] A prescription[186] is required unless the item is supplied to another professional person or dispensed for administering insulin to a diabetic or epinephrine to an asthmatic. Of course, the pharmacist is morally bound to ensure as far as possible the legitimacy of sales without prescription.

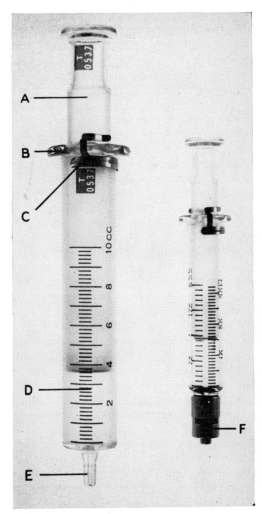

Fig. 13-26. Hypodermic syringes. (*Left*) Syringe which has plunger and barrel ground to fit together. A, plunger; B, barrel flange; C, plunger guard; D, barrel; E, tapered Luer tip. (*Right*) Interchangeable type. The syringe has both metric and apothecary graduations; it also has a Luer-Lok tip (F).

Diversion of these articles into illicit use with narcotics is the principal danger.

Description of Syringe. Basically, the hypodermic syringe (Fig. 13-26) consists of a barrel and a plunger, both of which are usually made of a borosilicate glass resistant to thermal shock and low in alkalinity. The all-glass syringe is known as the Luer syringe, after its inventor. The barrel is a tube open at one end and closed at the other except for a hollow tip. The open end is thickened and extended radially outward to form a flange to prevent slipping of the barrel through the fingers. The plunger is a glass rod with a flat distal end and a proximal end shaped into a button-type knob. The relative dimensions of the barrel and the plunger for a given syringe are such that the plunger will move freely throughout the barrel, yet the surfaces of the plunger and barrel must so closely approximate each other that fluid cannot pass between them even when under considerable pressure. Suitable fit has been achieved in two ways. In one, both the barrel inner surface and the plunger outer surface are ground with abrasives; then the two parts are placed together and further ground to make a matching pair. The two components are marked with identical serial numbers and must always be used only together since they are uniquely fitted. If one part is lost or broken, the other must be discarded. The second method makes use of unground barrels made of a glass tubing which has so uniform and constant an internal diameter that plungers can be precision ground to given dimensions to fit it. Consequently, both barrels and plungers are interchangeable.* Broken components can be replaced without difficulty because of this standardization. Syringes are usually supplied with a spring metal retaining clip which presses gently against the plunger so as to keep it from accidentally slipping out of the barrel. Users often prefer to remove this plunger guard, since it tends to interfere with manipulation of the syringe.

The tip of the syringe barrel provides the point of attachment for a hollow steel needle, the part of the instrument designed to penetrate into the body. The tip may be glass with the exterior surface ground, or it may be formed from a metal cylinder welded to the glass. The usual Luer metal or glass tip has a taper with standardized dimensions,† which allows the needle hub to be slipped over it and to be held on by friction. When this method of holding is used, the needle is reasonably secure, but it may slip off if it is not properly seated or if there is need for much manipulation of the needle after insertion. A more positive grip is assured with the Luer-Lok tip.* This is a patented metal collar (Fig. 13-26) with a circular internal groove into which a flange on the needle hub may be inserted. A half-turn locks the needle in place. The syringe tip is usually concentric to the barrel axis, but syringes with eccentric tips are available for situations (as in intravenous work) where it may be desirable to introduce the needle as nearly parallel to the surface as possible.

Syringe Graduations. The range of capacities for general-purpose syringes is from 2 to 100 ml.; larger and smaller ones are available for specialized uses. All markings on the syringe, including graduation lines and numerals, should be applied with pigments capable of withstanding repeated autoclaving. They may be fused in, fused on or etched and fused. Scales (Fig. 13-26) may be double (in minims as well as ml. and fractions thereof), or single (metric only) or may be specialized. Two basic factors affect the accuracy of syringe dosage.[101] One is the built-in accuracy of the syringe and the other is the accuracy of the administration. Federal specifications† which are generally followed by the industry require syringes to be tested (with water) for accuracy at each main graduation mark with a calibrated burette. Syringes must deliver ± 5 per cent of the capacity indicated at each mark. Each conventional ground-glass syringe must be individually graduated, since internal diameters of the barrels vary unpredictably. Precision sizing of tubing used for interchangeable syringes allows graduation en masse. To facilitate accurate readings, the plunger may be made of colored glass (usually blue) or it may have a narrow black or colored precision line near the bottom. It is estimated[101] that most of the available glass syringes are accurate to ± 3 per cent. Pharmacists tend to overlook the possibility of

---

* Multifit Syringe, Becton, Dickinson and Company, Rutherford, N. J.

† American Standard Dimensions of Glass and Metal Luer Tapers for Medical Applications, ASA, Z70.1-1955, American Standards Association, Inc., New York.

* Becton, Dickinson and Company, Rutherford, N. J.

† GG-S-921b, Federal Specification, Syringe, Luer (All-glass), August 7, 1958, General Services Administration Regional Offices, Federal Supply Service, New York, San Francisco and elsewhere. No charge.

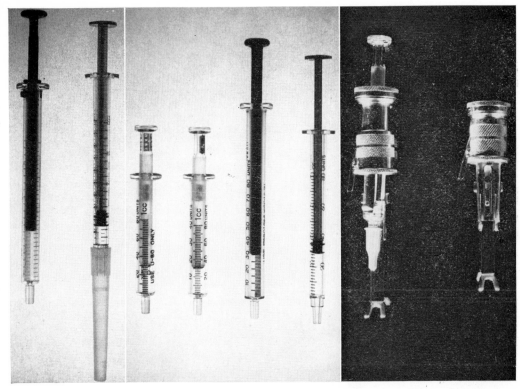

FIG. 13-27. (*Left*) Tuberculin syringes. Disposable syringe. Each syringe has two scales—one graduated to 0.01 cc. units, and one to ½ minim units. The plungers are colored blue. (*Center*) Insulin syringes. The plungers have been pulled back to the mark for 30 units of U 80 insulin. Short-type U 80 syringe; short-type double-scale syringe; long-type U 80 syringe with blue plunger; disposable U 80 plastic syringe. (*Right*) The Busher Automatic Injector. The injector at the left is loaded with a syringe and has been cocked so that touching the lever will move the syringe ahead and inject the needle.

using hypodermic syringes to measure small volumes when compounding.

Special-purpose syringes (Fig. 13-27) are named according to the usual intended use. These include the "vaccine," the "tuberculin" and the "insulin" syringes. They may differ from usual syringes in scale graduations, in over-all capacity and, perhaps, in length relative to capacity. A typical vaccine syringe may have a capacity of 1 ml. with graduations to 0.05 ml. It is intended for use also with epinephrine and other medications for which doses are 1 ml. or less. Tuberculin syringes are 0.25, 0.5 or 1.0 ml. in capacity and have long barrels with narrow internal diameters to allow precision in graduation to 0.01 ml. The thin plunger is colored blue typically. This design was developed for the intracutaneous injection of very small doses of

tuberculins for diagnostic purposes. Insulin syringes are shown in Figure 13-27, *center*.

Disposable Syringes. Sterile syringes which are to be discarded after being used once have advantages that have led to their acceptance in some quarters. These disposable syringes are convenient to use and lessen hazards of cross-infection. Institutions tend to convert to using them if cost-studies show that the change is justified by savings resulting from freeing personnel, equipment and space needed to clean, sterilize, assemble and store reusable syringes.[76] Individual physicians choose to carry them in their bags on the basis of convenience. Disposable syringes are made of glass or plastic or both. Some have metal parts also. The plastics used include polystyrene, polyethylene, polymethylmethacrylate, polypropylene and

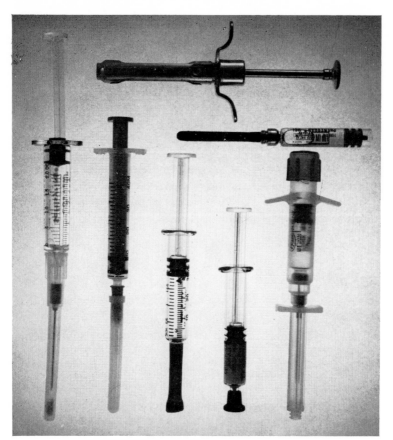

Fig. 13-28. Disposable syringes. (*Across*) Clear polystyrene barrel with removable needle; translucent polyethylene barrel, needle not supplied; glass barrel, needle permanently attached; polystyrene syringe supplied with medication (penicillin suspension) and a separately packaged needle; translucent barrel supplied with medication in glass container. The needle guard is used also as the piston when the syringe is assembled for use. (*Top*) Metal barrel and piston with rubber-sealed glass cartridge containing medication.

nylon.[235] Polystyrene (possibly the most used) and polymethylmethacrylate are glass-like in appearance, while the others lack optical clarity but are more flexible. A major deterrent to a wholehearted acceptance of plastic syringes has been the demonstration that, contrary to original expectations, plastics have been shown to be incompatible with a number of medications.[40,41] Users also have been disenchanted on occasion by poorly made syringes which were difficult to assemble or faulty in operation owing to ill-fit of barrels and plungers or to loose needles.

Disposable syringes are marketed in a variety of designs (Fig. 13-28). Some resemble conventional syringes in appearance and are supplied in an assembled form ready for use in individual sterilized paper envelopes or polyethylene bags. These may be all plastic or they may have a glass barrel with a plastic plunger. They are available with or without needles. Needles, when attached, are usually covered by a separate plastic sleeve. Some

forms of single-use units are supplied only with a cartridge of an injectable agent contained within the syringe barrel. A syringe of this type has to be taken apart and reassembled in order to insert the shaft of the piston into a rubber plunger. The cartridges have attached needles and are usually made of glass so that contact with the plastic of the syringe is avoided. In yet another type of disposable product, a rubber-sealed glass cartridge with selected sterile medication and needle is provided for insertion into a reusable metal syringelike device. The uses, evaluation, advantages and disadvantages of pre-filled disposable syringe systems have been reviewed.[150] The need to destroy disposable syringes to prevent discarded ones from falling into the hands of children or narcotic addicts has been documented.[114]

Dispensing of Syringes. Syringes are supplied in individual boxes or, for large users such as hospitals, in bulk packages. The community pharmacist is well advised to

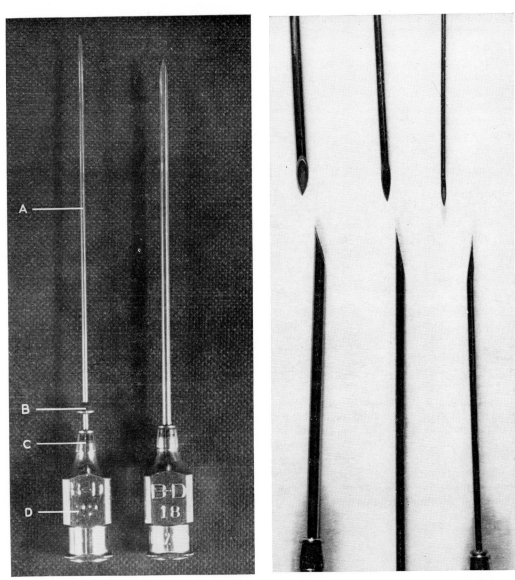

FIG. 13-29. (*Left*) Hypodermic needles. These are the same length, since the shaft of the security-bead needle (*left*) is measured from the bead. A, shaft; B, security bead; C, hub; D, gauge number. (*Right*) Variations in hypodermic needle points. (*Top*) Underside views. (*Bottom*) Side views. (*Across*) Short-bevel regular point; long bevel regular point; Huber point. In the side views the points are turned so that the openings into the canals face toward the right.

inspect each syringe before he releases it to his client, because these easily broken instruments are sometimes unjustifiably returned as having been defective when purchased. The proper fit of syringe components can be tested by covering the hole at the tip with a finger and pulling back on the plunger. The vacuum produced should be sufficient to make retraction of the plunger difficult. Before the plunger is released, the vacuum should be broken by uncovering the hole in the tip; otherwise, the plunger may shoot back to its initial position with sufficient force to knock out the bottom of the barrel.

Hypodermic Needle Construction. The parts of the hypodermic needle are illustrated in Figure 13-29. Needles are made from various special steels chosen for strength, flexibility and rust resistance. Needle size is designated by two numbers, the gauge and the shaft length in inches. Gauge numbers represent the outside diameter of the shaft expressed according to the Stubb's English wire gauge system. They run from 27 (the finest) to 13 (the thickest). The shaft, or cannula, is measured from its juncture with the hub to the tip of the point. As an exception, the "security" needle is measured from the small metal bead that is fastened ⅛ inch from the hub (for easy withdrawal in case of accidental breakage). Lengths range from ½ inch to 3½ inches. The gauge number is often stamped on the needle hub; the length is not.

Selection of Needle. The choice of needle size for a given use is governed by factors such as the desired depth of penetration, the fluidity of the injection, and the safety and comfort of the patient. Fine needles may be suitable for thin mobile liquids, whereas thicker ones may be needed for oils or suspensions. Short needles may be adequate for thin persons, while longer shafts will be needed for similar injections into obese patients. Table 13-6 presents suggestions for needle sizes to be used for several common types of injections. It should be recognized that physicians, nurses or patients may express individual preferences on occasion. Specialized needles for particular uses such as tissue biopsy, or spinal, hemorrhoidal and tonsilar injections are not usually stocked by the community pharmacist. This is also true for needles with gold or silver cannulae.

Several designs for needle points have been developed (Fig. 13-29). All are tapered with front and side bevels to minimize the amount of force needed for insertion and to reduce pain and trauma.[99] Needles with the regular long front bevel are generally used for hypodermoclysis and subcutaneous and intramuscular injections. Those with short bevels are preferred for intravenous injections and transfusions. Needles with a very short bevel are used intradermally. As it is being inserted, the regular point sometimes punches out a plug of tissue that may occlude the cannula. Because of its closed front bevel, which places the opening parallel to the shaft, the Huber point (Fig. 13-29) pierces rather than punches. Most users do not seem to discriminate in favor of either regular or Huber points. Aldous[2] has shown that dentists may more accurately place local anesthetics at the intended nerve site by using a larger gauge needle with a Huber point because this has the least deflection on insertion.

Needle Sources; Packaging. Needles obtained from reliable sources in the United States vary little in quality. A number of simple but effective quality tests the phar-

TABLE 13-6. SUGGESTED NEEDLE SIZES

INJECTION	GAUGE	LENGTH (inches)	BEVEL*	EXAMPLES
Intradermal	26G	¼ or ⅜	v. s. b.	Schick, Dick, allergic tests
Subcutaneous	26G	½ to ¾	r. b.	Insulin, immunizations
	25G	½ to ¾	r. b.	
	22G	1½	r. b.	Hypodermoclysis
Intramuscular	24G	¾ or 1	r. b.	Polio vaccine
	23G	1	r. b.	Hormones, bismuth
	22G	1	r. b.	
	22G	1¼ or 1½	r. b.	Penicillin
	20G	1½	r. b.	
Intravenous	22G	1¼ or 1½	s. b.	Penicillins, transfusions
	20G	1½	s. b.	Glucose, blood tests

*r.b., regular (long) bevel; s.b., short bevel; v.s.b., very short bevel.

macist can apply without elaborate equipment have been described.[49] Needles are supplied to the community pharmacy in boxes of 12 of the same size, or less frequently, of assorted sizes. Hospital packs may be gross lots. To protect the points, the needles may be encased in small plastic tubes or mounted on thin cardboard.

Needle Wires. A needle wire is a thin stainless steel rod of such diameter and length that it may be fitted through the hub into the cannula and extend for a short distance beyond the point. These wires are useful in protecting needle points and in preventing clogging of cannulae when the needles are not in use. For example, diabetics find that prior insertion of needle wires reduce the incidence of bent points in needles sterilized in a pan of boiling water. Wires may be supplied in the boxes of needles or may be obtained separately. The pharmacist should supply a wire with each needle and should explain its function.

Disposable Needles. It is difficult to maintain sharp points on needles when they are reused several times. Grinding them on smooth oil stones (Arkansas stones) restores bevels and removes burrs or fishhooks, but this requires considerable skill. Because dull points make for painful injections, sterile disposable needles (Fig. 13-30) have been developed. One-time use of these needles not only eliminates problems of sharpening but also does away with costly, time-consuming cleaning and sterilization procedures and with the transmission of serum hepatitis. Because reusability is not a factor, disposable needles can be made of less expensive steels. Plastic hubs that cannot be boiled or autoclaved may be used. Packages are designed to maintain sterility and to permit the needles to be removed without contamination. Cost studies in hospitals appear to justify the use of disposable needles in place of reusable ones.[234]

Use and Maintenance of Syringes and Needles. Pharmacists should be able to answer questions about the use and care of hypodermic syringes, needles and related items. Although the pharmacist does not inject drugs, he should be sufficiently informed about all parenteral technics to answer questions about hypodermic devices

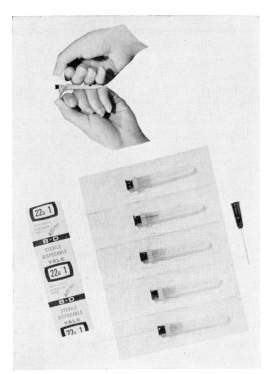

Fig. 13-30. Disposable needles, packed in sterile units.

in common use. Reviews[231] of common technics should be utilized. Care and handling of syringes has been well-described and published in a form* convenient to distribute to users. Immediately after use the syringe and the attached needle should be flushed several times with cool water. The disassembled components should be soaked in mild detergent solution for 15 to 90 minutes, the longer times being advocated if oily medications are to be removed. Prolonged soaking or the use of a cleaning solution that is alkaline, concentrated or hot may remove the pigment or destroy fit of plunger and barrel. After rinsing, the syringe and the needle may be sterilized by one of the several standard technics.[138]

If syringes and needles are not rinsed and disassembled immediately as suggested, the parts later may be found to be stuck together. Soaking overnight or longer in a detergent solution frequently releases the ad-

* Glass syringes: recommended care and handling, Leaflet supplied by Becton, Dickinson and Company, Rutherford, N. J.

herent surfaces, but may damage the glass. Boiling for 10 minutes in a 25 per cent aqueous solution of glycerin is said to be effective if the parts are separated while still hot.[112] As a service to his clientele, the pharmacist may wish to equip himself with a syringe opener. This is an all-metal syringe* with a female Luer-Lok tip. In use, the syringe opener is filled with warm water or cleaning solution and attached to the tip of the stuck syringe. Steadily increasing pressure is applied until the stuck plunger is expelled from the barrel.

Stains and deposits which develop on syringes may be removed by swabbing with cotton moistened with an appropriate reagent. Alkali deposits and blood are removed with 10 per cent nitric acid, iron stains by 10 per cent hydrochloric acid. Concentrated ammonia, sodium citrate solution, alcohol and organic solvents are sometimes used successfully.

Jet-injectors. Numerous attempts[242] have been made to develop injection devices superior to the hypodermic syringe and needle. Prominent among these are high-pressure instruments that force a fine jet of medication through the dermis into the underlying tissues. Experience[45,71,238] with large groups indicates several advantages of jet-injection for mass inoculation with vaccines. These include relatively less pain, less time required per injection, decreased personnel needs, release from need to sterilize between injections and lower cost per injection. Jet-injection of insulin[243] and of corticosteroids[191] also shows considerable promise. Intradermal, subcutaneous or intramuscular injections can be made, depending on the type of nozzle used. Penetration into veins is not possible. Dosages of 0.1 cc. to 1.0 cc. can be administered from multidose vials. Several models† are available. Manufacturers' brochures should be consulted for details of design and use. Although the high original cost may seem to be a deterrent, the evident usefulness of this system for mass inoculation should encourage the pharmacist to bring it to the attention of local public

health and school officials and physicians. The visually handicapped find the smaller models very suitable for self-injection.

DIABETIC SUPPLIES

Diabetes is an incurable condition that may demand rigorous diet control or continued medication or both in order to maintain life. The pharmacist must be prepared to render complete and expert service to the more than $3\frac{1}{2}$ million diabetics in this country. Notwithstanding the utility of oral hypoglycemics, insulin injections are required to control diabetes in many cases. This section deals mainly with the specialized equipment and technics used to inject insulin.

Syringes and Needles. The usual insulin syringes (Fig. 13-27) have a capacity of 1 cc., but syringes able to hold 2 or 3 cc. are also available. In order to facilitate self-administration by the diabetic, syringes are graduated in units of insulin, viz. the top scale line is marked either 40 or 80 (units) rather than 1 (cc.). The diabetic needs only to draw up the volume of insulin preparation that equals the number of units he is to inject. The pharmacist must be certain to dispense the syringe commensurate with the strength of insulin being used by the patient, and to advise him how to read the scale. The 40-unit scale markings are red and those of the 80-unit scale are green to correspond with the identifying colors specified for the boxes, labels and rubber stoppers of the containers for these strengths of insulin. A study[21] revealed that even with these aids to self-administration, 35 per cent of 112 diabetic patients observed during daily self-injection made serious errors in that they administered an amount of insulin at least 15 per cent different from the prescribed dose. The fact that 29 per cent of those using a dual-scale syringe (one with both 40 and 80 units) measured either half or double the prescribed dose because they used the wrong scale reinforces the oft made suggestion that only single-scale insulin syringes should be marketed. Packages of sterile disposable U-40 or U-80 syringe and 26 G $\times$ $\frac{1}{2}$" needle combination units* offer the advan-

---

* Becton, Dickinson and Company, Rutherford, N. J.

† Hypospray Injector, Professional Model & Model K-3, R. P. Scherer Corp., Detroit, Mich.; Dermo-Jet, Robbins Instrument Co., Chatham, N.J.

* Becton, Dickinson and Company, Rutherford, N.J.

tages of convenience, safety and a sharp needle for each injection, but the cost may limit the use to special circumstances such as emergencies or traveling. Some diabetics may prefer disposable needles, which are available sterilized and individually packaged for their use. The sizes of needles suitable for subcutaneous injection of insulin are given in Table 13-6. Either the regular point with a long bevel or the Huber point is preferred.

Sterilization technics[84] practiced by diabetics are quite simply carried out. The disassembled syringe and the wired needle are placed in a metal strainer (the common household type), which is then immersed in water and boiled for at least 5 to 10 minutes. The parts are assembled after cooling in the strainer removed from the water. Contamination is avoided by holding the plunger by the knob, the barrel by the sides and the needle by the hub. Immediately after use, the syringe and the needle should be rinsed with cool tap water and then with a small amount of rubbing alcohol. Between injections, the equipment may be stored in a container* filled with rubbing alcohol, where it will remain sterile for perhaps 1 or 2 weeks.[223] The practice of relying on a simple rinsing with alcohol as the only routine means of preventing contamination should be discouraged. A study[21] of procedures used by diabetics at home showed that only one-fifth of them used acceptable insulin equipment and sterilization practices.

Special Accessories. Pocket kits containing syringes, needles and various accessories are available. The Busher Automatic Injector† is a spring-loaded device that can be set to insert the needle at the proper angle and depth when the trigger is released (Fig. 13-27). It may be suggested as an aid for children or timid adults. The diabetic may be unduly concerned about the need to protect his insulin against deterioration when he travels. Insulin loses potency so gradually at room temperature that there is no cause to anticipate a significant change over the short time interval during which a vial

* B-D Steritube, Becton, Dickinson and Company.
† Becton, Dickinson and Company, Rutherford, N.J.

would normally be used up once started.[226] Specially-designed vacuum bottles that support an insulin vial in a packing of ice may be useful for long trips.

Diet Factors. In order to manage his condition properly the diabetic frequently requires special diet foods and diet information, sugar-free medication,[33] diagnostic aids and guidance. The pharmacist should be prepared to offer all of these. Liquid medications[124,146] suitable for diabetics can be compounded by the pharmacist as a distinctive individual contribution to the welfare of his diabetic clientele.

SURGICAL DRESSINGS AND RELATED SUPPLIES

Surgical dressings are materials applied over sores, wounds and other lesions. They have a long history of usage.[53] These and related supplies are appropriately available through the pharmacy to physicians and laymen. Surgical supply houses are the major outlet for specialized items in this category, such as surgical instruments, sutures and bulk packages of dressings. In terms of retail dollar value, nonpharmacy outlets such as supermarkets and variety stores now sell about 45 per cent of the first aid items purchased by the general public.[140] This is evidence that pharmacists in general have failed to demonstrate to the public a unique ability to advise in the selection and the use of these items.

Surgical dressings have multiple functions. Protection of wounds from bacterial or other contamination and from further injury is a prime one. Uses which sometimes may assume paramount importance are the partial or the complete immobilization of an injured area, the support of damaged tissues, the control of bleeding, the absorption of exudations and the holding of medication in place. These and other functions will be brought out as various forms of dressings are discussed. Items referred to by brand name have been selected only on the basis of the author's familiarity with them; no attempt has been made to be all-inclusive.

Cotton is the major raw material from which dressings are made. Rayon, cellulose, plastics and a host of adjunctive agents are also used. The production and the processing of cotton for medicinal uses has been described.[153] Cotton is naturally nonabsorbent because it contains waxes, resins and fatty substances which prevent water from wetting it. It is made absorbent when these substances are removed by boiling the previously cleaned cotton for several hours in dilute sodium hydroxide solution under steam pressure in a closed tank (kier). Subsequent bleaching with sodium hypochlorite converts the cotton from its natural gray color to a more appealing white. Nonabsorbent cotton has relatively limited medicinal uses as paddings and as moisture-resistant backings for dressings, for example. Absorbent cotton as such and also woven into fabrics is the form which is more widely used.

Official standards[240] for purified (absorbent) cotton provide specifications for purity and absorbency and impose other requirements as well. Cotton fibers are uncellular cellulose hairs with a spiral twist that makes them especially valuable for spinning. They vary in length from a few millimeters up to 50 mm. or slightly more. Short-staple cotton fibers average less than 25 mm., medium-staple fibers average from 25 to 30 mm. and long fibers from 30 to 40 mm. Each grade is employed in some form of dressing.

Small pieces of cotton have been found to be so useful as swabs that machine-made cotton balls have been marketed in three or four sizes. They are used to wipe off fluids, exudations and medications and to apply liquids, cleansers, antiseptics and medications. Similar balls made of rayon are said to be softer, smoother, more lint-free and more absorbent and to offer less hazard from static electricity. Bulk packages containing one to several thousand nonsterile cotton or rayon balls are supplied to institutions. Smaller packages containing sterile cotton balls are stocked in pharmacies. These are used mainly for cosmetic uses or for baby care.

Cotton-tipped applicators also make useful swabs for applying medications, cleaning wounds, noses and ears and taking cultures. They are made by winding long-fiber cotton on the end of smooth birch sticks. A binder which is insoluble in alcohol and common

medications and not affected by sterilization may be used to hold the cotton on. Applicators may be 3 or 6 inches long; tips may be small or large. Bulk packages are nonsterile. Small packages of sterile applicators are familiar first-aid items in pharmacies. Short double-tipped sterile applicators are marketed under several brand names for home uses, especially for baby care. These should have flexible, nonsplintering stems such as those made of rolled paper.

Cotton Gauze. Absorbent gauze is cotton in the form of a plain woven cloth conforming to standards set forth in the *U.S.P.*[240] It is an open meshwork of threads spun from long-staple cotton fibers. After the cloth is woven, it is rendered absorbent and bleached by kiering in processes similar to those used in making surgical cotton. Gauze is classified into types according to its mesh. Mesh is denoted by two figures, the first being the number of warp or lengthwise threads per inch and the second the number of fill or lateral threads per inch. There are eight official types.[240] Type I, the most closely woven, has a 44 x 36 mesh; Type VIII has a loose mesh, 14 x 10 (Fig. 13-31, *left*). Close weaves are stronger and more protective, open ones are softer and more absorbent. Gauze is used alone or along with more effective absorbents such as surgical cotton, rayon and cellulose. It is filmated, for example, by distributing a thin even layer of cotton between folds of gauze.

Rayon and Cellulose. Rayon, one of the earliest of the synthetic fibers, is becoming more widely used for surgical dressings. Most used is that made by the viscose process in which either wood pulp or short fiber cotton (linters) is dissolved in caustic soda and carbon disulfide and then forced through spinnerets into an acid salt bath to form filaments of cellulose. In comparison with cotton, rayon is claimed to be more absorbent and to absorb more quickly, have less lint, better shelf life and present no static hazard. Cellulose derived from bleached sulphite wood pulp and made into thin layers of creped paper* is used to replace cotton as an absorbent filler in some dressings.

Primary and secondary dressings are the two major categories of surgical dressings.

* Cellucotton, Bauer and Black, Chicago, Ill.

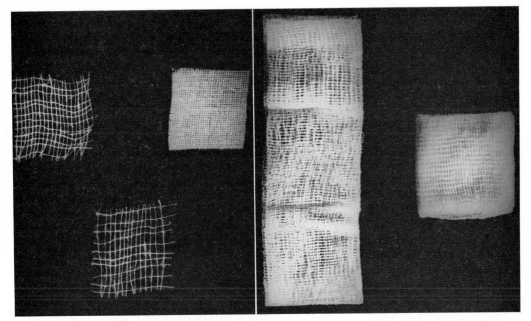

Fig. 13-31. (*Left*) Examples of cotton gauze mesh. (*Top*) Type VII, 20 x 12 mesh; Type I, 44 x 36 mesh. (*Bottom*) Type VIII, 14 x 10 mesh. (*Right*) gauze pads. The 2 inch x 2 inch pad can be unfolded to a 2 inch x 6 inch rectangle without exposing loose ends.

Primary dressings are intended for direct contact with wounds. Secondary dressings are applied over primary ones or to areas where no wounds exist. Dressings with which the community pharmacist should be familiar in each category will be described.

PRIMARY DRESSINGS

Gauze Dressings. Primary dressings must be sterile and absorbent. Cotton gauze is the basic cloth for most of these dressings. Gauze is manufactured in a variety of meshes in bolts, 100 yards by 36 inches. Bulk supplies are not sterile and are used chiefly by hospitals and other consumers who have facilities for sterilization. Usual packages contain 28 x 24-mesh or 24 x 20-mesh gauze cut into 1-yard or 5-yard lengths, folded to 4½-inch widths (8 plies or layers), wrapped in paper, rolled, placed in sealed cartons and sterilized. These are used chiefly in outpatient and emergency rooms and in doctors' offices.

Gauze Pads. Gauze pads or sponges are made by folding 20 x 12-mesh surgical gauze into squares or rectangles with 8 to 32 layers (Fig. 13-31, *right*). The folding pattern is such that all cut edges are inside and the pad may

be unfolded lengthwise without exposing cut edges or loose threads. Twelve-ply pads ranging from 2 x 2 inches to 4 x 4 inches, placed in individual sealed glassine envelopes and then sterilized and packaged in cartons of 12, 25 or 100, are supplied to pharmacies under a variety of trade names.* Sponges are also made of filmated gauze which is softer, has increased absorptive power and tends to carry drainage away from the wound. Pads may be filmated with cotton, rayon or either of these plus a center layer of cellulose. Bulk packages, sterile or otherwise, are supplied to hospitals.

Gauze dressings may adhere to wounds, in effect being glued on as the absorbed exudate dries within the network of gauze threads. Removal is painful and damaging. Attempts have been made to provide nonadherent dressings by modifying the surface to be placed in contact with the wound. Polyethylene or other plastic films† are used, for

* Steri-Pad, Johnson and Johnson, New Brunswick, N.J.; Readi-Pads, Parke, Davis and Co., Detroit, Mich.

† Telfa Pads, Bauer and Black, Chicago, Ill.; Non-Stick First Aid Pads, Johnson and Johnson, New Brunswick, N.J.

example. The film is pierced with multiple perforations or with slits to allow ventilation. Gauze, cotton or cellulose, alone or combined, are used as absorbent backings. Another form of nonadherent pad* is made from a rayon gauze impregnated with a bland water-in-oil emulsion in such a way as to leave open pores in the dressing. This type is said to be less adherent and less macerating than that faced with plastic.[153] A new single-layer dressing† woven of three different sizes of cellulose fiber is said to be nonadherent and aerating because it lifts itself from the wound, owing to a differential shrinkage of the warp threads. Gauze saturated with white petrolatum is available in various shapes and sizes for use as a protective, nonadherent dressing.‡ Specifications for petrolatum gauze are provided in the *U.S.P.*[240] Sterile dressings are individually packaged in sealed aluminum foil envelopes, or in the case of selvage strips, in a sealed plastic tube. The occlusive action of this dressing may or may not be desirable in a given situation. Clinical trials of nonadherent dressings have resulted in conflicting reports[50,214] as to their effectiveness. In vitro and animal experiments[214,245] showed the least adhesion to nontreated cotton, and they suggest that best results are obtained with materials that allow wounds to dry most rapidly. A new dressing§ with a facing of nonwoven fabric and an absorbent filler appears to be designed to keep wounds in a semi-dry condition.

Special Gauze Dressings. Specialized primary gauze dressings, which are usually supplied in bulk by surgical supply houses, include sponges that have radiopaque inserts incorporated in the gauze to permit detection by roentgenography if they should be left in a body cavity during surgery. Laparotomy packs, which are essentially oversize roentgenographically detectable sponges, fall into this category. Selvage-edge gauze strips are ½ inch to 2 inches wide with both edges woven to prevent shredding. These sterile strips, either plain or medicated with 5 per cent iodoform, are used as packing for wounds and cavities, mastoids, tooth sockets and the like to stop bleeding or to act as drainage wicks. The strips are packaged in sterile glass jars. Dressing combines are designed for absorption of large volumes of blood and exudations from wounds. The basic type consists of a layer of absorbent cotton about 1 inch thick backed up by a layer of nonabsorbent cotton. The cotton is enclosed in a gauze cover. The absorbent side is placed next to the wound, and the backing protects clothing or bedding against flow-through. A number of sizes are made. A modified type, with a layer of cellulose between two layers of absorbent cotton, is intended for use when topped by still a second pad. A sheeting* with a microporous, nonwoven, polypropylene facing, a cellulose acetate batting filler and a rayon fiber backing has been shown useful in preventing burn wounds from sticking.[39] The same material is now also available as surgical dressing pads edged with adhesive tape.

Adhesive Bandage *U.S.P.*[240] is well known under a variety of trade names,† since this handy form of compress is widely used as a dressing for small wounds. Each bandage is an individual sterile dressing composed of a small pad of folded gauze affixed to the center of an overlapping piece of adhesive plaster. The adhesive surfaces and the face of the pad are protected by coverings of crinoline, polyethylene or similar materials arranged so that they can be easily peeled off without touching the pad. The adhesive plaster backing of the pad is perforated to permit ventilation of the wound. Plasters may be cloth-backed, sometimes waterproofed, white or flesh-colored. Currently, plastic-backed tapes are more popular because they are thinner, waterproof and less conspicuous when applied. Elastic tapes‡ are also used. Some brands have nonadherent pads surfaced with perforated plastic films. Pads impregnated with merbromin, tyrothricin, nitrofura-

---

* Adaptic Non-Adhering Dressing, Johnson and Johnson.

† Notrauma, Seamless Rubber Company, New Haven, Conn.

‡ Vaseline Gauze, Chesebrough-Pond's Inc., New York, N.Y.

§ Dermicel Sterile Pads, Johnson and Johnson.

* Microdon Nonadherent Sheeting, 3M Company, St. Paul, Minn.

† Readi-Bandages, Parke, Davis and Co.; Curad Plastic Bandages, Bauer and Black; Band-Aid Adhesive Bandages, Johnson and Johnson.

‡ Elastoplast, Duke Laboratories, Inc., S. Norwalk, Conn.

zone and other anti-infective agents are sup-plied, but the need for medication applied this way is questionable. Severe competition among manufacturers has led to a prolifera-tion of sizes, shapes and even of colors. In-dividual bandages are sealed in paper en-velopes and sterilized. These are packaged in tins or boxes which may contain all one size and shape of bandage or an assortment of sizes or shapes.

Eye pads are oval-shaped, about 1¾ x 2⅝ inches, and are made of absorbent cotton covered by a fine-mesh gauze. They are applied as dressings to protect injured eyes, usually being held in place by clear plastic tapes. The pads are sealed in indi-vidual glassine envelopes, then sterilized. Fifty envelopes are packaged in a carton. A differently shaped and larger pad with a non-woven cotton fabric cover is also available.

SECONDARY DRESSINGS

Secondary dressings are used to hold pri-mary dressings in place, give additional sup-port and protection to the injured area, supply compression when needed and splint or immobilize portions of the body. Since they are not intended to contact wounds directly, secondary dressings need not be sterile.

Adhesive Plasters. Adhesive tape[240] con-sists of a fabric or a film evenly coated on one side with a pressure-sensitive adhesive mix-ture. The foundation may be a plain-weave cotton cloth, a resin-coated cloth for water-re-pellency, a napped flannel for moleskin, felt for chiropodist's tape, elastic woven cloth or films of plastics such as polyvinyl chloride.[7] The two principal components of the ad-hesive mass are the elastomer base and a resin. The latter component adds tackiness or "quick-stick" properties. Antioxidants, plasticizers, coloring agents and fillers such as zinc oxide are added to create a balanced blend of adhesion, cohesion, stretchiness and elasticity. Unvulcanized crepe rubber is a common elastomer, but synthetics such as polyisobutylene are beginning to be used. In the process of manufacturing cloth-backed tapes, the adhesive mass is heat-softened, laid on the backing and then spread over the sur-face and into the interstices of the cloth by passing the tape between rolls of a calender stack. Plastic film backing cannot be cal-endered but is coated by a solvent-spreading process.[7] With the exception of some types with specialized backings, tapes are cut into widths from ¼ to 4 inches. Lengths of 1 to 10 yards are wound into rolls on spools. Individual metal spools with protective snap-on metal sleeves are stocked in most phar-macies. Specialized plastic dispensers with built-in cutters are recent innovations. Rolls, 12 inches by 10 yards, uncut or precut into widths with uniform or assorted widths on a single roll, are packed in metal-capped, stiff cardboard cylinders for the use of hospitals or physicians. Inexpensive tapes usually have lighter-weight cloth backings but are quite adequate for most purposes. Tapes with an extra-heavy cloth backing should be recom-mended for strapping and other bandaging procedures requiring high tensile strength. Water-repellent tapes are needed when the bandaged part must be protected from water. Plastic tapes are strong, thin, waterproof, un-affected by soap or grease and may be slightly elastic. Clear plastic tapes are least visible on skin surfaces. Adhesive tapes which have elastic cloth backs are described in the section on elastic bandages (page 511).

Moleskin is a thick, soft, napped cotton used for cushioning purposes. Moleskin ad-hesive is used in orthopedic conditions where soft-tissue traction is required or where an extremity is to be supported and cushioned at the same time. It can be cut to provide padding for corns, calluses, bunions and the like. Chiropodist Adhesive Felt* is used for the same foot disorders. It is, perhaps, more resilient and pliable than moleskin. Both moleskin and felt-backed adhesives are pack-aged in wide rolls faced with crinoline or other protective coverings.

Adhesive tape has multiple uses.[12] It serves to hold primary dressings in place and pro-tect them. In orthopedic work, adhesive tape, plain and elastic, is applied to immobilize injured limbs and joints. Strapping the chest with adhesive tape when the ribs are broken reduces discomfort and hastens healing. Coaches and trainers of athletes make liberal

---

* Felt is a fabric produced by the matting or felting together of fibrous materials such as wool, hair or furs; Chiropodist Adhesive Felt (Parke-Davis) is 83 per cent wool, 17 per cent rayon.

use of support by adhesive tape to treat and prevent injuries. When cut into butter-fly shapes, adhesive tape can be used in place of skin sutures to close small wounds or to reinforce healing wounds after sutures are removed. Individually wrapped sterile butter-fly-type closures are available.

In general, proper ways to apply and re-move adhesive tapes are not known to lay people who, instead, rely on misconceptions passed along from others. The pharmacist can ascertain readily the intended use of the tape and should offer advice with respect to best procedures to follow.[12] Tape should be applied only to a clean, dry surface; moisture, oils, grease and powders interfere with ad-hesion. Improvement of adhesive masses has removed the need for prior application of compound benzoin tincture to skin as a tackifier. Tape should not be used to cover iodine tincture or counterirritant liniments. Adhesive tape may be removed without pain or trauma if done slowly and with the aid of solvents capable of dissolving or loosen-ing the adhesive mass. Carbon tetrachloride, ether, benzine or mineral oil can be applied with cotton to the back of the tape and al-lowed to soak through. In a few moments the edge of the tape can be peeled back and removal started. It is often more satisfactory to hold the tape tightly and to push the skin away from it rather than to pull on the tape. More solvent can be applied along the edge as necessary. Ripping the tape off rapidly is no longer recommended. To prevent pain and strain on a wound, the tape should be pulled toward the wound rather than away from it.[156] Tape that passes across a dressing should be cut at the edge of the dressing and the remainder removed from the skin separately. Remnants of the adhesive should be swabbed off with solvents. The skin should be washed and dried after solvents have been used.

Reactivity to Adhesive Tapes. The esti-mate that the incidence of skin reactions to adhesive tapes lies between 1 and 5 per cent is probably too low.[210] Some investigators have shown that nearly 50 per cent of their test subjects developed skin changes after the application of ordinary adhesive tapes.[122,209] Complaints about skin reactions are voiced to the pharmacist who, therefore,

should be informed concerning them. He also should be able to evaluate claims that one tape is less likely than another to pro-duce untoward reactions.

While there is not complete agreement on the etiology of the reactions, Russell and Thorne[201] suggest that reactions of at least five types may develop, owing variously to the following causes: trauma of removal; irritation by the adhesive; maceration of the horny layer after retention of sweat and serous discharges; disturbance of balance of skin bacterial flora; and eczematous sensitiza-tion. Reaction due to removal develops a minute or two after removal of tapes, espe-cially at hairy sites. It generally disappears quickly also. The reaction is greatest with more tacky tapes. It can be prevented almost completely by using a solvent or a detacki-fier such as ether or mineral oil to assist in removing the tape.

Irritation by the adhesive arises from mechanical or chemical stimulation of kera-tin formation, interference with desquama-tion, plugging of pilosebaceous follicles and probably also from unrecognized causes. It is more pronounced with people who per-spire heavily and in hot, humid surround-ings, and appears clinically 5 days or more after application. The more adhesive the tape, the greater the irritation. Waterproof and ordinary tapes with similar adhesiveness produce equivalent irritation, suggesting that the operative factor lies with the physico-chemical properties of the tapes, not with the degree of permeability of the backing.[201]

Although sweat retention and maceration of the horny layer may lead to infection or infectious eczema, tapes with porous back-ings are not always found to be less irritating than nonporous ones.[201] However, lack of irritation by newly developed surgical tapes, which are discussed later, is attributed in part to porosity of the backing and conse-quent absence of skin maceration. Distur-bance of the balance of bacterial flora on the skin assumes importance only when anti-bacterial agents are incorporated in the ad-hesive mass, in which case there is some possibility of an "ecologic" drug eruption.

The incidence of eczematous sensitization is much smaller than that of reactions due to direct irritation.[209,210] However, Kiel[133] has pointed out that allergic contact due to adhesive tape is by no means rare in the absolute sense. It develops after a latent period of 10 days on the first exposure or after a few hours on subsequent ones. Many of the constituents of the usually complex adhesive mass have been implicated, among them colophony resin (rosin), chloroxylenol (an antiseptic sometimes used) and the proteins in rubber.[201] Sensitivity to terpene structures in resins and rubber has been suggested as initiating the reaction.[210]

Hyporeactive Tapes. In attempts to eliminate skin irritation, tapes have been prepared using specially purified ingredients and a minimally complex adhesive mass of natural rubber. More recently, synthetic copolymers have been used as single-ingredient adhesive masses, which are thinly spread on backings that are microporous as constructed or else multiply punctured with small holes. These hyporeactive tapes (also called hypoallergenic) seem to offer the advantages of lessened occlusion and skin reaction without sacrifice of adhesiveness.[14,105,177] In one brand* an acrylate adhesive is thinly spread on a nonwoven rayon backing[14,239] so as to leave numerous small openings (micropores) for escape of moisture and for aeration. When smoothed down firmly on clean dry skin, the tape adheres tightly. It can be peeled off easily without trauma partly because hairs are not entrapped owing to the thinness of the adhesive layer. The tape is not dislodged by secretions, perspiration or soaking, and it does not leave a sticky residue on the skin. Complete lack of skin irritation or maceration is claimed.[105] Because the tape unwinds readily and rips easily, special dispensers are not necessary, but the manufacturer has found it necessary to use them as a competitive sales feature. It is available in widths of ½ to 3 inches in bulk packages for hospitals and ½ or 1 inch for home use. A similar tape† with a woven rayon backing appears to have equivalent attributes.[177] Other tapes with hypoallergenic adhesive masses and continuous plastic film backings‡ appear to overhydrate underlying skin and may cause skin stripping on removal, while

tapes with macropunctured plastic or fabric backings* do likewise to some degree because of the solid sections between the holes.[98]

Other Adhesives. An alert pharmacist will find opportunities to inform his patrons about less familiar adhesive materials that they may use to their advantage. For instance, a liquid adhesive mass† is sometimes more convenient than the conventional tapes for adhering small dressings over minor wounds or skin eruptions in areas that are difficult to bandage. It may be applied directly from the tube to form an elastic ring around the area to be protected. For example, boils on the back of the neck can be covered with a small piece of sterile gauze, a ring of liquid adhesive placed around the gauze and a slightly larger piece of soft flannel placed over all so that its outer edges are affixed to the skin. Cellulose film products such as Scotch tape‡ are well known for household uses. They may also be used to hold face dressings and eye pads in place when a product less conspicuous than ordinary tape is desirable. Perhaps it is not premature for the pharmacist to watch for developments in cyanoacrylate adhesives which are both tissue adhesives and hemostatic agents.[51,98] The cyanoacrylate monomer—general formula $CH_2{=}C(CN)COOR$—is sprayed on the surface to be treated, whereupon rapid polymerization occurs to form a thin film. Butyl cyanoacrylate has shown promise as a surface dressing in the oral cavity[51] and in the nose.[98]

Gauze Bandage. Most bandage rolls stocked by pharmacists for use by the general public are made of Type I gauze (44 × 36 mesh) to conform to *U.S.P.* standards for gauze bandage.[240] They are available in widths of 1 to 4 inches × 10 yards. Edges are treated to minimize raveling. Individual rolls are paper-wrapped, sealed in boxes and sterilized after packaging. Bandage rolls of looser meshes, as well as of unbleached muslin (56 × 60 mesh), are also made primarily for institutions and physicians. These rolls are nonsterile. They may be cut

---

* Micropore, 3M Company, St. Paul, Minn.
† Dermicel, Johnson and Johnson, New Brunswick, N.J.
‡ Blenderm, 3M Company.

*Polyvent, The Kendall Co., Chicago, Ill.; Band-Aid Air-Vent Tape, Johnson and Johnson, New Brunswick, N.J.
† Duo Adhesive, Thayer-Knomark, Inc., Jamaica, N.Y.
‡ 3M Company, St. Paul, Minn.

into standard widths and packaged by paper-banding a number of rolls together. Uncut rolls, 36 inches wide or more, are also supplied.

Gauze bandages are used to hold on dressings and occasionally to supply slight pressure or support. They are not intended for direct application to wounds. Muslin roller bandages are stronger than gauze and are used to hold splints or bulky dressings in place. Wrapping with roller bandage is an art requiring much practice if neat results are to be obtained. First-aid manuals and other sources[156] illustrate desirable technics. The pharmacist called on to render first aid is well advised to use one of the more easily applied bandages described in the following paragraphs.

Triangular Bandages. The Esmarch triangular bandage has numerous uses in first aid[156] because it is quickly and easily applied by one reasonably acquainted with its capabilities. Head dressings, binders for splints for broken bones, and arm slings are readily made from these bandages. They are isosceles right triangles of bleached muslin approximately 54 inches in length at the base. Nonsterile packages of various sorts are available.

Tubular Bandage. The pharmacist may enhance his stature as an advisor about first-aid supplies by informing his clients about unique products that have advantages over the highly promoted conventional ones that are readily obtainable from self-service racks in nonprofessional outlets. For example, a seamless tubular gauze bandage* can be recommended instead of the usual roller bandage to hold dressings on finger or toe wounds. The tube is applied more quickly and makes a neater and more comfortable covering. Sizes 1 and 2, which are for small and large fingers and toes, are packed with an applicator and instructions for use (Fig. 13-32). There are larger sizes that can be fitted over the hands, feet, elbows and head. Both white and flesh-colored rolls are made. The bandage as supplied is not sterile. A ready-made finger-toe cot† of the

* Surgitube, Surgitube Products, Corp., New York, N.Y.; Tubegauz, Scholl Mfg. Co., Inc., Chicago, Ill.
† Surgitube Roll-on Instant, Surgitube Products Corp.

same material has been marketed recently in four sizes and three colors. This appears to offer further advantages in bandaging speed and convenience.

Conforming Bandage. The discovery that preshrunk cotton gauze fibers become kinky and stick to each other[8] led to the development of a new form of roller bandage.* A 14×10 mesh gauze is used and the edges are folded to the center (Fig. 13-33). Owing to the loose mesh and the crimped threads, the bandage is soft and conforms readily to body contours, and overlapped layers grip one another, thus decreasing slippage. Because of its two-way stretch, it is less likely

*Red Cross Improved Gauze Bandage; Kling Elastic Gauze Bandage, Johnson and Johnson, New Brunswick, N.J.

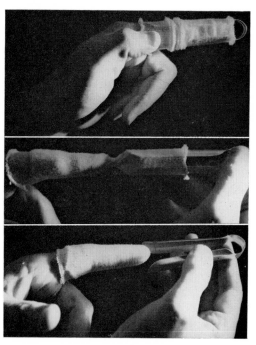

FIG. 13-32. Applying tubular gauze to a finger. (*Top*) A length of gauze slightly longer than twice the length of the finger is threaded over the applicator and placed on the finger. Breaks in the skin should first be covered with a sterile dressing. (*Center*) The applicator is pulled off the finger and twisted one full turn. (*Bottom*) The applicator is pushed forward again to apply a second layer of gauze and seal the tip end. The base of the bandage should be fastened down with adhesive tape.

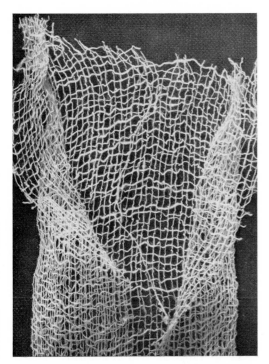

Fig. 13-33. Conforming bandage. The edges have been turned back so that the 2-ply construction and the individual threads can be seen.

to constrict swelling areas. The two-ply construction gives the bandage greater absorbency. The conforming bandage should be recommended for household use, because even a novice can make a neat covering with it. Individual sterile rolls are marketed in sizes from 1 to 4 inches $\times$ 5 yards. Bags containing nonsterile rolls up to 6-inch widths are also available. This gauze with a filler of rayon is used in institutions as a highly absorbent elastic compression dressing* for breasts, amputee stumps of limbs, and burns.

Self-adhering Bandage. Self-adhering gauze† is a useful form of bandage about which the lay public is not well informed. This is bleached absorbent gauze (32 $\times$ 28 mesh) impregnated with natural rubber latex so that the gauze sticks only to itself, not to skin or hair. The bandage is dry to the touch. It can replace adhesive tape as a

mild support for strains[156] or can function as a bandage for holding on dressings. Its advantage is that overlapping layers can be pressed together and made to cohere. The bandage is nonocclusive, because the gauze meshes are not filled in. Water does not materially affect the cohesiveness. An oil-resistant form impregnated with synthetic resins is available. Individually boxed sterile rolls of $\frac{1}{2}$ to 2 inches by $7\frac{1}{2}$ yards are supplied for pharmacies, and rolls 12 inches by 10 yards are cut to order for institutions.

Plaster of Paris bandages are used in orthopedic work to make plaster casts for fractures and for other conditions in which immobilization and support are necessary. Plaster of Paris ($CaSO_4 \bullet \frac{1}{2}H_2O$) is a white amorphous powder made by partial dehydration of gypsum ($CaSO_4 \bullet 2H_2O$). The plaster reacts exothermically with water to form crystals of gypsum, which interlock to form a hard, rigid mass on drying. The plaster can be molded to fit the contours of the area to which it is being applied, but after a certain critical point, known as the setting time, at which crystallization occurs in the hardening process, further movement of the plaster causes it to crumble.[104]

Bandages are made by rolling and rubbing the plaster into meshes of crinoline.* Although this may be done by hand, machine-made proprietary bandages are much more frequently used. The two main kinds of plaster bandages differ in the manner in which the plaster is present in the bandage. The loose plaster bandages are made by sprinkling the dry powder in a smooth, even layer on the crinoline and rolling the crinoline over on itself so as to hold in the powder. The hard-coated plaster bandages are made by applying a paste or an emulsion of the plaster to the crinoline and then baking it. The second type is preferred by most orthopedic men because it is less messy to handle, wets more rapidly and loses less plaster in the wetting process. The hardcoated form† is supplied in rolls of 2 to 8 inches $\times$ 3 or 5 yards. It is also supplied as straight board-like splints† made by cutting 3-inch, 4-inch

* K-S Compression Roll, Johnson and Johnson.
† Gauztex Bandage, General Bandages, Inc., Morton Grove, Ill.

*Crinoline is a loosely woven, bleached gauze stiffened by starch.
† Specialist Plaster of Paris Bandages, Specialist Plaster of Paris Splints; Johnson and Johnson, New Brunswick, N.J.

and 5-inch widths of hardcoated bandage into 15-inch, 30-inch or 45-inch lengths. Splints are used to reinforce casts and speed up cast making. Plaster of Paris bandages are sometimes packaged individually in sealed polyethylene bags* or in waterproof polyethylene papers† to protect against moisture.

The time required for the plaster to set after it is wetted depends on several factors. These are controlled to a degree in the manufacture of the bandages and the splints, most of which fall into one of two ranges of setting time. The extra-fast-setting, which crystallizes in 2 to 4 minutes, is useful for foot plasters on very small children. The fast-setting, which crystallizes in 5 to 8 minutes, is used for most cast work.[55] Setting can be hastened by adding either sodium chloride or alum, or delayed by adding borax, but the plaster is made brittle.[104] Experienced workers modify setting times while they are making the cast by controlling the temperature of the water used. Warm water accelerates setting; cool water delays it.

Formalin resins have been found to add waterproofing and strength to plaster of Paris casts, being especially useful for walking casts, for example. Casts may be made one half the thickness and the weight of an ordinary cast and about 4 times as strong.[55] The resin may be used as a powder to which water and a catalyst, usually ammonium chloride, are added. The regular fast-setting plaster bandages are wetted with this solution and applied as usual. Polymerization of the resin in situ forms a hard, waterproof, easily cleaned cast. Bandages‡ containing resin, plaster and catalyst as one unit ready for wetting are marketed also. Casts can be made entirely of synthetic resins, but this is not commonly done in this country.

Because plaster of Paris bandages are used by specialists trained in making casts, pharmacists are not often asked about technics of application. An interesting movie[188] depicts preparation, application and removal of splints.

Equipment[156] such as stainless steel buckets, plaster knives, spreaders, benders and cast cutters are generally obtained from surgical supply houses. However, pharmacies may stock materials such as stockinette and surgical (sheet) wadding, both of which are used as paddings under casts. Stockinette, which is slipped on directly over the skin, is a seamless tubular material knit of unbleached nonabsorbent cotton yarn. The knitted weave confers elasticity to allow the stockinette to adapt itself to body conformations. The 25-yard rolls come in widths ranging from 2 to 12 inches. It is not recommended for use over acute fractures or immediately postoperatively, because it acts as a constricting bandage and may impair circulation.[55] Sheet wadding is used for almost all casts, usually being wound over stockinette. It is made from bleached nonabsorbent cotton that has been glazed on both sides to give it tensile strength and to avoid matting or lumping. It is supplied in 6-yard lengths as uncut sheets 36 inches wide, as well as rolls 3 to 8 inches wide. A nonwoven cotton felt fabric,* available in rolls 2 to 6 inches × 4 yards, has properties of softness, elasticity, conformability and strength, which make it suitable for orthopedic cast padding.

Two materials that may replace plaster of Paris for limb splints have recently been marketed. One† is a lightweight thermoplastic material (isoprene) supplied in sheets that can be cut to any shape required, heated to a molding temperature of 150-170°F. and then formed into a splint around the limb. The material remains workable for about 5 minutes and can be reheated to make alterations or adjustments. The cast is washable, hypoallergenic and radiolucent. Velcro strips are used as fasteners. The second‡ is an inflatable plastic splint that comes in a variety of sizes so as to fit part or whole limbs. The double-walled sheet is wrapped arounds the injured limb, zippered shut and inflated by mouth. The rigidity immoblizes the limb, while the pressure can help control venous bleeding, hold pressure-point compresses in place for arterial bleeding

---

* Readi-Cast, Parke, Davis and Co., Detroit, Mich.

† Ostic, Bauer and Black, Chicago, Ill.

‡ ZOROC Resin-Plaster Bandages, Johnson and Johnson, New Brunswick, N.J.

*Webril Bandages, Bauer and Black, Chicago, Ill.

† Orthoplast Isoprene Splints, Johnson and Johnson, New Brunswick, N.J.

‡ Readisplints, Parke, Davis and Co., Detroit Mich.

control and help to control swelling. Transparency permits a ready visual check of the limb, as well as x-ray. The utility of such splints for emergency first aid has been demonstrated.[89] Ginsberg *et al.*[103] have pointed out that too high an air pressure may occlude the lumen of small blood vessels of the digits and lead to necrosis. Pharmacists providing these splints should advise that the air pressure be kept below 20 mm. Hg. This is roughly equivalent to inflating by mouth until the creases in the outer surface of the plastic are obliterated and a resistance to further inflation is felt.[103] Also the splint should not be left on the skin for longer than 12 hours because maceration may result owing to lack of ventilation.[103] Husni *et al.*[123] have shown that an air splint inflated to a pressure of 15 to 20 mm. Hg does not retard venous circulation and is therefore preferred to pressure bandaging of the knee with an elastic bandage.

PACKAGING AND STORAGE OF SURGICAL DRESSINGS

Surgical dressings are labeled to identify them either as sterile or as nonsterilized. Each sterile item is sealed in an individual package labeled to the effect that sterility is not guaranteed if the package bears evidence of damage or has been opened previously. Because opening the packages usually destroys the resale value, pharmacists tend to dispense surgical dressing without examining their construction or establishing their quality. For the sake of obtaining this necessary information, small packages should be opened or samples should be obtained. Surgical dressings should be stored in closed cabinets that protect them from dust in order to be consistent with the concept of sterility. When placed on open shelves, frequent dusting is mandatory. These items should not be stored near sources of heat because absorbency, color or adhesiveness may be affected adversely by elevated temperatures.

RELATED SUPPLIES

A number of items are related to surgical dressings in the sense that there is a similarity in construction and an association in use. Into this category fall obstetrical pads or sanitary napkins, vaginal tampons, medicated plasters, cellulose tissues, spray-on wound dressings, underpads, disposable diapers and surgical masks, for example. The last three on this list are described in the following sections.

Disposable Underpads. By preventing soilage of bed linens, disposable underpads save both time and energy for those engaged in home and institutional nursing.[196] These pads are usually constructed with a highly absorbent filler sandwiched between a soft fabric facing and a water-repellent backing. The more efficient styles* have a nonwoven fabric facing, a cellulose filler and a polyethylene or polypropylene backing. The less expensive ones† have a paper facing, a pulp or cellulose filler and a backing of paper made moisture repellent by coating with polyethylene or by other technics. Standard dimensions are $17\frac{1}{2} \times 24$ inches with both larger and smaller sizes available. Usually 200 or 300 pads are packed in a case for institutional use. Packages‡ with smaller quantities are marketed for home use.

Disposable diapers are basically similar to disposable underpads in design. They may be complete diapers, the whole pad being discarded when soiled or wet, or they may be single-use absorbent pads, which are inserted into a reusable plastic or nylon holder. Several brands are marketed, each in a range of sizes. Their major appeal is in convenience when traveling. Their use may also lessen the potential for contagion with impetigo. Following the near suffocation of a 4-month-old baby, whose nostrils and mouth became covered by the impermeable plastic backing,[34] the American Academy of Pediatrics has advised against the use of disposable diapers or underpads as crib sheets. The danger of this practice should certainly be pointed out by the pharmacist, if he has any reason to suspect this to be the intent of the purchaser.

Surgical Masks. Face masks of various

---

* Loress Linen Savers, Johnson and Johnson, New Brunswick, N.J.; Incontinent Pads, Bauer and Black, Chicago, Ill.; DeLuxe Disposable Underpads, Parke, Davis and Co., Detroit, Mich.

† Bed Pads, Johnson and Johnson; Disposable Underpads, Parke, Davis and Co., Detroit, Mich.

‡ Chux Disposable Underpads, Johnson and Johnson, New Brunswick, N.J.

types are used in operating rooms and elsewhere with the intent of filtering both inspired and expired air in order to prevent passage of pathogenic organisms either from or to the wearers. Masks are made to fit over the mouth and nose, and also to extend under the chin to keep perspiration from dropping into the work area. They are held in place by tie-tapes. A flexible metal strip in the upper seam is often provided to allow the mask to be molded over the nose. A close fit is necessary to prevent the breath from blowing up over the upper margin. However, wearers often complain that their eyeglasses are fogged by condensation of moisture from the breath. Interference with breathing, muffling of the voice and wetness of the mask after short periods of use are other discomforts that must be endured. The simplest conventional masks are made from a single layer of finely woven fabric or of 4-ply fine mesh surgical gauze. A gauze mask was found to be only 30 to 40 per cent efficient in bacterial filtration in a 2-minute test with a drop to 8 to 10 per cent efficiency at the end of 30 minutes.[167] Newer designs, which are one-time-use disposable units, incorporate filtering mats of synthetic fibers to achieve greater effectiveness in retention of bacteria. A study[154] of several such masks showed the following efficiencies in filtering bacteria from a simulated sneeze: a polypropylene fiber mask* retained 98.8 per cent of the bacteria; a polyester-rayon fiber mask,† 98.4 per cent; a glass fiber mask,‡ 97.3 per cent; a cellulose fiber (paper) mask§ less than 92.7 per cent. The polyester-rayon mask is unique in having a rigid molded contour shape. Added comfort is claimed because the mask does not make contact with the mouth or nostrils. These masks are furnished only in hospital multipacks. Despite the recognized importance of preventing spread of upper respiratory infections from ailing mother to infant, only the relatively inefficient gauze masks are available for home use.

* Filtron Surgical Mask, 3M Company, St. Paul, Minn.
† Aseptex Surgical Mask, 3M Company.
‡ Bardic Deseret Filtermask, Deseret Pharmaceutical Co., Inc., Sandy, Utah.
§ Paper Mask, R. C. Bard, Inc., Murray Hill, N.J.

HEARING AIDS

Some community pharmacists have successfully established a service to supply hearing aids and accessories to clients with loss of hearing.[176,227] The simpler supplies such as batteries and standardized replacement cords can readily be handled. To do more requires training such as that provided by some manufacturers of hearing aids, as well as a considerable investment in inventory, personnel and time. Careful review of the market involved and of the potential complications is warranted before undertaking to encompass this difficult area. It is not feasible within this short chapter to discuss hearing problems and the complex instrumentation needed to detect and to correct them.

AMBULATION AIDS

Wheelchairs. The wheelchair is designed to substitute wheels for lower extremities in order to give mobility to persons deprived of normal ambulation.[139] Amputees, hemiplegics, paraplegics, quadriplegics, arthritics, cerebral palsy victims and those disabled by accidents are major users. The prevalence of wheelchair users in the United States is now 1.5 per 1000 population.[139] Currently, almost 300,000 individuals in this country have permanent need of wheelchairs and thousands more are temporary users. As the number of aged increases, so also does the incidence of chronic disease and disabilities that necessitate using wheelchairs. A change[63] in the voluntary medical insurance plan of Medicare (Title 18B) in 1968 permits government payment toward purchase of durable medical equipment needed for use in the home. Presumably this will further stimulate wheelchair sales.

Selection of the correct wheelchair for a disabled person requires thorough knowledge both of the patient's needs and of available equipment.[91] An unsuitable chair can cause trauma, secondary deformities and disabilities, and other complications that may be irreversible. Some authorities[91,139] believe that wheelchairs should be supplied only on prescription orders written by physicians (Fig. 13-34). However, it is estimated that 80 to 95 per cent of the wheelchairs sold

NAME:_____AGE:_____DATE:_____

ADDRESS:_____

TYPE
☐ Outdoor—large wheel in rear   ☐ Amputee
☐ Indoor—large wheel in front

CONSTRUCTION
☐ Standard   ☐ Heavy duty

SIZE
☐ Adult—seat width 18″   ☐ Child—seat width 13″
☐ Narrow adult—seat width 16″   ☐ Extra width 20″
☐ Junior—seat width 16″   ☐ Extra width 22″

WHEELS AND CASTERS
☐ Standard   ☐ 8″ casters
☐ Balloon   ☐ 8″   ☐ 5″ solid

HANDRIMS
☐ Standard   ☐ Knobs
☐ Pegs—upright   ☐ Rt.   ☐ Lt. One-arm drive

BRAKES
☐ Lever   ☐ Rt.   ☐ Lt. extension
☐ Toggle   ☐ Bilateral extension

BACK
☐ Standard   ☐ Semi-reclining
☐ Rt.   ☐ Lt. back opening   ☐ Full reclining
☐ Screw stud   ☐ Zipper   ☐ Head extension
☐ Solid insert—contoured

SEAT
☐ Sling   hammock   ☐ Commode
☐ Solid   ☐ Hydraulic

CUSHIONS
☐ Seat _____inches   ☐ Back _____inches

ARMRESTS
☐ Standard upholstered   ☐ Offset
☐ Full   ☐ Desk removable   ☐ Locks

FOOTRESTS AND LEGRESTS
☐ Standard   ☐ Swinging detachable elevating legrests
☐ Elevating legrests
☐ Swinging detachable footrests   ☐ Heel loops
☐ No footrests   ☐ Toe loops

ACCESSORIES OPTIONAL
☐ Tray   ☐ Safety belt
☐ Rt.   ☐ Lt. Crutch holder   ☐ Front   ☐ Rear anti-tip

Signature _____M.D.

Address_____

FIG. 13-34. Wheelchair prescription. (From: Lee, M. H. M., *et al.*: Wheelchair Prescription. Washington, D.C., Gov't Printing Office, 1967)

TABLE 13-7. CLASSIFICATION OF
WHEELCHAIRS

Fixed back
  Basic or outdoor—drive wheels in back
  Reverse or indoor—drive wheels in front
  Amputee—drive wheels in back, long wheel-
    base
Reclining back
  Semireclining—adjustable from almost verti-
    cal to a 30-degree recline.
  Full-reclining—adjustable to any degree of
    recline between horizontal and nearly ver-
    tical.
Collapsible or folding—all the above types
Noncollapsible or hospital—generally reverse
  type only
By size—in most of above types
  Adult size
    Regular or average
    Narrow
    Wide
  Junior size
  Children size
    Large—for children 6 to 12
    Small—for children 2 to 6
By special feature
  Lightweight collapsible—about 30 lb. rather
    than 45 lb. or more
  Heavy duty collapsible—for individuals over
    180 lb.
  Motorized
  Customized—special sizes or accessories

are not so prescribed. That pharmacists have recognized an opportunity for specialized service is evidenced by the recent rapid increase in the number of pharmacies that can supply wheelchairs. In 1965, there were 8,166 pharmacies[29] stocking them; there were 15,361 in 1967. As close a physician-patient-pharmacist relationship should develop in this aspect of health care as it has with prescription drugs.

Specialized publications* and suppliers' catalogs should be examined for details of wheelchair construction and selection. These

* Wheelchair Selection: More than Choosing a Chair with Wheels, Minneapolis, Minn., Publications Office, American Rehabilitation Foundation ($1.25), 1967. Wheelchair Prescription, Public Health Service Publication No. 1666, Washington, D.C., Superintendent of Documents, Government Printing Office ($.20), 1967.

are acknowledged as the prime sources for the material herein. Several pharmacists with long experience in the field have also been consulted with benefit. The major types of wheelchairs are given in Table 13-7. Figure 13-35 illustrates the components of the basic collapsible wheelchair.

The wheelchair is selected after consideration of disability-related factors, physical measurements and mode of living. Table 13-8 is a general guide to selecting wheelchairs according to disability. A few specific examples are brought out here. How the person gets in and out of the wheelchair can determine the types of arms and footrests that are needed. If the person can come to a standing position on one or both feet, either alone or with assistance, then he can use fixed (standard) arms to push down on when arising, and the chair should have removable footrests that can be moved out of the way as necessary. If the person cannot stand but transfers by lifting himself with his upper extremities while in a sitting position, removable arms and removable footrests are best. This will allow for transfer out the side of the chair. If the person must be lifted to transfer him, then removable arms and removable footrests facilitate manual lifting by an attendant, but fixed arms may be satisfactory if a mechanical or hydraulic lift is used.

The usual chair can be readily propelled by an individual who has both hands and normal strength. If the hands have limited function, as in arthritis, the handrims may be equipped with knobs or pegs to compensate for a weak grip. As an alternative, a piece of garden hose may be slit lengthwise and taped to the rim so as to reduce hand slippage. For a person with one functional hand, the one-arm drive modification may be needed. This consists of two handrims, both attached to the wheel on the patient's unaffected side. One, the normal size rim, operates the wheel to which it is attached and the second rim, which has a smaller diameter, operates the opposite wheel. Simultaneous moving of both rims with the one hand propels the chair forward or backward in a straight line. Moving either rim separately turns the chair in the direction of the wheel that is moved. The one-arm

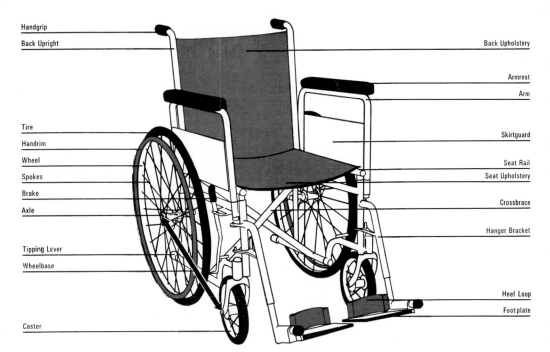

Handgrip

Back Upright

Back Upholstery

Armrest

Arm

Tire

Handrim

Wheel

Spokes

Brake

Axle

Skirtguard

Seat Rail

Seat Upholstery

Crossbrace

Hanger Bracket

Tipping Lever

Wheelbase

Heel Loop

Footplate

Caster

Arm: Frame which forms portion of chair providing side support and to which armrest is attached.

Armrest: Support for the upper extremity. **The person's forearms should be supported so that his shoulders are level. Padded armrests provide added comfort; for the person who uses his forearms to do push-ups in the wheelchair, the padding aids in preventing pressure areas.**

Axle: Shaft on which large or drive wheel revolves.

Back upholstery: Fabric which supports wheelchair user's back.

Back upright: Main frame of wheelchair perpendicular to seat.

Brake: Device which immobilizes wheelchair by stopping movement of drive wheel.

Caster: Small wheel which swivels as the chair is turned. **For maneuverability, 8-inch size is preferred to 5-inch.**

Crossbrace: Supporting underframe generally formed of steel tubing.

Footplate: Surface which supports the foot.

Footrest (legrest): Unit consisting of hanger bracket and footplate. **Length of the unit should be adjusted so that the person's weight is equally divided over the sitting area and thighs. Footrests should be removable to permit a close approach for transfers and to allow adequate foot space for the wheelchair user, plus an attendant when needed, during transfers.**

Handgrip: Molded rubber or plastic grip on end of back upright which attendant grasps to push chair.

Handrim: Metal rim attached to drive wheel which permits occupant to propel chair without touching tire.

Hanger bracket: Upright to which footplate is attached.

Heel loop: Strip of material fastened across back of footplate to prevent person's foot from slipping off backward.

Seat rail: Fixed horizontal bar to which seat upholstery is attached.

Seat upholstery: Fabric which forms sitting surface.

Skirtguard: Panel attached to arm tubing which protects wheelchair user's clothing from contact with large wheel.

Spokes: Round wires radiating from axle which support rim of wheel.

Tipping lever: Rearward projection from base of frame on which attendant applies force with foot to tilt chair backward and to permit gradually returning chair to horizontal position.

Tire: Continuous solid or pneumatic rubber cushion encircling wheel.

Wheel: Circular frame of metal, covered with tire and supported by spokes, that turns on axle. **Placement of the large or drive wheels in back and the casters in front permits the wheelchair user to maintain body balance and sit in good posture when wheeling the chair. Maneuverability of the chair also is greater with the large wheels in back than with the reverse arrangement.**

Wheelbase: Distance between axles of large wheel and caster.

FIG. 13-35.   (From Lee, M. H. M., *et al.*: Wheelchair Prescription. Washington, D.C. Gov't Printing Office, 1967)

drive chair requires good muscles in the sound arm, good coordination and good learning ability. A severely disabled person may require a motorized chair.

The arthritic with limited shoulder or elbow extension may prefer the reverse (indoor) chair, because he can reach a front drive wheel with less straining. However, when a patient's physical condition mandates an erect sitting posture as in emphysema, paraplegia or quadriplegia, only the basic (outdoor) chair should be supplied because self-operation of the reverse type tends to cause the body to slump forward. A person

TABLE 13-8. GUIDE TO WHEELCHAIR SELECTION ACCORDING TO DISABILITY*

Wheelchair	Hemiplegia	Paraplegia	Quadriplegia	Cerebral Palsy	Arthritis	Amputee
Type						
Basic	++	++	++	++		
Reverse	++					
Amputee				+	++	++
Handrims						
Standard	++	++	++	++	++	++
One-arm drive	++		+			
Pegs or knobs			+	+	+	
Brakes						
Toggle	++	++	++	++	++	++
Lever	++	++		++		++
Brake extension	++	+	+		+	
Back						
Standard	++	++	++	++	++	++
Back opening		++			++	++
Back insert			+	++	++	
Semireclining			++			
Full-reclining			++			
Head extension	+	+	+	+	+	+
Seat						
Sling	++	++	++	++		++
Solid	++	+	++	++	++	++
Commode			+	+		
Hydraulic					+	
Armrests						
Standard	++	++	++	++	++	++
Removable—full		++	++	++	++	
—desk				++		
Foot and Legrests						
Standard	++	++	++	++	++	
Elevating	++			+	++	
Swing, detachable		++	++	+	++	++
Swing, detachable, elevating		++	++	++	++	++
Heel loops	+	+	++			
Toe loops		+	+	+		+

*Modified from Lee, M. H. M. *et al.*: Wheelchair Prescription, Washington, D. C., Government Printing Office, 1967.
++ = preferred; + = consider.

with trunk muscle weakness and trunk instability may be adequately provided for by a head extension and a safety belt on a basic chair or else may require either a semireclining or a full-reclining chair, depending on the severity of the disability. The reclining chair may be useful for respiratory patients who must remain supine much of the time. A solid seat or a seat board is advocated for patients with tight adductors, for spastic paraplegics and quadriplegics, and cerebral palsy patients because the usual sling seat aggravates their tendency to be in a position of internal rotation at the hip joint. Hemiplegics may find it easier to rise from a seat made solid and higher by addition of a seat board. Seat boards should be padded or else covered with a suitable cushion. A 2-inch-thick back cushion may make a chair more comfortable for a person with bony or protruding scapulae. Persons with circulatory disturbances in the lower extremities, with lower limb casts, or with limited knee flexion or extension require elevating legrests. A cane and crutch holder should be attached to the back of the chair for a person who uses a cane or crutches to ambulate or to transfer. Antitipping brackets may be attached to the rear of a full-reclining chair to prevent the spastic patient from tipping the chair over backwards.

The wheelchair dimensions that may be selected to fit the physical measurements of the patient are seat height, seat depth, back height, seat and back width, and height of arm with armrest. The adult-size chair fits the adult of average height and weight, while the junior-size chair may suit a small adult or a teenager. Narrow, average and wide adult chairs are available. It is probably generally safest to take actual measurements of the patient whenever possible. Figure 13-36 illustrates and correlates the significant dimensions of patient and wheelchair. The wrong size wheelchair may be more than simply uncomfortable. For example, if there is excess room at the sides of the seat, the individual has to strain or sit unnaturally in order to reach the wheels, and in addition, may develop skin abrasions from rubbing against the armrest. When a too short back fails to give adequate support, the top edge of the back fabric will curl and sag. This further reduces support and also causes an uncomfortable ridge that presses against the patient's back. To get relief from fatigue and irritation, the patient slides down in the chair or slumps forward. A head extension added to the chair back may solve the problem.

The places where the chair will be used and the forms of activity in which the person normally engages should be considered. The patient who is going to school or working may prefer a chair equipped with desk arms. Desk arms are shorter than full armrests because the frontal portion (about 6 inches) has been lowered (about 4½ inches) so as to permit a close approach to the desk or work area. When narrow doorways in the home present a problem, a narrowing device may be attached to the sling seat of the wheelchair. By turning a crank the patient can then narrow the chair 2 or 3 inches when needed. Air tires may be better than the usual hard tires if the chair will be used frequently out-of-doors or on rough surfaces. If the person is especially active, heavy-duty features may be needed. A commode seat may be necessary for the patient who is unable to get into his home bathroom because of the physical arrangements of the room. A lightweight model could be desirable when there is frequent need to move the chair in and out of an automobile.

A reasonable approach to obtaining information necessary to make the best recommendations when getting a telephoned inquiry about wheelchairs is reported by Higbee.[116] He suggests keeping a cue card near the telephone to prompt asking about the patient's height, weight, sex, disability, special needs, width of doorways in home, special conditions such as traveling often in car, need for related equipment, and for the name of the physician or physical therapist who may be involved.

The multiplicity of available options presents an inventory problem. A minimum variety of wheelchairs and accessories calculated to meet a wide range of patient needs has been suggested:[91] (1) "all-purpose" chair, adult-size, fixed back, removable arms with padded armrests, swinging removable footrests, heel loops; (2) junior-size chair with same features as preceding type; (3)

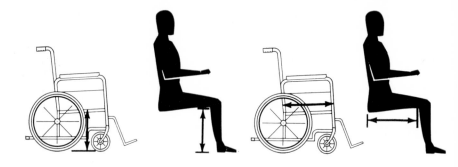

	Seat Height		Seat Depth	
Adult	19″ to 20″	Bottom of heel to inner bend of knee plus 3″ clearance	16″	1″ less than length from inner bend of knee to posterior bend of hip
Junior	17″ to 20″		16″, 14″, 13″	
Semireclining	Same as above		Same as above	
Full reclining	Same as above		Same as above	

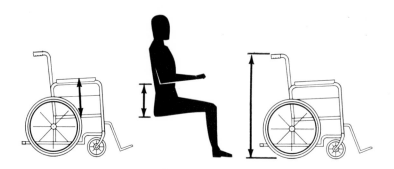

	Height of Arm with Armrest		Overall Height	
Adult	9″ to 9½″	Bottom of buttocks to outer bend of elbow	35″	
Junior	9″ to 10″		32″ to 37″	
Semireclining	Same as above		39″	plus about 10″ for removable headrest panel
Full reclining	Same as above		42″	

Check the manufacturer's catalog for specific dimensions.

FIG. 13-36.   (From Lee, M. H. M., et al.: Wheelchair Prescription. Washington, D.C., Gov't Printing Office, 1967)

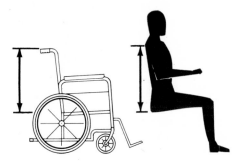
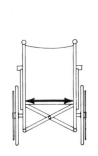
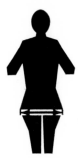

Back Height		Seat and Back Width	
16" to 17"	Bottom of buttocks to level of shoulders	18" (16" for narrow adult; 20" for wide adult)	Widest area of
16"		16"	hips and shoulders
20" to 21"	plus about 10" for removable	Same as above	
21½" to 22½"	headrest panel	Same as above	

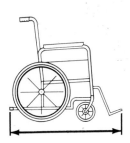
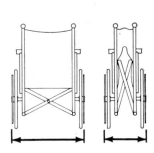

Overall Length	Width	Open	Closed	Weight
40" to 41"		24" to 25"	10"	44 to 50 lb. (24 to 30 lb. for lightweight)
38" to 41"		(22" to 23" for narrow adult; 27" for wide adult)		41 to 45 lb.
46" to 47"		22"	9" to 10"	55 to 62 lb.
49" to 50"		Same as above		57 to 64 lb.

Figures given are the approximate measurements for chairs made by several companies.

Figure 13-36 (*Continued*)

adult-size chair with semireclining back, removable arms with padded armrests and swinging removable legrests with heel loops; (4) Adult-size chair with fixed back, fixed arms with padded armrests and removable footrests with heel loops; (5) One pair each of removable desk arms with padded armrests, adjustable arms, and handrims with vertical pegs to interchange with comparable parts as needed.

A patient may need a chair for only a relatively short time, or he may for economic or psychologic reasons be unwilling to purchase one outright, so rental of wheelchairs is a common practice. Suggestions for good rental practices and a form of rental agreement have been drawn up.[126] A typical monthly rental charge is one-sixth of the cost of the chair to the pharmacist. The pharmacist who rents out chairs must be prepared for maintenance problems. Upholstery can be washed with mild soap and water followed by thorough drying. Metal parts should be kept dry and protected against rusting. Loose or broken parts should be repaired immediately. The pharmacist who supplies a faulty used chair as a rental runs the risk of a civil suit for damages.

The pharmacist has the responsibility also to instruct the patient and his family in the use and care of the wheelchair. For example, a collapsed wheelchair should be opened by pushing down on the seat rails (Fig. 13-35), not by trying to pull it apart by the arms. To close the basic chair, push heel loops forward on the foot plates, raise the foot plates until they are vertical to the floor, lift up on seat upholstery at front and back to almost close the chair, tuck the upholstery down between the seat rails, and then squeeze chair to complete fold. The closed wheelchair may be placed inside a car by tilting the chair back onto its large wheels and rolling it forward into the car, maintaining the tilted position until the casters clear the center hump in the floorboard. Another method is to put the wheelchair in the open car doorway with the large wheels next to the car and then to pull the chair backwards up and in on its large wheels from inside the car. To go up and down curbs, the attendant helping with the wheelchair manipulates it in much the same way

he would a baby carriage or a grocery cart. To descend, tilt the wheelchair back onto the large wheels, step on tipping lever (Fig. 13-35) and slowly roll the chair forward off the curb. To ascend, tilt the chair back onto the large wheels, place the casters up on the curb, lift the chair up by the handgrips and roll it forward onto the sidewalk. Two helpers are needed to maneuver stairs. The one at the back of the chair tilts the chair backward while the other at the front grasps the front frame beneath the seat or the fixed footrest. One step at a time, the chair is rolled backwards up the stairs or forward down the stairs.

Walkers. Walkers, crutches and canes serve as extensions that enable the upper extremities to transmit force to the floor so as to provide support and protection for the lower extremities and to improve balance. As a disabled person's condition improves, he may progress from requiring a wheelchair to getting about with the aid of a walker, then crutches, then a cane. Walkers are frequently used for balance by the very elderly and by apprehensive persons too fearful of falling to try to use the less supportive aids. The conventional walker[126] provides stability because the handgrips are attached to each other and to a rigid four-legged frame with a wide base. It has been likened to a set of portable parallel bars.

Suppliers' catalogs should be inspected for information about types of walkers. Walkers are available as simple rigid frames, as lightweight models, in folding styles, with legs adjustable to desired heights, with seats, with wheels, with underarm rests and with other modifications as well. Frames are generally made of stainless steel, chrome-plated steel, or chrome-plated steel or aluminum tubing. Heights range from 32 to 36 inches. The proper height for the handgrip may generally be ascertained by measuring from the patient's greater trochanter (the large bony prominence on the hip) straight down to the floor.[217] It may be difficult to find a walker high enough for a tall patient. Underarm rests, if present, should reach to 2 inches below the axilla.

Several gaits are possible with a pick-up walker.[126,217] The patient can advance the walker 8 to 12 inches forward, step in with

FIG. 13-37. (*Left*) Forms of crutches. Left to right: standard wooden double upright; adjustable wooden double upright; Canadian wooden; adjustable Lofstrand aluminum; and adjustable double upright aluminum with wooden axillary rest and hand grip. (*Right*) The tripod position.

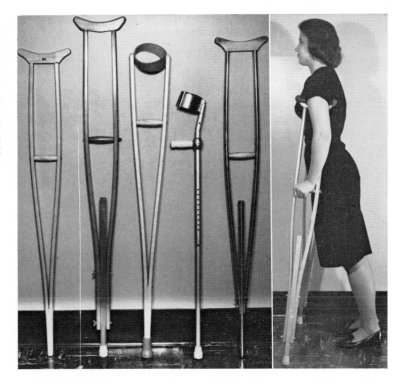

each leg and advance the walker again. If one leg is disabled, the patient steps in first with the disabled leg. In another gait, the patient advances the walker, steps in with one foot, advances the walker, steps in with the other foot, etc. The usual walker is useless on stairs.

Crutches. Pharmacists often sell or rent crutches without consultation with physicians to persons who are temporarily disabled from a broken leg, a sprained ankle or other crippling injury. This service entails selecting crutches appropriate to an individual's needs and instructing in their proper use. Amputees who wear prostheses, paraplegics and hemiplegics generally are supplied with crutches as a part of an institution-based rehabililation program. In these cases, pharmacists are called on for replacement or adjunct components and for advice about specific problems.

Several styles of crutches are shown in Fig. 13-37. Aluminum crutches are lighter and stronger but more expensive than hardwood crutches. The standard double upright, underarm crutch is fixed in length whereas an adjustable crutch may be set to several lengths. The double upright, under-arm crutch is best for short-term use by novices inasmuch as considerable strength and skill are needed to handle most of the others.

Standard wooden underarm crutches come in lengths of 26 to 60 inches in increments of 2 inches. About a dozen sizes are needed to take care of most youths and adults (Table 13-9). The pharmacist may prefer to stock the adjustable crutch in this style because he would then need to keep only four different sizes on hand. In the usual adjustable crutch, the center post is perforated along its length by a number of holes spaced 2 inches apart. Two of these holes are lined up with holes through the uprights, long bolts are passed through, and wing nuts are securely attached to fasten the center post in position and to make the crutch the desired overall length. Handgrips may be set at four or five positions by a similar bolt-and-nut arrangement. Crutch sizes are adjustable as follows: adult, 48 to 60 inches; youth, 36 to 48 inches; child, 30 to 36 inches; and infant, 24 to 30 inches. Brands vary slightly in these ranges of adjustment. Aluminum crutches are supplied only as adjustable models.

TABLE 13-9. STANDARD CRUTCH CHART

HEIGHT OF PERSON (inches)	CRUTCH SIZE*
52 53	36
54 55	38
56 57	40
58 59	42
60 61	44
62 63	46
64 65	48
66 67	50
68 69	52
70 71	54
72 73	56
74 75	58
76 77	60

* If height in inches is an odd number, subtract 17 to get crutch length; if even, subtract 16.

To estimate the correct size for an individual, measure from 2 inches below the axilla to a point about 4 inches to the side of one foot while the patient is standing erect, shoulders and pelvis in line, but slightly apart.[37] If the patient is still bedridden, measure to the heel and add 4 inches. A standard crutch chart (Table 13-9) posted in the crutch department is a helpful guide. The desired length is obtained by moving the center post as necessary. The position of the handgrip may be approximated by asking the patient to hold his arm as if he were using the crutch—i.e., fist clenched, wrist slightly hyperextended, elbow flexed to 30°—and then measuring from the level of the clenched fist to the point 4 inches to the side of the foot. The handgrip is placed at this distance from the crutch tip. When adjusting the crutch, measure it with crutch tips on and also with axillary pads if they are to be used. To determine if the selected or adjusted size is correct, have the patient assume the tripod position (Fig. 13-37, *right*), which will be used in walking. With the hands placed on the handgrips and the crutch tips about 4 inches in front of and to the side of the feet, the axillary rests should be about the width of three fingers below the axilla as the weight is borne on the wrists and palms. The wrist should be bent and the elbow flexed so that the forearm makes a 20° to 30° angle with the upper arm. An aluminum crutch, which is adjusted to length by sliding the telescope-like arrangement of its tubular shaft, is handy to have in the department although it is relatively costly, because it may be quickly and easily set to the estimated dimensions, checked against the patient, and then used as the model by which to adjust the crutches supplied to the patient.

Patients who require continued use of crutches frequently prefer the forearm crutch (Fig. 13-37), which is shorter, lighter, and more maneuverable than the underarm type once the technic is mastered. Good upper extremity strength and balance are required because there is no axillary bar to brace against the chest. A single forearm crutch used in a cane-like fashion can support 40 to 50 per cent of the body weight.[126] In this style, the forearm is gripped lightly by the strap or pivoting cradle at the top of the crutch so that the handgrip can be released without dropping the crutch or losing its support. Two measurements are necessary to fit the crutch. Measure the handgrip height from clenched fist to floor point as with the underarm crutch. Measure from the clenched fist to 1 inch below the elbow to determine the height of the forearm cuff.[3] Nonadjustable wooden crutches ranging from 30 to 42 inches are available, but the adjustable aluminum crutch is more commonly used.

Pharmacists too often supply crutches without being certain that the recipient knows how to use them. Instruction in how to walk with crutches should be an integral part of the service.[80] There are several gaits for crutch walking,[3,37] three of which are

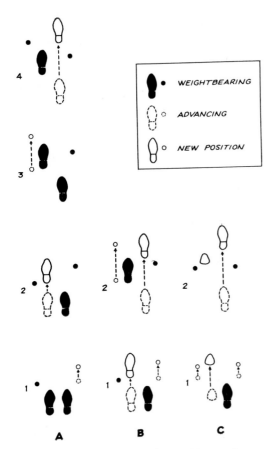

●	WEIGHTBEARING
◐ ○	ADVANCING
◌ ○	NEW POSITION

FIG. 13-38. Crutch gaits. A. Four-point gait: easiest and safest, useful when patient can bear some weight on both legs. The patient puts one crutch forward, then the opposite foot, the other crutch, the opposite foot; three weight-bearing points at all times. B. Two-point gait: weight on one leg and opposite crutch, bring other leg and crutch forward together and shift weight to them; faster than the four-point. C. Three-point gait: used when one leg is unable to bear weight (symbolized by toe only), but the other is strong enough to bear all of the patient's weight; weak leg and both crutches are advanced together and the weight is balanced on them as the good leg is moved forward.

easily learned (Fig. 13-38). Negotiating stairs presents problems (Table 13-10), as does going through doors or getting in and out of chairs. A special publication* that

* Ambulation: A Manual for Nurses, Minneapolis, Minn., Publications Office, American Rehabilitation Foundation ($1.25), 1966.

TABLE 13-10. HANDLING CRUTCHES ON STAIRS*

1. Hold railing with one hand.†
2. Place both crutches under opposite arm.†

A. Patient with one good leg, other can bear partial weight

To ascend:	To descend:
3. Step up with good leg.	3. Lower crutches and bad leg to the step below.
4. Lift bad leg and crutches to this level.	4. Bring good leg down to this level.

B. Patient with one good leg, other cannot bear weight

To ascend:	To descend:
3. Push on crutches and railing to lift body so that good leg can be placed on the step above.	3. Lower crutches to the step below.
4. Lift bad leg and crutches to this level.	4. Bend good knee, shifting weight to crutches and railing.
	5. Step down with good foot.

* Modified from Arje, F. B.: How to teach crutch walking, RN 24:38, 1961 (March).
† The first 2 steps apply to all 4 procedures.

details gait patterns and other technics for manipulating crutches should be consulted.

Crutch Accessories. Crutch arm pads, handgrip cushions and crutch tips are used to "dress" the crutch. Arm pads are generally made of sponge rubber, sometimes reinforced by fabric linings. Only one size is made because this can be stretched over the axillary bars of all standard adult crutches. The pad is attached in order to protect the axilla and rib cage against friction and pressure, but its presence gives the erroneous impression that the crutch user is supposed to bear his weight on the bars. The true purpose of the axillary bar is to provide lateral stability of the crutch by pressure against the chest wall.[126] The weight must be carried on the wrists and elbows; flexing the elbow allows the arm to lengthen or shorten at different phases of gait and also permits the triceps to act as a shock absorber.[126] Leaning on the axillary bar may cause compression of the radial nerve or even of the entire brachial plexus resulting in muscle paralysis. Weakness in the forearm, the wrist or the hand signifies the onset of this "crutch paralysis."

Rubber handgrip cushions may either be split lengthwise to permit slipping on over the crutch handgrip or may be a closed style. Some are made of a soft sponge rubber. Others are made of plastic or rubber molded into a pistol-grip shape. The cushion provides a broader surface for weight bearing and a larger grasping surface for patients with large hands or limited grip, as well as simply being softer than the regular wooden or metal bar.

Crutch tips are used to cushion against jarring and to prevent sliding. They are made

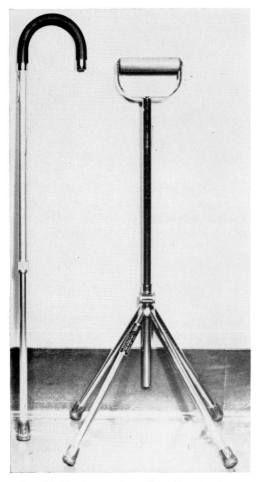

Fig. 13-39. Canes. An adjustable aluminum cane and a four-legged cane are shown.

of a rubber high in mineral filler content to make them resistant to abrasion. They may be fabric-lined to delay wearing through by the crutch. Tips have a characteristic shape with a concave suction-cup design on the bottom. Several sizes, with internal diameters ranging from $\frac{1}{2}$ to $1\frac{1}{4}$ inches are made. The crutch tip should fit tightly. A little talcum powder sprinkled inside makes the tip easier to slide onto the crutch. Lubricating with grease or oil damages the rubber. If used on dusty or waxed surfaces, the grooves should be scraped free of dirt and wax, and the tip should be wiped clean in order to prevent slippage. Crutch tips that are cracked, worn thin, worn unevenly or that have worn-over rounded edges are unsafe and should be replaced. Crutches should not be dispensed unless dressed with arm pads and tips, but the use of handgrips is somewhat less common.

Canes. Canes are used primarily for balance when walking. A cane does not provide much support[126] and has a tendency to be wobbly and unstable because it has only a single point of contact with the upper extremity—i.e., the handgrip. The cane is not the aid to use if it is to be required to bear more than 20 to 25 per cent of the body weight.[126] Three-legged and four-legged canes (Fig. 13-39) have uses of support and balance intermediate to those of crutches and walking canes. The blind man's cane (42 inches long, white at the top, red at the bottom and metal tipped) has an obvious specialized purpose.

Canes are made of wood or aluminum. Wooden canes vary greatly in quality of wood and degree of ornateness. The familiar rounded handle is sometimes modified to a pistol-grip or a T-handle for ease of grasping, especially by arthritics. The correct length for a cane is estimated by measuring from the person's greater trochanter straight to the floor.[217] The cane should permit a 15° to 30° flexion of the elbow during use. The elbow should be slightly bent when the individual is standing, with some weight borne on the cane and the tip placed about 6 inches to the side of the foot. The cane should be dressed with a rubber tip similar to a crutch tip in design and purpose. The standard cane length is 36 inches with lengths up to 44 inches available in some brands. Cane height may be adjusted by sawing an appropriate amount from the distal end of an overlong cane. Aluminum canes adjustable from 22 inches to 38 inches are available and may be used to ascertain the correct length for a wooden cane before irrevocably sawing off the tip.

When a cane is used for weight bearing, it may be carried beside the disabled leg.[3] In the more usual case where improved balance is desired, the cane is carried beside the sound leg.[3] This provides a wide base for balance. Also, because the center of gravity does not shift from side to side with each step, pelvic stability is increased and compressive forces on the hip joint of the affected leg are lessened.[3] One walking pattern[126] with the cane held in the hand opposite the weak leg is: start with feet comfortably apart, cane tip on floor at level of toe of shoe and 4 to 6 inches off to the side; advance cane a comfortable distance; bring involved leg forward so that the toe is in line with the cane tip; repeat. In going up stairs, hook the cane in belt or pocket and proceed as described in Table 13-10, *part A*. Note that the normal leg goes first when ascending and the disabled leg first when descending. In this way, the major strain of lifting and flexing is always placed on the good leg.

REFERENCES

1. Abramson, H. A.: Principles and practice of aerosol therapy of the lungs and bronchi. Ann. Allergy, 4:440, 1946.
2. Aldous, J. A.: Needle deflection: a factor in the administration of local anesthetics. J.A.D.A., 77:602, 1968.
3. Allgire, M., and Denney, R. R.: Nurses Can Give and Teach Rehabilitation. p. 60. New York, Springer, 1960.
4. AMA Committee on Human Reproduction: Evaluation of intrauterine contraceptive devices. J.A.M.A., 199:647, 1967.
5. Amphyl Booklet, Montvale, N. J., Lehn and Fink Products Corp.
6. Anon.: Prescription department move over. Rutherford, N. J., Becton, Dickinson and Co., Sept. 1, 1950.
7. Anon.: As waterproof as a fish. Rohm and Haas Rep. p. 7. Nov.-Dec., 1952.
8. Anon.: Non-slip bandage, Sci. N.L., 69:342, 1956.
9. Anon.: Probably no medical instrument is so widely used. Prescriptionist, 3:17, 1956.
10. Anon.: Mercury in the intestine. J.A.M.A., 163:1309, 1957.
11. Anon.: Temperature and activity of rheumatic fever. J.A.M.A., 163:1565, 1957.
12. Anon.: Therapeutic Uses of Adhesive Tape. ed. 2. New Brunswick, N. J., Johnson and Johnson, 1958.
13. Anon.: Electric heating pads. Consumer Rep., 25:32, 1960.
14. Anon.: Novel adhesive key to new tape. Chem. Eng. News, 38:36, Nov. 7, 1960.
15. Anon.: Selected Equipment Useful in the Hospital, Home or Nursing Home. Minneapolis, American Rehabilitation Foundation, 1962.
16. Anon.: Ear temperature appears more reliable than rectal-reading. J.A.M.A., 192:43, June 7, 1965.
17. Anon.: Clinical thermometers. Consumer Rep., 31:388, 1966.
18. Anon.: Clues to mysterious fevers. J.A.M.A., 197:29, July 11, 1966.
19. Anon.: Disposable enema kits. Med. Letter, 8:23, 1966.
20. Anon.: Electric heating pads. Consumer Rep., 31:492, 1966.
21. Anon.: Fifty-nine per cent of diabetics make dosage errors. Am. Drug., 155:35, Aug. 1, 1966.
22. Anon.: Natural rubber producers update technology. Chem. Eng. News, 44:56, May 9, 1966.
23. Anon.: Deaths from asthma. J.A.M.A., 199:31, 1967.
24. Anon.: 11,534 broach home health agencies; 8 per cent are accepted. Am. Drug., 155:11, April 10, 1967.
25. Anon.: Nursing Care of the Skin. pp. 10-12. Minneapolis, American Rehabilitation Foundation, 1967.
26. Anon.: Sickroom boom? Pharmacy News (SKF), 8:2, 1967.
27. Anon.: The pharmacist's role in expanding medical care. NARD J., 89:14, Jan. 2, 1967.
28. Anon.: Bronchodilator aerosols for asthma. Med. Letter, 10:29, 1968.
29. Anon.: Convalescent aids are now getting big ticket emphasis. Am. Drug., 157:13, Feb. 26, 1968.
30. Anon.: Electric vaporizers. Consumer Rep., 33:39, 1968.
31. Anon.: FDA-proposed device law criticized. F-D-C Rep., 30:21, 1968.
32. Anon.: Important home health care facts. NARD J., 90:31, July 15, 1968.

33. Anon.: Sugar-free liquids now total 129. Am. Drug., *161*:69, Apr. 6, 1970.

34. Anon.: Warning on disposable absorbent pads. Med. World News, *9*:75, Oct. 25, 1968.

35. Ansell, J.: Care of urinary retention catheters. Northwest Med., *64*:349, 1965.

36. Archambault, G. F.: Conceptual design of pharmaceutical practice in health care facilities. p. 57. Ann Arbor, Mich., Proc. Pharm.-Med.-Nursing Conf. on Health Ed., 1967.

37. Arje, F. B.: How to teach crutch walking. RN, *24*:38, Mar., 1961.

38. Arronet, G. H.: Studies on ovulation in the normal menstrual cycle. Fertil. Steril., *8*:301, 1957.

39. Artz, C. P., Fitts, C. T., and Hargest, T. S.: Use of a new nonadherent dressing. Am. J. Surg., *114*:973, 1967.

40. Autian, J.: Drug packaging in plastics. Drug Cosmet. Ind., *102*:79, May, 1968.

41. ———: Need for an ASHP certification program for plastic devices used in hospitals. Am. J. Hosp. Pharm., *25*:344, 1968.

42. Banyai, A. L., and Levine, E. R.: Dyspnea Diagnosis and Treatment. pp. 6-25, 96, 107-109, 188-193, 263-266. Philadelphia, F. A. Davis, 1963.

43. Barach, A. L.: Inhalation therapy, advances and retreats. Anesthesiology, *22*:367, 1961.

44. Barach, A. L., and Beckerman, H. A.: Pulmonary Emphysema. p. 225. Baltimore, Williams & Wilkins, 1956.

45. Barrett, C. D., Jr., and Molner, J. G.: Experiences with the Hypospray as the instrument of injection. J. School Health, *32*:49, 1962.

46. Beck, W. C.: Holes in rubber gloves. Am. J. Surg., *100*:363, 1960.

47. Benton, J. G., Brown, H., and Rusk, H. A.: Energy expended by patients on the bedpan and bedside commode. J.A.M.A., *144*:1443, 1950.

48. Bergman, L. V., and Silson, J. E.: Particle size produced by various instruments for inhalation therapy. Ann. Allergy, *19*:735, 1961.

49. Berke, M.: What to look for in purchasing hypodermic needles. Hosp., *31*:60, Jan. 16, 1957.

50. Betts, T. J., and Whittet, T. D.: A new non-adherent—its uses and identification. Pharm. J., *194*:25, 1965.

51. Bhaskar, S. N., and Frisch, J.: Use of cyanoacrylate adhesives in dentistry. J.A.D.A., *77*:831, 1968.

52. Bierman, W. J.: Therapeutic use of cold. J.A.M.A., *157*:1189, 1955.

53. Bishop, W. J.: A History of Surgical Dressings. Chesterfield, Robinson, 1959.

54. Blaug, S. M., and Karig, A. W.: Oral inhalation aerosols. Am. J. Hosp. Pharm., *24*:603, 1967.

55. Bleck, E. E., Duckworth, N., and Hunter, N.: Atlas of Plaster Cast Techniques, pp. 11, 12, 19. Chicago, Year Book Pub., 1956.

56. Bloomberg, M. H.: Orthopedic Braces: Rationale, Classification and Prescription. Philadelphia, J. B. Lippincott, 1964.

57. Borison, H. L., and Clark, W. G.: Drug actions in thermoregulatory mechanisms. Adv. Pharmacol., *5*:129, 1967.

58. Boyd, E. M., and Sheppard, E. P.: Friar's Balsam and respiratory tract fluid. Am. J. Dis. Child., *111*:630, 1966.

59. Boyland, H. L.: Surgical Appliance Handbook. ed. 2. pp. 134-160. Cincinnati, Surgical Appliance Industries, 1968.

60. Brieger, H.: Spillage of mercury. J.A.M.A., *199*:682, 1967.

61. Brody, G. S., McCorriston, J. R., and Skoryna, S. C.: Observations on fecal continence mechanisms. J.A.M.A., *173*:226, 1960.

62. Buxton, C. L.: In: discussion of Siegler, S. L., and Siegler, A. M.: Fertil. Steril., *2*:287, 1951.

63. Cain, R. W.: Medicare payments for durable goods. A.C.A. Sec. Newsletter, *26*:1, Feb. 25, 1968.

64. Cantor, M. O.: Mercury: its role in intestinal decompression tubes. Am. J. Surg., *73*:690, 1947.

65. ———: Mercury lost in the gastrointestinal tract. J.A.M.A., *146*:560, 1951.

66. Care and Processing of Surgical Gloves. New Haven, Conn., The Seamless Rubber Co.

67. Caswell, G. A.: The history of fever thermometers and modern developments. A.S.T.A. Journal, May, 1952.

68. Cherniack, R. M., and Hakimpour, K.: The rational use of oxygen in respiratory insufficiency, J.A.M.A., *199*:178, 1967.

69. Collins, V. J.: Inhalation therapy education and training programs. J.A.M.A., *207*:329, 1969.

70. Comarr, A. E.: In defense of the intraurethral catheter. Am. J. Surg., *111*:157, 1966.

71. Cooper, C., Morley, D. C., Weeks, M. C., and Beale, A. J.: Administration of measles vaccine by dermojet. Lancet, *1*:1076, 1966.

72. Cooper, P.: Ward Procedures and Techniques. pp. 105-118, 220-229. New York, Appleton-Century-Crofts, 1967.

73. Cozen, L.: Peroneal palsy caused by elastic bandages with traction. Ind. Med. Surg. 34:407, 1965.

74. Cravitz, L., and Tyler, V.: Gas sterilization adds to life of surgical gloves, tests show. Mod. Hosp., 96:106, 1961.

75. Creevy, C. D.: Use and abuse of urethral catheters. Northw. Med., 57:1427, 1958.

76. Crohn, L. B.: Hospital preferences in disposable syringes. Bull. Parent. Drug Ass., 14:18, 1960.

77. D'Amelio, C.: Rxmen can fit surgical appliances. Am. Prof. Pharm., 33:52, Aug., 1967.

78. Day, R. L.: O-t-c medications for menstrual problems. J. Am. Pharm., Ass. NS8:477, 1968.

79. Dease, J. C.: Expanding surgical appliances in your pharmacy. J. Am. Pharm. Ass., NS4:72, 1964.

80. Deaver, G. G.: What every physician should know about the teaching of crutch walking. J.A.M.A., 142:470, 1950.

81. Diglio, V. A., and Munch, J. C.: Pressor drugs. IV. The safety of inhalation therapy in human patients. Ann. Allergy, 13:257, 1955.

82. Dimond, E. G., and Andrews, M. H.: Clinical thermometers and urinometers. J.A.M.A., 156:125, 1954.

83. Doershuk, C. F., and Matthews, L. W.: Cystic fibrosis comprehensive therapy. Postgrad. Med., 40:550, 1966.

84. Dolger, H., and Seeman, B.: How To Live With Diabetes. ed. 4. pp. 79, 81, 158. New York, Pyramid, 1966.

85. Doyle, J. B., Ewers, F. J., Jr., and Sapit, D.: The new fertility testing tape. J.A.M.A., 172:1744, 1960.

86. Druss, R. G., O'Connor, J. F., Prudden, J. F., and Stern, L. O.: Psychologic response to colectomy. Arch. Gen. Psych., 18:53, 1968.

87. DuBois, E. F.: Fever. p. 7. Springfield, Ill., Charles C Thomas, 1948.

88. Dykes, E. R.: Technic for putting on elastic stockings. Am. J. Surg., 109:260, 1965.

89. Earle, A. S., Moritz, J. R., and Saviers, G. B.: Inflatable splint for ski injuries. J.A.M.A., 192:1094, 1965.

90. Ewing, M. R., Garrow, C., and McHugh, N.: Use of sheepskins as an aid to nursing. Lancet, 2:1447, 1961.

91. Fahland, B., and Grendahl, B. C.: Wheelchair Selection: More Than Choosing a Chair With Wheels. pp. 1, 16. Minneapolis, American Rehabilitation Foundation, 1967.

92. Fedder, D. O.: A 4-point yardstick for surgical appliances. Am. Prof. Pharm., 33:62, Aug., 1967.

93. Fedor, W. S.: Elastomers. Chem. Eng. News, 40:88, Mar. 12, 1962.

94. Fever thermometers, some helpful questions and answers; Facts about fever. Becton, Dickinson & Co.; Facts on fever, E. Kesseling Thermometer Co., Inc.; Fever, Taylor Instrument Co.

95. Findeisen, W.: Ueber das Absetzen kleiner, in der Luft suspendierter Teilchen in der menschlichen Lunge bei der Atmung. Pfluger's Arch. ges. Physiol., 236:367, 1935, quoted by Segal, M. S.

96. Fisher, H. L.: Chemistry of Natural and Synthetic Rubbers. New York, Reinhold, 1957.

97. Flaherty, P. T.: Braces: A Primer for Nurses. Minneapolis, American Rehabilitation Foundation, 1968.

98. Frable, M. A.: Cyanoacrylate plastics for epistaxis. J.A.M.A., 204:1198, 1968.

99. Franz, F., and Tovell, R. M.: A study of hypodermic needle points. Anesthesiology, 17:724, 1956.

100. Gant, J. Q., Jr.: An evaluation of a new cerumenolytic agent. A.M.A. Arch. Derm., 79:651, 1959.

101. Garrison, H. H.: Factors affecting syringe dosage accuracy. Bull. Parent. Drug Ass., 13:21, 1959.

102. Gershenfeld, L., Greene, A., and Witlin, B.: Disinfection of clinical thermometers. J. Am. Pharm. Ass. (Sci.), 40:457, 1951.

103. Ginsberg, M., Miller, J. M., and McElfatrick, G. C.: The use of inflatable plastic splint. J.A.M.A., 200:180, 1967.

104. Gleckler, E. O.: Plaster of Paris Technic. pp. 1, 14. Baltimore, Williams & Wilkins, 1944.

105. Golden, T.: Non-irritating, multipurpose surgical adhesive tape. Am. J. Surg., 100:789, 1960.

106. Greenberg, M. J., and Pines, A.: Pressurized aerosols in asthma. Brit. Med. J., 1:563, 1967.

107. Gregg, J. B., and Anderson, W. R.: The importance of environment control in the prevention of upper respiratory infections. So. Dakota J. Med., 21:21, Feb., 1968.

108. Griffiths, B., Becton, Dickinson and Co.: Personal communication.

109. Guyton, A. C.: Textbook of Medical Physiology. ed. 3. pp. 985-1000. Philadelphia, W. B. Saunders, 1966.

110. Hall, R. E.: A reappraisal of intrauterine contraceptive devices. Am. J. Obstet. Gynec., 99:808, 1967.

111. Halpern, S. R., and Sellars, W. A.: Practical tips in aerosol therapy in asthma. Am. J. Dis. Child., 107:280, 1964.

112. Harmer, B., and Henderson, V.: Textbook of the Principles and Practices of Nursing. ed. 5. pp. 251, 462, 637, 647, 652, 705, 712-765, 911, 915, 974. New York, Macmillan, 1955.

113. Harris, R. L., and Riley, H. D., Jr.: Reactions to aerosol medication in infants and children. J.A.M.A., 201:953, 1967.

114. Healy, J. J.: Disposable hypodermic syringes and needles. J.A.M.A., 191:57, 1965.

115. Henderson, J.: A Parents' Guide to Children's Illnesses. New York, Bantam, 1957.

116. Higbee, R. K.: How to handle convalescent aid customers. NARD J., 90:59, July 15, 1968.

117. Higgs, H.: Utilizing space in space age pharmacy. Apothecary, 80:38, May, 1968.

118. Hipps, H. E.: Back braces: types, functions and how to order and use them. Med. Clinics No. Am., 51:1315, 1967.

119. Hopkins, G. H.: Elastomeric closures for pharmaceutical packaging. J. Pharm. Sci., 54:138, 1965.

120. Horvath, S. M., Menduke, H., and Piersol, G. M.: Oral and rectal temperatures of man. J.A.M.A., 144:1562, 1950.

121. House, R. J., and Henderson, R. J.: Disinfecting the clinical thermometer. Brit. Med. J., 2:1414, 1965.

122. Humphries, R. E.: New factors in adhesive formulas which lessen irritation. J. Invest. Derm., 9:219, 1947.

123. Husni, E. A., Ximenes, J. O. C., and Hamilton, F. G.: Pressure bandaging of the lower extremity. J.A.M.A., 206:2715, 1968.

124. Huyck, C. L., and Maxwell, J. L.: Diabetic syrups. J. Am. Pharm. Ass., (Pract.) 19:142, 1958.

125. Incontinence a challenge to understanding. Part II. Providence, R.I., Davol Rubber Co.

126. Jebsen, R. H.: Use and abuse of ambulation aids. J.A.M.A., 199:5, 1967.

127. Jeter, K.: Management of children with ileal conduits. Hosp. Topics, 46:91, Feb., 1968.

128. Johnson, H. R. M., and Koumides, O.: Unusual case of mercury poisoning, Brit. Med. J., 1:340, 1967.

129. Kalant, N., Pattee, C. J., Simpson, G. W., and Hendleman, M.: Timing of ovulation. Fertil. Steril., 7:57, 1956.

130. Kaminetsky, H. A.: Vaginal biology and the douche. J.A.M.A., 191:950, 1965.

131. Kanig, J. L.: Pharmaceutical aerosols. J. Pharm. Sci., 52:513, 1963.

132. Katona, E. A: Learning colostomy control. Am. J. Nursing, 67:534, 1967.

133. Keil, H.: Further studies on the mechanism of adhesive tape dermatitis. A.M.A. Arch. Derm., 64:68, 1951.

134. Kory, R. C., Bergmann, J. C., Sweet, R. D., and Smith, J. R.: Comparative evaluation of oxygen therapy techniques. J.A.M.A., 179:767, 1962.

135. Kravitz, H.: Temperatures of the umbilicus. J. Pediat., 68:418, 1966.

136. Lange, W. R.: Experiences in a vaginitis clinic. J.A.M.A., 174:1814, 1960.

137. Large, P. C., and Mukheiber, W. J.: Injury to rectum and anal canal by enema syringes. Lancet, 2:596, 1956.

138. Lawrence, C. A., and Block, S. S.: Disinfection, Sterilization and Preservation. pp. 517-531. Philadelphia, Lea & Febiger, 1968.

139. Lee, M. H. M., Pezenik, D. P., and Dasco, M. M.: Wheelchair Prescription. P.H.S. Pub. No. 1666. pp. 1, 26. Washington, D.C., U. S. G.P.O., 1967.

140. Liebson, R. A.: How drugstores scored on 340 product lines. Drug Topics, 113:29, Sept. 29, 1969.

141. Levine, I., and Kirschner, C.: How we boosted surgical supplies' sales by 800% in one year. Am. Prof. Pharm., 33:36, May, 1967.

142. Lich, R., Jr.: Therapy of present day recalcitrant urinary tract infections. J. Arkansas Med. Soc., 52:271, 1956.

143. Little, L. D., and Wise, R. A., General Electric Co., Asheboro, N. Carolina: Personal communication.

144. Loraine, J. A., and Bell, E. T.: Fertility and Contraception in the Human Female. pp. 315-335. Edinburgh, Livingstone, 1968.

145. Lyght, C. E. (ed.): Merck Manual. ed. 11. pp. 418, 430-432, 1684, 1690. Rahway, N. J., Merck & Co., Inc., 1966.

146. Lynch, M. J., and Gross, H. M.: Artificial sweetening of liquid preparations. Drug Cosmet. Ind., 87:324, 1960.

147. McAuliffe, P. J.: Expanding pharmacy's health services. J. Am. Pharm. Ass., *NS4*: 66, 1964.

148. McDermott, C. G.: Expanding surgical supplies natural for your pharmacy. J. Am. Pharm. Ass., *NS4*:78, 1964.

149. McDonnell, J. N.: Professional services. In: Martin, E. W. (ed.): Remington's Pharmaceutical Sciences. ed. 13. Chap. 90. p. 1633. Easton, Pa., Mack, 1965.

150. McLeod, D. C.: Single unit packages of drugs available today. Am. J. Hosp. Pharm., *24*:696, 1967.

151. McNamara, R. J., Farber, E. M., and Roland, S. I.: Problems and treatment of the circumileostomy skin. J.A.M.A., *171*:1066, 1959.

152. Margulies, L. C.: Intrauterine contraception: a new approach. Obstet. Gynec., *24*:515, 1964.

153. Martin, E. W. (ed.): Remington's Pharmaceutical Sciences. ed. 13, pp. 1644, 1660, 1748, 1749. Easton, Mack, 1965.

154. Masden, P. O., and Masden, R. E.: A study of disposable surgical masks. Am. J. Surg., *114*:431, 1967.

155. Mehnert, J. H.: Broken thermometer bulb penetrating the submaxillary duct. Am. J. Surg., *98*:743, 1959.

156. Meyer, S. W.: Functional Bandaging. pp. 155-187, 219, 255-265, 270. New York, American Elsevier, 1967.

157. Miles, G.: Prevention of injury to urethra by Foley catheter. J.A.M.A., *202*:989, 1967.

158. Milles, G.: Catheter-induced hemorrhagic pseudopolyps of the urinary bladder. J.A.M.A., *193*:968, 1965.

159. Modell, J. H., Giammona, S. T., and Alvarez, L. A.: Effect of ultrasonic nebulized suspensions on pulmonary surfactant. Dis. Chest, *50*:627, 1966.

160. Modell, W. (ed.): Drugs of Choice, 1968-69. pp. 421, 436, 509. St. Louis, C. V. Mosby, 1967.

161. Modern Medical Methods for the Control of Contraception. pp. 17-21. Raritan, N.J., Ortho Pharmaceutical Corp., 1961.

162. Montag, M. L., and Swenson, R. P. S.: Fundamentals in Nursing Care, ed. 3, pp. 316, 318, 371, Philadelphia, Saunders, 1959.

163. Moore, F. T., Wallace, H., and Freundlich, C.: A protocol for ileostomy management. Am. J. Surg., *111*:687, 1966.

164. Mothes, W., and Hecker, W. C.: Iatrogenic perforation of alimentary tract in children. München med. Wschr., *109*: 643, 1967 (from J.A.M.A., *200*:205, 1967).

165. Munch, J. C.: Pressor drugs. III. Safety of inhalation therapy. J. Am. Pharm. Ass. (Sci.), *44*:208, 1955.

166. Murphy, D. J., and Fernekes, R. J., Casco Products Corp., Bridgeport, Conn.: Personal communication.

167. Musselman, M. M., McFadden, W. H., Jr., Cosand, M. R., and Porter, J. W.: Experience with a new surgical mask. Hosp. Topics, *39*:87, 1961.

168. Myers, R. D., and Sharpe, L. G.: Temperature in the monkey: transmitter factors released from the brain during thermoregulation. Science, *161*:572, 1968.

169. Neuroth, M. L.: Aerosols newest of old therapy. Am. Prof. Pharm., *26*:233, 1960.

170. Nichols, G. A.: Measurements of oral temperature in children. J. Pediat., *72*: 253, 1968.

171. Nichols, G. A., and Glor, B. A. K.: Temperature taking times in Vietnam. Mil. Med., *133*:154, 1968.

172. Nichols, G. A., Ruskin, M. M., Glor, B. A. K., and Kelly, W. H.: Oral, axillary and rectal temperature determinations and relationships. Nurs. Res., *15*:307, 1966.

173. Notter, L. E.: Disinfection of clinical thermometers. Nurs. Outlook, *1*:569, 1953.

174. Olsen, P. C.: Pharmacies up five million dollars in first aid sales. Drug Topics, *107*:40, July 1, 1963.

175. ———: What customers spent for all products sold in drug stores. Drug Topics, *107*:6, July 15, 1963.

176. Omhart, L. M.: Hearing Aids on ℞ only. Am. Prof. Pharm., *33*:26, Aug., 1967.

177. Orentreich, N., Berger, R. A., and Auerbach, R.: Anhidrotic effects of adhesive tapes and occlusive film. Arch. Derm., *94*:709, 1966.

178. Orloff, M. J.: Odor from colostomy. J.A.M.A., *192*:1112, 1965.

179. Ostomy Training Manual and Catalog. ed. 10. Largo, Fla., United Surgical Corp., 1967.

180. Page, S. G., Jr., Riley, C. R., and Hoag, H. B.: A comparative clinical study of several enemas. J.A.M.A., *157*:1208, 1955.

181. Palmer, F., and Kingsbury, S. S.: Particle size in nebulized aerosols. Am. J. Pharm., *124*:112, 1952.

182. Pecorella, P. J.: The basic 130 steps required for making the clinical thermom-

eter. Brooklyn, Pecorella Mfg. Co. (undated).

183. Perkin, G. W.: Intrauterine Contraception. Canad. M. A. J., *94*:431, 1966.

184. Petty, T. L., and Broughton, J. O.: A new, simple IPPB device for hospital and home use. J.A.M.A., *203*:871, 1968.

185. Petty, T. L., and Nett, L. M.: Home inhalation equipment for less than $10. J.A.M.A., *196*:1027, 1966.

186. Pharmacy Laws of California, pp. 34, 48, 75. Sacramento, Dept. of Professional and Vocational Standards, 1969.

187. Pierce, V. M. (ed.): Ostomy Quarterly. Los Angeles, United Ostomy Association, Inc. [This journal is a good general source of information about ostomies. Au.]

188. Plaster Casts and Splints—Preparation, Application, Removal. 16 mm. color, sound movie. Chicago, A.M.A. Motion Picture Library, 1965.

189. Postlethwait, R. W.: Microenema as evacuant before proctoscopy. Curr. Ther. Res., *7*:7, 1965.

190. Prigal, S. J.: Fundamentals of Modern Allergy. pp. 560, 561, 565. New York, McGraw-Hill, 1960.

191. Rankin, T. J., and Good, A. E.: Corticosteroid injection of small joints by hypospray. Arth. Rheum., *9*:611, 1966.

192. Rehfuss, M. E., and Price, A. H.: Practical Therapeutics. ed. 3. p. 92. Baltimore, Williams & Wilkins, 1956.

193. Reif, A. E., and Holcomb, M. P.: Operation characteristics of commercial nebulizers and their adaptation to produce closely sized aerosols. Ann. Allergy, *16*: 626, 1958.

194. Reif, A. E., and Mitchell, C.: Size analysis of water aerosols. Ann. Allergy, *17*: 157, 1959.

195. Rhoads, J. E.: The use and abuse of the Miller-Abbott tube. Surg. Gynec. Obstet., *92*:244, 1951.

196. Roberts, G. W., and Mann, L.: Disposable underpants for incontinent patients nursed at home. Lancet, *2*:208, 1960.

197. Robillard, E., Lepine, C., and Dautrebande, L.: Influence of particle size on systemic effects after breathing potent medicated aerosols. Canad. M. A. J., *86*: 362, 1962.

198. Roland, C. G., and Rogers, A. G.: Rectal perforations after enema administration. Canad. M. A. J., *81*:815, 1959.

199. Roland, M.: Intrauterine contraceptive device. J.A.M.A., *193*:1127, 1965.

200. Rowbotham, J. L.: Stomal care. New Eng. J. Med., *279*:90, 1968.

201. Russell, B., and Thorne, N. A.: Skin reactions beneath adhesive plasters. Lancet, *268*:67, 1955.

202. Sachs, N. R.: Surgical appliances: the beginning of the greatest section in your pharmacy. Am. Prof. Pharm., *34*:36, Aug., 1968.

203. Safar, P. (ed.): Inhalation Therapy. Clinical Anesthesia. Vol. 1. pp. 14-27, 140-164, 170-202, 203-241. Philadelphia, F. A. Davis, 1965.

204. Samp, R. J.: Results of a questionnaire survey of colostomy patients. Surg. Gynec. Obstet., *105*:491, 1957.

205. Secor, S. M.: New hope for colostomy patients. Nurs. Outlook, *2*:643, 1954.

206. Seedor, M. M.: Therapy with Oxygen and Other Gases. Philadelphia, J. B. Lippincott, 1966.

207. Segal, M. S.: The Management of the Patient with Severe Bronchial Asthma. pp. 99, 100. Springfield, Charles C Thomas, 1950.

208. Seide, D.: Caring for colostomy and ileostomy patients. RN, *23*:37, Sept., 1960.

209. Sheldon, J. M., Hensel, H. M., and Blumenthal, F.: Adhesive tape irritation. J. Invest. Derm., *4*:295, 1941.

210. Sidi, E., and Hincky, M.: Allergic sensitization to adhesive tape: experimental study with a hypoallergenic tape. J. Invest. Derm., *29*:81, 1957.

211. Siegler, S. L., and Siegler, A. M.: Evaluation of the basal body temperature. Fertil. Steril., *2*:287, 1951.

212. Silver, H. K., Kempe, C. H., and Kempe, R. S.: Healthy Babies, Happy Parents. ed. 2. pp. 40, 192. New York, McGraw-Hill, 1960.

213. Silver, H. M., and Fuchs, M.: Aspiration of nebulizer cork. J.A.M.A., *205*:187, 1968.

214. Slome, D. (ed.): Wound Healing. p. 54. New York, Pergamon, 1961.

215. Sommermeyer, L., and Frobisher, M., Jr.: Laboratory studies on disinfection of oral thermometers. Nurs. Res., *1*:32, 1952.

216. Sommermeyer, L., and Frobisher, M., Jr.: Laboratory studies on disinfection of rectal thermometers, Nurs. Res., *2*:85, 1953.

217. Sorenson, L., and Ulrich, P. G.: Ambulation: A Manual for Nurses. pp. 10, 11, 20, 33, 34, 38. Minneapolis, American Rehabilitation Foundation, 1966.

218. Sparberg, M., Prohaska, J. V., and Kirsner, J. B.: Solid state karaya gum for use in disposable and permanent ileostomy appliances. Am. J. Surg., *111*:610, 1966.

219. Spence, W.: Artificial fat for prevention of decubitus ulcers. Clin. Med., *74*:25, 1967.

220. Spence, W., Burk, R. D., and Rae, J. W.: Gel support for prevention of pressure necrosis. Arch. Phys. Med. Rehab., *48*:283, 1967.

221. Spock, B.: The Pocket Book of Baby and Child Care. p. 354. New York, Pocket Books, 1951.

222. Sprowls, J. B., Jr., and Beal, H. M. (eds.): American Pharmacy. ed. 6. pp. 397-402. Philadelphia, J. B. Lippincott, 1966.

223. Staub, W. A.: Facts about syringes and needles. Apothecary, *79*:38, Oct. 1967.

224. Stevens, H. R., and Albregt, H. B.: Assessment of ultrasonic nebulization. Anesthesiology, *27*:648, 1966.

225. Stone, H. M.: The technique of the vaginal diaphragm. Hum. Fertil., *6*:97, 1941.

226. Storvick, W. O., and Henry, H. J.: The effect of storage temperature on stability of commercial insulin preparations. Diabetes, *17*:499, 1968.

227. Stuart, R. C.: Hearing aids in the pharmacy. J. Am. Pharm. Ass., *NS4*:83, 1964.

228. Surgical Business, Lancaster, Pa., Cassack.

229. Tanenbaum, M. H.: Spandex dermatitis. J.A.M.A., *200*:899, 1967.

230. The Faultless Way. Ashland, Ohio, The Faultless Rubber Co.

231. Thompson, E. M., and Murphy, C.: Textbook of Basic Nursing. ed. 8, pp. 267, 302, 322, 343-352, 556. Philadelphia, J. B. Lippincott, 1966.

232. Tietze, C.: The Condom as a Contraceptive. pp. 6, 8. New York, National Committee on Maternal Health, 1960.

233. Tietze, C., Lehfeldt, H., and Liebmann, H. G.: The effectiveness of the cervical cap as a contraceptive method. Am. J. Obstet. Gynec., *66*:904, 1953.

234. Tinker, R. B.: Disposable hypodermic needles. Bull. Am. Soc. Hosp. Pharm., *13*:319, 1956.

235. Title, M. M.: Disposables up to date. Hosp., *34*:73, Dec. 13, 1960.

236. Today's Horizon in Health. 16 mm., sound, 23 min., New York, N.Y., Young Drug Prod. Corp.

237. Tompkins, P.: The use of basal temperature graphs in determining the date of ovulation. J.A.M.A., *124*:698, 1944.

238. Towle, R. L.: New horizons in mass inoculation. Public Health Rep., *75*:471, 1960.

239. Ulrich, E. W.: Pressure-sensitive adhesive sheet material. U.S. Patent 2,884,126, issued April 28, 1959, assigned to 3M Co.

240. United States Pharmacopeia. 17th Revision. pp. 58, 59, 150, 260, 263, 696, 778. Easton, Mack, 1965.

241. Van Itallie, P. H.: No one man invented the hypodermic syringe. Pulse of Pharm., *19*:6, 1965.

242. Warren, J., Ziherl, F. A., Kish, A. W., and Ziherl, L. A.: Large-scale administration of vaccines by means of an automatic jet injection syringe. J.A.M.A., *157*:633, 1955.

243. Weller, C., and Linder, M.: Jet injection of insulin vs. the syringe-and-needle method. J.A.M.A., *195*:844, 1966.

244. Winter, C., and Roehm, M. M.: Sawyer's Nursing Care of Patients with Urologic Diseases. ed. 2. pp. 55, 72, 75, 77, 80, 130-135. St. Louis, C. V. Mosby, 1968.

245. Winter, G. D.: Note on wound healing under dressings with special reference to perforated film dressings. J. Invest. Derm., *45*:299, 1965.

246. Wolfson, J. J.: Rectal perforation in infant by thermometer. Am. J. Dis. Child., *111*:197, 1966.

247. Wollmann, H., and Dripps, R. D.: *In*: Goodman L., and Gilman, A.: The Pharmacological Basis of Therapeutics. ed. 3. pp. 893-914. New York, Macmillan, 1965.

248. Wright, E. S., and Mundy, R. A.: Studies on disinfection of clinical thermometers. 1, 2. Appl. Microbiol., *6*:381, 1958; *9*:508, 1961.

249. Yunis, E. J., and Landes, R. R.: Hazards of glove powder in renal angiography. J.A.M.A., *193*:304, 1965.

Chapter 14

Hospital Pharmacy

Victor A. Yanchick, Ph.D., Assistant Professor of Pharmacy,
University of Texas College of Pharmacy, and
George F. Archambault, Ph.C., LL.B., LL.D., Sc.D., Pharm.D.

OBJECTIVES

This chapter is intended to provide a broad introduction to the practice of pharmacy in hospitals. In general, it follows the proposed syllabus for a course in hospital pharmacy administration as presented by the special Committee on Education of the American Society of Hospital Pharmacists. Although many aspects of hospital pharmacy practice resemble the general practice of pharmacy, there are many unique administrative functions and procedures found in hospitals that merit special study.

In general, three objectives have been proposed for this section on hospital pharmacy:

1. To acquaint the individual with the basic concepts of the practice of hospital pharmacy administration;

2. To familiarize the individual with the responsibilities, functions and scope of the practice of hospital pharmacy and

3. To explore the areas in which pharmacists may relate effectively with other members of the health professions to provide efficient and sound health care to all patients.

INTRODUCTION

The providing of pharmaceutical services in hospitals is emerging as one of the most dynamic and challenging areas within the profession of pharmacy. Today, nearly 10,000 pharmacists are employed in hospitals and, as the shift of total health services swings more and more to institutional practice, it is estimated that an additional 10,000 pharmacists will be needed by 1980.

The trend in institutional growth is reflected in a recent survey by the American Hospital Association which reveals that there were 7,137 hospitals registered in 1968. These institutions had 1,663,203 beds, admitted 29,765,683 inpatients and spent over 19 billion dollars to provide services at the inpatient and outpatient levels. Thus, in 1968 there was one admission for every seven citizens in the United States. Also reported in this survey was the fact that approximately 29 per cent of these hospitals did not offer the services or facility of a pharmacy department. This figure may be misleading, since well over 95 per cent of all hospitals with over 100-bed capacity did offer some type of pharmacy service. A good idea of the rapid improvements that have been made in the providing of hospital pharmacy services can be made by comparing the 29 per cent figure for 1968 with the 1956 statistics, in which 45.8 per cent of all hospitals were reported as not having a functioning pharmacy department.

Hospital pharmacy practice traditionally involves the supplying of medications for inpatient and outpatient use, the preparing of sterile medications, bulk compounding, prepackaging, drug formulation, research, and serving as the focal point in the dissemination of information relating to drug therapy to the entire hospital staff. Additionally, the pharmacist is now beginning to utilize his professional judgement and expertise not only within his department but also in previously unexplored areas such as the nursing station, the medical laboratory and at the patient's bedside. These emerging new roles as a vital member of the health care team not only allow the pharmacist to utilize his knowledge of drugs to the highest degree but also makes clear the importance of sound pharmacy service to the total care of the patient.

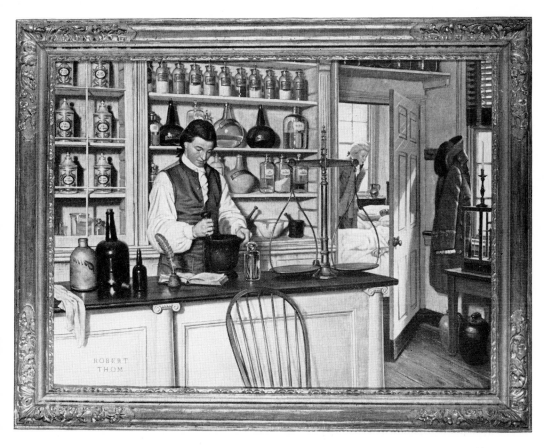

FIG. 14-1. Picturization of the first hospital pharmacy in Colonial America (c. 1755).
(Copyright, 1954, Parke, Davis and Co.)

HISTORY

The separation of pharmacy from medicine first took place in the early charity institutions engaged in caring for the sick and the injured. History records the fact that pharmacies were important segments of hospital activities as long ago as the 4th century, this era, at a time when hospitals were part of many of the monasteries. After the plague in the 14th century, the separation of pharmacy from medicine became an established fact, and hospitals of that era are reported to have had well-equipped pharmaceutical services.

The first hospital pharmacist in colonial America is believed to have been Jonathan Roberts, pharmacist of the Pennsylvania Hospital in Philadelphia (1752) (Fig. 14-1).

Benjamin Franklin, who aided in the establishment of this hospital, wrote:

The practitioners charitably supplied the medicine gratis till December, 1752, when the managers, having procured an assortment of drugs from London, opened an apothecary's shop in the hospital, and it being found necessary, appointed an apothecary to attend and make up the medicines daily, according to the prescription, with an allowance of fifteen pounds per annum for his care and trouble, he giving bond, with two sufficient sureties, for the faithful performance of his trust.

Prior to 1920, for a period of approximately 170 years, the recorded history of hospital pharmacy in the United States is quite brief. The majority of pharmacists engaged in this specialty of the profession reported little in the literature and received little recorded recognition from American pharmacy.

Not until the American College of Surgeons began its hospital standardization program in 1918 was there any notable change in this apathy.

Starting in the early twenties and continuing strongly thereafter, hospital pharmacy began to attract attention as an important element in hospital patient care.

AMERICAN SOCIETY OF HOSPITAL PHARMACISTS

The national society for hospital pharmacists was founded in 1942 and incorporated in 1955. The society, an affiliate of the American Pharmaceutical Association, is devoted to the profession of hospital pharmacy and dedicated to the improvement of pharmaceutical service in the interest of better patient care in hospitals. Over 6,000 hospital-pharmacy practitioners hold membership in this organization, many belonging to one of the 73 regional or state and local chapters. The journal of the society, American Journal of Hospital Pharmacy, is well known internationally in hospital and pharmaceutical circles.

The objectives of the American Society of Hospital Pharmacists as stated in the constitution and bylaws (1969 revision) are:

The objectives of the Society shall be: (1) to provide the benefits and protection of a qualified hospital pharmacist to the patient, to the institution which he serves, to the members of the allied health professions with whom he is associated, and to the profession of pharmacy; (2) to assist in providing an adequate supply of such qualified hospital pharmacists; (3) to assure a high quality of professional practice through the establishment and maintenance of standards of professional ethics and education; (4) to promote research in hospital pharmacy practices and in the pharmaceutical sciences in general; (5) to disseminate pharmaceutical knowledge by providing for interchange of information among hospital pharmacists and members of allied specialties and professions.

RESPONSIBILITIES AND DUTIES OF THE HOSPITAL PHARMACIST

The responsibilities of the Director of Pharmacy Service are set forth clearly in the Minimum Standard for Pharmacies in Hospitals of the American Society of Hospital Pharmacists as amended November 8, 1962. These duties are stated to be as follows:

(a) The preparation and sterilization of injectable medications when manufactured in the hospital; (b) the manufacturing of pharmaceuticals; (c) the dispensing of drugs, chemicals, and pharmaceutical preparations; (d) the filling and labeling of all drug containers issued to services from which medication is to be administered; (e) necessary inspection of all pharmaceutical supplies on all services and at nursing medication stations; (f) the maintenance of an approved stock of antidotes and other emergency drugs; (g) the dispensing of all narcotics, hypnotics, and alcohol and the maintenance of a perpetual inventory of them; (h) the development of specifications both as to quality and source for the purchase of all drugs, chemicals, antibiotics, biologicals, and pharmaceutical preparations used in the treatment of patients; (i) furnishing information concerning medications to physicians; interns and nurses; (j) the establishment and maintenance, in cooperation with the accounting department, of a satisfactory system of records and boookkeeping in accordance with the policies of the hospital for: (1) charging patients for drugs and pharmaceutical supplies, and (2) maintaining adequate control over the requisitioning and dispensing of all drugs and pharmaceutical supplies; (k) the planning, organizing, and directing pharmacy policies and procedures in accordance with the established policies of the hospital; (l) the maintenance of the facilities of the department; (m) cooperation in teaching courses to students in the school of nursing and in the medical and dental intern training programs; (n) implementing the decisions of the Pharmacy and Therapeutics committee and serving as secretary to the committee; and (o) the preparation of periodic reports on the progress of the department for submission to the administrator of the hospital.

To the Administration. Directly or indirectly, these responsibilities and functions are aimed to provide the best in pharmaceutical service for the patient at the most economical cost. Not only is it the duty of the hospital pharmacist to provide good pharmaceutical service to the patient, it is also his responsibility to operate the pharmacy department efficiently and economically. This the competent pharmacist does by providing quality medications and services at the most favorable prevailing prices.

To the Clinicians. It is often said that the hospital pharmacist is the drug-therapy consultant to the staff; this is one of his prime responsibilities. As an integral part of the system for drug utilization in health care, the hospital pharmacist is well acquainted with the increasingly complex problems of pharmacotherapy, the biomedical community's difficulty in trying to cope with an overwhelming drug literature, and the limitations of existing drug experience surveillance systems for assessing efficacy and safety of investigational as well as newly marketed drugs. Recognizing the implications for professional responsibility in this situation, many hospital pharmacists are exploring new service roles through which they can contribute more effectively to the resolution of these patient care problems. Drug information programs and centers are being developed in this regard and are being utilized not only by clinicians but by virtually all members of the health sciences.

To the Nursing Profession and Other Members of the Health Care Team.   The hospital pharmacist has professional responsibilities to the nurse, the dietitian, the laboratory technologist, the X-ray technician and the medical record librarian. In his periodic inspections of the nursing medication stations, he should be alert to prevent labeling and packaging by nursing personnel; detect outdated biologicals, antibiotics and other dated medications; spot excess and obsolete stocks as well as check on narcotic and hypnotic violations. The pharmacist can also assist the nurse and physician by identifying all drugs brought to the hospital by the patient. He should also provide written policies and procedures to the nurse for securing drugs from the pharmacy when not covered by the pharmacist and help nursing service design unit drug stations for efficient administration and storage of all drugs. The hospital pharmacist fulfills his teaching responsibilities by periodic lectures to hospital personnel on timely information on drugs, posology and toxicology. It is strongly urged that all pharmacists assume complete control over the preparation of all antibiotic solutions and suspensions, surgical fluids and the preparation and control of parenteral fluids and admixtures.

The pharmacist's responsibilities to the dietetic department lies in his knowledge of vitamins, essential and non-essential amino acids, minerals and other food supplements. Current research has documented many serious and sometimes fatal reactions with certain drugs and the diet. Also, his skill in the preparation of elegant flavoring extracts for patient consumption can be utilized very effectively.

The laboratory department may benefit from the pharmacist's knowledge of drug-induced modifications of laboratory test values. These interactions are being recognized as quite significant in providing explanations for many abnormal test results. Also, the pharmacist may assist the technologist in the compounding of stock solutions and buffers used in routine laboratory analysis.

The pharmacist can assist the X-ray department in the proper storage and distribution of radioisotopes and diagnostic agents. The pharmacist may also utilize his talents in the preparation of palatable and more elegant preparations for use in certain X-ray examinations.

To the medical record librarian, as well as to all members of the health care team, the pharmacist has the responsibility to teach, among other things, scientific drug nomenclature and generic names of drugs, as well as of being the main source of reference on all aspects of drug use.

To the Department.   To the pharmacy itself, the hospital pharmacist is responsible, of course, for adequate inventories of quality drugs; the periodic inspection of equipment and its maintenance; the general appearance of the department; the standardization of medication containers for pharmacy and nursing-station dispensing units; and the giving of prompt, efficient service.

Also, under this brief discussion of responsibilities should be mentioned the necessity for adopting a policy relative to interviewing "detail men," the professional service pharmacists of the drug manufacturers (see under Pharmacy and Therapeutics Committee, p. 572, for details).

ORGANIZATION AND POLICIES

The statements in the Minimum Standard for Pharmacies in Hospitals on this subject read:

Organization. There shall be a properly organized pharmacy department under the direction of a professionally competent, legally qualified pharmacist whose training in hospital pharmacy conforms to the standards herein established by the American Society of Hospital Pharmacists.

Policies. The Director of Pharmacy Service, with the approval and cooperation of the director of the hospital, shall initiate and develop rules and regulations pertaining to the administrative policies of the department. The pharmacist in charge, with the approval and cooperation of the Pharmacy and Therapeutics Committee, shall initiate and develop rules and regulations pertaining to the professional policies of the department.

ORGANIZATIONAL CHARTS AND HOSPITAL PHARMACEUTICAL SERVICE

The organizational charts reproduced in Figures 14-2 and 14-3 illustrate sound organizational and administrative principles. Each hospital pharmacy should have organizational charts indicating its activities, responsibilities and relationship to the other departments in the hospital.

POLICY STATEMENT

A hospital pharmacy should have a definite statement of policy of objective by which it may be evaluated administratively. Obviously, the objective statement of each institution must be tailored to its individual needs, depending on whether the hospital is large or small, teaching or nonteaching, research or nonresearch.

*Sample Outline of Policy or Objective Statement**

In the development and conduct of the Pharmacy Service (Department) of . . . . Hospital, it shall be the primary purpose of the Sisters of . . . ., their associates and assistants in this department, to render efficient professional service motivated at all times by

* Prepared by Mr. Ray Kneifl, Sister Mary Berenice and associates, Catholic Hospital Association, Institute on Hospital Pharmacy, July, 1952.

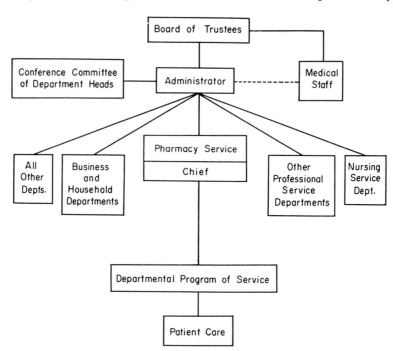

FIG. 14-2. The pharmacy service in relation to the administrator and to all other departmental services of the "X" Hospital. (Developed by Mr. Ray Kneifl, Sister Mary Berenice and others for the Catholic Hospital Association in connection with the Point-Rating Plan for Hospital Pharmacy Service in the *Bulletin* of the American Society of Hospital Pharmacists, *9*: No. 4)

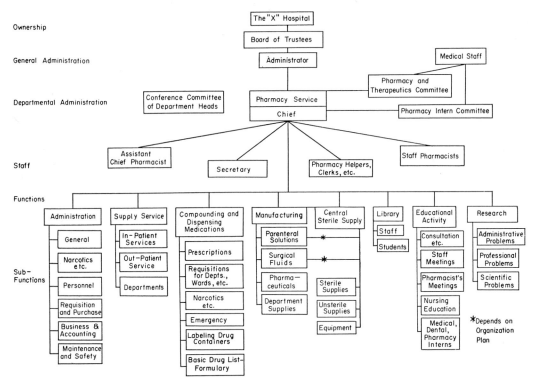

FIG. 14-3. Organization chart of the pharmacy. (Developed by Mr. Ray Kneifl, Sister Mary Berenice and others for the Catholic Hospital Association in connection with the Point-Rating Plan for Hospital Pharmacy Service in the *Bulletin* of the American Society of Hospital Pharmacists, *9*: No. 4)

Christian charity to in- and out-patients of all economic levels; to this end, the chief pharmacist and staff pharmacists will cooperate wholeheartedly with medical staff members, and especially with the Pharmacy and Therapeutics Committee, in the development of sound policies governing this service. The program of service shall include . . . .
. . . .

To achieve the desired measure of efficiency throughout the hospital, this department will at all times cooperate with other special departments in . . . . Hospital harmoniously and effectively to assure continuity of service to patients, providing the educational guidance and materials relating to scientific advances in drug therapy for other professional groups as well as for pharmacists. The Pharmacist will cooperate with the Director of the School of Nursing in her teaching program for student nurses.

In realizing this goal, the administrator of the hospital and the chief pharmacist are guided by the "Minimum Standard for Hospital Phar-

macies" of the American Society of Hospital Pharmacists in the organization, staffing, equipment and administration of the pharmacy. In complying with the Standard, the Pharmacy Service of . . . . Hospital attempts to qualify for recognition by appropriate accrediting agencies in Medical, Pharmacy and hospital fields as providing a service of professional quality adequate to safeguard the health of the people.

(Paragraphs may be added or developed for special services (functions) if desired.)

PHARMACY AND THERAPEUTICS COMMITTEE

The Minimum Standard for Pharmacies in Hospitals in reference to the Pharmacy and Therapeutics Committee states:

Pharmacy and Therapeutics Committee. There shall be a Pharmacy and Therapeutics Committee, which shall hold at least two regular meetings annually and such additional meetings as may be required. The members of the committee shall be chosen from the several divisions of the medical staff. *The Director of Pharmacy Service shall be a member of the committee and shall serve as its secretary.* He shall keep a transcript of proceedings and shall forward a copy to the proper governing authority of the hospital. The *purpose* of the committee shall be (A) to develop a formulary of accepted drugs for use in the hospital, (B) to serve as an advisory group to the hospital pharmacist on matters pertaining to the choice of drugs to be stocked, (C) to evaluate clinical data concerning drugs requested for use in the hospital, (D) to add to and to delete from the list of drugs accepted for use in the hospital, (E) to prevent unnecessary duplication in the stock of the same basic drug and its preparations and (F) to make recommendations concerning drugs to be stocked on the nursing units and other services.

To this role, another important item has been added recently—the periodic review of patient's charts for inconsistencies in medication orders, possible adverse drug reactions, therapeutic incompatibilities and medication errors, with report on findings made at least once annually at staff meetings. Names of patients and physicians are, of course, not revealed.

The role of the chief pharmacist on this committee, as its recorder or secretary and as one of its voting members, is an important one. Among the more important functions are:

1. Maintenance of an adequate, up-to-date library and a drug-therapy reference file for the use of the committee and the staff

2. Interviewing and screening of professional medical representatives ("detail men") of pharmaceutical firms, and arranging for departmental interviews with them when indicated. This is an important function of the secretary inasmuch as it keeps him informed of the latest drug-therapy agents being detailed by the pharmaceutical firms to physicians on the staff, either at the hospital or in their offices. This function is administratively valuable to the hospital in that it conserves the time of staff members without the loss of the valuable information that the detail representatives have for members of the various services.

Arranging with the detail representative for the presentation of exhibits to the staff at optimum times. At such meetings, the detail representative of a pharmaceutical firm has the opportunity to discuss the pharmacology, the biochemistry, the microbiology or the pharmacy of his product with all interested staff members.

3.(a) Prompt preparation and dissemination of accurate minutes of committee activities. This responsibility cannot be emphasized too strongly. The proper custody of the minutes is equally important. The surveyor for the Joint Commission on Accreditation of Hospitals may ask to inspect the record of pharmacy committee meetings. In evaluating the hospital pharmacy, the inspector considers the recorded activities of the pharmacy committee as well as the hospital formulary.

(b) Seeing that the minutes of the committee and the format of the formulary are more than a mere recording of decisions to add and delete drugs and a list of drugs currently stocked. The minutes should contain the pharmacologic basis for a drug's selection or rejection. The formulary should contain a format on each drug consisting of its generic or official name, all important trade names, its identifying characteristics, actions, contraindications, side effects, toxicology, posology, size and strengths available.

4. Preparation of the agenda for each meeting after approval by the chairman and releasing it to committee members sufficiently in advance of the meeting to allow time for intelligent preparation

5. Editing of the formulary (after review by all pharmacy committee members and final review and approval by the medical and the dental staffs), as well as maintaining custody of and issuance of formulary and supplements to medical staff members, residents, interns and other authorized personnel such as nurses and medical-record librarians.

6. Encouraging of individual staff members to present requests for drugs to the committee, and assisting of staff members to collect proper and adequate information to cover the request (see Fig. 14-4).

7. Serving as a drug-therapy consultant to the staff, especially the residents, the interns and the nurses. These services usually are given in private conferences, but much value is obtained from formal lectures to medical and dental interns and the nursing staff.

Also, as a voting member on this committee, the pharmacist must:

PHS. 1689
REV. 6-55
REQUEST FOR NON-BASIC DRUG

HOSPITAL OR CLINIC	DATE

TO: PHARMACY COMMITTEE through Chief Pharmacist

NAME OF DRUG

NAME OF MANUFACTURER

DOSAGE FORM WANTED (Check one)

☐ TABLET   ☐ CAPSULE   ☐ LIQUID   ☐ OINTMENT   ☐ POWDER

☐ AMPULE   ☐ OTHER (Specify)_____

MINIMUM SUPPLY REQUESTED   ☐ ROUTINE   ☐ EMERGENCY

NAME OF PATIENT OR SERVICE FOR WHOM DRUG IS REQUIRED

DESCRIBE PHARMACOLOGICAL ACTION NEEDED

IS THERE A SIMILAR-ACTING DRUG STOCKED IN THE PHARMACY WHICH MAY BE USED?

☐ NO   ☐ YES (If "YES," what advantage does this drug have?)

REMARKS

SIGNATURE OF MEDICAL OR DENTAL OFFICER REQUESTING   SIGNATURE OF CHIEF OF SERVICE
APPROVED:

PHARMACEUTICAL SERVICE REPORT ON DRUG

AVAILABILITY OF DRUG	INDICATE IF DRUG REQUESTED IS RECOGNIZED BY U.S.P., N.F., N.N.D., OR A.D.R.
COST OF DRUG	COST OF SIMILAR-ACTING ITEM STOCKED

REMARKS

SIGNATURE OF CHIEF, PHARMACEUTICAL SERVICE	DATE

PHARMACY COMMITTEE REPORT

DRUG ☐ APPROVED   ☐ REJECTED

REASONS

PHARMACY COMMITTEE RECORDER (Signature)	DATE

FIG. 14-4. Request for nonbasic drug to pharmacy commtitee through the chief pharmacist. (U.S.P.H.S.)

1. Prepare himself by sufficient study to intelligently discuss and participate in making decisions on the subjects placed on the agenda for consideration.

2. Attend all meetings regularly and promptly.

3. Place the medical needs of the patients and the hospital above his personal scientific interests and desires in making recommendations and decisions.

4. Disseminate the committee's thinking and aims among his colleagues as well as bring his colleagues' problems and suggestions to the attention of the committee.

5. Stress the use of generic and official names when working with the staff or the teaching residents, the interns, the nurses and the medical-record librarians.

6. Favor the policy of using "double-blind tests" in controversial areas. In other words, drugs to be studied should be so labeled that only the chairman and the secretary of the committee know the exact identity of a drug until the committee has had time to evaluate all the clinical and pharmacologic evidence presented to it.

7. Keep himself appraised not only of the pharmacologic merits of drugs but also of their comparative costs in relation to their efficacy.

8. Weigh his decisions not only in the light of providing the best drug therapy for patients but also of preventing needless and wasteful duplication in the same class of drugs.

9. Work for the establishment of meaningful drug terminology. Discourage unsafe practices in drug identification such as the use of synonyms, codes, numbers or letters, and the use of trade names without knowledge of the generic or the official name; also promote and advocate the use of the metric system in ward prescribing, nursing station medication labeling and formularies.

10. Advocate and work for the establishment of *Restricted Drug Lists*. Because of their complex action, potency and toxicity, certain modern-day drugs, in the interest of better patient care, should be restricted to use by those staff members with special competency in their administration.

THE HOSPITAL FORMULARY

A formulary has the following purposes and goals:

1. To provide the patient with the best possible drug therapy

2. To provide the physician and the dentist with carefully selected agents of proved effectiveness, which will be a basis for flexible drug therapy

3. To provide a standard of comparison for the evaluation of new therapeutic agents

4. To provide the physician, the dentist, the pharmacist and the nurse with a ready reference on the essential pharmacology of the basic drugs

5. To provide for simplification of all drug-therapy record keeping

Pharmacy and therapeutic committees are now in operation in many of the nation's hospitals. These committees have individually developed criteria for the evaluation of drugs. Essentially, these criteria all aim at selecting for the formularies of the hospitals the best among approximately 2,500 available drug-therapy agents. Criteria used by many committees are as follows:

1. The therapeutic efficacy of the drug should be well established.

2. Quality of all drugs should not be compromised for economic considerations. When applicable, such products should meet the standards of quality of the *U.S.P.* or *N.F.*

3. Unnecessary duplication of action should be avoided.

4. Drugs of secret composition should be rejected.

5. Unless they provide a real advantage in combination form, mixtures of drugs should be avoided.

Formularies should be revised periodically or be loose-leaf manuals that can be kept up-to-date by sheet replacements. The use of the formulary system should never be so restrictive as to prevent the physician from obtaining any desired drug in an emergency. The use of the formulary system has many advantages. Foremost, of course, is the bringing to the patient those drug-therapy agents considered by the committee to be the best available. Other advantages are reduction in inventories and in the number of orders processed. This is brought about by the elimination of many duplications in basic drugs. The formulary is a valuable reference for the staff, especially the busy intern and resident, as to the drugs stocked by the pharmacy, their preparations, strengths, forms, dosage and dispensing sizes.

It cannot be stated too strongly that the formulary of a hospital and the use of the formulary system is a medical staff responsibility and not a function or a responsibility of the hospital administrator or pharmacist. These individuals implement the system and the decisions of the Pharmacy Committee as ratified by the medical staff as a whole. Further, "current" or "present" consent of the prescriber is involved in the dispensing of a nonproprietary medication irrespective of whether it is or is not of the same brand referred to in the prescription or medication order. For the legal protection of the pharmacist and the hospital, all medication containers dispensed under the formulary system should carry the strip label approved by the American Hospital Association and the American Society of Hospital Pharmacists and reproduced below.

> Note for information of staff: Contents may be used,—per formulary policy, to fill prescriptions or orders for any of the following brands of the same basic drug.

Further, prescription order forms and patient progress or medication charts should carry the following footnote: "☐ Authorization is given for dispensing by nonproprietary name unless checked here."

It must be borne in mind by hospital pharmacists and administrators, relative to the Formulary System Concept, that this is an accepted and approved method whereby the *medical staff* of a hospital, working through a Pharmacy and Therapeutics Committee *selected by it,* evaluates, appraises and selects from among the various medicinal agents available those that are considered to be most useful in patient care, together with the pharmaceutical preparations in which they may be administered most effectively.

FIVE-POINT STATEMENT OF OPERATION FOR THE HOSPITAL FORMULARY SYSTEM

(Adopted January 10, 1964 by the American Society of Hospital Pharmacists, the American Pharmaceutical Association, the American Hospital Association and the American Medical Association.)

To promote the adoption of a Formulary System by the hospital medical staff with the understanding that the administration of such a program will:

1. Be initiated and operated within the individual hospital through regulations promulgated by its medical staff

2. Insure the maintenance of the responsibility and prerogatives of the physician in the exercise of his professional judgment

3. Provide for final determination by physicians and pharmacists of medications to be included in the formulary

4. Authorize the physician to prescribe medications not included in the formulary if in his judgment individual patients require special treatment and

5. Permit the physician, at the time of prescribing medications, to approve or disapprove the dispensing or administration of medications in accordance with the Hospital Formulary System.

PERSONNEL

Again referring to the Minimum Standard, it is noted:

Personnel. The Director of Pharmacy Service shall be well trained in the specialized functions of hospital pharmacy and shall be a graduate of an accredited college of pharmacy or meet an equivalent standard of training and experience as set forth in the supplement to these standards. He shall have such assistants as the volume of work in the pharmacy may dictate. These assistants shall include an adequate number of additional licensed pharmacists and such other personnel as the activities of the pharmacy may require to supply pharmaceutical service of the highest quality. All members of the staff of the pharmacy shall be competent, of good moral character and mentally and physically fit to perform their duties acceptably.

Specifically, the properly qualified hospital pharmacist should be well versed in his knowledge of medications and their actions including side effects and contraindications; he should have the ability to develop and conduct a pharmaceutical bulk-compounding program; he should have intimate knowledge of control procedures including technics to ensure quality control and distribution control. He also must have the ability to conduct and participate in research, teaching and in-service training programs. Finally, he must have the ability to administer and manage a pharmacy service in a hospital that devotes itself to patient care, research and teaching.

Proper manpower in terms of quantity and quality is necessary in operating any type of service. Sound personnel practice requires that the personnel office recruit for specific vacancies, screen out those applicants who manifestly do not meet the requirements of the proposed position, and refer, when available, no less than 3 qualified applicants to the chief pharmacist for interview, discussion of the work and final selection. In referring these applicants, it should be the responsibility of the personnel office of the hospital to make whatever pertinent recommendations may be indicated to guide the pharmacist in making his selection. The chief pharmacist makes the final selection based on such factors as ability of the candidate to work with the present personnel and his degree of efficiency. This is usually standard procedure for interviewing of hospital pharmacy personnel. Obviously, proof of licensure should be demanded. Further, references concerning the professional and moral character of the applicant should be made only of individuals who have *current* knowledge of the subject.

USE OF NONPROFESSIONAL PERSONNEL

Nonprofessional personnel (pharmacy helpers) should be utilized wherever possible, but never in activities requiring the skills or the knowledge of a pharmacist. Many activities, such as the collection and the delivery of nursing station pharmacy baskets, stock checking, storeroom arrangements, perpetual-inventory record keeping, dusting and cleaning, and prepackaging (under direct and immediate supervision) may be allocated properly to helpers. Floor collection and delivery of baskets should be on a definite schedule. Some hospitals find, on experimentation, that Monday, Wednesday and Friday "basket days" serve the hospital adequately and allow the remaining days of the week for bulk-compounding, prepackaging and other pharmaceutical or administrative activities.

PHYSICAL FACILITIES

Facilities. Adequate pharmaceutical and administrative facilities shall be provided for the pharmacy department, including especially: (A) the necessary equipment for the compounding, dispensing and manufacturing of pharmaceuticals and parenteral preparations, (B) bookkeeping supplies and related materials and equipment necessary for the proper administration of the department, (C) an adequate library and filing equipment to make information concerning drugs readily available to both pharmacists and physicians, (D) special locked storage space to meet the legal requirements for storage of narcotics, alcohol and other prescribed drugs, (E) a refrigerator for the storage of thermolabile products, (F) adequate floor space for all pharmacy operations and the storage of pharmaceuticals at a satisfactory location provided with proper lighting and ventilation.*

THE COMPLETE DEPARTMENT

The current concept of a complete hospital pharmacy department consists of the following areas: (1) a waiting area, (2) an office for the Chief of Service, (3) the outpatient dispensing unit, (4) the manufacturing or bulk-compounding unit, (5) the sterile preparations unit with facilities for an IV-additive service, (6) the "in-house," ward basket and prepackaging units, (7) the pharmacy storeroom, (8) the research, analysis and control unit, (9) the special technics area, (10) the alcohol and volatile liquid area, (11) the narcotic vaults, (12) the allergy preparation unit, (13) a radioactive isotope dispensing unit, (14) the central sterile supply area and (15) a "cold" storage room with a regulated temperature range of 12° C. to 15° C. Items 1, 2, 5, 8, 12, 13, 14 and 15 depend on the size of the institution and the need and the desirability for inclusion.

When one considers the progress made in patient care since 1945 and the facilities needed to give this modern care, one recognizes the dire need for expansion space for many of the old-line hospital departments. Until recently, pharmacies, by and large, were "drug or dispensing rooms," located in the basement or some other out-of-the-way

* From "Minimum Standard for Pharmacies in Hospitals," with guide to application, as amended November 8, 1962.

place in the hospital. Today, because of its many and varied activities, the department is considered a "service," not unlike the outpatient, the dietetic, the radiology or the nursing service. The pharmacy may have several subdepartments such as outpatient, pharmacy proper for house issues, manufacturing, prepackaging, bulk-pharmacy storage, drug-security vault; research, control and analysis area, parenteral and surgical fluid area, special technics area, allergy department, and, more and more of late, central sterile supply, an IV additives area, and, in some instances, a radioisotope prescription dispensing unit. These subdepartments all demand certain minimum square footage for their proper functioning. Furthermore, where patients present themselves to the pharmacy for prescriptions, the department must be no less presentable than other patient areas, and must be located functionally. Today, hospital administrators favor the concept that a pharmaceutical service should be located in a central place on the first floor, adjacent to outpatient activities and elevator facilities—in other words located functionally in relationship to "traffic flows."

LAWS AND REGULATIONS

Space does not permit a discussion of the laws and the codes applicable to hospitals and hospital pharmacy. The hospital pharmacist should be familiar with Federal, state and local laws as well as the common law as they apply to the charitable trust doctrine—present legal trend; the hiring of hospital pharmacists; the degree of skill and care required of the hospital pharmacist; the state hospital licensing acts and regulations; the legal aspects of P.R.N. orders; the liability of the hospital for acts of the pharmacist; the law concerning the compounding and the manufacturing of pharmaceutical preparations covered by patent rights; prescriptions as privileged communications; the statute of limitation on suits for negligence; the laws on substitution and duplication; the fire and safety codes and regulations; the fair trade laws; the Federal Caustic Poison Act; the Federal Insecticide Act; the Federal Food and Drug Laws; the Therapeutics Trials Committee (the Research Committee of the Council on Pharmacy and Chemistry) of the American Medical Association guide lines on procedures for the clinical testing of investigational drugs; Federal laws and regulations relative to industrial alcohol, tax-free and tax-paid (Regulation No. 3); registration of stills; the Federal Harrison Narcotic Act (Regulation No. 5); and state and local pharmacy and hospital laws and regulations. The hospital-pharmacy aspects of these laws are to be found in hospital and pharmaceutical jurisprudence texts (see Bibliography) and Journals. This chapter discusses the highlights of the major Federal laws.

NARCOTIC AND OTHER RECORDS IN HOSPITALS

One of the more important legal responsibilities of the hospital pharmacist is that of supervision and control of *narcotics, hypnotics, ethyl alcohol and spirituous liquors* in the hospital. Several systems have been developed to provide sound internal checks on these items. The system in use in the hospitals of the U.S. Public Health Service throughout the country is presented (in form manner) as one method of handling this activity. The 8 forms are numbered to show the flow of the controlled drug from the time of arrival at the hospital to their actual administration to the patient or the release of the drug to an outpatient.

One should note in particular that this type of control system provides "checks" hospitalwise as well as pharmacy-wise. This is essential in hospital narcotic control. The chief pharmacist who does not protect his hospital by assuming responsibility for this item from the time of its arrival at the hospital to the time of consumption or release to the patient is not fulfilling his duty in this area. It is of special importance that security controls be in operation that check transfers of supplies from the pharmacy through the nursing medication stations. In the system illustrated, the pharmacist prepares these audits monthly and ascertains the status of all outstanding certificates of disposition (Fig. 14-8: Form 1435-2, No. 4).

HARRISON NARCOTIC ACT

Registration. Hospitals are registered in class 4 (authority to *administer* narcotics);

classes 4 and 5 (class 5 gives authority to *deal* in *"exempt"* narcotics); or classes 3, 4 and 5 (class 3 is for retail dealers and is used for hospitals dispensing narcotic prescriptions to outpatients). Physicians attached to a hospital may not use the narcotic registration number of the hospital, the so-called narcotic number, to write prescriptions or orders for an individual patient.

Practitioners who prescribe narcotics for, or order narcotics dispensed to, patients in a hospital must be entitled under the laws of the state, the territory or the district (Medical Practice Act) to prescribe or order dispensed narcotic drugs and must be registered with the Director of Internal Revenue for this purpose.

Interns, residents and medical officers who

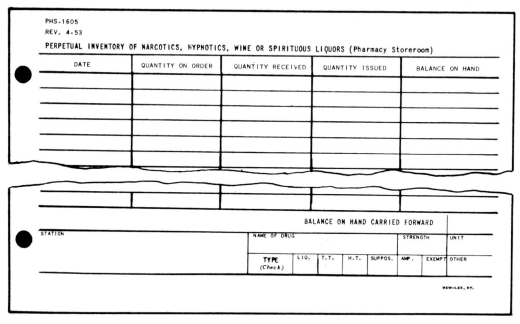

FIGURE 14-5

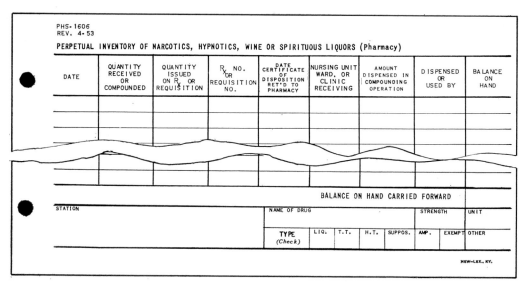

FIGURE 14-6

are attending patients in hospitals, *if entitled under the State, Territorial or District Medical Practice Act* to prescribe or dispense narcotic drugs to patients *in the hospital,* may obtain the requisite registration from the Treasury Department, Director of Internal Revenue, to complete their qualifications to write prescriptions for, or order narcotics dispensed to, hospital patients in the course of their professional practice. However, this authority is limited to the patients assigned to the intern, resident or medical officer, *and no others.*

Usually, the State, Territorial or District Medical Practice Act sets forth the requirements for the professional right to prescribe and dispense narcotic drugs. The licensed physician, dentist or veterinarian in good standing has this right. However, there may be a question as to whether an intern or a resident has such a right, even as limited to hospital patients, unless the Medical Practice Act or other statute confers this authority. If it is determined authoritatively that the intern has such a legal right limited to hospital patients, he may apply for a registration

Fig. 14-7. (U.S.P.H.S.)

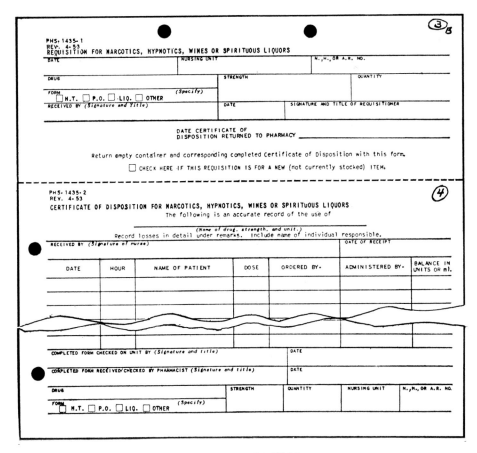

Fig. 14-8. (U.S.P.H.S.)

under the Federal Narcotic Act. This is a matter which must be determined in each state. Some authorities on this subject believe that the laws of most states do not authorize the intern to prescribe for, or dispense narcotic drugs to, a patient on his own independent professional judgment. In such instances, the intern cannot be authorized to prescribe narcotics by the Bureau of Narcotics because the intern is an unlicensed practitioner. In the former instance, qualified or restricted licensing gives the authority.

The administrative head of the hospital as a registrant is responsible for the proper safeguarding and handling of narcotics within the hospital. Responsibility for storage, accountability and proper dispensing of narcotics from the pharmacy usually is delegated to the pharmacist. Likewise, the director of nursing usually is responsible for the proper storage at nursing stations and use as directed by physician orders. However, delegation of authority does not relieve the administrative head of the hospital of supervisory responsibility to ensure detection and correction of any diversion or mishandling. The administrator should be certain that all possible internal control measures are observed.

A doctor's narcotic orders for patients normally appear on the doctor's order sheets; no prescription is required. The nursing floor stock used in administering narcotics is ac-

EIGHT (8) HOUR NURSE AUDIT RECORD

(5)

(Losses and Extended Disposition Record should also be noted. Attach another Form (PHS-1435-2) should more space be needed)

DATE	TIME	SIGNATURE ON-COMING NURSE	INITIALS OFF-GOING NURSE	DATE	TIME	SIGNATURE ON-COMING NURSE	INITIALS OFF-GOING NURSE	DATE	TIME	SIGNATURE ON-COMING NURSE	INITIALS OFF-GOING, NURSE

REMARKS

(Signature)

GPO 83-49497

FIG. 14-9. (U.S.P.H.S.)

(6)

PHS-1435-3
6-53

EMERGENCY TRANSFER OF NARCOTICS, HYPNOTICS, WINES OR SPIRITUOUS LIQUORS

INSTRUCTIONS: *(EMERGENCY USE ONLY during hours Pharmaceutical Service is not available)*. For emergency transfer of Drug and Certificate of Disposition (PHS-1435-2) between Nursing Units. Complete form in duplicate, forward original to Pharmacy and attach duplicate to Certificate of Disposition.

DATE	TIME AM PM	NURSING UNIT RECEIVING ITEM	N.H., OR A.R. NO.
DRUG		STRENGTH	QUANTITY
FORM ☐ H.T. ☐ P.O. ☐ LIQ. ☐ AMP. ☐ OTHER *(Specify)*			
TRANSFERRED BY *(Signature and Title)*		RECEIVED BY *(Signature and Title)*	

FIG. 14-10. (U.S.P.H.S.)

counted for on the narcotic Certificate of Disposition.

The doctor's full name or initials must appear on the doctor's sheet. His registry number is *not* needed.

Telephone orders are permissible only in absolute necessity. The nurse will write the order on the doctor's order sheet, stating "Telephone Order," and sign the doctor's name and her own initials. The narcotic may be administered *once*. The doctor must verify on the patient's chart within 24 hours.

Verbal orders are permitted in a bona fide emergency. They should be handled as telephone narcotic orders.

Procedure in case of waste, destruction and contamination:

1. ALIQUOT PART OF NARCOTIC SOLUTIONS USED FOR DOSE. The nurse should use the proper number of tablets or ampuls from the nursing unit stock. She should expel into the sink that portion of the narcotic solution that is not to be used. She should record the number of tablets or ampuls used and the dose given in the proper columns on the Narcotic Administration Sheet (the Certificate of Disposition).

2. PREPARED DOSE REFUSED BY PATIENT OR CANCELED BY DOCTOR. When a narcotic dose has been prepared for a patient but not used due to refusal by the patient or cancellation by the doctor, the nurse should expel the solution into the sink and record on the back of the Narcotic Administration Sheet the reason why the narcotic was not administered. (*Example:* "Discarded: Refused by patient or order canceled by Dr. A. Jones.") The head nurse of the unit should sign the statement and the director of nursing or her assistant countersign it.

3. ACCIDENTAL DESTRUCTION OF NARCOTICS. When a narcotic solution, tablet, ampul or substance is destroyed accidentally on a Nursing Unit, the person responsible should indicate the accidental loss by a check in the spaces allowed for the record on the Narcotic Administration Sheet of that narcotic. The person should write on the back of that Narcotic Administration Sheet a complete report of the accident and sign the statement. The head nurse of the unit should sign the statement when complete. Then the director of nursing or her assistant should sign the statement also.

PHS-1603
REV. 10-51   ⑦

To: Medical Officer in Charge
Through: Clinical Director

Subject: Narcotic Audit Report
        I certify that on _____ an audit of narcotic inventories was made
                          day   month   year
and the physical inventories checked against the perpetual inventory records. This audit included:

    1. A check of the prescriptions and requisitions as to authenticity and correct postings;
    2. A check as to the accuracy of the posting procedures; and
    3. An actual count of physical stocks and reconciliation with the pharmacy narcotic records.

The following discrepancies were noted; *(if none, write none)*

ITEM	OVERAGE	SHORTAGE	COMMENTS:

IT is recommended that a survey be made to determine the reason for the apparently excessive uses of: *(if none, write none)*

ITEM	WARD OR PATIENT	REMARKS:

SIGNATURE OF AUDITOR	DATE

FIG. 14-11. (U.S.P.H.S.)

4. Contaminated or Broken Hypodermic Tablets and Contaminated Narcotic Solutions. When a narcotic hypodermic tablet is contaminated or broken or a narcotic solution is contaminated, the person responsible, or the head nurse, should place the tablets, the particles or the solution in a suitable container and label them. The person responsible, or the head nurse, should indicate the contaminated narcotic by a check in the space or spaces allowed for the record on the Narcotic Administration Sheet of that narcotic. She should write on the back of the sheet a complete report of the accident and sign the statement. The head nurse should sign the statement when complete. The director of nursing or her assistant should then sign the statement. The container with the contaminated narcotic should be returned to the pharmacy. The pharmacist will receive it and note on the Narcotic Administration Sheet covering that particular narcotic that it has been returned. The hospital should return the material either by itself or with similar narcotic material at a convenient time to the Narcotic Bureau in the proper manner.

In using the above procedures, the head nurse should sign entries as a witness. In addition, a professionally responsible supervisory official should initial the entries to assure an awareness on the part of supervisory professional personnel of all matters relating to narcotics.

Procedure in case of loss and theft:

1. Discrepancies in narcotics count involving small amounts (such as single doses) should be reported to a responsible supervisory official. An investigation should be made to determine the cause of the loss. A copy of the report of investigation, signed by the responsible supervisory official, should be filed with the hospital narcotic records and appropriate action taken to prevent recurrence.

2. In cases of recurring shortages, or loss of significant quantities of narcotics (several doses), a thorough investigation should be made, making every effort to determine the reason for the shortage and the person responsible, if possible, with a complete report of the incident and findings made to the administrative authority of the hospital. Appropriate action should be taken *immediately* to prevent recurrence. A copy of the report, including any findings resulting from the local investigation, should be forwarded to the District Supervisor of the Bureau of Narcotics, in accordance with Article 194, Bureau of Narcotics Regulation No. 5.

Questions concerning interpretation of the law and regulations as they apply to hospitals should be directed to the Commissioner of Narcotics in Washington, D.C.

Questions on law and regulations violations should be directed to the local narcotic agents.

Two significant changes involving hospitals and related institutions took place during 1968 in connection with the control of narcotics and drugs of abuse. Institutional registrants of classes 3 and 4 are now permitted to order narcotics on a single form and to use a single file system and physical inventory. Previously, separate records, inventories and orders had to be maintained for both inpatient and outpatient stocks.

Secondly, the Bureau of Narcotics was moved from the Department of Treasury and joined with the Bureau of Narcotics and Dangerous Drugs, as a part of the Department of Justice.

The Multiple-Dose Vial Problem. It is claimed that nurses seldom obtain the theoretically possible number of doses from a multiple-dose vial. The Bureau of Narcotics has suggested that hospitals use the *U.S.P.* and *N.F.* limit of tolerances as a guidepost —i.e., 2 to 20 per cent, depending on the size of the vial and the number of doses withdrawn.

In order to minimize this problem, many hospitals have switched to supplying the nurses' station with single doses of narcotic preparations such as individual ampuls or tablets, or to utilizing prepacked single-dose disposable parenteral units, such as the Tubex products available from Wyeth Laboratories. This system greatly helps the pharmacist maintain an accurate narcotic inventory at all times, assures the patient of a sterile uncontaminated and accurate dose and assists the nurse in her narcotic accounting records.

"Standing" and "P.R.N." orders for narcotics are permissible, but they should not

PHS-1604(HSP)
REV. 9-51
MONTHLY NARCOTIC REPORT (For Medical Officer in Charge and Clinical Director)   ⑧

STATION _____   REPORT PERIOD   FROM _____ TO _____

ITEM	PERPETUAL INVENTORY RECORD 1/					PHYSICAL INVENTORY		
	BALANCE START OF PERIOD	QUANTITY RECEIVED	TOTAL QUANTITY AVAILABLE FOR ISSUE	QUANTITY ISSUED	BALANCE ON HAND END OF PERIOD	BALANCE ON HAND [Actual Count]	OVER	SHORT
Acetoph., Acetylsal. Ac., caff., & cod., 15 mg. tab.								
Acetoph., Acetylsal. Ac., caff., & cod., 30 mg. tab.								
Apomorphine HCl HT, 6 mg.								
Camphorated Tincture of Opium								
Cocaine alkaloid hydrochloride								
Codiene phosphate								
phos. amp. 30 mg./cc								
sulf. HT, 15 mg.								
sulf. HT, 30 mg.								
sulf. HT, 60 mg.								
Ethylmorphine HCl								
Meperidine HCl amp. 100 mg.								
HCl tab. 50 mg.								
Morphine sulf. amp. 50 mg./cc								
sulf. HT, 8 mg.								
sulf. HT, 10 mg.								
sulf. HT. 15 mg.								
Opium Tincture								
Papaverine HCl amp. 65 mg./2cc								
HCl tab. 0.1 Gm.								

1/Figures taken from perpetual inventory record of narcotics in pharmacy.

REMARKS: (Appreciable increases to individual wards or clinics, or any continuous or unusually large-quantity prescribing should be noted.)

SIGNATURE - Chief, Pharmacy Service   DATE

Fig. 14-12. (U.S.P.H.S.)

be given for periods exceeding 72 hours, *regardless of the type of case*—terminal, cancer or otherwise. This helps to eliminate the chances of drugs being diverted illicitly after the death of a patient.

Storage. Narcotics must be kept in a locked, secure place. Reserve stocks should be kept in a *"strong safe,* substantial enough to deter entry and heavy enough to prevent their being carried away."* Other valuable property may be kept in the safe. A chest or safe meeting Underwriters Laboratories requirements for an X-60 rating is designed to offer protection against attack by tools or explosives for a period of 1 hour; one with a TR-60 rating protects against tools or torch; one with a TX-60 rating protects against tools, torch or explosives for the same period of time. A safe with any of these ratings, or of equivalent construction, is considered a *"strong safe"* by the Bureau.

For small stocks, the Bureau of Narcotics has occasionally, though reluctantly, accepted lighter safes with only a T-20 rating. This type of safe is built to resist attack by ordinary burglar's tools only, and only for a period of 20 minutes. While better than no safe at all, it offers a bare minimum of protection. Although sometimes insisted on as a minimum requirement, it is never recommended as adequate and certainly is not adequate for safekeeping of a narcotic stock of any appreciable size or value.

Any safe weighing less than 750 pounds should be securely anchored in concrete to the floor or the wall to prevent its being carried away. If bolts are used, they should be imbedded completely so that they cannot readily be reached and cut, sawed or unbolted (see General Circular 195, Bureau of Narcotics).

The president of the hospital corporation is usually the individual in whose name the narcotic registration is issued. However, he may delegate certain authority to proper employees of the hospital; for example, he may delegate to the registered pharmacist authority to sign forms. He may not delegate the right to sign the application for registration. Applications of corporations must be signed by an officer duly authorized to act (Article 8 of Regulation 5). Supposedly, this refers to the president, the vice-president or the secretary.

The hospital license must be renewed annually on or before July first.

A physician may not replenish his office narcotic supply or his physician's bag supplies from the hospital pharmacy narcotic supplies. He must order from a drug wholesaler on a special narcotic order form. An exception rarely, if ever, used is the single ounce of an aqueous or oleaginous solution of not over 20 per cent when ordered on the physician's official Federal narcotic order blank, *not* on his prescription blank (Article XV of the Act).

Though not discussed here, the regulations that apply to the handling of narcotics in community pharmacies apply also to hospital pharmacy.

Classes of Narcotics. General Circular No. 262 classifies narcotics into four categories:

Class A—fully controlled narcotics that require a written signed prescription

Class B—narcotic drugs authorized for oral prescription

Class X—exempted preparations which may be sold without a prescription by a registered pharmacist only.

Class M—specially exempted preparations which may be sold without a prescription

It is of special interest to hospital pharmacists to note that Class M narcotics are exempt from record keeping at the hospital. Examples of Class M drugs are Papaverine and Nalorphine (Nalline) preparations. It is only the original sale by the manufacturer that need be recorded for Class M preparations.

FEDERAL FOOD AND DRUG CODE AND REGULATIONS

Prescriptions for prescription legend drugs *may not be refilled* unless authorized by the physician or the dentist.

Prescriptions for prescription legend drugs must contain on the label (1) the name of the prescriber, (2) the serial number and the date of filling, (3) the name of the patient, if on the prescription, (4) any directions or warnings given in the prescription (signa) and (5) the name and the address of the store or the hospital.

Oral prescriptions from physicians and dentists for such items should be noted in writing by the pharmacist and filed. The pharmacist must record (1) the date and the serial number, (2) the names of the doctor and the patient, (3) the items and the quantities prescribed, (4) directions and cautions, if any and (5) refill directions, if any.

The doctor's oral refill authorization should be noted on the original prescription. While the Act may not specifically require the exact procedure as indicated in this and the preceding paragraph, the adoption of such procedures meets in full the requirements of the law.

The Statute of Limitations for violations of the Durham-Humphrey Act is 5 years. During this period prescriptions, medication orders and purchase orders should be kept as evidence of compliance with the Act. (1954 Amendment, U.S.C.A. Title 18, Crimes and Criminal Procedure, 1959 Annual Pocket Pact for use during 1960, Title 18, Chapter 231. Limitations, Section 3282, Offenses not Capital; The Prescription Legend, a F.D.A. Manual for Pharmacists, p. 12).

FEDERAL CODE AND REGULATIONS PERTAINING TO ETHYL ALCOHOL

Nonprofit hospitals and clinics may obtain tax-free alcohol for use *in* the hospital or the clinic, including use in the compounding of bona fide medicines for treatment of clinic patients outside the clinic, but such medicines may *not* be sold (Section 3108 (C) of the Internal Revenue Code of 1939 and Section 5310 (C) of the Internal Revenue Code of 1954).

Hospitals operating outpatient departments and charging for prescriptions containing alcohol (such as phenobarbital elixir, terpin hydrate elixir, terpin hydrate elixir with codeine and belladonna tincture), dispensed to outpatients may not use tax-free alcohol in these preparations.

Tax-free alcohol may not be used in the preparation of condiments, culinary extracts, flavoring or other preparations used in food products. This exception specifically prohibits the use of tax-free alcohol in the making of vanilla, lemon, maple or other flavoring extracts by the pharmacy for the dietetic service of the hospital.

FEDERAL CODE AND REGULATIONS PERTAINING TO STILLS

Stills must be registered with the Assistant Regional Commissioner, Alcohol and Tax Division of the Region (Regulation 23, Internal Revenue Service).

This regulation applies only to stills used or intended to be used for the distillation, the redistillation or the recovery of distilled spirits, including alcohol or any dilution or mixture thereof (Section 5174, Internal Revenue Code). Prior to the Internal Revenue Code of 1954, stills used for distilling water or the preparation of drugs or chemicals or for recovering cleaning fluids were required to be registered. This is no longer a requirement.

INVESTIGATIONAL DRUGS

STATEMENT OF PRINCIPLES INVOLVED IN THE USE OF INVESTIGATIONAL DRUGS IN HOSPITALS*

Hospitals are the primary centers for clinical investigations on new drugs. By definition these are drugs which have not yet been released by the Federal Food and Drug Administration for general use.

Since investigational drugs have not been certified as being for general use and have not been cleared for sale in interstate commerce by the Federal Food and Drug Administration, hospitals and their medical staffs have an obligation to their patients to see that proper procedures for their use are established.

Procedures for the control of investigational drugs should be based upon the following principles:

1. Investigational drugs should be used only under the direct supervision of the principal investigator who should be a member of the medical staff and who should assume the burden of securing the necessary consent.

2. The hospital should do all in its power to foster research consistent with adequate safeguard for the patient.

3. When nurses are called upon to administer investigational drugs, they should have available to them basic information concerning such drugs—including dosage forms, strengths available, actions and uses, side effects, and symptoms of toxicity, etc.

* Developed by the American Hospital Association and the American Society of Hospital Pharmacists Joint Committee.

4. The hospital should establish, preferably through the pharmacy and therapeutics committee, a central unit where essential information on investigational drugs is maintained and whence it may be made available to authorized personnel.

5. The pharmacy department is the appropriate area for the storage of investigational drugs, as it is for all other drugs. This will also provide for the proper labeling and dispensing in accord with the investigator's written orders.

It will be noted that the statement ensures that the hospital, its nurses and pharmacists, as well as the physicians evaluating an investigational drug in clinical practice, will have complete information available to them *within the institution*. In this connection, the *code* to break the "double blind" and other studies is available in the event of an adverse or unexpected reaction from the administration of an investigational drug to a patient. Theoretically, similar information is readily available in "remote coding" programs by telephoning the central point and breaking the code there; however, communication difficulties may result in dangerous delays.

SAFETY PRACTICES

Keep narcotics, hypnotics, amphetamines and poisons stored separately in locked cabinets.

Keep narcotics in as small supply as is expedient.

Keep volatile liquids in a cool place.

Store acids and other irritating liquids below knee level.

Verify the accuracy of pharmaceutical calculations with a mental estimate of the answer.

Where possible, have a second person check the pharmaceutical calculations on preparations requiring weights and measures.

Check each prescription with a second pharmacist, if possible.

Check labels 3 times: first as the item is taken from the shelf, secondly when used and lastly when returned to the shelf.

Verify the accuracy of the label by careful macroscopic examination of the material in the container.

Use every precaution to prevent a prescription-label or a stock-container-label switch.

Permit no unidentified substance to remain in the pharmacy.

Pour below eye level and avoid splashing; handle strong chemicals with care.

Give close attention to materials being heated. Do not leave process unattended.

Be certain that you have fulfilled the intent of the prescriber before dispensing the prescription.

Use the check system to ensure delivery of the proper prescription to the patient.

Include the patient's full name on the label of each prescription.

Use "strip labels" when indicated, such as "eyedrops," "nosedrops," "Do not use after ————," etc.

Make certain that the patient fully understands how to take the medication.

Where the prescription calls for a pharmaceutical specialty, a basic drug or biological, place the name of the manufacturer, the trade name of the product (if any) and the manufacturer's lot control number on the reverse side or face of the prescription. (See Fig. 14-7.)

Use dual code labels in prepackaging. Leave one label on the container, affix the other to the prescription being filed.

Also, the use of a code number on all prepackaged and floor stock containers which identifies the entry of that item in the chronological log is highly desirable to ensure quality control. For example, Code No. 1169105 indicates that the item was prepackaged in November 1969 and was the 105th item packaged. With this information, it is possible to find in the log (1) the name of the pharmacist responsible for the packaging, (2) the name of the manufacturer and (3) the manufacturer's lot or control number.

VOLUME COMPOUNDING

Volume compounding or bulk compounding are terms applied by hospital pharmacists to the manufacturing of pharmaceuticals in hospitals. The *Mirror to Hospital Pharmacy** reports that approximately 40 per cent of

*Francke, D. E., Latiolais, C-J., Francke, G. N., and Ho, N. F. H.: *Mirror to Hospital Pharmacy,* American Society of Hospital Pharmacists, Washington, D.C., 1964, p. 122.

hospital pharmacies conduct some type of bulk compounding program: 75 per cent of all short-term general hospitals with greater than 500 beds and a similar figure for all long-term hospitals engage in some type of manufacturing.

When to manufacture is often a difficult problem to decide. A simple rule-of-thumb

NAME OF ITEM					SOURCE				
CONTROL NO.	QUANTITY	BULK COMPOUNDED BY	CHECKED BY	DATE	CONTROL NO.	QUANTITY	BULK COMPOUNDED BY	CHECKED BY	DATE

PHS-1687
REV. 5-55   PHARMACEUTICAL FORMULATION CONTROL RECORD

NAME OF ITEM	SOURCE

ITEM	SOURCE OF FORMULA

FORMULA:

PHS-1687 (BACK)

FIG. 14-13. (*Top*) Pharmaceutical formulation control record. (*Bottom*) Reverse side. (**U.S.P.H.S.**)

used by many pharmacists is to manufacture only those items that may be prepared in as good or better quality at a cost less than or equal to the purchased item. Obviously, items not commercially available must be manufactured.

The problem of when to bulk compound becomes more complex in the teaching hospital. Here, the hospital has teaching obligations as well as patient care responsibilities, and, while a high-quality medication standard must be adhered to, an increased cost can be justified for bulk compounding on the grounds that it is necessary for the intern to become familiar with manufacturing technics and with the operation of equipment such as blenders, filter pumps, homogenizers, ointment mills,

tanks, mixers, bacterial filters, sterilizers, prepackaging and labeling equipment and similar items.

An important factor in bulk compounding over and above formulation, research and actual compounding problems (subjects discussed in other chapters) is that of controls.

Reproduced in Figures 14-13 and 14-14 are 2 forms used in the Public Health Service Hospitals bulk-compounding activities. These are self-explanatory of the system involved. It will be noted that the manufacturing worksheet (Fig. 14-14) carries not only the name of the drug or the chemical but also its source and the manufacturer's or supplier's package control number.

Many items in the hospital pharmacy ob-

PHS-1688
REV. 4-56

PHARMACEUTICAL BULK COMPOUNDING WORKSHEET

STATION   PREPARATION

QUANTITY   SOURCE OF FORMULA   DATE PREPARED

INGREDIENTS AND QUALITY	AMOUNT	MANUFACTURER	MANUFACTURER'S LOT CONTROL NO.	REMARKS
1.				
2.				
11.				
12.				

CALCULATIONS AND PROOF

NARCOTICS USED   ALCOHOL USED

APPROXIMATE TIME TO COMPLETE PREPARATION   PREPARED BY

CHECK   REMARKS

CALCULATIONS

FORMULA

INGREDIENTS

WEIGHTS

CHECKED BY *(Pharmacist)*   CONTROL NO.

HEW-LEX., KY.

FIG. 14-14. (U.S.P.H.S.)

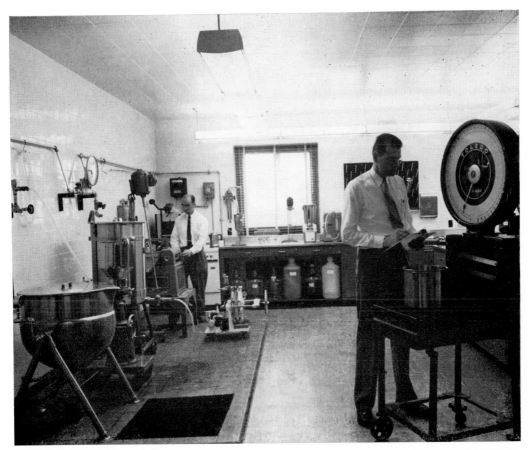

FIG. 14-15. Bulk compounding unit in a hospital pharmacy. (Clinical Center, N.I.H., U.S.P.H.S.)

viously lend themselves to bulk compounding at considerable savings to the institution.

PREPACKAGING

The larger hospital pharmacies with heavy nursing-station medication orders (basket-filling duties) and outpatient-prescription activities find it good management practice to prepackage the heavy repeating items.

Prepackaging consists of packaging in dispensing-size units large quantities of fast-moving items in advance of actual need. The time saved is considerable inasmuch as the pharmacist merely replaces the empty container returned from the floors with filled ones or need concern himself only with individual outpatient-prescription labeling for the pre-packaged prescription item. The prepackaging process places the preparation of these items at off-peak periods. This type of oper-

ation ensures neat, clean containers with properly shellacked or varnished labels, moving to the floors at all times, as well as an adequate prepackaged stock of individual patient-size prescription items.

Obviously, a control system must be applied also to prepackaging because of the shelf life of the items. A self-explanatory 2-form control system is illustrated in Figures 14-16 and 14-17.

STANDARDIZATION OF PRESCRIPTION AND WARD-ISSUE MEDICATION CONTAINERS

While it is realized that medications for ward, clinic and outpatient use are consumed normally in relatively short periods of time after being dispensed from the pharmacy, it is known also that many such medications have long "shelf life." Adequate protection

P. I. C. C.
MEDICATION

CONTROL NO.	DATE	MANUFACTURER	MFG'S CONTROL OR LOT. NO.	AMOUNT IN CONTAINER	BAL. ON HAND	NUMBER PACKAGED	NEW BALANCE	CHECK IP	OP	PACKAGED BY	LABELED BY	CHECKED BY

PHS-1686
Rev. 2-59   PREPACKAGED PHARMACEUTICAL ITEM CONTROL RECORD   (*Affix label on back in each instance.*)

P. I. C. C.
MEDICATION   16—74311-1 **GPO**

FIG. 14-16. (U.S.P.H.S.)

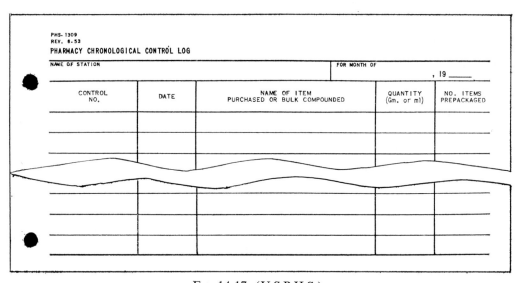

FIG. 14-17. (U.S.P.H.S.)

should be provided to maintain the full therapeutic effectiveness of these preparations. It is for this reason that many hospital pharmacists standardize their prepackaged ward, clinic and prescription containers to the amber-type containers used by manufacturers in complying with *U.S.P.* and *N.F.* requirements to "store and preserve in tight light-resistant containers."

METHODS OF TRANSMITTING PRESCRIPTION ORDERS TO THE PHARMACIST

Although hospitals vary in their total drug distribution systems, three commonly used procedures are available for the transmission of the physician's drug order from the nursing station to the pharmacist. They are:

1. The prescription order is written on a separate blank by the physician.

2. A carbon copy or other copy of the physician's order sheet is sent to the pharmacist.

3. Drug orders are transcribed by the nurse or other hospital personnel assigned to the nursing station and sent to the pharmacist.

Individual prescription orders are written by the physician, particularly in the smaller institutions. This system established the same professional relationship and practice that exists in community pharmacy services. Although the pharmacist is allowed to interpret the physician's order in most cases, this system has the distinct drawback of an increased risk of misplaced orders, since the hospital patient typically receives a sizeable number of drugs at one time. Additionally, many physicians do not favor this method, since most doctors are accustomed to writing all orders on the patient's chart and leaving all further details to the hospital personnel.

The second method of transmitting drug orders using some type of copy of the physician's order sheet is a relatively new develop-ment in hospital pharmacy practice and represents a great improvement in the reduction of medication errors. In this system, the pharmacist receives a copy of the original drug order in the physician's own handwriting. Many different types of forms have been developed utilizing either a carbon copy or an NCR* copy. One example of this type of form is illustrated in Figure 14-18. Although Xerox copies of the original order may also be used, the cost of such an operation is usually prohibitive.

A physician's order sheet that has a specific area for all drug orders contributes to the success of such an operation. The pharmacist must educate the physician to limit the writing of drug orders only to the assigned areas of the patient's chart; moreover, unless the copy sheets are promptly removed and sent to the pharmacy immediately after the order is written, delays in dispensing may occur. Although this system eliminates nursing personnel from transcribing drug orders and thus conserves valuable nursing time, consideration must be made of the additional time it takes the pharmacist to review every

* National Cash Register Company, Dayton, Ohio. (A trademark for No-Carbon Required.)

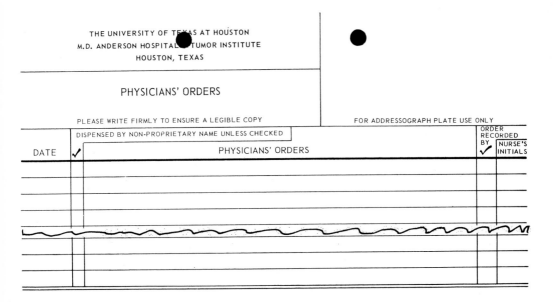

A Red Dot Indicates Pharmacy Copy Available

FIG. 14-18. Physicians' Order Form with series of three NCR copies for pharmacy use. (The University of Texas at Houston, M. D. Anderson Hospital and Tumor Institute)

drug order written, including those for floor items. Naturally, matters of patient safety are paramount rather than the saving of time.

Some hospitals have designed these order sheets so that a copy is made for the nurse's Kardex, thus saving additional time in transcribing by the nurse.

In the method most generally employed at present the registered nurse or other ward personnel transcribes the physician's written order to another form and sends it to the pharmacist for dispensing. The transcribed order may also be used by the parmacist to initiate the medication charge. In addition to involving the nurse in unnecessary paper work, this system has the obvious disadvantage of permitting non-pharmacists to interpret the drug order as well as to indicate what drugs are to be used by the patient. The pharmacist has little chance of discovering a wrong transcription unless a really obvious mistake has occurred. This system also promotes the rather common practice of storing sizable quantities of drugs at the nursing station, a practice purported to improve nursing service —but at the expense of good drug control.

METHODS OF DRUG DISTRIBUTION IN HOSPITALS

The distribution of drugs to inpatients varies considerably from institution to institution, depending on the size of the hospital, its classification, the types of services offered, the administrative policies, and the qualification of the director of pharmacy service. The Minimum Standard for Pharmacies in Hospitals and the Statement on Guiding Principles on the Operation of the Hospital Formulary System emphasize the responsibility of pharmacy service in the establishment and maintenance of an adequate system of drug control in the hospital.

Systems of drug dispensing now in general use in hospitals include:
1. Individual prescription order system
2. Complete ward stock system
3. Combination of (1) and (2)

The first system directs that virtually all drugs be dispensed by the pharmacist on individual prescription orders via any one of the methods of drug order transmission described previously. The filling of orders may be as simple as having a courier deliver a drug order to the pharmacy for dispensing (as might be the case in a small hospital), or it may involve more elaborate systems such as pneumatic tubes or elevator service. The most sophisticated application of the individual prescription order system is the unit dose method of drug distribution in which each dose is dispensed to the patient at the proper time in a form that is ready to administer. More will be said about the concepts of unit dose later in the chapter.

Pharmacies that operate under the individual prescription system customarily dispense the drugs in multiple doses, usually a three- or four-day supply. Because revenue from medication services is frequently very important to hospitals using this system, detailed methods have been developed for charging the proper account. This system is used most frequently in private hospitals because of its revenue production and in smaller rather than in larger hospitals because of the manpower requirements for individualized service.

Some advantages that may exist with the individual prescription order system are:
1. The reduction of medication errors by having the pharmacist review and interpret at least a transcription of each prescription order *before* the drug is dispensed
2. Coordination of the patient's drug program through closer contact between physician, nurse and pharmacist in medication matters
3. Close control of revenue
4. More rigid control of inventory

Some disadvantages which may exist with the individual prescription order system are:
1. Possible delay in obtaining medication for administration to the patient
2. Increased personnel expense
3. Increased amount of credits for unused drugs (unit dose dispensing is the exception)

In the second system, complete ward stock, all but the most unusual drugs are stocked at the nursing station. This system is utilized predominantly in governmental hospitals or other hospitals in which charges for drugs are not made to the patient or when an all-inclusive daily room rate is used for charging. Drugs that are particularly expensive, rarely used, or require special control or handling are omitted from the ward stock. Such drugs are dispensed on a prescription-only basis and are indicated for use only by the individual patient. Probably the most common feature in this system is the presence of large stocks of drugs on nursing wards. These stocks often consist of bulk packages of the most commonly used medications, and it is from these stocks that the nurse dispenses medications to the patient.

A system of complete ward stock places the responsibilities of drug distribution on the nurse, who generally is not qualified to accept them. There is no check or interpretation of orders from the patient's chart and no check on what drugs are being dispensed. Under these conditions, the pharmacist has an obligation to maintain these stocks of drugs in the most efficient way possible in order to minimize medication errors. There are some hospitals that use the "complete ward stock" system but still wish to charge the patient for individual medication. Various systems have been devised for this procedure, but, in each case, nursing service must initiate some report or charge form to be successful. Some advantages that may be cited with this system are:

1. Ready availability of most drugs to the nurse and physician assigned to the nursing station

2. Reduction in the number of inpatient prescription orders

3. Reduction in the number of medications returned to the pharmacy for credit

4. Reduction in pharmacy personnel requirements

Among the disadvantages of a complete ward stock system are:

1. An increased potential for medication errors resulting from the lack of review by the pharmacist of each individual prescription order

2. Financial loss due to misappropriation of medicine by hospital personnel and the administration of medication to patients without initiating charges (estimated to run from $30 to $120 per bed per year)

3. Increased drug inventory

4. Increased cost of drug losses due to obsolescence, deterioration or misplacement

5. Improper storage facilities and limited capacity on many nursing stations

6. Increased danger of unnoticed drug deterioration, jeopardizing patient safety

The third system is a combination of the individual prescription order system and the ward stock system and is probably the most widely used method of drug distribution in hospitals today. These institutions use the individual order system as their primary method of dispensing, but have at least twenty drug items (in addition to the narcotic and hypnotics) on ward stock. Although this system varies considerably among institutions, it starts with a basic list of floor stock drugs. Included are the common non-prescription drugs such as aspirin, magnesia magma, Clinitest tablets and enemas, and certain legend drugs that are used routinely by patients. Also, drugs not suited for individual prescription order and charges such as multiple dose vials used only once or twice per patient may be included. A typical example of a standard floor stock requisition form is illustrated in Figure 14-19.

The advantages and disadvantages of this combined system are a composite of those of each of the two systems previously discussed, in proportion to the ratio of floor stock to individual prescription orders. When properly coordinated, the best features of each may be realized.

EXPERIMENTAL AND DEVELOPMENTAL SYSTEMS

In recent years many hospital pharmacists have initiated new and innovative methods of drug distribution in order to improve specific deficiencies in their present systems. Much of the research that is being carried out in hospital pharmacy concerns improved and streamlined patterns of drug distribution with emphasis on improved record keeping, physical distribution, ordering and billing.

One such system tried by a number of hospitals is the Brewer System of drug control which employs a mechanical storage and dispensing device at the nursing station. This machine is designed to hold eight containers of as many as 96 different items.

The drugs to be dispensed in this system are placed in cardboard boxes specially designed to fit in each compartment. The containers are fitted with a plastic sleeve to prevent loss of drug from the container and the

STANDARD FLOOR STOCK REQUISITION
FOR NURSING UNITS
BRACKENRIDGE HOSPITAL PHARMACY

Ordered by_____

Date_____   Issued by_____

Nursing Unit_____   Received by_____

Directions:
1. One copy of this requisition should accompany your drug basket.
2. Note the unit size for each item and write in quantity needed.
3. Each nursing unit should have a master copy listing the maximum allowable quantities for each item. Use this as a guide when preparing orders.
4. Return only empty containers to the Pharmacy. If necessary keep a reserve supply on hand.
5. Each of the nursing units listed below should order according to the following schedule:

Mon. & Thurs.	Tues. & Fri.	Wednesday
6N WW	Nursery	Formula Room
5N 4S	Delivery Room	
4N 2S	2 North	

6. **Floor Stock Charging Procedures:**
   a. Items preceded by an asterisk (*), are free to the patient and will be charged to the nursing unit.
   b. Items not preceded by an asterisk are to be charged to the patient.
   c. Items not listed on this requisition are not floor stock and should be ordered on the patient's drug chart.

QUANTITY NEEDED	NAME & STRENGTH OF MEDICATION	UNIT SIZE	QUANTITY ISSUED	TEMPORARILY OUT-REORDER	QUANTITY NEEDED	NAME & STRENGTH OF MEDICATION	UNIT SIZE	QUANTITY ISSUED	TEMPORARILY OUT-REORDER
	INJECTABLES					Penicillin G Potassium 5 mil. units	vial		
	Adrenalin Chloride Solution 1:1000	1 ml				Penicillin G Potassium 20 mil. units	vial		
	Adrenalin in Oil 1:500	1 ml				Penicillin G 100,000 u + Procaine Penicillin			
	Adrenal Cortex (Eschatin)	10 ml				300,000 u/ml	10 ml		
	Aminophylline—I.M. 0.5 Gm (7½ gr)/2 ml	2 ml				Penicillin G Procaine 600,000 units/1.2 ml	12 ml		
	Aminophylline—I.V. 0.5 Gm (7½ gr)/20 ml	20 ml				Penicillin G 400,000 units + Streptomycin			
	Aminophylline I.V. 0.25 Gm (3¾ gr)/10 ml	10 ml				0.5 Gm/2 ml	10 ml		
	Amytal Sodium 0.5 Gm (7½ gr)/10 ml	10 ml				Phenergan 25 mg/ml	10 ml		
	Amytal Sodium 0.25 Gm (3¾ gr)/5 ml	5 ml				Phenobarbital (Luminal) 130 mg (2 gr)/ml	1 ml		
	Aqua Mephyton 10 mg/ml	1 ml				Phenobarbital (Luminal) 320 mg (5 gr)/2 ml	2 ml		
	Aramine 10 mg/ml	10 ml				Phenol sulfonphthalein (PSP) Dye	1 ml		
	Atropine Sulfate 0.4 mg (1/150 gr)/ml	20 ml				Pitocin 10 units/ml	1 ml		
	Benadryl HCl 10 mg/ml	10 ml				Potassium Chloride 20 meq. (1.49 Gm)/10 ml	10 ml		
	Benadryl HCl 50 mg/ml	1 ml				Potassium Chloride 20 meq. (2.98 Gm)/20 ml	20 ml		
	Berroca—C	20 ml				*Procaine HCl 1%	30 ml		
	Bronkephrine	10 ml				*Procaine HCl 2%	30 ml		
	Caffeine & Sodium Benzoate 500 mg/2 ml	2 ml				Prostigmin 1:4000	1 ml		
	Calcium Chloride 1 Gm/10 ml	10 ml				Prostigmin 1:2000	1 ml		
	Calcium Gluconate 1 Gm/10 ml	10 ml				Reserpine (Serpasil) 2.5 mg/ml	10 ml		
	Cedilanid—D 0.4 mg/2 ml	2 ml				Scopolamine 0.65 mg (1/100 gr)/ml	1 ml		
	Deladumone-OB	2 ml				Scopolamine 0.43 mg (1/150 gr)/ml	1 ml		
	Dextrose 50%	50 ml				Scopolamine 0.32 mg (1/200 gr)/ml	1 ml		
	Digifortis 1 units/ml	1 ml				Seconal Sodium 50 mg/ml	20 ml		
	Digoxin (Lanoxin) 0.5 mg/2 ml	2 ml				Sodium Bicarbonate 3.75 Gm/50 ml	50 ml		
	Dramamine 50 mg/ml	5 ml				*Sodium Chloride, Isotonic	30 ml		
	Ephedrine Sulfate 50 mg/ml	1 ml				Streptomycin 0.5 Gm/ml	12.5 ml		
	Ergotrate Maleate 0.2 mg (1/320 gr)/ml	1 ml				Tetanus Toxoid Fluid	7.5 ml		
	Insulin, Regular 40 units/ml	10 ml				Thiomerin	10 ml		
	Insulin, Regular 80 units/ml	10 ml				Vasoxyl 15 mg/ml	1 ml		
	Insulin, N.P.H. 40 units/ml	10 ml				Vasoxyl 15 mg/ml with Procaine 1%	1 ml		
	Insulin, N.P.H. 80 units/ml	10 ml				Vistaril 50 mg/ml	2 ml		
	Largon 20 mg/ml	1 ml				Vitamin K (Synkayvite) 5 mg/ml	1 ml		
	Librium 100 mg/2 ml	2 ml				Vitamin K (Synkayvite) 10 mg/ml	1 ml		
	Lorfan Tartrate 1 mg/ml	1 ml				Vitamin K (Synkayvite) 75 mg/2 ml	2 ml		
	Lyo-B-C Forte c̄ B₁₂	vial				*Water, Sterile Distilled	30 ml		
	Magnesium Sulfate 50%	2 ml				Wydase 150 units/ml	1 ml		
	Marezine 50 mg/ml	1 ml				*Xylocaine 1%	50 ml		
	Methergine 0.2 mg (1/320 gr)/ml	1 ml				*Xylocaine 1% c̄ Epinephrine	50 ml		
	Nembutal Sodium 50 mg (¾ gr)/ml	20 ml				*Xylocaine 2%	50 ml		
	Neo-Synephrine 10 mg/ml	5 ml				*Xylocaine 2% c̄ Epinephrine	50 ml		
	Penicillin G Potassium 1 mil. units	vial							

65-281   11-65

FIG. 14-19. Standard floor stock requisition for nursing units. (Brackenridge Hospital, Austin, Texas)

QUANTITY NEEDED	NAME & STRENGTH OF MEDICATION	UNIT SIZE	QUANTITY ISSUED	TEMPORARILY OUT-REORDER	QUANTITY NEEDED	NAME & STRENGTH OF MEDICATION	UNIT SIZE	QUANTITY ISSUED	TEMPORARILY OUT REORDER
	TABLETS & CAPSULES					**LIQUIDS, EXTERNAL**			
	*Acetest	100				*Acetone	8 oz		
	*Aspirin 0.3 Gm (5 gr)	200				*Ammonia, Aromatic Spirits	2 oz		
	*Aspirin 0.1 Gm (1¼ gr)	50				*Collodion, Flexible	8 oz		
	*Aspirin Compound (APC)	200				*Hand Lotion	pt		
	*Atropine 0.43 mg (1/150 gr)	20				Merthiolate Tincture	8 oz		
	*Atropine 0.65 mg (1/100 gr)	20				*Zephiran Chloride 1:750 Solution	gal		
	*Benadryl 25 mg	50				*Zephiran Chloride 1:750 with Anti Rust	gal		
	*Benadryl 50 mg	50							
	*Clinitest	100							
	Coumadin 2 mg	20							
	Coumadin 2½ mg	20							
	Coumadin 5 mg	50							
	Coumadin 7½ mg	20							
	Coumadin 10 mg	50				**SUPPOSITORIES**			
	Coumadin 25 mg	20				Aminophylline 0.5 Gm (7½ gr)	12		
	Diethylstilbestrol 5 mg	50				Aminophylline 0.25 Gm (3¾ gr)	12		
	Diethylstilbestrol 25 mg	20				Aspirin 600 mg (10 gr)	12		
	*Digitalis Leaf 0.1 Gm (1½ gr)	50				Aspirin 300 mg (5 gr)	12		
	*Digitoxin 0.1 mg	20				Aspirin (Supprettes) 65 mg (1 gr)	12		
	*Digitoxin 0.15 mg	20				Aspirin (Supprettes) 200 mg (3 gr)	12		
	*Digitoxin 0.2 mg	20				Dulcolax 10 mg	24		
	*Digoxin (Lanoxin) 0.25 mg	50				Glycerin, Adult	12		
	*Digoxin (Lanoxin) 0.5 mg	50				Glycerin, Infant	12		
	Ergotrate 0.2 mg (1/320 gr)	20				Nembutal 32 mg (½ gr)	12		
	Methergine 0.2 mg (1/320 gr)	100				Nembutal 65 mg (1 gr)	12		
	*Nitroglycerin 0.65 mg (1/100 gr)	20				Nembutal 120 mg (2 gr)	12		
	*Nitroglycerin 0.43 mg (1/150 gr)	20				Nembutal 200 mg (3 gr)	12		
	*Nitroglycerin 0.32 mg (1/200 gr)	20				Seconal 32 mg (½ gr)	12		
	Peri-Colace	100				Seconal 65 mg (1 gr)	12		
	*Phenobarbital 16 mg (¼ gr)	20				Seconal 120 mg (2 gr)	12		
	*Phenobarbital 32 mg (½ gr)	50				Seconal 200 mg (3 gr)	12		
	Prenatal Vitamin Formula	100							
	Telepaque	6							
						MISCELLANEOUS			
	LIQUIDS, ORAL								
	*Bellabarb Elixir	8 oz				Dermoplast Spray	3 oz		
	*Benylin Expectorant	8 oz				*Kerodex "71"	4 oz		
	*Cascara Sagrada, Aromatic	8 oz				*Lubricating Jelly 2.7 Gm Foil pkg	144		
	*Glycerin	pt				*Lubricating Jelly 5 Gm Tube	48		
	*Kaopectate	pt				*Lubricating Jelly	5 oz		
	*Magnesium Sulfate Sat. Solution	pt				*Magnesium Sulfate Crystals	8 oz		
	*Milk of Magnesia	pt				*Petrolatum,	8 oz		
	*Mineral Oil	pt				*Petrolatum, Tube	3/5 oz		
	*Mouth Wash	pt				*Silver Nitrate Applicators	100		
	Neoloid	4 oz				Syringe Detergent	4 oz		
	*Paregoric (Camphorated Opium Tinc.)	4 oz							
	*Phenobarbital Elixir	8 oz							
	*Phospho Soda, Fleets	8 oz							
	*Terpin Hydrate c̄ Codeine Elixir	8 oz							
	X-Prep	2½ oz							

FIG. 14-19 (*Continued*)

box is labeled and placed in the storage bins within the machine.

The procuring of drugs by the nurse is quite simple. The nurse must use three separate plates: her identification plate which is coded specifically for each nurse operating the machine, the drug plate which identifies the drug which is to be dispensed, and the patient's identification plate. These plates are inserted in shuttle together with the charge voucher set. The shuttle is pushed in, the activator button pressed, and the box containing the desired drug is released from the storage bin and into the drug delivery outlet. After receiving the pharmacy pre-packed medication box, the nurse returns the drug plate to its proper slot and deposits the medication box in the individual patient drawer in the medication cart.

The Brewer System makes four records of the nurse's medication withdrawal; three on the charge voucher and one on a continuous roll inside the machine. These four records are designed to be utilized by the pharmacist, the nurse and the business office in order to provide needed information on drug flow from the individual machine.

The Brewer Corporation also supplies a medication cart designed for use with the Brewer System. The cart usually contains 35 to 56 drawers under one central lock. Each drawer is labeled with patient information and has room inside for medications.

This method of drug distribution is designed to improve on the ward-stock type of drug distribution and is said to have certain advantages over the latter. It is claimed that the Brewer System reduces pharmacy inventory, extends the pharmacist's control of drug flow at the nurses' station, gives complete and effective control of inventory (thus assuring the proper handling of drugs), relieves the pharmacist of much paper work (pricing, labeling, typing, etc.) and reduces loss of charges.

The utilization of the Brewer System represents a considerable financial investment in the distribution of drugs to patients. Although this system has been successful in certain hospitals and can lead to the reduction of medication errors when full time pharmacy service is unavailable, it does not provide the full depth control services that a pharmacist is able to offer. Some hospitals have utilized a Brewer machine as an emergency drug station for use when the pharmacy department is closed and have reported considerable success in this respect.

Automated data processing (ADP) and other electronic devices are being utilized to a great extent in order to improve efficiency of areas associated with drug distribution. Areas that are most likely to be improved with this method are inventory control, purchasing, narcotic control, accounting functions and drug information.

Unit Dose Drug Distribution. The search for improved pharmacy services and reduction of medication errors led to the development of the concept of unit-dose drug dispensing. The results of extensive research at The University of Arkansas, The University of Iowa and The University of Kentucky and other institutions provided valuable information on the feasibility and practicality of this system for application, at least in part or with modifications, in most hospitals.

In the unit-dose system, the major portion of drugs are dispensed from either a centralized or decentralized pharmacy. In the centralized pharmacy, all dispensing originates from a single pharmacy department. In the decentralized system satellite pharmacies or pharmacy substations designed to serve a specific number of patients are located at strategic points throughout the hospital. In both cases, the drugs are dispensed in single doses that are properly labeled and ready for administration.

Because of the increased use of unit-dose systems in hospitals, many drug firms now package a rather complete line of products—generally through contract packagers—in single-dose form. Additionally, many hospitals utilizing the unit-dose concept repackage a great number of drugs within their own departments so that virtually all medications can be dispensed in individual doses.

The unit-dose system of drug distribution offers some distinct advantages, such as: reduction in medication errors; reduction in nurse's time spent on drug-related activities, making available more patient-care time; improvement in narcotic and inventory control; decreased loss of drugs through pilferage and missed charges; elimination of credits; improvement in record keeping; effective utilization of nonprofessional personnel in dispensing; use of distribution methods that enable better use of automated data processing; increased opportunity for pharmacists to become more involved in direct patient care. Disadvantages include: higher initial cost of individual doses; increased demand for pharmacy space, more personnel; need for hospitals to engage in their own unit packaging activity to some degree.

The following outlines offer a comparison of a centralized unit dose dispensing system as originally developed at the University of Arkansas and a decentralized unit dose operation as developed at the University of Iowa.

Centralized Unit Dose Dispensing

1. Physician writes medication order on order form, producing a duplicate copy.

2. Duplicate copy of drug order is sent directly to the pharmacy.

3. Orders are punched into IBM cards by trained keypunch operator.

4. Pharmacist checks IBM cards against duplicate order.

5. Print-out sheet containing all information from new and previous IBM cards for patient is received by teletypewriter at the nursing station.

6. IBM cards are duplicated and used as a requisition in pharmacy for unit-dose medication.

7. Medications and IBM cards are checked by pharmacist.

8. Medications and brief descriptions of each drug are sent to nursing station at appropriate times.

9. Duplicate IBM cards, signed and dated by pharmacist, are sent to accounting office for billing and inventory control.

10. Medication is received by nurse and checked against print-out sheet in Kardex file.

11. Unit dose is given to the patient.

12. Administration of dose is recorded on print-out sheet.

Decentralized Unit-Dose Dispensing

1. Physician writes medication order on physician's order form, producing duplicate copy.

2. Duplicate copy of drug order is sent to pharmacy substation in nursing area.

3. Order is checked by pharmacist.

4. Order is entered in Kardex file in pharmacy substation on nursing floor.

5. Unit-dose medication is prepared and sent to nurse with individual "med note" at appropriate time.

6. Nurse checks medication with record in nurses' Kardex file (obtained from original order).

7. Medication in unit dose is given to patient.

8. Administration of dose is recorded in Kardex file.

9. Billing is accomplished through observation of completed record in Kardex file.

A complete in-depth description of unit dose is not within the scope of this chapter. The reader is urged to consult the literature for a more complete study of this system.

Since hospitals that utilize the unit-dose system of drug distribution must repackage many drugs in a unit-dose package, certain guidelines should be kept in mind. The most important requirements for hospital single-unit packages are summarized in Figure 14-20.

Unit-dose Packaging Requirements. The package should be designed to improve the safety and efficiency of the hospital drug distribution system. Therefore, the package must ensure the stability, the purity and the efficacy of the drug from packaging to administration. Additionally, it must be compatible with the existing systems or promote the development of better systems of storing, dispensing, delivering, administering, record keeping and inventorying. It should also promote the establishment of efficient packaging system to enable its production at a cost that is within reason, and it must conform to legal requirements as established by federal and state government.

In response to the growing interest in unit-dose systems and single-unit packages, the American Society of Hospital Pharmacists introduced a set of guidelines for single-unit packages of drugs. In this set of guidelines, a differentiation is made between "unit-dose packages" and "single-unit packages." "A unit-dose package contains the ordered amount of drug in a dosage form ready for administration to a particular patient by the prescribed route at the prescribed time." A single-unit package is described as "one which

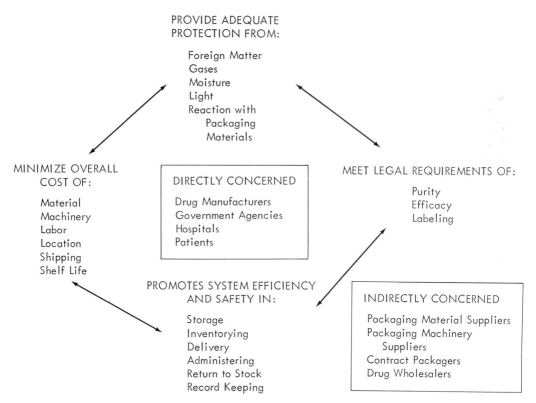

FIG. 14-20. Requirements for hospital inpatient single unit packages. (Reynolds Metals Company, Richmond, Virginia, Market Research Department)

contains one discrete pharmaceutical dosage form, i.e., one tablet, one capsule, or one 2 ml. quantity of a liquid, etc." Therefore, a single-dose package is a unit-dose package only when the dose ordered is the same as the dose packaged as a single dose. In both cases the package is properly labeled and its contents can be administered directly from the package. The package should be easy to open, easy to use, and require little additional training or experience in learning its use.

Each individual container should be labeled properly in a form that is easy to read and is highly legible. The ASHP proposes the following recommendations:

NONPROPRIETARY NAME
(dosage form if special)
STRENGTH
Trade Mark
Control Number
(any applicable special notes)

A. The nonproprietary name (generic, public, or established name) and the strength should be the most prominent part of the label. It is suggested that 6 point type be considered the minimum and that the style of type be chosen to provide maximum legibility.

B. Special characteristics of the dosage form should be part of the label. In a transparent package containing a tablet, for instance, it should be labeled that it is delayed release, extended release, enteric coated, etc.

C. Strength should be stated in accordance with the terminology in the *American Hospital Formulary Service*. The metric system should be used, and ml. (milliliters) is preferred to cc. (cubic centimeters).

D. It is not necessary to have the trade name, if any, on the package.

E. The name of the manufacturer and the control number should be on the package. It is also desirable that the date of manufacture be obvious from the control number.

F. Special instructions, conditions of storage and administration are to be included on the bottom of the label.

The dispensing container is to be completely labeled as required by law and with such information as the manufacturer believed might be helpful. The ASHP also states that the dispensing package be relatively narrow and not tall and should be designed to make maximum use of the back of the shelf or depth of the drawer space.

To facilitate inventory taking, it is desirable that master containers be designed so that (1) it is evident that the container has not been opened and (2) if opened, it is easy to count the remaining units. Some strip packing is reversed in number for this purpose.

In summary, the concept of unit-dose drug dispensing has opened up a whole new field in the search for better methods of drug distribution. Perhaps the most far-reaching effects have been on the development of single-unit drug packaging which has found use not in hospitals alone but in all areas of drug distribution. It is estimated that the unit-packaged share of proprietary drugs will have increased from 6 per cent in 1967 to 12 per cent in 1970 and to about 38 per cent in 1975.

Certain guidelines, as proposed by the ASHP in their Statement on Hospital Drug Distribution Systems, should be given primary consideration when evaluating the design of new hospital drug distribution systems as well as in the modifying of existing ones (particularly if the proposed changes would commit a hospital to considerable financial investment in a system that does not include or could not easily be altered to include the recommended practices).

1. Before the initial dose of medication is administered, the pharmacist should review the prescriber's original order or direct copy.

2. Drugs dispensed should be as ready for administration to the patient as the current status of pharmaceutical technology permits and must bear adequate identification including (but not limited to): name or names of drug, strength or potency, route(s) of administration, expiration date, control number, and such other special instructions as may be indicated.

3. Facilities and equipment used to store drugs should be so designed that the drugs are accessible only to medical practitioners authorized to prescribe, to pharmacists auth-

orized to dispense, or to nurses authorized to administer such drugs.

4. Facilities and equipment used to store drugs should be designed to facilitate routine inspection of the drug prior to the time of administration.

5. When utilizing automated (mechanical and/or electronic) devices as pharmaceutical tools, it is mandatory that provision be made to provide suitable pharmaceutical services in the event of a failure of the device.

6. Such mechanical or electronic drug storage and dispensing devices as require or encourage the repackaging of drug dosage forms from the manufacturer's original container should permit and facilitate the use of a new package that assures the stability of each drug and meets the USP standards for the packaging and storage of drugs, in addition to meeting all other standards of good pharmacy practice.

7. In evaluating automated (mechanical and/or electronic) devices as pharmaceutical tools, distinction must be made between the grade of accuracy as required in accounting practices and that required in dispensing practices.

INTRAVENOUS ADDITIVE SERVICE BY THE HOSPITAL PHARMACIST

Since total drug control within the hospital is the responsibility of the pharmacist, it follows that it is his professional and legal duty to supervise the extemporaneous preparation of all intravenous fluid admixtures.

An intravenous additive service is concerned with "the preparation of intravenous fluids with additives by individuals other than those who will administer them or who will assume the responsibility for monitoring the effects on the patient once the administration has been initiated."*

Certain objectives should be considered when attempting to implement an IV additive service. They are:

1. To minimize the possibility of incompatibilities, chemical, physical or therapeutic

2. To provide a controlled "clean" environment for the addition of drugs to sterile IV fluids

* Ravin, R. S.: Hosp. Form. Management, 3: 35, 1968 (Oct.).

THE UNIVERSITY OF TEXAS AT HOUSTON
M.D. ANDERSON HOSPITAL AND TUMOR INSTITUTE
PHARMACY DEPARTMENT

NURSING UNIT STOCK SOLUTIONS
CHARGE VOUCHER

TO: CENTRALIZED I.V. PREPARATION AREA

TIME SOLN.
ADMINISTERED _____ DATE _____

FOR ADDRESSOGRAPH IMPRINT

SOLUTION ADMINISTERED: (_____ML. VOLUME)

☐ DEXTROSE 5% IN WATER
☐ DEXTROSE 5% IN 1/4 STR. SALINE
☐ NORMAL SALINE
☐ LACTATED RINGER'S SOLUTION
☐ IONOSOL-T
☐ NORMOSOL-M

☐ OTHER _____

SOLUTION CHARGE: $_____

PSF(AA-32)

THE UNIVERSITY OF TEXAS AT HOUSTON
M.D. ANDERSON HOSPITAL & TUMOR INSTITUTE
PHARMACY DEPARTMENT

SOLUTION RETURN FORM

TO: I.V. PREPARATION AREA OF PHARMACY

FROM: _____ DATE: _____

FOR ADDRESSOGRAPH IMPRINT

SOLUTION NOT ADMINISTERED DUE TO:

INCORRECT PATIENT ☐
INCORRECT SOLUTION ☐
CONTAMINATED SOLUTION ☐
ORDER DISCONTINUED ☐

INCOMPATIBILITY OF SOLUTION ☐
OTHER: _____

PLEASE INDICATE ONE OF THE ABOVE REASONS.

BOTTLE NO. _____

PSF(AA-28)

MEDICATION ORDER REVISION

TO THE NURSE - ATTN: PLEASE ENTER "NEW" ORDER IN THE PATIENT RECORD FOR HANDLING AS A VERBAL ORDER AND PHYSICIANS' COUNTER SIGNATURE. RETAIN THIS COPY UNTIL THE ORDER IS VERIFIED.	DATE	PATIENT IDENTIFICATION
	TIME	

ORIGINAL ORDER: _____
_____
_____
_____
_____
_____
_____

NEW ORDER: _____
_____
_____
_____
_____
_____
_____

THE UNIVERSITY OF TEXAS AT HOUSTON
M.D. ANDERSON HOSPITAL & TUMOR INSTITUTE
PHARMACY DEPARTMENT

VERBAL ORDER RECORDED BY-
PSF(AA-31)   R.PH.

FIG. 14-21. (*Caption on facing page*)

THE UNIVERSITY OF TEXAS AT HOUSTON
M.D. ANDERSON HOSPITAL & TUMOR INSTITUTE
PHARMACY DEPARTMENT

EMERGENCY ORDER
INTRAVENOUS SOLUTION

PATIENT NAME- _____

PATIENT NO. _____   ROOM No. _____

VOLUMES			SOLUTIONS
50cc	/	/	1. DEXTROSE _____ % IN WATER.
100cc	/	/	2. DEXTROSE _____ % IN _____
150cc	/	/	3. INVERT SUGAR _____ % IN _____
200cc	/	/	4. IONOSOL ____ WITH _____ %
250cc	/	/	5. SODIUM CHLORIDE _____ % INJECTION
500cc	/	/	6. LACTATED RINGERS INJECTION
1,000cc	/	/	7. RINGERS INJECTION
/ / OTHER _____ CC.			8. NORMOSOL ____ WITH _____
			9. OTHER- _____

ADDITIVES   CONC.

1. POT. CHLORIDE INJ.   _____ MEQ.   RATE OF
2. SOD. BICARBONATE INJ.   _____   ADMINISTRATION
3. SOLU-B _____   _____
4. HEPARIN _____ UNITS   _____
5. SOLU-CORTEF _____ MG.   _____   _____ CC/HR.
6. KEFLIN _____ GMS.   _____
7. KANAMYCIN _____ MGS.   _____   OR
8. PEN G OR K _____ U.   _____ UNITS   _____ GTTS./MIN.
9. AMPICILLIN _____ MGS.   _____
10. CYTOXAN _____ MGS.   _____ MGS.
11. CYTOSINE ARAB. ____ MG.   _____ MGS.
12. XYLOCAINE _____ %   _____
13. OTHER - _____

PSF(AA-29)

FIG. 14-21. Nursing forms for Intravenous Additive Service. *Facing Page:* (*Top*) Nursing unit stock solutions charge voucher. (*Center*) Solution return form. (*Bottom*) Medication order revision. *Above:* Intravenous solution emergency order. (University of Texas at Houston, M. D. Anderson Hospital and Tumor Institute)

3. To provide properly labeled admixtures with regard to uniformity of contents, stability, flow rate desired, etc.

Before such a program is undertaken, extensive groundwork must be carried out to assure its success. Initial investigation of present hospital policies and procedures in regard to IV fluid administration should be made. Additionally, surveys of the number of intravenous fluids to which drugs are added and

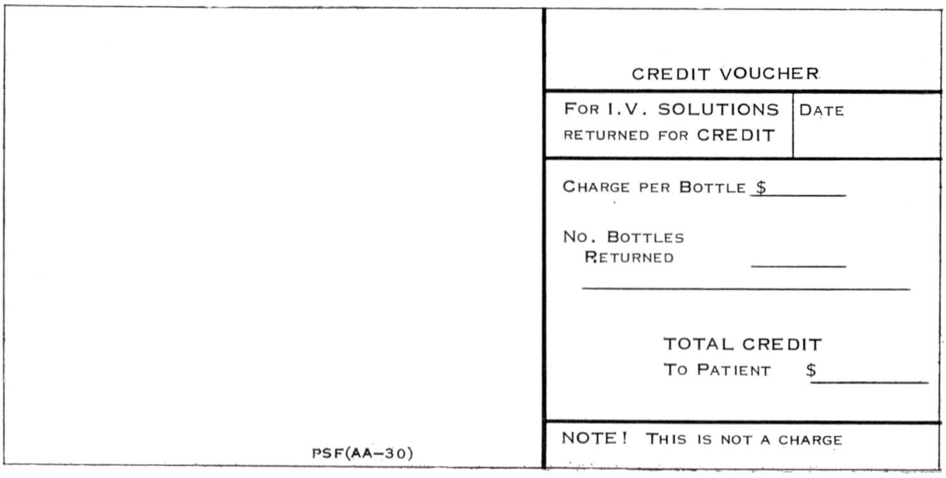

CREDIT VOUCHER

| For I.V. SOLUTIONS RETURNED FOR CREDIT | Date |

CHARGE PER BOTTLE $ _____

No. BOTTLES
RETURNED   _____

TOTAL CREDIT
To Patient $ _____

NOTE! THIS IS NOT A CHARGE

PSF(AA-30)

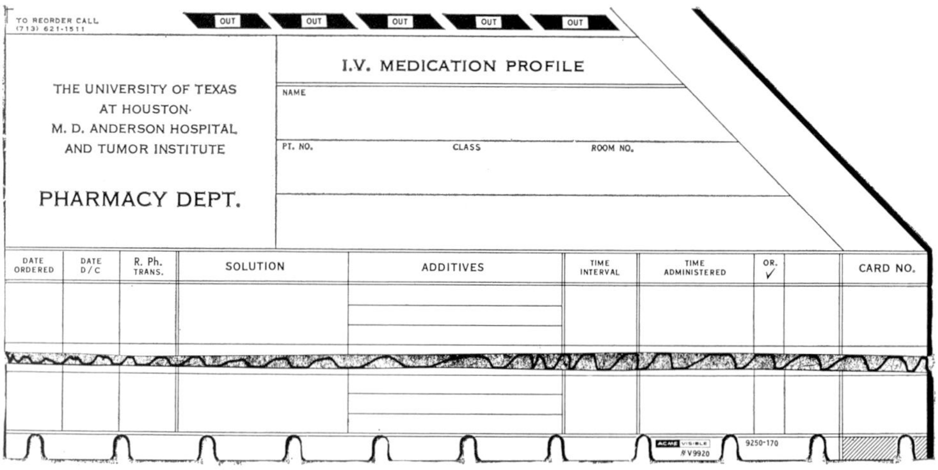

TO REORDER CALL
(713) 621-1511

| OUT | OUT | OUT | OUT | OUT |

I.V. MEDICATION PROFILE

THE UNIVERSITY OF TEXAS
AT HOUSTON·
M. D. ANDERSON HOSPITAL
AND TUMOR INSTITUTE

NAME

PT. NO.   CLASS   ROOM NO.

PHARMACY DEPT.

DATE ORDERED	DATE D/C	R. Ph. TRANS.	SOLUTION	ADDITIVES	TIME INTERVAL	TIME ADMINISTERED	OR. ✓	CARD NO.

ACME VISIBLE
V 9920   9250-170

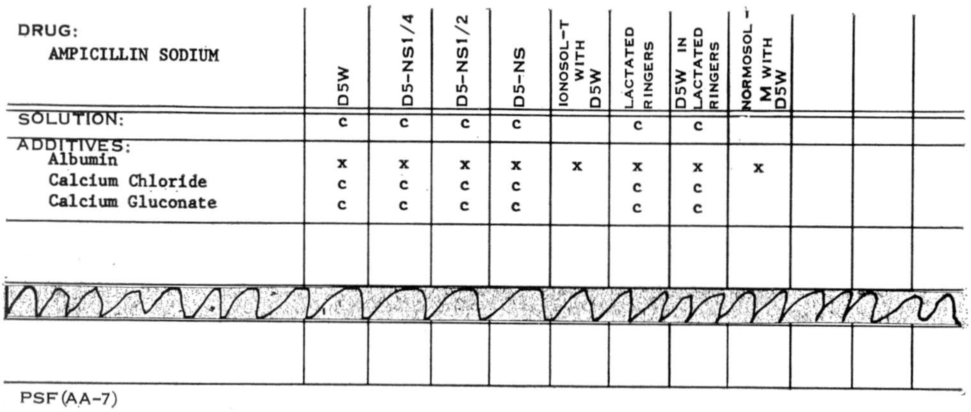

DRUG: AMPICILLIN SODIUM	D5W	D5-NS1/4	D5-NS1/2	D5-NS	IONOSOL-T WITH D5W	LACTATED RINGERS	D5W IN LACTATED RINGERS	NORMOSOL-M WITH D5W			
SOLUTION:	c	c	c	c		c	c				
ADDITIVES: Albumin	x	x	x	x	x	x	x	x			
Calcium Chloride	c	c	c	c		c	c				
Calcium Gluconate	c	c	c	c		c	c				

PSF(AA-7)

FIG. 14-22. Various forms for use by the pharmacy department for the Intravenous Additive Service program. (*Top*) Credit voucher. (*Center*) I.V. medication profile. (*Bottom*) Individual drug incompatibility chart. (The University of Texas at Houston, M. D. Anderson Hospital and Tumor Institute)

the number of venous punctures performed are necessary to determine the pattern and scope of the service.

In establishing an IV additive service, several administrative and logistical problems must be solved. For example:

1. What special forms are needed for both nursing service and pharmacy service to requisition and control?

An example of a set of forms that can be used is shown in Figures 14-21 and 14-22. The forms designed for such an operation should be easy to use, specific in nature and compatible with other existing forms.

2. How are the requisitions to be transmitted to the pharmacy?

Most hospitals utilize their present method of order transmission with certain modifications such as the use of a telephone for each new additive order. This method permits the initial IV order to be prepared at the earliest possible time so that there is little delay in the start of therapy. The transcribed telephone order is compared with the written order before the admixture leaves the pharmacy. These procedures should be outlined explicitly in writing and presented to all involved personnel before the system begins its operation.

3. Will the prepared IV fluids be available for use when needed?

To minimize the problem of late or lost orders, all IV drug requisitions should be divided into two classes: those needed for immediate treatment of life-threatening emergencies and those representing the routine or "non-emergency" solutions. Since it is common practice for physicians to indicate the time period for which they expect a specified volume to run, it is relatively easy for the pharmacist to plan ahead for additional doses.

4. What type facilities should be available for this type of service?

It is strongly recommended that a clean air center be established for all procedures in the reconstituting and adding of parenteral fluids. The most common method of providing this type of environment is through the use of either a horizontal or a vertical laminar flow work area that utilizes a HEPA (high efficiency particulate air) filter. The laminar flow hoods are available from a num-

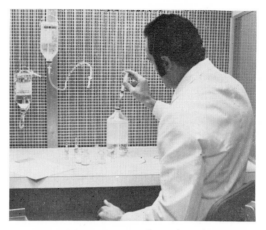

Fig. 14-23. Preparation of an intravenous admixture, utilizing a laminar flow hood. (Bexar County Hospital, San Antonio, Texas)

ber of companies varying from compact counter-top models to large flow units.

Additional equipment recommended for this area are storage carts or cabinets for stock solutions, additives, and other necessary items, a small refrigerator (between 1 and 2 cubic feet capacity), a Purdum-Gregorek soluter for mass reconstitution of lyophilized injectables, a B-D Cornwall pipette, a Fermpress hand-operated decapper and a Fermpress hand-operated crimper, a pH meter, empty vials of various capacities and rubber closures and caps.

INSPECTION OF NURSING-STATION MEDICATION UNITS

The monthly inspection of each nursing-station medication unit by the chief pharmacist and the director of nursing as part of their supervisory duties has been discussed previously. Outdated and surplus stock is kept to a minimum by this routine inspection. Label and container condition is detected quickly; also, violations of hospital regulations relative to narcotics, hypnotics and other controlled drugs are subject to exposure by alert inspections.

OUTPATIENT DEPARTMENT

The outpatient prescription service is another vital activity performed by the hospital pharmacist. Inasmuch as many of the factors to be considered here are the same as those involved in the dispensing of prescriptions at the community pharmacy, this topic will be treated by mention of only those key points to be observed in maintaining a well-operated department.

Labels should be typed neatly and should carry the prescription number, the date, the patient's full name, the signa and the physician's name as well as the name and the address of the hospital and the initials or name of the pharmacist. (Some hospitals require that the prescription contents (medication identification and strength) also be typed on the label unless prescriber requests otherwise.)

Proper "strip" or "supplementary" labels should be used.

The pharmacist should present the patient with the prescription and should be willing to discuss the directions for use as well as any other information relevant to the safety of the patient.

"Counter prescribing," attempts to diagnose, discussion of prescriptions in a derogatory manner with a patient, or discussion of the disease or the ailment for which the pharmacist believes the prescription is intended, are, of course, prohibited by ethics.

EMERGENCY AND ANTIDOTAL DRUGS CABINET

Most hospital pharmacies maintain an emergency cabinet stocked with ready-to-use emergency and antidotal drugs and information on clinical toxicology. This is especially important today with the increased number of household and economic poison cases entering the hospital. The contents of such kits is properly the responsibility of the pharmacy committee of the hospital. Periodic inspection and replenishment of these supplies is the duty of the pharmacist.

DRUG CHARGES

The hospital should have an approved uniform schedule for the charging of drugs. There are several systems in use. They may be classified as:

1. The all-inclusive or no-special-charge

TABLE 14-1. TYPICAL LIST OF EMERGENCY AND ANTIDOTAL DRUGS

PARENTERALS
Aminophylline 250 mg./10 ml.
Amyl nitrite, ampuls
Atropine Sulfate 0.4 mg./ml.
BAL in oil, 10%, 4.5 ml.
Caffeine sodium benzoate 500 mg./2 ml.
Calcium gluconate 1 Gm./10 ml.
Digoxin 0.25 mg./ml.
Diphenhydramine hydrochloride 50 mg./ml.
Diphenylhydantoin sodium 250 mg. vial
Epinephrine hydrochloride 1 : 1000
Heparin sodium 10,000 u./ml.
Hydrocortisone-21-phosphate 100 mg.
Isoproterenol 1 mg./ml.
Lidocaine 4%
Magnesium sulfate ampuls 10% and 50%
Metaraminol bitartrate 10 mg./ml.
Mannitol 25%
Methylphenidate hydrochloride 10 mg./ml.
Nalorphine hydrochloride 5 mg./ml.
Neostigmine methylsulfate 0.25 mg./ml.
Norepinephrine 0.2%
Pentobarbital sodium 50 mg./ml.
Pentylenetetrazole hydrochloride 100 mg./ml.
Phenobarbital sodium 120 mg./ml.
Phenylephrine hydrochloride 10 mg./ml.
Phytonadione 50 mg./ml.
Picrotoxin 3 mg./ml.
Procainamide hydrochloride 100 mg./ml.
Protamine sulfate 10 mg./ml.
Propranolol 1 mg./ml.
Quinidine sulfate 200 mg./ml.
Sodium bicarbonate 3.75 Gm.
Sodium chloride for injection
Sodium lactate
Water for injection

ORAL PREPARATIONS
Cornstarch
Cottonseed oil
Magnesium sulfate
Milk of magnesia
Mineral oil
Sodium bicarbonate
Universal antidote

rate. The cost of medications is absorbed in the all-inclusive day rate.

2. A part-inclusive rate. Charges are made for medications not on the "free" or "supplied" list.

3. A cost-plus rate (see Zugich system in Table 14-2)

4. A flat rate for each outpatient prescription

5. The suggested list or fair-trade price

6. Actual cost of medication plus a professional fee (the preferred system and one that is growing in acceptance).

TABLE 14-2. ZUGICH SYSTEM FOR DETERMINING DRUG CHARGES*

A hospital can use this equation as one basis for reasonable, consistent drug charges. Cost fluctuations and differences in dollar value thus may be adjusted and the pharmacist may maintain better control of his department, its surplus earnings, its financial needs and its fairness to hospital and patient.

$$\frac{\text{Desired income from drugs}}{\text{Cost of prescription drugs}} \times 100 = \frac{\text{per cent above cost to be charged for prescriptions}}$$

1. Determine desired income from drugs.
2. Divide desired income by cost of prescription drugs.
3. Multiply the result by 100.

In one hospital, where no profit from prescription drugs was desired, the formula was used in this manner:

1. Desired income, based on cost of medications issued without charge to patients:

Total nursing-unit expense ...	3,153.06
Auxiliary professional-unit expense	280.83
Narcotics	80.00
Nuisance prescriptions	215.38
Pharmacy salaries and other expense	1,284.62
Desired income (tabulation)..	5,013.89
Desired surplus earnings	00.00
Desired income to meet expenses	5,013.89

2. Cost of prescription drugs $6,430.00
3. Above cost percentage

$$\frac{\$5,013.89 \text{ (desired income)}}{\$6,430 \text{ (prescription cost)}} \times 100 = 78 \frac{\text{(per cent above cost to be charged for prescriptions)}}$$

The 78 per cent represents the mark-up necessary to meet all pharmacy costs and to place the pharmacy on a self-paying basis with no desired profit.

*From John Zugich. University Hospitals, University of Michigan, Ann Arbor.

PURCHASING

Normally, drug supplies for hospitals are purchased in one of the following ways: (1) by bid, (2) by direct order to the pharmaceutical or the chemical house or (3) from the local wholesaler. However, the subjects of drug buying and pharmacy administration —in general like subjects such as the manufacture of sterile and nonsterile preparations, ophthalmic solutions, formulation studies, pharmaceutical research and kindred technical problems common to the profession— are not within the scope of this chapter. Much of this material is to be found either in this volume or in Sprowls' *American Pharmacy*.

CENTRAL STERILE SUPPLY

Some of the larger pharmacies operate as subdepartments the central sterile supply service of the hospital. This department is responsible for providing sterile items such as dressings, syringes, needles, sterile solutions (parenteral and surgical), trays and similar items. The smooth functioning of this activity is accomplished best by bringing problems in this area to the pharmacy committee and a special procedure committee representing nursing and pharmacy.

MANAGEMENT RESPONSIBILITIES

Good management on the part of a department head presupposes his ability to combine the factors of men and money, time and "tools" to produce an efficient, economical end product—in this instance, a good pharmaceutical service.

No department head can expect to perform this feat without the management tools of responsibility and accountability. The tools of management, other than men and money, needed for sound hospital pharmacy administration are:

1. An inventory policy
   A. Storage
   B. Perpetual inventory records
2. A monthly or quarterly and an annual reporting system of workloads and costs

INVENTORY POLICY—STORES

The first point usually considered in discussing inventories is one of location. Where

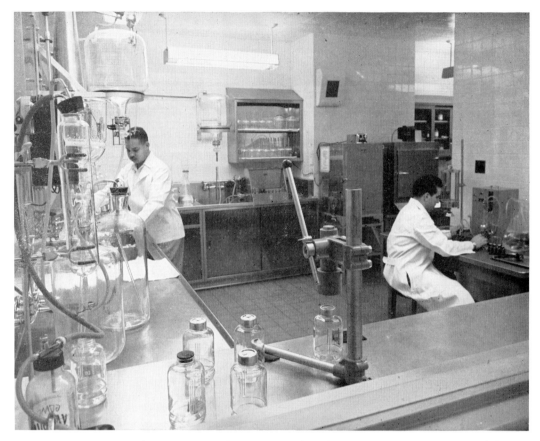

Fig. 14-24. Section of the central sterile supply service of the pharmaceutical service of the Clinical Center of the National Institutes of Health. (U.S.P.H.S.)

should the bulk-drug inventory items be stored? What is the best storage place for pharmacy supplies—in a general storeroom or in a separate storeroom attached to and part of the pharmacy?

Management experts all agree that, in general, a common or central storeroom is ideal. Inventory is controlled and labor and record keeping are lessened by such a procedure. However, many well-founded rules have exceptions, and pharmacy is the exception here —there is no question that, in the interest of economy and efficiency, there should be a separate pharmacy storeroom under the complete control of the Pharmacy Department and as close to it as possible.

In arriving at the policy that drug supplies should be stored in *separate* pharmacy storerooms under the jurisdiction of the chief pharmacist as against any dichotomous ar-

rangement involving general supplies, an analysis is made of the factors of public health and safety as well as those of efficiency and economy. A few of these fundamental considerations are the 4 following:

1. Responsibility for storage of drugs, many of which deteriorate by improper storage, is given to those who by their education and training are best qualified to assume this responsibility.

2. Rapid changes in drug-therapy trends and the prescribing habits of physicians and dentists usually are known immediately by the pharmacist. This information is not commonly held by other persons involved with supplies; it is necessary in properly determining reorder amounts and/or the addition and the deletion of items in the drug inventory.

3. Such a system of operation gives im-

mediate availability and knowledge of persons of supplies to the department which has the sole authority to use the stock—the pharmacy department. This ensures more efficient service and lowers the amount of capital invested in drug supplies as contrasted with the amount of investment required in any other system. It also couples with the responsibility of maintenance of vital drug inventories the necessary management companion—accountability.

4. Stock-control and inventory-cost records are made by pharmacy personnel at or close to the time of the action; thus, lengthy delays in posting and preparation of requisitions, as well as duplication of effort, are avoided.

This basic pattern for the control of drug supplies and stores follows principles laid down by Malcolm T. MacEachern, M.D., former associate director of the American College of Surgeons. Dr. MacEachern, in his text on *Hospital Organization and Management,* states that:

. . . in selecting a location it must not be forgotten that ample space is required for bulk storage and that this storeroom (pharmacy) is preferably located on the ground floor *close to the pharmacy* . . . that the purchase of drugs and pharmaceuticals is a specialty which can be carried out to the best advantage by a pharmacist trained in managing a hospital pharmacy. . . . This is the only department in the hospital in which it is usually *not* advisable to have purchasing done by a general purchasing agent.

STOREROOM ARRANGEMENT AND CONTROL OF STOCK

Dating of Stocks. Sound business management indicates that money invested in drug supplies be turned over 4 to 5 times yearly. This is called "stock turn." Normally, a stock turn of less than 4 indicates an over-inventory and of over 5, "outs" and shortages.

Therefore, as the first step in a program of sound inventory control, all expendable drug items, when received into stores, should be marked or stamped with the month and the year of receipt. For example, an item received on February 15, 1970, should be marked or stamped in small print "2/70."

The introduction of such a dating system

ensures the use of old stocks first and makes more noticeable any overbuying on a particular item.

Drug-Stock Arrangement. Drug supplies maintained as stores (not expended to the pharmacy proper, but kept in the pharmacy storeroom) should be arranged in simple alphabetical order with 5 exceptions:

1. GALLONAGE. Gallon containers should be arranged and maintained *in alphabetical order* in a separate section or stored on bottom shelves.

2. PERISHABLES such as biologicals, antibiotics and others should be stored in properly refrigerated units.

3. NARCOTICS. These should be stored in properly locked containers that satisfy the regulations of the Harrison Narcotic Act and local authorities.

4. ALCOHOL, SPIRITUOUS LIQUORS AND WINES. These should be stored in properly locked, fireproof cabinets that meet the requirements of the Federal codes and the local laws, including fire regulations.

5. LARGE BULK ITEMS. Liter parenterals, plasma, gases and others.

"Shelf-Stripping." This consists of applying tape (the width of the rim of the shelf), capable of carrying writing, to the upper front edge of shelves. The information and the rulings on the tape indicate the "home" of each particular item. Each item is allotted a definite width of the shelf for its accommodation. *Example:*

Acetylsalicylic Acid Tablets 325 mg. (4) 5,000	Acid Fuchsin (1) 10 g.	Agar (2) LB.

Information on the tape may give the name (acetylsalicylic acid tablets), the strength, if any (325 mg.), the unit quantity (5,000), as well as the minimum level (4) or reorder point. "Shelf-stripping," besides providing a double check against shortages, ensures a definite width of space on the shelf as the "home" for the item. The item is set directly back of the tape in the space designated. The markings on the tape may be erased and changed several times before a new tape is required.

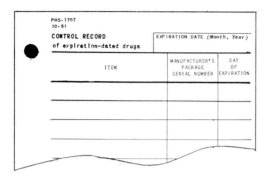

FIG. 14-25. Biological stock control form.
(U.S.P.H.S.)

PERPETUAL INVENTORY RECORDS

With drug stock systematically arranged in a pharmacy storeroom, the task of setting up and maintaining a perpetual inventory system becomes fairly simple. For this purpose, use of a visible Kardex or similar type drawer file appears to offer the ideal solution.

This system provides a standard method of controlling stock levels, ensuring availability of supplies, the reporting of drug-usage rates and a monthly inventory value on each item stocked. Inasmuch as current statistics indicate that 25 to 33 per cent of every supply dollar at a hospital goes into drug purchases, the value of sound records in the pharmacy department cannot be underestimated.

Operation of Inventory Control System. Normally, the chief pharmacist places the responsibility of posting to the stock cards and the accuracy of the records, including the accuracy of inventory and the correction of extensions, on one person, usually a competent pharmacy helper. This person is given the responsibility for drug receipts, withdrawals, perpetual inventory records and storeroom arrangement in addition to his other duties. In practice, it has been found that, when the pharmacy helper has been properly selected and trained, he is well qualified to assume this responsibility. Obviously, in one-man pharmacies, this responsibility must rest on the pharmacist himself.

The person made responsible for the periodic checking of physical stocks against the perpetual inventory records should be instructed to check items in at least 2 letters of the alphabet weekly, i.e., A and B items one week, C and D items the next week and so on. Neat stock arrangement; clean, dust-free storeroom; and accurate unit and extension cost records in the perpetual inventory usually result when such a check system is employed. Furthermore, such a check system gives, annually, 4 complete physical checks of supplies against records plus the usual official physical inventory taken at the close of the fiscal year.

Some hospitals have found it convenient to locate the stock-control records just inside the entrance of the pharmacy storeroom where postings of inflow and outflow of stock may be made at the time of the action.

Purchase requests for supplies usually are prepared when the minimum or reorder point is reached on the stock-control cards; however, in determining reorder amounts and/or the addition and deletion of items from the drug inventory, such factors as drug-therapy trends and changes in medical and dental staffs also must be taken into consideration. As a rule, except in emergencies, purchase requests for supplies are submitted to the Purchasing Department on certain designated days. Purchase requests should be dated and prepared in duplicate with the carbon retained in a "requisitions pending" file in the pharmacy. Copies of purchase orders issued for pharmacy supplies by the hospital should be routed to the pharmacy where they are stapled to copies of the requisitions. This material is kept in an "orders pending" file until receipt of the stock, at which time it is filed for the duration of the fiscal year in the contractor's folder on file in the pharmacy.

It will be noted that items expended from the storeroom to the pharmacy proper are not included in the inventory value. The value of such items may be kept at a constant figure for a 12-month period, when a new physical inventory provides the adjustment factor. While it is admitted that this is not an accurate inventory figure, for 11 months out of the 12, it is correct as of the last month of each fiscal year and does not impose the cost of an expensive physical inventory of open stock each month.

A QUARTERLY AND ANNUAL REPORTING SYSTEM FOR COSTS AND WORKLOADS

It is the responsibility of chiefs of pharmaceutical services to provide the administrator with a quarterly or monthly and yearly yardstick with which to measure departmental activity and progress.

This report is one of the major tools of management. Through it, a department head documents his needs for a larger or a smaller budget, for increased or decreased personnel, for equipment and for other needs.

A hospital might well adopt a combination professional–business-type report. In such a report, the quarterly or monthly professional workload factors could be divided into inpatient and outpatient activities. The workload might be broken also into various categories, such as those requiring special accounting as made necessary by Federal and state laws (narcotics and ethyl alcohol), and those categories not entailing extra manhours of bookkeeping.

In brief, the workload of the pharmacy is presented as a report of specific areas of major activity. Each prescription, requisition or issue to a ward or a clinic and each manufactured item and item prepackaged is tabulated.

Space may be provided in the quarterly or monthly workload report for reporting pharmacy committee meetings and their activities, as well as space for remarks on pharmacy activities of the quarter or the month, such as clinical-pharmaceutical research, new equipment received, papers prepared for publication, drug-therapy consultant activities and other matters.

Finally, the reporting system should provide for noting the number of group meetings, both intramural and extramural. This is a valued part of the report inasmuch as it covers "nonmeasurable workloads." In hospital pharmacy, considerable time is devoted to "nonmeasurable" loads such as individual consultations on drug-therapy problems with medical, dental and allied personnel; hospital pharmacy indoctrination and teaching schedules for medical and dental interns, nurses and hospital aides; also man hours are consumed in the requisitioning or purchasing of

supplies, the keeping of perpetual narcotic, hypnotic, grain-alcohol and spirituous-liquor inventories; the preparation of the quarterly or monthly reports on stock control, drug costs, workloads, indoctrination and teaching of junior hospital pharmacists and, in some instances, senior pharmacy students; as well as time spent in attendance and preparation for staff and pharmacy committee meetings.

Total personnel is reported in Part III of the monthly or quarterly report form (Fig. 14-26, *top* and *bottom*) used to illustrate the reporting system described. All personnel assigned to the department, even though part of their time is spent in other areas, are reported with this system. This serves to bring to the attention of the administrator the added responsibilities of pharmacy personnel in nonpharmaceutical duties.

Value of Reports. In the quarterly or monthly report, the hospital administrator has a yardstick or measurement tool of the pharmacy department; he knows quarterly or monthly and annually (see annual "recap" sheet, Fig. 14-27, *top* and *bottom*) the professional workload, the committee activities and the personnel structure, as well as the pharmacy's inventory status, inventory or "stock turn," the average cost of medications per outpatient visit, the average cost or value of inpatient medications per inpatient day and the average cost of each prescription. Nothing is left to guess or estimates. Should a department need increased manpower, one has documented proof of the need. Should the administrator be required to cut back on budgeted funds, one again has proof of actual drug needs based on usage rates— proof that the pharmacy budget fund can be released to other areas or that pharmacy funds cannot be cut if normal service flow is to be maintained. To aid in the recording of the statistics indicated in this type report, a daily worksheet is utilized (see Fig. 14-28).

DRUG DISPENSING AS DRUG ADMINISTRATION

Drug administration is a nursing activity by which a single dose is administered to the patient by the nurse on the order of a physician or a dentist.

The filling or the refilling of a nursing sta-

Name of Reporting Station | Location | Report for

(Quarter)　(Fiscal Year)

PART I - PHARMACEUTICAL ACTIVITIES

Description	Number of Items		
	Inpatient	Outpatient	Total
1. Prescriptions and Requisitions			
(a) Ethyl Alcohol, Wines, and Spirituous Liquors			
(b) Narcotics			
(c) Hypnotics			
(d) Regular			
(e) Total - Prescriptions and Requisitions			
2. Issues to Nursing Units, Clinics, and Outpatient Services (Includes issues to Outpatient Services of reporting hospital)			
3. Issues to Other Facilities (Includes all items - clinic drugs, prepackaged patient medication, etc.)			
4. Bulk Compounded Items (Considered as inpatient activity in Hospitals)			
5. Prepackaged Units			
6. Total Workload Units (Items 1 through 5)			

PART II - INVENTORY STATUS

Description	Pharmacy Supplies - Dollar Value		
(Figures for Items 2 and 4 are to be taken from Pharmacy Storeroom Stock Control Records)	(a) Special - Item A Antibiotics	(b) Special - Item B	(c) All other Pharmacy Supplies
			(d) Total - All Items
1. Beginning Inventory (Beginning of each quarter)			
2. Purchases Received (During Quarter)			
3. Available Inventory (Item 1 plus Item 2)			
4. Closing Inventory (End of Quarter)			
5. Supplies Issued (Total during Quarter) (Item 3 minus Item 4)			
6. Supplies Issued to Other Facilities (If applicable)			
7. Supplies Issued for Station Use (Item 5 minus Item 6)			
8. Annual Stock Turn Estimated (Item 5d X 4 divided by Item 4d)			

Remarks

PART III - UNIT VALUE OF DRUGS ISSUED

1. Value of Drugs Issued During Quarter (Part II, Item 7, Column (d))	
2. Outpatient Visits During Quarter (To be Supplied by Medical Record Office)	
3. Cost per Outpatient Visit (Cost for Clinics = Item 1 ÷ Item 2; Cost for Hospitals = January or July Costs of all Medications and Containers Issued for Outpatient purposes divided by number of Outpatient Visits for that Month, to be computed by Chief Pharmacist each January and July)	
4. Number of Outpatient Prescriptions Dispensed during Quarter, Clinics only (Part I, Item 1e, Outpatient Column)	
5. Cost per Outpatient Prescription (Cost for Clinics = Item 1 ÷ Item 4; Cost for Hospitals = January or July Costs of all Medications and containers issued for Outpatient Prescriptions divided by the number of Outpatient Prescriptions for the month, to be computed by Chief Pharmacist each January and July)	
(Items 6, 7, and 8 for hospitals only)	
6. Estimated Value of Outpatient Medications (Item 2 X Item 3)	100%
7. Estimated Value of Inpatient Medications (Item 1 – Item 6)	%
8. Inpatient Days During Quarter (To be supplied by Medical Record Office)	%
9. Average Cost of Inpatient Medications per Inpatient Day (Item 7 – Item 8)	

PHS-1310-1 (REV. 4-62)　PHARMACY OPERATIONS - QUARTERLY REPORT

FIG. 14-26. Quarterly report of pharmacy operations, parts I, II and III. (U.S.P.H.S.)

PART IV - MEETINGS AND COMMENTS

1. Number of Pharmacy Committee meetings held during Quarter? ____________

2. (A) Remarks on Pharmacy activities during the quarter. *(Research; formula development; significant changes in inventory and/or workload; equipment received; papers published; attach separate statement if necessary, etc.)*

   (B) If pertinent, have you attached a list of drugs *(1)* added; *(2)* deleted; *(3)* in investigational status this period? ☐ Yes ☐ No

3. Special Studies Report
   (a) ____________ *(b)* ____________ *(c)* ____________

4. Number of group conferences held
   (a) Intramural ____________ *(b)* Extramural ____________

PART V - PERSONNEL CURRENTLY ON DUTY *(Show all Positions By Grade And Number In Grade)*

Position Title	Grade or Rank	No.	Position Title	Grade or Rank	No.
1. Pharmacist, Chief			5. Clerical		
2. Pharmacist, Ass't. Chief			6. Pharmacy Helper - Storekeeper		
3. Pharmacists, Staff			7. Pharmacy Helper		
4. Pharmacy Interne			8. Other *(Specify)*		
			9. Total		

Other Duties *(Indicate percent of time spent on other duties by Pharmacy personnel and type of such duties)*

Position	Percent	Type of Duty

PART VI - ISSUES TO OTHER FACILITIES *(Exclusive of direct Station Activity)*

Name of Installation	No. of Units	Value	Name of Installation	No. of Units	Value
1.			5.		
2.			6.		
3.			7.		
4.			Total		

PART VII - MEDICARE PRESCRIPTIONS

1. Number of Prescriptions	
2. Total Cost of Prescriptions	
3. Average Cost per Prescription *(Item 2 ÷ Item 1)*	
4. Number of Outpatients Served by this Service	

REMARKS

DISTRIBUTION OF COPIES *(one each to)*

Division Headquarters, c/o Pharmacy Branch
Medical Officer in Charge
Pharmacy
Medical Records Office
Fiscal Office

Prepared by *(Signature of Chief Pharmacist)*	Date Prepared	Approved by *(Signature of Medical Officer in Charge)*

FIG. 14-26 (*Continued*). Quarterly report of pharmacy operations, parts IV, V and VI. (U.S.P.H.S.)

PHARMACY OPERATIONS SUMMARY

LOCATION OF STATION

FOR FISCAL YEAR

PART I – PHARMACEUTICAL ACTIVITIES

1. Prescriptions and Requisitions

QUARTER	(a) Ethyl Alcohol, etc.	(b) Narcotics	(c) Hypnotics	(d) Regular	(e) Total	2. Issues to Nursing Units, Clinics and Outpatient Services	3. Issues to Other Facilities	4. Bulk Compounded Items	5. Prepackaged Units	6. Total Workload Units (Items 1, 2, 3, 4 and 5)
1st										
2nd										
3rd										
4th										
Total										

PART II – INVENTORY STATUS

2. Purchases Received

QUARTER	(a) Special – Item A Antibiotics	(b) Special – Item B	(c) All Other Pharmacy Supplies	(d) Total All Items	4. Closing Inventory (a) Special – Item A Antibiotics	(b) Special – Item B	(c) All Other Pharmacy Supplies	(d) Total All Items	5. Total Supplies Issued (a) Special – Item A Antibiotics	(b) Special – Item B	(c) All Other Pharmacy Supplies	(d) Total All Items
1st												
2nd												
3rd												
4th												
Total					(Average)	(Average)	(Average)	(Average)				

6. Supplies Issued to Other Facilities (If applicable)

QUARTER	(a) Special – Item A Antibiotics	(b) Special – Item B	(c) All Other Pharmacy Supplies	(d) Total All Items	7. Supplies Issued for Station Use (a) Special – Item A Antibiotics	(b) Special – Item B	(c) All Other Pharmacy Supplies	(d) Total All Items
1st								
2nd								
3rd								
4th								
Total								

8. ACTUAL STOCK TURN (Annual)

A. Total supplies issued for year (5d) _____
B. Average closing inventory (4d) _____
C. Stock turn (A ÷ B) (carry to one decimal place) _____

INVENTORY STATUS (June 30 – End of F.Y.)
1. No. of items (cards) on perpetual inventory June 30 _____
2. No. of items (cards) showing no activity during the last 12 months _____
3. Dollar value of item 1 above _____
4. Dollar value of item 2 above _____
5. No. of items (cards) having issues during last 12 months but with more than 12 months supply on hand _____
6. Dollar value of item 5 above _____
7. Stock turn end of F.Y. based on closing inventory (A above ÷ item 3 above) (carry to one decimal place) _____

PHS-1330-2
REV. 2-62

Fig. 14-27. Annual "recap" sheet, parts I and II. (U.S.P.H.S.)

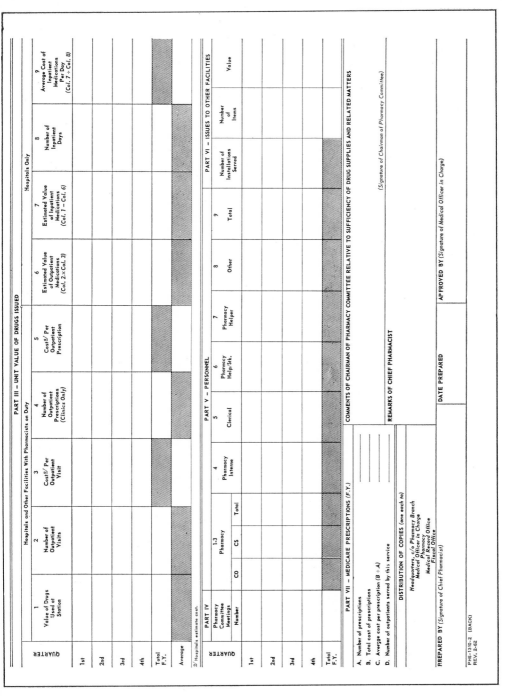

Fig. 14-27. (*Continued*). Annual "recap" sheet, parts III, IV, V, VI and VII. (U.S.P.H.S.)

[613]

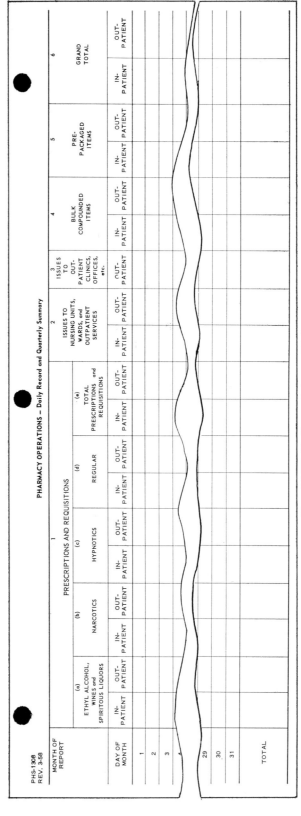

Fig. 14-28. Daily worksheet. (U.S.P.H.S.)

tion medication container with the drug called for is "drug dispensing" and can be engaged in legally only by a licensed pharmacist under the Pharmacy Practice Act and the regulations of the several states.

The public health point at issue concerns patient safety and error control. Should a nurse remove a single dose from a wrong container the damage is confined to the patient in her charge. However, should the nurse perform an act restricted by law to trained pharmacists (drug dispensing), such as the refilling of a patient's prescription or a floor stock medication container, it is possible that an error may injure *all* patients who subsequently receive medication from that container, whether the medication is "administered" by the nurse making the error or other nurses on duty at the medication center where the container is housed.

One must study automation activities in this light: automation equipment that bestows "drug dispensing" responsibilities on nurses, or "drug administration" activities on pharmacists is, quite likely, illegal under the laws of the states. Such equipment places in the hands of individuals responsibilities which they have not been trained to handle. For example, nurses are trained by formal study and experience in "drug administration," i.e., to observe in the giving of a medication the outward signs of reactions such as changes in respiration, pulse and myotic or mydriatic reactions. Pharmacists, on the other hand, are trained in drug evaluation, selection, storage, *identification,* compounding and dispensing characteristics. The following practice would quite likely be in violation of state laws and regulations: if a nurse should place a label on a medication container or otherwise identify the container as prepared for a particular patient when the amount of the medication is in excess of the number of doses to be administered by that nurse during her 8-hour tour of duty, such an act would be drug "dispensing" and not drug "administration."

HOSPITAL PHARMACY RESIDENCIES

A pharmacy residency in a hospital is a postgraduate program of organized training that meets the requirements set forth and ap-

proved by the American Society of Hospital Pharmacists. The resident participates in a predetermined and regular schedule supervised in all of the activities of pharmacy service as indicated in Table 14-3. The training covers a minimum of 2,000 hours training time and extends over a period of at least 50 weeks.

Residencies approved by the American Society of Hospital Pharmacists may be given only in general hospitals accredited by the Joint Commission on Accreditation or the American Osteopathic Association. Furthermore, pharmacy residencies are to be conducted only in those hospitals in which the educational benefits to the resident are considered to be of paramount importance in relation to the service benefits that the hospital may obtain from the resident.

Hospitals wishing information regarding accreditation regulations are urged to write to The American Society of Hospital Pharmacists, Washington, D.C., for the *Guide to Interpretation and Use for Accreditation Standard For Residency in Hospital Pharmacy.*

TABLE 14-3. ACTIVITIES OF PHARMACY SERVICE AND MINIMUM TIME TO BE SPENT BY A RESIDENT IN HOSPITAL PHARMACY

ACTIVITY	HOURS
Departmental Administration	200
Outpatient Dispensing and Control	100
Inpatient Drug Distribution and Control	300
Formulation, Preparation and Control of Sterile Dosage Forms ..	100
Formulation, Preparation and Control of Non-sterile Products	100
Drug Information Services	100
Clinical Services in Patient Care Areas	100
Collateral and Interdepartmental Activities	100
Lectures, Conferences and Seminars	100

BIBLIOGRAPHY

American College of Surgeons: Manual of Hospital Standardization, 1946.
American Hospital Association: The Magic Key to Hospital Literature.

————: Statement of principles on the use of investigational drugs in hospitals, Hospitals, January 1, 1958.

————: The hospital formulary system, Hospitals, October 16, 1960.

————: Editorial Notes—Formula for formulary Hospitals, July 1, 1963, p. 23.

————: Guide Issue, Hospitals, August 1, 1969, Vol. 43, Part 2.

American Society of Hospital Pharmacists: Minimum standards for pharmacy internships in hospitals with guide to application, as amended Jan. 1, 1966.

————: Accreditation standard for residency in hospital pharmacy, April 11, 1970, Am. J. Hosp. Pharm.

————: Statement on the abilities required of hospital pharmacists, Am. J. Hosp. Pharm. 19:493, 1962.

————: Constitution and bylaws, as revised 1969.

————: Goals for Hospital Pharmacy, Am. J. Hosp. Pharm., 21:535, 1964.

————: Guidelines for Single-Unit Packages, Am. J. Hosp. Pharm., 24:79, 1967.

————: Statement on Research in Hospital Pharmacy, Am. J. Hosp. Pharm., 21:537, 1964.

————: Statement on Hospital Drug Distribution Systems, Am. J. Hosp. Pharm., 21:535, 1964.

————: The Hospital Pharmacist and Drug Information Services, Am. J. Hosp. Pharm., 25:381, 1968.

Archambault, G. F.: Hospital pharmacy as a career, Sci. Counselor 17:61, 1954.

————: A narcotic control system for the general hospital, Hospitals 28:112, 1954.

————: Procedural manuals for hospital pharmacies, Am. Prof. Pharmacist 19:42, 1953.

————: Hermetically packaged surgical fluids, Pharm. Internat. 6:35, 1952.

————: Practical applications of minimum standards (in 3 parts), Hosp. Prog. 33:90; 33:80; 33:84, 1952.

————: The business side of hospital pharmacy, Bull. Am. Soc. Hosp. Pharmacists 9: 102, 1952.

————: Standards for prescription containers, Bull. Am. Soc. Hosp. Pharmacists 8:108, 1951.

Arthur, W. R.: Law of Drugs and Druggists, ed. 3, St. Paul, Minn., West, 1947.

Barker, K. N., and Heller, W. M.: The development of a centralized unit dose dispensing system, part I, Am. J. Hosp. Pharm., 20: 568, 1963.

Bierman, C. H., and Archambault, G. F.: The hospital pharmacy from the administrator's point of view, Hosp. Management 57:86, 1944.

Black, H. J., and Tester, W. W.: Decentralized pharmacy operations utilizing the unit dose concept. part I, Am. J. Hosp. Pharm., 21: 345, 1964; part III, Am. J. Hosp. Pharm., 24:120, 1967.

Drawback on Tax on Distilled Spirits Used in Manufacturing of Non-Beverage Products—Regulation No. 29, U.S. Treasury Department, Bureau of Internal Revenue, 1947.

FitzGerald, E. J., and Archambault, G. F.: The Public Health Service, Bull. Am. Soc. Hosp. Pharmacists 9:270, 1952.

Food and Drug Administration: Service and Regulatory Announcements—Food, Drug and Cosmetic No. 1, Revision No. 3, Department of Health, Education, and Welfare.

Francke, D.: Evaluation of management guides, Hosp. Progress, p. 94, September, 1954.

Francke, D. E., Latiolais, C. J., Francke, G. N., and Ho, N. F. H.: Mirror to Hospital Pharmacy, Easton, Pennsylvania, Mack, 1964.

Freund, R. G. A.: A centralized unit dose dispensing program, Hosp. Pharm., 3:13, 1968 (Sept.)

Goodness, J. H.: Personal communications.

Guild of Public Pharmacists: Hospital Pharmacy Planning, ed. 2, London, 1961.

Harrison Narcotic Act—Regulation No. 5 and Supplements (1969), U.S. Treasury Department, Bureau of Narcotics.

Hauser, J.: Federal regulation of unit dose drug packages, Hosp. Pharm., 5:17, 1970.

Himmelsbach, C. K., and Nelson, K.: The Responsibilities and Functions of the Individual Pharmacy Committee Members, U.S. Public Health Service, Division of Hospitals Circular Memorandum No. 54-130, March. 1954.

Hogan, T. J., and Archambault, G. F.: Meeting problems of design in hospital pharmacy, Bull. Am. Soc. Hosp. Pharmacists 10:293, 1953.

Hope, M. C.: The hospital survey and construction program, Am. J. Publ. Health 39:7, 1949.

Hyatt, Hyatt, and Groeschel: Law of Hospital, Physician and Patient, ed. 2, New York, Hospital Text Book, 1952.

Industrial Alcohol: U.S. Treasury Department, Bureau of Internal Revenue, Regulation No. 3 (1942) and Supplements.

Jeffries, S. B.: A new approach to costing and pricing prescriptions in the hospital pharmacy, Bull. Am. Soc. Hosp. Pharmacists 11: 455, 1954.

Joint Commission on Accreditation of Hospitals —Standards for Hospital Accreditation, December, 1953.

Lamy, P. P.: Laminar flow and environmental control, Hosp. Form. Management, *3*:29, 1968 (Oct.)

MacEachern, M. T.: Hospital Organization and Management, Chicago, Physician's Record Co., 1940.

McGibony: Principles of Hospital Administration, New York, Putnam, 1952.

Marihuana Act—Regulation No. 1 (1937), U.S. Treasury Department, Bureau of Narcotics.

Oddis, J. A.: Hospital pharmacy: present tasks, and future challenges, Hospitals, J.A.H.A. *42*:106, 1968.

Oddis, J. A.: Hospital Pharmacy—A Rewarding Career, The Squibb Review.

Parker, P. F.: Unit-dose systems reduce error, increase efficiency, Hospitals: J.A.H.A., *42*: 65, 1968 (Dec. 1).

Petit, W.: Manual of Pharmaceutical Law, New York, Macmillan, 1951.

Ravin, R. L.: An I.V. additive program—suggested procedures, Hosp. Form. Management, *3*:35, 1968 (Oct.).

Regan, L. J.: Doctor and Patient and the Law, ed. 2, St. Louis, Mosby, 1949.

Registration of Stills—Regulation No. 23, U.S. Treasury Department, Bureau of Internal Revenue.

Shoup, L. K., Anderson, R. D., and Latiolais, C. J.: Stability of drugs after reconstitution, Am. J. Hosp. Pharm., *24*:666, 1967.

Skolaut, M., Scigiliano, J., and Salvina, J.: The central sterile supply of a pharmacy department, Bull. Am. Soc. Hosp. Pharmacists 2: 114, 1954.

Sloan, R. P.: This Hospital Business of Ours, New York, Putnam, 1952.

Trautman, J., Masur, J., and Archambault, G. F.: Facilities for pharmaceutical service, Clinical Center, National Institutes of Health, Bull. Am. Soc. Hosp. Pharmacists *9*:38, 1952.

Unit Dose Packaging Report, Richmond, Va., Reynolds Metals Company, 1968.

U.S. Government Printing Office: Operations of the United States Marine-Hospital Service, 1896.

U.S. Public Health Service: Hospital Services, 1953, Pharmacy, Bull. Div. Hosp. Facilities.

Williams, R. C.: The United States Public Health Service, 1798-1950, Bethesda, Md., U.S. Publ. Health Service, 1951.

Zugich, J. J.: Pharmacy, Hospitals *27,* No. 6, Part II, June, 1953.

———: Monthly reports emphasize value of pharmacist to hospital, Bull. Am. Soc. Hosp. Pharmacists *2*:64, 1945.

Note: A comprehensive indexed bibliography on hospital pharmacy has been prepared by the American Society of Hospital Pharmacists; it covers all facets of hospital pharmacy. The student is referred to this bibliography for additional reference material (see Heller, W. M., and Francke, G. N.: Comprehensive bibliography on hospital pharmacy, Am. J. Hosp. Pharm. *22*:213, 1965.)

Chapter 15

Radiopharmaceuticals

William H. Briner*

HISTORY

Although the use of radioactive materials to study and treat some of the ills of mankind is not particularly new, the emergence of radiopharmaceutical products as an important part of the American medical scene has come about largely as a direct result of the weapons technology of World War II. Radium-226 and its radioactive daughter radon-222 had been widely used to treat a variety of pathologic states both in this country and abroad for nearly 40 years before the beginning of World War II. In addition, early in 1936 Dr. Joseph G. Hamilton undertook the first studies of sodium movement in the body using the radionuclide sodium-22, which had been produced in the cyclotron at the Berkeley campus of the University of California.[65] Following this, a number of investigators throughout the world performed studies of thyroid metabolism and the treatment of hyperthyroidism using radioactive iodine derived from particle accelerators.

Then, in December of 1942, occurred an event so remarkably significant that its importance is not understood by many people even today. The incident was, of course, the production of the first controlled chain reaction. This took place in an atomic pile composed of graphite bricks, fueled with natural uranium, located on a squash court beneath Stagg Field at the University of Chicago. This first successful experiment in the criticality of piles, or reactors, was directed by the Italian-born physicist, Enrico

Fermi. The ultrasecret Manhattan District then developed more sophisticated nuclear reactors for the production of fissionable material to be used in atomic bombs.

Large quantities of highly radioactive waste were formed as a result of reactor operations. This by-product material consisted of a number of different radionuclides characterized as "mixed fission products." Appropriate chemical separation processes were developed, and after the cessation of hostilities, some of these radioactive species were diverted to civilian uses, including a number of medical applications.

In those earlier days, the Oak Ridge National Laboratory, a contractor of the U.S. Atomic Energy Commission, served as the primary supplier of all reactor-produced radioactive materials released for nonmilitary use. During the period 1946-1947, the first year in which these substances became available for civilian uses, approximately 280 shipments were made from the Oak Ridge facility to users of all types, including medical.[46] In 1948, the first of the major radiopharmaceutical manufacturers began marketing radioactive pharmaceutical products. Fewer than 1000 shipments were made by this firm during their first year of operation,[71] and an early price sheet listed fewer than 10 radioactive compounds that were then available for diagnostic or therapeutic purposes.[72]

It is interesting to contrast this rather meager beginning with the situation as it exists today. In November, 1965, the Atomic Energy Commission listed more than 6,000 licensees in the medical or medical institutional category.[31] Catalogues of major radiopharmaceutical suppliers list from 40 to 60

* Captain, United States Public Health Service; Chief, Radiopharmaceutical Service, The Clinical Center, National Institutes of Health, Bethesda, Md.

dosage forms available for sale to authorized clinicians and hospitals, and industry shipments in excess of 100,000 annually have been estimated.[53]

PHILOSOPHY OF A RADIOPHARMACEUTICAL SERVICE

In the early days of research in nuclear medicine, it was extremely difficult for a pharmacist to participate or assist in this new area of biomedical investigation, and indeed, few pharmacists expressed any interest in these problems. This is not to say that the need for pharmaceutical expertise was not recognized during this period. The entrance of the first major pharmaceutical manufacturer into the production and distribution of radioactive pharmaceuticals in 1948 signaled the beginning of this era. Two years later, the Vice-Chairman of the Joint Committee on Atomic Energy of the Congress of the United States suggested that atomic energy ought to be a matter of concern to pharmacists,[34] and a professor of pharmaceutical chemistry in a school of pharmacy stated unequivocally that the hospital pharmacist should be prepared to provide information and assistance in radioisotope programs in hospitals.[25] Nevertheless, pharmacists were not involved in this type of practice in the immediate post-war period. Scientists who were engaged in clinical and research activities in this field at that time included physicians, physicists, chemists, engineers and a number of veterinarians.

However, in the ensuing years, during which time radiopharmaceutical products have become firmly established in value and use, pharmacists have become more acutely aware of their abilities and responsibilities in this area of practice. Numerous monographs for radiopharmaceutical dosage forms now appear in the current revision of the *United States Pharmacopeia*[54] and the *National Formulary*.[51] Many schools of pharmacy now include courses of instruction in radiopharmaceutical topics, both at the undergraduate and the graduate level. Thus, certain professional deficiencies formerly evident in the curricula of many schools of pharmacy are fast disappearing, although in reality, these deficiencies in the past were frequently given too much emphasis by non-pharmacy personnel in evaluating the abilities of pharmacists in these areas. For example, it is true that very few pharmacists, even today, are also nuclear physicists or radiation chemists. It is also true that most pharmacists are not doctors of medicine. However, this fact does not prohibit some of them from engaging in professional practice involving the formulation of injectable products used by physicians in their practice.

The important point to remember is that some additional training is usually required no matter what facet of specialized practice a pharmacist may choose, whether it be injectable formulation in industrial or hospital pharmacy practice, teaching, radiopharmaceutical practice, or any one of a myriad avenues of specialization open to a graduate pharmacist. Additional training requirements are not limited to the profession of pharmacy, because physicians, too, are obligated to obtain specialized training in nuclear medicine before they can be authorized to use radiopharmaceuticals in their practice.

Perhaps the most meaningful justification for pharmacists participating in radiopharmaceutical practice is on the basis of need. When radioactive materials first became available in substantial quantities for use in medicine, the primary concern was directed toward protecting personnel and patients from the potentially harmful effects of the radiation emanating from these products, and perhaps rightfully so. A combination of circumstances made this approach a valid one. First, in the early days, much of the emphasis in this field was in the area of therapeutic use of radionuclidic materials, involving relatively large amounts of radioactivity. The sophistication of instrumentation available then was quite limited, by present-day standards, so that larger doses of radioactive drugs were required, even for diagnostic or tracer purposes. With the advent of exceedingly more sensitive radiation-detection systems, and with the rapid advances in diagnostic applications in which radiopharmaceutical products are being utilized, doses of radiation have become significantly lower. Thus, the nuclear medicine community, as well as regulatory agencies concerned with such matters, is directing considerably more attention to the pharmaceutical quality of this class of drugs than had previously been the case. The contributions that pharmacists with adequate training and experience can make in this field are now well recognized, and radiopharmacy is indeed now emerging as an acknowledged specialty.[20]

TYPES OF RADIOACTIVITY

Radioactivity is customarily divided into two different types: these are natural radioactivity and artificial radioactivity. Radioactivity itself has been defined[14] as the several processes by which atomic nuclei spontaneously decay or disintegrate by one or more discrete energy levels or transitions until, ultimately, a stable state is reached. When such events take place in a material without the addition of energy, the substance is said to be naturally radioactive. Artificial radioactivity, often called "man-made radioactivity," may be described[58] as the property of radioactivity produced by particle bombardment or electromagnetic irradiation—the radioactivity of synthetic nuclides.

Natural Radioactivity

The first reported evidence of natural radioactivity appeared in 1896, as a result of Henri Becquerel's discovery that a shielded photographic plate is darkened when exposed to uranium ore, in much the same way as a film reacts when exposed to x-rays.[8-10] There are more than 50 known naturally occurring radionuclides, examples of which include uranium-238, thorium-232, radium-226, actinium-237, lead-210, and potassium-40.

Artificial Radioactivity

Artificial radioactivity may be produced in a variety of ways, and in any of several devices, depending on what bombarding particle or ray is utilized. In general, these nuclear reactions are categorized as charged particle, photon or neutron-induced reactions. In the examples of each that follow, the subscript refers to the atomic number of the element, often called the Z number, while the superscript denotes the atomic mass number of the isotope, and is often referred to as the A number. It should be noted that the subscripts and the superscripts on each side of the equations balance, in much the same manner as ordinary chemical equations are balanced.

Charged-Particle Reactions. Reactions of these types may be produced with protons (illustrated symbolically as $_1^1H$ or p); deuterons ($_1^2H$ or d); alpha particles ($_2^4He$ or α); or occasionally by electrons or beta particles ($_{-1}^0e$ or $_{-1}^0\beta$).

A proton-initiated reaction:

$$_1^1H + _{11}^{23}Na \rightarrow _{12}^{23}Mg + _0^1n$$

In this reaction, nonradioactive sodium is bombarded with protons to form magnesium-23, the reaction also yielding a neutron ($_0^1n$).

A deuteron-induced reaction:

$$_{13}^{27}Al + _1^2H \rightarrow _{12}^{25}Mg + _2^4He$$

An alpha-particle-initiated reaction:

$$_7^{14}N + _2^4He \rightarrow _8^{17}O + _1^1H$$

Photon-Induced Reactions. Electromagnetic radiations or photons of high energy may also induce nuclear reactions, as the following example illustrates:

$$\gamma + _4^9Be \rightarrow _4^8Be + _0^1n$$

The source of electromagnetic energy utilized in this type of reaction may be a gamma-emitting radionuclide, as in the example cited, or a high voltage x-ray generator.

Neutron-Induced Reactions. One of the most important and also most widely used methods of producing artificially radioactive nuclides is the bombardment of a nonradioactive target nucleus with a source of thermal neutrons. An example of such a reaction is the production of radioactive sodium-24 by neutron capture in sodium-23:

$$_{11}^{23}Na + _0^1n \rightarrow _{11}^{24}Na + \gamma$$

Another extremely important use of this type of reaction is in the relatively new method of chemical analysis known as activation analysis. In this application, radioactivity is induced in a sample of unknown chemical composition by exposing the sample

TABLE 15-1. ELEMENTS DETERMINED IN TRACE QUANTITIES BY
NEUTRON ACTIVATION ANALYSIS*

ELEMENT	SENSITIVITY OF DETECTION (g)	ELEMENT	SENSITIVITY OF DETECTION (g)
Bismuth		Potassium	
Calcium		Rubidium	
Iron		Selenium	10^{-8}
Magnesium		Thorium	
Nickel	10^{-6}	Yttrium	
Niobium		Zinc	
Silicon			
Sulfur		Antimony	
Titanium		Arsenic	
		Bromine	
Cerium		Copper	
Chromium		Gallium	
Mercury		Gold	
Molybdenum		Iodine	
Neodymium		Lanthanum	
Platinum		Palladium	
Ruthenium	10^{-7}	Praseodymium	10^{-9}
Silver		Scandium	
Strontium		Sodium	
Tellurium		Tantalum	
Thallium		Terbium	
Tin		Thulium	
Zirconium		Tungsten	
		Uranium	
Aluminum		Vanadium	
Barium		Ytterbium	
Cadmium			
Cesium		Holmium	
Chlorine		Indium	
Cobalt		Iridium	
Erbium	10^{-8}	Lutetium	10^{-10}
Gadolinium		Manganese	
Germanium		Rhenium	
Hafnium		Samarium	
Osmium		Europium	10^{-11}
Phosphorus		Dysprosium	

* From Radioisotopes—Special Materials and Services, 3rd revision, 1960. Oak Ridge National Laboratory, operated by Union Carbide Corporation for the U. S. Atomic Energy Commission.

for a given period to a neutron flux. At the conclusion of the exposure period, the sample is removed from the neutron source, and the induced radioactivity is analyzed both qualitatively and quantitatively by means of suitable radiation analyzers. As is apparent from Table 15-1, this is an extremely sensitive method of analysis.

Activation analysis also has important biomedical applications, particularly in the area of trace element determinations in human tissue or body fluid samples. Babb and others have suggested the use of neutron activation analysis in the early diagnosis of cystic fibrosis.[5] The content of trace elements in leukocytes has been determined using this method by Frischauf,[38] and Fell has compared copper levels in patients suffering from hepatolenticular degeneration, using both chemical methods and activation analysis.[35] Kanabrocki and associates studied manganese and copper levels in serum and urine in patients with myocardial infarction,[47,48] and Barak and Beckenhauer reported on trace element composition of fatty and cirrhotic livers, using activation analytical methods.[6] From these few examples, it should be obvious that this method of analysis has a great deal of potential in a number of rather difficult areas. It is safe to assume that, just as is the case in many other facets of nuclear medicine and radiopharmacy, this rather unique tool will become much more widely used in the future.

RADIOACTIVE DECAY

Radioactive species by definition exist in a highly excited, unstable state, characterized by an energy excess. These nuclides ultimately achieve stability through the process of radioactive decay and the release of large amounts of energy, either kinetic or electromagnetic or both of these types simultaneously. In this process of decay there are three parameters which are characteristic of a given radioisotope. Indeed, identification of unknown radionuclides is based on these three properties: the rate of decay, the type(s) of radiation exhibited in the decay scheme, and the energies of these radiations.

The rate of decay of a radioisotope is indicated by the number of atoms of the nuclide which are disintegrating per unit time. This number is proportional to the total number of radioactive atoms present in the sample, as is evident from the following relationship: $\Delta N = -\lambda N \Delta t$, where ΔN is the number of atoms disintegrating per unit time Δt, and N is the number of radioactive atoms present. The symbol λ is the decay constant. The negative sign in the equation is used to indicate that the number of atoms is decreasing with the passage of time. By integrating this equation, the more familiar mathematical relationship often known as the decay equation is derived:

$$N = N_0 e^{-\lambda t}$$

where N is the number of radioactive atoms present at time t, and N_0 is the number of atoms originally present at time zero. The decay constant, lambda, may be defined as the fraction of the number of atoms of a radionuclide which decay in unit time.[58] The use of the decay equation is appropriate only if there is a sufficiently large number of radioactive atoms present at $t = 0$ to make the relationship statistically valid. That is to say, it is impossible to determine when any one radioactive atom in a given sample will disintegrate, but, if there is a statistically large number of such atoms present, the fraction of the total which is disintegrating per unit time can be predicted with a high degree of accuracy. In actuality, the statistical reliability of an observation is given by the standard deviation, s, where

$$s = N^{1/2}$$

in which N is the number of observed disintegrations. Thus, radioactive decay is a typical first-order reaction.

The physical half-life of a radioisotope, noted symbolically as $T^{1/2}$, is defined as the time interval during which half the radioactive atoms originally present in a sample will have decayed. There is a close relationship, both theoretically and mathematically, between physical half-life and decay constant, for they both indicate rates of radioactive decay, although in a somewhat different manner. Their mathematical relationship is shown by the equation

$$T^{1/2} = \frac{0.693}{\lambda}$$

The basic decay equation is extremely useful, for, by substituting in the basic equation as follows, both the activity (A) remaining in a sample after a given time and the intensity of radiation (I) after time t can be determined:

$$A = A_0 e^{-0.693t/T^{1/2}} \text{ or } I = I_0 e^{-0.693t/T^{1/2}}$$

While these values can always be computed using the relationships given above, decay tables for all of the commonly used medical radionuclides are reproduced in standard reference books. Table 15-2 shows a typical table, indicating the decay of gold-198.

Modes of Radioactive Decay

There are a number of methods by which radionuclides decay or disintegrate to ground state. These modes include alpha particle decay, beta particle (negatron) emission, positron (positive beta particle) emission,

TABLE 15-2. DECAY TABLE FOR ^{198}Au*

(λ factor (30 minutes) = 0.00537; $T^{\frac{1}{2}}$ = 2.69 days or 64.6 hours)

Hours	0	0.5	1.0	1.5	2.0	2.5	3.0	3.5	4.0	4.5
0	....	.9946	.9893	.9840	.9787	.9735	.9683	.9631	.9579	.9528
5	.9477	.9427	.9376	.9326	.9276	.9226	.9177	.9128	.9079	.9030
10	.8982	.8934	.8886	.8838	.8791	.8744	.8697	.8650	.8604	.8558
15	.8512	.8466	.8421	.8376	.8331	.8287	.8242	.8198	.8154	.8110
20	.8067	.8024	.7981	.7938	.7896	.7853	.7811	.7769	.7728	.7686
25	.7645	.7604	.7564	.7523	.7483	.7443	.7403	.7363	.7324	.7285
30	.7246	.7207	.7168	.7130	.7092	.7054	.7016	.6978	.6941	.6904
35	.6867	.6830	.6793	.6757	.6721	.6685	.6649	.6613	.6578	.6543
40	.6508	.6473	.6438	.6404	.6369	.6335	.6301	.6268	.6234	.6201
45	.6167	.6134	.6102	.6069	.6036	.6004	.5972	.5940	.5908	.5876
50	.5845	.5814	.5783	.5752	.5721	.5690	.5660	.5629	.5599	.5569
55	.5539	.5510	.5480	.5451	.5422	.5393	.5364	.5335	.5306	.5278
60	.5250	.5222	.5194	.5166	.5138	.5111	.5083	.5056	.5029	.5002
65	.4975	.4949	.4922	.4896	.4870	.4844	.4818	.4792	.4766	.4741
70	.4715	.4690	.4665	.4640	.4615	.4590	.4566	.4541	.4517	.4493
75	.4469	.4445	.4421	.4397	.4374	.4350	.4327	.4304	.4281	.4258
80	.4235	.4212	.4190	.4167	.4145	.4123	.4101	.4079	.4057	.4035
85	.4014	.3992	.3971	.3949	.3928	.3907	.3886	.3866	.3845	.3824
90	.3804	.3783	.3763	.3743	.3723	.3703	.3683	.3663	.3644	.3624
95	.3605	.3586	.3566	.3547	.3528	.3509	.3491	.3472	.3453	.3435
100	.3416	.3398	.3380	.3362	.3344	.3326	.3308	.3290	.3273	.3255
105	.3238	.3220	.3203	.3186	.3169	.3152	.3135	.3118	.3102	.3085
110	.3068	.3052	.3036	.3019	.3003	.2987	.2971	.2955	.2939	.2924
115	.2908	.2892	.2877	.2862	.2846	.2831	.2816	.2801	.2786	.2771
120	.2756	.2741	.2727	.2712	.2697	.2683	.2669	.2654	.2640	.2626
125	.2612	.2598	.2584	.2570	.2556	.2543	.2529	.2516	.2502	.2489
130	.2475	....	.2449	....	.2423	....	.2397	....	.2371	....
135	.2346	....	.2321	....	.2296	....	.2272	....	.2247	....
140	.2223	....	.2200	....	.2176	....	.2153	....	.2130	....
145	.2107	....	.2085	....	.2062	....	.2040	....	.2018	....
150	.1997	....	.1976	....	.1955	....	.1934	....	.1913	....
155	.1892	....	.1872	....	.1852	....	.1832	....	.1813	....
160	.1794	....	.1774	....	.1755	....	.1737	....	.1718	....
165	.1700	....	.1682	....	.1664	....	.1646	....	.1628	....
170	.1611	....	.1594	....	.1577	....	.1560	....	.1543	....
175	.1527	....	.1510	....	.1494	....	.1478	....	.1462	....
180	.1447	....	.1431	....	.1416	....	.1401	....	.1386	....
185	.1371	....	.1357	....	.1342	....	.1328	....	.1314	....
190	.1300	....	.1286	....	.1272	....	.1258	....	.1245	....
195	.1232	....	.1218	....	.1205	....	.1193	....	.1180	....
200	.1167	....	.1155	....	.1142	....	.1130	....	.1118	....
205	.1106	....	.1094	....	.1083	....	.1071	....	.1060	....

* From Radiological Health Handbook, PB 121784R, U. S. Department of Health, Education and Welfare, U.S.P.H.S., Washington, 1960.

electron capture, isomeric transition and certain conversion processes.

Alpha Particle Decay. Alpha decay occurs only in isotopes of the heavier elements. An alpha particle is composed of two protons and two neutrons and has been identified as a helium nucleus. Symbolically, an alpha particle is written $^{4}_{2}$He, and because there are two protons present, the particle has a double positive charge. The general equation defining alpha decay is:

$$_Z^A X \rightarrow {}_{Z-2}^{A-4} Y + {}_2^4 He + Q$$

where X is the parent radionuclide, Y the daughter resulting from that decay, and Q the energy required to make the reaction go, or the energy released as a result of the reaction. Substituting actual elements in the equation, we can indicate the process by which the uranium isotope of mass 238 decays:

$$_{92}^{238} U \rightarrow {}_{90}^{234} Th + {}_2^4 He + Q$$

In alpha decay, because two protons are lost, the atomic number is decreased by two, and because four atomic mass units are also emitted, the mass number of the daughter is also decreased by four. It can be derived mathematically that the magnitude of Q in this equation is in excess of 4 million electron volts (MeV).

Alpha particles are the heaviest of the particles emitted from the nuclei of radioactive atoms; they also have the greatest kinetic energy of any of the particulate radiations.

Beta Particle Decay. When beta particle emission is mentioned without further qualification, it can be assumed that negative beta particles, or negatrons, are being considered. However, in the strictest sense, beta emissions also include positive beta particles, or positrons, which are considered in the next section.

Negatrons have often been compared with, or indeed identified as, electrons that originate in the nucleus. This definition may be satisfactory for purposes of diagrammatic representation of certain nuclear reactions, but it implies that there are free electrons present in the nucleus, a condition known not to exist. A negative beta particle is emitted when a nuclear neutron is spontaneously converted to a proton, just before the emission occurs, according to the equation:

$$_0^1 n \rightarrow {}_1^1 p + {}_{-1}^0 \beta$$

As is apparent, this reaction increases the atomic number by one, while leaving the total number of nuclear particles unchanged —conditions known to be present in negative beta emission.

The general equation for beta decay is:

$$_Z^A X \rightarrow {}_{Z+1}^A Y + {}_{-1}^0 \beta + Q$$

Substituting the isotope of phosphorus with a mass of 32 in this equation, we have an example of pure beta decay:

$$_{15}^{32} P \rightarrow {}_{16}^{32} S + {}_{-1}^0 \beta + Q$$

Positron Decay. The general equation denoting decay by positron emission is:

$$_Z^A X \rightarrow {}_{Z-1}^A Y + {}_{+1}^0 \beta + Q$$

The daughter product of such a reaction is less positive by one unit of charge, and the mass number remains unchanged. An example of a radionuclide that decays by positron emission is:

$$_{28}^{57} Ni \rightarrow {}_{27}^{57} Fe + {}_{+1}^0 \beta + Q$$

In both negative and positive beta decay reactions, it can be shown that an apparent energy discrepancy results in the simple equations shown for these reactions, unless some other particulate emanation is present in these transitions. This is in fact the case, for in negative beta emission, a particle identified as a neutrino (electrically neutral and of extremely small mass when compared with the mass of the beta particle) is present in the reaction shown below:

$$_Z^A X \rightarrow {}_{Z+1}^A Y + {}_{+1}^0 \beta + \nu + Q$$

where the Greek letter Nu (ν) indicates the presence of the neutrino in the reaction.

In the case of the positron emitter, the equation becomes:

$$_Z^A X \rightarrow {}_{Z-1}^A Y + {}_{+1}^0 \beta + \nu + Q$$

where Nu again indicates the presence of an additional particle, this time known as an antineutrino. The antineutrino, like its counterpart the neutrino, accounts for the energy surplus in the reaction, has no charge and has a very small rest mass.

Although only pure beta emitters have been outlined in the examples cited for positron and negatron decay, a mixed beta-gamma decay scheme is frequently encountered in actual practice. An excellent example of this type of decay scheme is that of sodium-24. This radionuclide decays by negative beta emission to magnesium-24, with the concurrent emission of two energetic gamma rays of 1.38 and 2.76 MeV, respectively, as shown in the following general equation:

$$^{24}_{11}\text{Na} \rightarrow {}^{24}_{12}\text{Mg} + {}^{0}_{-1}\beta + \gamma + Q$$

In the case of either positive or negative beta decay, particles are emitted from unstable nuclei with a continuous energy spectrum, ranging from nearly zero kinetic energy to a maximum beta energy listed in isotope tables for each radionuclide. A rule of thumb, in cases where the mean beta energy for a given transition is not known, is to assume the mean beta energy to be one third that of the maximum listed in the tables. In actuality, these means range in value from 0.2 to 0.4 of the maximum.

Orbital Electron Capture. The most frequent electron capture reactions involve the K shell. In this case, a nuclear proton is transformed into a neutron by capturing within the nucleus an electron from the K shell and emitting a neutrino. This results in the formation of a decay product in which the Z number has been reduced by one and in which there is a vacancy in the K shell of orbital electrons. After a rearrangement of electrons, and the emission of characteristic x-rays resulting from this rearrangement, the products of such a reaction are the same as if a positron had been emitted:

$$^{A}_{Z}\text{X} + {}^{0}_{-1}\text{e} \rightarrow {}^{A}_{Z-1}\text{Y} + \text{hv}$$

As previously mentioned, the equation indicates that one of the products of this reaction (hv) is electromagnetic radiation (or photons) that can be produced either as gamma rays or as x-rays. An example of a frequently used radioisotope that decays by orbital electron capture is the radionuclide chromium-51, whose decay equation is:

$$^{51}_{24}\text{Cr} + {}^{0}_{-1}\text{e} \rightarrow {}^{51}_{23}\text{V} + \text{hv}$$

Radionuclides that decay by positron emission or by electron capture are artificially produced (man-made). Naturally occurring radionuclides decay by negatron or alpha emission.

Isomeric Transition. Isomeric transition is defined[58] as the process by which a nuclide decays to an isomeric nuclide (one with the same mass number and atomic number) of lower quantum energy. There are certain well defined ways in which neutrons and protons may be arranged within the nucleus.[64] In each of these configurations, a different amount of energy is stored in the nucleus. The excited nucleus attains a more stable configuration either by gamma ray emission or by a competing process known as internal conversion, in which the excitation energy of the nucleus is transferred to an orbital electron which is then ejected from the atom. The energy spectrum of such a nuclide is frequently a mixture of gamma rays and of these conversion electrons.

The more excited (or upper isomeric) state is called the *metastable state* or level, and is indicated by adding the letter m to the mass number of the nuclide. Examples of radionuclides that decay by isomeric transition are technetium-99m and bromine-80m.

Another useful means of indicating the decay reactions that take place with a given radionuclide is in the diagrammatic representation of the decay scheme. In the case of chromium-51, the decay scheme can be diagrammed as follows:

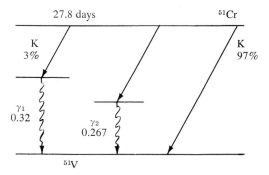

UNITS OF RADIOACTIVITY

It is difficult to describe anything without having the means with which to describe it and some baseline with which it can be compared. In the case of radioactivity, one must become thoroughly familiar with the systems of units which are used to characterize nuclear radiations and their effects in media through which they traverse and with which they react.

Of greatest interest to the biological sciences are perhaps two systems of units. One of these is used to indicate the amount or the quantity of radioactivity which is represented by a given sample, and the other system is utilized to define the dose which a given amount of radioactivity delivers to the system of interest. This system of interest may take the form of air, tissue or any material of interest, depending on the units one uses to delineate the dose.

QUANTITY UNITS

The Curie. It is possible to indicate the amount of radioactive material present in a given sample as a function of the mass of the radionuclide present. In fact, for many years this was the means utilized to define the amount of activity present. The amount of radon in equilibrium with 1 Gm. of radium was adopted as one Curie of activity.

Usually, we are not concerned as much with the mass of the radioisotope as with the rate of radioactive decay of the radionuclide. Therefore, the Curie unit was defined more precisely as that amount of any radioactive material which is decaying at the rate of 3.700×10^{10} disintegrating atoms per second. In medicine, sub-units of the Curie are more frequently used, such as the millicurie (3.7×10^7 disintegrating atoms per second), and the microcurie (3.7×10^4 disintegrating atoms per second).

Specific Activity. Another unit of activity frequently encountered is known as specific activity, which may be defined as the amount of radioactivity contained in 1 Gm. of a substance. However, some sort of qualifying statement must be made if one is dealing with a compound rather than an element, in order to avoid confusion. For example, if the radioisotope sodium-24 is present in sodium carbonate ($^{24}Na_2CO_3$) and one states merely that the specific activity is 40 millicuries per Gm., it is not known whether the mass indicated is for sodium carbonate or for sodium only. Therefore, it is less confusing if one speaks of specific activity (compound), specific activity (element) or specific activity (isotope).

DOSE UNITS

The estimation of the dose delivered to or, at times, absorbed by a material of interest is an extremely complex task, and the result is, at best, only a good estimate when compared with the results of other more accurate and precise methods of dose determination used in nonradioactive medicinal products. Further complicating the measurement is the fact that, with certain radioactive materials, the dose can be administered to the body even though the material is located outside and at some distance from the body. This, of course, is the case wih a gamma-emitting radionuclide. Thus, it is necessary to consider both external and internal dose, due to both electromagnetic and particulate radiations, in order to cover the general topic of radiation dosage adequately. A thorough understanding of the various units used to assess dosage is absolutely necessary if one is to comprehend the meaning of these terms. The units most frequently used to indicate the magnitude of radiation dose are the roentgen and the radiation absorbed dose.

The roentgen (abbreviated r) is the fundamental unit of radiation dosage from which all other units are derived. As it was originally defined at the Stockholm Congress of Radiology in 1928, it was applicable only to x-ray dose. However, the Chicago Congress of Radiology (1937) modified this definition to its present form so that it can be used for either x-ray or gamma-ray dose estimation. Thus, the roentgen is defined as the quantity of x-radiation or gamma-radiation such that the associated corpuscular emission per 0.001293 Gm. of air produces in air ions carrying one electrostatic unit of quantity of electricity of either sign. This definition was given international standing by the International Commission on Radiological Units and Measurements (ICRU) in 1956[61] and again in 1959.[62] Although the definition suggested by this Commission in 1962 was stated in somewhat different terms, the unit is numerically identical with that previously mentioned.[57] Thus, the unit of exposure is the roentgen.

The radiation absorbed dose (abbreviated rad), as the name indicates, is the unit of absorbed dose. It may be defined[57] as the dose of ionizing radiation that results in an absorption of 100 ergs per Gm. or 1/100 Joule per Kg. of any material. The rad is the more recently derived unit that replaced the older roentgen equivalent physical (rep). The basic difference between the two is that the rep specifies tissue as the material in which the radiation dose is absorbed, whereas the rad may be used for any material of interest. In contradistinction to the roentgen, which is an *exposure* unit used only for electromagnetic radiations, the rad is a unit of *absorbed dose,* which may be used for any type of electromagnetic or particulate radiation.

The roentgen equivalent man (rem) until rather recently had been used to express human biological doses as a result of exposure to one or several types of ionizing radiation, as the following equation indicates:

$$\text{rem} = \text{rad} \times \text{R.B.E.}$$

where R.B.E. is a factor known as the "relative biological effectiveness." However, because it proved difficult to reach agreement on the magnitude of R.B.E. for various types of particulate and electromagnetic radiations, this unit of dose equivalent has largely fallen into disuse in nuclear medicine and radiopharmacy practice. Nevertheless, Handbook 84[57] continues to use the rem in both radiobiological dosimetry and in radiation protection, although the use of R.B.E. is restricted in this report to radiobiology.

RADIATION PROTECTION

From the standpoint of the practicing radiopharmacist, there can be no more important facet of his daily practice than radiation protection, for it concerns not only the safety of his patients but his own health as well. Anyone who works with radioactive materials must have a fundamental knowledge of radiologic health if he is to fulfill his responsibility in this important area. However, in a discussion of so broad and complex a subject as radiation safety, comprehensiveness must be sacrificed to some extent in the interests of brevity. Therefore, the discussion here is confined to those aspects of radiation protection and radiologic health of concern to the occupationally exposed individual (as opposed to the general population) who in the course of his daily practice works with radioactive materials that are either pure beta, pure gamma, or mixed beta-gamma emitters. We thus have ruled out consideration of machine-generated radiation (from x-ray machines, for example), as well as nuclear reactors and alpha emitters, in order to shorten our discussion.

This compromise or limitation is not so serious as it may seem. There would seldom be a situation in which a radiopharmacist would be called on to serve as the one who is responsible for the overall safety program, as it relates to radiation, in his institution. Generally, this person—usually called the Radiation Safety Officer—is chosen because of his strong background in radiation physics, or, in some cases, he may be a physician knowledgeable in such areas as nuclear physics, radiation hazard evaluation and radiation chemistry. In any case, it is seldom a good policy to assign radiation safety responsibilities to one who customarily uses radioactive materials in his daily work, just as it would be unwise to allow the production department of a pharmaceutical manufacturer to carry out the quality control procedures on the products this same department formulates. The radiopharmacist has no real need to know every detail of the extremely specialized practice of radiation safety, or health physics, as it is often called. His need is to comprehend enough to allow him to function in a manner compatible with the safety of his patients, his environment, and himself. Actually, it matters little to whom the overall responsibility is given, assuming that person has adequate training, for it is the direct and inescapable obligation of all who work or are in anyway associated with radioactive materials to do so in the safest possible manner for all concerned. The real problem is to induce personnel to accept this responsibility.

Maximum Permissible Exposure

In the absence of any definitive evidence that there is a tolerance level below which no possible harm can evolve from radiation dose of such magnitude, reason dictates that exposure levels be kept at the lowest possible level which will permit a given procedure to be accomplished. Further, the physician, in determining whether or not to use a radioactive material in a patient, must weigh the possible harm to the patient against the benefits to be derived from the administration of the radiopharmaceutical product. In any case, except in cases of therapeutic dosage (as opposed to diagnostic or tracer use), it is prudent to keep patient exposures below the maximum permissible levels for occupationally exposed personnel, and the radiopharmacist must develop a method that permits him to accomplish the task within these limits.

Maximum permissible exposures for occupationally exposed individuals in the United States are recommended by the National Committee on Radiation Protection (N.C.R.P.).[49] These exposure levels are categorized and reproduced in part below.*

A. *External exposure to critical organs. Whole body; head and trunk; active blood-forming organs; eyes or gonads.* The maximum permissible dose (MPD) to the most critical organs, accumulated at any age, shall not exceed 5 rems multiplied by the number of years the worker is beyond age 18, and the dose in any consecutive 13 weeks shall not exceed 3 rems. The accumulated maximum permissible dose may be calculated from the relationship: MPD = (N − 18) × 5 rems, where N is the age in years and is greater than 18. In arriving at these values, it is assumed that one does not have occupational exposure to radiation prior to age 18. The maximum permissible weekly dose that is used most frequently remains at 300 millirems, but exposures of this magnitude each week of the year obviously would be in excess of the recommended value.

B. *External exposure to other organs. Skin of whole body.* MPD = 10(N − 18) rems, and the dose in any 13 consecutive weeks shall not exceed 6 rems. This rule applies to radiation of low penetrating power. *Hands and forearms; feet and ankles:* MPD = 75 rems per year, and the dose in any 13 consecutive weeks shall not exceed 25 rems.

C. *Internal exposures.* The permissible levels from internal emitters shall be consistent as far as possible with the age-proration and the dose principles given in the preceding paragraphs.

* Maximum Permissible Body Burdens and Maximum Permissible Concentrations in Air and in Water for Occupational Exposure, Handbook 69, Washington, D.C., National Bureau of Standards, U.S. Department of Commerce, 1959.

Control of the internal dose is achieved by limiting the body burden of radioisotopes. This is generally accomplished by control of the average concentration of radioactive materials in the air, the water or the food taken into the body. Since it would be impractical to set different maximum permissible concentration (MPC) values for air, water and food for radiation workers as a function of age, the MPC values are selected in such a manner that they conform to the established limits when applied to the most restrictive case. In other words, they are applicable to radiation workers of any age, assuming that there is no occupational exposure to radiation permitted at age less than 18.

The maximum permissible average concentrations of radionuclides in air and water are determined from biologic data when such data are available, or they are calculated on the basis of an averaged annual dose of 15 rems for most individual organs of the body, 30 rems when the critical organ is the thyroid or the skin, and 5 rems when the gonads or the whole body is the critical organ. For bone-seekers (radionuclides which tend to accumulate in bony tissues), the maximum permissible limit is based on the distribution of the deposit, the Relative Biological Effectiveness and comparison of the energy release in the bone with the energy release delivered by a maximum permissible body burden of 0.1 mcg. ^{226}Ra plus daughters. A comprehensive listing of maximum permissible body burdens and maximum permissible concentrations of radionuclides in air and water for occupational exposure, in which body organs of reference are tabulated, may be found in the I.C.R.P. Internal Radiation Report.[60]

METHODS OF PROTECTION

The means of protecting oneself from the harmful effects of ionizing radiation must be considered from the standpoints of those radiations that present a hazard even when they remain outside the body and those which are likely to be harmful only when the radionuclide is in the body.

There are, basically, only three rules to keep in mind when working with externally hazardous radioisotopes. These are expressed in terms of time, distance and shielding. That is to say, make exposure to a source of ionizing radiation as brief as possible; increase as much as possible one's distance from the source; and make use of suitable absorbers or shields to diminish to a reasonable level the amount of radiation reaching the body.

It is frequently necessary to make use of all three of these methods.

Insofar as the radiopharmacist is concerned, radionuclides which are considered to be hazardous externally are those which emit gamma rays, as well as certain beta-emitting radioisotopes of relatively high energy. The dose rate from a point source* of a gamma-emitter varies inversely with the square of the distance from that source.

This relationship may be expressed mathematically by equation (1):

$$\frac{I_1}{I_2} = \frac{(R_2)^2}{(R_1)^2} \tag{1}$$

where I_1 is the gamma intensity at distance R_1 from the source and I_2 is the gamma intensity at distance R_2. For example, it is known that the dose rate from a 1-millicurie point source of ^{24}Na at a distance of 1 cm. is 18.4 r per hour. If one wished to find the dose rate at a distance of 10 centimeters, the answer may be conveniently calculated from the equation (2):

$$\frac{18.4}{I_2} = \frac{(10)^2}{(1)^2} \tag{2}$$

and I_2 is found to equal 184 milliroentgens per hour. It should be emphasized again that the inverse square law is valid only for point sources with no shielding or attenuation considerations; it does not apply to radiation fields due to multiple sources, beams of radiation or to extended sources. However, the law is approximately correct as long as the distance from the detector or point of interest is at least three times the physical dimensions of the source.

Beta-emitting radionuclides of relatively high energy may constitute an external hazard in a number of situations. If the radioactive substance comes into physical contact with the skin or the eyes and is not removed immediately, a radiation burn may result. In addition, the external radiation dose from an energetic beta-emitter may be considerable. For example, it has been estimated[39] that the dose delivered by a 1-mc. ^{32}P source with an area of 1 sq. cm. approxi-

* A point source is a source which is small in physical dimensions when compared with the distance from the detector.

mates 200,000 mrad/hr. when that source is 1 cm. from the target. When one considers that the maximum permissible hand exposure from any radioactive source is 18,750 mrem per quarter (3 months), it becomes quite evident that somewhat extreme precautions against even microcurie levels of contamination are required to avoid serious exposures. And finally, energetic beta-emitters may release x-rays when the beta particles impinge on and are stopped by certain materials. These x-rays are known as bremsstrahlung, or "braking radiations." The number and character of these x-rays are functions of the kinetic energy of the beta particles and the atomic number of the absorber, or target. This phenomenon is analogous to that existing in an x-ray tube, in which electrons are accelerated across a large difference in potential to impinge on a target material of high atomic number, such as tungsten.

Plastic formulations of low atomic number are frequently used to shield syringes in which large doses of such nuclides as ^{32}P are to be administered, and a thin sheet of lead is added to the syringe holder to shield against any bremsstrahlung produced (Fig. 15-1).

Internal Hazards. Protection against radionuclides that are hazardous only if they gain entrance to the body is generally afforded by good laboratory procedure and acceptable personal hygiene. Many sets of rules for conduct in radioisotope laboratories have been advanced by radionuclide workers, all of which are intended to reduce to a minimum the hazard of radioisotope work. A representative set of rules appears in the Radiation Safety Guide in current use at the National Institutes of Health[52] and is quoted in part below.

Each individual at the NIH who has any contact with radioactive materials is responsible for:

1. Keeping his exposure to radiation as low as possible, and specifically below the Maximum Permissible Exposure as listed in Appendix Table 1. Laboratory air and water concentrations shall be maintained below the levels in Appendix Table 2.

2. Wearing the prescribed monitoring equipment such as film badges and pocket dosimeters

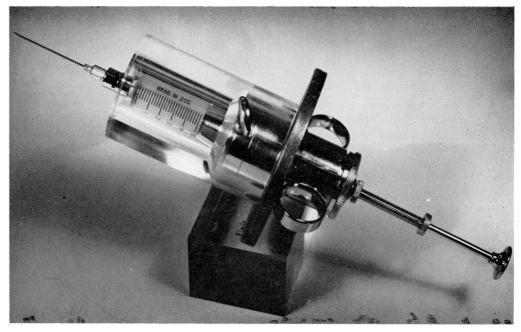

FIG. 15-1. Radioisotope syringe with plastic and lead shields. (National Institutes of Health, **U.S.P.H.S.**)

in radiation areas. Personnel who work only with pure alpha emitters or only with pure beta emitters having a maximum energy of less than 0.2 Mev will not be required to wear film badges.

3. Surveying his hands, shoes and body for radioactivity, and removing all loose contamination before leaving the laboratory to smoke, eat, etc.

4. Utilizing all appropriate protective measures such as:

(a) Wearing protective clothing whenever contamination is possible, and not wearing such clothing outside the laboratory area.

(b) Wearing gloves and respiratory protection where necessary.

(c) Using protective barriers and other shields wherever possible.

(d) Using mechanical devices whenever their aid will assist in reducing exposure.

(e) Using pipet filling devices. NEVER PIPET RADIOACTIVE SOLUTIONS BY MOUTH.

(f) Performing radioactive work within confines of an approved hood or glove box unless serious consideration has indicated the safety of working in the open.

5. Avoiding smoking or eating in isotope laboratories. It is recommended that eating be done in the cafeterias whenever possible.

Smoking or eating may be permitted in an office area of the laboratory that has been demonstrated to be free of contamination. Refrigerators should not be used jointly for foods and radioactive materials.

6. Maintaining good personal hygiene.

(a) Keep fingernails short and clean.

(b) Do not work with radioactive materials if there is a break in the skin below the wrist.

(c) Wash hands and arms thoroughly before handling any object which goes to the mouth, nose or eyes.

7. Checking the immediate areas, e.g., hoods, benches, etc., in which radioactive materials are being used, at least once daily for contamination. Any contamination observed should be removed immediately. If such removal is not possible, the area shall be clearly marked and the Radiation Safety Office notified.

8. Keeping the laboratory neat and clean. The work area should be free from equipment and materials not required for the immediate procedure. Keep or transport materials in such a manner as to prevent breakage or spillage (double containers), and to ensure adequate shielding. Wherever practical, keep work surfaces covered with absorbent material, preferably in a stainless steel tray or pan, to limit and collect spillage in case of an accident.

9. Labeling and isolating radioactive waste and equipment, such as glassware, used in laboratories for radioactive materials. Once used for radioactive substances, equipment should not be used for other work, or sent from the area to cleaning facilities, repair shops, or to surplus, until demonstrated to be free of contamination.

10. Requesting Radiation Safety supervision of any emergency repair of contaminated equipment in the laboratory by shop personnel or by commercial service contractors. At no time shall servicing personnel be permitted to work on equipment in radiation areas without the presence of a member of the laboratory staff to provide specific information.

11. Reporting accidental inhalation, ingestion, or injury involving radioactive materials to his supervisor and the Radiation Safety Office, and carrying out their recommended corrective measures. The individual shall cooperate in any and all attempts to evaluate his exposure.

12. Carrying out decontamination procedures when necessary, and for taking the necessary steps to prevent the spread of contamination to other areas.*

The extremes to which one must go to protect oneself from a source of radioactivity depend on many things. Among such considerations are the quantity of radioactivity with which one is to work, the type and energy of the radiation emitted by the source, the complexity of the radiopharmaceutical procedure with which one is faced, the physical and biological half-lives of the compound, and the physiologic behavior of the compound should it gain entrance to the body. However, it is important to recognize that *all* radioactive contaminants, regardless of their type of emission, may be hazardous if they are absorbed or are ingested in sufficient amounts; they differ only in the degree of that hazard.

Chemical Radioprotective Agents. While, in the author's experience, the use of chemical radioprotective agents has never been indicated in the practice of radiopharmacy, some mention of these compounds should be made in any discussion of radiation protection. Presumably, these compounds might be used when the probability exists of receiving

a single, relatively large dose of radiation. In general, these compounds should be administered prior to or during the period of irradiation; little beneficial effect is to be expected from administration of these compounds after exposure.

Since radiation damage to biologic tissue probably results from the ionization of certain tissue constituents and, in certain cases, the production of free radicals, a number of mechanisms of action of protective agents may be suggested. These chemical compounds may react directly with the ions and the free radicals to neutralize or reduce their toxic effects; they may exert some purely physical shielding effect to protect against the products of ionization, or they may reduce the oxygen tension in the tissue environment to diminish the production of strong oxidizing agents resulting from the reaction of the ions and the free radicals with oxygen.

The early work of Patt and his associates at Argonne National Laboratory indicated that the prior ingestion or injection of compounds containing a sulfhydryl group, such as certain amino acids, significantly reduced the number of deaths in animals that were given lethal doses of radiation. Through a systematic approach to the problem, Doherty and his co-workers at Oak Ridge National Laboratory discovered a modified amino acid configuration which showed great promise in its protective effect on laboratory animals. This substance is S-(2-aminoethyl) isothiuronium bromide hydrobromide, commonly called AET, which breaks down in the body to the compound 2-mercaptoethylguanidine hydrobromide (MEG); it is the latter compound which exerts the protective effect.[37,66]

While, on theoretical grounds, these compounds should be effective in preventing acute radiation sickness in patients receiving large therapy doses of radiation, the results thus far have been far from uniformly successful. However, the search goes on in many laboratories throughout the world.

Other means may occasionally be used to minimize the radiation-induced damage that may result from the inadvertent administration of excessively large doses of radioactive compounds to patients, or, in other cases, to reduce the magnitude of the absorbed dose in certain diagnostic applica-

* Brown, J. M., and Cool, W. S.: National Institutes of Health Radiation Safety Guide, Washington, D.C., U.S. Department of Health, Education and Welfare, Public Health Service, 1962.

tions of radiopharmaceutical products. In general, these methods are based on in vivo exchange reactions between the radioactive compound and a stable, or nonradioactive chemical entity of similar or identical composition. In other instances, further uptake of a radioactive compound by a target organ or tissue is prevented by administering a "blocking" dose of a similarly organ-specific nonradioactive compound followed by suitable isotope exchange procedures. Frequently, there is also an attempt made to promote and hasten the excretion of the radioactive compound released by the exchange.

For example, Cobau, Simons, and Meyers reported[27] the apparently successful treatment of a patient who had received approximately twice the intended dose of phosphorus-32 in a radiation therapy procedure. This was accomplished by administering large amounts of stable phosphate and calcium ions, followed by substantial quantities of parathyroid extract to promote the excretion of phosphate ion by diuresis. Calcium ion was administered in this case to prevent concurrent calcium depletion in the body, a concomitant effect of parathyroid extract.

Another example of an in vivo isotope exchange to diminish tissue irradiation is the use of potassium iodide to reduce thyroid irradiation from [131]I.[13] If a 100 to 200 mg. dose of potassium iodide is given prophylactically in anticipation of iodine-131 exposure, the irradiation dose to the thyroid may be decreased by as much as 98 percent. The same dose of potassium iodide given at intervals after ^{131}I absorption is less effective, but still reduces uptake to less than half after a delay of 3 hours. It must be emphasized that this suppressive effect of potassium iodide for such purposes is of short duration. Thus, the 100 to 200 mg. dose of stable iodide must be repeated at daily intervals for prolonged protection. These are but two examples of the use of chemical radioprotective agents in the practice of nuclear medicine.

ACCEPTABLE RISK

It may seem quite logical to question the wisdom of engaging in radiopharmaceutical practice in view of the possible hazards of radiation exposure. In fact why should not one avoid *all* exposure to radiation? The fundamental impracticality of this proposition is apparent when one considers that man has been bathed in a field of radiation since time immemorial—an exposure over which he has, at best, only a limited control. This is, of course, the natural background radiation from the cosmic rays and from certain naturally occurring radionuclides which are widely dispersed throughout our environment (and, indeed, throughout our body as well). It has been estimated[45] that the total amount of external background radiation to which a man is subjected every day of his life is of the order of 0.3 mr. per day; internally, there are at least three naturally occurring radioisotopes which administer to a man weighing 70 Kg. a radiation dose equivalent to approximately 0.1 mr. per day. These radionuclides are potassium-40, carbon-14 and radium-226.

Consideration of radiation exposure in this context leads inevitably to the concept of "acceptable risk." This has been defined[14] as a risk that is made so small that it is readily acceptable to the average individual; that is, the risk is essentially the same as that present in ordinary occupations not involving exposure to radiation. The concept of acceptable risk obviously implies that those who work with radionuclides have had sufficient training and experience to allow them to do so safely. Most authorities today are in agreement concerning the validity of this concept.

ABSORBED DOSE CALCULATIONS

When one speaks of absorbed dose in radiopharmacy, the connotation is somewhat different from that encountered in classic pharmacology and therapeutics. In this newer context, it is the quantity of *energy* deposited in the organ or tissue of interest with which we are concerned, rather than the *mass* of a particular drug in the more familiar situation involving a nonradioactive drug product. Several factors affect the absorbed dose of a radiopharmaceutical product, including the activity of the administered radiopharmaceutical, its chemical and physical state, the route of administration, its metabolic fate, and the energy released per disintegrating atom.[69] It is difficult to overestimate the importance of accurately determining absorbed dose values in nuclear medicine procedures; without such data, it is impossible for a physician to weigh the expected benefits against the potential harm that may result from these procedures.

In order to serve the needs of the nuclear medicine community in the determination of the radiation absorbed dose to patients who are administered radiopharmaceuticals, in October, 1964, the President of The Society of Nuclear Medicine appointed an ad hoc committee known as the Medical Internal Radiation Dose (MIRD) Committee. The objective of this committee is to provide the best possible estimate of the absorbed dose to patients resulting from the diagnostic or therapeutic use of internally administered radiopharmaceuticals. The work of this committee has continued, and the preliminary report of their work has already been published as a supplement to the *Journal of Nuclear Medicine* in February, 1968.[50] This supplement can be heartily recommended for the reader who desires a somewhat more detailed discussion of this subject than is presented here. The supplement consists of three extremely important titles:

Pamphlet No. 1: Loevinger, R., and Berman, M.: A Schema for Absorbed Dose Calculations for Biologically-Distributed Radionuclides. Pamphlet No. 2: Berger, M. J.: Energy Deposition in Water by Photons from Point Isotropic Sources. Pamphlet No. 3: Brownell, G. L., Ellett, W. H., and Reddy, A. R.: Absorbed Fractions for Photon Dosimetry.

In addition to the schema mentioned above, several others have been used in making absorbed dose calculations. In actuality, the results of calculations by any of these recognized methods do not differ greatly, regardless of the method employed. With respect to the types of computations usually encountered in the use of radiopharmaceutical products, these equations may be categorized as beta dosimetry, gamma dosimetry and beta plus gamma dosimetry equations.

Beta Dosimetry. Equation (3) is used to compute the beta dose in rads, D_β, for complete disintegration of the radionuclide (∞):

$$D_\beta (\infty) = 73.8\ \overline{E}_\beta C_0 T^{1/2}(\text{eff.}) \quad (3)$$

where $\overline{E}_\beta$ is the *average* beta particle energy in MeV, C_0 is the initial concentration of the radionuclide in $\mu c/Gm.$ of tissue, and $T^{1/2}(\text{eff.})$ is the effective half-life. Effective half-life is defined as the time required for a radionuclide fixed in tissues to be diminished by a factor of 50 per cent, due to the combined effects of radioactive decay and biological elimination. Effective half-life may be computed from equation (4):

$$T^{1/2}(\text{eff.}) = \frac{\text{Biological half life} \times \text{Radioactive half life}}{\text{Biological half life} + \text{Radioactive half life}} \quad (4)$$

It should again be emphasized that tables of beta energies found in the literature are tables of *maximum* beta energies for a given radionuclide. The average beta energy used in most calculations is approximately 1/3 the maximum listed in the reference tables.

If one wishes to determine the beta dose in rads for any time, t, after the administration of a given radioisotope, where t is in days, Equation (5) may be used:

$$D_\beta = \overline{E}_\beta C_0 T^{1/2}(\text{eff.}) \times (1 - e^{-0.693t/T^{1/2}\ (\text{eff.})}) \quad (5)$$

Gamma Dosimetry. There are a number of reasons why gamma ray dosimetry is not so simple a procedure as is beta particle dosimetry. In the case of beta particles, although it may not be apparent, an assumption is made that the energy dissipated per gram of tissue is the same as the energy absorbed in the same mass of tissue. Because of the much longer range and the infinitely greater ability of a gamma ray to penetrate materials, no such assumption can be made in this case. The dose delivered by a gamma emitter depends on a number of parameters, such as the effective half-life of the radionuclide, its concentration in the tissue, and also, to a large extent, the energy of the gamma ray. A relationship which is frequently used to determine the gamma dose in roentgens for complete disintegration of the isotope (∞) is given by equation:

$$D\gamma\ (\infty) = 0.0346\Gamma\rho\bar{g}C_0T^{\frac{1}{2}}(\text{eff.})\quad(6)$$

where:

$\rho =$ Density of tissue in Gm./cm.³
$\Gamma =$ Emission constant (r/mc./hr. at 1 cm.)
$\bar{g} =$ geometry factor, which is a function of size and shape of the tissue volume and the penetration of the radiation (tables available)
$C_0 =$ initial concentration of the isotope in μc/gram of tissue
$T^{\frac{1}{2}}(\text{eff.}) =$ effective half-life of the isotope in days

If one wishes to know the gamma dose for any time (t) when t is in days, equation (7) may be used:

$$D_\gamma\ (t) = 0.0346\bar{g}C_0T^{\frac{1}{2}}(\text{eff.})(1 - e^{-0.693t/T^{\frac{1}{2}}\ (\text{eff.})})\qquad(7)$$

RADIATION DETECTION INSTRUMENTS

Since human sensory perception is incapable of detecting either the presence or the magnitude of a radiation field, instruments have been developed to make these determinations. It is customary to classify radiation detection instruments according to the use to which they are put or with respect to the type of medium in which the determination is made. When categorized according to use or function, they may be classified as survey instruments, personnel monitoring instruments and laboratory instruments.

SURVEY INSTRUMENTS

Survey instruments are usually portable, relatively simple in design, and may display a reading in roentgen units or counts per unit time. They are used for gross determinations of the presence and the magnitude of a radioactive source or contamination. Two of the most frequently used survey instruments are the portable Geiger counter (Fig. 15-2) and the ionization chamber instrument (Fig. 15-3), often referred to as "Cutie-Pie" in the literature.

PERSONNEL MONITORING INSTRUMENTS

The function of instruments in this category is to afford a reasonably reliable estimate of the radiation dose which an occupationally exposed individual receives in his daily work. Since these devices are concerned with the health and the welfare of radiation workers and, thus, may serve a legal function should a claim for radiation injury arise, they are among the most important of all radiation detection instruments to both the worker and management. However, unless they are of good quality and are used properly in a well-founded health physics program, the results may be something less than satisfactory.

Two of the most important personnel monitoring devices are the film badge (Fig. 15-4) and the pocket dosimeter (Fig. 15-5). A film badge is an opaque packet containing a photographic film which varies in known sensitivity to radiation of diverse energies and types. After exposure to radiation, it will be found, on developing, that a darkening of the film has occurred as a result of the interaction of the incident radiation particles or rays with the silver halide granules in the photographic emulsion. The degree of dark-

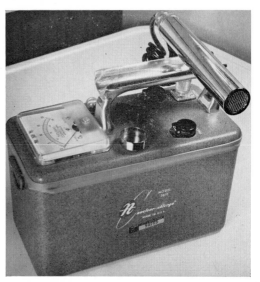

FIG. 15-2. Portable Geiger-Mueller survey meter. (National Institutes of Health, U.S.P.H.S.)

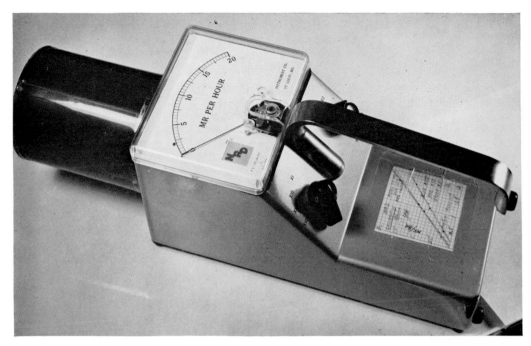

Fig. 15-3. Portable ionization chamber survey meter (Cutie-Pie). (National Institutes of Health, U.S.P.H.S.)

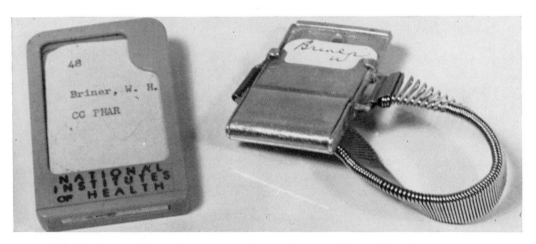

Fig. 15-4. Film badges, standard and wrist. (National Institutes of Health, U.S.P.H.S.)

ening of the films, as determined by measuring the transmittance of light through the film on a densitometer, gives a fairly accurate indication of the amount of radiation striking (and reacting with) the badge. In order to make this determination, standard or "control" films from the same emulsion number as the batch worn by workers are exposed to known amounts of radiation of various types and energies. The control films are then developed at the same time as the "unknown" films, or those actually worn by the radiation workers, using the same developing technics and chemicals. The densitometer readings from the control films versus the dose administered are plotted on graph

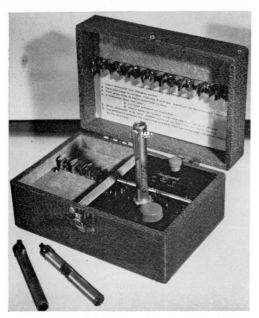

FIG. 15-5. Pocket dosimeters and charger. (National Institutes of Health, U.S.P.H.S.)

paper, and then the exposure of the unknown films may be read from the graph. While this procedure seems simple and forthright, it must be emphasized that an exceptionally fine system of quality control on the part of the group providing the film badge service and a sincere, conscientious attitude in the radiation worker who wears the badge are necessary if results are to be meaningful. Neither a haphazard calibration procedure nor a film badge which should be worn on the person of the worker but which is placed, soon to be forgotten, in his desk drawer will provide significant records of radiation exposure.

Pocket dosimeters, or pocket ionization chambers, resemble fountain pens in outward appearance. In actuality, these instruments are self-contained electrometers in which the amount of ionization in a sensitive volume of gas within the electrometer is measured. This ionization then can be related to the amount of radiation which has reacted with the electrometer. Both the film badge and the pocket dosimeter indicate a cumulative dose of radiation, rather than a dose rate.

LABORATORY INSTRUMENTS

These are the most sensitive of all radiation detection devices. This kind of instru-

ment is employed when an assay or calibration of a source of radioactivity is necessary. The conditions under which these instruments are used lend themselves well to reproducibility of results, a factor which is seldom, if ever, attainable with other types of instruments or devices.

It is obviously impracticable to discuss or even list the considerable number of laboratory instruments currently available in the United States. However, it may be convenient to classify such devices in terms of the detector utilized in the particular system. Those in general use include ionization chambers, proportional counters, Geiger-Mueller counters and scintillation counters. The first three types are known as gas-filled detectors (although, in certain instances, the "gas" is merely the atmosphere around us) and include some of the oldest—yet most widely used—radiation detectors devised. Scintillation detectors, while relatively new, are extremely valuable and, perhaps, the most versatile of all.

Ionization Chamber Detectors. Basically a detector of this type is designed to measure quantity of ionizing radiation in terms of the charge of electricity associated with ions produced within a defined volume. Thus, in the strictest sense, Geiger-Mueller counters and proportional counters should also be included in this group. However, it is customary to qualify this definition by considering detectors as ionization chambers only if there is no gas amplification factor involved. If one plots the number of ions collected versus the applied voltage, five regions of instrument response will be noted as the voltage applied is increased above zero (Fig. 15-6). In the first region, known as the region of recombination, the ions which are formed are under so low a voltage gradient that they tend to recombine with each other rather than migrate to the electrodes and be collected. As the voltage is increased, this recombination phenomenon decreases and actually disappears at the start of the second region. It is obvious that radiation detection instruments cannot be operated in this region.

The second region is known as the ionization region and represents a point at which all of the ions formed are collected. The

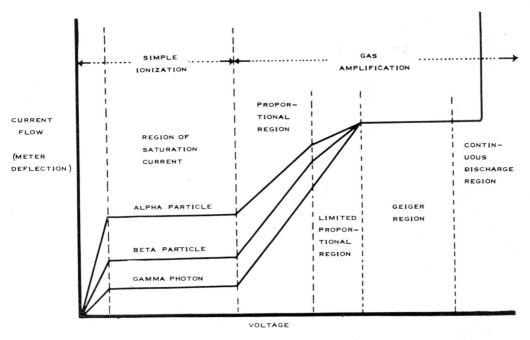

Fig. 15-6. Regions of instrument response. (From Chase, G. D.: Principles of Radioiostope Methodology, Minneapolis, Burgess)

electron portion of the primary ion pair which is formed is accelerated toward the anode of the chamber, while the positive ion moves somewhat more slowly toward the cathode. At some large voltage increment above the region of recombination, there is a saturation point at which all of the ions formed are collected. This is known as the saturation current region, or ionization chamber region. An excellent example of an ionization chamber instrument is the Lauritsen electroscope, which is widely used in the measurement of gamma radiation. Another ionization chamber instrument which has been used to measure beta and gamma radiation is the Landsverk electrometer.

If one applies still higher voltage to the detector, the number of ions collected will also increase. This apparent ambiguity (more ions being collected than are formed by the primary radiation source) is due to the increased force with which the electrons are accelerated toward the anode. With a sufficiently high voltage—and resultant velocity—these migrating electrons produce a secondary ionization of the gas in the detector, resulting in an amplification of the primary ion

current produced by the radiation. As the applied voltage increases, the gas amplification factor also increases. Since the size of the current pulse which results is proportional to the applied voltage and to the number of primary ions formed, this region is known as the proportional region. It should be noted that the number of primary ion pairs formed is a function of the specific ionization of the radiation. Thus, an alpha particle, with its relatively high specific ionization, will produce a larger current pulse than will a beta particle, of a correspondingly lower specific ionization. Proportional counters are extremely versatile in that it is possible to distinguish between alpha and beta-gamma radiations.

If the voltage is increased still further, gas amplification is also increased; this is due to an even greater acceleration of electrons than that observed in the proportional region. In this, the fourth region of instrument response (known as the Geiger-Mueller region), a veritable avalanche of ions is produced, and gas amplification factors as high as 10^{10} are not uncommon. Over a relatively narrow range known as the operating plateau,

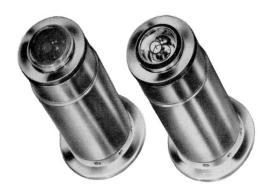

FIG. 15-7. Gas flow detector for solid beta-emitting samples (may be used as a windowless or an ultra-thin window detector). (Nuclear-Chicago Corp.)

the count rate produced by this avalanche of ions is nearly independent of applied voltage in a good detector. That is to say, small changes in either line voltage or applied voltage will have a relatively small effect on count rate. The instrument also is relatively independent of the specific ionization of the triggering particle or photon within this plateau. The Geiger-Mueller region is sensitive to any radiation event which produces even a single ion pair, which means that individual ionizing events may be detected. An obvious example of an instrument which operates within this region is the Geiger-Mueller counter, which is one of the oldest of all radiation detection instruments. These detection devices may be of the older "end window" type, in which the gas is enclosed within a Geiger tube which the ionizing radia-

tion must penetrate to be detected, or of the more recent variety of windowless flow Geiger counter (Fig. 15-7). In the latter case, the radioactive source is literally bathed in the detecting gas, resulting in a much higher detection efficiency. In the past, Geiger-Mueller counters were widely used to detect both beta and gamma radiation. There are now much more efficient detectors for use with gamma emitters, so that beta counting is the most frequent function of a laboratory instrument of this type.

The fifth region of instrument response is attained when the applied voltage is increased beyond the Geiger-Mueller region. Like the first region (that of recombination), this level is not utilized in radiation detection instruments, for, in this instance, the gas arcs and a state of continuous discharge results. This is the region of continuous discharge.

Scintillation Detectors. The most recently devised method of detection which is in wide use is that of scintillation. Systems employing this detection medium may be of either the solid crystal or the liquid type. Both types have been used successfully to detect and measure alpha, beta and gamma radiations. Whatever the detection medium, whether solid or liquid in nature, the basic principle is similar. When radiation, of either electromagnetic or particulate nature, interacts with a detector of suitable material, photons, or quanta of visible light, are emitted by the molecules of the detector. These light pulses are then observed, multiplied and amplified by a photomultiplier tube and, finally, after additional amplification, counted by an electronic adding machine known as a scaler. The

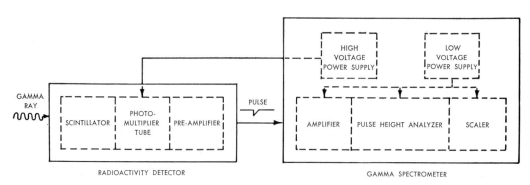

FIG. 15-8. Block diagram of gamma ray spectrometer. (National Institutes of Health, U.S.P.H.S.)

process is essentially one in which the energy of the radioactive material is transformed into visible light energy in the detector and into electrical energy in the photomultiplier tube. It is this electrical energy which ultimately is counted in some suitable device.

Solid Detectors. If one utilizes the proper solid crystal, it is possible to detect alpha, beta or gamma radiation. However, in this section we shall consider only those solid detectors which are used to measure gamma radiation. In most cases, a thallium-activated sodium iodide crystal is used as the phosphor. A block diagram of such a counting system is shown (Fig. 15-8). When gamma rays impinge on the crystal detector, the intensity of the resultant scintillation is substantially proportional to the energy of the gamma radia-

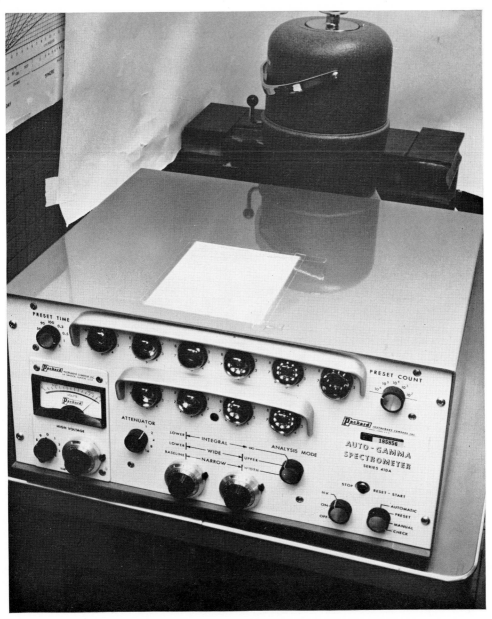

Fig. 15-9. Gamma ray spectrometer with scintillation well detector. (National Institutes of Health, U.S.P.H.S.)

tion. The number of pulses which are caused in the crystal by the impinging radiation is a measure of the disintegration rate of the sample when compared with a known standard of the same radioactive species. The amplification factor in a photomultiplier tube is dependent on the number of stages in the tube; as light pulses from the crystal cause the emission of photoelectrons from the light-sensitive photocathode within the tube, these photoelectrons are accelerated by the difference in potential applied to the tube. The photoelectrons, in this acceleration through the tube, strike a succession of other surfaces, or stages, known as dynodes, with secondary emission of electrons occurring at each surface. For each incident electron hitting one of the dynodes, there are approximately four secondary electrons emitted in a conventional photomultiplier tube.[36] More recently, a photomultiplier tube of greatly increased performance has been marketed[2] that may enhance even further this method of detection. By using gallium phosphide in the first stage, the efficiency of secondary emission has been increased markedly. For an applied field of 600 volts, gallium phosphide can multiply one primary electron into an average of 30 secondary electrons.

The pulse leaving the photomultiplier is given additional amplification and then fed into the spectrometer, or pulse height analyzer. Using the discrimination inherent in the spectrometer, the instrument can be adjusted to a given discrete energy of a particular gamma-emitting nuclide, and only pulses caused by impinging radiation of that energy are counted. This technic, known as "counting on the peak," is utilized when other radioactive materials in the vicinity of the detector may give false count rates or, in other cases, when the daughter, or decay product, of the radionuclide of interest is also a gamma-emitting isotope. Figure 15-9 illustrates a typical single-channel gamma scintillation spectrometer.

In more sophisticated gamma spectrometers, additional channels may be added to assist in identifying and quantitating gamma-emitting radionuclides. Figure 15-10 illustrates a multichannel instrument of this type. By calibrating the system so that each of the 100 channels spans a known number of electron volts, identification of an unknown gamma emitter is considerably simplified. The cathode ray tube mounted on the front panel of the instrument presents a visual display of the gamma spectrum, in this case cesium-137. Thus, energy peaks resulting from the decay of the nuclear species under observation may be read directly by observing the channel numbers in

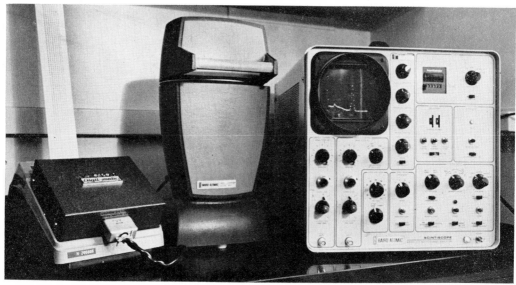

FIG. 15-10. A 100-channel gamma ray spectrometer with scintillation well detector and digital printer. (National Institutes of Health, U.S.P.H.S.)

which they are located. A permanent record of the total number of counts in each channel is afforded by the high-speed digital printer that is also a part of the system.

Liquid Detectors. In the 1950's, there appeared on the American commercial market a system in which beta-emitting nuclides, particularly those of low energy such as ^{14}C and ^{3}H, may be counted with reasonably good efficiency. This system, also a scintillation method, is known as liquid scintillation counting, and as the name implies, the detection medium in this case in liquid in nature. There is an intrinsic advantage in this method of detection, for the sample containing the radioactive material is usually dissolved in the detecting medium, thus placing the atoms of the radionuclide in intimate contact with those of the detector. In so doing, essentially 100 per cent geometry is obtained, and self-absorption is kept to a minimum.

While there are certain similarities between solid and liquid scintillation counters, there are certain important differences also. These differences are largely due to three factors:

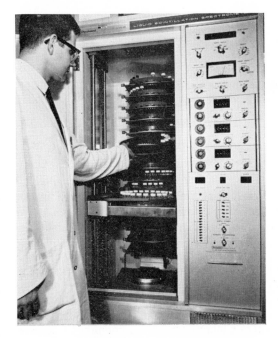

FIG. 15-11. Three-channel liquid scintillation counting system showing freezer and sample trays. (National Institutes of Health, U.S.P.H.S.)

(1) beta energies under observation are usually of much lower magnitude than the gamma energies previously considered; (2) the efficiency of liquid scintillators in emitting light is much less than that of solid crystals; and (3) all photomultiplier tubes produce a considerable and variable number of thermal pulses. The amplitude of these thermal pulses is quite similar to the amplitude of the beta decay events which one wishes to measure.

Thus, discrimination against the thermal pulses, as in the gamma spectrometer, is not possible, for the instrument is incapable of distinguishing between legitimate pulses originating in the radioactive source and thermal pulses from the photomultiplier tube, without the presence of additional components in the system. The operation of the photomultipliers and the detector at reduced temperatures in a freezer greatly diminishes the rate of thermal pulses occurring in the photomultiplier (Fig. 15-11).

To limit the acceptance of the remaining thermal pulses by the spectrometer, a coincidence arrangement of photomultipliers is used. Two photomultiplier tubes view the sample simultaneously, and any scintillation occurring in the sample will be "seen" by both tubes at essentially the same instant. The coincidence circuit allows such an event to pass, but blocks any random event which occurs in only one photomultiplier. Thus, unwanted thermal pulses (often termed "accidentals" in the literature) are practically eliminated from the background in a good liquid scintillation counting system.

While it is sometimes necessary to count samples in a suspended state (even a thixotropic gel has been utilized), it is the usual practice to dissolve the sample in a suitable solvent which also contains the phosphor, or scintillator. The liquid scintillator consists of a solute and a solvent. The solute emits a burst of photons for each radioactive event that deposits energy in the solution, and the solvent absorbs energy and transfers it to the solute.

For a solute to be useful in liquid scintillation counting, at least three criteria must be met: (1) It must be an efficient light emitter; (2) it must produce a photon spectrum that, in a conventional scintillation detector, will be efficiently transmitted and reflected in

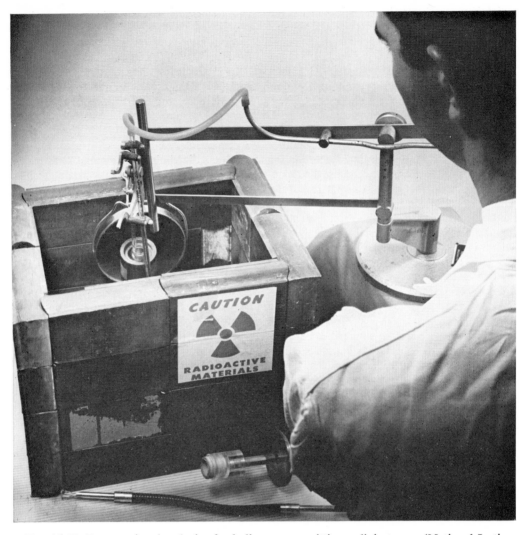

FIG. 15-12. Remote pipetting device for bulk gamma-emitting radioisotopes. (National Institutes of Health, U.S.P.H.S.)

the optical system and converted into electrical energy by the photomultiplier; and (3) it must be compatible with solubility restrictions imposed by the nature of the counting solution and by the temperature at which the counting is performed.[43] Since the most efficient light emitters have emission spectra which lie within a very narrow range of wavelengths, it is common practice to employ a combination of two solutes in a given counting "cocktail"—a primary scintillator to provide a large number of photons, and a secondary scintillator to shift the emission spectrum of these photons to a more

convenient wavelength for detection by the optics in the system.

There are many different liquid scintillation counting solutions used to count a variety of sample types, and the reader is directed to other references for a more comprehensive discussion and listing of these substances.[11,43] A representative example of a "cocktail" used (and modified) in the author's laboratory for the counting of aqueous samples, and originally described by Bruno and Christian,[24] is listed below to illustrate the types of chemical entities used as solutes and solvents in liquid scintillation counting.

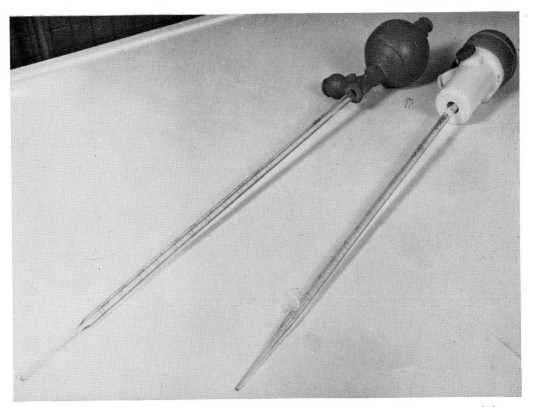

FIG. 15-13. Remote pipetting devices for beta-emitting and low-activity gamma-emitting radionuclides. (National Institutes of Health, U.S.P.H.S.)

Dimethyl POPOP, 1,4-bis-2-(4-methyl-5-phenyloxazolyl)-benzene	0.100 Gm.	
PPO, 2,5-diphenyloxazole	4.000 Gm.	
Cellosolve* (ethylene glycol monoethyl ether)	500.0	ml.
Toluene	500.0	ml.

It is interesting to note that the designations dimethyl POPOP, PPO, and others are much more frequently noted in the literature than are the chemical names also listed above. All chemicals used in preparing "cocktails" should be of scintillation grade.

OTHER EQUIPMENT

Much of the equipment used in radio-pharmaceutical practice is quite similar to that utilized in more familiar areas of pharmaceutical practice. However, because of

* Cellosolve (Carbide and Carbon Chemicals Company)

the inherent hazard involved in working with radioactive materials, several somewhat specialized pieces of equipment should be mentioned.

For example, there are various remote pipetting devices in common use in radio-pharmaceutical laboratories. Figure 15-12 shows an instrument used to withdraw aliquots of a gamma-emitting radionuclide from a bulk bottle in such a way as to prevent the operator from receiving an unnecessary radiation dose during the procedure. Note that the bulk bottle is stored behind a barricade composed of interlocking lead bricks; the mirror facilitates placing the pipet in the bottle without looking over the lead shielding.

When it is necessary to pipet beta emitters or relatively small amounts of gamma emitters, two other remote pipettors (Fig. 15-13) may be used to avoid pipetting by mouth.

Glove boxes, or hoods (Fig. 15-14) are also frequently used in this specialized area

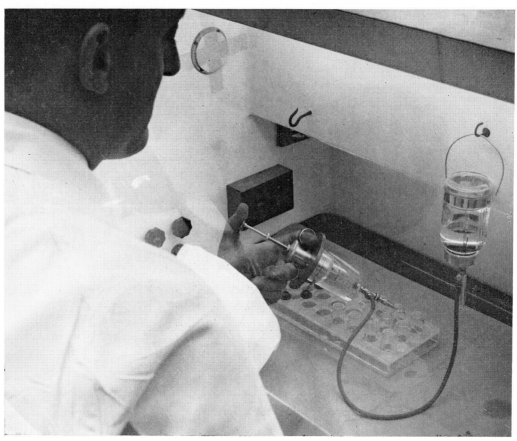

FIG. 15-14. Radioisotope gloved box, with aseptic transfer in progress. (National Institutes of Health, U.S.P.H.S.)

TABLE 15-3. GENERATOR SYSTEMS*

DAUGHTER ISOTOPE	HALF-LIFE	PARENT ISOTOPE	HALF-LIFE	APPLICATIONS
^{28}Al	2.3 min	^{28}Mg	21.3 hr.	Aluminum tracer
^{137}Ba	2.6 min.	^{137}Cs	30 yr.	Dynamic studies
^{68}Ga	68 min	^{68}Ge	280 days	Positron scanning and bone studies
^{113m}In	1.7 hr.	^{113}Sn	118 days	Scanning: brain, lung, liver, heart, etc.
^{132}I	2.3 hr.	^{132}Te	3.2 days	Thyroid studies, double tagging
^{87m}Sr	2.8 hr.	^{87}Y	80 hr.	Bone scanning
^{99m}Tc	6 hr.	^{99}Mo	67 hr.	Scanning: brain, thyroid, etc.
^{90}Y	64 hr.	^{90}Sr	28 yr.	Therapy

* As modified, from Richards, P.: Nuclide Generators, in Andrews, G. A., Kniseley, R. M., and Wagner, H. N., Jr. (eds.): Radioactive Pharmaceuticals, Washington, D.C., U.S. Atomic Energy Commission, CONF-651111, 1966.

of practice. These enclosures serve to confine contamination during a given procedure and may have ultraviolet lights within them to provide an aseptic environment for sterile procedures. Because these boxes should be maintained at a negative pressure with respect to the laboratory air, in order to prevent the outflow of air-borne contaminants, a bacterial-retentive filter is necessary in the air intake line. Customary laboratory utilities, such as air, gas and vacuum, are usually incorporated in gloved boxes for the convenience of the operator.

DOSAGE FORMS AND USES OF RADIOPHARMACEUTICALS

Dosage Forms. Commercially available radiopharmaceuticals are limited at present to oral dosage forms and a variety of injectable products. Those in the oral category are supplied as either an oral solution or as capsules. Injectable products include those that may be administered by the intravenous or the intracavitary routes of injection. In certain investigational applications involving dosage forms, the intrathecal and intracisternal,[33] inhalation by aerosol,[56,73] and nasal instillation[55] routes of administration have also been utilized.

Nuclide Generators. Although not a new concept, the use of nuclide generators, more commercially available radiopharmaceutical familiarly known as "isotope cows," has become widespread in nuclear medicine and radiopharmacy in recent years. For example, radiologists have been familiar for many years with the method of separating ^{222}Rn (half-life, 3.8 days) from the parent ^{226}Ra (half-life 1620 years) in the preparation of radon seeds. Of more current interest, however, is the use of these generators for making short-lived radionuclides continuously available at hospitals and clinics that are great distances from the source of production. Table 15-3 lists a number of generator systems that are either commercially available or that have been used for investigational purposes.

In theory, the use of such generators involves a scheme in which a daughter radionuclide can be readily and repeatedly separated from its longer-lived parent nuclide.[63]

Ion exchange is the most frequently used method of separation. Thus, the parent is bound to a suitable adsorbent medium packed in a column. As the parent decays, there occurs a simultaneous build-up of the daughter on the column. At appropriate intervals, as determined by the growth-decay curves for the particular system of nuclides being used, the column is eluted, or "milked," with an eluent in which the parent has essentially no solubility, but in which the daughter is readily soluble. The generator must provide an eluate with exceedingly high chemical, radiochemical, and microbiological purity if its use is to be safe and efficacious.

In nuclear medicine, the ^{99}Mo-^{99m}Tc generator currently enjoys the widest use of any of the available systems. The decay scheme of this parent-daughter system may be shown as follows:

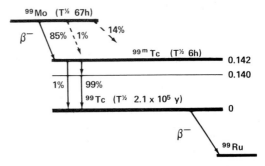

An example of a commercially available ^{99m}Tc generator is shown diagrammatically in Figure 15-15. The generator is supplied in a pyrogen-free and sterile state by the manufacturer. Elution of the system is carried out by the user in an aseptic fashion by attaching a sterile, evacuated collecting vial to the milking tube. The vacuum in the collecting vial pulls 30 ml. of pyrogen-free and sterile eluent (Sodium Chloride Injection, 0.9 per cent) through the column and into the vial. A separate milking tube and collecting vial is provided by the manufacturer for each elution. Figure 15-16 shows an actual generator of this type. Because substantial quantities of molybdenum-99 are present in the generator, adequate shielding must be provided around the column itself. In addition, the collecting vial must be shielded as a further protection to the opera-

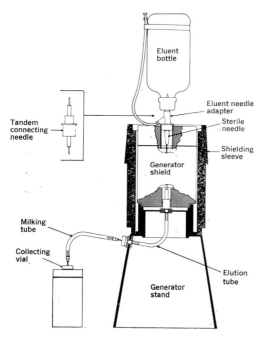

FIG. 15-15. Diagrammatic representation of ^{99}Mo-^{99m}Tc nuclide generator. (From E. R. Squibb and Sons, Inc.)

tor. A ^{99}Mo-^{99m}Tc "cow" has a useful life of approximately 1 week. Daily elutions are usually carried out for maximal yields, although more frequent milkings are possible if the need arises. After an elution has been performed, ^{99m}Tc again builds up on the column, reaching a maximum in 23 hours; however, the growth of technetium reaches approximately 50 per cent of maximum in approximately 6 hours, thus making feasible several elutions each day if necessary.

^{99m}Tc is eluted from the generator as sodium pertechnetate, Na^{99m}TcO$_4$, when Sodium Chloride Injection is used as the eluent. Appropriate tests to indicate the amount of ^{99}Mo and alumina present in the eluate must be completed prior to its use in patients. The upper limits of both of these contaminants are prescribed, at present, by USAEC regulations.

USES OF RADIOPHARMACEUTICALS

A comprehensive listing of the multitude of uses to which radiopharmaceutical products are put is beyond the scope of this text. As mentioned previously, both the *United*

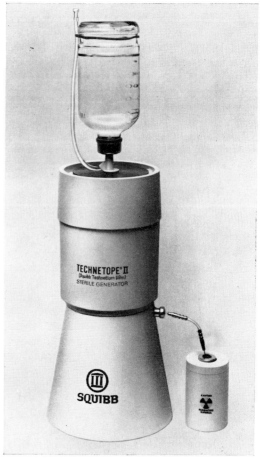

FIG. 15-16. Sterile, pyrogen-free technetium-99m generator system. (From E. R. Squibb and Sons, Inc.)

States Pharmacopeia[54] and the *National Formulary*[51] contain monographs for radioactive drugs. Other national pharmacopeias, such as the *British Pharmacopoeia 1968,*[23] as well as the *International Pharmacopoeia*[70] also contain radiopharmaceutical monographs. Excellent review articles by Silver[68] and Wolf and Tubis[77] describe in some detail these broad areas of use. The proceedings of two symposia held at the Oak Ridge Associated Universities can also be highly recommended as sources of information, the first covering the topic of radiopharmaceuticals,[1] and the second presenting a detailed discussion of many in vitro uses of radionuclides in medicine.[44] Williams and Sutton[76] presented a preliminary report on a comprehensive survey of the use of radio-

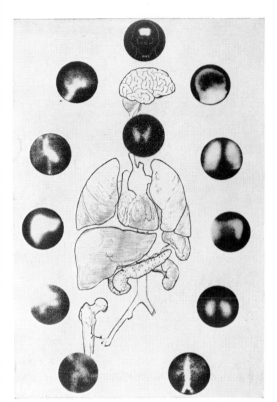

FIG. 15-17. Panoramic presentation of the organ systems it is now possible to scan routinely with radiopharmaceutical products. Actual visualizations of these organs by means of a gamma scintillation camera are seen in the black circles on the periphery. (National Institutes of Health, U.S.P.H.S.)

nuclides in medicine. This is the first phase of a broad study undertaken by the U.S. Public Health Service to determine the current use of radioactive materials in medicine. The quantitative data presented in this document represent procedures performed during the year 1966 and are based solely on the nearly 3,900 responses to a questionnaire sent to 7,200 physicians known to devote at least a part of their practice to nuclear medicine.

The intent of use of radiopharmaceutical products may be either diagnostic or therapeutic. However, it is in the area of diagnostics that the progress of nuclear medicine and the use of radiopharmaceuticals has been more dramatic, for there are even today

relatively few indications for the therapeutic use of internally administered radionuclides. Diagnostic uses include both function studies and scanning procedures.

Function Studies. Many examples of diagnostic function studies in which radiopharmaceuticals are employed may be found in even a cursory examination of current medical literature. These include: thyroid function (uptake) studies with ^{131}I as iodide; blood volume determinations with iodinated (^{131}I or ^{125}I) human serum albumin; renal function studies (renograms) with sodium iodohippurate ^{131}I; vitamin B_{12} absorption studies (Schilling tests) using ^{57}Co labeled cyanocobalamin, as a diagnostic aid in pernicious anemia; erythrocyte survival times, using ^{51}Cr labeled red blood cells; cardiac output studies, using either iodinated (^{131}I) human serum albumin or sodium pertechnetate (^{99m}Tc); and studies of fat absorption and pancreatic lipase activity using iodinated (^{131}I) triolein and iodinated (^{125}I) labeled oleic acid (Fig. 15-17).

Scanning Procedures. Nuclear medicine scanning procedures depend primarily on a selective localization, for even brief periods, of the radiopharmaceutical in the organ or tissue of interest. An automated and very sensitive scintillation detector is then moved mechanically over the area of interest, and data is automatically recorded by the scanning instrument. Figure 15-18 shows three brain scans performed on the same patient with three different radiopharmaceuticals: ^{197}Hg-chlormerodrin, ^{99m}Tc-human serum albumin and sodium ^{99m}Tc pertechnetate. The AV-malformation from which this patient suffered was most clearly visualized with the technetium-labeled albumin. Other scanning procedures include: thyroid scanning with ^{131}I iodide or sodium pertechnetate (^{99m}Tc); kidney scanning with ^{197}Hg-chlormerodrin; liver scanning with ^{131}I rose bengal, ^{198}Au colloid, or ^{99m}Tc sulfide colloid; lung scanning, using ^{131}I labeled macroaggregated human serum albumin; and placental scanning, with ^{99m}Tc labeled human serum albumin.

The reader is directed to the references cited, as well as any textbook on nuclear medicine, for more detailed information on these and other uses that are becoming in-

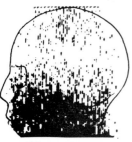
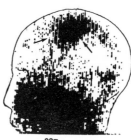
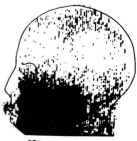
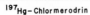

^{197}Hg-Chlormerodrin ^{99m}Tc-Albumin ^{99m}Tc-Pertechnetate

FIG. 15-18. Lateral brain scans obtained separately in the same patient with three different radiopharmaceuticals. The large arteriovenous malformation (*arrows, center view*) is most clearly visualized with ^{99m}Tc Albumin. (National Institutes of Health, U.S.P.H.S.)

creasingly popular in the diagnosis and treatment of a variety of pathologic states.

THE PRACTICE OF RADIOPHARMACY

It is fortunate indeed that there is no longer any evidence of the type of professional jealousy on the part of physical and biological scientists and physicians in the practice of nuclear medicine that was formerly a rather substantial impediment to any pharmacist who wished to engage in radiopharmacy practice.[15] The acute need for radiopharmacists is well documented[75] and widely recognized by the entire nuclear medicine community. In general, the professional practice of a hospital pharmacist who has specialized in radiopharmacy may be categorized into formulation and dispensing, product development, quality control and consultation functions.[18]

Formulation and Dispensing. Into this category one can place a variety of procedures that range from the relatively simple to the rather complex type of task. For example, it is usually much less expensive to purchase radiopharmaceutical injectable products in a bulk or multiple dose package. In many cases, the concentration of radioactive material in such products is somewhat higher than would allow a clinician to withdraw accurately a single dose of the product. A radiopharmacist is called on to prepare an aseptic dilution of the required medication for administration to one or several patients.

The advent of radionuclide generators in

hospitals has also emphasized the need for a radiopharmacist to assist the nuclear medicine department. The elution of a generator, or "cow," constitutes aseptic repackaging of an injectable product, and thus should be done under the supervision of or by a radiopharmacist.

Under certain circumstances, it may be necessary for a radiopharmacist to compound radioactive medications from basic radionuclide solutions or salts, in much the same manner as a hospital or community pharmacist compounds extemporaneous prescriptions for patients. However, in radiopharmaceutical compounding, a considerable amount of quality control testing is required on the finished product, for Federal regulations specify that byproduct material shall not be administered to humans until its pharmaceutical quality and assay have been established.[40]

It is also advisable, in a busy nuclear medicine facility, to have a radiopharmacist available for unit dose dispensing, even if no dilutions or other modifications of a commercially procured product are involved. It is not infrequent in a busy department to have numerous patients in the area awaiting the administration of various radiopharmaceuticals by the medical staff. In order to avoid medication errors, it is obviously desirable to have these medications dispensed and adequately labeled by a radiopharmacist who has been trained to avoid such errors.

Product Development. The extent to which a radiopharmacist is required to function in this area is, of course, dependent on the complexity of the nuclear medicine department that utilizes his services. If a significant amount of clinical research is carried out, product development can become an exceedingly important aspect of the practice of radiopharmacy. The dynamic nature of nuclear medicine has made it exceedingly difficult for radiopharmaceutical manufacturers to provide every product required in this medical specialty. Thus, an adequately trained radiopharmacist is able to contribute a great deal in an area in which there is this recognized void. The advantage that results from having a professional who is trained in product development and formulation procedures is obvious. An example of the type product development activity carried out in the Radiopharmaceutical Service of the National Institutes of Health that resulted in a very useful clinical product is discussed in some detail. Additional references are cited for other examples of this type of activity.

The first product to be considered is ^{99m}Tc-Human Serum Albumin Injection. In considering the attributes of routinely available brain scanning agents, two factors became abundantly clear. Albumin is a biologically favorable tumor-localizing agent[59,74] and the physical characteristics of ^{99m}Tc as a radionuclidic tag, or marker, are nearly ideal.[42] Thus, it was decided to combine the favorable physical characteristics of the radionuclide with the advantageous biological behavior of albumin in developing a brain scanning agent.[3] After a considerable research and development effort, the following protocol was established:

1. *Reagents and Materials Required*

A. Sodium ^{99m}Tc-Pertechnetate Injection
B. Ferric chloride, hexahydrated, analytical reagent grade
C. Ascorbic acid, analytical reagent grade
D. Sodium hydroxide, 1.0N and 0.1N, analytical reagent grade
E. Hydrochloric acid, 1.0N and 0.1N, analytical reagent grade
F. Normal Human Serum Albumin, *U.S.P.*
G. Biorad* AG 1×8, chloride form, 50-100 mesh, anion exchange resin

* Bio-Rad Laboratories, Richmond, Calif.

H. Sodium Chloride Injection *U.S.P.* (without preservative)
I. Membrane filter, 0.22μ pore size, sterile
J. Magnetic stirrer with Teflon stirring bar

2. *Procedure*

A. To a 30 ml. beaker, add 5 ml. Sodium ^{99m}Tc-Pertechnetate Injection; place stirring bar in beaker, which is then placed on magnetic stirrer.
B. While stirring, add 0.5 ml. HCl, 1.0N, in which 2 to 4 mg. ferric chloride hexahydrated has been dissolved (results in pH approximately 1.2).
C. Add 10 mg. ascorbic acid (dry powder).
D. Titrate to pH 9.0-9.5 with NaOH (check with pH meter).
E. Titrate to pH 4.5-5.0 with HCl (check with pH meter).
F. Add 5 mg. Normal Human Serum Albumin *U.S.P.*
G. Titrate to pH 2.1-2.5 with HCl (check with pH meter).
H. Pass solution through Biorad AG 1×8 ion exchange column; pretreat column by passing 25 ml. Sodium Chloride Injection *U.S.P.* (without preservative) through the column. Adjust flow rate of column to 10 to 20 drops per minute.
I. Titrate product to pH 4.5-5.0 with NaOH (check with pH meter).
J. Sterilize product by filtration through a 0.22μ membrane filter, positive pressure type.

3. *Control Testing*

A. Pyrogen test (*U.S.P.* method).
  a. 0.5 ml. product diluted to 10 ml. with Sodium Chloride Injection *U.S.P.*; rabbit dose, 1.5 ml. per kilogram.
B. Sterility Test (*U.S.P.* method).
C. Assay for activity.
D. Radiochemical purity determination.
  a. Paper chromatography vs. methanol, 85%
    (1) >97% of activity at origin.

^{99m}Tc-Human Serum Albumin Injection not only proved to be a clinically useful product in brain scanning, but it also became the agent of choice in the diagnosis and follow-up of cerebrospinal fluid rhinorrhea using isotope cisternographic procedures as well.[4,32]

The next example of a product development effort that led to the design of a valuable clinical tool is that of ^{125}I-Labeled Microaggregated Human Serum Albumin Injection for use in studies of reticuloendothelial function. It had been demonstrated that an estimate of the phagocytic capacity of the reticuloendothelial system (RES) can yield information quite useful in the clinical management of a variety of pathologic states.[7,12,41] For example, it has been suggested that RES function may be a valuable indicator in patients of the extent of Hodgkin's disease.[67] Therefore, it seemed appropriate to develop a product that was safe from an immunologic and microbiologic standpoint, and one that exhibits a predictable and uniform plasma clearance in normal states. ^{125}I-Labeled Microaggregated Human Serum Albumin Injection met these criteria.[21]

Other examples of product development activities include ^{51}Cr-Labeled Human Serum Albumin Injection and ^{131}I-Labeled Polyvinylpyrrolidone Injection, which proved useful in detecting a number of protein-leaking gastroenteropathies;[17,22] the development of a [85]Kr Injection for the detection of congenital cardiac shunts;[16] and a number of others as well. Thus, these examples serve to illustrate the contributions a radiopharmacist can make to a nuclear medicine program in his hospital.

Quality Control. As it applies to radiopharmaceuticals, quality control consists of a series of tests, observations, and analyses that indicate beyond a reasonable doubt the identity, quality, and quantity of all ingredients present in a product. In addition, these procedures should demonstrate that the technology employed in the formulation or manufacture of the product will yield a dosage form of the highest possible safety, reliability and efficacy. In general, quality control considerations may be grouped into those of a strictly pharmaceutical character and those related to the radiation characteristics of the product.

The extent to which an individual radiopharmaceutical product should be tested by a hospital radiopharmacy depends on a number of things. For example, it should not be necessary to subject a commercially procured radiopharmaceutical product to the same full scale quality control program that is incumbent on the primary manufacturer. On the other hand, experience has shown that it is advisable to perform certain tests on all radiopharmaceutical products, regardless of the source of supply.[19,26]

The use to which the radiopharmaceutical is to be put is also a determining factor in quality control decisions. For example, if ^{99m}Tc-Sulfide Colloid Injection is to be used for routine liver scans, the allowable limit of ^{99m}Tc present in the product as pertechnetate ion is somewhat higher than would be permissible if the product were intended for bone marrow scans. In the latter case, some reliable method for estimating the amount of pertechnetate in the product would be required, if definitive marrow scans were to be obtained.

It should be obvious, however, that as complete a quality control program as it is possible to provide should prevail. Further, if a considerable amount of extemporaneous or scheduled manufacturing is carried out by a radiopharmacy or nuclear medicine facility, a broad and comprehensive quality control plan is mandatory, approaching even that of a commercial radiopharmaceutical manufacturer. To provide any less is neither fair to the patients who entrust themselves to the care of that department, nor a defensible condition from the medicolegal standpoint if a challenge is entered in a court of law. Therefore, an outline of many of the matters of concern in radiopharmaceutical quality control is presented. Certain of these are considered in greater detail in the sections following the outline. It should be emphasized again, however, that the extent to which this listing is utilized by a specific radiopharmacy or nuclear medicine department depends on the scope of that particular department. In addition, the list is not intended to be all-inclusive. Other tests and observations may be required under certain circumstances.

RADIOPHARMACEUTICAL QUALITY CONTROL

1. *Pharmaceutical Considerations*
    A. Inspection of label content

a. Product identity
b. Manufacturer—name and address
c. Product list and lot numbers
d. Total radioactivity (time and date)
e. Concentration (time and date)
f. Specific activity (activity per unit mass)
g. Diluent
h. Additives
i. Expiration date
j. Recommended storage conditions
B. Appearance
a. Color
b. Clarity (if product is a true solution)
c. Particle size (if product is a suspension)
C. pH Determination of liquid formulations
a. Preferably obtained by pH meter
D. Biological testing or certification
a. Apyrogenicity and sterility (parenterals)
b. Acute toxicity and safety
c. Chronic toxicity
d. Efficacy

2. *Radiation Considerations*
(assuming product contains mixed beta-gamma or pure gamma emitters)
A. Radionuclidic assay
a. Gross, or total, activity in container
b. Activity per unit volume
c. Dose calibration
B. Radiochemical purity
a. Radiochromatography
a. Paper strip
b. Thin layer
b. Autoradiography
c. Electrophoretic behavior
d. Dialysis
C. Removable contamination
a. Smear of surface of container

PHARMACEUTICAL CONSIDERATIONS

The aspects of a radiopharmaceutical product considered under this section are well understood by all pharmacists, for certainly these are matters of concern in all pharmaceuticals. However, many nuclear medicine practitioners have little appreciation of the importance of these data. An excellent example of a pitfall an unsuspecting physician may encounter, if he fails to note certain things on a radiopharmaceutical label, is the presence of a bacterial preservative. If a product containing benzyl alcohol were chosen for a procedure in which regional blood flow measurements were to be made, the vasodilating action of this bacterial preservative may well invalidate the results —particularly if the product were to be used near the date of expiration when a relatively large volume of the material would have to be administered to obtain the required activity.

Pyrogen testing and sterility testing frequently must be explained to other scientists involved in nuclear medicine. For example, one frequently encounters otherwise well-informed professionals who believe that sterility connotes freedom from pyrogens, when, of course, this is entirely false.

RADIATION CONSIDERATIONS

Radionuclidic Assay. It has previously been mentioned that assays of all radiopharmaceutical products should be performed by the radiopharmacy or by the nuclear medicine department in which they are to be used, regardless of where these products have been procured.[26] If the product is an in-house formulation, one formulated by a radiopharmacy, this procedure is mandatory before the product may be administered to patients. Two different radionuclidic assays have been cited—a gross assay, and an assay to indicate the concentration of the radionuclide. The advisability of performing both is indicated by Table 15-4. The data in this table compares the information printed on the label of a commercially procured product with that established by assays performed after receipt of the product from the manufacturer.

It became evident, after further investigation, that a significant amount of the ^{99m}Tc-sulfide colloid in the formulation was adsorbed to the wall of the vial in which it was packaged, and thus was unavailable for use. The adsorption process was dynamic, as indicated by the disparity between the two activity per unit volume assays. In this case, the patient would have received far less of the product than the physician had intended to administer if the information on the sup-

TABLE 15-4. ^{99m}Tc-Sulfide Colloid RP 9758 092167*

Type of Assay	Supplier's Value	NIH Value	% Agreement
Gross, total vial	7.53 mc.	7.20 mc.	96
Activity/unit volume	2.51 mc./ml.	0.78 mc./ml.	31
		†0.50 mc./ml.	20

* All values normalized to 1200 EDT 9/21/67.
† Actual calibration performed 3 hours after initial activity/unit volume calibration, value corrected to same time and date as initial calibration.

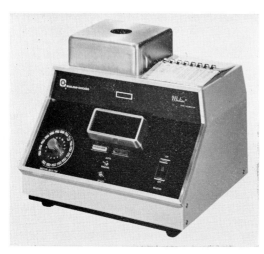

Fig. 15-19. Ion chamber dose calibrator for gamma-emitting radiopharmaceuticals. (From Nuclear-Chicago Corp.)

plier's label had not been questioned.

These two types of assay may be performed either by some gamma spectroscopic means or by means of an ion chamber type of instrument, such as that illustrated by Figure 15-19. This type of instrument may also be utilized for individual dose calibration for any radiopharmaceutical, for either the whole vial or a syringe containing the dose may be calibrated.

If radionuclidic purity must be determined, gamma spectroscopic technics must be employed. Radionuclidic purity is defined as the proportion of total activity that is present as the stated radionuclide. It is self-evident that a radionuclidic identification is also accomplished while the purity is being established. Radionuclidic identity and purity are extremely important considerations. In-

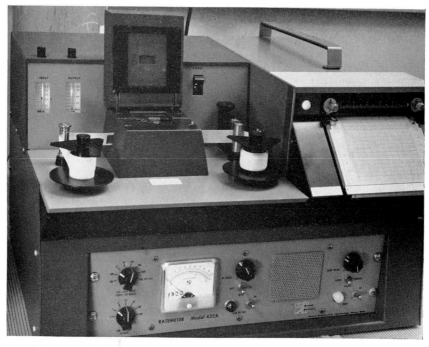

Fig. 15-20. Radiochromatogram scanner, with count rate meter and strip chart recorder. (National Institutes of Health, U.S.P.H.S.)

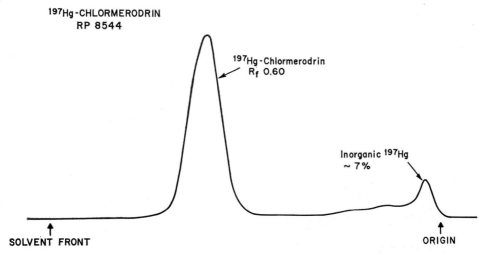

FIG. 15-21. Radiochromatogram scan of ^{197}Hg-Chlormerodrin Injection, showing excessive inorganic ^{197}Hg. Solvent system: benzene:glacial acetic acid:water, 2:2:1, descending paper. (National Institutes of Health, U.S.P.H.S.)

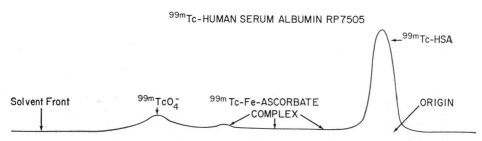

FIG. 15-22. Radiochromatogram scan of impure ^{99m}Tc-Human Serum Albumin Injection. Solvent system: methanol, 85 percent in water, descending paper. (National Institutes of Health, U.S.P.H.S.)

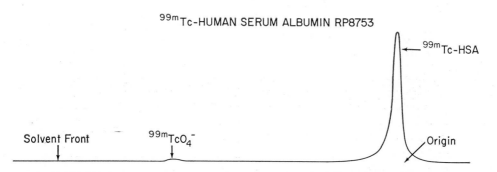

FIG. 15-23. Radiochromatogram scan of clinically usable ^{99m}Tc-Human Serum Albumin Injection. Note small amount of pertechnetate contaminant. Solvent system: methanol 85 per cent in water, descending paper. (National Institutes of Health, U.S.P.H.S.)

deed, in certain circumstances, it is mandatory that the user establish these values prior to the use of even commercially procured dosage forms. This is the case in the use of ^{99}Mo-^{99m}Tc generators, in which the USAEC has established an upper limit of 1 μc. of ^{99}Mo per millicurie of ^{99m}Tc in the eluate, and has further stipulated that no more than 5 μc. of ^{99}Mo may be administered to any patient.

Radiochemical Purity. This term may be defined as the fraction of the stated radionuclide present in the stated chemical form. Although several methods of determining radiochemical purity have been cited, radiochromatographic methods are most frequently used. Radiochromatography is quite similar to other chromatographic technics not involving radionuclides; the differences arise chiefly in the methods employed to localize areas of activity on the chromatogram. In radiochromatography, this is usually accomplished through the use of a radiochromatogram scanner, such as that illustrated in Figure 15-20. In this device, the paper strip, or the thin layer plate, is mechanically moved through a system of continuous flow Geiger detectors. These detectors, when suitably collimated, reflect the passage of an area of activity in their field of view by a deflection of the needle on the rate meter on the front panel, by an audio signal generated within the instrument, and by a deflection of the writing pen of the strip chart recorder, which is also a part of the instrument. The speed with which the strip or plate is drawn through the detection system and the speed at which the chart moves are the same, so that localization of an area of radioactivity on the strip or plate is simply a matter of measuring from some reference point (such as the origin or the solvent front) marked on both the strip (or plate) and the chart recording. It is not necessary to apply reagents to the strip to develop a color, although this is frequently done when an aliquot of a nonradioactive reference standard is also spotted along with the radiopharmaceutical. Figure 15-21 illustrates a radiochromatogram scan of a commercially obtained ^{197}Hg-Chlormerodrin Injection. In this case, approximately 7 per cent of the total ^{197}Hg present in the product was found to be in the inorganic ionic form. Had this product been used, an excessive "blood background" would have resulted, owing to the pronounced affinity of inorganic mercurials for sulfhydryl groups found in erythrocyte membranes. Thus, a brain scan in which this product might have been employed would have been extremely difficult, if not impossible, to interpret. Figure 15-22 illustrates a radiochromatogram scan of ^{99m}-Tc-Albumin Injection in which excessive amounts of a ^{99m}Tc-iron-ascorbate complex were found to have occurred. This complex would have localized in the kidney, thus subjecting that organ to a useless radiation dose. In addition, excessive nonorganically bound technetium is evident. Figure 15-23 shows a scan of a much more clinically satisfactory product, with no complex formation and very little pertechnetate.

Records. Although not usually considered a part of quality control, the need to keep adequate records in any scientific discipline cannot be overemphasized. If no records

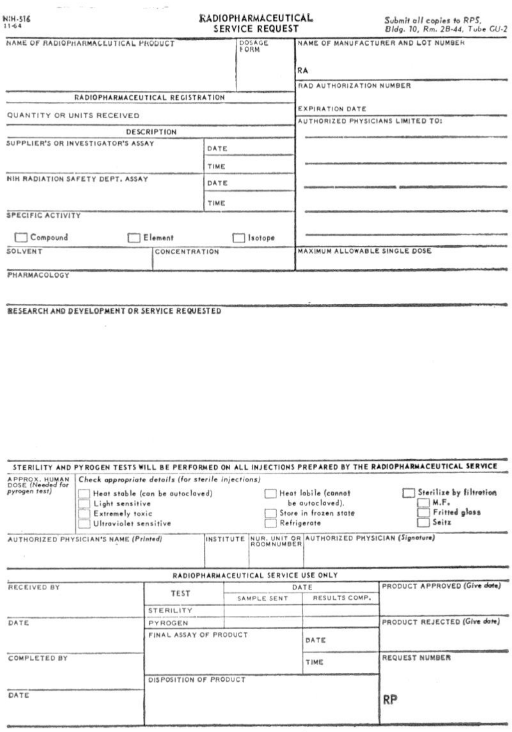
NIH-516
11-64
RADIOPHARMACEUTICAL
SERVICE REQUEST
Submit all copies to RPS, Bldg. 10, Rm. 2B-44, Tube GU-2
NAME OF RADIOPHARMACEUTICAL PRODUCT
DOSAGE FORM
NAME OF MANUFACTURER AND LOT NUMBER
RA
RAD AUTHORIZATION NUMBER
RADIOPHARMACEUTICAL REGISTRATION
EXPIRATION DATE
QUANTITY OR UNITS RECEIVED
AUTHORIZED PHYSICIANS LIMITED TO:
DESCRIPTION
SUPPLIER'S OR INVESTIGATOR'S ASSAY
DATE
TIME
NIH RADIATION SAFETY DEPT. ASSAY
DATE
TIME
SPECIFIC ACTIVITY
☐ Compound ☐ Element ☐ Isotope
SOLVENT
CONCENTRATION
MAXIMUM ALLOWABLE SINGLE DOSE
PHARMACOLOGY
RESEARCH AND DEVELOPMENT OR SERVICE REQUESTED
STERILITY AND PYROGEN TESTS WILL BE PERFORMED ON ALL INJECTIONS PREPARED BY THE RADIOPHARMACEUTICAL SERVICE
APPROX. HUMAN DOSE *(Needed for pyrogen test)*
Check appropriate details (for sterile injections)
☐ Heat stable (can be autoclaved)
☐ Light sensitive
☐ Extremely toxic
☐ Ultraviolet sensitive
☐ Heat labile (cannot be autoclaved).
☐ Store in frozen state
☐ Refrigerate
☐ Sterilize by filtration
☐ M.F.
☐ Fritted glass
☐ Seitz
AUTHORIZED PHYSICIAN'S NAME *(Printed)*
INSTITUTE
NUR. UNIT OR ROOMNUMBER
AUTHORIZED PHYSICIAN *(Signature)*
RADIOPHARMACEUTICAL SERVICE USE ONLY
RECEIVED BY
TEST
DATE
SAMPLE SENT
RESULTS COMP.
PRODUCT APPROVED *(Give date)*
STERILITY
DATE
PYROGEN
PRODUCT REJECTED *(Give date)*
FINAL ASSAY OF PRODUCT
DATE
COMPLETED BY
TIME
REQUEST NUMBER
DISPOSITION OF PRODUCT
DATE
RP

FIG. 15-24. Radiopharmaceutical Service Request (front). (National Institutes of Health, U.S.P.H.S.)

FORMULATION DATA		
CHEMICAL AND QUALITY	QUANTITY	NAME OF MANUFACTURER AND LOT NUMBER

PROCEDURE AND CALCULATIONS

AFFIX
LABEL HERE

WORK UNITS	UNITS COMPLETED

CATEGORY	(Check one) ☐ R & D ☐ Service ☐ Control

NIH-516
11-64

FIG. 15-25. Radiopharmaceutical Service Request (reverse side). (National Institutes of Health, U.S.P.H.S.)

are kept, the documentation of the identity and amount of a radiopharmaceutical a patient receives is impossible.

In addition, if a radiopharmacy engages in any manufacturing or formulation work, it is imperative that proper records concerning the product constituents and the formulation method be maintained. This is necessary if reproducibility of succeeding batches of the product is to be accomplished. Data concerning biological testing of products must also be maintained under these circumstances.

Figures 15-24 and 15-25 show the front and back of a Radiopharmaceutical Service Request utilized for a number of years in recording appropriate information concerning individual products, whether these are the result of a research and development, routine formulation, or a commercial procurement action. Figure 15-26 illustrates the Pyrogen Test Record form and Figure 15-27 indicates the Radiopharmaceutical Products Examination Request form that have also been used.

Thus, these few examples of quality control technics show the value of such pro-

MANUFACTURER	TEST NO.

RADIOPHARMACEUTICAL SERVICE, PHARMACY DEPARTMENT, CLINICAL CENTER

PRODUCT

LOT NUMBER RP-	DATE OF TEST	INJECTION METHOD

REMARKS

RABBIT NUMBER	DOSE/KG RABBIT	VARIATION IN DEGREES CENTIGRADE AT POST-INJECTION HOURS								MAXIMUM RISE		IMMEDIATE REACTION	DILUTION	REMARKS
		1 HOURS	2 HOURS	3 HOURS	4 HOURS	5 HOURS	6 HOURS	3 HOURS	HOURS					
ROOM TEMPERATURE														

RESULTS

NIH-323-1 (Formerly PHS-3979)
Rev. 6-64

PYROGEN TEST RECORD

FIG. 15-26. Pyrogen Test Record. (National Institutes of Health, U.S.P.H.S.)

PRODUCT·		LOT NO.
		RP-

STATED POTENCY OR COMPOSITION	PHYSICAL AND CHEMICAL CHARACTERISTICS

DATE MANUFACTURED	EXPIRATION DATE	PRESERVATIVE	DOSE

PACKAGING *(Check)*:
☐ AMPUL   ☐ TRAY   ☐ OTHER
☐ BOTTLE ☐ VIAL   *(Specify)* _____

TEST *(Check)*:
☐ CHEMICAL   ☐ STERILITY
☐ PYROGEN   ☐ OTHER *(Specify)* _____

REMARKS

DATE:	RECEIVED	ISSUED	REPORTED

TESTS	RESULTS

SIGNATURE

NIH-324-1
Rev. 6-64

PHARMACY DEPARTMENT – RADIOPHARMACEUTICAL SERVICE
CLINICAL CENTER, N.I.H.
RADIOPHARMACEUTICAL PRODUCTS EXAMINATION

FIG. 15-27. Radiopharmaceutical Products Examination Request. (National Institutes of Health, U.S.P.H.S.)

cedures, as well as the important contributions to patient safety a radiopharmacist can offer.

Consultation. This function is possible for a pharmacist to fulfill even if he has had little or no training or experience in radiopharmacy. He is, nonetheless, the recognized expert on drugs in his hospital. In a strictly pharmaceutical frame of reference, he is thus able to advise medical and paramedical personnel on packaging and administration methods and supplies, chemical stability of various pharmaceutical and chemical systems, and a whole host of other necessary information. In addition, pharmacological and chemical incompatibilities are areas in which a pharmacist is competent. Experience has shown that in these matters a pharmacist can be extremely helpful to the nuclear medicine community, and advice on such subjects should be freely offered.

REGULATORY CONTROL OF RADIO-PHARMACEUTICAL PRODUCTS

A comprehensive discussion of the many intricacies of regulatory control over this class of drugs and those who use them is beyond the scope of this text. It will suffice to point out that there are three Federal agencies involved in the regulatory program. These agencies, with references to the statutory authority under which they operate in this area, are: the United States Atomic Energy Commission,[28] the U.S. Food and Drug Administration,[29] and the United States Public Health Service.[30] In addition, the USAEC has delegated their responsibility in this area to a number of Agreement States.

SUMMARY

Information has been presented to give the reader a better understanding of the practice of radiopharmacy. The text is not intended to be comprehensive, and detailed explanations of the medical uses of radiopharmaceuticals have been purposely avoided. The reader is encouraged to examine the references cited for more detailed information on these matters.

REFERENCES

1. Andrews, G. A., Kniseley, R. M., and Wagner, H. N., Jr. (eds.): Radioactive

Pharmaceuticals. Washington, D.C., U.S. Atomic Energy Commission, CONF-651111, 1966.

2. Anon.: RCA achieves marked increase in photomultiplier performance. Res. Devel. *19*:10, 1968.

3. Ashburn, W. L., DiChiro, G., Briner, W. H., and Harbert, J. C.: ^{99m}Tc-Albumin for brain scanning. Drug Intell., *1*:314-316, 1967.

4. Ashburn, W. L., Harbert, J. C., Briner, W. H., and DiChiro, G.: Cerebrospinal fluid rhinorrhea studies with the gamma scintillation camera. J. Nucl. Med., *9*:523-529, 1968.

5. Babb, A. L., *et al.*: The use of neutron activation analysis in the early diagnosis of cystic fibrosis in children. Trans. Am. Nuc. Soc., *9*:591, 1966.

6. Barak, A. J., and Beckenhauer, H. C.: Liver and serum manganese, magnesium, and zinc in fatty cirrhosis. J. Nucl. Med., *7*:358, 1966.

7. Bases, R. E. and Krakoff, I. H.: Enhanced reticuloendothelial phagocytic activity in myeloproliferative diseases. J. Reticuloendothel. Soc., *2*:1, 1965.

8. Becquerel, H.: Physique—Sur les radiations émises par phosphorescence. Compt. Rend., *122*:420, 1896.

9. ————: Physique—Sur quelques propriétés novelles des radiations invisibles émises par divers corps phosphorescents. Compt. Rend., *122*:559, 1896.

10. ————: Physique—Émission des radiations nouvelles par l'uranium métallique. Compt. Rend., *122*:1086, 1896.

11. Bell, C. G., Jr., and Hayes, F. N.: Liquid Scintillation Counting—Proceedings of a Conference Held at Northwestern University, August 1957. Oxford, Pergamon, 1958.

12. Biozzi, G. Benacerraf, B., Halpern, B. N., Stiffel, C., and Hillemand, B.: Exploration of the phagocytic function of the reticuloendothelial system with heat denatured human serum albumin labeled with I-131 and application to the measurement of liver blood flow in normal man and in some pathologic conditions. J. Lab. Clin. Med., *51*:230, 1958.

13. Blum, M., and Eisenbud, M.: Reduction of thyroid irradiation from ^{131}I by potassium iodide. J.A.M.A., *200*:112-116, 1967.

14. Briner, W. H.: Certain aspects of radiological health. Am. J. Hosp. Pharm., *15*:44-51, 1958.

15. ————: Radiopharmaceuticals are drugs. Mod. Hosp., *95*:110-114, 1960.

16. ————: The formulation of radioactive Krypton-85 for intravenous use. Am. J. Hosp. Pharm., *18*:170-175, 1961.

17. ————: A note on the formulation of Iodine-131 labelled polyvinylpyrolidone for intravenous administration. J. Nucl. Med., *2*:94-98, 1961.

18. ————: Radioactive materials—new dimensions for pharmacy. Hosp. Topics, *43*:79-90, 1965.

19. ————: Quality control, pyrogen testing, and sterilization of radioactive pharmaceuticals. *In*: Andrews, G. A., Kniseley, R. M., and Wagner, H. N., Jr. (eds.): Radioactive Pharmaceuticals. pp. 93-111. Washington, D.C., U.S. Atomic Energy Commission, CONF-651111, 1966.

20. ————: Radiopharmacy—the emerging young specialty. Drug Intell., *2*:8-13, 1968.

21. ————: Preparation of ^{125}I-labeled microaggregated human serum albumin for use in studies of reticuloendothelial function in man. J. Nucl. Med., *9*:482-485, 1968.

22. Briner, W. H., Gordon, R. S., Jr., and Waldmann, T.: Principles in the production and formulation of I-131 labeled polyvinylpyrrolidone and Cr-51 labeled serum albumin for parenteral use. *In*: Schwartz, M., and Vesin, P. (eds.): Plasma Proteins and Gastrointestinal Tract in Health and Disease. Copenhagen, Munksgaard, 1961.

23. British Pharmacopoeia 1968. London, The Pharmaceutical Press, 1968.

24. Bruno, G. A., and Christian, J. E.: Determination of carbon-14 in aqueous bicarbonate solutions by liquid scintillation counting techniques. Analyt. Chem., *33*:9, 1961.

25. Christian, J. E.: Radioactive isotopes in hospital pharmacy. Bull. Am. Soc. Hosp. Pharm., *7*:178-183, 1950.

26. Cliggett, P. A., and Brown, J. M., Jr.: Assays of radioactive materials for use in patients—a five year study. J. Nucl. Med., *9*:236-240, 1968.

27. Cobau, C. D., Simons, C. S., and Meyers, M. C.: Accidental overdosage with radiophosphorus: therapy by induced phosphate diuresis. Am. J. Med. Sci., *254*:85/451-97/463, 1967.

28. Code of Federal Regulations (CFR), Title 10: Part 20 (Standards for Protection Against Radiation), Part 30 (Byproduct Material), and Part 35 (Human Uses of Byproduct Material), as amended, Washington, D.C.

29. Code of Federal Regulations (CFR), Title 21: Part 130 (Investigational Drug Regu-

lations), Part 133 (Drugs: Current Good Manufacturing Practice in Manufacture, Processing, Packing, or Holding), as amended, Washington, D.C.

30. Code of Federal Regulations (CFR), Title 42: Part 73 (Public Health Service Regulations—Biological Products), as amended, Washington, D.C.

31. Cunningham, R. E.: U.S. Atomic Energy Commission Licensing and Regulation of Radiopharmaceuticals. In: Andrews, G. A., Kniseley, R. M., and Wagner, H. N., Jr. (eds.): Radioactive Pharmaceuticals. Washington, D.C., U.S. Atomic Energy Commission, CONF-651111, 1966.

32. DiChiro, G., Ashburn, W. L., and Briner, W. H.: Technetium Tc 99m serum albumin for cisternography. Arch. Neurol., 19:218-227, 1968.

33. DiChiro, G., Ommaya, A. K., Ashburn, W. L., and Briner, W. H.: Isotope cisternography in the diagnosis and follow-up of cerebrospinal fluid rhinorrhea. J. Neurosurg., 28:522-529, 1968.

34. Durham, C. T.: Pharmaceutical aspects of atomic energy. J. Am. Pharm. Ass. (Pract. ed.), 11:346-350, 1950.

35. Fell, G. S.: Wilson's disease: comparison of copper levels by neutron activation and chemical methods. Proc. Ass. Clin. Biochem., 3:287, 1965.

36. Fields, T., and Seed, L.: Clinical Use of Radioisotopes. Chicago, Year Book Pub., 1961.

37. Fowler, J. M., et al.: Fallout—A Study of Superbombs, Strontium-90, and Survival. New York, Basic Books, 1960.

38. Frischauf, H.: Studies on the content of trace elements in leukocytes with neutron activation analysis. Folia Haemat. (Frankfurt), 7:291, 1963.

39. Gruverman, I. J., and Davidson, J. D.: Phosphorus-32 and Phosphorus-33—A Danger and an Opportunity. Atomlight No. 66, Boston, New England Nuclear Corporation, 1968.

40. A Guide for the Preparation of Applications for the Medical Use of Radioisotopes. Washington, D.C., U.S. Atomic Energy Commission, Mar. 1965.

41. Halpern, B. N.: The role and function of the reticuloendothelial system in immunological processes. J. Pharm. Pharmacol., 11:321, 1959.

42. Harper, P. V., Lathrop, K. A., McCardle, R. J., and Andros, G.: The use of technetium-99m as a clinical scanning agent for thyroid, liver and brain. Medical Radioisotope Scanning, I.A.E.A. Symposium,

Athens 2:33, April 1964.

43. Hayes, F. N.: Solutes and Solvents for Liquid Scintillation Counting. Packard Technical Bulletin No. 1, La Grange, Ill., Packard Instrument Co., Inc., Jan. 1962.

44. Hayes, R. L., Goswitz, F. A., and Murphy, B. E. P. (eds.): Radioisotopes in Medicine—In Vitro Studies. Washington, D.C., U.S. Atomic Energy Commission, CONF-671111, 1968.

45. Hine, G. J., and Brownell, G. L.: Radiation Dosimetry. New York, Academic Press, 1958.

46. Isotopes—An Eight Year Summary of U. S. Distribution and Utilization. USAEC, Washington, D.C., Superintendent of Documents, March 1955.

47. Kanabrocki, E. L.: Manganese and copper levels in human urine. J. Nucl. Med., 6: 780, 1965.

48. Kanabrocki, E. L., et al.: Neutron activation studies of biological fluids: manganese and copper. Int. J. Appl. Radiat., 15:175, 1964.

49. Maximum Permissible Body Burdens and Maximum Permissible Concentrations of Radionuclides in Air and Water for Occupational Exposure. Handbook 69, Washington, D.C., National Bureau of Standards, U.S. Department of Commerce, 1959.

50. MIRD Supplement Number 1, J. Nucl. Med. Vol. 9, No. 2, Supplement 1, Feb. 1968.

51. The National Formulary. ed. 13. Washington, American Pharmaceutical Association, 1965.

52. National Institutes of Health Radiation Safety Guide. Washington, D.C., U.S. Department of Health, Education and Welfare, Public Health Service, 1962.

53. Numerof, P.: Personal communication.

54. The Pharmacopeia of the United States of America, Eighteenth Revision. New York, U.S. Pharmacopeial Convention, Inc., 1965.

55. Proctor, D. F., and Wagner, H. N., Jr.: Clearance of particles from the human nose. Arch Environ. Health, 11:366, 1965.

56. Quinn, J. L., III, and Head, L. R.: Radioisotope photoscanning in pulmonary disease. J. Nucl. Med. 7:1-7, 1966.

57. Radiation Quantities and Units. International Commission on Radiological Units and Measurements (ICRU), Report 10a, Handbook 84. Washington, D.C., National Bureau of Standards, U.S. Department of Commerce, 1962.

58. Radiological Health Handbook. PB121-

784R, DHEW, Washington, D.C., U.S. Public Health Service, 1960.

59. Raimondi, A. J.: Localization of radio-iodinated serum albumin in human glioma —an electron microscopic study. Arch. Neurol. (Chicago), *11*:173-184, 1964.

60. Recommendations of the ICRP. Report of the Committee on Permissible Dose for Internal Radiation, London, Pergamon, 1958.

61. Report of the International Commission on Radiological Units and Measurements (ICRU). Handbook 62, Washington, D. C., National Bureau of Standards, U.S. Department of Commerce, 1956.

62. Report of the International Commission on Radiological Units and Measurements (ICRU). Handbook 78, Washington, D. C., National Bureau of Standards, U.S. Department of Commerce, 1959.

63. Richards, P.: Nuclide generators. *In*: Andrews, G. A., Kniseley, R. M., and Wagner, H. N., Jr. (eds.): Radioactive Pharmaceuticals. Washington, D.C., U.S. Atomic Energy Commission, CONF-651111, 1966.

64. Rohrer, R. H.: Basic Physics of Nuclear Medicine. *In*: Wagner, H. N., Jr. (ed.): Principles of Nuclear Medicine. Philadelphia, W. B. Saunders, 1968.

65. Seaborg, G. T.: Third Annual Nuclear Pioneer Lecture. Dallas, Texas, The Society of Nuclear Medicine, June, 1962.

66. Shapiro, B.: USAF School of Aviation Medicine, 59-30, 1-12, 1959.

67. Sheagren, J. N., Block, J. B., and Wolff, S. M.: Reticuloendothelial system phagocytic function in patients with Hodgkin's disease. J. Clin. Invest., *46*:855, 1967.

68. Silver, S.: Uses of radioisotopes in medicine. Nucleonics *23*:106-111, 1965.

69. Smith, E. M., Brownell, G. L., and Ellett, W. H.: Radiation Dosimetry. *In*: Wagner, H. N., Jr. (ed.): Principles of Nuclear Medicine. Philadelphia, W. B. Saunders, 1968.

70. Specifications for the Quality Control of Pharmaceutical Preparations. International Pharmacopoeia. ed. 2. Geneva, World Health Organization, 1967.

71. Storey, R. H.: Personal communication.

72. Tabern, D. L.: Radioactively Tagged Compounds Available from Abbott Laboratories, December 1, 1950.

73. Taplin, G. V., *et al.*: Lung perfusion and bronchial patency evaluation by radioisotope scanning. Picker *Scintillator,* March 14, 1966.

74. Tator, C. H., Morley, T. P., and Olszewski, J.: A study of the factors responsible for the accumulation of radioactive iodinated human serum albumin (RIHSA) by intracranial tumors and other lesions. J. Neurosurg., *22*:60-76, 1965.

75. Williams, K. D., Cooper, J. F., Moore, R. T., and Hilberg, A. W. (eds.): Reduction of Radiation Exposure in Nuclear Medicine—Proceedings of a Symposium held at Michigan State University, Aug. 7-9, 1967. Rockville, Md., U.S. Department of Health, Education and Welfare, Public Health Service, National Center for Radiological Health, PHS No. 999-RH-30, Dec. 1967.

76. Williams, K. D., and Sutton, J. D.: Survey of the Use of Radionuclides in Medicine—Preliminary Report. Rockville, Md., U.S. Department of Health, Education and Welfare, Public Health Service, National Center for Radiological Health MORP 68-10, 1968.

77. Wolf, W., and Tubis, M.: Radiopharmaceuticals. J. Pharm. Sci., *56*:1-17, 1967.

Appendix

Therapeutic Incompatibilities

There is no question that information about drug interactions is increasing at an almost exponential rate. There also is no question that the traditional sources of information for physicians—colleagues, medical representatives, medical journals, and direct mail advertisements—will not be able to keep the physician abreast of these developments nor will these sources serve to separate the "important" from the "less important" interactions. Finally, there is no question that both the institutional and the community pharmacist are admirably situated to assume this role for both the physician and the patient. However, for the pharmacist to be able to fulfill this function, a rational, categorized approach is needed.

Drugs, of course, are the cause of many effects, desirable and undesirable. In prior years, any untoward effect was known as a side-effect. Now that the basis for many of these untoward effects has been established, it is no longer possible to dump all of these effects under one heading. Terms such as interaction, reaction, therapeutic incompatibility, adverse reaction, side effect, untoward effect, allergic reaction, idiosyncrasy, iatrogenic, teratogenic, contraindication, and many others abound in the literature and serve so to overwhelm the pharmacist that significant information may well be lost.

To overcome this development and to make a rational approach to the problem of unsuspected drug action possible, it is suggested that the scheme shown in table A-1, which is somewhat similar to a recent suggestion in the literature,* be adopted and be used in future reports on drug interaction.†

The following examples illustrate the usefulness of this classification scheme:

Side effects
Xerostomia with anticholinergic antispasmodic (e.g., atropine, belladonna, propantheline)

Extension effects
Hemorrhage with anticoagulants

Hypersensitivity
Succinylcholine apnea

Adverse reaction
Teratogenic activity of thalidomide

Allergic reaction
Allergic hematologic cytopenias
    Aplastic anemia—chloramphenicol
Non-hematologic
    Hepatitis—methyldopa

Therapeutic incompatibilities
Propranolol with sympathomimetic bronchodilators

Therapeutic interactions
Alcohol with CNS depressants

Contraindications
Barbiturates in patients with porphyria

---

*Borda, T., Slone, D., and Jick, H.: J.A.M.A. 205:645, 1958.

†Lamy, P. P., and Blake, D. A.: J. Am. Pharm. Ass. NS10:72, 1970.

Table A-1. Classification of Untoward Effects of Drugs*

Category	Definition	Correction
Side effect	Undesirable but unavoidable effect which occurs at the proper therapeutic dose level in most individuals	Palliative treatment, patient will adapt or in severe instances drug must be withdrawn
Extension effect	Undesirable effect which occurs only at a dose level in excess of the required therapeutic dose or an excessive duration of therapy (unintentional overdose)	Decrease amount of dose or frequency of dosage based on blood level of drug or clinical evaluation
Hypersensitivity	Excessive pharmacologic or toxic response caused by unusual susceptibility (usually of genetic origin)	Drug history of patient and relatives and diagnostic tests are of prime importance in prevention of occurrence
Adverse reaction	A direct undesirable cytotoxic action which does not involve immunologic mechanisms	Immediate withdrawal of the drug. Initiate appropriate corrective treatment
Allergic reaction	Undesirable reaction requiring previous exposure to the drug or a cogener, where the existence of antibodies is known or presumed	Immediate withdrawal of the drug. Initiate symptomatic treatment for allergic manifestations. Drug history of patient and relatives and sensitivity tests of prime importance in prevention of occurrence
Idiosyncrasy	Unsuspected response to a drug which occurs in rare instances and the mechanism is unknown (does not fit into other categories)	Immediate withdrawal of drug or reduction of dosage
Therapeutic incompatibility	Hazardous interaction of two or more drugs or other therapeutic measures	Withdrawal of one or all drugs
Therapeutic interaction	Interaction of two or more drugs or other therapeutic measures resulting in a decrease or increase in pharmacologic activity	May necessitate alteration of dose level or careful monitoring of patient but not the withdrawal of the drugs involved
Contraindication	Pre-existing condition which may be aggravated by a drug	Immediate withdrawal of drug. Patient's history should serve as a guide to prevent the use of certain drugs

*Lamy, P. P., and Blake, D. A.: J. Am. Pharm. Ass. *NS10*:72, 1970.

Index